SEVENTEENTH
EDITION

MATERNITY NURSING

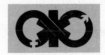

Family, Newborn, and Women's Health Care

We have chosen the signs for woman, man, birth, and infinity for our logo. As woman and man combine their corporal and spiritual energy in the drama of birth, new beings are brought into existence which have, in turn, their own energy and existence. We know from principles of physics that once matter and energy exist they can never be destroyed, although their forms may change. Hence, once an individual's substance and energy are created, they exist infinitely. Indeed, the phenomenon of birth is the most awe-inspiring and dramatic episode of a lifetime and beyond.

SEVENTEENTH
EDITION

MATERNITY NURSING

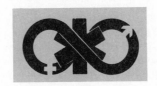

Family, Newborn, and Women's Health Care

SHARON J. REEDER RN, PhD, FAAN

Professor of Nursing and Chair, Maternal Child Health/Primary Ambulatory Care Section
School of Nursing
University of California
Los Angeles, California

LEONIDE L. MARTIN RN, MS, DrPH

Professor, Department of Nursing
Director, Family Nurse Practitioner Program,
Sonoma State University
Rohnert Park, California

DEBORAH KONIAK RN, EdD

Associate Professor
School of Nursing
University of California
Los Angeles, California

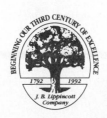

J.B. Lippincott Company
Philadelphia
New York   London   Hagerstown

Sponsoring Editor: Barbara Cullen
Coordinating Editorial Assistant:
  Jennifer E. Brogan
Project Editor: Melissa McGrath
Indexer: Barbara Littlewood

Designer: Susan Hess Blaker
Design Coordinator: Susan Hermansen
Production Manager: Helen Ewan
Production Coordinator: Kathryn Rule
Compositor: Tapsco, Incorporated
Printer/Binder: Courier Book Company/Westford

17th Edition

1 3 5 6 4 2

Library of Congress Cataloging-in-Publication Data

Reeder, Sharon J.
    Maternity nursing: family, newborn, and women's health care/
Sharon J. Reeder, Leonide L. Martin, Deborah Koniak-Griffin.—17th ed.
        p.   cm.
    Includes bibliographical references and index.
    ISBN 0-397-54813-3
    1. Maternity nursing.   I. Martin, Leonide L.   II. Koniak-Griffin,
Deborah.   III. Title.
    [DNLM: 1. Gynecology—nurses' instruction.   2. Obstetrical
Nursing.   3. Perinatology—nurses' instruction.   WY 157 R325m]
RG951.Z3   1992
618.2—dc20
DNLM/DLC
for Library of Congress   91-25799
                                                                                CIP

*The 17th edition of **Maternity Nursing: Family, Newborn, and Women's Health Care** is dedicated to our students and all the challenges and excitement in nursing that they will face.*

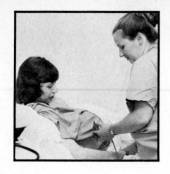

Contributors

Ida Stanley Bird, RN, MN
Assistant Clinical Professor
UCLA School of Nursing
UCLA Center for the Health Sciences
Childbirth Educator in Private Practice
Los Angeles, California

Chapters 17, 23, and Appendix C: Education for Pregnancy and Parenthood; The Nurse's Contribution to Pain Relief During Labor; Prenatal and Postpartum Exercises

Scot D. Foster, CRNA, PhD
Assistant Professor of Clinical Anesthesiology
School of Medicine
University of California, Los Angeles
Los Angeles, California

Co-author, Chapter 24: Analgesia and Anesthesia During Childbirth

Roberta J. Gerds, RN, MN
Associate Professor, Department of Nursing
California State University, Bakersfield
Bakersfield, California

Chapters 18, 25, 29, 30, 32, and 38: Nutritional Care in Pregnancy; Immediate Care of the Newborn; Assessment of the Newborn; Nursing Care of the Normal Newborn; Nutritional Care of the Infant; Complications of Labor

Susan M. Ludington, RN, CNM, PhD
Associate Professor of Nursing
School of Nursing
University of California, Los Angeles
Los Angeles, California

Chapter 31: Sensory Enrichment With the Newborn

Jane McAteer, RN, MN
Associate Professor
College of San Mateo
San Mateo, California

Chapters 44, 45, and 46: Disorders of Gestational Age and Birth Weight; The High-Risk Infant: Developmental Disorders; The High-Risk Infant: Acquired Disorders

Mary E. Sheridan, RN, MN
Coordinator, Perinatal Outreach Education Program
Long Beach Memorial Medical Center
Long Beach, California

Chapter 22: Management of Normal Labor

Catherine Walla, RN, MA, MN
Assistant Clinical Professor
School of Nursing
University of California, Los Angeles
Research Coordinator
Department of Obstetrics and Gynecology
Cedars-Sinai Medical Center
Los Angeles, California

Chapters 42 and 43: Fetal Diagnosis and Treatment; Intrapartum Fetal Monitoring and Care

Wynne Waugaman, CRNA, PhD
Associate Professor of Clinical Anesthesiology
School of Medicine
University of California, Los Angeles
Los Angeles, California

Co-author, Chapter 24: Analgesia and Anesthesia During Childbirth

Wendy S. Wetzel, RN, MSN, FNP
Nurse Practitioner, Private Practice
Fairfield, California
Instructor
California State University

Chapters 13, 14, and 39: Management of Infertility; Genetic Counseling and Diagnosis During Pregnancy; Operative Obstetrics

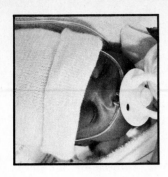

Preface

The 17th edition of Maternity Nursing: Family, Newborn, and Women's Health Care has been extensively revised. All chapters have been reorganized and rewritten, and several chapters have been consolidated to provide continuity and decrease overlap. Three new chapters have been added. The nursing process has been delineated in detail and diagnoses are illustrated according to the current NANDA recommendations. As in the previous edition, the nursing process provides a unifying conceptual basis for the nursing care throughout the book. All nursing care plans and clinical chapters reflect the nursing process.

Society continues to change at a phenomenal pace, and the institutions in our society continue to reorganize. This is especially true for the family and health-care systems. As society changes, clients change their orientations, values, and behavior; consequently, health-care providers must also change in order to keep pace. The provision of health care has become part of the medical–industrial complex with concomitant skyrocketing costs and necessary attempts at cost containment. Health providers too often try to provide quality care in the face of severe economic constraints and personnel shortages. They must change their attitudes and practices to maintain a synchrony in their newer roles.

The demographics of the nation are changing considerably, and family life-styles are continuing to evolve. With these various life-styles come a melange of attitudes and behaviors regarding reproduction, sexuality, and childrearing. A large amount of immigration continues with all the health-care problems that accrue during large-scale moves. More women and mothers are entering the work force, some without a choice in the matter. These factors broaden the scope of maternal and perinatal care. Moreover, the continuing innovations that are occurring in the health-care delivery system in response to health-care economics are having a profound impact on the maternity–perinatal specialty. These current issues are examined in depth to enable students to understand their importance so that this knowledge can be incorporated into the care they provide.

Unit I has been reorganized to present a variety of fundamental concepts regarding the structure and function of the modern family and health-care systems, emerging multiple life-styles, and various social factors relating to health. The chapter on the nursing process serves as a basis for implementing nursing care throughout the book. Ethical and legal considerations in reproduction have been updated to reflect current changes in thinking and legislation that applies to perinatal care. Chapter 6, Culture, Society, and Maternal Care, and Chapter 8, Social Risk Factors and Reproductive Outcomes, have been combined into a new chapter, Sociocultural Influences on Reproduction. In this chapter, we examine the effects of culture and society on motivations for childbearing and the use of health services by clients and the delivery of maternity–perinatal care by providers.

Again, there is an in-depth discussion regarding sexuality, changing role relationships in the family, nursing and parenting, reproductive behavior, and the use of maternity services. This information provides a broad conceptual base that the student can use to deliver comprehensive perinatal nursing care to families.

In Unit 11, the chapters dealing with conception and the development and physiology of the embryo and fetus have been combined. Sections on the development and physiology of the embryo and fetus have been revised to reflect current data and thinking. This unit supplies the basic anatomy, physiology, and development necessary for the study of nursing care.

Unit III continues an in-depth examination of areas of sexuality and various facets of reproduction. Common concerns of individuals regarding sexuality are addressed as well as the affectional and relational aspects of sexuality. Common concerns centering around sexuality and family planning management have been combined into a new chapter, Sexual Health and Management of Family Planning. Nursing intervention together with medical management is stressed in these (and all) chapters. This section provides a further elaboration of the concepts introduced in Unit I and provides the student with a sound knowledge base in this area.

The chapters dealing with pregnancy termination, infertility, and genetic counseling provide additional necessary information for the delivery of quality maternity care. We welcome the nurses who have contributed these chapters. Content has been extensively revised to focus on the assessment and management of nursing care as well as medical management.

Units IV through VI deal with the normal reproductive cycle from conception through the postpartum period. Again, we welcome the nurse anesthesiologists to our contributor list. All content has been extensively revised and updated. These chapters will enable the student to gain a knowledge of the total normal reproductive cycle and its management. Throughout these chapters and others in the book, dimensions of effective nursing care for each phase of the reproductive cycle have been expanded, based on recent research and conceptual developments in nursing practice and related disciplines. The nursing process is used throughout as a basis for care.

Units VII and VIII reflect current research and practice regarding the assessment and management of maternal and infant high-risk conditions and disorders. Three new chapters appear in Unit VII: Infectious Diseases in Pregnancy, Addictive Disorders in Pregnancy, and Adolescent Pregnancy. All have the most current research and thinking about these salient topics and all address nursing assessment and management. Emergencies in perinatal nursing, such as precipitous delivery, are considered in this unit. Numerous nursing care plans based on the nursing process have been developed for these chapters to guide students in planning and implementing care. One chapter has been devoted to fetal monitoring and its appropriate use. Nursing care in this area has been expanded. Fetal diagnosis and the management of the high-risk infant have been extensively updated to reflect current thinking and nursing management.

Three chapters are devoted to management of the infant with neonatal disorders. These chapters provide the student with the basic knowledge necessary to observe who is at risk and to provide care for those newborns and their families. The information in these chapters is essential as the field of perinatal nursing burgeons.

Unit IX examines the issue of women's health promotion and the assessment and management of women's health problems. These two chapters focus on those areas of gynecology that a maternity–perinatal nurse is likely to encounter. The maternity nurse is probably the most important individual many women will ever consult on health matters. Therefore, one chapter deals with gynecological health promotion, and another chapter discusses menstrual and bleeding disorders.

This edition of Maternity Nursing: Family, Newborn, and Women's Health Care has been reformatted to provide greater readability. New photographs, drawings, illustrations, tables, and boxed highlights have been added to reinforce points made in the text and to provide the student with quick reference information. Again, at our readers' request, we have included study questions and conference material at the end of each of the units. In this edition, we have placed answers to the questions at the back of the book, immediately preceding the Index. All of the suggested readings have been updated with references from current professional literature.

Sharon J. Reeder, RN, PhD, FAAN
Leonide L. Martin, RN, MS, DrPH
Deborah Koniak, RN, EdD

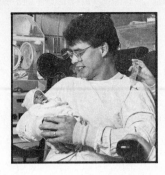

Acknowledgments

Once again, we wish to thank our contributors who have given a special dimension to the 17th edition of Maternity Nursing: Family, Newborn, and Women's Health Care with their varied expertise. In this edition, all of the contributors are nurses, which broadens and deepens each chapter's content and nursing orientation. We wish to express our gratitude for the help and encouragement of our many colleagues and friends in the revision of this edition. In particular, we would like to thank Rudy Martinez, Dee Ann Naylor, Marion Heller, and Antoinetta A. Russo for their scholarly and meticulous pursuit of the literature searches and for their general assistance. We especially appreciate the assistance of Wendy Phelan and Juan Ton with the various computer-related activities needed by the authors. Mrs. Bunny Lewis was extremely helpful in providing input for the production and revision of the care plans. We are also indebted to Carmen Methange for her expert word processing and editorial services.

We would like to extend our thanks to the Maternity Center Association of New York for permission to publish the exercises taught by the Center in its prepared childbirth program. We would also like to express our appreciation to colleagues, publishers, and organizations for the use of illustrations, assessment tools, and other tools that are found in the text. We are especially appreciative of the many parents, nursing students, and staff members who granted their permission for photographs appearing in Maternity Nursing: Family, Newborn, and Women's Health Care.

Finally, we take this opportunity to thank the people of J.B. Lippincott Company for their suggestions and cooperation through the production of this edition. Most especially, we are indebted to Diana Intenzo, Publisher, for all of her considerable expertise in bringing about this edition. We would also like to thank Barbara Cullen, Editor, Dave Carroll, Senior Editor, and Carole Wonsiewicz, Developmental Editor, for their steadfast assistance to the authors and contributors in the preparation of this edition.

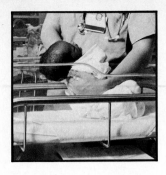

Contents

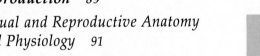

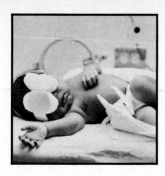

Expanded Contents

UNIT VI
Assessment and Management in the Postpartum Period 583

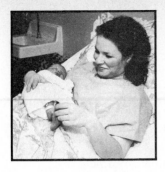

Nursing Care Plans

Seventeenth
Edition

MATERNITY NURSING

Family, Newborn, and Women's Health Care

UNIT I

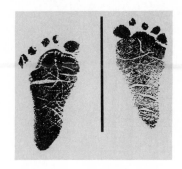

Nursing,
Family Health,
and
Reproduction

1

Philosophy of Family-Centered Care

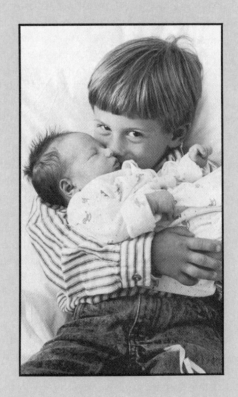

Of all the phenomena that humans experience, birth is perhaps the most emotional, dramatic, and awe inspiring. Birth is a family affair, and the reproductive health of the total family is the cornerstone on which a healthy society rests. Thus, the study of obstetrics and nursing care of women and their families during childbearing includes the study not only of anatomical and physiological adaptations to human reproduction but also of human growth and development and the many complex, interdependent relationships to the total society.

Knowledge of the anatomy and physiology of the reproductive organs and of the development of the unborn child from conception to birth is basic to the understanding required by everyone who participates in maternity care. The physiological mechanism by which conception takes place and the new human being develops is a fascinating story that has far-reaching implications for the family. All that a person becomes depends on many factors—his or her heritage, the prenatal environment, the care at birth, and the care thereafter throughout infancy and childhood. Thus, it becomes apparent that the health, well-being, and safety of each mother, father, and infant must be protected and, simultaneously, that the highest level of wellness possible for every childbearing family be achieved in the broadest sense of physical, emotional, and social well-being. Moreover, it is also important to understand the extent to which the structure and function of the family, as it relates to the larger society, influence the reproductive behavior and health of the childbearing family.

This chapter orients the student to maternity nursing. The philosophy and assumptions underlying care for the family during reproduction are given, and basic concepts of care are examined. In the remainder of the unit, information and concepts relating to childbearing families and how they intermesh with society are explored (Table 1-1).

■ EVOLUTION OF THE CONCEPT OF MATERNITY CARE

All definitions and modes of health care have a history. Maternity care is no exception. For the moment, we will concern ourselves with a brief overview of some terms and the concepts of care that have become associated with them.

Obstetrics

Obstetrics is defined as that branch of medicine that deals with parturition, its antecedents, and its sequelae. Thus, obstetrics is concerned principally with the phenomena and the management of pregnancy, labor, and the puerperium under both normal and abnormal circumstances.[1]

The word *obstetrics* is derived from the Latin, *obstetricia*, or *obstetrix*, meaning *midwife*. The verb form *obsto* (*ob*, before; *sto*, stand) means to stand by. Thus, in ancient Rome a person who cared for women at childbirth was known as an *obstetrix*, or a person who *stood by* the woman in labor. In both the United States and Great Britain, this branch of medicine was called *midwifery* until the latter part of the 19th century. The term *obstetrics* really came into use little more than a century ago, although reference to a variety of words of common derivation can be found occasionally in earlier writings.

The post–World War II era brought dramatic changes in the care of childbearing women and concomitant changes in terminology relating to them. In the then-current frame of reference, it seemed more appropriate to use the term *maternity care* because it focuses on the *recipient* of care rather than on the *provider*. Moreover, it has come to imply a broader meaning of the care of the mother and her offspring; it emphasizes the importance of interpersonal relationships that are significant in the family and takes into consideration all the factors that are crucial in promoting the general health and well-being of the entire expanding family group.

More than 30 years ago, the World Health Organization Expert Committee on Maternity Care[2] defined and delineated the goals of maternity care. The proper objectives of this care, they said, were to ensure that every expectant mother bore healthy children, maintained good health, and learned the art of child care. Not only did care consist of the mother's personal care, which included a safe delivery, a postnatal examination, maintenance of lactation, and care of the neonate, but also, in a far wider sense, it included care begun much earlier in the reproductive cycle. Promoting the health of young people, including personal health, family planning, and infertility counseling, together with helping couples develop appropriate approaches to family life and a knowledge of the family's place in society, were cornerstones in this concept.[2]

Thus, from the rather narrow definition that focused primarily on the provider of care, we expanded our concept of obstetrics to include not only the childbearing woman but all those significant persons in her social

TABLE 1-1. CHARACTERISTICS OF MATERNITY CARE AND EMERGENCE OF MATERNITY NURSING

Maternity Care	Maternity Nursing
Birth a family and community event, integrated into everyday life	Midwives usual birth attendants, precursors to maternity nurse
Development of scientific medicine and physician participation in childbirth	Gradual replacement of midwives by physicians as birth attendants
Increasing understanding of asepsis and increased technology in obstetrics	Nursing emerged as women's occupation, paralleling growth of scientific medicine
Growing emphasis on hospital deliveries rather than on home births	Nurses in obstetrics taught by medical (pathological) model
Increasing numbers of women delivering in the hospital	Nursing students focused upon technical competence and physical care of clients in hospitals
Necessity for efficient, organized aseptic care in hospitals, due to organizational structure	Nursing students provided service to hospitals where trained
Borrowing of timesaving approaches and work-efficient procedures from industry	Nursing orientation was toward efficient care of a number of clients, without in-depth nursing therapy (as there was no theoretical foundation)
"Assembly-line care" in hospitals	Institution-oreinted nurses became the physician's "right arm"
Ritualistic practices, rigid adherence to rules and procedures	Development of the humanistic-supportive nursing model as distinct from the pathological-intervention medical model
Impersonal, routine care	Expansion of the maternity nurse's role to include personalized care, parent education, counseling and psychosocial support, advocacy, alternative-care services to childbearing families
Resurgence of family and participant focus in childbearing, through natural childbirth and consumer movements	Emergence of new roles (nurse practitioner, clinical specialist) and resurgence of nurse-midwifery
Pressure for change in hospital routines and procedures, alternative birth approaches	
Development of family-centered maternity care, participant childbirth, rooming-in, alternate birth centers	

network. More recently, as the concept of high risk and regionalization have evolved, the term *perinatal care* has come into usage. All terms, however, relate to maternity care in some aspect (Fig. 1-1).

Maternal–Child Health

The term *maternal–child health* has been used for more than 70 years. In 1912, the US Children's Bureau was created by an act of Congress for the purpose of promoting maternal and child health "among all classes of people." Until its reorganization into the National Institutes of Health, the Children's Bureau continued to make significant contributions to the promotion of maternal–child health in this country.

Perinatal Care

During the past decade, as knowledge and technology have continued to burgeon, an effort has been made to provide a conceptual umbrella to encompass maternal-fetal health care as a unit. Consequently, the term *perinatal care* has evolved. By definition, the word *perinatal* means the 6-week period preceding or following birth; however, in actual use the connotation is much more encompassing. All of the definitions imply that both an obstetric and pediatric orientation are involved. Hence, perinatal care is a method of health-care delivery that would serve to decrease the segmentation and fragmentation of care for the mother and infant.[3,4]

Perinatal care has also become associated with the high-risk mother and infant in those hospitals desig-

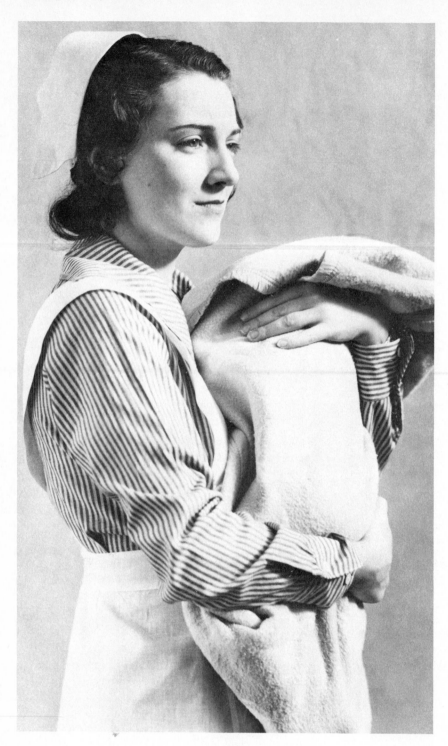

■ *Figure 1–1*
Obstetric nursing has evolved from being physician- and nurse-centered to family-centered maternity nursing.

nated as tertiary care, or Level III. These hospitals have the resources and expertise to manage any complication of pregnancy or the newborn. The personnel in Level III institutions provide care for normal patients and for all types of maternal-fetal and neonatal illnesses and abnormalities. By contrast, Level I hospitals provide for management of uncomplicated maternal and neonatal

patients, and in these institutions there should be a strong component of preventive services and early detection of existing or potential problems, which then may be referred to the Level III institutions. Level II hospitals provide the same services as the Level I hospitals; however, they can provide for some high-risk obstetric problems and certain types of neonatal illnesses that do not require the wide array of expertise and technology that is found in the Level III hospitals (Tables 1-2 and 1-3).[3]

Perinatal nursing has emerged as a subspecialty of professional maternity nursing. It has evolved in response to a need that arose from past gaps, failures, and successes in the delivery of quality nursing care during the reproductive process. It encompasses many of the best features of the above roles, and the knowledge base is not significantly different from that of the midwife or master's-prepared maternity nurse.

TRENDS IN PERINATAL CARE

There are several major trends apparent in society and the health-care industry today that will have both direct and indirect effects on perinatal care, particularly perinatal nursing. The settings in which health care is delivered, the practitioners who deliver care, and the manner in which reimbursement is provided will all be transformed by economic, demographic, social, and health-status changes.

Trends Affecting Future Health Care Delivery. The following trends will have a major impact on the future of American health-care delivery and will therefore affect all health-care providers, including perinatal nurses.

AGING OF THE POPULATION. By the year 2040, it is projected that the proportion of individuals over 65 will be 21%. The "graying of America" will probably be the *single* most important trend affecting the health-care delivery system between the years 2010 and 2030, when the "baby boomers" are expected to reach age 65.[5]

Perinatal nursing professionals will feel the impact of the growing number of elderly persons in the form of decreased resources for infants and women in their childbearing years. It is expected that the elderly will continue to use a disproportionate share of health resources, and health care will become increasingly focused on the long-term care and rehabilitation of older patients, with the availability of health resources diminishing for the nonelderly population subgroups. Moreover, it is anticipated that the older population, with their growing numbers, together with the use of their economic and political power, will wield consid-

TABLE 1-2. SERVICES PROVIDED IN LEVEL I, II, AND III HOSPITALS

Level I

- Surveillance and care of all patients admitted to the obstetric service, with an established triage system for identifying high-risk mothers who should be transferred to a level II or III facility prior to delivery
- Proper detection and supportive care of unanticipated maternal–fetal problems that occur during labor and delivery
- Performance of cesarean delivery
- Care of postpartum conditions
- Resuscitation of all neonates born in their delivery facilities
- Stabilization of unexpected small or sick neonates before transfer to a level II or III facility
- Evaluation of the condition of healthy neonates and continuing care of these neonates until their discharge

Level II

- Performance of level I services
- Management of high-risk mothers and neonates admitted and transferred

Level III

- Provision of perinatal service for all mothers and neonates
- Research support
- Compilation, analysis, and evaluation of regional data

Reprinted with permission from *Guidelines for Perinatal Care,* 2nd ed. 1988. The American Academy of Pediatrics and the American College of Obstetricians and Gynecologists.

TABLE 1-3. RECOMMENDED NURSE/PATIENT RATIOS FOR PERINATAL SERVICES

Nurse/Patient Ratio	Care Provided
1:2	Antepartum testing
1:2	Laboring patients
1:1	Patients in second stage of labor
1:1	Ill patients with complications
1:2	Oxytocin induction or augmentation of labor
1.1	Coverage of epidural anesthesia
1:1	Circulation for cesarean delivery
1:6	Antepartum/postpartum patients without complications
1:2	Postoperative recovery
1:3	Patients with complications, but in stable condition
1:4	Recently born infants and those needing close observation
1:6	Newborns needing only routine care
1:3	Mother–newborn care
1:1	Newborns requiring multisystem support
1:3–4	Newborns requiring intermediate care
1:1–2	Newborns needing intensive care

Reprinted with permission from *Guidelines for Perinatal Care,* 2nd ed. 1988. The American Academy of Pediatrics and the American College of Obstetricians and Gynecologists.

erable influence in tailoring health-care policy, services, and resources to the needs of the elderly. This, in turn, may obscure the needs of the young, which are the focus of perinatal nursing.[5]

CHANGING ECONOMICS. The economic forces influencing health-care delivery come from both escalating health-care costs and the resultant attempts at cost-containment programs, as well as from reduced government support of social and health programs. These measures limit the ability of consumers to afford health services. As a result of the escalating cost of health care, the United States spends approximately $1 billion a day on health care, which is about 10.8% of the gross national product, and this proportion is expected to keep rising.[6]

Several cost-containment programs have been developed that have been somewhat successful. These include limiting reimbursement, as with the Medicare diagnosis-related group model, and lowering costs through contract agreements that provide discounts for consumers who use the services of selected practitioners or institutions. One outcome of these cost-containment efforts has been the rapid growth of nontraditional health-care settings, such as freestanding centers, health maintenance organizations (HMOs), prospective payment organizations, and business consortia. The impact of these changes on the quality of care has not been determined, although there is substantial evidence to indicate that although hospital occupancy rates have decreased, patients are being released from acute care settings more quickly with more serious illnesses.[7]

Although budget restrictions are changing the health-care industry internally, external factors are diminishing clients' ability to pay for services, including perinatal care. Sixteen percent of women in their childbearing years are without health insurance coverage.[8] Medicaid and Aid to Families with Dependent Children benefits have both been cut. Overall funding for maternal–child health programs was cut 27% when programs were reorganized into a federal block program. Similarly, the WIC program, a supplemental food program for women, children, and infants was cut, and other restrictions are apparent on the horizon. This climate will have a negative effect on the use of perinatal services and will be manifested in the health of women and their infants.[5]

As the health-care system becomes more fiscally austere, perinatal nurses will be increasingly pressured to demonstrate cost as well as quality consciousness. Accounting systems that "cost out" nursing care are one attempt to formalize this effort. Restraints on equipment purchases and constraints on the development and use of perinatal technology are other possible outcomes. Thirty percent of all women who had live births in 1980 had at least one ultrasound examination, and almost 50% had electronic fetal monitoring during

their pregnancy—given this current high level of use of technology in perinatology, the possibility of the reduction of either the use or the development of technology could be of concern to those nurses who work in very high-risk settings.[5,9]

Perinatal nurses will be required to move increasingly into nontraditional settings, such as freestanding birthing centers, HMOs, and homes. New skills will be required to ensure no loss in quality of care.

PHYSICIAN SURPLUS. The number of physicians practicing medicine in the United States is expected to exceed 700,000 by the year 2000, a growth rate of 54% or more from the 455,000 in 1980. It has been estimated that by 1990, there will be a 45% oversupply in the fields of obstetrics and gynecology.[10] It is anticipated that with more physicians than necessary in the marketplace, independent practice will be limited and hospitals, HMOs, and the like will experience an increase in physician employees. This trend has already been seen.[5] There has been speculation that physicians may attempt to take over many of the expanded role functions that nurses have assumed, such as teaching, counseling, and follow-up. However, as hospitals continue cost containment, there should be minimal effect in the long term. The District of Columbia has passed a comprehensive clinical privileges bill that prohibits hospital and other licensed institutions from denying clinical privileges to five nonphysician practitioners, including nurse–midwives, nurse practitioners, and nurse anesthetists.[11] This gives some indication that nurses are able to maintain their roles in competitive situations.

Trends with Direct Impact on Perinatal Nursing

DEMOGRAPHIC TRENDS. Three demographic trends significantly affecting perinatal nursing practice are the declining birth rate, changes in childbearing patterns, and the increasing number of women working outside the home. The U.S. birthrate declined from 1957 to 1976 and showed a slight increase from 1977 to the present. This small increase is a reflection of the baby boom cohort having their children. The average number of children has dropped from 2.1 in 1977 (a replacement rate) to 1.9 per family in 1983. As the size of the population in need of perinatal services decreases, so will the need for providers of those services.[12]

A second demographic trend affecting perinatal nursing is the changing pattern of childbirth among American women. More babies are being born to women at the extremes of the childbearing years. More women are choosing to have their first baby in their 30s and, at the same time, teenage pregnancies are increasing at an alarming rate.[5,12] Both younger and older mothers face a variety of medical complications during pregnancy for themselves and their infant. These risks are discussed in subsequent chapters.

The final demographic trend affecting perinatal

nursing practice is the increase in the number of women employed outside the home while pregnant and immediately following birth. One of the major concerns is the exposure these women and their fetuses face from toxic chemicals, excessive noise, radiation, and stress in the workplace. Moreover, women working in nontraditional jobs use tools, machinery, and surfaces that have been designed to meet the average male worker's requirements, a fact that has the potential for jeopardizing the safety of the female worker.[5,12]

HEALTH STATUS TRENDS. The high incidence of low-birth-weight newborns in the United States and the increasing rate of sexually transmitted diseases are health-status trends that have implications for perinatal practice. The high proportion of low-birth-weight infants is in a large degree responsible for the slowing in the decline in the national infant mortality rate. Most low-birth-weight infants are born prematurely, and this condition accounts for two thirds of the yearly 39,000 infant deaths nationally. A variety of risk factors contribute to low birth weight and prematurity. These are discussed in detail in other chapters. It is important to remember, however, that the other factors we have previously mentioned, particularly the changing health-care economics, will contribute to the incidence of these conditions. In 1984, 24% of all pregnant women received no prenatal care, and many others received inadequate care because they began care later or terminated care early.[9]

The collision of societal trends, changing client needs, and consequent changes in the provider role can lead to confusion about practice standards for maternity/perinatal nursing. To clarify basic standards of practice, The Nurses' Association of the American College of Obstetricians and Gynecologists (NAACOG) has developed standards for obstetric, gynecologic, and neonatal nursing.[3] These standards are not meant to limit innovation in nursing care but should be viewed as part of an ongoing process being constantly revised as the need arises. Students are advised to familiarize themselves with these important standards of practice and the Pregnant Patient's Bill of Rights (see Appendix A).

■ PHILOSOPHY ABOUT MATERNITY CARE

Health providers' responses to their client's needs in both health maintenance and illness management must take into consideration current attitudinal, social, and cultural changes. Health care is not delivered in a vacuum; it takes place in a larger social context and is greatly influenced by current thinking and change manifested by the host society. Philosophies of care evolve from this thinking and change.

We believe maternity care to be a philosophy of client care rather than a special area of medical services or nursing. We believe that begetting children is a family affair; thus, the medical and nursing care of maternity clients is properly a family-centered activity.

In almost no other normal physiological process does one find such individual extremes of reactions within a normal context. For both the woman and her partner, these reactions may be based on events going back to childhood or experienced as an adolescent and adult. Certainly, they are influenced by the immediate home environments from which the couple come. Moreover, the expectant parents' level of satisfaction and the level of contentment of the newly delivered mother and infant are modified by the interpersonal relationships of those most significant to them in the health-care environment.

Recommendations for Perinatal Nurses Regarding Trends

- Become knowledgeable and active in the political arena; utilize national health policy fellowships, Robert Wood Johnson fellowships and so forth to prepare to contribute.
- Voice support for continued resources for perinatal services.
- Stand in the forefront to maintain a balance between technology and humanized care.
- Conduct market surveys to determine need for services and tailor services accordingly. Conduct clinical nursing research to determine relevant problems in the health care of women and their fetuses and infants and the relationship of these problems to clinical nursing practice.
- Expand the leadership and practice roles to nontraditional practice settings, such as ambulatory care settings, home. The perinatal home care aspect will become increasingly important.

■ ASSUMPTIONS ABOUT MATERNITY CARE

Underlying the philosophy about maternity care are the following assumptions:

- All individuals have the right to be born healthy, and, to ensure this right, every pregnant woman and every fetus has the right to quality health care.

- The sexuality of individuals is inextricably bound to reproduction but not subordinate to it; changing societal attitudes toward sexuality, role relationships, and childbearing, together with technological advances in fertility control, have combined to make parenthood increasingly a voluntary state.
- Reproduction is not experienced alone; whatever the circumstances, it involves one or more individuals.
- Reproduction is part of a normal psychophysiological process and can be physically and emotionally rewarding for the individuals involved.
- The childbearing experience is a developmental opportunity; it can also be a situational crisis during which family members benefit from the solidarity of the family unit.
- The profound physiological changes and adjustment that both the mother and her offspring experience during the childbearing process make them particularly vulnerable to changeable and noxious environments and situations that would ordinarily not prove hazardous.
- Each individual's attitudes, values, and health behavior are influenced by the culture and society from which he or she comes; thus, each individual's reproductive outcomes and childbearing experience will be influenced by his or her cultural heritage.

■ MATERNITY NURSING AND FAMILY-CENTERED CARE

Definition

Maternity nursing can be defined as the delivery of professional-quality health care while recognizing, focusing on, and adapting to the physical and psychosocial needs of the childbearing woman, the family, and the newly born offspring.

Implicit in this definition is the notion of a family-centered approach. This approach assumes that the family is the basic unit of society and, as such, is to be viewed as a total unit within which each member is a distinct individual. It is further assumed that childbearing and the rearing and socialization of children are unique and important functions of the family. Therefore, the experience of childbearing is appropriate and beneficial to share as a unit.

When we speak of the "family," we do not necessarily mean the traditional nuclear family composed of a married pair and their children. In Chapters 4 and 5, we examine the various definitions and emerging family forms.

Maternity nursing involves direct, personal care to the childbearing woman and her infant, as well as the related activities of teaching, counseling, and supervising during the various phases of the childbearing experience. A cornerstone of care is client/consumer education with respect to health maintenance and reproductive health. It differs from the practice of nursing in other areas in that the clinical focus involves, primarily, the care of the childbearing unit (the mother, father, and infant) in contrast, for example, to the care of surgical or psychiatric patients. It is unique in that the nurse is called on to attend, educate, and counsel all age groups, from the fetal period through childhood, adolescence, and adulthood, because the childbearing unit may span all those stages in the life cycle.

How the maternity nurse meets the needs of members of the childbearing unit cannot be spelled out in stereotyped activities. The nurse will intervene to relieve or reduce problems caused by physiological, psychological, or social stress. In addition, the nurse will make clients aware of the principles of health maintenance so that they may incorporate these into their preventive health-behavior patterns.

A significant aspect of maternity nursing on the professional level is that the nursing care involves purposeful, sustained interaction during which the nurse makes an assessment of the client's problems and resources and then takes action to relieve the problem and support the strengths with appropriate nursing measures. If the condition requires additional services from the other members of the health team, referral or consultation is given.

Implementation

The successful implementation of family-centered nursing care includes recognition that the provision of high-caliber care requires a team effort by the woman and her family, the health-care providers, and the community. The composition of the team may vary from setting to setting and includes obstetricians, pediatricians, family physicians, certified nurse–midwives, nurse practitioners, and maternity clinical nurse specialists. Although physicians are responsible for providing direction for medical management, other team members share appropriately in managing the health care of the family, and each team member must be individually accountable for the performance of his or her facet of care. The team concept includes the cooperative interrelationships of hospitals, providers, and the community in an organized care system so as to provide for the total spectrum of maternity/newborn care within a particular geographic region.[13]

Expanding Roles in Maternity Nursing

In the mid-1960s, experiments began to expand nursing roles to include greater responsibility for primary-care treatment of common problems and health needs. Early programs were started by physician–nurse teams (Ford, RN, and Silver, MD, in Denver; Resnick, RN, and Lewis, MD, in Los Angeles) to expand nursing roles in pediatrics[14] and adult health.[15] In 1971, the National Commission for the Study of Nursing and Nursing Education (Jerome Lysaught, Director) reported a study of nursing roles and recommended that nursing roles be expanded, educational systems repatterned, and nursing input into health care increased.[16] Also during that year, the American Nurses Association (ANA) and the American Academy of Pediatrics jointly developed guidelines for training pediatric nurse associates and held a national conference to implement these. The ANA and the American College of Obstetricians and Gynecologists also met to draw up guidelines for training clinical nurse specialists in obstetrics and gynecology.

In 1972, the Committee to Study Extended Roles for Nurses reported to the Secretary of the Department of Health, Education, and Welfare that functions of nurses "need to be broadened [so they can] assume broader responsibility in primary care, acute care, and long-term care."[17] The new nurse practitioner was functioning in expanded nursing roles in many areas, including obstetrics, pediatrics, psychiatry, and medical-surgical nursing.

In 1973, Lysaught's National Commission[16] reported on the implementation phase of its study. To encourage the expansion of nursing practice, it conducted educational and informational activities aimed at nursing professionals and the public, developed a national joint practice commission between medicine and nursing with state counterparts, and developed statewide planning committees to generate changes in patterns of education and practice (see Appendix B).

These expanded nursing roles developed in two general directions. The nurse practitioner role focused mainly on primary ambulatory care, and the nurse clinical specialist role focused on secondary and tertiary hospital care.

NURSE PRACTITIONER

As the nurse practitioner role evolved, it encompassed additional skills in the techniques of physical diagnosis that were formerly in the realm of medicine, as well as the knowledge base to diagnose and treat common problems and minor illness. Health prevention and maintenance, including examination, testing, and education, as well as management of stabilized chronic illness, are also included in nurse practitioner functions. The nurse practitioner combines the nurse's sensitivity to emotional needs and focus on adaptation and social aspects of client care with the techniques and knowledge of medicine to diagnose and treat pathophysiological problems. These nurses usually practice in a primary-care setting, defined as the first contact with the health-care system in any given episode of illness, and are responsible for continuance of care, including maintenance of health, evaluation and management of symptoms, and appropriate referrals.[16,17]

Maternity Nurse Practitioner. The maternity nurse practitioner, or ob-gyn nurse practitioner, provides prenatal care for uncomplicated pregnancies in conjunction with a physician consultant. The nurse takes a health and pregnancy history, performs the physical and obstetric examination, orders and interprets laboratory and other diagnostic studies, plans for necessary treatments and medications in conjunction with the physician, and assesses family relationships and psychosocial needs.

Throughout the pregnancy, the maternity nurse practitioner sees the woman on antepartal visits, sometimes alternating with the physician, evaluates the progress of the pregnancy, and manages minor physical problems. Information and counseling related to pregnancy and childbirth and assessment of the couple's adjustments and family problems are also part of the nurse practitioner's role. Referrals to community agencies, prepared childbirth classes, and other medical specialties may also be made. Most maternity nurse practitioners are skilled in provision of contraception and can select appropriate methods for the client, including oral contraceptives, intrauterine devices, and diaphragms, and teach about their use and about other methods.

Family Nurse Practitioner. Family nurse practitioners also provide care during pregnancy. They are generalists who care for all family members similarly to family-practice physicians. In addition to the functions described above for maternity nurse practitioners, family nurse practitioners provide postdelivery care for the baby as it grows, thus providing continuity throughout the reproductive process except during the intrapartum phase.

MATERNITY CLINICAL SPECIALIST

Maternity clinical specialists undergo advanced study of maternity nursing at the graduate level and are able to provide in-depth intervention for many of the adaptational and physiological problems encountered in maternity care. Frequently, clinical specialists have an area of expertise within the specialty field, such as a maternity clinical specialist with special expertise in the care of pregnant diabetics, breast-feeding mothers, parents experiencing neonatal death or abnormalities, Rh-sensitized mothers, and so on. These nurses with master's degrees also serve as consultants to other maternity nursing staff, assisting them to plan care for difficult problems or special situations encountered in the unit.

Although clinical specialists also may be involved in staff education, their primary function is direct client services using a high degree of knowledge, skill, and competence in their area of specialty.

Critical Care Obstetrics. This subspecialty is only recently emerging and relates primarily to high-risk delivery room and critical care postpartum. There has been little in the literature regarding this type of practice.

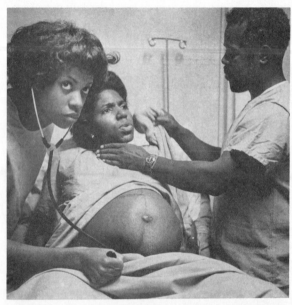

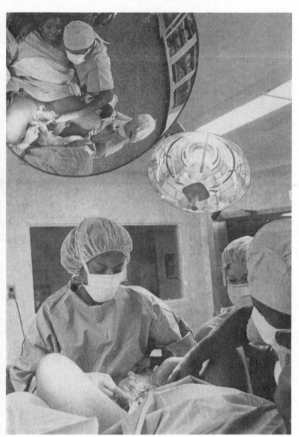

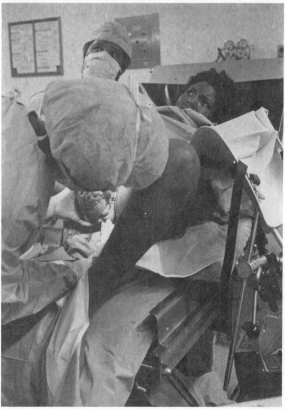

■ *Figure 1–2*
Labor conducted by a nurse–midwife. (A) The nurse–midwife monitors the fetal heart, while the father coaches the mother to keep her Lamaze breathing light and high in the chest. (B) The nurse–midwife delivers the baby with the mother out of stirrups in the semi-upright position. The parents watch the birth in the overhead mirror. (C) The nurse–midwife supervises the father as he cuts the umbilical cord. (Photos by Allison Wachstein.)

However, with the increasing number of high-risk clients and the burgeoning of hi-tech equipment, it is expected that this specialty will become prominent.

NURSE–MIDWIFE

The "expanded" role known as nurse–midwife has been around for centuries. Modern obstetrics requires certification and special education. Certified nurse–midwives are registered nurses who have completed a specific program of study and clinical experience recognized by the American College of Nurse Midwives. They must also pass a certification test before beginning practice. They are qualified to take complete health histories and perform complete physical examinations for their clients. They can provide complete antepartal care, including teaching and counseling. They are qualified to give comprehensive care during the intrapartal period, including delivery of the infant (Fig. 1-2). They are able to deliver care to the mother and infant in the postpartum period, including family-planning information and devices. Thus, they attend both the mother and the infant throughout the maternity cycle as long as the mother's progress is considered normal and uncomplicated.

Nurse–Midwifery

What Is a Certified Nurse-Midwife?

A certified nurse–midwife (CNM) is an individual educated in the two disciplines of nursing and midwifery, who possesses evidence of certification according to the requirements of the American College of Nurse–Midwives.

What Is Nurse-Midwifery Practice?

Nurse–midwifery is the independent management of care of essentially normal newborns and women, antepartally, intrapartally, postpartally, and/or gynecologically, occurring within a health-care system that provides for medical consultation, collaborative management, or referral and is in accord with the *Functions, Standards, and Qualifications for Nurse–Midwifery Practice* as defined by the American College of Nurse–Midwives.

The nurse–midwife provides care for the normal mother during pregnancy and stays with her during labor, providing continuous physical and emotional support. She evaluates progress and manages the labor and delivery. She evaluates and provides immediate care for the normal newborn. She helps the mother to care for herself and for her infant, to adjust the home situation to the new child, and to lay a healthful foundation for future pregnancies through family planning and gynecologic services. The nurse–midwife is prepared to teach, interpret, and provide support as an integral part of her services.

(J Nurse–Midwifery 26(2):42, March/April 1981)

■ SOCIAL CONTEXT OF MATERNITY CARE

Maternity care is practiced in the context of the total society and, as such, is influenced by the values, attitudes, and practices of that society. Of late, society is adopting a new stance, particularly with regard to women. At least half of the maternity nurse's clientele will be women, and attitudes and practices regarding these women have great relevance for nursing practice. The maelstrom of social change this country has experienced, particularly in the last 25 years, has greatly expanded the options of behavior.

Growing numbers of women and men no longer accept the traditional definitions of "feminine" and "masculine" identities and roles. They are seeking more individualized definitions of self that offer wider ranges of expression of their unique characteristics as *persons* rather than simply as *women* or *men*. Indeed, the common qualities shared by both women and men are believed to far outweigh their sex-related differences. Hence, social roles are developing that provide each sex with a much broader repertoire of behaviors.

Women, in particular, expect more choices of lifestyle. They may choose whether to marry, to have children, or to pursue any career or employment. They expect to have a voice in the determination of their lives and well-being. And, increasingly, they are demanding a large decision-making role regarding economic and social policies that affect their lives and the larger society in which they live.

At one time, women had to make a choice between a family or a career; now, women are increasingly combining the two. Moreover, many types of occupations and professions formerly closed to women are becoming more accessible. Federal legislation now supports equal treatment of working women, and more mechanisms to challenge discrimination and unfair employment practices against women are being developed at the state level. Antidiscrimination laws have also had an impact on educational institutions. This is forcing a gradual change in the social biases toward a male privilege, perpetuated through values taught in primary and secondary schools and culminating in the sex-linked admissions practices and career choices fostered by colleges and universities.

Women who choose to rear families spend significantly less of their lifetime in childbearing and child-rearing. This fact, of course, has a direct impact on the structure and function of the family. Today's families are smaller, and for those who start childbearing early, the last child is often born when the mother is in her mid- to late 20s or early 30s. The high degree of technology in the majority of American households has freed the woman from hours of household chores; thus, homemaking does not provide the full-time occupation that it once did. With her life span lengthened and her health improved, the 35- to 40-year-old woman can be healthy and vigorous and can look ahead to at least another 25 years of productivity in a sphere outside the home.

It has been said that roles are differentiated in pairs; that is, every role has its complementary role. Thus, as women's roles change and broaden, so too must men's. More egalitarian relationships are slowly developing between the two sexes. Increasingly, men are assuming more responsibility in childrearing and running the household as their partners are forging ahead with careers. When both parties are pursuing a career, there is a growing tendency for household management, chores, and child-related activities to be shared equally. Thus, social power is very slowly being equalized, and sex-linked exploitation is very gradually being diminished. However, there is still a long way to go before true equality can be achieved.

7. Medicare patients discharged sicker, state survey shows. Am J Nurs 17:3–5, 1985
8. Gold RB, Kenny A-M, Singh S: Financing Maternity Care in the United States. New York, The Alan Guttmacher Institute, 1987
9. US Department of Health and Human Services: Health, Education, Welfare, United States, 1983. Washington, DC, US Government Printing Office, 1983
10. Crozier DA, Iglehart JK: Datawatch: Trends in health manpower. Health Affairs 3:122, 1984
11. Solomon SB: DC regulatory battle proves our fight is far from over. Nurs Health Care 6:242–244, 1985
12. Adams CJ: Women in their reproductive years. In Adams CJ (ed): Nurse–Midwifery for Women and Newborns. New York, Grune & Stratton, 1983
13. Lauver EB: Where will the money go? Economic forecasting and nursing's future. Nurs Health Care 6:133–135, March 1985
14. Silver HK, Ford L: The pediatric nurse practitioner program: Expanding the role of the nurse to provide increased health care for children. JAMA 204:298–302, April 22, 1968
15. Lewis CE, Resnick BA: Nurse clinics and progressive ambulatory patient care. N Engl J Med 227:1236–1241, December 7, 1967
16. National Commission on the Study of Nursing and Nursing Education, Jerome Lysaught, Director: An Abstract for Action. New York, McGraw-Hill, 1971
17. Extending the Scope of Nursing Practice: A Report of the Secretary's Committee to Study Extended Roles for Nurses. Washington DC, Department of Health, Education, and Welfare, November 1972

■ REFERENCES

1. Cunningham FG, McDonald PC, Gant NF: Williams' Obstetrics, 18th ed. Norwalk, CT, Appleton & Lange, 1989
2. World Health Organization: Technical Report Series No. 51. Geneva, Switzerland, World Health Organization, 1952
3. NAACOG: Standards for Obstetric, Gynecologic, and Neonatal Nursing, 3rd ed. Washington DC, NAACOG, 1986
4. NAACOG: Nursing Practice Resource: Considerations for Professional Nurse Staffing in Perinatal Units. Washington, DC, NAACOG, October 1988
5. Andreoli KG, Musser LA: Major trends shaping the future of perinatal nursing. J Perinatol 6:325–330, Fall 1986
6. Grier P: US health care costs still ballooning: The question is how high can they soar before something pops? Houston Post, September 20, 1983

■ SUGGESTED READINGS

Adams C: Nurse–Midwifery practice in the United States, 1982 and 1987. Am J Public Health 79:1038–1039, August 1989
Gleeson RM, Bowen AG, Fain WL et al: Advanced practice nursing: A model of collaborative care. MCN 15:9–12, January/February 1990
Jacox A, Pillar B, Redman BK: A classification of nursing technology. Nurs Outlook 38:81–85, March/April 1990
Kaufman K, McDonald H: A retrospective evaluation of a model of midwifery care. Birth 15:95–99, June 1988
Myers ST, Stolte K: Nurses' responses to changes in maternity care. Part II. Technologic revolution, legal climate, and economic changes. Birth 14:87–90, June 1987
Phillips CR: Rehumanizing maternal-child nursing. MCN 13:313–318, September/October 1988
Sherwen LN: Maternal-infant competencies for new nurses: A joint effort by educators and practitioners. J Perinatol 9:173–177, June 1989

2

The Nursing Process in Maternity Care

COMPONENTS OF THE PROCESS
Assessment
Nursing Diagnosis

Planning and Intervention
Evaluation and Reassessment
KNOWLEDGE AND SKILLS IN IMPLEMENTING THE PROCESS

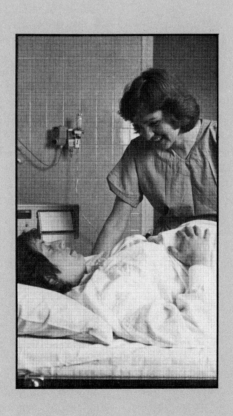

mplicit in the delivery of effective, professional nursing care is the ability to use a method that helps the nurse arrive at informed judgments about clients that have a sound data base. With the data base and these appropriate clinical judgments, nursing care can be planned and implemented so as to enable clients to maintain or return to a state of high-level wellness. This method has been conceptualized as the *nursing process* by a variety of authors in an effort to describe a lucid, organized, scientifically based, problem-solving approach to professional nursing practice.[1-4]

Nursing process is the organizing conceptual framework used throughout this text to help the student learn to make nursing judgments appropriate to nursing care. It supplies a mechanism that enables the nurse to arrive at a responsible, valid judgment about clients from which to assess, diagnose, plan, implement, and evaluate nursing care that is responsive to the client's varied needs.

■ COMPONENTS OF THE PROCESS

It is important to point out that, in the midst of the press and crush of everyday practice, when human lives may be at stake, calm fact-finding and judicious deliberation become increasingly difficult. Some of our most crucial nursing problems arise from conflicts between principle and expediency. Hence, we need to have a method so internalized as to be second nature so that we can arrive quickly at appropriate decisions and conclusions about our patients.

The components of the process also can help the student understand how nursing practice can be made operational. The various operations have been classified under headings derived over time by nurse theorists, practitioners, and researchers. One is not to assume that these categories are mutually exclusive or stand alone. Rather, there are constant feedback loops in the process.

The scientific method is used by other disciplines to provide a way of problem solving for their members and as a basis from which to formulate research that will expand the theoretical base of the discipline. Because nursing also has the concern of expanding its theoretical knowledge to provide a sound basis for its practice, it is important that the nursing process be scientifically grounded (see the chart on Relationship of the Scientific Method to the Nursing Process).

Over time, the nursing process has come to comprise five stages: assessment, nursing diagnosis, planning, intervention, and evaluation.[4] Various authors have conceptualized the process using different terminology, including assessment, problem identification, diagnostic phase, validation, action, and evaluation.[5,6] New conceptualizations and new terminology have evolved over the years, and as nursing science develops, other terminology will no doubt be employed. Although the components may be elaborated in slightly different ways by various authors, it is generally agreed that the process is as follows: in *assessment*, data are gathered on the state of the client's health, and *nursing diagnoses* are made from these data. Following the construction of the diagnoses, the nurse *plans* for intervention, based on assessment data and diagnoses. After *planning*, the nurse implements *interventions*. As the client's condition changes, *evaluations* are made of the outcomes of the interventions. Additional assessments, diagnoses, plans, and interventions are made as indicated by the evaluation of the outcomes. Thus, a continuous feedback loop is in operation (Fig. 2-1).

The use of the nursing process is twofold: (1) to provide a method that becomes second nature for quick but appropriate nursing decisions and conclusions; and (2) to provide a scientific approach to problem solving, which is essential to any profession. For clarity and ease, we use the four-step format for nursing process and care plans in this book: assessment, nursing diagnosis, planning and intervention (combining these two components), and evaluation.

We use the North American Nursing Diagnosis Association (NANDA) classification taxonomy for nursing diagnoses (see list in Appendix I). For those who are unfamiliar with NANDA, it is a group that evolved from a series of national conferences on nursing diagnosis made up of representatives from all areas of the nursing profession: clinical practice, education, and research.[4] The first conference was held in 1973, with eight subsequent meetings, and from those meetings the nursing diagnoses (see list in Appendix I). For those who are extremely important by most members of the profession and is viewed as a major advancement toward nursing professionalism.[7]

Some controversy has existed within the nursing profession as to the practicality of using a method such as nursing process in contrast to a more holistic approach to patient care.[7,8] Some nurses have suggested alternatives to the extant classification taxonomies such as NANDA's.[8] Whatever the concerns of those who have conflicting opinions and whatever the data show, it is crucial that this discussion and alternatives be aired. It is only through such informed discussion and debate that the profession will advance.

Assessment

Assessing is the act of reviewing a human situation based on information from the client and a variety of

Relationship of the Scientific Method to the Nursing Method

	Components of the Nursing Process	Scientific Method
Assessment	1. Collect data (subjective, objective). a. Gather information on the physical, social, and psychological aspects of the health status of the individual and family. b. Construct the data base by observation, interview, history taking, physical examination, and role taking. c. Develop impressions.	1. Recognize general problem area. a. Survey pertinent information (literature, past experience, observation). b. Construct data base (organize, select). c. Develop "hunches."
Nursing Diagnosis	2. Define the problem. a. Make decisions regarding deficits or potential deficits in health status of the individual and family assigning resources. b. Make nursing diagnoses based on clinical judgment and inference and review of related information, that is, theoretical formulations and research.	2. Define specific problem. a. Make decisions about relevance. b. Review related information (research already done, theoretical formulations).
Planning/Intervention	3. Plan the intervention. a. Make decisions regarding the actions believed to be appropriate to effect a solution of defined problems. b. Decisions include goal setting, priority setting, and nursing prescriptions. 4. Implement the intervention. a. Execute a nursing regimen by adminstering a prescribed medication or treatment, executing a medical regimen, providing comfort measures and physical care, providing counseling, providing referral services, coordinating services for the patient, and providing health education.	3. Propose hypotheses. 4. Test hypotheses. a. Establish baseline data. b. State criteria for acceptance or rejection. c. Collect data.
Evaluation and Reassessment	5. Evaluate the intervention. This in turn may lead to further reassessments. a. Determine the degree of effectiveness of the actions	5. Analyze data and interpret results.

(continued)

	Components of the Nursing Process	Scientific Method
	taken in solving the defined problems by observation, interview of patient status and conditions, physical examination, and reading of current records. b. Predict future nursing action and patient potential for change. 6. Terminate or modify relationship.	6. Terminate or modify study. a. Make recommendations and predictions for future research.

other sources. The information gathered forms a crucial data base. Assessing is done to affirm the degree of wellness of the client and to diagnose potential problems; one may also affirm an illness state.[3,10] The assessment phase of the process incorporates a variety of data-gathering efforts and activities, including the following:

- Taking a nursing history and utilizing records
- Performing a health assessment
- Using a variety of data-gathering tools: thermometer, sphygmomanometer, stethoscope, and other tools
- Using the techniques of physical examination: palpation, auscultation, percussion
- Using the five senses[3,10]

If these activities are used systematically, they will provide the information to make valid nursing judgments and diagnoses. Thus, it becomes clear that the purpose of the assessment phase is to identify and obtain data on the client's needs that enable the nurse, client, and family to assess their degree of wellness, recognize actual and potential problems, and plan care that will ensure that the client and family will arrive at appropriate solutions.

In her assessments, the nurse will consider the interrelationships of such factors as the client's age, sex, education, stage of growth and development, and socioeconomic status. These factors are discussed more fully in Chapter 6

Specific data can be obtained by interviewing the client and performing a health examination. The interview and examination incorporate both physical and psychosocial dimensions, and a systematic format needs to be used. Previous records and charts should be considered to ensure completeness of information and to avoid fragmentation of information with consequent impact on continuity of care.

While the nurse collects data, inferences are validated to ensure accuracy in interpretation. When the existence of a problem, condition, or situation is inferred from the accumulated facts, it will be confirmed with the client. The mother then has the opportunity to confirm or deny the perceptions or diagnosis.[3,10]

Carpenito has pointed out that after the data are gathered and examined, alternative explanations need to be tested and ruled out.[4] At this time the nurse will have reached one of four conclusions:

- No problem is evident at the present time; hence, no health promotion or intervention is indicated.
- No problem is evident, but health promotion activities are indicated to ensure and maintain the present level of wellness and to prevent health alterations.
- Actual or potential clinical problems are evident requiring medical referral or implementation of the medical regimen by the nurse.
- Actual or potential nursing problems are apparent that are within the legal and educational domain of the nurse and that require nursing orders.

Nursing Diagnosis

The assessment phase concludes with the nurse making one or more nursing diagnoses. In the care plans in this text, we refer to "possible nursing diagnoses," because

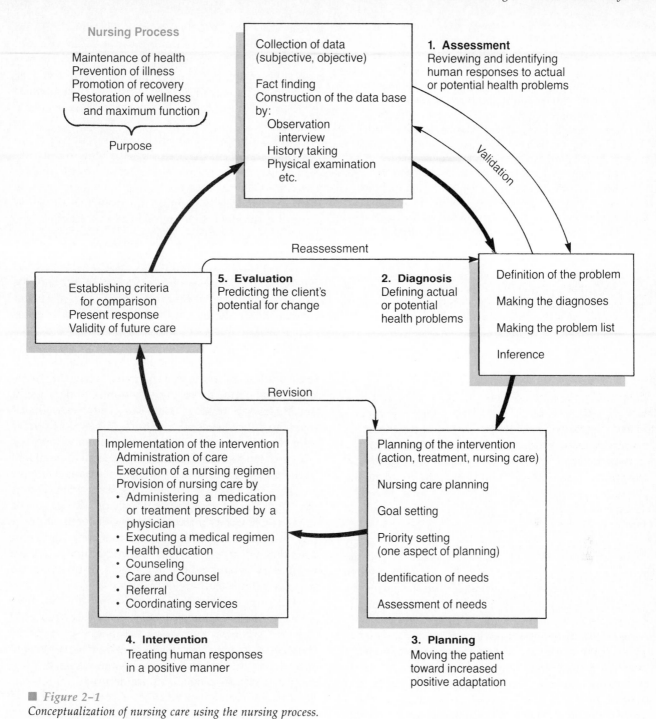

■ *Figure 2–1*
Conceptualization of nursing care using the nursing process.

without having an actual situation from which to extrapolate, it would be impossible to state what the diagnoses might actually be. We also use the basic classification categories developed by NANDA. Although we based our diagnoses on these categories, we have made them more specific to maternity when appropriate to make them more understandable to the student. We also couch them in a two- or three-part statement, as recommended by Carpenito, thereby showing clearly

that the diagnoses describe the human response, contributing factors, and signs and symptoms when appropriate.[4]

Potential and *possible* nursing diagnoses have two parts. The first part is a diagnostic label or statement, which is followed by the second part, a statement regarding the presence of risk factors. Thus, an example of a two-part statement (*potential nursing diagnosis* related to *risk factors*) might be "Possible self-care deficit

---

Definitions of Nursing Diagnosis

- The actual or potential health problems that nurses, by virtue of their education and experience, are capable and licensed to treat.[12]
- The judgment or conclusion that occurs as a result of nursing assessment.[2]
- A clinical judgment about an individual, family, or community that is derived through a systematic process of data collection and analysis and that provides the basis for prescription for definitive therapy for which the nurse is accountable. The diagnosis is expressed concisely and includes the etiology when known.[13]
- A statement that describes the human response (health state or actual/potential altered interaction pattern) of an individual or group that the nurse can legally identify and for which the nurse can order the definitive interventions to maintain the health state or to reduce, eliminate, or prevent alterations.[4]

---

related to impaired ambulation due to cesarean section." An *actual* nursing diagnosis consists of three parts, the diagnostic label + contributing factors + signs and symptoms.[11] An example might be, "Anxiety related to the long, dysfunctional, painful labor as manifested by statements of 'I'm afraid I'm not going to be able to deliver my baby.'"

As we acquire our data, we become able to decide on the existence and extent of a problem. We can say in the most general terms that a problem does exist when there is a health goal to be obtained, but the client sees no well-defined, well-established means of attaining it. For instance, she may be too ill or too weak to help herself. Again, the goal may be so vaguely defined or unclear that the client cannot determine relevant means of achieving it. Thus, she may not understand or know how to accept conditions and instruction for achieving the goal of health.

As previously stated, a decision about the existence and extent of the problem or need initiates a diagnosis. The student will note that over the years, various definitions have been offered. See the chart listing some of these.

A review of the literature also reveals that the term *nursing diagnosis* has taken on two somewhat different meanings. In some situations, the term is used to describe the process of problem solving; in other situations, it is used to mean an actual statement of the problem. This dual use has created a good deal of confusion. When the term is used to define the process of analyzing data and identifying a problem, the outcome of this process can be the delineation of both medical and nursing problems. The former must be referred to the physician, and the nurse may participate in the implementation of the medical regimen. Nursing problems, on the other hand, can be treated by the nurse, because they are within the nurse's legal and educational purview.[4]

For our purposes, we shall define a nursing diagnosis as a statement that describes the human response (which may be a health state or actual or potential altered interaction pattern) of an individual or group that the nurse can legally identify and for which the nurse can order the definitive interventions to maintain the health state or to reduce, eliminate, or prevent alterations.[4]

As we said, Carpenito (and others) advise that the diagnosis be a two- or three-part statement, and she cautions about the importance of not linking the statements with words that imply cause and effect, because such a relationship can result in legal and professional difficulty for the nurse. The use of the phrase *related to* rather than *caused by* or *due to* obviates this problem. Thus, additional potential diagnoses that the nurse might make while attending a maternity patient might be "Anxiety about labor related to a knowledge deficit about the labor process," "Extreme discomfort during labor related to inefficient but painful contractions," or "Elevated temperature related to inadequate hydration." Sometimes it is impossible to ascertain any etiologic factors despite a complete assessment. In this instance, one might have a diagnosis: "Fear of caring for the newborn related to unknown factors." Moreover, there may be several diagnoses relating to a constellation of interrelated problems the client has. The three diagnoses given above could conceivably apply to one client at any given time.

Finally, one can have the same nursing diagnosis but have different etiologic factors. In the case of a newly delivered infant, for instance, the diagnosis might be "Inadequate oxygenation related to a possible congenital heart defect" or "Inadequate oxygenation related to immature lungs associated with prematurity."

The student is referred to the Carpenito reference[4] for in-depth information about nursing diagnosis.

Planning and Intervention

The third component of nursing diagnosis involves the planning and implementation of knowledgeable intervention in the form of nursing activities that encompass everything from the administration of comfort measures to counseling and health education. These activities are directed at moving the client toward increased positive adaptation to the environment and high-level wellness.

Nursing prescriptions or orders are given here.

Example of Nursing Orders and Interventions in a Given Situation

Nursing Prescriptions/Orders	*Nursing Planning/Intervention*

Increase fluids to at least 2400 ml/24 hr.
   1000 ml 7–3
    700 ml 3–11
    100 ml 11–7
	Increase fluid intake.

Likes all juices and carbonated beverages	
Do not count coffee or tea in above amount.	
Nurse infant on each breast at each feeding.	Ensure that breasts are emptied.
Time on each breast as tolerated	
Nurse q2h or on demand; do not allow longer intervals than q4h between feedings.	Ensure that breasts are stimulated frequently.
Can nurse sitting or lying down	

These are required to prevent, reduce, or eliminate the alteration in the client's health–illness continuum. Carnevali[1] states that nursing orders should be composed of the following: the date when written; a directive verb; what, when, how often, how long, and where the order is to be executed; and, finally, the signature of the nurse who wrote the order. The objective of the nursing prescription or order is to direct individualized care to the client. Orders differ from nursing actions in that the latter are broad interventions that can apply to any number of persons sharing a similar problem or health alteration.[4] For instance, we might have nursing orders and interventions for a mother who is recovering from dehydration and is having some difficulty establishing breast-feeding, as given in the Example of Nursing Orders and Interventions in a Given Situation.

Remember that the implementation phase is fluid because it is based on a diagnosis or diagnoses that may be reassessed at any point in the process. Moreover, as we administer care, the client's condition will be expected to change, which, on evaluation, will necessitate possible new diagnoses and modification of care. Therefore, continuous feedback loops are built into the process.

TABLE 2-1. PRIMARY KNOWLEDGE AND SKILLS NEEDED TO IMPLEMENT THE NURSING PROCESS

Theoretical Knowledge	Communication Skills	Technical Skills	Therapeutic Use of Self
Basic science	Interviewing	Organization	Goal setting for self and others
General physiology	Mutual sharing	Use of equipment	Ability to use past experiences and role take
General pathophysiology	Writing	Knowledge of general and specific:	
Nursing research	Nonverbal	Techniques	Ability to appreciate others' value systems
Social science	Listening	Safety	
Ethical/religious		Physics	Ability to recognize limitations in self and others
Family systems		Asepsis	

Reproductive:
  Physiology
  Pathophysiology
  Psychosocial			

Pharmacology			

Nutrition:
  Basic
  Relating to reproduction			

(Adapted form Carpenito, LJ: Nursing Diagnosis Application to Clinical Practice, 3rd ed. Philadelphia, JB Lippincott, 1989)

TABLE 2–2. SECONDARY KNOWLEDGE AND SKILLS NEEDED TO IMPLEMENT THE NURSING PROCESS

Assessment	Nursing Diagnosis	Planning and Implementation	Evaluation
Ability to • Differentiate cues and inferences • Observe systematically • Perform a nursing health assessment • Identify patterns of problems • Validate impressions	Ability to • Differentiate nursing problems from medical clinical problems • Identify and test alternatives • Recognize patterns of problems • Correctly label patterns	Ability to • Identify goals • Identify interventions • Write nursing orders Management skills Communication skills Teaching skills Ability to implement change theory	Knowledge of • Process criteria • Outcome criteria

(Adapted from Carpenito LJ: Nursing Diagnosis: Application to Clinical Practice, 3rd ed. Philadelphia, JB Lippincott, 1989)

In this phase, the nurse has the responsibility to disseminate her plan of care to her medical and nursing colleagues so that comprehensive care for the client can be attained. This can be done by means of the Kardex, verbal reporting, charting, and nursing-assessment care plans. Most hospitals have instituted these care-plan forms, and they provide a thorough but brief summary of pertinent patient data together with space to write and record nursing prescriptions, interventions, evaluations, and client response to care.

Evaluation and Reassessment

The fourth component includes both evaluation and prediction facets. A worthwhile evaluation includes an estimation of the results of our past nursing care activities to help predict the validity of our future care. Carpenito suggests that appropriate evaluations consist of the following:[4]

- Establishing criteria to observe and measure
- Assessing the present response for evidence
- Comparing the present response to the established criteria

Any statement of the effectiveness and reliability of our actions is best made with qualifications indicating the degree or amount of effectiveness and the reliability claimed:

- What is the present state of the client?
- Were all symptoms relieved?
- What was the extent of the results?
- On what evidence (observation of self, others, verbal response, cessation of symptoms)?
- Who was involved (nurse, client, others)?
- In what context (what else was happening when the action was performed)?

When these points are established, we can begin to build categories of nursing action that are effective under certain circumstances, for certain patients, given certain conditions. As we ascertain the extent of our effectiveness, we are then in a better position to predict the client's potential for change toward stability or a wellness condition.

■ KNOWLEDGE AND SKILLS IN IMPLEMENTING THE PROCESS

There are certain basic knowledge and skills that the nurse must have to implement the nursing process. Tables 2-1 and 2-2 give the student a handy referent for the knowledge and skills needed as the nursing process is used with the maternity client and her family. As the student increases in expertise in these areas and becomes increasingly proficient in using the nursing process, relationships with clients will develop more quickly and will be on a greater empathic level.[4]

■ REFERENCES

1. Carnevali DL: Nursing Care Planning: Diagnosis and Management, 3rd ed. Philadelphia, JB Lippincott, 1983
2. Gebbie K: Toward the theory development for nursing diagnoses classification. In Kim MJ, Moritz DA (eds): Classification of Nursing Diagnoses. New York, McGraw-Hill, 1982
3. McLane A: Measurement and validation of diagnostic concepts: A decade of progress. Heart Lung 16:616–624, 1987

4. Carpenito LJ: Nursing Diagnosis: Application to Clinical Practice, 3rd ed. Philadelphia, JB Lippincott, 1989
5. Little D, Carnevali DL: Nursing Care Planning, 2nd ed. Philadelphia, JB Lippincott, 1976
6. Aspinall MJ, Tanner C: Decision Making for Patient Care. New York, Appleton-Century-Crofts, 1981
7. Korbert L, Folan M: Coming of age in nursing. Nurs Health Care 11:308–312, June 1990
8. Turkoski BB: Nursing diagnoses in print, 1950–1985. Nurs Outlook 36:142–144, May/June 1988
9. Jenny J: Classifying nursing diagnoses: A self care approach. Nurs Health Care 10:83–88, February 1989
10. McCann/Flynn JB, Heffron PB: Nursing: From Concept to Practice. Bowie, MD, Robert J Brady, 1984
11. Carpenito LJ: Handbook of Nursing Diagnosis 1989–1990. Philadelphia, JB Lippincott, 1989
12. Gordon M: Nursing Diagnosis: Process and Application. New York, McGraw Hill, 1982
13. Shoemaker J: Characteristics of a nursing diagnosis. Occup Health Nurs 33:387–389, 1985

■ SUGGESTED READINGS

Carpenito LJ: Nursing Diagnosis: Application to Clinical Practice, 3rd ed. Philadelphia, JB Lippincott, 1989
Korbert L, Folan M: Coming of age in nursing: Rethinking the philosophies behind holism and nursing process. Nurs Health Care 11:308–312, June 1990
Levin RF, et al: Diagnostic content validity of nursing diagnoses. Image 21:40–44, Spring 1989
NAACOG: Nursing Diagnosis: OGN Nursing Practice Resource. Washington, DC, NAACOG, December 1989
Vincent KG, Coler MS: A unified nursing diagnostic model. Image 22:93–95, Spring 1990

3

Vital Statistics

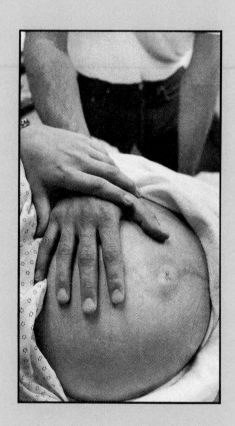

Statistical profiles are useful because they summarize a large amount of data about various populations and therefore supply health-care providers and policymakers with a valuable overview of needs and gaps in care.

■ VITAL STATISTICS

In the United States, vital statistics reports are published officially by the U.S. Public Health Service, National Center for Health Statistics (NCHS), Vital Statistics Division. The terms listed in Definitions Pertaining to Vital Statistics have been defined by the NCHS. Mortality and morbidity terminology are classified according to the World Health Organization's (WHO) *Manual of International Classification of Diseases, Injuries, and Causes of Death* (ICD).

■ NATALITY

Overall, the number of registered births in the United States has decreased in the past three decades from over 4 million live births in 1957 to 3.5 million in 1968 and 3.15 million in 1975. However, there was a small 1% rise in the number of live births in 1976 and again in 1981. Provisional data from the NCHS indicate that there were 3.82 million live births for the year ending February 1988. This was the largest number of births recorded since 1964 and indicates a consistent increase.[1]

Birthrates

The increase in the number of births is the result of the increase in the number of women in the childbearing ages (15–44). This number has risen rapidly owing to the high birthrates of the 1940s and the 1950s—the "baby boom" of the post–World War II era. Although the fertility rate reached a record low in 1976 for the fifth consecutive year, the decline was not enough to offset the 2% increase in the number of women of childbearing age. Provisional data for 1988 indicate that for the 12-month period ending with October 1988, there was a 3% increase in the rate over that of the previous year.[1]

Thus, an important consideration that influences the number of children being born annually is the size and the age composition of the female population of childbearing age. Although the fertility rate is computed on the basis of births per 1000 women between ages 15 and 44, most of the childbearing continues to be

---

Definitions Pertaining to Vital Statistics

Birthrate. The number of births per 1000 population; also known as the crude birthrate

Marriage rate. The number of marriages per 1000 total population

Fertility rate. The number of births per 1000 women aged 15 through 44 years

Neonatal. The period from birth through the 28th day of life

Neonatal death rate. The number of neonatal deaths per 1000 live births

Stillbirth or fetal death. A death in which the infant of 20 weeks or more gestational age dies *in utero* prior to birth

Perinatal mortality. All stillborn infants whose gestational age is 28 weeks or more, plus all neonatal deaths under 7 days per 1000 births.* The 1979 revision of the ICD, however, uses birth weight rather than gestational age as a criterion. It also recommends two different categories of reporting. (For national data collection, the recommendation is that 500 g be used as the minimum weight of stillborn and live-born infants. For international comparisons, however, the weight should be 1000 g or more. When weight is unknown, either gestational age [28 weeks] or body length corresponding to 1000 g may be used.) Obviously, these different criteria will make comparisons with previous data impossible and will also make national and international statistical comparisons difficult. There is current debate as to the efficacy of using the newly developed criteria.

Infant mortality rate. The number of deaths before the first birthday per 1000 live births

Maternal mortality rate. The number of maternal deaths resulting from the reproductive process per 100,000 live births

Race and color. Births in the United States are classified for vital statistics according to the race of the parents in the categories of white, black, American Indian, Chinese, Japanese, Aleut and Eskimo combined, Hawaiian and part-Hawaiian combined, and "other nonwhite." In most tables a less detailed classification of "white" and "nonwhite" is used. The white category includes births to parents classified as white, Mexican, Puerto Rican, or "not stated."

* Current definition approved by WHO.

---

concentrated among women in their 20s.[2] There has been a slight rise in the rate of marriages since 1968. However, more married couples are electing not to have children, and there are children being born more often from social contract and other nonlegal unions.

Multiple Births

There has been a slight decline in the frequency of multiple births in the United States.[2,3] Changes in age and the racial composition of the population, as well as the use of certain ovulation-producing drugs for infertility, contribute to fluctuations in the rate over time. There are differences, for instance, in the occurrence of twins, depending on the number of births the mother has had before delivery of the multiple birth. There are differences between the rate of monozygotic or identical twins and dizygotic or fraternal twins, and the relative proportions of monozygotic and dizygotic twins are not the same for all races.

The Birth Certificate

All 50 states and the District of Columbia demand that a birth certificate be filled out on every birth and that the certificate be submitted promptly to the local registrar. After the birth has been registered, the local registrar sends a notification to the parents of the child. Also, a complete report is forwarded from the local registrar to the state authorities and then to the National Office of Vital Statistics in Washington.

Complete and accurate registration of births is a legal responsibility (Fig. 3-1). The birth certificate gives evidence of age, citizenship, and family relationships and, as such, is often required for military service and

H105.142 Rev. 5-78

COMMONWEALTH OF PENNSYLVANIA
DEPARTMENT OF HEALTH
VITAL STATISTICS
CERTIFICATE OF LIVE BIRTH

TYPE OR PRINT IN PERMANENT INK

PRIMARY DIST. NO. ____________ STATE FILE NO.

A. ____________
B. ____________
C. ____________
D. ____________
E. ____________
F. ____________
G. ____________
H. ____________
I. ____________

CHILD–NAME FIRST MIDDLE LAST 1. | SEX 2. | DATE OF BIRTH (Mo. Day Year) 3a. | HOUR 3b. ______ AM PM

HOSPITAL NAME (If not in Hospital, Give Street and Number) 4a. | City, Boro, or Twp. of Birth 4b. | COUNTY OF BIRTH 4c.

I CERTIFY THAT THE STATED INFORMATION CONCERNING THIS CHILD IS TRUE TO THE BEST OF MY KNOWLEDGE AND BELIEF 5a. (Signature) ▶ | DATE SIGNED (Mo, Day, Year) 5b. | CERTIFIER–NAME AND TITLE (Type or Print) 5c.

Name and Title of Attendant at Birth if other than Certifier (Type or Print) 5d. | CERTIFIER'S MAILING ADDRESS (Street or R.F.D. No., City or Town, State, Zip) 5e.

MOTHER–MAIDEN NAME FIRST MIDDLE LAST 6a. | AGE (At time of this Birth) 6b. | STATE OF BIRTH (If not in U.S.A., Name Country) 6c.

MAILING ADDRESS STREET AND NUMBER CITY AND STATE ZIP CODE 7.

WHERE DOES MOTHER ACTUALLY LIVE? STATE COUNTY CITY, BORO, TWP. (Specify) 8.

FATHER–NAME FIRST MIDDLE LAST 9a. | AGE (At time of this Birth) 9b. | STATE OF BIRTH (If not in U.S.A., Name Country) 9c.

INFORMANT 10a. | Relation to Child 10b. | REGISTRAR'S SIGNATURE AND DATE RECEIVED 11. ▶

CONFIDENTIAL INFORMATION FOR MEDICAL AND HEALTH USE ONLY

Death Under One Year Of Age – Number of Death Certificate For This Child

RACE–MOTHER (e.g., White, Black, American Indian, etc. – Specify) 12. | RACE–FATHER (e.g., White, Black, American Indian, etc. – Specify) 13. | EDUCATION–MOTHER (Specify only highest grade completed) ELEMENTARY OR SECONDARY (0-12) | COLLEGE (1-4 or 5+) 14. | EDUCATION–FATHER (Specify only highest grade completed) ELEMENTARY OR SECONDARY (0-12) | COLLEGE (1-4 or 5+) 15. | IS MOTHER MARRIED TO FATHER? ☐ Yes ☐ No 16.

PREGNANCY HISTORY (Complete each section)
LIVE BIRTHS (Do not include this child): 17a. Now living Number___ None ☐ | 17b. Now dead Number___ None ☐ | 17c. Date of Last Live Birth (Mo. Year)
OTHER TERMINATIONS (Spontaneous and Induced): 17d. Before 16 wks. Number___ None ☐ | 17e. After 16 wks. Number___ None ☐ | 17f. Date of Last Other Termination (Mo. Year)

Date Last Normal Menses Began (Mo. Day, Year) 18. | Month of Pregnancy Pre-Natal Care Began (1st, 2nd, etc.) (Specify) 19a. | Pre-Natal Visits – Total (If none, so state) 19b. | Length of Pregnancy in weeks. 20.

Multiple Births Enter State File Number for Mate(s)

BIRTH WEIGHT 21. | THIS BIRTH–Single, Twin, Triplet, etc. (Specify) 22a. | If NOT Single Birth – Born First, Second, Third etc. (Specify) 22b. | APGAR SCORE 1 Min. 23a. | 5 Min. 23b.

Method of Delivery 24. | COMPLICATIONS OF PREGNANCY (Describe or write "none") 25.

Live Birth(s)

CONCURRENT ILLNESSES OR CONDITIONS AFFECTING THE PREGNANCY (Describe or write "none") 26. | COMPLICATIONS OF LABOR AND/OR DELIVERY (Describe or write "none") 27.

Fetal Death(s)

BIRTH INJURIES OF CHILD (Describe or write "none") 28. | CONGENITAL MALFORMATIONS OR ANOMALIES OF CHILD (Describe or write "none") 29.

■ *Figure 3-1*
Certificate of live birth used by Pennsylvania Department of Health. Similar forms are used by other cities and states.

passports and to collect benefits on retirement and insurance.

A new revision of the U.S. Standard Certificate of Live Birth will soon be adopted by all but three states in the early 1990s. The new revision will change drastically in both form and content. Check boxes will be used to obtain detailed medical, health, and life-style information as well as obstetric procedures, medical conditions of the newborn, birth attendant, and place of birth (Figs. 3-2 and 3-3). When these data are combined with other socioeconomic and health data, it is anticipated that a wealth of new information can be accumulated relevant to the etiology of neonatal health problems and adverse pregnancy outcomes.[4]

```
┌─────────────────────────────────────────────────┐
│  OBSTETRIC PROCEDURES                            │
│  (Check all that apply)                          │
│  Amniocentesis ...........................  01 □  │
│  Electronic fetal monitoring .............  02 □  │
│  Induction of labor ......................  03 □  │
│  Stimulation of labor ....................  04 □  │
│  Tocolysis ...............................  05 □  │
│  Ultrasound ..............................  06 □  │
│  None ....................................  00 □  │
│  Other_____   07 □  │
│       (Specify)                                  │
└─────────────────────────────────────────────────┘
```

■ *Figure 3–3*
Obstetric procedures. (Reproduced from the 1989 US Standard Certificate of Live Birth.)

■ POPULATION

The population of the United States more than doubled during the first half of this century and has continued to grow in tremendous proportions as was predicted.

Three vital factors determine the rate at which population grows: births, deaths, and migration. The decline in the death rate that was so apparent in the first half of this century has fluctuated near the same relatively low level. Recent modifications in immigration practices will undoubtedly exert an influence on this factor in our population growth.

The former decline in the annual number of births was partly related to the age and sex structure of the population. The majority of Americans are young. More than half are under 28 years of age, but the proportion is shifting because of the fluctuating birth rates. The young-adult group, composed of persons between ages 18 and 34, remains the fastest growing portion of the population, reflecting the high birth rates that followed World War II. Moderately large increases are anticipated in the 65-year-and-over age group. It is projected that by the year 2040, approximately 21% of the population will be over 65.

According to population projections made by the Bureau of the Census, during the next 10 years the number of women of childbearing age will probably rise in this country. The uncertainty as to how much the population will grow rises from the unpredictable number of children who will be born to contemporary young couples. Although their fertility potential is huge, much will depend on their choice in family size. That size has dropped from a replacement rate of 2.1 in 1980 to 1.9 in 1983.[5]

```
┌─────────────────────────────────────────────────┐
│  MEDICAL RISK FACTORS FOR THIS PREGNANCY         │
│  (Check all that apply)                          │
│                                                  │
│  Anemia (Hct. < 30/Hgb. < 10)............  01 □   │
│  Cardiac disease ........................  02 □   │
│  Acute or chronic lung disease ..........  03 □   │
│  Diabetes ...............................  04 □   │
│  Genital herpes .........................  05 □   │
│  Hydramnios/Oligohydramnios .............  06 □   │
│  Hemoglobinopathy .......................  07 □   │
│  Hypertension, chronic ..................  08 □   │
│  Hypertension, pregnancy-associated .....  09 □   │
│  Eclampsia ..............................  10 □   │
│  Incompetent cervix .....................  11 □   │
│  Previous infant 4000+ grams ............  12 □   │
│  Previous preterm or small-for-gestational-age   │
│      infant .............................  13 □   │
│  Renal disease ..........................  14 □   │
│  Rh sensitization .......................  15 □   │
│  Uterine bleeding .......................  16 □   │
│  None ...................................  00 □   │
│  Other_____   17 □   │
│       (Specify)                                  │
└─────────────────────────────────────────────────┘
```

```
┌─────────────────────────────────────────────────┐
│  OTHER RISK FACTORS FOR THIS PREGNANCY           │
│  (Complete all items)                            │
│                                                  │
│  Tobacco use during pregnancy ....... Yes □ No □  │
│      Average number cigarettes per day_____   │
│  Alcohol use during pregnancy ....... Yes □ No □  │
│      Average number drinks per week _____      │
│  Weight gained during pregnancy _____ lbs.   │
└─────────────────────────────────────────────────┘
```

■ *Figure 3–2*
Medical and other risk factors for the pregnancy are listed on the new US Standard Certificate of Live Birth that will help give new information and statistics regarding the etiology of neonatal health problems and adverse pregnancy outcomes. (Reproduced from 1989 US Standard Certificate of Live Birth.)

■ MORTALITY

Maternal Mortality

Maternal mortality refers to deaths that result from childbearing, that is, the underlying cause of the woman's death is the result of complications of pregnancy, childbirth, or the puerperium.

The reduction in maternal mortality rates has been rather consistent since 1951. The dramatic decline in these rates began about the mid-1930s and continued until 1956. During the succeeding 5 years, the maternal mortality rate declined more slowly, reaching the all-time low in 1962. In 1963 the rate rose slightly but resumed its decline. Since then, the decline has been slow but steady, culminating in a 7.8 rate per 1000 births in 1985 and a 7.2 rate in 1986.[6] The risk of maternal death for all mothers is lowest at ages 20 to 24. It is slightly higher under age 20 and from age 25 on. Increasing age is associated with a steep rise in maternal mortality. At 40 to 44 years of age, the mortality rate is six times greater than at 20 to 24. At the oldest age in the reproductive age span, 45 years or older, the mortality is about 12 times greater than the low figure.

CAUSES OF MATERNAL MORTALITY

The reduction in maternal mortality from the hemorrhagic disorders of pregnancy and childbirth was the largest single factor responsible for the reduction in the total maternal mortality rate (from 82.7 per 100,000 live births in 1949–1951 to 9.6 in 1978). The hypertensive disorders and sepsis (cases other than abortion) were next in importance as conditions affecting the mortality rate. The rate in 1987 was 6.6 per 1000 births (Fig. 3-4). These three conditions will be discussed later in more detail, but it is important to stress that deaths from these causes are now largely preventable.

Although *hemorrhage* is no longer the primary cause of maternal death, it still remains an important factor in the morbidity of mothers and in the underlying cause of death. According to the official classification, only the direct cause of death is considered, although predisposing causes may be just as important factors. For example, in a case in which the mother has a massive hemorrhage and in her weakened condition develops a puerperal infection that eventually causes her death, the death is classified as a result of puerperal infection. Hemorrhage is often a predisposing factor, and its toll in maternal mortality should not be underestimated.

Puerperal infection is a wound infection of the birth canal after childbirth, which sometimes extends to cause phlebitis or peritonitis. The nurse can play an important

Causes of Maternal Mortality

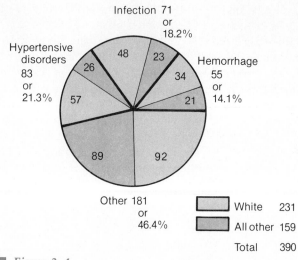

■ *Figure 3–4*

Annual summary of births, deaths, marriages and divorces: United States, 1988 DHHS Pub. No. (PHS) 110–111. Monthly Vital Statistics Report 37:59, January 19, 1989.

role in helping to prevent such infections by maintaining flawless technique in performing nursing procedures.

The *hypertensive disorders of pregnancy* are certain disturbances peculiar to gravid women, characterized mainly by hypertensive edema and albuminuria and, in some severe cases, by convulsions and coma. Antepartal care is an important part of prevention or early detection of symptoms, and, with suitable treatment, the disturbance often can be allayed.

REDUCTION IN MATERNAL MORTALITY

Many factors are responsible for achieving the overall reduction in maternal mortality in this country during the past 25 years.

Medical management has improved. The widespread use of blood and plasma transfusions and antibiotics, together with careful maintenance of fluid and electrolyte balance and sophisticated anesthesia management, has changed obstetric practice substantially. Access to abortion has also helped reduce the number of maternal deaths associated with abortion.

Perhaps more important is the development of widespread *training and education programs* in obstetrics and maternity care, which have provided more and better qualified specialists, professional nurses, and other personnel to deliver care in this area. *Better hospital facilities* and the development of *alternative hospital facilities* to meet consumer demands for a more homelike setting for parturition may also prove to be a helpful factor.

The distinct change in *attitudes of physicians, nurses, and parents* has also contributed to this progressive saving of mothers. Childbirth is no longer an event to be awaited helplessly by the expectant mother with what fortitude she is able to muster; instead, it is the climax of a period of preparation—a true state of preparedness attained through the cooperation of the physician, the nurse, and the expectant parents.

Antepartal care has been an important achievement in maternity care during the present century. This contribution to the mother's welfare was initiated by the nursing profession in 1901 when the Instructive Nursing Association in Boston began to pay antepartal visits to some of the expectant mothers who were to deliver at the Boston Lying-In Hospital. This work gradually spread until, in 1906, all of these women were visited at least once prior to confinement by a nurse from the association. By 1912 this association was making about three antepartal visits to each client. In 1907, another pioneer effort in prenatal work was instituted when George H.F. Schrader gave the Association for Improving the Condition of the Poor, New York City, funds to pay the salary of two nurses to do this work. In 1909, the Committee on Infant Social Service of the Women's Municipal League in Boston organized an experiment of antepartal work. Pregnant women were visited every 10 days, more often if necessary. This began the movement for antepartal care that has been extremely important in promoting the health and well-being of many pregnant women.

Another important factor in the reduction of maternal mortality has been the development of maternal and child health programs in state departments of public health, particularly the work of community-health nurses. These nurses visit a large number of the mothers who otherwise would receive little or no medical care, bringing them much-needed aid in pregnancy, labor, and the puerperium. This service fills a great need not only in rural areas but also in metropolitan centers.

Perinatal Mortality

The two groups of problems in infant mortality that are of chief concern in maternity are those in which the fetus dies in the uterus prior to birth and those in which it dies within a short time after birth (neonatal death). The term *perinatal mortality* is used to designate the deaths in these two categories.

FETAL DEATH

In an effort to end confusion arising from the use of a variety of terms, such as *stillbirth, abortion,* and *miscarriage,* WHO recommended the adoption of the following definition of fetal death:

> Fetal death is a death before complete expulsion or extraction from its mother of a product of conception, irrespective of duration of pregnancy; the death is indicated by the fact that after such separation, the fetus does not breathe or show any other evidence of life, such as beating of the heart, pulsation of the umbilical cord, or definite movement of voluntary muscles.[7]

WHO further defined fetal death by indicating four subgroups, according to gestational age in weeks.

Infant Mortality

Two decades ago, a total of 103,390 infant deaths before the first birthday were reported. Figure 3-5 indicates how the rate has dropped in the 1970s and 1980s. Several factors are believed to have effected this decline in infant mortality, including a declining fertility rate, better contraceptive practices, the availability of safe clinical abortions, and a higher standard of living in the general population. However, it has been shown that these national statistics do not accurately reflect trends in the

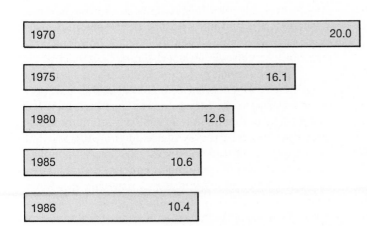

Year	Rate
1970	20.0
1975	16.1
1980	12.6
1985	10.6
1986	10.4

■ *Figure 3–5*
Infant mortality rates per 1000 live births, 1970–1986 (National Center for Health Statistics). Statistical Abstracts of the United States. Washington, DC, US Department of Commerce, Bureau of the Census, pp 57–83, 1985.

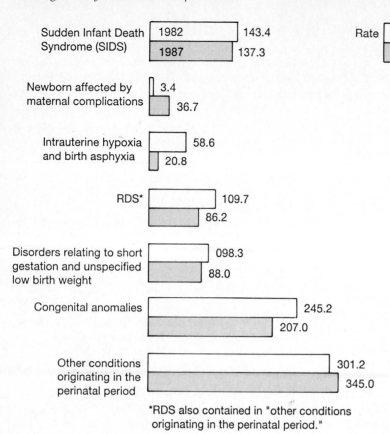

| | 1982 | 143.4 |
Sudden Infant Death Syndrome (SIDS) — 1982: 143.4, 1987: 137.3

Rate — 1982: 1100.2, 1987: 1008.2

Newborn affected by maternal complications — 3.4 / 36.7

Intrauterine hypoxia and birth asphyxia — 58.6 / 20.8

RDS* — 109.7 / 86.2

Disorders relating to short gestation and unspecified low birth weight — 098.3 / 88.0

Congenital anomalies — 245.2 / 207.0

Other conditions originating in the perinatal period — 301.2 / 345.0

*RDS also contained in "other conditions originating in the perinatal period."

■ *Figure 3–6*
Causes of infant mortality per 100,000 live births in 1979 and 1987 (National Center for Health Statistics) Statistical Abstracts of the United States. Washington, DC, US Department of Commerce, Bureau of the Census, pp 57–83, 1985.

large urban areas and the southern states, where the decline has been much less.

Many factors are responsible for infant mortality. The leading causes of infant mortality are listed in Figure 3-6 and include respiratory distress syndrome, preterm birth, asphyxia and atelectasis, congenital malformations, and birth injuries.

These recent national statistics also reflect a startling increase in the category of "newborns affected by maternal complications," showing an increase from 3.4 per 100,000 births in 1982 to 36.7 per 100,000 births in 1987. These maternal complications often relate to the mother's lifestyle or habits, including substance abuse, smoking, or poor prenatal care. This category has now eclipsed the "birth trauma" category, which is no longer considered a major cause of mortality.

During the first 4 weeks of life, early gestational age and low birth weight are the chief causes of death. Birth injuries of infant loss still remain a cause. Almost one third of these deaths are due to intracranial and spinal injury at birth. In the vast majority of these cases, death occurred within less than 7 days of life. These conditions will be discussed in detail later. It suffices to say that one of the first and most important of them, immaturity, is largely a nursing management problem.

The welfare of approximately 3,500,000 babies born annually in the United States is very much the concern of maternity nurses and obstetricians and one of the main objectives of the entire field of maternity care. To reduce the enormous loss of newborn lives, to protect the infant not only at birth but also in the prenatal period and during the early days of life, and to lay a solid foundation for the infant's health throughout life are the problems and the challenge of maternity care.

■ REPRODUCTIVE WASTAGE

The large number of infants lost by spontaneous abortion is a matter of grave concern. About 10% of all pregnancies terminate in spontaneous abortion because of such factors as faulty genetic development, unsatisfactory environmental conditions, and hormonal and many other unknown etiologic causes.[8]

Today, the concerns for the United States stemming from the overall problem of maternal and fetal reproductive wastage reflect a symptom of far-reaching social change. The reduction in maternal and infant mortality rates presents concrete evidence of the progress that has been achieved in maternity care in this country. Nevertheless, the current major concern is that a large segment of our population is not receiving maternity care.

The needs resulting from problems of maternal and child health in rural areas continue today, but what is alarming is that now there is a parallel situation in the larger cities. The population still includes a large segment of disadvantaged, low-income families, as well as foreign immigrants, who recently have concentrated in the major cities. With the increased cost of health services in general and the cost of hospital care in particular, these low-income families are straining the local resources of the communities in which they reside. The most serious problem by far is that many of these women are receiving poor or, often, no antepartal care, owing in part to dissatisfaction with the kind of care provided. Inadequate care during pregnancy has been demonstrated to bear a direct relationship to the rate of immaturity.

Moreover, with the recent economic fluctuations, middle-class couples are feeling the impact of not being able to afford adequate health care. They are not eligible for welfare coverage yet are not affluent enough to seek appropriate care.

Much of the difficulty in providing adequate care is due to an artificial shortage of professional personnel in the maternity field. The rapid growth of the population in certain sections, such as rural and inner city areas, has not been accompanied by a proportionate increase in the number of physicians and nurses willing to staff these underserved areas.

■ REFERENCES

1. National Center for Health Statistics: Annual summary of births, deaths, marriages and divorces: United States, 1988. DHHS Pub. No. (PHS) 110–111. Monthly Vital Statistics Report 37:59, January 19, 1989

2. Statistical Abstracts of the United States, 1985. U.S. Department of Commerce, Bureau of the Census, pp 57–83

3. United States Department of Health, Education and Welfare: Characteristics of births: United States, 1973–1975. DHEW Publication No. (PHS) 78-1908, September 1980

4. Taffel SM, Ventura SJ, Gay GA: Revised US certificate of birth: New opportunities for research on birth outcome. Birth 16:188–193, December 1989

5. Andreoli KG, Musser LA: Major trends shaping the future of perinatal nursing. J Perinatol 6:325–330, Fall 1986

6. Statistical Abstracts of the United States, 1990. U.S. Department of Commerce, Bureau of the Census. Based on data from NCHS, Vital Statistics of the United States, Tables 110–112, 1988

7. National Summaries: Fetal Deaths, US, 1954. National Office of Vital Statistics 44:11, August 1956

8. Wallace HM, et al: Infant mortality in Sweden and Finland: Implications for the United States. J Perinatal 10: 3–11, March 1990

■ SUGGESTED READINGS

Arnold LS, et al: Lessons from the Past. MCN 14:75, March/April 1989

Mayfield J, et al: The relation of obstetrical volume and nursery level to perinatal mortality. Am J Public Health 80:819–828, July 1990

Nesbitt TS, et al: Access to obstetric care in rural areas: Effect on birth outcomes. Am J Public Health 80:814–818, July 1990

Salmon ME, Peoples-Sheps M: Infant mortality and public health nursing. Nurs Outlook 37:6, January/February 1989

4

The Family and Nursing Practice

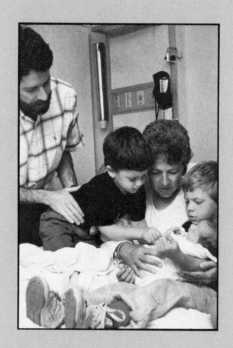

■ WHAT IS THE FAMILY?

Most people know intuitively what they mean by "the family." They have known families throughout their lifetime, and intuitive definitions are sufficient for everyday conversation and action. However, when we begin to define what constitutes a family, to analyze the unit as a social institution, or to attempt to deliver comprehensive care to its members, it becomes apparent that what we have considered as the family is inappropriate for systematic treatment. The characteristics of the families of our own personal experience often do not fit "families" of other segments of society or other cultures.

The family has been defined in a variety of ways. The U.S. Census Bureau's definition, for instance, is simple and straightforward. According to this definition, a family is a group of two or more persons who are related by blood, marriage, or adoption and are residing together.[1] The concept of residing together is important for purposes of census enumeration, but, in fact, there are times and situations in which members do not share the same household. Other authors have defined the family as a system of roles or as a unit of interacting personalities who may not necessarily be sanctioned by law but have some commitment to each other.[2,3] Generally, we can define the family as a group of kin united by blood, marriage, or adoption who share a common residence for some part of their lives, assume reciprocal rights and obligations with regard to one another, and are the principal source of socialization of its members.[4]

Common to all these definitions is the fact that the members relate to each other in some way, that is, they interact with specified patterns of behavior and, in so doing, differentiate and structure roles for themselves, thus providing valuable functions for the unit as well as society as a whole.

■ FUNCTIONS OF THE MODERN FAMILY

It has been said that the modern family has lost many of its former socialization functions. Protective services are now provided by law enforcement, the fire department, child protective services, and the like. Education and religious training are now entrusted to schools and churches. Even the production, preservation, and preparation of food have become largely the domain of industry. Duvall and Miller state that there are still at

---

> ### *Functions of the Modern Family*
>
> - Generating affection
> - Ensuring continuity of companionship
> - Providing personal security and acceptance
> - Giving satisfaction and a sense of purpose
> - Providing social placement and socialization
> - Inculcating controls and a sense of what is right

least six basic functions left to the family, and they are crucial for producing competent persons who must survive in a complex, ever-changing world.[5]

Generating Affection. This is a phenomenon that must go on between all members of the unit as well as among members of the different generations. Love, then, is a product of family living. In Western societies, couples generally marry for love and have children as an expression of that love. In the ideal situation, both parents and children grow in a climate of mutual affection that contributes to a healthy development of all concerned. In actual fact, however, we know that the ideal is often not achieved.

Ensuring Continuity of Companionship. In today's highly mobile world, often only family associations endure. One's friends, colleagues, neighbors, and acquaintances enter and leave one's social network; jobs change, neighborhoods expand and contract, and social mobility continues. The family unit provides a continuing presence of sympathetic companions who encourage family members to share both disappointments and successes.

Providing Personal Security and Acceptance. Most persons look to their family for the security and acceptance they need to make their lives dignified and worthwhile. It is within the family's protective security that the members can make mistakes, learn from them, and form complementary rather than competitive relationships. These relationships allow the members to develop naturally and at their own pace.

Giving Satisfaction and a Sense of Purpose. The family, at its best, can give its members a basic sense of satisfaction and worth that the other arenas in a person's life often do not fulfill. Family rituals, celebrations, gatherings, and the like serve to act as cohesive factors to dilute the frustrations and problems found in the larger society.

contract sense, but rather as it exists by virtue of the interaction of its members. Thus, a single parent with a child is a family unit, as is an unmarried couple with or without children.

Within the family, each member occupies a position or positions to which a number of roles are assigned or allocated. Through socialization and role differentiation (structuring a role), the individual perceives certain norms (rules) or role expectations that the other members of the family have set for his or her behavior in role performance. The response of the others in the family reinforces or challenges this conception that the individual is developing. Thus, people define their role expectations in a given situation in terms of a reference group (others who are important to them) and also by means of their own self-concept.

Implicit in this formulation is the fact that human beings interpret or define one another's actions instead of merely reacting to them. For instance, a woman's response to her mate is not made merely on the basis of his actions; it also depends on the meaning that both partners attach to such actions. Thus, the family members act and react by using symbols, and the key concept involved in the use of symbols is communication.

Interpersonal relations among family members based on communication is one of the major distinguishing aspects of the interactional approach. The emphasis in this framework is on the development of competence in interpersonal relations, and as such it describes a process rather than a state.[10,13]

FAMILY INTERACTION AND STRESS

Several problems for investigation have grown out of these concerns and emphases on family unity, communication, and interpersonal competence. The one that is particularly important for health practitioners is that of the study of discontinuities in family life, particularly family crises or stress. This includes the impact of the reproductive process and parenthood on the family, stress created by acute or chronic illness of the various family members at any time during the life cycle, and the crisis brought about by death of a family member, particularly during the reproductive years.

Using a family interaction perspective, the nurse can get inside the family group and analyze its coping as far as it involves interaction among members. Each family member, therefore, can be viewed as a developing member in a changing group. This approach can be particularly useful to the helping professions not only because it provides a practical way of inspecting the family, but also because it allows the professional to isolate and specify the potential sources of difficulty as family members relate to one another and to their society.[2,10]

◼ RELATIONSHIP OF FAMILY THEORY TO NURSING PRACTICE

The structure and function of the family help determine their use of health services. Hence, all members of the health team need to be aware of a variety of theories regarding human behavior and how families develop their various patterns of behavior. This awareness necessitates using knowledge from other specific disciplines when it is appropriate.

Family-Centered Care

The concept of family-centered care and its logical extension, family nursing, has always been a part of nursing. Some areas of practice, notably that of community health, have traditionally claimed more interest, expertise, and responsibility for total family care than others. Delivering care in the client's home has allowed the nurse more insights into the family and its workings and the implications its structure and function have for the health of its members. Moreover, it has allowed the nurse to assess the problems and progress of the family members as a whole.

However, other nursing specialists, notably those in maternal-child health, have also demonstrated interest in family care, focusing initially on the mother–child dyad and later, on parenting. In addition, midwifery has used a family-centered approach to home delivery services by using family resources to prepare for care of the mother–infant couple in the home setting.[10] Antepartal and postpartal parents' classes have also become popular. As nursing has evolved to keep pace with today's health needs, it is apparent that concepts from other disciplines can be useful to supply a total picture of the family unit for which high-quality care is to be provided.

As more nurses acquire research expertise, the profession is increasingly able to join with other related disciplines whose basic interests and expertise in the family may some day ensure team approaches to research in clinical matters, multidisciplinary educational programs, and, most important, team effort in family care.

◼ ROLES, ROLE THEORY, AND IMPLICATIONS FOR NURSING PRACTICE

As background for understanding the family, we must deal with another concept that permeates both lay and professional language today. That concept is role, and it is an integral part of the structure and function of the family.

As with the concept of family, we have an intuitive sense of what a "role" is, but when attempts are made to study systematically the construct, we find a broad latitude in definitions and understandings of it. Personality develops within a social system, which in our culture is the family. Therefore roles, which are crucial to personality development, may be viewed from a psychosocial viewpoint, which enables us to focus on the individual and how he or she integrates role relationships, and also from a sociological viewpoint, which guides us in focusing on group or social relationships, primarily those within the family. We must also deal with culture, for the self can be viewed as the unit of personality, a person's status, or position in a unit of society, or as a role enacted in the culture.[2,3]

Roles and Status

Basic to any discussion of role is the definitions of role and status. Status, or position, generally refers to a person's location in a system of interaction. On the other hand, role applies to behavior that reflects the goals, values, and sentiments operating in a given situation.

From an interactionist frame of reference, role is more than a series of dos and don'ts (the structuralist position) for the behavior expected of a person occupying a given position. Rather, it is a constellation of behaviors that emerges from interaction between the self and others that constitutes a meaningful unit and is an expression of the values, goals, or sentiments that provide direction for that interaction. It is true that these constellations of behaviors become patterned over time and that the actors proceed as if there were prescriptions for performance.[2,3]

However, there is much more latitude in the symbolic interaction conception of role rather than the structuralist, because it allows for innovative, individualistic designing of a person's role performance on the basis of assignment of some sentiment or goal to the behavior of relevant others.

This conception of role is particularly salient for nursing practice as it allows for a broader interpretation of the behavior of all actors than do more traditional concepts. Moreover, it does not limit either the interpretation of the behavior or the nurse's response to the behavior to a prescribed set of dos and don'ts. Hence, it permits creativity and innovation in interaction with clients.

COMPLEMENTARY ROLES

Another basic concept in role theory is that of the complementary roles, or the fact that all roles are learned in pairs. Thus, a role does not exist in isolation but is patterned to mesh with that of a role partner. For instance, the nurse's role meshes with the client's role, the husband's with the wife's, the child's with the parent's, and so on. Some of these roles that are basic in society, such as husband, wife, child, and so on, have become more patterned in the various cultures than others, and, thus, firmer expectations have come about. But we need only look at the innovative variation in recent family lifestyles to appreciate how traditional role prescriptions and expectations can, and often must, be modified.[2,10,14]

Whether there be firm or loose expectations, this pairing or complementarity of roles provides for reciprocal arrangements in interaction and therefore allows social interaction to proceed in an orderly fashion, because there emerges a predictability in interaction (Fig. 4-1). The actors "know" what they are to do. Without this complementarity, it would be difficult to maintain stable interaction networks such as exist in the family system. Indeed, the family's equilibrium depends on this role pairing.[2]

ROLE SOCIALIZATION AND ROLE MODELS

Roles are learned through the process of socialization. In socialization, individuals learn the ways of social groups so that they can function within these groups. Socialization takes place through both intentional and incidental instruction, that is, by providing specific instruction regarding a certain facet of behavior and by providing examples of desired behavior, in other words, role modeling. All of the various socialization agencies the family in the beginning and, later, the church and schools, teach the child certain role behaviors through intentional programs of learning and study. Operating conjointly may be incidental learning in which the child adopts the ways of others in his environment through play acting, peer-group relations, and observations of adult and peer role models.

Thus, the significant others in the child's world teach him or her, both by defining the world and by serving as models for attitudes and behavior (Fig. 4-2). The child learns through a system of rewards and punishment, and if that child behaves as the significant others desire, he or she receives positive attention and invitations to continue his participation and interaction. If, on the other hand, the child behaves otherwise, he or she is refused attention, reprimanded, or physically punished.[13]

It is important to remember that much of the role learning that takes place in the family is indirect. The child learns by observing and participating in the interpersonal relations patterns established by the family, the examples set by the other family members, and the role that the child develops within the family. Hence,

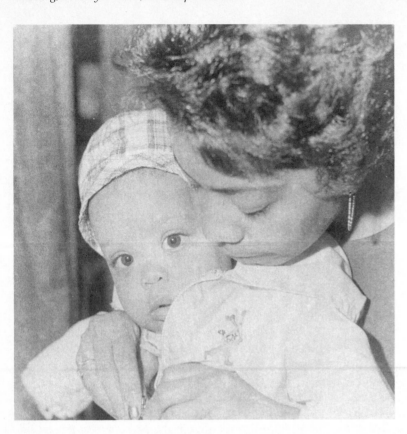

■ *Figure 4-1*
In our culture, the ideal mother has traditionally been the nurturer.

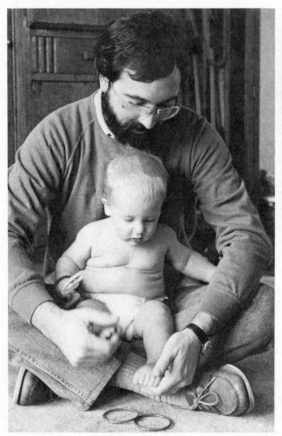

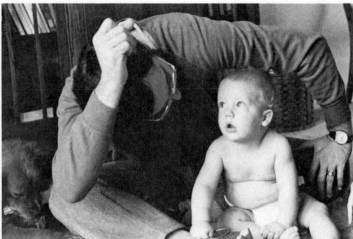

■ *Figure 4-2*
Although the father has traditionally been viewed as an authority figure and breadwinner, attachment to his infant must also involve feelings of tenderness and gentleness and a gratifying personal involvement with his children.

the child learns and adopts basic role skills from family members and concurrently adapts to the roles of the other family members.[13]

SOCIALIZATION OF THE CHILD

There are many techniques of socialization, and the evidence indicates that no one technique is better than another. Rather, each set of parents must choose and modify what is best for them, and this will depend on the many factors that we have previously alluded to. Spiegel[15] has attempted to delineate the various steps in the maintenance of role complementarity so that the family can balance the demands that society's expectations place on it, the family's attitudes, and the child's needs and eventually arrive at a progressively healthier family role equilibrium. These steps are conceived along the route of socialization as comprising two major groups of five steps, each linked by a sixth, or middle, step (Fig. 4-3).[15]

Role Induction. The first group consists of *role induction procedures* that elicit compliance of the child. These are primarily manipulative and ensure that the child gradually realizes that he or she must learn and that his parents are the chief source of learning.

The first and second steps are *coercion* and *coaxing*, in which punishment and rewards are used, respectively, to focus the child's attention on the fact that there are rules that must be observed and that the parents are the enactors of these rules.

The third step is *evaluation*, in which a value judgment of good or bad is placed on the behavior and implies or directly gives praise or blame to ensure appropriate behavior.

The fourth step is *masking*, or withholding correct information or giving wrong information for the sake of settling a conflict. This can be pernicious, and a crisis may occur if the child uncovers the truth; trust can be lost and reality is distorted.

Fifth is the technique of *postponing*, which can be useful because it puts off dealing with a conflict until a fresher look can be taken at the situation. Of course, if this maneuver is overused, it will intensify and prolong the difficulty.

The sixth step is the transitional step and has been called *role reversal* or *role taking*, that is, putting oneself in the role or position of the other and looking at the situation from the point of view of another. Some call this *empathic ability*. It is the first glimmer of adult thinking and requires a well-developed understanding of self and reality. The ability to perform this maneuver early and successfully depends on the degree of masking that goes on in the family. The less the extent of masking, the better the success of role taking.[15]

Role Modification. The second group of procedures has been called *role modification* maneuvers. The basic characteristic of this group is communication and how persons learn to complement each other in role change.

Role modification begins with the seventh step of *joking*, or *humor*, in which persons develop the ability

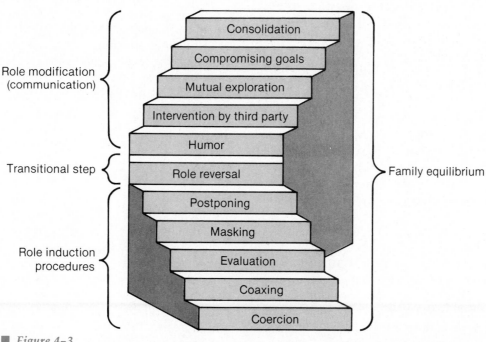

■ *Figure 4–3*

to laugh at themselves and each other (but affectionately). It is felt to be an outgrowth of role taking and the first of several tension-relieving mechanisms that families employ.

The eighth step employs the *intervention of a third party* (not necessarily a professional), who brings to the situation certain skills, a point of view, or knowledge that is not available to the parents or child within the family unit.

Mutual exploration is the ninth step, in which each person probes the capacity of the other to come to a solution regarding a conflict or problem. Here, trust and regard are expressed and invested in all members, including the children (to the extent of their capacity).

The tenth step, *compromising goals*, is an extension of mutual exploration. Here, goals are altered, but to no single person's detriment.

Similarly, the last step, *consolidation*, is the refined, integrated effort of learning to compromise successfully. It is associated with adjustment, redistribution of rewards, and role clarification.

Needless to say, the evolution through these various steps does not necessarily proceed smoothly, nor at times are all accomplished, especially steps 8 to 10. However, the more frequently they can be used, the easier each subsequent role adaptation and transition will become.[15]

EMOTIONAL BASIS OF ROLE LEARNING

Another important aspect of role learning for adults as well as children is that it is not merely a cognitive process. It is associated with multiple emotional or affective ties that the individual makes with others. These attachments begin with the mother and gradually include increasing numbers of persons with whom the child interacts and comes to identify with. As these attachments grow, the child develops a sense of self, in that he or she can take a position from the outside and view his or her own thoughts, feelings, and actions. In this way, the behavior that is expected is gradually internalized as the child figuratively stands back and looks at himself or herself. The child guides, judges, and reflects on his or her own behavior according to the child's perceptions of others' expectations for his or her behavior.

It has been noted that, although individuals learn role behavior in much the same way, there are differences in respective role performances. This differential role performance may be due to differences in the ways persons respond in interpersonal situations, their knowledge of the role in general, their motivation to perform specific roles, their attitude toward themselves and, finally, their response to the behavior of other persons in the interaction.[3,13]

TENSION IN ROLE RELATIONS

Tension and discontinuities in role relations must also be considered when considering the concept of role. Many terms have been used to illustrate the idea of tension or interruptions in a smooth process of interaction. Terms such as *role conflict, role strain, role change,* and *role transition* have been used to convey the various aspects of tension that can occur in a role system.

We have made the point that role interaction is dynamic. As theories of the development of human nature change, so do socialization patterns. As these latter change, variant family life systems evolve that, in turn, redefine reciprocal role relationships. Tensions and disruptions in smooth and rewarding role interaction may occur at any point.

Use of Social Power in the Family

As roles become differentiated (structured) and allocated (who gets what role), the element of social power comes into play. Various authors have defined this concept as the ability to influence a decision, to influence the emotions and behavior of others, or to achieve intended outcomes or goals.[14] It is a dynamic concept, and decision making is one indicator of power in the family. Moreover, several bases of power have been delineated[16] (see Bases of Social Power).

Families tend to use one type of power predominantly, although each may be used at different times and several may be used simultaneously.

Decision making in the family is a key indicator of social power and hence dominance in the family.[17] Decision making reflects how the family meets the needs of its members, including its health needs; it has implications for family cohesiveness. There are several areas that can be assessed that will give the nurse needed information in this area (see Assessment of Family Decision Making).

Adjustment to the Role

The major determinants of the degree of adjustment a person makes to a role are summarized in the box, Determinants of Role Adjustment. When there is a high degree of adjustment, the enactment of a person's set of roles can be rewarding in that they define a self-concept anchorage and a sense of belongingness and purpose. They provide social recognition and support, which, in turn, allow individuals to buy or earn desired conditions or things in the world and to view themselves as worthwhile, contributing members of society.

Feeth
i
Gene
V
la

Bases of Social Power

- *Legitimate power.* The shared belief that one person in the family system has the right to make decisions for others in the system. The basis for such power is traditional; thus, parents exert legitimate power over their children. In some families it is the father's traditional prerogative to make most of the decisions. When role relationships are egalitarian, legitimate power is a more shared phenomenon.
- *Expert power.* The perception that a family member or group has particular knowledge or skills. Thus, nurses are often seen by their clients as having expert knowledge to effect a change in behavior.
- *Referent power.* The influence of one person over another. Occurs through positive identification with the more powerful person, and there is the adoption of the behaviors, values, and attitudes of the powerful person. Role modeling is an example.
- *Reward power.* The expectation that the person has the resources to reward others. Parents are invested with this type of power. The hierarchical structure of nursing also carries this power.
- *Coercive power.* The expectation that punishment will occur if certain things are done or not done, certain behavior is exhibited or not exhibited, or certain expectations are met or not met. Examples include abuse in the family; denying a child access to school if not immunized.
- *Informational power.* Conveying a message that change is necessary. The media is an example. Families use this power when providing instruction to the members; often used in conjunction with expert power.

Assessment of Family Decision Making

- Who usually instigates a decision-making process?
- Who decides who will be involved in the decision?
- Who actually is involved and how did this come about?
- What processes are used in making decisions? For instance, are control, negotiation, persuasion, or authoritativeness modes employed, and how frequently?
- Who seems to exert the most power during decision making?
- Who makes the final decision?
- How is it implemented?
- What is the significance of the decision for the family, and what are the effects on family interaction?

If we in maternity nursing define the family as the unit to be served, we must have a thorough knowledge of its dynamics, and that includes much more than the physiological and psychological stages the mother passes through during pregnancy, labor, delivery, and the postpartum period. The use of role theory provides a vehicle to tie all of these disparate aspects of childbearing into related units, making them amenable for study and practice.

Considerations in the Nurse's Role

There are multiple facets or aspects to be considered in the nurse's role (Fig. 4-4).

■ FAMILY ROLES AND THE NURSE

The understanding and application of role theory in nursing practice provides a conceptual base for understanding the populations that we serve and gives some anchorage to our therapeutic method. It increases our capacity to view the forces of personality, family interaction, social systems, the health condition, and nursing intervention as a unit. It provides a needed framework for studying motivations for childbearing, reproductive behavior, childrearing techniques, and cultural goals. In addition, it provides a basis for understanding ourselves and our colleagues who provide health care.

Nursing is an applied science. The broad implications of its scientific nature challenge its practitioners to document this aspect with intellectual experimentation, innovations in practice, and constant research.

Determinants of Role Adjustment

- The clarity with which a specific role and its complementarity are defined and demonstrated
- The clarity or definiteness of the transitional procedures in the acquisition of a new role
- How well the role is learned and enacted; partly dependent on the first two determinants and the strength of the socialization process to the new role
- The consistency of the responses a role evokes
- A role's compatibility with the other roles in the person's set of roles
- A role's congruity with the emotional needs of the person
- The degree of complementarity that exists between reciprocal roles
- The bases and use of social power in the family

Research Highlight

The increased number of childbearing women in the work force has led to consideration of the relationship between pregnancy outcome and work. In a well designed, longitudinal study from 1979 to 1982, 786 pregnant women from 14 to 21 years of age were interviewed. Questions focused on family and social relationships, education, reproductive experiences, health care during pregnancy, work history, and attitudes toward working. Work-related stress was defined and measured. Preterm delivery and low birth weight were studied as indicators of work-related stress. The study indicated that job stressors did not negatively effect pregnancy outcome in women who were motivated to remain in the work force. However, there was an increase in the number of preterm deliveries and/or low-birth-weight babies when the woman was not motivated to work. Further study is needed to measure the impact of work on pregnancy across all ages of women, as well as to examine motivation factors more closely.

Utilizing these findings, nurses should be aware of the motivation component and assess women during pregnancy for their response to job stress. Work satisfaction and physical stress should be evaluated in the working pregnant woman. Women who are not motivated to work may need closer monitoring throughout their pregnancy.

Homer C, James S, Siegel E: Work-related psychosocial stress and risk of preterm, low birthweight delivery. Am J Public Health 80(2):173–177, 1990.

---

remarriage, partners may shift, but the monogamous ideal remains.[2]

Some of the more startling changes in the family are highlighted below (Dramatic Changes in the Family) and in Figure 5-5.

Many persons experience a variety of family structures in their lifetime.

Traditional Family Structures

Although it may seem that the traditional family structure is on the wane, there are a variety of traditional family forms extant. The most prominent among these are the following:

- *Nuclear family* (husband, wife, and children live in a common household). A single or a dual career may be pursued, and the wife's career may be continuous or interrupted as the children are born.
- *Nuclear dyad* (husband and wife live alone). They may be childless or not have children living at home. Again, there may be a single or dual career or a "second career" for the wife after the children have left home.
- *Single-parent family* (one head as a consequence of death, divorce, abandonment, or separation). Children are usually present. A career may be pursued. When financial aid is not forthcoming from the absent spouse, the parenting spouse usually engages in some form of occupation.
- *Single adult*. One person lives alone.

- *Three-generation family or extended family.*
- *Kin network*. Nuclear households or unmarried members live in close geographic proximity and operate within a reciprocal system of exchange of goods and services.[5,6]

Dramatic Changes in the Family

- Thirty million new households established since 1960. This constitutes a 58% increase.[3]
- In 1960, 52% of the 53 million U.S. households had no children under 18. By 1983, this proportion had grown to 63% of 84 million households. This has been due to increasing rates of childlessness and because older persons, especially women, are able to maintain their own households.[2]
- More women are expecting to be childless.[2,3]
- Since 1960 the overall rate of married-couple households has increased slowly; in 1983 they accounted for six in ten households. Cohabitation, on the other hand, has skyrocketed, primarily since 1970, increasing by 331%![2,3]
- There has been a 175% increase in one-parent households compared with a 26% increase in married families. This rise was most accelerated during the 1970s, when divorce rates greatly increased and the number of out-of-wedlock births was also greatest.[3]
- Nearly one half of all marriages in the 1980s ended in divorce; one in every three marriages is a remarriage.[1,5]

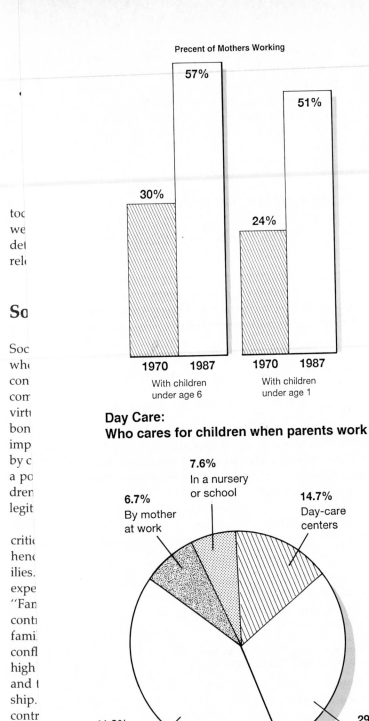

Precent of Mothers Working

57%

51%

30%

24%

| 1970 | 1987 | | 1970 | 1987 |

With children under age 6

With children under age 1

Day Care:
Who cares for children when parents work

7.6%
In a nursery or school

6.7%
By mother at work

14.7%
Day-care centers

41.3%
In another's home

29.7%
In own home

■ *Figure 5–2*
Even with the sharp rise in working mothers, most children are still cared for at home—their own or someone else's.

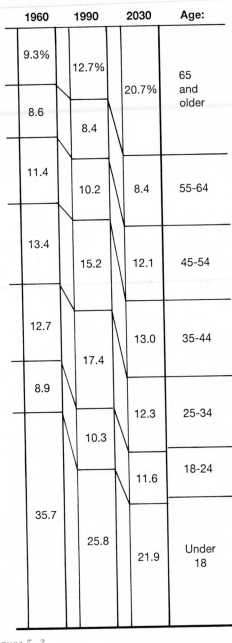

Age Distribution

1960	1990	2030	Age:
9.3%	12.7%	20.7%	65 and older
8.6	8.4		
11.4	10.2	8.4	55-64
13.4	15.2	12.1	45-54
12.7	13.0		35-44
	17.4		
8.9		12.3	25-34
	10.3		
		11.6	18-24
35.7	25.8	21.9	Under 18

■ *Figure 5–3*
As the old get older, the percentage of young gets dramatically smaller.

toc
we
del
rel

So

Soc
wh
con
com
virt
bon
imp
by c
a po
dren
legit

critic
hen
ilies.
expe
"Fan
conti
fami
confl
high
and t
ship.
contr
ing to
one h
invol
event
The s
child'
highe
Paren
and th
childr
ever, t
the tir
lowest

Each of these will have its problems and resources with respect to health needs and utilization of services. Generally, traditional households are looked on more favorably by society because they are considered stable and provide a legitimating anchorage for the children born of these unions.

It has been said that nuclear families suffer from isolation and cannot cope with illness, repeated pregnancy, or reproductive wastage; hence, they must turn to professionals for sustenance and care. However, research indicates that the nuclear family probably has less isolation and better coping ability than formerly was thought. This is because there appears to be great role adaptability and flexibility in time of stress as well as a greater utilization of kin and other social networks for advice and sustenance during childbearing as well as for other health conditions.[4,5]

family must be assessed with care tailored to their needs, some basic principles remain. Families today, especially those of the middle class, regardless of ethnicity, may assume a more questioning attitude. Rationales for treatment plans are questioned, and prognoses and alternatives are requested. This may prove disconcerting to some health providers, but clients' questions should be answered and options discussed.

Evaluating Health Information

Health professionals often expect clients to accept their information as true because it is drawn from a scientific body of knowledge. However, some intelligent clients may regard modern science as attempting to bring forth more and more "laws" aimed at finding absolute truth in a relative world. On the other hand, information from other sources is also subjected to scrutiny and evaluation before acceptance. This questioning attitude does not preclude interest in what the nurse has to say.

Expectant parents will have many questions, and when the nurse responds to their inquiries, they may go on to relate information that they have gathered from other sources. It becomes important to discuss this information seriously and with respect because it is valuable to the parent. Health teaching documented with rational explanation is much more readily accepted. The advice and teaching must be practical, also. To insist that a vegetarian eat meat, even if she may have anemia, is simply too impractical, especially if there are others in the family to consider. Similarly, ethnic food preferences and preparation, often dictated by the culture, no matter how repugnant to the nurse, must be taken into consideration.

Families today also expect a fuller and more complete explanation than previously, particularly if they are well educated. If a mother prefers a vegetarian diet and wants to know the food values of the foods she wishes to include in her diet, she may not be satisfied with only a suggested menu. Exchanges and equivalents must be discussed. Similarly, it is not sufficient to tell a mother in an antepartal clinic to return in so many weeks for another blood test without telling her the reason for returning and the purpose of the procedure. If clients reject some of the advice, this, too, is to be treated with respect.

Choosing Reproductive Services

The factors that influence the choice of antepartal services include past experience with health personnel, geographic location, economics, feelings about the pregnancy, the influence of significant others, and the parents' physical condition. These areas will need assessment.

Increasingly, high priority is placed on ambience and interpersonal relations during the pregnancy and at the time of delivery. Selection of services is made on the basis of consultation with friends, referrals from professionals, and past experience with health providers. In general, couples are taking a more active role in the planning and execution of their care and tend to seek out health professionals who allow them this right. This is true for the immigrant families as well, who tend to select professionals who are sensitive to their cultural needs. It then becomes important in planning care with the client to be sure that the couple is duly informed about the nature of their care, including their right to sign themselves out of the hospital. This information, together with a genuine indication of regard for the couple, is usually sufficient to lessen the apprehension about the particular service.

Selecting a hospital or choosing between a hospital or home delivery involves many of the same factors as those considered in the selection of antepartal services. For most couples today, childbirth is regarded as a natural process; thus, alternative birth centers may be sought. Modern equipment and technological expertise may be much less important than an environment that simulates the home.

Today, parents come to their deliveries much more knowledgeable than previously. This is due, in part, to the large variety of books now available dealing with nutrition in pregnancy and the physiology of pregnancy, labor, and delivery; there are even "how to" books on home delivery. Parents, therefore, expect their requests to be considered. Hospitals that have the reputation for having a great deal of restrictions are avoided.

The need for control over one's own life may also be a strong motivating factor in the choice of a home delivery. These types of deliveries remain controversial. Safety of the mother and infant continues to be a grave concern for the health professionals, and there are data that indicate that this concern is well founded. Birth carries a strong symbolic meaning, however, and the home typifies this meaning. The traditional hospital setting is seen by many couples as a sterile place with little room for intimacy and family integration. Many hospitals have instituted birthing rooms or birth centers that simulate a homelike atmosphere free from many of the restrictions and rigidities imposed by the traditional delivery suite. Couples enjoy and utilize these services, and data indicate that the risk to the infant and mother is minimal when the mother and infant are low risk.

■ REFERENCES

1. Thornton A: Changing attitudes toward family issues in the United States. J Marr Fam 51:873–893, November 1989
2. The 21st century family. Newsweek, Special Issue, 3–108, Winter/Spring 1990
3. Glick PC: American household structure in transition. Fam Plan Perspect 16(5):204–211, Sept/Oct 1984
4. Reeder SJ: The Impact of Disabling Health Conditions on Family Interaction [dissertation]. Los Angeles, University of California at Los Angeles, 1974
5. McCubbin H, Dahl BB: Marriage and Family, Individuals and Life Cycles. New York, Wiley, 1985
6. St. Clair PA, et al: Social network structure and prenatal care utilization. Med Care 27:823–831, August 1989
7. Alexander J, Kornfein M: Changes in family functioning amongst nonconventional families. Am J Orthopsychiatry 53:408–417, July 1983
8. Zimmerman IL, Bernstein M: Parental work patterns in alternative families: Influence on child development. Am J Orthopsychiatry 53:418–425, July 1983
9. Eiduson B: Conflict and stress in nontraditional families: Impact on children. Am J Orthopsychiatry 5:426–435, July 1983
10. Glick PC, Norton AJ: Marrying, divorcing and living together in the US today. Population Bulletin 32(5). Washington, DC, Population Reference Bureau, 1982
11. Gelman D, et al: The single parent's family albums. Newsweek, July 15, 1985
12. Gersick KE: Fathers by choice: Divorced men who received custody of their children. In Levinger G, Moles OC (eds): Divorce and Separation: Context, Causes and Consequences, pp 303–323. New York, Basic Books, 1979
13. Mackey WC: Fathering Behaviors: The Dynamics of the Man–Child Bond. New York, Plenum Press, 1985
14. Greif GL: Single fathers rearing children. J Marr Fam 47(1):185–191, February 1985
15. Greif GL: Custodial dads and their ex-wives. Single Parent 27:17–20, January/February 1984
16. Greif GL: Single Fathers. Lexington, MA, Lexington Books, 1985
17. Riley D, Cochran MM: Naturally occurring childbearing advice for fathers: Utilization of the personal social network. J Marr Fam 47:275–286, May 1985
18. Klinman DG: Fatherhood USA. New York, Garland Publishing, 1984
19. Eiduson B, et al: Comparative socialization practices in alternative family settings. In Lamb M (ed): Nontraditional Families. New York, Plenum Press, 1981
20. Lamarine R: The dilemma of Native American health. Health Educ 20:15–18, December 1989
21. Bullough VL, Bullough B: Health Care for the Other Americans. New York, Appleton Century Crofts, 1982
22. Queen SA, Habenstein RW, Quadagno JS: The Family In Various Cultures. New York, Harper & Row, 1985
23. Moore LG, Van Arsdale PW, Glittenberg JE, Aldrich RA: The Biocultural Basis of Health. St. Louis, CV Mosby, 1980
24. Hofferth SL: Kin networks, race, and family structure. J Marr Fam 46:791–806, November 1984
25. Dawkins C, Ervin N, Wiessfeld L, Yan A: Health orientations, beliefs and use of health services among minority, high-risk expectant mothers. Public Health Nurs 5: 7–11, March 1988
26. Galli N, Greenberg JS, Tobin F: Health education and sensitivity to cultural, religious and ethnic beliefs. J School Health 57:177–180, May 1987
27. U.S. Bureau of the Census: Statistical Abstracts of the United States. Washington, DC, Government Printing Office, p 32, 1982
28. Henderson G, Primeaux M: Transcultural Health Care. Menlo Park, CA, Addison-Wesley, 1981
29. Refugee Resettlement Program: 1988 Report to Congress. Washington, DC, U.S. Department of Health and Human Services, Social Security Administration, 1988
30. Thomas RG, Tumminia PA: Maternity care for Vietnamese in America. Birth 9(3):187–190, Fall 1982
31. Poss JE: Providing health care for southeast Asian refugees. J NY State Nurs Assoc 20:4–6, June 1989

■ SUGGESTED READING

Choi EC: Unique aspects of Korean-American mothers. JOGNN 15: 394–400, September/October 1986

Collins C, Tiedje LB: A program for women returning to work after childbirth. JOGNN 17:246–253, July/August 1987

Glenn ND, Supancic M: The social and demographic correlates of divorce and separation in the United States: An update and reconsideration. J Marr Fam 46:563–575, August 1984

Greif GL: Single Fathers. Lexington, KY, DC Heath, 1985

Klinman DG, Kohl R: Fatherhood USA. New York, Garland Publishing, 1984

Lazarus ES, Phillpson EH: A longitudinal study comparing the prenatal care of Puerto Rican and white women. Birth 17:6–11, March 1990

Poss JE: Providing health care for southeast Asian refugees. J NY State Nurs Assoc 20:4–6, June 1989

Reinert BR: The health care beliefs and values of Mexican-Americans. Home Healthcare Nurse 4(5):23–31, 1987

6

Sociocultural Influences on Reproductive Care

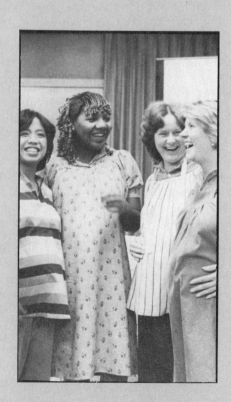

Values, attitudes, perspectives, and behavior are formed and conditioned by the social groups in which we participate from earliest childhood. Consequently, there are differing orientations to health and health care, reflecting memberships in differing ethnic, racial, religious, and social-class groups. These varying health orientations become manifest both in the behavior of individuals and in the institutions that are organized to deliver health services.

In recent years, there has been a heightened awareness of the importance of social and cultural factors in health status, specifically maternal care. Although Americans are accustomed to thinking of their health status as being the best in the world, their health care is still far short of its potential. Large segments of the population either do not have access to adequate medical care or are deprived of quality care in the services that they do receive. There has been a great stimulus to improve the prenatal care system to improve reproductive outcomes. There has been some expansion and elaboration of the existing system of maternity services. Whether this will have the desired effects depends on a variety of factors.

This chapter focuses on those forces in society that influence the field of maternity services and reproductive outcomes. It examines the social and cultural meaning of pregnancy (i.e., the current social, cultural, and economic forces that influence motivations for childbearing). It also discusses some of the critical issues in the use of maternity services, social risk factors associated with in reproductive outcomes, and aspects of the nurse's role in these matters.

■ SOCIAL AND CULTURAL MEANING OF CHILDBEARING

As discussed in Chapter 1, pregnancy itself needs to be considered in terms of the social context in which it occurs, namely, the family and the larger society. Pregnancy and childbearing generally have different meanings in various societies and even within any given society.

Childbearing Motivations

No biologic event has greater significance for society than reproduction and its outcome, because it is important in family and population dynamics and therefore has a heavy impact on individual and national welfare. Women begin their preparation for childbearing early in life. In a sense, they begin at the time of their own conception.

As mentioned previously, society is organized primarily for families with children, and the argument for having children can be very persuasive. Even in this newer era of voluntary childbearing, couples without children can still be made to feel "out of place," especially if they have been married for a time. Research has indicated that the value of having children remains generally accepted by the majority of Americans.[1] The availability of acceptable means for preventing conception should theoretically permit childbearing today to be a consequence of motivated human action rather than mere biologic happenstance. However, regardless of when pregnancies occur or if they are planned, the number of children that a couple has and the time at which they have them are, to a large extent, a function of the couple's childbearing motivations, which, in turn, are influenced by cultural imperatives.

CHILDBEARING WITHIN A CULTURAL SYSTEM

Griffith suggests that childbearing concepts can focus on four components of a cultural system:[2]

- Mores and value systems, involving notions of duty, obligation, and desirability
- Kinship system, prescribing reciprocal rights, duties, and obligations in relationships resulting from marriage and family descent
- Knowledge and belief system, defining conception, labor, and childbearing
- Ceremonial and ritual systems, providing reenactment of symbolic elements and allowing for their incorporation into daily lives

In attempting to understand the patterns of belief surrounding childbearing in other cultures, the nurse can keep in mind the Questions Involving Belief Systems Surrounding Childbearing, listed on the following pages, when using the nursing process in assessing, planning, implementing, and evaluating care for clients.

PRESENT SOCIETAL TRENDS AFFECTING CHILDBEARING MOTIVATIONS

Fertility Control. In Chapter 11, techniques of contraception and family planning are discussed. In this chapter we highlight certain implications of fertility control. We have discussed the trends that have resulted in lower fertility in previous chapters. Middle-class families are restricting their families to one to two children. Thus, in the opinion of many demographers, a revolution in the fertility regimen of American women is taking place. At the core is an apparent reassessment of the values associated with fertility control. Improvement in the number and reliability of contraceptive de-

Research Highlight

Previous research that has shown significant relationships between life stress, social support, or anxiety and complications of pregnancy failed to control for preexisting medical risks, parity, or age and focused on primarily white middle-class women. Norbeck and Anderson studied a population of lower socioeconomic women from three ethnic groups: black, Hispanic, and white.

After controlling for preexisting complications, illnesses, and known drug abuse, 208 women participated in this study. Life stress, social support, and anxiety were measured and analyzed. Norton and Anderson found that life stress had no significant effect on pregnancy outcome. Separate analyses showed significant differences between the ethnic groups. Blacks disclosed partner support as the highest predictor of gestation complications and mother's support for all labor-related complications. Surprisingly, high friend support was an indication of increased complications in labor. In whites, drug use accounted for the variance in cesarean sections and smoking for the birth weight, each being connected with high stress/high support, whereas high levels of maternal support were associated with longer labors. Hispanic outcomes were never significantly predictive of complications, having very low life stress, substance use, or complications, except for prolonged labor.

Considering the questionable validity of the tools used on the lower socioeconomic groups, further research is needed to support or refute these findings. Despite conflicting conclusions, nurses should continue to assess the patient's response to stress and her reactions to social support during pregnancy, while observing the effects on the pregnancy. Ethnic differences continue to be important in assessing who is the supportive person, the woman's perception of support, and the relationship to pregnancy outcomes.

Norbeck JS, Anderson NJ: Psychosocial predictors of pregnancy outcomes in low-income black, Hispanic, and white women. Nurs Res 38(4): 204–209, July/August 1989.

vices has resulted not only in a more effective means of fertility control but also in an apparent change in the rules under which fertility decisions are made.[3,4]

The widespread use of the pill has facilitated the adoption of other effective contraceptive methods, including sterilization and abortion. More reliable contraceptives have also separated contraception from sexual activity. Now, childbearing can be voluntary in a radically different sense than ever before. Under the previous fertility regimen, because women could not confidently plan the prevention of unwanted pregnancies, the role expectations of women were structured around motherhood and became, in fact, rationalizations of the inevitable.[3]

Competing Social Roles. These new fertility-control values have given more support to the equal opportunity concept by making nonfamilial roles a realistic and viable option for women. Motherhood itself can now become more a matter of rational evaluation.[5] One of the consequences has been to place motherhood more directly in competition with alternative, socially desirable career roles. When there is choice for motherhood, emphasis is placed on planning. Among the factors that must be taken into account are the direct social, psychological, and economic costs of children themselves, and also the loss of the wife's earnings and intrinsic satisfaction with her occupation (Fig. 6-1).

This is no small matter. Modern life-styles are significantly dependent on the wife's earnings. In a majority of the families in which both the husband and wife have incomes, the wife's income represents over one fifth of the total family income.[3]

IMPACT ON MATERNITY SERVICES

The implications of all this are enormous, for fertility statistics influence almost every facet of our lives. Two trends in particular are worth mentioning. First, some hospitals are closing or merging their maternity units; thus, regionalization is an accomplished fact. It is anticipated that this will improve the quality of obstetrical care in addition to controlling costs and avoiding duplication of services. Second, the experience of fertility control may make women more sensitive and aware of the need for better maternal care during pregnancy. Indeed, the increased availability of safe abortion after 1970 has been associated with a reduction in pregnancy-associated maternal mortality. There is also good reason

■ SOCIOCULTURAL FACTORS AFFECTING CHILDBEARING

Sociodemographic Factors and the Use of Maternity Services

SOCIOECONOMIC STATUS

Socioeconomic status is an important determinant of maternal reproductive behavior and maternal use of services. Because socioeconomic status, or social class, as it is sometimes called, has such a pervasive influence on health and health care, it is important to describe briefly its central features.

Socioeconomic status is a complex concept referring to a theoretical formulation of relationships between subgroups in our society. It is a term frequently used by sociologists and epidemiologists in medical research in an effort to subdivide populations into a few descriptive categories that differ in a variety of social and economic characteristics, background, and behavior.[6-8]

To determine socioeconomic status, the usual procedure is to select as indicators of social differences one or several characteristics, each of which is closely related to income, education, occupation, housing and place of residence, social values, and the general life-style of population subgroups. By far the most widely used indicator of socioeconomic status is occupation. It is the best indicator of a person's income, education, standard of living, social values, and a variety of other attributes.[6,7]

Not all social differences stem from socioeconomic status, however. Dividing a population along one social dimension does not automatically provide categories that are socially meaningful in other respects. It can be demonstrated that such social variables as age, geographic region, height, parity, and ethnicity each contribute independently to the total picture of social variation in pregnancy outcome. The same may be said of other more complex social influences.[8,9]

It is generally accepted that adequate medical care during pregnancy, particularly in the early stages, reduces the incidence of neonatal and maternal mortality, congenital malformations or other birth defects, prematurity, and so on. The relationship between low socioeconomic status and failure to receive adequate antenatal care has been well documented. The data appear to be similar in the United States, Great Britain, and various other Western nations. Not only do women of lower socioeconomic status typically comprise the highest proportion of those who have not received antenatal care, but they are also the women, as a group, who contribute to the highest proportion of underusers

---

Questions Involving Belief Systems Surrounding Childbearing

Antepartum

Who may have a child?

At what age?

By whom may one have a child?

How many children can one have?

Can one space pregnancies?

What should be the behavior during pregnancy?

Are there restrictions on the father?

Are there any restrictions on sexual activity?

Who may see and touch certain body parts?

How is a fetus formed?

What are the beliefs regarding conception?

Intrapartum

What causes labor?

How does one behave during labor?

How should one respond to pain?

Should one take medication?

Where should labor take place?

Postpartum

What general behavior is expected?

What behavior is expected of the father and others?

Are there restrictions on food or activity?

Care of the Newborn

When is he recognized?

What are the rules for his care?

Who cares for him?

(Adapted from Griffith S: Childbearing and the concept of culture. JOGN Nurs 11(3):181, May/June 1982.)

---

to connect the trends in fertility control to the decline in infant mortality.[3,5]

It should be recognized that it is not certain that the current pattern of fertility control will continue indefinitely. Nevertheless, it is important to remember that the baby boom children of the 1950s have formed their own families. Consequently, there will be an increase of approximately 20% in the number of women in the childbearing age groups of 15 to 44 years. Thus, the absolute number of births is rising even if the birth rate may not be.[3]

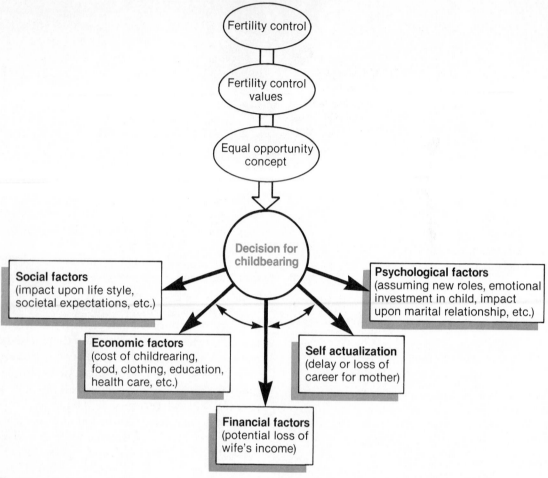

■ *Figure 6–1*
Fertility control has made childbearing a matter of choice. This illustration shows some of the factors that may be included in the decision for childbearing.

of antenatal care.[7,9–11] According to data for the United States, the average white mother had 60% more visits for medical care than the average nonwhite mother. This is undoubtedly related more to the influence of socioeconomic status than to the ethnicity of the mother. According to these data, as family income increased, the number of visits for medical care also increased, and when income rose above the poverty line, the number of visits jumped significantly. On the average, women living in families below the poverty level made 9.3 visits for medical care; women from middle-income families averaged 13.7 visits. Most of the women in the lowest income group visited medical facilities (clinics, hospitals) for their care, as contrasted to the women in the highest-income group, the majority of whom visited physicians for medical care.[11–13]

PROBLEMS WITH HEALTH-CARE ORGANIZATION

There are a variety of features characteristic of the organization of health care that hinder some clients from receiving appropriate use of care. The major issues correlated with underutilization are discussed below.

Inadequate Outreach Programs. In the 1970s, there was a national commitment for equality of health care for all citizens, which led to a variety of important legislative acts whose aims were to extend and improve the system of health organization so that care could be offered more efficiently to the poor and economically advantaged. For example, the federally subsidized maternal- and infant-care (MIC) projects were instituted to help reduce the incidence of mental retardation and other handicapping conditions caused by complications associated with childbearing and to help reduce infant and maternal mortality. These programs have been concentrated in the low-income areas of large and small cities and have emphasized early, comprehensive prenatal care for all clients in the geographic area served. The results, however have been only partially successful, and with the current era of economic austerity in governmental subsidies, it remains to be seen whether there will continue to be a national commitment to quality health services for all strata of society.[12,13]

Size. The massiveness of medical organization itself can be very intimidating. Most lower-income women tend to visit medical facilities such as hospitals and clinics, which are often large and complex, very specialized, and often impersonal. Poorly educated clients are ill equipped to cope with these complexities.[13] Moreover, they often lack confidence in the community facilities for their care. They find that two kinds of care exist: one for those who can pay and another for those who cannot. Because so many people now feel that proper health care is a right of citizenship, the provision of adequate health services for all requires a restructuring of present national priorities and an escalation of the public's social consciousness. Most health professionals agree that any worthwhile program should provide financial support and maintain the mother's dignity as well. The concept of comprehensive health planning by states and localities, including area health education centers, community clinics, and innovative programs in hospital clinics, has been an attempt to provide a higher caliber of care for all segments of society.

Within the past 10 years, the focus of service in many outpatient departments and clinics has changed from dispensing first aid to giving ambulatory care with a dynamic, change-oriented focus. Similarly, nurses now function in these settings in a care-centered, more independent role in which they are expanding their functions of educating clients, providing supportive guidance, and making observations. In this role, the professional nurse becomes primarily responsible for maintaining continuity of health care for a specific client population. Increasingly, expanded nursing roles are used to provide routine prenatal care in outpatient, ambulatory settings.[14,15]

Skills and Education Needed to Cope With the High Degree of Professionalization. Professionalization in health care demands a certain degree of communication skills and good understanding and compliance with appointment schedules and prescribed regimens. Many regimens that are ordered are impossible for low-income clients to follow. The simple order to take medication "with each meal" may be difficult for many lower-income families who eat irregularly and may not eat three meals a day.[7] Lower-income people may be less skilled in obtaining information and explanations from professionals regarding care. Higher-income clients have greater aggressive and interactional skills and can cope more effectively with the professional's failure to communicate.

Middle-Class Bias. Another characteristic of medical organization that influences the quality of medical care is the middle-class bias of most professional health workers. That is, middle-class clients are preferred by most providers and are viewed as more treatable. Thus, there may be a distinct bias expressed against the lower-income client, based honestly on professional conceptions. Typically, the staff members do not understand the perspectives, attitudes, customs, and life-styles of the lower-income clients. They often take for granted that the clients have the same attitudes about health as they do. Hence, they tend to issue orders that are not understood or cannot be followed easily. Often there is a tendency to think of lower-income people in stereotyped terms: they cannot keep appointments, they have little sense of time or responsibility, and so on. Lower-income clients may perceive these class biases, and this can affect utilization of services.

The many hours of waiting, the impersonal routines of institutional care in large hospitals or clinics, particularly in the municipal and county hospitals, and the real or imagined perceptions of racial and class bias all tend to maximize dissatisfactions of lower-income clients and reduce use. Moreover, the distances that clients must travel to the facilities and the cost of transportation are realistic matters. Customarily, poorer people organize their lives so as not to go far for the necessities of living. This is one of the factors in the relative success of the MIC program and the neighborhood health centers that reached into the lower-income communities and brought clinic facilities into the neighborhood.[13–15]

Maldistribution of Health Personnel and Manpower. The urban specialty orientation in health care contributes to the disparity in outcomes noted among various population groups. Rural and geographically isolated communities, as well as the inner cities, have traditionally experienced difficulties obtaining adequate health care because *professional socialization and economic considerations* promote practice in desirable metropolitan areas.

Lack of coordination and overlap in agencies presents another dimension of maldistribution of health services. For example, there may be several community-health nursing services in one area, such as the health department, a voluntary nursing agency, and school nursing services. They may all serve one family, but they seldom communicate with one another. Similarly, some hospitals may be overcrowded, while others have empty beds.

It is believed that quality maternity care in the future will be provided by a closely integrated team of physicians, professional nurses, nurse–midwives or nurse practitioners, laboratory technicians, social workers, nutritionists, health educators, and homemakers. None of these except physicians is available in sufficient numbers at the present. However, the development of expanded roles for nurses is proving to be a viable effort to deliver quality care. Research has indicated that when nurses are used in expanded roles and are integral members of the health-care team, there are considerably fewer broken antepartal appointments, better postpartal clinic attendance, better use of family-planning services and techniques, and reduction of infant mortality.[15–17]

Government programs have been developed to encourage health professionals to enter practice in medically underserved rural or inner-city urban areas. Efforts such as the National Health Service Corps, which supports team practices between physicians and nurse practitioners in rural communities, Medicare reimbursement of nurse practitioners and physicians' assistants in rural clinics, scholarships and educational subsidies for primary-care providers, and program grants for primary care to schools of nursing and medicine are steps toward ensuring greater availability and appropriate distribution of health personnel.

The training of *indigenous community members* through decentralized educational programs has been a most effective method of providing quality care to underserved populations. Their familiarity with the lifestyles of childbearing families, their knowledge of the socioeconomic factors to be considered, and their willingness to provide whatever service is needed, be it transportation or referral for counseling, are salient factors in their success. Programs planned by outsiders that do not consider the involvement of those whom they serve are doomed to failure and in no way deliver quality care.

The development of *innovations*, such as community clinics and alternative birth centers (Fig. 6-2), are attempts by the health system to respond to consumer needs. Community clinics are initiated and organized by the indigenous population and are staffed largely by local people. Supported largely by federal and state funds, which are in increasingly short supply, community clinics can be very effective in responding to specific health-care needs.

HEALTH INSURANCE COVERAGE FOR MATERNAL CARE

Although the stated goals for health care on the national level include ensuring quality, access, and control of costs, methods of financing services continue to support disparities among population groups. The chief protection for the health needs of most young parents lies in voluntary and commercial prepayment insurance. Maternity benefits traditionally have been distressingly low. Young low-income families are frequently saddled with a large medical and hospital bill at a time when they can least afford to pay. Many professionals feel that maternity care should be entirely covered, but the actuaries believe that the rates for this kind of coverage would be prohibitive. However, it might be noted that insurance companies have had this opinion about other forms of coverage and under public pressure have increased benefits. Many community-health leaders believe that the resources of this country are so vast that

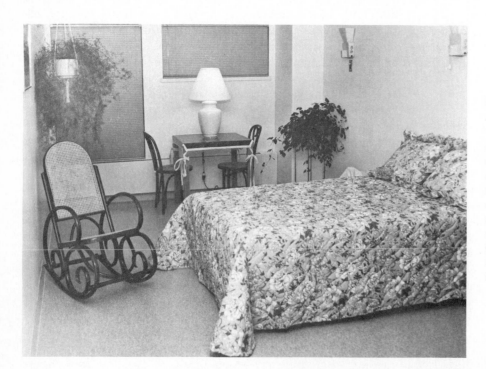

■ *Figure 6–2*
Alternative birth centers are special units associated with an acute hospital that offer a more homelike atmosphere for labor and delivery. Low-risk mothers undergo labor in a comfortable room without the usual equipment and requirements of standard labor rooms and deliver in a natural position in the same bed. Companions may be present, and there is as little intervention by the health provider as possible.[18]

full coverage is feasible if there is a public mandate to provide it.[11,17,18]

Various bills for national health insurance have been introduced in the U.S. Congress, but conflicting goals continue to make it very difficult for legislators to develop a comprehensive, widely acceptable plan. Many question the commitment of the majority to the concept that equitable health care is a right of all people. Certainly our values supporting individual rights and minimum government interference provide significant obstacles to a sense of national social purpose. The involvement of concerned nurses in the governmental processes can help promote an equitable health-care system (Fig. 6-3).

■ CHANGING RELATIONSHIPS BETWEEN CLIENTS AND PROVIDERS

Consumer Satisfaction

Consumers complain that it is more and more difficult to find a primary-care physician who will give them the personal attention they want. Regardless of the socioeconomic status of the woman, it is very difficult for her to receive continuity of care from the providers of maternity services. Group practice, regardless of its other

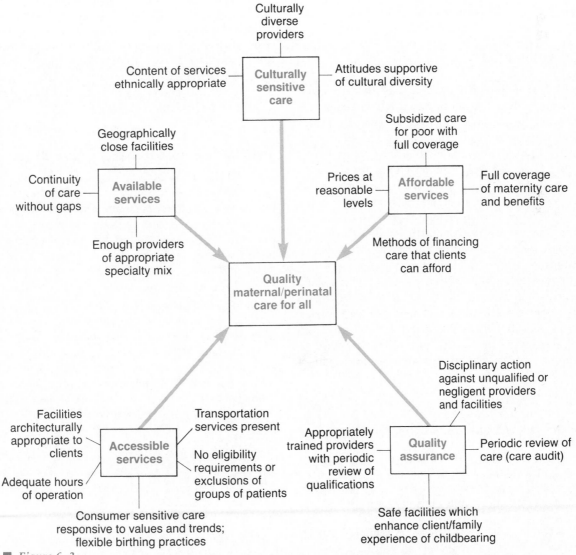

■ *Figure 6–3*
Health-care system requirements for providing quality maternity/perinatal care for all.

merits, sometimes disrupts the relationship between patient and physician; hospital structure requires nursing personnel to change with shift changes; clients have difficulty determining the status of the person in the medical office to whom they are speaking on the telephone. Patients feel that obstetricians seem to relinquish their responsibility for the neonate during the postpartum period. Similarly, in this period, pediatricians (from the mother's perspective) do not appear to be centrally involved with the needs of the mother. These features of the medical-care system are reflected in the concept of fragmented health care and consumer dissatisfaction.[18,19]

Consumer satisfaction refers to the attitudes toward the health-care system of those who have experienced contact with the system. It is concerned with the satisfaction of the client with the quantity or quality of care actually received and relates to several dimensions (see Dimensions of Consumer Satisfaction).

Communication

One of the more important transactions that occurs in the provider–client relationship is effective communication from the provider to the client concerning the nature of her condition and the actions to be taken. The degree to which she has understood the physician and nurse and can verbalize the advice and instructions depends on the quality of the relationship. Similarly, good health care results in communication from the client to the providers. In particular, the degree to which the woman's concerns, worries, and fears about her condition have been perceived by the provider are equally important.

Commentators on the physician–client relationship frequently have discussed the social-class and value differences between providers and clients as one barrier to communication and, ultimately, to utilization of health services. Numerous studies indicate that middle-class clients tend to obtain most of their information about illness by asking their physicians and nurses direct questions. In contrast, working-class clients receive their information from a passive process in which they are given information without asking; they also tended to receive less information.[17,19] Despite their reluctance to request information, working-class maternity clients are not much different from upper-class clients in their desire for information.[7] Although upper-class clients may desire more technical details regarding their health condition, there is no general social-class difference in clients' desires for as much information as possible presented in nontechnical language.

Part of the issue of better communication between provider and client results from a reflection of a general social-class difference in language use, which was alluded to earlier. Working-class clients sense that physicians do not expect them to ask questions, and there is social distance. But even middle-class clients hesitate to communicate freely with their physician about troublesome problems or symptoms. A virtual legend has been created and accepted about the hard-working, busy physician. Thus, although there may be some apparent social-class differences in the quantity and quality of communication with physicians, it is a matter of degree of communication.

Implications for the Nurse as Communicator

Given this situation, the maternity nurse has a crucial role to play. Generally, the nurse is not perceived by the client in the same manner as the physician. Thus, the nurse has an opportunity to fill a much-needed role in the delivery of health care by seizing the initiative and by closing the communication gap in the client–provider relationship. Such action would be congruent with client expectations; moreover, several studies have indicated that the nurse can perform roles involving the receiving and giving of information to clients far more effectively than can physicians.[12,17,18] Because communication problems have a significant effect on the appropriate use of services, the nurse's contribution to facilitating communication becomes crucial.

■ SOCIAL RISK FACTORS AND REPRODUCTIVE OUTCOMES

In this section, we discuss the risk factors that may jeopardize the health of the maternity client. Some of these factors, such as age, may be beyond the client's control; others, however, such as behavioral risk factors, are mutable.

Dimensions of Consumer Satisfaction

- Accessibility/convenience of services: convenience of care and emergency care
- Availability: family physicians, hospitals, specialists
- Continuity: regular family physician, same physician
- Physician conduct: consideration of feelings, explanations
- Financial aspects: cost of services, insurance coverage, payment mechanisms

Sociodemographic Risk Factors

MATERNAL AGE AND PARITY RELATED TO UTILIZATION OF HEALTH-CARE SERVICES

There is also differential use of health-care services by age and parity; women in the younger age group tend to come to prenatal care later than women in the other age groups. This may be due partly to the fact that the highest rates of unwed pregnancies are in the youngest age groups. Both the young mother and the unwed mother tend to be latecomers to prenatal care. Multiparas who have had little trouble with previous pregnancies also tend to come later and be more lax in keeping appointments.

MATERNAL AGE AND PARITY RELATED TO MORBIDITY AND MORTALITY

Findings indicate that mortality and morbidity are higher among infants of the older primipara and multipara mothers and among those of very young mothers. There is also a strong correlation between socioeconomic status and age of the mother. In births to parents with more education or higher family income, the mothers tend to be older. The lower the socioeconomic status, the greater the tendency for the mother to be younger.[20,21]

Although women age 35 and older account for only about 5% to 6% of all births in the United States, births to these women are viewed with interest and apprehension because they have come to be viewed as high risk both for the primigravida as well as the multipara. Multiparity is also associated with less successful outcomes when it is associated with advanced age.[20,22] Heretofore, attention has usually been focused on the maternal rather than the fetal results. More recently, because of the availability of sophisticated antenatal fetal assessment technology, the focus has gravitated to fetal risk.

Pregnancy in the adolescent is also fraught with maternal and neonatal morbidity and mortality. The complications, both obstetrical and social, are so enormous that we will discuss the phenomenon of adolescent pregnancy in detail in Chapter 37.

Thus, age and parity are two biologic categories that have specific social significance, because they contribute to a general picture of poor reproductive outcomes for both mother and infant.

Nursing Implications. The role of the maternity nurse becomes particularly important in counseling of women with respect to the problems they may encounter in such pregnancies and the risks associated with some of the antenatal diagnostic techniques. Some popular articles have given the impression that these diagnostic tests somehow cure fetal defects and can make pregnancy safer. This is erroneous, and the mother and father need to be appraised of the limitations associated with these tests. They are not a panacea for a safe pregnancy outcome. They are useful because they can determine if some fetal defects do exist and, thus, the parents may decide to have an abortion. They can also give a good indication of the age and well-being of the fetus, which helps if early delivery is indicated. Thus, these parents need meticulous antepartal care, particularly from the nurse.

SOCIODEMOGRAPHIC AND ETHNIC INDICATORS OF RISK

Certain indicators of socioeconomic status, such as family income, education of mother and father, and ethnicity can be risk factors in pregnancy. Low-income individuals are considerably more predisposed to lowered health status and obstetrical complications during pregnancy. Low birth weight is particularly prevalent in the low-income African-American population. The role of ethnicity becomes readily apparent when one analyzes data that have accrued since 1935 on racial background.

Throughout this period, marked differences have occurred on the basis of racial background, with nonwhites faring much worse than whites. Indeed, the relative differential has actually risen during this period. The racially related differentials in mortality have also been noted beyond the first year of life. It should be stressed that virtually all of the race-related differentials in mortality are socioeconomically related.[9,10,17]

Factors Placing Mother or Fetus at Risk

- Sociodemographic risk factors
  >35 years of age
  Adolescence
- Socioeconomic and ethnic factors
  Education of parent
  Ethnicity
  Family income
  Undernutrition
- Behavioral risk factors
  Addictive habits: smoking, alcohol, drugs
  Teratogenic foods and additives
- Life events and life stress
  High life stress and low social support
  Attitudes and emotions

EARLY PRENATAL CARE RELATED TO ETHNICITY AND GEOGRAPHIC AREA

Evidence indicates that white mothers receive care earlier in pregnancy than nonwhite mothers. There is a consistent difference between white and nonwhite mothers in the receipt of medical care during each of the trimesters of pregnancy. There is evidence that women living in metropolitan areas receive care earlier than those outside metropolitan areas; this holds true for both white and nonwhite women. Furthermore, more nonwhite women in metropolitan areas receive care than do nonwhite women residing outside metropolitan areas. It is worth noting, though, that within any given income or educational group, there is an insignificant difference regarding when mothers first receive medical care between those who live in metropolitan and those who live in nonmetropolitan areas.[7]

Undernutrition. One of the most important sequelae of low socioeconomic status is undernutrition. Studies have revealed that, compared with more affluent persons, the poor are twice as deficient in four essential diet ingredients. Most striking, poor persons had about four times as much clear-cut iron deficiency anemia and twice as many borderline cases as had the nonpoor. In three categories of essential diet ingredients—vitamin A, vitamin C, and riboflavin—the poor were found to have about twice as much of a clear-cut deficiency as the nonpoor. The survey also found a greater percentage of low height and weight measurements for children living below the poverty line than for those who were more affluent.[23]

Obviously, there is a complex interaction between undernutrition, poverty, and other environmental and genetic factors.

EFFECTS ON FETAL BRAIN DEVELOPMENT. Studies have found that deficiencies in the diet of a pregnant woman can have profound effects on a number of pregnancy outcomes (Fig. 6-4). For example, it has been shown that nutritional and genetic factors may interact during prenatal development with consequent irreversible results on the development of the baby's brain. This is one of the most important recent discoveries in the field of mental retardation. It is estimated that 10% of the children born today are seriously affected as a consequence of malnutrition. Research at the National Institutes of Health suggests that there is a correlation between the level of the amino acids in the blood of a pregnant woman and the subsequent intelligence of her baby.[24–26]

LOW BIRTH WEIGHT. Undernutrition has been identified as one of the causes of low-birth-weight infants born to poor urban mothers. Extremely low birth weights have been reported among poorly fed groups in Asia and Africa. The relationship between low birth weight and malnourished populations may have a more complex explanation than simple nutrition. Rather than dietary deficiency in pregnancy, the size of the baby may reflect long-term maternal undernutrition dating back to the early childhood of the woman, as well as severe deprivation in the social environment.[24–26]

HYPERTENSIVE DISORDERS. The effect of socioeconomic influences on disease was most dramatically illustrated during World War II in Great Britain. During this period, the mortality from the pregnancy hyper-

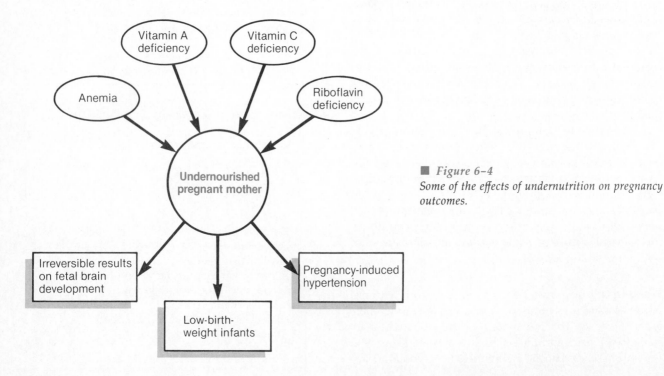

■ *Figure 6–4*
Some of the effects of undernutrition on pregnancy outcomes.

tensive disorders fell dramatically. The underlying reason for the drop in mortality resulting from this condition in England and Wales was that, during the evacuation of many women from the cities to the country, pregnant and nursing mothers were given preferential treatment in rationing. For the first time, women of the lower socioeconomic groups were fed as well as other population groups. Thus, there is some evidence that the incidence of these conditions can be modified by environmental changes, either situational or behavioral.[23,24,27]

NURSING IMPLICATIONS. The nurse can be a force in the community and in the clinic setting to help improve preventive services to those at highest risk because of situational factors. Health education that includes clear nutritional counseling, together with other environmental risk factors and their solutions, needs to be incorporated into all prenatal counseling. Moreover, the nurse can be a positive force in the community to exert influence on other institutions, such as the schools, health departments, government agencies, and voluntary agencies, to provide preventive measures to the population at greatest risk.

Behavioral Risk Factors and Life Events

In the previous section, the client's social position and factors that are not easily controlled by the client or the providers were discussed. As the following section will show, however, there are certain behavioral factors that result in certain life-styles that can be changed, albeit with difficulty; the concepts of healthy living and stress management associated with life events has particular relevance in pregnancy.

ADDICTIVE DISORDERS

The great reliance of Americans on various substances that, although they give momentary pleasure, have been found to be addictive and harmful to the user's health, particularly in pregnancy, has been a much-publicized topic. These substances include cigarettes, alcohol, and drugs. Because these substances can cause grave harm to both the mother and fetus, they will be discussed in depth in Chapter 36. Suffice it to say here that clients who continue to participate in such behaviors need prompt counseling and possibly referral to treatment programs if the pregnancy is to result in a positive outcome.

LIFE-STYLES

It is important to take into account the characteristic life-styles of clients, particularly those of the econom-

ically disadvantaged. *Life-style* refers to a way of living that can have implications for health. The experiences of the lower-income person and his or her world is distinctive for its problems and crisis-dominated character. Health concerns are minor to those who feel they confront much more pressing troubles; health problems are just one crisis among many with which they must try to cope.

The middle-class value orientations, activistic, rational mastery, and future-time, tend to result in a specific outlook on life that is reflected in health beliefs and behavior. Preventive health practices are used; illness is remedied, not endured.

Conversely, the lower classes, whose position in the social structure does not support a belief in the rational mastery of the world, may have a different orientation based on fatalism and lack of control over events. Planning, education, and involvement in organized activity are less important in this framework; they seek help from those in their social network rather than from "experts" or professionals.[28]

In addition, many lower-income households are often much more understaffed than those of higher incomes. Understaffing of households may mean that each individual's health receives relatively little attention as far as preventive measures are concerned, and when someone is sick, it is more difficult to obtain appropriate care. Hence, illnesses are "lived with" rather than remedied.

TERATOGENIC FOODS AND ADDITIVES

In the early years of the 20th century, concern for the safety and quality of the food supply in the United States prompted the enactment of the Food and Drug Act, which prevented the addition of poisonous or other deleterious ingredients to foods. As technology has advanced and food production and processing, as well as advertising, have become increasingly sophisticated, concern has mounted as to the safety of foods and additives. It has been found that many heretofore unsuspected substances, both naturally occurring and artificially added, are, in fact, mutagens, teratogens, or embryotoxins. Mutagens change the inherited chromosomal structure of cells; teratogens produce congenitally malformed infants; and embryotoxins kill or alter the embryo.[29-32]

There are problems associated with the study of teratogens, particularly those relating to methodology; hence, we do not have the definitive data that we have for smoking and fetal morbidity. These problems revolve around the choice, dosage, and amount of the experimental substance; the choice of the subject animals (humans cannot be experimented on); the difficulty in isolating variables and, hence, measuring results; the difficulty in determining preconditioning factors; and the need for multigenerational studies.[30,31] Some authors, in fact, maintain that there is little evidence that rates of human malformations have increased in the past few decades.[31] Nevertheless, consumer and health-provider concern has increased recently. Militant consumers feel that the Food and Drug Administration is too politically responsive to the demands of the food and drug industries. They also cite the hundreds of additives that have never been tested and that have been designated as "generally recognized as safe." Thus, it is particularly important that the prospective mother be made aware of the potential hazards, because ingesting

---

Potential Hazards of Foods and Additives

Nitrosamines (N-nitroso Compounds)

These compounds are potent carcinogens in all tested species, including amphibians, birds, fish, and mammals. Although nitrosamines themselves are rarely found in foods, their precursors, nitrites (which combine with other nitrogen-containing compounds) are common. Sodium nitrite and sodium nitrate are added to most smoked and cured meat and fish to act as an antioxidant to ensure preserving the foodstuff. Nitrate, which may break down to nitrite, is found in soybean oil and naturally in leafy vegetables such as cauliflower, broccoli, lettuce, cabbage, and beets, especially when high levels of nitrate fertilizers are used. Drinking water in areas experiencing fertilizer runoff may also contain high levels. Ascorbic acid (vitamin C) can be used in place of nitrites as an antioxidant.

Aflatoxins

These substances are related to mycotoxins and are produced by fungal growths on a wide range of foodstuffs. Contamination is usually caused by excessive moisture before harvest or during storage. Aflatoxins are quite toxic to humans. For instance, the mycotoxin ergotism of rye can induce abortion as well as gangrene and other ills of the vascular system. Peanuts are particularly susceptible to infection, as are cereal grains, legumes, cocoa, cassava, sweet potatoes, improperly fermented foods and alcoholic beverages, and dairy products from animals fed contaminated feed. These toxins are not destroyed by home cooking or freezing, but milling is effective because the infected outer shells are removed. Regulation of harvest, storage, and marketing protects the consumer to a great extent.

U.S.-Certified Food Colorings

These are the "azo" dyes, which include red #2 (amaranth), red #4, yellow #6 (tartrazine), green (ferrous gluconate), and some others. Red #2 was found to be embryotoxic to rats and also to cause small litters in the same species; it has been banned since 1976. There is no clear-cut carcinogenic or teratogenic evidence regarding the other dyes; hence, Public Law 86-618 provides for setting "safe limits" for these and other food substances.

Artificial Sweeteners

Again there is no clear evidence of a carcinogenic or teratogenic effect with sodium cyclamate, saccharin, mannitol, and xylitol. Researchers have found that mothers who had taken cyclamates during pregnancy had children who suffered from hyperactivity and learning disabilities.[30] At present, research is continuing on these products, because the studies to date suffer from the methodologic problems mentioned previously.

Caffeine

This substance is of concern because of its chemical structure, purine, one of the constituent groups of DNA. Moreover, it crosses the human placenta and is known to penetrate the preimplantation blastocyte in mammals. In addition, it has been found to cause chromosomal rearrangements in the sperm of mice. The data on human populations are not conclusive, and conflicting evidence is given. A recent large study in Finland, the country that leads the world in coffee consumption, did not produce any definitive data or recommendations.[32]

Thus, although there is reason for caution in using caffeine during pregnancy (and excessively in general), there is yet insufficient evidence to implicate it as a teratogen.

Trace Elements and Metallic and Chemical Contaminants

Such trace elements and metallic contaminants as lead, selenium, arsenic, cadmium, mercury, and methylmercury occur in the ground; in fish and crustaceans, especially when they come from contaminated waters; and in some fruits, cheeses, cereals, and other foodstuffs. When taken in large quantities they are known to be teratogenic, producing a variety of symptoms from congenital malformations to central nervous system problems.

Similarly, chemical contaminants, including pesticides, space sprays (DDVP, dichloros, vapona), herbicides, and fungicides are embryotoxic, mutagenic, and teratogenic in mammals. The pesticide DVCP has been banned because of the occurrence of sterility in farm workers who used the substance in their work. Ingestion of these in pregnancy should be avoided.

large quantities of these substances may be harmful to her fetus. The groups of foods and additives are summarized in Potential Hazards of Foods and Additives.[30]

Life Events and Life Stress as Risks

Life events and *life stress*, in the sense used here, refer to such events as divorce, illness, death of a significant other, such as a family member, and job loss rather than to the occurrence of the actual pregnancy itself, although this, too, may be a factor in pregnancy outcome. Appropriate intervention by nursing staff can be especially effective in meeting the needs and reducing the risks associated with such life stress. The interest in the relationship between the psychological and social world of the individual and human disorders and disease has a long history. Even the findings of carefully designed and conducted investigations have not always yielded clear-cut and unambiguous results concerning this relationship.[9,33,34] This is in sharp contrast to the dramatic results that have been obtained with animal experiments in which the various elements in the social environment have been correlated. Nevertheless, there is accumulating evidence of the intimate interaction between the social environment, physiological reactions, and pathological outcome in the individual. This is particularly true of the chronic diseases, such as heart disease and cancer.[35,36]

Data on the relationship between disorders of pregnancy and life changes and experiences that may be stressful are relatively scanty.

HIGH LIFE STRESS AND LOW SOCIAL SUPPORT

Norbeck and Tilden have looked at the relationship of life stress, social support, and emotional disequilibrium to complications in pregnancy outcomes.[33] In a prospective study, they found that high life stress and low social support were significantly related to high emotional disequilibrium; social support and life stress were not significantly related to each other, however. They also found a relationship between high life stress, social support, and gestational complications, as well as infant condition complications. Social support appeared to play a mediating role. In a separate study, Tilden documented a significant relationship of life stress and social support to emotional disequilibrium during pregnancy.[34] However, she was not able to discern what contribution the pregnancy itself might have made to the overall relationship.

As these and other investigators point out, additional research is needed, but their data help to explain some of the discrepant results in the literature.[35–37] In short, the research and the approach cast serious doubt

on the utility of specificity (as far as current clinical syndromes are concerned) in research concerned with psychosocial factors in disease etiology. Similar psychosocial factors may be related to different disease syndromes. Currently, this research approach is very promising, and additional work needs to be done using this approach.

ATTITUDES AND EMOTIONS

Much has been written in recent years on the role of emotional and attitudinal factors and psychological stress during pregnancy, as these may be related to pregnancy outcomes. The evidence is inconclusive, but, more important, much of it is based on poorly designed research and on inadequate samples of the population at risk. Despite this poor state of affairs, there is a general consensus in medical science that psychological factors are in some way associated with various aspects of the maternity cycle. Indeed, some investigators have asserted that early psychological assessment of pregnant women holds promise of being predictive of the course and outcome of pregnancy. Most of the literature attempts to measure the attitudes of the woman toward her pregnancy, her perception of herself as mother, and other psychosocial factors, as these may influence the outcome.[37–39] Surely there are attitudinal differences among women toward their individual pregnancies. There also may be intimate interaction between the psychosocial stress experienced by the person, the buffering effects of social supports, and psychological reactions.[39] Complications of pregnancy, labor, and delivery can be obscured by this interaction. Thus, physiological changes and discomfort may trigger psychologically negative attitudes toward the pregnancy, and, conversely, life stress may precipitate somatic problems.[37]

Nursing Implications. There is no doubt that many women experience some psychological stress during pregnancy. However, the literature in medical and nursing journals alike tends to assume that some of these conditions are psychosomatic or emotional in origin. In an article that has become a classic, Lennane and Lennane criticize the cloudy thinking that has characterized such conditions as menstrual pain, nausea of pregnancy, and pain in labor as caused or aggravated by psychogenic factors. They suggest sexual prejudice as the basis for such thinking. Such scientific evidence as exists clearly suggests organic causes for these conditions.[40]

The point is that nurses must not unwittingly and uncritically accept long-established attitudes that are rooted in prejudice rather than in scientific evidence. Stereotypical thinking is not only poor in scientific terms, but also more importantly, it tends to influence the course and quality of treatment of female clients. Nurses

Assessment Tool

High-Risk Pregnancy Factors

Prenatal Factors

1. Maternal disease
   a. Diabetes mellitus
   b. Preeclampsia and eclampsia
   c. Hypertension
   d. Cardiopulmonary disease
   e. Renal disease
   f. Infection: syphilis, rubella, tuberculosis
   g. Drug addiction
   h. Alcoholism
   i. Endocrinopathy
   j. Severe anemia and blood dyscrasias
   k. Malnutrition
   l. Malignancy during pregnancy
2. Maternal practices
   a. Taking of medications associated with adverse fetal effects
   b. Smoking
   c. Excessive exposure to radiation
   d. Less than three prenatal visits
3. Age: <16 years and >35 years
4. Short maternal stature
5. Severe isoimmunization (Rh or other)
6. Multiple gestation (e.g., particularly second of twins, third of triplets)
7. Premature rupture of the membranes (PROM): >37–38 weeks (not considered here as a high-risk factor because all preterm infants are PROM)

8. Prolonged rupture of membranes: >18–24 hr (predisposes to neonatal sepsis, intrauterine pneumonia, and infections)
9. Polyhydramnios, oligohydramnios
10. Evidence of intrauterine growth retardation
11. Previous perinatal and neonatal deaths, preterm or low-birth-weight deliveries
12. Lower socioeconomic status

Previous Labor and Delivery Factors

1. Placental accident or hemorrhage
   a. Abruptio placentae
   b. Placenta previa
2. Cesarean section
3. Mechanical factors
   a. Abnormal presentation (i.e., breech, transverse)
   b. Anatomy of the birth canal: cephalopelvic disproportion (CPD)
4. Fetal distress
5. Prolonged or obstructed labor that leads to fetal asphyxia (>24 hr for primigravidas; >18 hr for multigravidas)
6. Prolonged second stage of labor
7. Prolapsed, knotted, or entangled umbilical cord leading to fetal asphyxia
8. Maternal fever
9. Depressant drugs given to mother near delivery (e.g., meperidine [Demerol])

(Adapted from Trotter CW, Chang P-N, Thompson T: Appendix: High-risk pregnancy factors. JOGN Nurs 11:90, March/April 1982).

---

have an important role to play in assisting the pregnant woman to use her psychosocial assets to the fullest in coping with the fears, anxieties, somatic complaints, and other problems associated with the pregnancy in the prenatal and intrapartal periods. Emotional and social support during and following the pregnancy can be a comfort to the client and may also assist in reducing problematic outcomes.

■ ASSESSMENT AND NURSING CARE

The Assessment Tool provides a guide for assessing a variety of high-risk factors, both social and obstetrical, discussed in this chapter. Specific care plans can be found in those chapters dealing with complications of pregnancy and the high-risk infant.

■ REFERENCES

1. Skolnick AS: The Intimate Environment: Exploring Marriage and the Family, 4th ed. Boston, Little, Brown, 1987
2. Griffith S: Childbearing and the concept of culture. J Obstet Gynecol Neonatal Nurs 11(3):181–184, May/June 1982
3. Glick PC: American household structure in transition. Fam Plan Perspect 16(5):204–211, September/October 1984
4. Thornton A: Changing attitudes toward family issues in the United States. J Marr Fam 51:873–893, November 1980

5. Devore NE: Parenthood postponed. Am J Nurs 83(8): 1161–1163, August 1983

6. Hyman H: The value systems of different classes. In Bendix R, Lipset S (eds): Class Status and Power, pp 426–442. Glencoe, IL, Free Press, 1953

7. Nelson MK: The effect of childbirth preparation on women of different social classes. J Health Soc Behav 23:339–352, December 1982

8. Collins JW, David RJ: The differential effect of traditional risk factors on infant birthweight among blacks and whites in Chicago. Am J Public Health 80:679–681, June 1990

9. Norbeck JS, Anderson NJ: Psychosocial predictors of pregnancy outcomes in low-income black, Hispanic and white women. Nurs Res 38:204–209, July/August 1989

10. Geronimus AT: The effects of race, residence and prenatal care on the relationship of age to neonatal mortality. Am J Public Health 76:1414–1421, December 1986

11. McCormick MC, et al: Outreach case finding: Its effect on enrollment in prenatal care. Med Care 27:103–111, February 1989

12. Patterson ET, Freese MP, Goldenberg RL: Seeking safe passage: Utilizing health care during pregnancy. Image 22:27–31, Spring 1990

13. Wilner S, et al: A comparison of the quality of maternity care between a health maintenance organization and fee for service practices. N Engl J Med 304(13): 784–789, March 26, 1981

14. Lubic RW: Evidence that the childbearing center has influenced hospital maternity practice. Birth 10(3):179, Fall 1983

15. Baruffi G, et al: A study of pregnancy outcomes in a maternity center and a tertiary care hospital. Am J Public Health 74(9):973–978, September 1984

16. Norton K: Beyond ''choice'' in childbirth. Birth 10(3): 179–182, Fall 1983

17. Pettitti D, Coleman C, Binsacca D, Allen B: Early prenatal care in urban black and white women. Birth 17: 1–5, March 1990

18. May KA, Ditolla K: In-hospital alternative birth centers: Where do we go from here? MCN 9:48–59, Jan/Feb 1984

19. Finlay W, Mutran ES, Zeitler RR, Randall CS: Queues and care: How medical residents organize their work in a busy clinic. J Health Soc Behav 31:292–305, September 1990

20. National Center for Health Statistics: Annual Summary for the United States, 1979. DHHS Publ No (PHS) 81–1120, Monthly Vital Statistics Reports 28:13, November 13, 1980

21. McCormick L, Shapiro S, Starfield G: High-risk young mothers: Infant mortality and morbidity in four areas in the United States, 1973–1978. Am J Public Health 74(1):18–23, January 1984

22. Trotter CW, Chang P, Thompson T: Prenatal factors and the developmental outcome of preterm infants. JOGN Nurs 11(2):83–90, March/April 1982

23. Kotelchuck M, et al: WIC participation and pregnancy outcomes: Massachussetts Statewide Evaluation Project. Am J Public Health 74(10):1086–1092, 1984

24. Jacobson HN: Diet therapy and the improvement of pregnancy outcomes. Birth 10(1):29–31, Spring 1983

25. Committee on Nutrition of the Mother and the Preschool Child, Food and Nutrition Board, National Research Council: Nutrition Services in Perinatal Care. Washington, DC, National Academy Press, 1981

26. Super C, Herrara M, Mora J: Long term effects of food supplemental and psychosocial intervention on the physical growth of Colombian infants at risk for malnutrition. Child Dev 61:29–49, 1990

27. Lechtig A: Studies of nutrition intervention in pregnancy. Birth 9:115–121, 1982

28. Taylor RJ: Need for support among black Americans. J Marr Fam 52:584–589, August 1990

29. Stein Z, Kline J, Kharazzi M: What is a teratogen? Epidemiologic criteria. In Kalter H (ed): Issues and Reviews in Teratology. New York, Plenum Press, 1984

30. Streitfeld PP: Congenital malformation: Teratogenic foods and additives. Birth Fam J 5:7–19, Spring 1978

31. Wilson T (ed): Handbook of Teratology. New York, Plenum Press, 1987

32. Kurppa K, et al: Coffee consumption during pregnancy and selected congenital malformations: A nationwide case-control study. Am J Public Health 73:1397–1400, December 1983

33. Norbeck JS, Tilden VP: Life stress, social support and emotional disequilibrium during pregnancy: A prospective, multivariate study. J Health Soc Behav 24:30–46, March 1983

34. Tilden VP: The relation of life stress and social support to emotional disequilibrium during pregnancy. Res Nurs Health 6:167–173, 1983

35. LaRocco JM, House JS, French JR Jr: Social support, occupational stress and health. J Health Soc Behav 21: 202–218, 1980

36. Thoits PA: Conceptual, methodological and theoretical problems in studying social support as a buffer against life stress. J Health Soc Behav 23:145–159, 1982

37. Walker L: Longitudinal analysis of stress process among mothers and infants. Nurs Res 38:339–343, November/December 1989

38. Beck NC, et al: The prediction of pregnancy outcomes: Maternal preparation, anxiety and attitudinal sets. J Psychosom Res 24:343–351, 1980

39. Brown MA: Social support during pregnancy: A unidimensional or multidimensional construct. Nurs Res 35: 4–9, January/February 1986

40. Lennane KJ, Lennane RJ: Alleged psychogenic disorder in women: A possible manifestation of sexual prejudice. N Engl J Med 6:288–292, 1973

■ SUGGESTED READING

Bryant NB: Self help groups: An important strategy for perinatal health: J CA Perinatal Assoc IV(1):24–27, Winter 1984

Conger RD, Yang RK, Burgess RL: Mother's age as a predictor of observed maternal behavior in three independent samples of families. J Marr Fam 46:411–424, May 1984

Council on Scientific Affairs: Effects of toxic chemicals on the reproductive system. JAMA 253:3431–3437, June 21, 1985

Luegenbiehl DL: The birth system in Germany. JOGN Nurs 14(1):45–49, Jan/Feb 1985

Mercer RT, Hackley KC, Bostrom AG: Relationship of psychosocial and perinatal variables to perceptions of childbirth. Nurs Res 32(4):202–207, July/August 1983

Morris TM: Culturally sensitive family assessment: An evaluation of the family assessment device used with Hawaiian-American and Japanese-American families. Family Process 29:105–116, March 1990

Patterson ET, Freese MP, Goldenberg RL: Seeking safe passage: Utilizing health care during pregnancy. IMAGE 22:27–31, Spring 1990

Petitti D, Coleman C, Binsacca D, Allen B: Early prenatal care in urban black and white women. Birth 17:1–5, March, 1990

Richards MPM: The trouble with "choice" in childbirth. Birth 93(4):253–260, Winter 1982

Simons RL, Whitbeck RD, Conger RD, Melby JN: Husband and wife differences in determinants of parenting: A social learning and exchange model of prental behavior. J Marr Fam 52:375–392, May 1990

Strickland OL: The occurrence of symptoms in expectant fathers. Nurs Res 36:184–189, May/June, 1987

7

Ethical and Legal Considerations in Reproduction

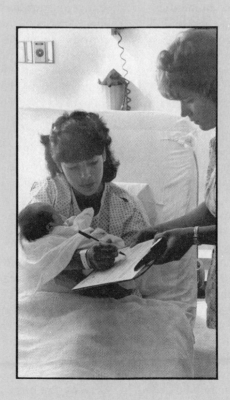

The direct personal encounters that an individual has with himself or herself and others constitute his life experience, which over time become reality to that person. As more encounters are experienced and data thought to be important are pursued and investigated, the individual's awareness and relationship to himself or herself and to others are expanded. Throughout this process, the person makes choices: what experiences to pursue, what data to discard, and so on. Rational choices are based on factual information, but they have a large subjective component that involves value judgments. The concept of choice necessarily involves freedom, that is, the ability to choose among alternatives, and the consequent responsibility for right or wrong action taken.[1] Thus, the combination of knowing and valuing is put to the test when we make difficult ethical choices.

Authors writing in the field of ethics make the point that not all choices or problems are ethical ones.[1,2] They outline several characteristics that make ethical problems unique:

- *The problem cannot be resolved entirely from empirical data.* For instance, should a healthy person be forced to donate an organ to someone who would otherwise die without the donor organ? Clearly, any of the sciences cannot answer that question definitely; the various sciences and humanities can contribute information, but the answer lies beyond the competence of the scientific disciplines.
- *The problem is inherently perplexing.* There are a variety of conflicts of values and uncertainties about the amount or type of information needed to make a decision. If an infant is born with repairable multiple congenital anomalies but has a chromosomal aberration that will eventually cause death at an early age, should aggressive efforts be made to keep the infant alive as long as possible, even if these efforts may cause pain and suffering for the parents as well as the neonate?
- *The answer to the ethical problem will have profound relevance for several areas of human concern.* It will have far-reaching effects on one's perception of fellow human beings, the relationships among human beings, the relationship of human beings to society, and the relationship of various societies to the world at large. If, for example, the decision is made to force a person to donate a body part to a family member, the decision is based on several premises and assumptions: a person's right to bodily integrity may be violated if someone else can benefit by it; one's right to life includes the right to require another to undergo painful surgery with the end result of permanent loss of body part and damage to general

body integrity; health professionals and others in authority can force or otherwise coerce a person to sacrifice body integrity for the well-being of another. The above choice involves the concepts of human rights, the limits of benevolence, and the power of those in authority. Although the above example was dramatic, other issues are less clear-cut, such as a woman's right to take drugs and alcohol during pregnancy or how long to prolong the life of an irreparably damaged neonate. It is suggested that the above criteria be applied when the nurse is determining whether a decision involves an ethical problem or not.[1,2]

■ LEGAL ASPECTS OF MATERNITY AND PERINATAL CARE

Hankanson and others have pointed out that the maternity and perinatal field has become especially high risk for malpractice suits for several reasons.[3–5] Some hospitals are facing financial exigencies that cause them to implement inadequate staffing patterns that can be dangerous for the client and nurse alike. An exceptionally high degree of technology has developed for monitoring the mother and fetus preconceptually, conceptually, and postconceptually, and many of the techniques carry with them the risk of producing iatrogenic effects that can damage the mother or fetus, sometimes irreversibly. Perhaps most importantly, there are potentially two claimants in any instance of mother–baby damage, and this doubles the risk to the nurse and other health providers. In the following section, we discuss several basic legal issues that can provide a foundation for viewing and evaluating nursing practice.

Nursing Practice and Accountability

Nursing practice today is legislated by each state in the form of nurse practice acts. These practice acts define the boundaries of nursing practice by setting certain requirements regarding education, licensure, and standards of care. Because these requirements vary among the states, it is the nurse's responsibility to be familiar with the acts of the states in which he or she practices.[4] Standards of care are developed by the nurse practice acts, by the hospitals or other institutions that employ the nurse, and by professional organizations such as the Nurses Association of the American College of Obstetricians and Gynecologists (NAACOG). It is important that nurses know and implement the accepted standards of care in their community, because not to do so would result in a *breach of duty* or a charge of *negligence*. A breach of duty is considered to occur if the nurse performs an unauthorized act, fails to act, or carries out an authorized act improperly. If the nurse is found guilty of a breach of duty, he or she may lose his or her license or be a defendant in a malpractice lawsuit.[4–6] To be found guilty of negligence, the following facts must be established: (1) that the nurse had a responsibility to the client; (2) that the nurse failed to carry out that responsibility; (3) that injury was sustained by the client; and (4) that there was a casual relationship between the client's injury and the nurse's breach of duty (proximate cause). See the box, Facts That Must Be Established to Prove Guilt of Negligence. Thus, it can be seen that in nursing practice today, nurses are accountable for their care, not only morally and ethically, but legally as well. In past decades, before health care became so complex and nurses expanded their roles, institutions and physicians were considered the primary responsible parties. However, with increasing independence in nursing came the responsibility to be accountable to the client for nursing care and. hence, to some degree, for the client's well-being. Accountability also extends beyond the nurse's individual sphere of care. If the nurse knows that the care given by other members of the health team is inappropriate or inferior, she also has the legal and ethical obligation to report such care to the appropriate authorities.[4,6]

One further point needs emphasis. Every nurse should carry professional liability insurance. This is in addition to any insurance provided by the institution that employs the nurse. Institutional insurance generally covers the nurse only for the hours that she is on duty at the institution, not at other times when she might practice. The legal costs of a lawsuit can be truly horrendous; moreover, it is becoming more common for an institution to sue the nurse involved if the institution loses a malpractice suit.[6] Because adequate coverage

usually can be purchased at a reasonable price, it is well worth the investment for the nurse's personal protection.

■ ETHICAL AND LEGAL CONSIDERATIONS PRIOR TO CONCEPTION

Often a couple will have difficulty in conceiving. The reasons for infertility are many and varied and are discussed in depth in Chapter 13.

In the last decade, medical engineering has been closing the circle of sex without reproduction by offering methods of reproduction without sex, including artificial insemination with husband (AIH) and donors (AID) and in vitro fertilization and embryo transfer (IVF/ET). As with contraception, artificial reproduction is defended by its proponents as life affirming and denounced as unnatural by its detractors.[7] In addition, there has arisen what one author had called a *"hucksterism,"* or hype, surrounding much of this technology, particularly that of IVF/ET assisted reproduction, which is seen by some as an exploitation of the infertile couple, with all of the attendant advertisement and hype about success rate that some centers employ. Those professionals urging caution point out that the incidence of *live births* (not pregnancy) is still low with these techniques.[7–11]

In the following section, we examine these techniques from an ethical–legal standpoint, because all have some element of controversy.

Artificial Insemination

As previously stated, artificial insemination employs two methods. In AIH, the wife is inseminated within her reproductive tract with sperm from her husband. This is perhaps the least controversial of all of the assisted reproductive methods, because it is clear who the genetic and sociological parents are. Some religious denominations object to masturbation as a means of sperm collection, but this method generally is without grave ethical or legal questions.

The second method, AID, is more problematical. The woman is inseminated with the sperm of an anonymous donor. This method, of course, separates the sociological parent (the woman's husband) from taking part in his offspring's conception. This method had become the preferred treatment when the husband has an absence or marked decrease in the amount of sperm. AID also is used when the husband suffers from a genetic defect or is Rh sensitized. This procedure has de-

---

Facts That Must Be Established to Prove Guilt of Negligence

1. The nurse had a responsibility to the client.
2. The nurse failed to carry out that responsibility.
3. Injury was sustained by the client.
4. There was a causal relationship between the client's injury and the nurse's breach of duty.

Breach of duty occurs if the nurse performs an unauthorized act, fails to act, or carries out an authorized act improperly.

creased in recent years because of the possibility of transmitting the human immunodeficiency virus (HIV). Currently, all donors and each specimen are screened for HIV. As long as the husband of the woman consents, the donor is not considered the legal father of the child. Thus, the husband replaces the genetic father as the legal father of the child. As can be seen, this therapeutic model places contracts among the parties ahead of genetic or "bloodline" considerations. This model has been suggested as a model for embryonic transfer, but there is a large question as to whether it fits.[7]

Legal obligations are satisfied by written, informed consent by all parties—wife, husband, and donor. It is recommended that the donor, husband, and wife all remain anonymous and that the physician be given the right to select the donor. This recommendation raises questions as to the limits of authority for the professional. The consent usually includes a clause removing liability from the health professionals if the child is born with abnormalities. The question of the child's legitimacy can be resolved by adoption.[7]

In Vitro Fertilization and Embryo Transfer

A variety of ethical and legal questions have been raised over time regarding IVF/ET. The first live birth using IVF occurred in 1978, and by January 1984 over 200 children had been born in the United States and abroad following IVF/ET.[12] In this procedure, an egg or eggs are removed from a woman's ovary, fertilized by sperm in a laboratory dish, cultured, and then transferred back into the uterus. IVF is the only method of reproduction for women whose fallopian tubes are damaged or missing. It is also used for wives whose husbands have low sperm counts, women whose cervical mucus is nonreceptive to sperm, and women with infertility of unknown causes.[13]

In 1984, gamete intrafallopian transfer (GIFT) was developed at the University of Texas Health Science Center, San Antonio. This procedure involves the transfer of sperm and eggs into the ampullary portion of the fallopian tubes after aspiration of the ovarian follicles at laparoscopy. It is the procedure of choice when there is at least one functional fallopian tube. Data suggest that the *pregnancy rate* is better than with IVF/ET alone, perhaps due to the timing of implantation.[14]

The demand for these procedures keeps growing. The National Center for Health Statistics estimates that almost half of currently married women aged 15 to 44 suffer from some degree of infertility, and 10% of married couples fail to conceive after 1 year of no contraceptive use.[15] According to the American Fertility Society, at least 46 centers in the United States have or

are planning to have IVF clinics. Practically every major city where Western medicine is practiced has at least one IVF/ET clinic, and there have been five World Congresses devoted to this topic.[12,13]

While these procedures move ahead clinically, there has been no federally funded research in humans since 1975 because of a de facto moratorium. Congress first imposed a temporary moratorium on fetal research on July 12, 1974 (Public Law 93-348). This was technically lifted on August 8, 1975, when regulations were issued by what was then the Department of Health, Education, and Welfare. These regulations required all proposals dealing with IVF and fetal research to be reviewed by a national Ethics Advisory Board (EAB) in addition to the usual Institutional Review Board (IRB) review and peer review for scientific merit. The EAB was duly but slowly constructed; it examined the topic of IVF thoroughly and concluded in a report on May 4, 1979, that although controversy was legitimate, IVF/ET was acceptable from an ethical standpoint.[12] The major conclusions of the EAB are listed in Recommendations of the EAB. However, at subsequent public hearings and presentations to Congress, the response was overwhelmingly negative and so a de facto moratorium set in.

The ethical–legal concerns have changed over the years. They can be summarized as follows:

Current Concerns Regarding In Vitro Fertilization and Embryo Transfer

1. *Concern over the moral status of the fetus.* The human embryo is entitled to profound respect, but this respect does not necessarily encompass the full array of legal and moral rights attributed to a person. Mainstream ethicists and theologians generally concur that IVF/ET is not problematical as long as the EAB's guidelines are followed. Conservative theologians, however, believe that any tampering with the procreative process is unnatural and should not be attempted. Thus, the research use of human embryos remains a problem.[12]
2. *Safety and efficacy.* During the late 1970s, there was only limited understanding about the risks involved in this procedure. As data have been collected over time, there is a good (but not conclusive) indication that there are no patterns of abnormality or short-term risks either in laboratory research with animals or in clinical experience with humans. Until further research is conducted, however, this concern will remain.[12]
3. *"The slippery slope."* This concern relates to the fear that research procedures performed on nonhuman mammalian species might be performed

on human embryos and the results could lead to undesirable clinical applications. Some ethicists are concerned about extending the procedure to unmarried persons, including surrogate mothers, third-party donors, and the like. They see the basic relationship between husband and wife and, indeed, the whole institution of marriage as being threatened. These were the same concerns that artificial insemination sparked decades ago.[12]

4. *Funding and cost.* There is general acknowledgment that the procedure is costly. Although some believe that it is ethical to federally fund research projects relating to IVF, it should have a low national priority, because there are many other national health problems that are far more pressing. Those who oppose the procedure say that efforts would be better spent finding and preventing the causes of infertility and tubal obstruction.[12]

Surrogate Mothers

Commercial surrogacy involves the contractual hiring of a woman to bear another couple's child. The father's sperm may be used to impregnate the surrogate or, in surrogate embryo transfer (SET), the surrogate is implanted with the genetic parent's embryo. When the fetus is born, the surrogate mother relinquishes to the couple her rights to the infant as per the terms of a contract that has been drawn up. Some people view this as yet another instance of collaborative reproduction such as AID and IVF, saying these methods are no different ethically and legally from adoption, which separates conception and gestation from childrearing.

However, ethical and legal issues remain. First there is the issue of "hiring" the surrogate mother. The mother typically receives a fee for carrying the child. Although this may seem only fair for the surrogate mother's efforts, some find the idea of the payment of money for producing a child repugnant and morally offensive. Children are reduced to commodities to be bought and sold, and some have suggested that mothers who need money may "sell" themselves as surrogates to keep their own families together.[16,17] Second, there is the stress of the complex relationship involving a stranger in such an intimate context, which may be entangling and disturbing to the parties. For instance, the surrogate may experience depression on giving up the child, or the couple may continue the relationship with the mother out of misplaced feelings of indebtedness. Third, the lineage of the children may become confused and the fabric of the marriage may be damaged. However, Robertson has argued that although these concerns are legitimate, they must be balanced against the deep desires of the infertile couple to have children.[18]

There are legal concerns surrounding the legality of the contractual arrangements. Gersz maintains that a well-drawn contract may obviate some of the difficulties in the three-way relationship.[16] This was not true for the Baby C case being litigated in California in 1990, wherein the surrogate mother abrogated the well-drawn contract with the parents by charging neglect by the parents during pregnancy as well as bonding to the infant she carried. The surrogate mother is suing for shared custody of the child.[19,20] In the Baby C case just described and in the famed Baby M case, it is evident that well-drawn contracts can be contested, causing a great deal of stress for all parties, including the infant.[19,20] Furrow also cites critics who are concerned about cases in which neither party wants a child born with impairments or cases in which the surrogate mother is reluctant to surrender the child.[17] The legality of such contracts remains a controversial issue, because the courts are still battling the extent to which these contracts are binding.

The issue of the amount of control the couple can exert over the surrogate is also a difficult one. Certainly the couple wishes to ensure the best possible "environment" for the fetus and may want to regulate the surrogate's nutrition and life-style. This brings into focus the issue of the surrogate mother's right to privacy and freedom of choice.[16,17] Because of these and other complexities, Great Britain has made it a criminal offense for third parties to benefit from commercial surrogacy, although voluntary surrogacy is still legal. However, because of the legal climate and hostile public and medical sentiment regarding surrogacy, the method is essentially banned in that country.[21] Jones cautions that the use of a surrogate mother, even for so short a time, together with the inconvenience of synchronizing the menstrual cycles of the donor and recipient and the medical risks to the donor, will make this method less appealing to many.[22]

Amniocentesis

Amniocentesis has been available for well over a decade and is discussed fully in Chapter 13. Legal issues relate to errors of omission or commission. For instance, if a woman is a candidate for the test because of age (over 35), has produced a child with a chromosomal anomaly, or has a history of genetic disease and is not made aware of the test, the physician may be culpable if she produces a defective infant. Risks and benefits of the test must also be given the patient in the form of a written consent. If the mother has the test and is told that her infant is normal and she subsequently produces a defective child, the physician and laboratory performing the test could be held accountable. If the physician has personal beliefs about either the efficacy of the test or whether the woman should abort if the test shows a defective fetus, and cannot perform the test based on moral, ethical, or religious grounds, the physician nevertheless has the obligation to inform the patient about the test and refer her elsewhere.[23]

■ ETHICAL AND LEGAL CONSIDERATIONS IN ABORTION

The current conflict between the pro-choice and the pro-life groups has rekindled the fires that have raged around the topic of abortion. It has been pointed out that nurses must understand their own ethical position on this matter if they are to render quality care to their clients.[24] Because the nurse is involved in counseling clients about abortions from a variety of standpoints, a brief review of the ethical and legal considerations is given in the following sections.

Ethical Considerations

The ethics involved in the abortion issue revolve around terminating the life of a fetus by removing it from the uterus, that is, from its life support system. It has been argued that if given a choice, humans would choose health and lack of suffering for themselves. Furthermore, the argument goes, humans do not have the right to inflict the tragic consequences of detectable diseases on a fetus. By aborting a defective fetus, "nothingness" is given rather than the pain of living with an abnormality, and the damaged fetus can be replaced with a normal one in a subsequent pregnancy. Although this line of reasoning supports aborting damaged fetuses, it does not address the ethics of aborting healthy (or undetermined) products of conception, and it raises the issue of who determines what is normal or healthy.[25,26]

Pro-choice advocates take the position that the mother has the ultimate responsibility and freedom of choice regarding her body. It is important to remember that pro-choice is not pro-abortion. Pro-choice advocates stress using abortion only as a last resort. They uphold responsible use of contraception, amniocentesis to determine fetal defects, and adoption whenever possible. Pro-life advocates believe that the fetus is human from the time of conception and that to destroy human life is murder and, hence, indefensible morally.

Legal Considerations

ABORTION MADE LEGAL

In 1973, in the historical *Roe v. Wade* case, the U.S. Supreme Court declared that abortion was legal anywhere in the United States. The decision rendered existing state laws prohibiting abortion as unconstitutional on the grounds that such laws invaded the mother's privacy. The decision also stipulated several other points: (1) a state *could not* prevent a woman from obtaining an abortion from a licensed physician any time during the first trimester; (2) the state *could* regulate the performance of an abortion to protect the woman's health during the second trimester; (3) the state *could* regulate and even prohibit abortions in the third trimester except in cases in which the mother's life or health might be jeopardized; and (4) the state also had the right to impose safeguards for the fetus in the last trimester. The decision did not provide "abortion on demand." It was the intent that physicians would still use their clinical judgment when clients requested abortion.

The law also did not consider pregnant minors. Some states allow pregnant minors to have an abortion without parental consent. A precedent of sorts was set in 1981, when the Supreme Court upheld the constitutionality of a Utah law that required physicians to inform parents of a minor's request for abortion.[27,28]

One major problem with the ruling is that there was no decision as to when life begins. The Court felt that because no other scholars or scientists were able to reach a consensus opinion on this matter, it would be presumptuous for the Court to do so. They did decide that the fetus was not a "person" for the purposes of the Fourteenth Amendment and that neither the father of the fetus nor the woman's husband had the right to interfere in or prevent the abortion.[29] The issue of when life actually begins and when the fetus becomes a person still continues to be debated.

In many states, there are laws that include "conscience clauses," which allow institutions, health providers, and others to refuse to assist in abortions without risk of reprisal if participation is against their moral, ethical, or religious beliefs. However, public hospitals must allow the use of their facilities for abortion because they are supported by public funds.

Reaffirmation of Women's Rights. Ethicists point out that abortion must remain a moral decision for the mother unless sexual inequality is to be governmentally institutionalized. The *Roe v. Wade* decision is somewhat of a technological decision, because it still relies on medical technology and expertise to ascertain the viability of the fetus and to determine at what stage of pregnancy abortion is safer for the mother. However, there are positive and negative sides to decisions based solely on available technology. For example, if advances in drug technology produce a safe method of allowing all women to self-induce early abortion by way of medication, then abortion decisions will be automatically removed from governmental interference. The danger of this is that such methods will confuse the distinction between methods of contraception and methods of abortion, thus allowing women to find the whole issue less morally troubling.[27–29]

ABORTION OPPONENTS CONTINUE TO SEEK LEGISLATION

Abortion opponents continue to seek laws and regulations that discourage or restrict abortions. The constitutionality of such requirements is usually tested before the Supreme Court by such advocates of legalized abortion as Planned Parenthood, the National Organization for Women, and the American Public Health Association.[30] The Supreme Court has, in the past, upheld the principle that a woman's right to choose may not be burdened with excessive or discouraging regu-

---

Legal Status of Abortion

In 1973 the United States Supreme Court ruled that abortion was legal. A summary of the decision follows:

1. The abortion decision and its implementation must be left to the judgment of the woman and her physician when pregnancy is in the first trimester.
2. After the first trimester and before the end of the second trimester, the state, in promoting its interest in the health of the pregnant woman, may choose to regulate abortions in ways that are reasonably related to health.
3. After pregnancy has reached the time of viability (defined as 24 to 26 weeks' gestation), the state, in promoting its interest in the potentiality of human life, may, if it chooses, regulate and even prescribe abortion, except where it is necessary, in medical judgment, to preserve the life or health of the pregnant woman.

In 1976, the Supreme Court further ruled that the state cannot impose the requirement of consent by a third party on the woman's right to abortion; thus, abortion cannot be denied if a spouse or parent objects.

In 1983, the Supreme Court struck down state restrictions that imposed waiting periods for first-trimester abortions, that required specific informed consents, and that require hospitalization for second-trimester abortions.

Although states can implement requirements for parental notification of abortion services to pregnant minors, this can be waived by a state court or administrative agency if the minor is judged mature enough to give informed consent.

Tactics to Restrict Abortion

- State laws that require physicians to take the same degree of care in aborting a possibly viable fetus as they would take in delivery of a live birth.
- Requiring physicians to use the abortion method most likely to result in fetal survival, unless this significantly increases risk to the woman. Impacts on second-trimester abortions and often involves fetuses with diagnosed genetic abnormalities.
- Increasing the burden to providers and the mother through reporting or lengthy information requirements, including filing the reports, which contain personal/social data, with state health departments.[30]

lations. However, the changing political composition of the Court leaves open the possibility of more conservative and restrictive interpretations.

■ ETHICAL AND LEGAL CONSIDERATIONS FOR THE FETUS AND SICK NEONATE

Perhaps the area in perinatology and neonatology that is most fraught with dissension, discussion, debate, and ethical and legal dilemmas is the areas of neonatal intensive care and fetal research and treatment. Ironically, many of the problems in this area are a result of the extraordinary technological advances developed in the field of neonatology and perinatology. Fetuses that would have naturally aborted or been stillborn 5 years ago now can often be sustained in utero until they are almost full term. Infants who had no chance of survival a decade ago now may look forward to a relatively healthy and productive life. What then, is the cause for debate?

As technology and expertise increase, there will certainly be more attempts to save fetuses at earlier and earlier stages, even those with severe conditions. In many of these cases, the saved infant will be severely handicapped either physically or mentally. Heroic efforts are made by health professionals to prolong life, when it is questionable whether it is in the best interest of the infant or family. Health providers and parents are often faced with these ethical and moral dilemmas because of federal regulations and guidelines. The major ethical and legal problems encountered in these areas are discussed in the following section.

The Fetus

The fetus has rights from the time of conception and can be the beneficiary of a trust and inherit property. Although not legally considered a person until born, the rights of the fetus have been upheld in the courts. For instance a woman was ordered to have a cesarean section by the courts because of fetal distress. The woman had refused the procedure and was adamant about leaving the hospital. After conferring with her, the legal staff of the hospital procured a court order and the woman had to undergo the cesarean. This was the first time a woman had legally been coerced into surgery. There was another case in which the courts ordered a mother who was a Jehovah's Witness to have a blood transfusion to save the life of her infant.[31]

FETAL RESEARCH

Although federal funding for fetal research is more or less at a standstill, there are still many advocates who believe the research has great potential for preventing costly diseases. However, many states have made fetal research illegal, especially when the fetus is an abortus or is still in utero. The ethics of fetal tissue transplants is hotly debated.[32,33] Several difficult questions have been raised regarding the rights of the mother versus the rights of the fetus:

Does the mother have the right to determine what will be done with fetal remains?
Does a mother who plans an abortion have the right to allow experimentation in utero?
Can an aborted fetus be kept alive for experimental purposes?

Federal guidelines require that fetal research be designed to meet the needs of the fetus, be of minimal risk, and have the potential to develop important medical knowledge. These global guidelines allow for rather wide interpretation. Experts seem to agree that we are on the threshold of great discoveries. However, with this progress will come even more difficult decisions for expectant parents and those who care for them.[33]

FETAL THERAPY

We now have the capacity to drain spinal fluid from the brain of a fetus (cephalocentesis), catheterize the fetus in utero, remove its lower body from the uterus to repair a urinary tract obstruction, transfuse the fetus in utero for erythroblastosis, repair gastroschisis, and surgically repair skeletal defects. Although these are certainly milestones in the area of therapy, investigators generally advise caution and note the experimental nature of many of the treatments.[32-34] Harrison and colleagues have stated that the only anatomical malformations that warrant consideration are those that interfere with fetal organ development and that, if alleviated, would allow normal fetal development to proceed.[35]

There are ethical and legal questions and possible conflicts that can emerge as these treatments become more used. What happens if a physician feels he or she can help a fetus, but the mother refuses consent or the surgical consent is ambiguous? If a court orders the mother to submit to fetal treatment, does this invade her right to privacy and her own body integrity? Could she be charged with fetus abuse if she refuses treatment? Is the risk to benefit ratio favorable enough to cause this very costly therapy to be a national priority?[34] Answers to these questions are not easy, and solutions are becoming difficult as technology improves.

The Neonate

How much should a child have to suffer for the sake of life? More importantly, which should be regarded more highly—the sanctity of life or the quality of life?

Doctors, nurses, and parents will increasingly continue to face these dilemmas as infant mortality rates continue to decline. Of the approximately 3.5 million babies delivered in the United States each year, about 250,000 are born with significant defects or are victimized by birth injury.[36] Clearly, medicine is advancing in its effort to save lives, but the long-range outcomes may be questionable.

EFFECTS OF INVASIVE PROCEDURES

Some of the procedures deemed necessary for a sick newborn can produce a disease or defect (an iatrogenic effect). Prolonged use of ventilators can scar respiratory passages. Oxygen therapy, if it is given at too high a concentration, can cause varying degrees of vision impairment (retrolental fibroplasia). Neonates are subjected to needles stuck into their heels, tubes down their throat, and catheters into their heart, bladder, and other orifices. Health-care providers often view the patient's suffering as justifiable, something that must be endured to make patients better in the long term. Although this point of view enables them to practice with less guilt and, indeed, is often required by current legal regulations, it may be dismal from the infant's point of view. The infant clearly has no choice, whereas adults have the option of refusing treatment; therefore, deciding what is reasonable treatment for infants is more difficult.[36] There is a growing consensus among both providers and ethicists that society must come to terms with several difficult questions in the next few years: should we be saving the lives of certain infants only to have them lead lives of pain, disability, and deprivation? Or should we let those die who would not otherwise survive without major intervention? And if so, who makes the decision? What is the family's role in these decisions, and how much power should they have? What kind of care does one deny or give an infant to allow death with comfort and dignity? Some of these questions have received partial, albeit ambiguous, answers in the controversial "Baby Doe" regulations.[37-42]

BABY DOE REGULATIONS

In March 1983 the first Baby Doe regulation was issued by the Secretary of the Department of Health and Human Services (DHHS). This was in response to a report that an infant with Down's syndrome had died in an Indiana hospital because her esophageal atresia was left uncorrected. The main thrust of the regulation was the threat to remove federal funding from hospitals that did not comply with a notice that was to be posted that stated that failure to feed or care for handicapped infants was against federal law. In addition, a Baby Doe hotline was established by which suspected hospital failures to comply could be reported. Some alleged failures were reported, and "Baby Doe squads" were dispatched to the suspected hospitals. Needless to say, there were major disruptions at all levels, including actual medical and nursing care, as charts were confiscated, providers interrogated, time taken from care, and the like. It was eventually proved that the hospitals in question were entirely blameless.

The American Academy of Pediatrics and others sought an injunction against the regulation. This was denied; however, a waiting period was granted in which public comment was to be solicited. Debate was heated, because health professionals felt the judiciary was interfering in a process of decision making that was in the purview of themselves and the parents and was insidiously labeling the parties "child abusers."[43] In September 1983, the regulation was reissued with little change. One change was that hotline notices were to be posted only in nurses' stations, assumedly to encourage nurses to report "abuse," because they often were "afraid of reprisal" otherwise. Annas and others state that this was a demeaning rationalization of nurses, because it deprecates nurses as intelligent, participating members of the health team.[43-45]

On October 11, 1983, an infant was born in Port Jefferson, New York, with multiple neural tube defects, including spina bifida, microcephaly, and hydrocephaly. After consulting with physicians and their Roman Catholic priest, the parents chose conservative medical rather than surgical treatment to reduce the chance of infection rather than to correct the defects. A lawyer in Vermont, unrelated to any of the above participants, managed to get a court order to appoint a guardian *ad latem* for the child (depriving the parents of their parental authority) to have the surgery performed. The trial court's ruling was struck down eventually by New York's State Court of Appeals. The court commented on the often "offensive activities of those who sought to displace parental responsibility for management of her medical care."[45] Nevertheless, fears were aroused once more as to the possibility of further interference in the provider–client relationship.[42] In January 1984, what were thought to be the final regulations pertaining to handicapped infants were issued by the Secretary of DHHS. They were entitled, "Nondiscrimination on the Basis of Handicap, 1984." Legal rights of handicapped infants were required to be posted, and state protective services were to develop procedures for protecting infants from medical neglect. The regulations did not require neonatal intensive care units to provide futile efforts to prolong the act of dying. Hospitals were encouraged (but not required) to set up infant-care review committees (ICRC) to review all cases of infants who might be deprived of care because of their health condition(s). The American Academy of Pediatrics has developed guidelines for the composition and duties of such a committee and regards these committees as viable alternatives to hotlines and squads of investigators.[45]

On May 15, 1985, the latest Baby Doe regulation went into effect as the Child Abuse Amendments of 1985 to Public Law 98-457—the Child Abuse Prevention and Treatment Act.[46] It provides for several more explicit definitions (see Further Regulations Resulting From the Child Abuse Amendments of 1985 to Public Law 98—The Child Abuse Prevention and Treatment Act) and describes a brief set of requirements that a state protective agency must fulfill to qualify for federal grants. The amendment has been called anticlimactic. It has had minimal impact on medical and ethical decision making, because the trend is toward aggressive treatment of nonlethal conditions and the narrowing of parents' and physicians' discretion on treatment decisions (the "best interest of the infant" standard). Moreover, although encouraging hospitals to form ICRCs, DHHS was careful to maintain that these are guidelines only and does not offer sanctions or rewards for their establishment.[46] There still remains confusion over the language, particularly the "chronically and irreversibly comatose" phrase, which tends to get interpreted in both narrow and broader senses depending on the judge and attorneys.[47,48] Thus, this aspect of care continues to be fraught with weighty ethical and legal issues.

■ ETHICAL AND LEGAL CONSIDERATIONS IN CARE OF THE MOTHER

Specific Ethical and Legal Issues in Maternal Care

One controversial legal and ethical issue is whether pregnant women should be compelled by law to receive medical or surgical treatment for benefit of the fetus. There have been several cases of unusual circumstances that have focused on these issues.[49] In one case, the ethical question revolved around the appropriateness of using life support systems on the mother for a short period to improve substantially the outcome of the fetus. An ethicist noted in a commentary that the use of the mother's body to serve the interest of her infant would be permissible if the mother had given prior consent or

---

Further Regulations Resulting From the Child Abuse Amendments of 1985 to Public Law 98—The Child Abuse Prevention and Treatment Act

Medical neglect: withholding of medically indicated treatment from a disabled infant with a life-threatening condition

Definition of *"withholding medically indicated treatment"*:

"The failure to respond to the infant's life-threatening conditions by providing treatment (including appropriate nutrition, hydration, and medication) which, in the treating physician's (or physicians') reasonable medical judgment, will be most likely to be effective in ameliorating or correcting all such conditions."

Withholding medical treatment is not *"medical neglect"* under three conditions:

1. The infant is chronically and irreversibly comatose;
2. The provision of such treatment would merely prolong dying, not be effective in ameliorating or correcting all of the infant's life-threatening conditions, or otherwise be futile in terms of the survival of the infant; or
3. The provision of such treatment would be virtually futile in terms of the survival of the infant and the treatment itself under such circumstances would be inhumane.

Definition of *"reasonable medical judgment"*:
"medical judgment that would be made by a reasonably prudent physician knowledgeable about the case and the treatment possibilities with respect to the medical condition involved."

(Adapted from Murray TH: The final anticlimactic rule on Baby Doe. Hastings Center Rep 15(3): 5–7, June 1985)

---

signed an anatomical donation card. Without the mother's consent, permission must be obtained from her next of kin. Such cases inevitably create controversy and conflicting opinions between relatives and the health-care providers and raise questions regarding the limits of benevolence and authority.[50] Such cases need to be reviewed by a multidisciplinary team of ethicists, lawyers, physicians, and clergy in conjunction with consultation with the family.

Unlike this extreme case noted above, there is much question regarding just how far laws should extend to compel women to accept even routine medical or surgical treatment for the benefit of the fetus during pregnancy. Such treatments could include attending frequent medical appointments, submitting to various tests and treatments, or even complying with medical recommendations to refrain from sexual intercourse, taking drugs, consuming alcohol, or exercise. If the mother refused to comply with the suggested regimen, she could be liable to criminal prosecution. Many ethicists and physicians believe that there is no legal, ethical, or moral basis that justifies requesting the courts to order a mother to undergo a given medical or surgical procedure for the benefit of the fetus when the pregnant mother objects to the procedure.[51,52]

Nurse's Responsibility

The nurse has certain obligations to the mother. She must have the knowledge and expertise to use the equipment necessary for the mother's care, particularly fetal monitors. She should be familiar with the guidelines for monitoring developed by the American College of Obstetrics and Gynecology. The nurse must be proficient in being able to read the monitor accurately, make appropriate notations, and report complications to the physician immediately. Another important area of responsibility is to observe the newborn carefully after delivery and report and record any sign of complication or problem. Monitoring tapes should be appropriately stored, as they are often important evidence in the event of a medical malpractice suit. Nurses can be held culpable in the event of maternal or newborn complications, so it is extremely important that they are knowledgeable regarding their appropriate responsibilities and care.

■ REFERENCES

1. Curtin L, Flaherty MJ: Nursing Ethics, Theories and Pragmatics. Bowie, MD, Robert J Brady, 1982
2. Bushy A, Randall R, Matt BF: Ethical principles: Applications to an obstetric case. JOGNN 18:207–212, May/June 1989
3. Hankanson EY: Reducing the risk involved in providing medical care for women. Malpractice Digest 24–32, July–August 1980
4. Fiesta J: The Law and Liability: A Guide for Nurses. New York, John Wiley & Sons, 1983
5. Greenfield VR: Wrongful birth: What is the damage? JAMA 248:926–932, 1982
6. Regan WA: Nursing malpractice: A giant leap on damages. RN 44(12):69–72, 1981
7. Annas GJ: Redefining parenthood and protecting embryos: Why we need new laws. Hastings Center Rep 14(5):50–52, October 1984
8. Shearer BH: Some effects of assisted reproduction on perinatal care. Birth 15:131–133, September 1988
9. Bonnicksen A: Some consumer aspects of in vitro fertilization. Birth 15:145–147, September 1988
10. Kola I: Commentary: Embryo and fetal abnormalities in IVF. Birth 15:145–147, September, 1988
11. Williams LS: It's going to work for me: Responses to failures of IVF. Birth 15:154–156, September 1988
12. Abramowitz S: A stalemate on test-tube baby research. Hastings Center Rep 14(1):5–9, February 1984
13. Holmes HB: In vitro fertilization: Reflections on the state of the art. Birth 15:134–145, September 1988
14. Pace-Owens S: Gamite intrafallopian transfer (GIFT). JOGNN 18:93–97, March/April 1989
15. Mosher WD, Pratt WF: Reproductive improvements among married couples: United States, pp 13, 32. Vital and Health Statistics, Series 23, No. 11, National Center for Health Statistics, December 1982
16. Gersz SR: The contract in surrogate motherhood: A review of the issues. Law Med Health Care 12(3):107–114, 1984
17. Furrow BR: Surrogate motherhood: A new option for parenting? Law Med Health Care 12(3):106, 1984
18. Robertson JA: Surrogate mothers: Not so novel after all. Hastings Center Rep 13(5):28–30, October 1983
19. Gewertz C: Surrogate-born baby now with genetic parents. Los Angeles Times, pp A1, A28, September 23, 1990
20. Gewertz C: Surrogate mother's visitation rights reduced by judge. Los Angeles Times, p A34, September 28, 1990
21. Brahams D: The hasty British ban on commercial surrogacy. Hastings Center Rep 17:16–19, February 1987
22. Jones HW: Variations on a theme (editorial). JAMA 250:2182, October 28, 1983
23. Stern L: On ethics, difficult choices and the responsibility of physicians. J Perinatol 8:81, Spring 1988
24. Cohen L: Whose right to life? MCN 13:83, March/April 1988
25. Cohen SS: Health care policy and abortion: A comparison. Nurs Outlook 38:20–25, January/February 1990
26. Overall C: Selective termination of pregnancy and women's reproductive autonomy. Hastings Center Rep 20:6–11, May/June 1990
27. Annas GJ: Roe vs. Wade reaffirmed, again. Hastings Center Rep 16:26–27, October 1986
28. Annas GJ: Webster and the politics of abortion. Hastings Center Rep 19:36–38, March/April 1989
29. Baron CH: "If you prick us, do we not bleed?" of Shylock, fetuses and the concept of person in the law. Law Med Health Care 2(2):52–61, 1983
30. APHA high court brief to oppose rules restricting abortions. Nation's Health 8(1):8, August 1985
31. Patterson P: Fetal therapy: Issues we face. AORN J 35(4):663–668, March 1982
32. Elias S, Annas GJ: Perspectives on fetal surgery. Am J Obstet Gynecol 145:807–815, 1983
33. Fine A: The ethics of fetal tissue transplants. Hastings Center Rep 18:5–8, June/July 1988
34. Ruddick W, Wilcox W: Operating on the fetus. Hastings Center Rep 12(5):10–13, 1982
35. Harrison MR, Golbus MS, Filly RA: Management of the fetus with a correctable congenital defect. JAMA 246:776–782, August 14, 1981

36. Lyon J: New treatments, new choices. Nurs Life 4(2): 48–52, 1984

37. Strong C: Defective infants and their impact on families: Ethical and legal considerations. Law Med Health Care 11(4):168–172; 181, 1983

38. Harrison H: Neonatal intensive care: Parents' role in ethical decision making. Birth 13:165–175, September 1986

39. Klaus MH: Ethical decision making in neonatal intensive care: Commentary with parents. Birth 13:175, September 1986

40. Hardwig J: What about the family? Hastings Center Rep 20:5–10, March/April 1990

41. Committee on the Legal and Ethical Aspects of Health Care for Children: Comments and recommendations on the ''Infant Doe'' proposed regulations. Law Med Health Care 11(5):203–209, 1983

42. Doudera AE: Section 504, handicapped newborns and ethics committees: An alternative to the hotline. Law Med Health Care 2(5):200–202, 1983

43. Annas GJ: Baby Doe redux: Doctors as child abusers. Hastings Center Rep 13(5):25–32, 1983

44. Murphy CP: The changing role of nurses in making ethical decisions. Law Med Health Care 12(4):173–175; 184, September 1984

45. Fleischman AR, Murray TH: Ethics committees for Infant Doe? Hastings Center Rep 13(6):5–9, December 1983

46. Murray TH: The final anticlimactic rule on Baby Doe. Hastings Center Rep 15(3):5–7, June 1985

47. Confusion over the language of the Baby Doe regulations. Hastings Center Rep 162, December 1986

48. Smith JB: Ethical issues raised by new treatment options. MCN 14:183–187, May/June 1989

49. Dillon WP, et al: Life support and maternal brain death during pregnancy. JAMA 248(9):1089–1091, September 3, 1982

50. Veach RM: Maternal brain death: An ethicist's thoughts. JAMA 248(9):1102–1103, September 3, 1982

51. Nelson LJ, Milliken N: Compelled medical treatment of pregnant women: Life, liberty and law in conflict. JAMA 259:1060, 1988.

52. Annas GJ: Pregnant women as fetal containers. Hastings Center Rep 16:13–14, December 1986

■ SUGGESTED READINGS

Annas GJ: Pregnant women as fetal containers. Hastings Center Rep 16:13–14, December 1986

Committee on Ethics: Ethical Dilemmas Confronting Nurses. Missouri, American Nurses Association, 1985

Committee on Ethics: Ethics In Nursing: Position Statements and Guidelines. Missouri, American Nurses Association, 1988

Fries ES: The ethical issues of transplanting organs from anencephalic newborns. MCN 14:412–414, November/December 1989

Infants' Bioethics Task Force and Consultants: Guidelines for infant bioethics committees. Pediatrics 72(2):306–310, August 1984

Milne BJ: Couples' experiences with in vitro fertilization. JOGNN 17:347–352, 1988

Myers ST, Stolte K: Nurses' responses to changes in maternity care. Part II: Technologic revolution, legal climate, and economic changes. Birth 14:87–90, 1987

Price FV: The risk of high multiparity with IVF/ET. Birth 15:157–163, 1988

Schifrin BS: Polemics in perinatology: The abortion thing. J Perinatol 10:81–83, March 1990

Smith JB: Ethical issues raised by new treatment options. MCN 14:183–187, May/June 1989

Thompson FE, Thompson HO: Living with ethical decisions with which you disagree. MCN 13:245–250, July/August 1988

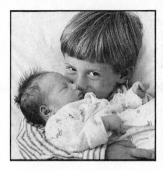

Unit I
Nursing, Family Health, and Reproduction

CONFERENCE MATERIAL

1. Discuss the expanding roles of the maternity/perinatal nurse. Is there a difference between these roles? If so, how do they differ? Include a discussion of the rationale of why/why not the roles differ.

2. How would you go about refining the nursing diagnoses related to maternity care? Include a discussion of the present categories of nursing diagnoses. How do they relate to maternity/perinatal care?

3. What are the types of families that you see in your geographic area? Discuss how these may have an impact on nursing care.

4. Discuss the social and behavioral risk factors that you see threatening the clientele you serve.

MULTIPLE CHOICE

1. The 1973 U.S. Supreme Court decision on abortions (and subsequent decisions) held that, in the first trimester of pregnancy
   A. The abortion decision must be left to the woman and her physician.
   B. The state may regulate abortions in ways reasonably related to health.
   C. The state may proscribe abortions except where necessary to preserve the life or health of the pregnant woman. ____

2. Which of the above is true until the time of fetal viability (defined as 24 to 26 weeks' gestation)?

3. Commercial surrogacy in the United States
   A. Has been made illegal
   B. Has no federal legal restrictions, but presents ethical and legal dilemmas to all parties
   C. Has been shown to be a safe, highly recommended alternate to adoption for infertile couples ____

UNIT II

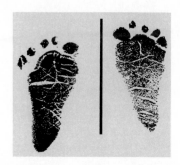

Biophysical Aspects of Human Reproduction

8

Sexual and Reproductive Anatomy and Physiology

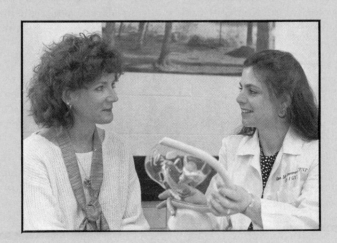

Women have a limited reproductive life span, beginning soon after the first menstrual period, declining somewhat in the late reproductive years, and finally terminating at the menopause. No more than 500 eggs or ova may be released during the course of reproductive life. In the male, sperm production is initiated at the time of puberty and continues well into old age. The number of mature spermatozoa produced by the testes during this very long interval are in the billions, and the reproductive capacity of a given fertile male is astounding.

Another important difference is that in the male, the capacity to reproduce is necessarily associated with sexual excitement, erection of the penis, and ejaculation. However, the capacity of the female to reproduce may be disassociated from sexual excitement and receptivity. Consider that conception can occur by mechanical placement of the ejaculate through artificial insemination. The capacity of the woman for sexual pleasure, however, is extremely important. There is no doubt that the physical aspects of a relationship play a critical role in the communication process that brings a couple closer together.

Anatomy and physiology of the reproductive organs are discussed in this chapter, whereas orgasm is discussed in Chapter 9 and ovum and sperm development and fertilization are discussed in Chapter 10.

■ MALE ORGANS OF REPRODUCTION

The male reproductive system consists of the penis, the testes, and an excretory duct system with their accessory structures (Fig. 8-1). Embryological development and genital differentiation of the male reproductive system are discussed in Chapter 10.

Penis

The penis, the male organ of copulation, consists of two lateral, cavernous bodies (*corpora cavernosa*) and a central core of erectile tissue (*corpus spongiosum*) that encloses the urethra. The enlarged conic structure at the free end of the penis, an extension of the corpus spongiosum, is called the *glans penis*. The glans contains the external orifice of the urethra and is covered by a fold of retractable skin called the *foreskin*, or prepuce. Sometimes the foreskin is removed by circumcision.

The two corpora cavernosa are surrounded by a thick but elastic fibrous envelope. They are intimately connected along their course but are separated at their base into two *crura*, strong tapering fibrous processes that are firmly attached to the pubic bone. The corpora cavernosa receive their blood supply from branches of the dorsal artery of the penis. These divide further and terminate in a capillary network, the branches of which open directly into the cavernous spaces. These are usually quite empty, and the organ is flaccid. When these spaces fill with blood, the organ becomes turgid. This is called an *erection*. The flow of blood is controlled by the autonomic nervous system (vasodilator fibers) and varies with sexual arousal. When the erect penis is stimulated further, impulses from the autonomic nervous system trigger pulsatile release of semen along the urethra.

Testes

The functional capacity of the male reproductive tract is governed principally by the *testes*. The testes are dependent on an interplay between the brain, the hypothalamus, and the pituitary gland. Like the ovary, the testes have two functions: secretion of *testosterone* (the male hormone), and *spermatogenesis* (the production and release of spermatozoa). Both are initiated at about the time of puberty and, under normal circumstances, continue well into senescence. Testosterone production can occur independently of spermatogenesis, but spermatogenesis cannot occur independently of testosterone production.

The testes are approximately 5 cm long and are contained in a fibrous protective covering, the *tunica albuginea*, which subdivides the testes into lobules (Fig. 8-2). Each lobule contains *seminiferous tubules*, coiled ducts in the walls of which spermatogenesis occurs. The testes also contain testosterone-producing cells, the *interstitial cells of Leydig*, as well as larger supporting cells, the *Sertoli cells*, which are important for sperm transport within the seminiferous tubules.

SCROTUM

Unlike the ovaries, the testes are located outside the abdominal cavity in the *scrotum*, which means "bag." During early fetal life, the testes are abdominal. As the fetus develops, the testes move downward and enter the scrotum through the inguinal canal shortly before birth. The scrotum is located between the penis and the anus. It is a saclike structure composed of fascial connective tissue containing smooth-muscle fibers (dartos fascia) with overlying corrugated skin. The skin of the scrotum is pigmented with scattered hairs and sebaceous glands. Its wrinkled appearance is produced by the dartos fascia that underlies it. The muscle contained in dartos fascia responds to cold by contracting, accentuating the wrinkled appearance as the scrotum is drawn closer to the body wall. The two testes are separated from

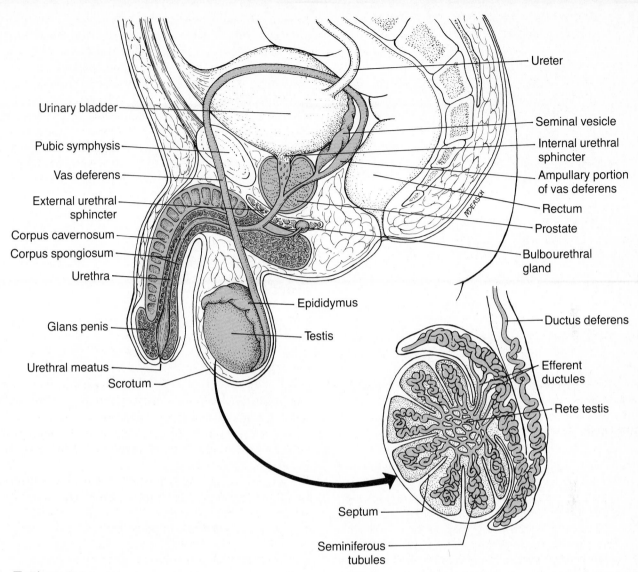

■ *Figure 8–1*
Organs of the male reproductive system.

each other by a medial septum within the scrotum, which is an extension of the dartos fascia. Its location in the midline is marked by a ridge on the external surface of the scrotum.

TESTICULAR HORMONE PRODUCTION

The adult testes produce a continuous supply of the male hormone, testosterone. Testosterone is synthesized and released by the interstitial cells, also referred to as *Leydig cells.* The interstitial cells are located in the interstitial connective tissue that surrounds and supports the seminiferous tubules. They are stimulated to produce testosterone by luteinizing hormone (LH), which is released from the anterior pituitary gland. This is identical to the LH that is released in large amounts at midcycle to trigger the onset of ovulation in the female.

In the male, LH is sometimes referred to by another name, *interstitial cell stimulating hormone* (ICHS). ICHS does not display the marked cyclic variation in concentration seen during the menstrual cycle; however, as in the female, its release from the pituitary gland is controlled by releasing hormones from the brain and hypothalamus. There is a reciprocal relationship between LH release and testosterone production by the interstitial cells.

Testosterone establishes and maintains the secondary sex characteristics of the male, such as development and maturation of the external genitalia, prostate, and seminal vesicles; growth of body and facial hair; and maturation of the larynx. It also contributes to body growth and general development.

The principal role of testosterone in terms of reproduction is maintenance of spermatogenesis. Unless this

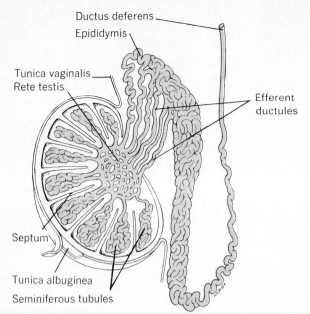

■ *Figure 8–2*
Diagram of structural features of the testis and epididymis.

hormone is present in normal amounts, fertility is impaired.

SPERMATOGENESIS

Production of spermatozoa is initiated and maintained in the seminiferous tubules of the testes (Fig. 8-3). The seminiferous tubules are long, coiled structures containing a lumen into which spermatozoa are released from the epithelial wall where they are produced. During this process, meiosis occurs, and the number of chromosomes in each cell is reduced to half, which is the haploid number (see Fig. 10-2). A structurally mature spermatozoon is produced, complete with head, midpiece, and tail (see Fig. 10-3). The maturation of the human spermatozoon occupies an interval of 60 days.

Spermatogenesis is a heat-sensitive process. The 2° to 3° difference between scrotal and abdominal temperatures allows spermatogenesis to proceed normally in the cooler environment. Testosterone production is not affected by temperature. When there has been failure of the testes to descend, spermatogenesis is severely impaired, but testosterone production remains unaffected.

TESTICULAR RELEASE OF SPERM

The wall of the seminiferous tubules is separated into two physiologically distinct compartments by specialized supporting cells, the Sertoli cells. These cells are large, easily identifiable structures that are joined to each other by firm cell-to-cell connections. They separate the epithelium into a basal and a luminal compartment.

This arrangement produces an effective separation of the basal compartment from the circulation and provides a blood–testes permeability barrier. In this way the early-developing sperm-forming elements are protected from harmful substances that may be circulating in the bloodstream.

The Sertoli cell plays an active role in the release of spermatozoa into the lumen of the seminiferous tubules. The tight junctions between the Sertoli cells break down transiently to permit upward movement of spermatocytes into the compartment adjacent to the lumen. They are then drawn into the cytoplasm of the Sertoli cell, moved upward toward the surface of the cell, and finally extruded by contractions of the cytoplasm of the apex of the Sertoli cells (Fig. 8-4).

Duct System

Leading from the testes are the transporting and storage ducts of the male reproductive tract.

EPIDIDYMIS

The seminiferous tubules coalesce at the rete testis (see Fig. 8-2) and enter the *epididymis*. This structure is located adjacent to the testis (see Fig. 8-1) and serves as a reservoir for sperm. It is divided into a head portion (caput) and a tail (cauda).

When spermatozoa are released into the seminiferous tubules, although endowed with tails, they are not yet capable of motility. They acquire motility as they pass along the epididymis.

VAS DEFERENS

The ducts of the epididymis lead to the *vas deferens*, the transporting passage along which spermatozoa traverse to the base of the penis (see Fig. 8-1). The ductus deferens, or vas deferens, has contractile power that allows it to propel the spermatozoa upward to the ejaculatory duct and through the urethra to the base of the penis.

Accessory Structures

The accessory structures consist of the *seminal vesicles*, the *prostate gland*, and the *bulbourethral glands* (see Fig. 8-1). The seminal vesicles are sacculated structures located behind the bladder and in front of the rectum: the prostate gland surrounds the base of the urethra and the ejaculatory duct; and the bulbourethral glands, or Cowper's glands, lie at the base of the prostate and on either side of the membranous urethra. The function of the accessory sex organs is maintained by testosterone. The bulbourethral glands produce a mucinous

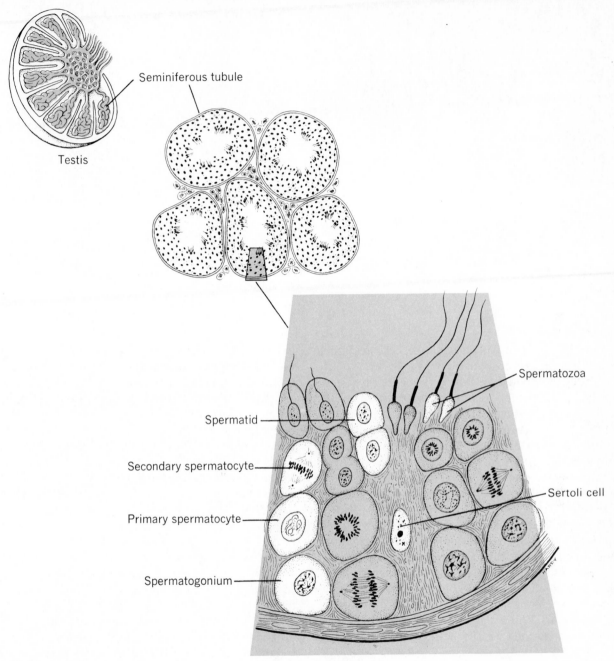

Seminiferous tubule

Testis

Spermatozoa

Spermatid

Secondary spermatocyte

Sertoli cell

Primary spermatocyte

Spermatogonium

■ *Figure 8–3*
Section of a seminiferous tubule, showing various stages of spermatogenesis.

substance that lubricates the urethra and coats its surface.

The prostate rests on the rectum, through which it can be felt, and in shape and size resembles a chestnut. It consists of two lateral lobes of equal size and a much smaller middle lobe. The ejaculatory ducts pass through the gland between the middle and lateral lobes, and the urethra traverses it. It sometimes becomes enlarged in men past middle age (benign prostatic hypertrophy) and causes urinary obstruction that requires surgical treatment.

SEMEN AND EJACULATION

During ejaculation, the semen receives contributions from the seminal vesicles and the prostate gland. The seminal vesicles deliver the secretions to the urethra through the ejaculatory ducts, discharging a fructose-rich product. The seminal vesicles are a major source of prostaglandins, substances that stimulate smooth-muscle contractions. The prostate transmits its contents into the urethra during ejaculation through a number of small ducts. It secretes a clear fluid with a slightly

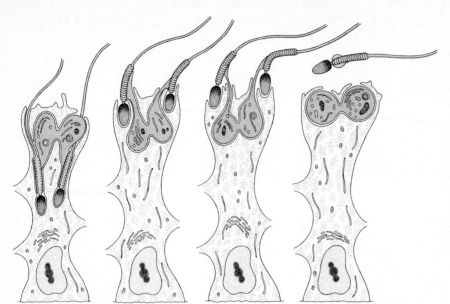

■ *Figure 8-4*
Diagram of the stages of sperm release. The conjoined cell bodies of the advanced spermatids are retained in the epithelium while the nucleus, neck region, and tail are gradually extruded into the lumen. The narrow stalk connecting the neck region with the cell body becomes increasingly attenuated and finally gives way. Individual spermatozoa are thus separated from the syncytial cell bodies. (Redrawn from Greep RO, Koblinsky MA [eds]: Frontiers in Reproduction and Fertility Control. Cambridge, MIT Press, 1977)

acid pH that is rich in acid phosphatase, citric acid, zinc, and a number of proteolytic enzymes.

The bulbourethral, or Cowper's, glands, are accessory glands that empty into the bulbous urethra. They produce a lubricating fluid that maintains moisture within the urethra. At the height of sexual excitement and full erection, their contents may be released, sometimes carrying with them a few spermatozoa. The functions of the secretions of the accessory glands are to facilitate transportation of spermatozoa along the urethra during the ejaculatory process and to provide a temporary milieu where spermatozoa can survive. Thus, the ejaculate or semen is made up of spermatozoa contained in seminal vesicular and prostatic secretions, with a small contribution from Cowper's glands. On intravaginal ejaculation, some spermatozoa leave the ejaculate almost immediately and begin to traverse the cervical mucus. Within a matter of minutes, some spermatozoa are on their way to the site of fertilization.

Male Sexual Maturity

The average male enters puberty at 11.6 years of age.[1] The hormonal changes associated with sexual maturation begin before the appearance of the physical signs of puberty. Increased production of adrenal sex steroids (adrenarche) occurs about 2 years before maturation of the hypothalamic-pituitary-gonadal axis. Three major adrenal steroids are produced: dehydroepiandrosterone, androstenedione, and estrone. A decreased sensitivity to the negative feedback system between the central nervous system and the testes is believed to cause the

hypothalamus and pituitary gland to begin secreting increased amounts of gonadotropin releasing hormone (GnRH), follicle-stimulating hormone (FSH), and LH.

Subsequent to the increased secretion of pituitary hormones, testosterone levels rise progressively during maturation. On the average, changes associated with puberty in the male occur 1 year later than in the female and span an interval of approximately 4 years. These include development of axillary, pubic, and body hair, as well as maturation and growth of the testes and penis, over a 2- to 3-year period, accompanied by a growth spurt and general muscular development. Development of the internal glands (prostate, bulbourethral, seminal vesicles) occurs synchronously with penile and testicular growth. Ejaculation of fluid with penile erection may occur within a year after the beginning of growth of the penis, even before it is of mature size.

Other somatic changes occur during puberty. Approximately 25% of adult height and 50% of adult weight is accrued during puberty.[2] The peak growth spurt occurs about 2 years after the onset of genital enlargement. Circulating testosterone affects muscle development, by increasing lean body mass (a percentage of body weight) from 80% or 85% to 90%. Generally, the ability to grow a full beard signifies the completion of male sexual maturity.

Tanner developed a staging system for describing and categorizing secondary sexual characteristics in boys and girls (sexual maturity ratings). The Tanner stages are displayed in Table 8-1. Although adolescents pass through a sequential series of pubertal events as they mature, the age at onset of events and the time interval between one event and the next is variable.[2]

TABLE 8-1. TANNER STAGING IN MALES

Stage	Testes	Penis	Pubic Hair	Other*	Range in Years
I	No change, testes 2.5 cm or less	Prepubertal	None		Birth to 15
II	Enlargement of testes, increased stippling and pigmentation of scrotal sac	Minimal or no enlargement	Long, downy, slightly pigmented hair often occurring several months after testicular growth; chiefly at base of penis		10–15
III	Further enlargement of testes and scrotum	Significant penile enlargement, especially in length	Increase in amount, now darker, coarser and curled at and lateral to the base of the penis	Peak growth spurt begins	10½–16½
IV	Further enlargement, increased pigmentation of scrotum	Further enlargement, especially in diameter	Adult type but not distribution, limited to pubic region	Axillary hair and some facial hair develop	Variable 12–17
V	Adult size and shape	Adult size and shape	Adult distribution and quality (medial aspects of thighs)	20% have peak height velocity; body hair development and increase in musculature may continue for several months to years	13–18

* Criteria not included in original Tanner stages. (Adapted from Wasserman G, Gromisch DS: Survey of Clinical Pediatrics, 7th ed. New York, McGraw-Hill, 1981; Tanner JM: Growth at Adolescence, 2nd ed. Oxford, Blackwell Scientific Publications, 1969; and Marshall WA, Tanner JM: Variations in pattern of pubertal changes in girls. Arch Dis Child 44:291–303, 1969)

■ FEMALE STRUCTURES AND ORGANS OF REPRODUCTION

Female Pelvis

The *pelvis*, so named because of its resemblance to a basin, is a bony ring interposed between the trunk and the thighs. The vertebral column, or backbone, passes into the pelvis from above and transmits the weight of the upper part of the body to it. Then the pelvis, in turn, transmits weight to the lower limbs. From an ob-

stetric point of view, however, it is the cavity that contains the generative organs and is the canal through which the fetus must pass during birth.

BONY STRUCTURE

The pelvis is made up of four united bones: the two hipbones (*os coxae*, or innominate), situated laterally and in front, and the *sacrum* and the *coccyx*, situated behind (Fig. 8-5).

Anatomically, the hipbones are divided into three parts: the *ilium*, the *ischium*, and the *pubis*. These bones

Female Organs of Reproduction

External	Internal
Vulva	Ovaries
Mons veneris	Fallopian tubes
Labia majora	Uterus
Labia minora	Corpus (body)
Clitoris	Cervix (neck)
Vestibule	
Perineum	

become firmly joined into one by the time the growth of the body is completed (between the ages of 20 and 25) so that when the pelvis is examined, no trace of the original edges or divisions of these three bones can be discovered. Each of these bones is briefly described below.

The *ilium*, the largest portion of the bones, forms the upper and back part of the pelvis. Its upper flaring border forms the prominence of the hip, or crest of the ilium (hipbone).

The *ischium* is the lower part below the hip joint, and from it projects the tuberosity of the ischium, on which the body rests when in a sitting position.

The *pubis* is the front part of the hipbone; it extends from the hip joint to the joint in front between the two hipbones, the symphysis pubis, and then turns down toward the ischial tuberosity, thus forming, with the bone of the opposite side, the arch below the symphysis, the pubic or subpubic arch. This articulation of the two pubic bones encloses the pelvic cavity anteriorly.

The *sacrum* and the *coccyx* form the lowest portions of the spinal column. The sacrum is a triangular wedge-shaped bone that consists of five vertebrae fused together. It serves as the back part of the pelvis. The coccyx forms a tail end to the spine. In the child, the coccyx consists of four or five very small, separate vertebrae; in the adult, these bones are fused into one. The coccyx is usually movable at the point of attachment to the sacrum, the sacrococcygeal joint, and may become pressed back during labor to allow more room for the passage of the fetal head.

The marked projection formed by the junction of the last lumbar vertebra with the sacrum is of special importance. This is the *sacral promontory*, one of the most important landmarks in obstetric anatomy.

ARTICULATION AND SURFACES

There are four *articulations*, or joints of the pelvis, that have obstetric importance. The two *sacroiliac articulations* are posterior, located between the sacrum and the ilia on either side; the *symphysis pubis* is in front, between the two pubic bones, and the *sacrococcygeal articulation* is located between the sacrum and the coccyx.

All of these articular surfaces are lined with fibrocartilage, which becomes thickened and softened during pregnancy; likewise, the ligaments that bind the pelvic joints together become softened, and as a result greater

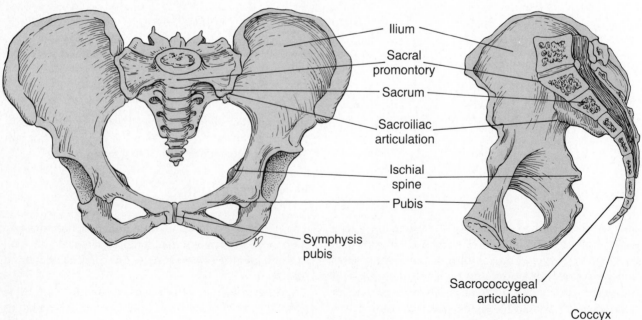

■ *Figure 8–5*
Front and lateral views of the pelvis, showing major bones and articulations.

mobility of the pelvic bones develops. A certain definite, although very limited, motion in the joints is desirable for a normal labor; however, there is no change in the actual size of the pelvis. The increased mobility that these joints develop in pregnancy produces a slight "wobbliness" in the pelvis and throws greater strain on the surrounding muscles and ligaments. This accounts for much of the backache and leg ache in the later months of pregnancy.

The pelvis is lined with muscular tissue that provides a smooth, somewhat cushioned surface for the fetus to pass over during labor. These muscles also help to support the abdominal contents.

TRUE AND FALSE PELVES

Regarded as a whole, the pelvis may be described as a two-story, bony basin that is divided into two parts by a natural line of division, the *inlet* or *brim*. The upper part is the false pelvis, and the lower part is the true pelvis (see Fig. 20-1).

The *false pelvis*, or upper flaring part, is much less implicated in the problems of labor than is the true pelvis. It supports the uterus during late pregnancy and directs the fetus into the true pelvis at the proper time.

The *true pelvis*, or lower part, forms the bony canal through which the fetus must pass during parturition. For descriptive purposes it is divided into three parts: an inlet or brim, a cavity, and an outlet. The importance of these parts and the various ways of assessing them during pregnancy and labor are discussed in Chapter 20.

External Organs

The external female reproductive organs are called the *vulva*, from the Latin word meaning *covering*. This includes everything that is visible externally from the lower margin of the pubis to the perineum, including the *mons veneris*, the *labia majora* and *minora*, the *clitoris*, the *vestibule*, the *hymen*, the *urethral opening*, and various glandular and vascular structures (Fig. 8-6). The term *vulva* has often been used to refer simply to the labia majora and minora.

The *mons veneris* is a firm, cushionlike formation over the symphysis pubis that is covered with crinkly hair.

The *labia majora* are two prominent longitudinal folds of adipose tissue that are covered with skin and extend downward and backward from the mons veneris and disappear in forming the anterior border of the perineal body. These two thick folds of skin are covered with hair on their outer surfaces after the age of puberty but are smooth and moist on their inner surfaces. At the bottom, they fade away into the perineum poste-

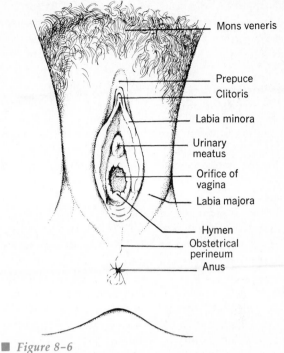

■ *Figure 8–6*
External genitalia of the female.

riorly, joining together to form a transverse fold, the posterior commissure, which is situated directly in front of the fourchette. This fatty tissue is supplied with an abundant plexus of veins that may rupture as the result of injury sustained during labor and give rise to an extravasation of blood, or hematoma.

The *labia minora* are two thin folds entirely covered with thin membrane that are situated between the labia majora. The outer surfaces join with the inner surfaces of the labia majora. The labia minora extend from the clitoris downward and backward on either side of the orifice of the vagina. In the upper extremity, each labium minus separates into two branches, which, when united with those of the opposite side, enclose the clitoris. The upper fold forms the prepuce, and the lower fold forms the frenum of the clitoris. At the bottom, the labia minora pass almost imperceptibly into the labia majora, blending together as a thin fold of skin, the fourchette, which forms the anterior edge of the perineum or perineal body.

The *clitoris* is a small, highly sensitive projection that is composed of erectile tissue, nerves, and blood vessels and is covered with a thin epidermis. It is analogous to the penis in the male and is regarded as the chief area of voluptuous sensation. The clitoris is partially hidden between the anterior ends of the labia minora.

The *vestibule* is the almond-shaped area that is enclosed by the labia minora and extends from the clitoris to the fourchette. It is perforated by four openings: the urethra, the vaginal opening, the ducts of Bartholin's glands, and the ducts of Skene's glands. *Bartholin's glands* are two small glands situated beneath the vestibule on either side of the vaginal opening. *Skene's glands* open on the vestibule on either side of the urethra.

The *hymen* marks the division between the internal and the external organs. It is a thin sheath of mucous membrane situated at the orifice of the vagina. It may be entirely absent, or it may form a complete septum across the lower end of the vagina.

The hymen changes in shape and consistency throughout the life cycle. In the newborn, it projects beyond the surrounding parts. In adult virgins, it is a membrane of varying thickness that presents an aperture that varies in size from a small opening to one that readily admits one or even two fingers. The opening is circular or crescent shaped. In rare instances, the hymen may be imperforate and cause retention of menstrual discharge if it occludes the vaginal orifice completely.

The *perineum* consists of muscles and fascia of the urogenital diaphragm and lies across the pubic arch and the pelvic diaphragm (Fig. 8-7). The pelvic diaphragm itself consists of the *coccygeus* and the *levator ani muscles*, together with the fascia covering their internal and external surfaces. It is the most inferior portion of the body wall and stretches across the pelvic cavity like a hammock. The levator ani forms a slinglike support for the pelvis. It can generally be separated into two parts, the *pubococcygeus* and the *iliococcygeus*. The pubococcygeus, as its name implies, arises from the dorsal sur-

face of the pubis. It is separated from its counterpart on the opposite side by the urethra, vagina, and rectum. Behind the rectum the two pubococcygeus muscles join, forming a loop or sling. The more superficial fibers of these muscles are attached to the perineal body. The iliococcygeus is the most lateral portion of the levator ani, arising from the ischial spine and inserting in the last two segments of the coccyx as well as in the perineal body. Between the anus and the vagina, the levator ani is reinforced by a central tendon of the perineum, where three pairs or muscles converge: the *bulbocavernous*, the *superficial transverse muscles of the perineum*, and the *external sphincter ani*. These structures, which constitute the perineal body, are also joined by fibers of the levator ani and together form the main support of the pelvic floor. They are often lacerated during delivery.

The *pubococcygeus muscle* is the muscle located immediately adjacent to the urethra, vagina, and rectum. Because it forms a sling around the structure, it is one of the most important muscles in terms of pelvic support. If this muscle becomes attenuated as a result of childbirth, the support of these structures is altered, with possible herniation of the bladder (cystocele) and rectum (rectocele), as well as descent into the vagina of the cervix and uterus. Associated symptoms of this condition include urinary stress incontinence (inability to retain urine with coughing or sudden movement). Correction of these conditions can sometimes be accomplished with the use of exercises designed to strengthen the pubococcygeus muscles. Patients can be

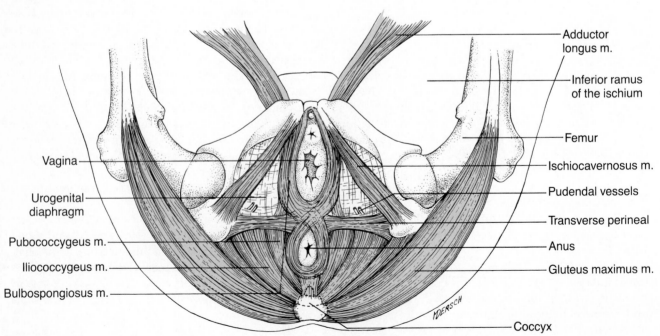

Vagina
Urogenital diaphragm
Pubococcygeus m.
Iliococcygeus m.
Bulbospongiosus m.

Adductor longus m.
Inferior ramus of the ischium
Femur
Ischiocavernosus m.
Pudendal vessels
Transverse perineal
Anus
Gluteus maximus m.
Coccyx

■ *Figure 8-7*
Muscles of the pelvic floor (female perineum).

instructed to contract these muscles, and successful use of such exercises can sometimes obviate the necessity for corrective surgical procedures.

Internal Organs

The internal organs of reproduction are the *vagina*, the *uterus*, the *fallopian* or *uterine tubes*, and the *ovaries* (Figs. 8-8 and 8-9).

OVARIES

The *ovaries* are two almond-shaped glandular organs that are situated in the upper part of the pelvic cavity on either side of the uterus. They are embedded in the posterior fold of the broad ligament of the uterus and are supported by the suspensory, the ovarian, and the mesovarium ligaments (see Fig. 8-9). The ovaries are composed of three layers: the tunica albuginea, serving a protective function; the cortex, containing the ova, graafian follicles, corpora lutea, corpora albicantia, and degenerated follicles; and the medulla, containing the

nerves and the blood and lympatic vessels. Although there is some variation in the size of the ovaries among women and with the phase of the menstrual cycle, each organ weighs approximately 6 to 19 g and is 1.5 to 3 cm wide and 2 to 5 cm long.

The chief functions of the ovaries are the development and the expulsion of ova and the provision of certain internal secretions, or hormones (estrogen and progesterone). The ovaries correspond to the testes in the male.

Each ovary contains a large number of germ cells, or primordial ova, in its substance at birth. This huge storage of primordial follicles present at birth more than suffices the woman for life. It is believed that no more are formed and that this large initial store is gradually exhausted during the period of sexual maturity. Beginning at puberty, one of the follicles that contain the ova enlarges each month and ruptures. The ovum and the fluid content of the follicle are released from the ovary; then they are swept into the tube. The absence of peritoneal covering on the ovaries aids eruption of the mature ovum. The development and the maturation of follicles containing the ova continue from puberty to menopause.

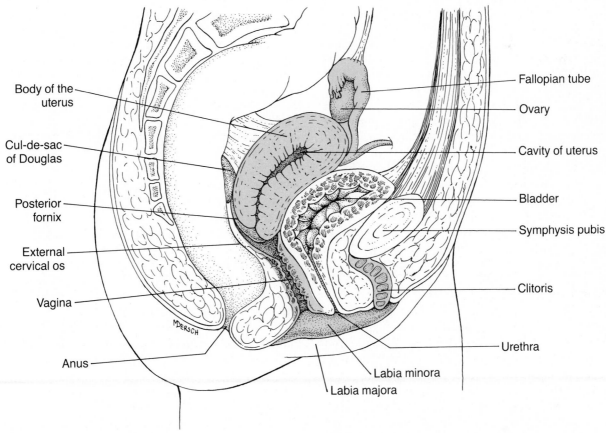

■ *Figure 8–8*
Female reproductive organs as seen in sagittal section.

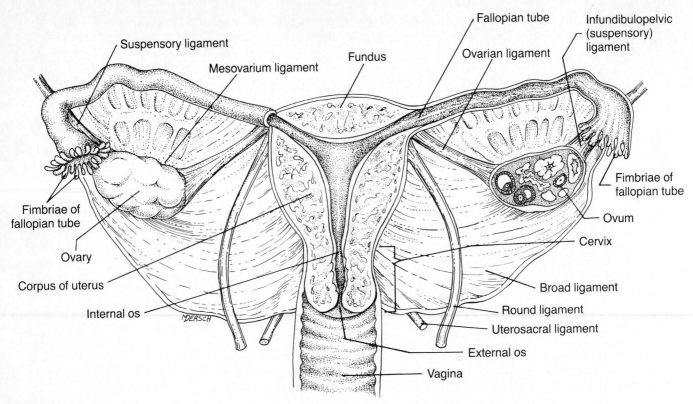

■ *Figure 8–9*
Anterior view of the uterus and related structures.

The arteries that supply the ovaries are four or five branches that arise from the anastomosis of the ovarian artery with the ovarian branch of the uterine artery (Fig. 8-10). The veins that drain the ovary become tributaries to both the uterine and the ovarian plexus. Superiorly, the ovarian vein drains into the inferior vena cava on the right and into the renal vein on the left.

The nerves supplying the ovaries are derived from the craniosacral and the thoracolumbar sympathetic systems. The postganglionic and visceral afferent fibers form a plexus that surrounds the ovarian artery, which is formed by contributions from the renal and the aortic plexuses and corresponds to the spermatic plexus in the male.

FALLOPIAN TUBES

The *fallopian tubes* are two trumpet-shaped, thin, flexible, muscular tubes that are about 12 cm long. They extend from the uterine cornua along the upper margin of the broad ligaments to the ovaries. Each tube is sectioned in three parts: the isthmus, the ampulla, and the infundibulum (fimbria). The straight and narrow isthmus has a thick, muscular wall and a lumen 2 to 3 mm in diameter. The curved ampulla contains the outer two thirds of the tube and is adjacent to the isthmus. It is the site of fertilization of the primary oocyte by a sper-

matozoon. The ampulla ends in the infundibulum, which is shaped like a funnel and is comprised of many fingerlike projections known as *fimbriae*. The fallopian tubes have two openings, one into the uterine cavity and the other into the abdominal cavity. The opening into the uterine cavity is minute and will admit only a fine bristle. The abdominal opening is larger and is surrounded by a large number of fimbriae. The fimbriated extremity lies near the ovary, but it is not necessarily in direct contact with it. It is generally believed that the cilia on the fimbriated end of the tube create a current in the layer of fluid that surrounds the various pelvic organs.

The tubes convey the ovum by ciliary action and peristalsis to the cavity of the uterus. The fimbriated ends of the tube convey the escaped ovum into the tube, where fertilization occurs.

The tubes are lined with mucous membrane that contains ciliated and secretory epithelium. The muscular layer is made up of longitudinal and circular fibers that provide peristaltic action. The serous membrane covering the tubes is a continuation of the peritoneum, which lines the whole abdominal cavity.

The fallopian tubes receive their blood supply from the ovarian and the uterine arteries (see Fig. 8-10). The veins of the tubes follow the course of these arteries and empty into the uterine and the ovarian trunks. The

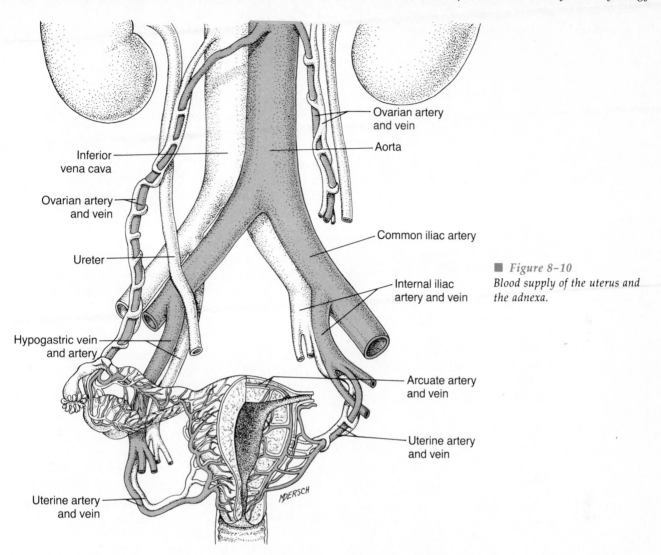

Inferior vena cava

Ovarian artery and vein

Ureter

Hypogastric vein and artery

Uterine artery and vein

Ovarian artery and vein

Aorta

Common iliac artery

Internal iliac artery and vein

Arcuate artery and vein

Uterine artery and vein

MDERSCH

■ *Figure 8–10*
Blood supply of the uterus and the adnexa.

fallopian tubes are innervated by parasympathetic and sympathetic motor and sensory nerves from the pelvic plexus and ovarian plexus.

UTERUS

The *uterus* is a hollow, thick-walled, muscular organ (see Fig. 8-9). It serves two important functions: (1) it is the organ of menstruation; and (2) during pregnancy, it receives the fertilized ovum and retains and nourishes it until it expels the fetus during labor.

The uterus varies in size and shape according to the age of the woman and whether or not she has borne children. The uterus of the adult nullipara weighs approximately 60 g and measures 5.5 to 8 cm in length.

It resembles a flattened pear in appearance and has two divisions, the upper triangular portion, the *corpus*, composed mainly of myometrium, and the lower constricted cylindrical portion, the *cervix*, which projects into the vagina. The fallopian tubes extend from the

cornu (the Latin word meaning *horn*) of the uterus at the upper outer margin on either side. The upper rounded portion of the uterus between the points of insertion of the tubes is the fundus (see Fig. 8-9).

The nonpregnant uterus is situated in the pelvic cavity between the bladder and the rectum. Almost the entire posterior wall and the upper portion of the anterior wall are covered by peritoneum. The lower portion of the anterior wall is united with the bladder wall by a layer of loose connective tissue. The lower posterior wall of the uterus and the upper portion of the vagina are separated from the rectum by the Douglas cul-de-sac, or pouch of Douglas.

Because of its muscular composition, the uterus is capable of enlarging to accommodate a growing fetus; at the termination of pregnancy it weighs about 1 kg, or 2 lbs. It is made up of involuntary muscle fibers that are arranged in all directions, making expansion possible in every direction to accommodate the products of conception. The arrangement of the uterus enables the fetus to be expelled at the end of a normal labor. Arranged between these muscular layers are many blood vessels, lymphatics, and nerves.

The cavity of the uterus is somewhat triangular. It is widest at the fundus, between the small openings into the fallopian tubes, and narrowest at the opening into the cervix. The anterior and posterior walls lie almost in contact, so that if a cross section of the uterus could be examined, the cavity between them would appear as a mere slit. The body of the uterus is lined with endometrium.

Cervix. The *cervix* is less movable than the body of the uterus. It is composed mainly of fibrous connective tissue with some muscle fibers and elastic tissue. The muscular wall of the cervix is not as thick, and its lining is different from the uterine body in that it is much folded and contains crypts that produce mucus; these are the chief source of the mucous secretion during the menstrual cycle and in pregnancy. The cervix has an upper opening, the *internal os*, leading from the cavity of the uterine body into the cervical canal, and a lower opening, the *external os*, opening into the vagina. The cervical canal is small (about 2 to 2.5 cm in external diameter) in the nonpregnant woman, barely admitting a probe. At the time of labor, the cervix dilates to a size sufficient to permit the passage of the fetus.

Ligaments. The uterus is supported by ligaments extending from either side of the uterus and by the muscles of the pelvic floor. The ligaments that support the uterus in the pelvic cavity are the broad ligaments, the round ligaments, and the uterosacral ligament (see Fig. 8-9).

The *broad ligaments* are two winglike structures that extend from the lateral margins of the uterus to the pelvic walls and divide the pelvic cavity into an anterior and a posterior compartment. Each consists of folds of peritoneum that envelope the fallopian tubes, the ovaries, and the round and ovarian ligaments. Its lower portion, the *cardinal ligament*, is composed of dense connective tissue that is firmly joined to the supravaginal portion of the cervix. The median margin is connected with the lateral margin of the uterus and encloses the uterine vessels.

The *round ligaments* are two fibrous cords that are attached on either side of the fundus, just below the fallopian tubes. They extend forward through the inguinal canal and terminate in the upper portion of the labia majora. These ligaments aid in holding the fundus forward.

The *uterosacral ligaments* are two cordlike structures that extend from the posterior cervical portion of the uterus to the sacrum. They help to support the cervix. The uterovesical ligament is merely a fold of the peritoneum that passes over the fundus and extends over the bladder. The rectovaginal ligament is a fold of the peritoneum that passes over the posterior surface of the uterus and is reflected on the rectum.

Uterine Blood Supply. The uterus receives its blood supply from the ovarian and the uterine arteries (see Fig. 8-10). The uterine artery, the principal source, is the main branch of the hypogastric artery, which enters the base of the broad ligament and makes its way to the side of the uterus. The ovarian artery is a branch of the aorta. It enters the broad ligament and, as it reaches the ovary, it breaks up into smaller branches that enter that organ, while its main stem makes its way to the upper margin of the uterus, where it anastomoses with the ovarian branch of the uterine artery.

The uterovaginal plexus returns the blood from the uterus and the vagina to the venous circulation. These veins form a plexus of thin-walled vessels that are embedded in the layers of the uterine muscle. Emerging from this plexus, the trunks join the uterine vein, which is a double vein. These veins follow on either side of the uterine artery and eventually form one trunk that empties into the hypogastric vein, which makes its way into the internal iliac.

Uterine Nerve Supply. The uterus possesses an abundant nerve supply that is principally derived from the sympathetic nervous system and partly from the cerebrospinal and parasympathetic system. Both the sympathetic and the parasympathetic nerve supplies contain motor and a few sensory fibers. The functions of the nerve supplies of the two systems are mostly antagonistic. The sympathetic system causes muscular contraction and vasoconstriction, and the parasympathetic system inhibits contraction and leads to vasodilatation.

Position of Uterus. Because the uterus is a freely movable organ that is suspended in the pelvic cavity between the bladder and the rectum, the position of the uterus may be influenced by a full bladder or full rectum. The uterus can be pushed backward or forward. The uterus also changes its position when the patient stands, lies flat, or turns on her side. Variations may exist in position, such as anteflexion, in which the fundus is tipped far forward; retroversion, in which the fundus is tipped far backward; and prolapse, which occurs when the muscles of the pelvic floor and the uterine ligaments are attenuated (Fig. 8-11).

Lymphatic Vessels. A complex lymphatic drainage system channels through the vagina, with vessels draining the upper, middle, and lower parts of the structure. The lymphatic vessels drain into several lymph nodes (e.g., inguinal, lumbar, and external iliac).

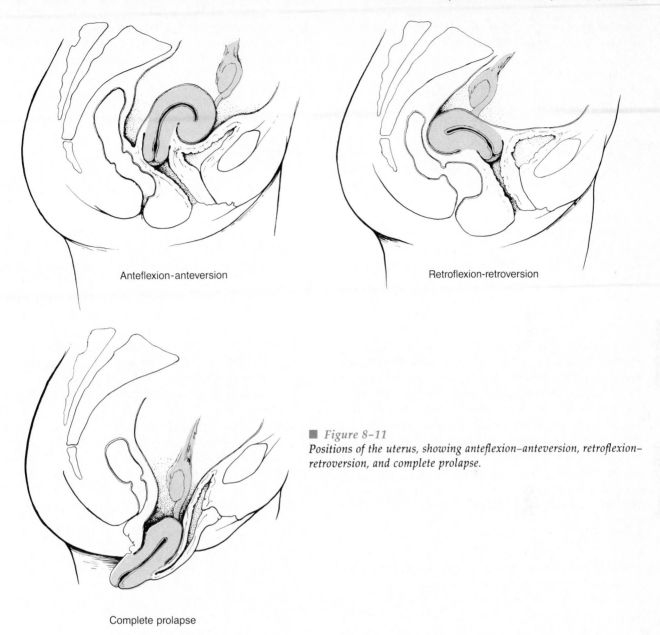

Anteflexion-anteversion

Retroflexion-retroversion

■ *Figure 8-11*
Positions of the uterus, showing anteflexion–anteversion, retroflexion–
retroversion, and complete prolapse.

Complete prolapse

VAGINA

The *vagina* is a dilatable, mucous membrane-lined passage between the bladder and the rectum (see Fig. 8-8). The vaginal opening occupies the lower portion of the vestibule. The vagina is from 8 to 12 cm long, and at the upper end is a blind vault, commonly called the *fornix*, into which the lower portion of the cervix projects.

The fornix is divided into four parts for descriptive purposes. The lateral fornices are the spaces between the vaginal wall on either side and the cervix; the anterior fornix is between the anterior vaginal wall and the cervix; and the posterior fornix is between the pos-

terior vaginal wall and the cervix. The posterior fornix is considerably deeper than the anterior fornix because the vagina is attached higher up on the posterior than the anterior wall of the cervix. The fornices are important for two reasons: they provide space for semen to collect after intercourse, thereby improving the chances of conception; and their thin walls usually enable the examiner to palpate the internal pelvic organs.

The vagina serves three important functions: (1) it represents the excretory duct of the uterus through which secretion and the menstrual flow escape; (2) it is the female organ of copulation; and (3) it forms part of the birth canal during labor. Its walls are arranged into thick folds, the columns of the vagina, and, in women who have not borne children, numerous ridges, or *rugae*, which extend outward and almost at right angles to the vaginal columns and give the surface a corrugated appearance. Normally, the anterior and the posterior walls of the vagina lie in contact, but they are capable of stretching to allow marked distention of the passage, as in the process of childbirth. In the anterior wall of the vagina and adjacent to the urethra is located a highly sensitive center named the *Grafenberg spot*, commonly known as the *G spot*. This area is surrounded by delicate erectile tissue similar to that found in the penis and clitoris.[3]

The vagina receives an abundant blood supply from branches of the uterine, the inferior vesical, the median hemorrhoidal, and the internal pudendal arteries. The passage is surrounded by a venous plexus; the vessels follow the course of the arteries and eventually empty into the hypogastric veins. The lymphatics empty into the inguinal, the hypogastric, and the iliac glands.

The acidic environment that exists in the vagina (pH 4–5) during the reproductive years is a result of the symbiotic relationship between the lactic acid-producing bacilli and the vaginal epithelial cells. The bacilli break down the glycogen produced by the vaginal epithelial cells into lactic acid. This delicate balance may be adversely effected by antibiotic therapy, alterations in the levels of ovarian hormones, douching, or use of vaginal suppositories, sprays, or deodorants.

Related Pelvic Organs

BLADDER

The *bladder* is a muscular sac that serves as a reservoir for urine. It is situated in front of the uterus and behind the symphysis pubis (see Fig. 8-8). When empty or moderately distended, it remains entirely in the pelvis, but if it becomes greatly distended, it rises into the abdomen. Urine is conducted into the bladder by the ureters, two tubes that extend down from the basin of the kidneys and over the brim of the pelvis beneath the uterine vessels to open into the bladder at about the level of the cervix. The bladder is emptied through the urethra, a short tube that terminates in the urethral meatus. Lying on either side of the urethra and almost parallel with it are two small glands, less than 2.5 cm long, known as *Skene's glands*. Their ducts empty into the urethra just above the meatus. Often in cases of gonorrhea, Skene's glands and ducts are involved.

ANUS

The *anus* is the entrance to the rectal canal. The rectal canal is surrounded at the opening or anus by its

sphincter muscle, which binds it to the coccyx behind and to the perineum in front. It is supported by the muscles passing into it; these are the muscles that help to support the pelvic floor (see Fig. 8-8). The rectum is considered here because of the proximity to the field of delivery.

Mammary Glands

Although the mammary glands are not actual organs of reproduction, they are discussed in this section because of their importance as accessory glands, especially in the female body, and because they are directly affected by the female hormones.

The *breasts*, or mammary glands, are two highly specialized cutaneous glands located on the anterior chest wall between the second and third ribs superiorly, the sixth and seventh costal cartilages inferiorly, the anterior axillary line laterally, and the sternal border medially (Fig. 8-12). They are abundantly supplied with nerves. The breasts contain tissue that responds to hormones. Thus, breast development at puberty and lactation during pregnancy occur as a result of endocrine influences.

The internal mammary and the intercostal arteries supply the breast glands, and the mammary veins follow these arteries. Also, there are many cutaneous veins that become dilated during lactation. The lymphatics are abundant, especially toward the axilla. These breast glands are present in the male but exist only in the rudimentary state.

INTERNAL STRUCTURE

The breasts of a woman who never has borne a child are conic or hemispheric in form, but they vary in size and shape at different ages and in different persons. In women who have borne one or more babies, the breasts may become pendulous. At the termination of pregnancy, certain exercises may aid in restoring the tone of the breast tissue.

The breasts are made up of glandular tissue and fat. Each organ is divided into 15 or 20 lobes, which are separated from each other by fibrous and fatty walls. Each lobe is subdivided into many lobules, which contain numerous acini cells. The *acini* are composed of a single layer of epithelium, beneath which is a small amount of connective tissue richly supplied with capillaries. The products necessary for the milk are filtered from the blood by the process of osmosis, but the secretion of the milk really begins in the acini cells. As the ducts leading from the lobules to the lobes approach the nipple, they are dilated to form little reservoirs in which the milk is stored; they narrow again as they pass into the nipple. The size of the breast depends on the

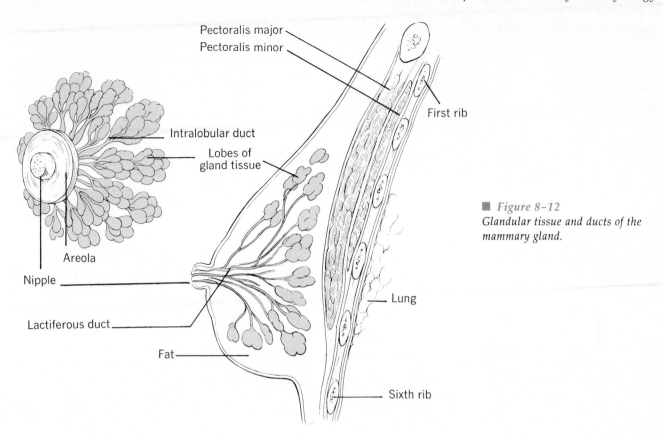

Pectoralis major
Pectoralis minor
First rib
Intralobular duct
Lobes of
gland tissue
Areola
Nipple
Lung
Lactiferous duct
Fat
Sixth rib

■ *Figure 8–12*
Glandular tissue and ducts of the mammary gland.

amount of fatty tissue present and in no way denotes the amount of lactation possible.

EXTERNAL STRUCTURE

The external surface of the breast is divided into three portions. The first is the smooth and soft area of skin extending from the circumference of the gland to the areola.

The second is the *areola*, which surrounds the nipple and is of a delicate pinkish hue in blondes and a darker rose color in brunettes. The surface of the areola is roughed by small fine lumps of papillae, known as *Montgomery's glands*. These enlarged sebaceous glands, which are white and are scattered over the areola, become more marked during pregnancy. Under the influence of gestation, the areola becomes darker, and, in many cases, this pigmentation constitutes a helpful sign of pregnancy in the primigravida.

The *nipple* is largely composed of sensitive, erectile tissue; it forms a large conic papilla projecting from the center of the areola; and its summit is at the openings of the milk ducts. There are 3 to 20 milk duct openings.

Breast care (see Chaps. 19 and 28) constitutes one of the important phases of the nursing care of the maternity patient throughout pregnancy and the puerperium.

Female Sexual Maturity

Sexual maturity in the female begins at the time of puberty, with the onset of dramatic bodily changes. The first sign of pubertal development is the onset of breast budding (*thelarche*), which occurs at about 10 years, with a range from approximately 8 to 13 years.[2] The whole process of puberty spans about 3 years. Early in the course of puberty, axillary and pubic hair appear. Shortly thereafter, there is a gradual change in the contour of the labia. The peak growth spurt in girls occurs approximately 1 year after the onset of puberty, and growth is largely completed by the age at which first menstruation begins, *menarche*. Establishment of the menstrual cycle is the most clearly identifiable sign of puberty and serves as an indication that the internal sex organs are approaching maturity. These physical changes are accompanied by emotional changes.

With maturation, fat deposition in girls increases, and their lean body mass decreases from 80% to 75%. The increase in body fat to a critical level of about 17% is believed by some to stimulate the onset of menses.[2] This theory, if correct, would explain the trend for earlier onset of menarche evident in Western countries since 1840, based on better nutrition among adolescents.[2]

Tanner's stages for the development of female secondary sex characteristics are displayed in Table 8-2. Girls are assigned a sexual maturity rating based on

TABLE 8–2. TANNER STAGING IN FEMALES

Stage	Breasts	Pubic Hair	Other*	Range in Years
I	None	None		Birth to 15
II	Breast budding (thelarche): areolar hyperplasia with small amount of breast tissue, erect papillae	Long, downy pubic hair over mons veneris or labia majora; may occur with breast budding or several weeks or months later (pubarche)	Thickening of vaginal epithelium tissue, lowering of vaginal pH	8½–15
III	Further enlargement of breast tissue and widening of areola with no separation of their contours	Increase in amount of hair (dark, coarse and curly) spread sparsely over junction of pubes	Peak height spurt begins; enlargement of uterus; axillary hair begins to appear	10–15
IV	Double contour form: areola and papillae form secondary mound on top of breast tissue	Adult appearance but less area covered, no spread to medial aspects of thighs	Axillary hair present, uterus enlarges, vaginal discharge	10–17
V	Larger, mature breast with single contour form	Adult distribution and quantity with spread to medial aspects of thighs	Adult characteristics present	12½–18

* Criteria not included in original Tanner stages.

(Adapted from Wasserman G, Gromisch DS: Survey of Clinical Pediatrics, 7th ed. New York, McGraw-Hill, 1981; Tanner JM: Growth at Adolescence, 2nd ed. Oxford, Blackwell Scientific Publications, 1969; and Marshall WA, Tanner JM: Variations in Pattern of Pubertal Changes in Girls. Arch Dis Child 44:291–303, 1969)

pubic hair and breast development. The time sequence of changes that culminates in the attainment of reproductive potential varies considerably from person to person. Bodily manifestations of puberty, such as the beginning of breast development, the appearance of pubic hair, and a spurt of growth, precede the actual onset of menstruation by a variable amount of time.

Throughout puberty there is an interplay of physiological and sociocultural forces, and often the nurse is called on to explain the bodily and psychological changes in puberty to mothers who have daughters approaching their teens. There is often anxiety about the onset of pubertal changes that are thought to be occurring too early or too late. Therefore, it is important to recognize the wide variability from one young woman to the next. The progression of puberty is considered abnormal if more than 5 years elapse between thelarche and menarche in the female.[4]

■ MENSTRUATION AND OVULATION

Menstruation is the periodic discharge of blood, mucus, and epithelial cells from the uterus. It usually occurs at monthly intervals throughout the reproductive period, except during pregnancy and lactation, when it is usually suppressed.

The monthly flow of blood is only one phase of a marvelous cyclic process that not only makes childbearing possible but also profoundly influences both body and mind. For this reason, the time of the onset of menstruation is a critical period in the life of a young woman.

The span of years during which childbearing is possible, that is, from about ages 12 to 45, corresponds to the period during which ovulation and menstruation occur. In general, a woman who menstruates is able to conceive, whereas one who does not is probably infertile. Ovulation and menstruation are closely interlinked, and because no process of nature is purposeless, menstruation must play some vital and indispensable role in childbearing.

Menarche

Puberty refers to the entire transitional period between childhood and sexual maturity. Menarche is one sign of puberty that usually occurs between the ages of 9 and 16. In the majority of girls, menarche begins during breast development (Tanner stage 3 or 4), but in some, it will not occur until their breasts are fully mature.[5] Heredity, race, state of nutrition, climate, and environment may influence the onset of menarche. For example, maturity tends to occur earlier in warm climates and later in cold regions. The age of onset of menarche has declined steadily until recent years; this decline has now ceased in the United States. Nutritional advances and an improved sedentary, agrarian lifestyle in women are believed to have led to earlier menarche.[5,6] The reproductive period spans about 35 years, from some point after the beginning of menstruation until its cessation during menopause.

Throughout childhood the *gonadotropins*, hormones produced by the pituitary gland to stimulate the ovaries, appear in very low concentrations. Estrogen, produced by the ovaries in the adult, remains undetectable. Puberty begins when there is a rise in the release of gonadotropins from the pituitary gland. These stimulate the ovary to secrete increasing amounts of *estrogen*, the hormone responsible for many of the bodily changes of puberty.

An orderly sequence of endocrinological events resulting in ovulation may not occur initially. The first few menstrual cycles following the menarche may not be associated with ovulation and are often irregular. However, once menstruation has occurred, it must be assumed that there is ovulation and, therefore, fertility and the potential for pregnancy.

Ovulation and the Ovarian Cycle

Each month, with considerable regularity, a blisterlike structure about 1 cm in diameter develops on the surface of one of the ovaries. Within this bubble, almost lost in the fluid and cells around it, lies a tiny speck, scarcely visible to the naked eye (a thimble would hold 3 million of these specks). This speck is the human ovum, a truly amazing structure. It not only has the potential to develop into a human being but it also embodies the mental as well as physical traits of the woman and her ancestry. These traits could be her own brown eyes, her father's tall stature, her mother's genius at mathematics, or her grandfather's love of music. These and a million other potentials are contained in the ovum, which is so small that it is about one fourth the size of the period at the end of this sentence.

In the process of ovulation, one blister on one ovary ruptures at a given time each month and discharges an ovum. The precise day on which ovulation occurs is a matter of no small significance. For instance, because the ovum can only be fertilized (impregnated by the spermatozoon, or male germ cell) within hours after its escape from the ovary, the day after ovulation a woman is no longer fertile. However, a woman is potentially fertile for a number of days preceding the actual time of ovulation because spermatozoa survive in the female reproductive tract for hours, even days, awaiting the arrival of the ovum.

In a given cycle, the time of ovulation is unpredictable. Even the woman who consistently has regular menstrual periods could experience a delayed or early ovulation in any one cycle. This possibility of irregularity, combined with the potential for fertility any time prior to ovulation due to the fact that spermatozoa retain their ability for fertilization, makes it difficult to identify accurately the fertile phase of a given cycle.

It should be remembered that the only really infertile interval is after ovulation has occurred. The time between ovulation and menstruation is relatively constant (14 ± 2 days); the time between menstruation and ovulation is variable enough that ovulation cannot be accurately predicted from one cycle to the next.

GRAAFIAN FOLLICLE

In delving further into the process of ovulation, we find that, at birth, each ovary contains a huge number of undeveloped ova, probably more than 400,000. These are rather large, round cells with clear cytoplasm and a good-sized nucleus occupying the center. Each ovum is surrounded by a layer of a few small, flattened or spindle-shaped cells. The whole structure, ovum and surrounding cells, is a *follicle*, but in its underdeveloped state at birth it is a *primordial follicle*.

The formation of primordial follicles ceases at birth or shortly after, and the large number contained in the ovaries of the newborn represents a lifetime supply. The majority have disappeared before puberty, so that there are then perhaps 30,000 left. This disintegration of follicles continues throughout reproductive life until menopause when, usually, none are found.

Meanwhile, from birth to the menopause, a few of these primordial follicles show signs of development. The surrounding granular layers of cells begin to multiply rapidly until they are several layers deep; at the same time, they become cuboid in shape. As this proliferation of cells continues, a very important fluid develops between them, the *follicular fluid*.

After puberty, the cells within the developing follicles produce estrogenic hormones, which in turn act on the reproductive organs and bring about cyclic bodily changes. During each menstrual cycle, several follicles develop further. One of these is finally selected, by a process not as yet completely understood, for complete maturation and ovulation.

Follicular fluid accumulates in such quantities that the multiplying follicle cells are pushed toward the margin; the ovum itself is almost surrounded by fluid and is suspended from the periphery of the follicle by only a small neck of cells. The structure is now known as the *graafian follicle*.

As it increases enormously in size, the graafian follicle naturally pushes aside other follicles that form each month, and a very noticeable, blisterlike projection appears on the surface of the ovary. At one point the follicular capsule becomes thin, and as the ovum reaches full maturity, it breaks free from the few cells attaching it to the periphery and floats in the follicular fluid. The thinned area of the capsule now ruptures, and the ovum is expelled from the ovary in the process of ovulation (Fig. 8-13).

CHANGES IN THE CORPUS LUTEUM

After the discharge of the ovum, the ruptured follicle undergoes a change. It becomes filled with large cells containing a special yellow matter. The follicle then is known as the *corpus luteum*, or yellow body. If pregnancy does not occur, the corpus luteum reaches full development in about 8 days, then retrogresses and is gradually replaced by fibrous tissue, the *corpus albicans*.

If pregnancy occurs, the corpus luteum enlarges somewhat and persists throughout the period of gestation, reaching its maximum size about the fourth or fifth month and retrogressing slowly thereafter. The corpus luteum secretes an extremely important substance, progesterone, which will be discussed later in this chapter.

In the absence of pregnancy, the corpus luteum remains active for about 2 weeks. The corpus luteum produces progesterone for the standard duration of the postovulatory phase of the menstrual cycle.

The Menstrual Cycle

If day by day we observed the *endometrium*, the lining membrane of the uterus, we would note some remarkable alterations (Fig. 8-14). These changes have only one purpose, to provide a suitable bed for the fertilized ovum to secure nourishment and to grow. If an ovum is not fertilized, these alterations serve no useful function.

The menstrual cycle is broken into three phases: proliferative, secretory, and menstrual. The menstrual cycle is related directly to the ovarian cycle, and both are under hormonal influences. Hormones are discussed after this section.

PROLIFERATIVE PHASE

Immediately following menstruation, the endometrium is very thin. During the subsequent week or so it proliferates markedly. The cells on the surface become

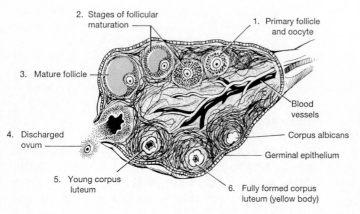

2. Stages of follicular maturation
1. Primary follicle and oocyte
3. Mature follicle
Blood vessels
4. Discharged ovum
Corpus albicans
Germinal epithelium
5. Young corpus luteum
6. Fully formed corpus luteum (yellow body)

■ *Figure 8–13*
Ovarian follicle development.

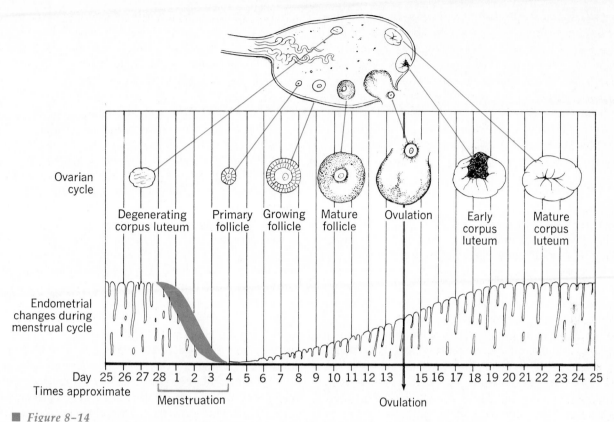

■ Figure 8–14

Schematic representation of one ovarian cycle and the corresponding changes in thickness of the endometrium. It is thickest just before the onset of menstruation and thinnest just as it ceases.

taller, while the glands that dip into the endometrium become longer and wider. As the result of these changes, the thickness of the endometrium increases sixfold or eightfold. Its glands become more and more active and secrete a rich, nutritive substance.

Each month during this phase of the menstrual cycle (from approximately the 5th to the 14th days), a graafian follicle is approaching its greatest development and is manufacturing increasing amounts of follicular fluid. This fluid contains the estrogenic hormone *estrogen*. Because estrogen causes the endometrium to grow or proliferate, this phase of the menstrual cycle is called the *proliferative phase*. Sometimes it is referred to as the *follicular*, or *estrogenic*, *phase*.

SECRETORY PHASE

Following the release of the ovum from the graafian follicle (ovulation), the cells that form the corpus luteum begin to secrete another important hormone, *progesterone*, in addition to estrogen. This supplements the action of estrogen on the endometrium in such a way that the glands become very tortuous or corkscrewed in appearance and are greatly dilated. This change occurs because the glands are swollen with a secretion.

Meanwhile, the blood supply of the endometrium is increased, and it becomes vascular and succulent. The process reaches its height; the endometrium is now of the thickness of heavy, downy velvet and has become soft and succulent with blood and glandular secretions. At this time the ovum, if it has been fertilized, is embedded into this luxuriant lining.

These effects are directed at providing a bed for the fertilized ovum. This phase of the cycle occupies the last 14 ± 2 days and is called the *secretory phase*. Sometimes it is referred to as the *progestational*, *luteal*, or *premenstrual phase*.

MENSTRUAL PHASE

Unless the ovum is fertilized, the corpus luteum is short lived. Because corpus luteum cells secrete both progesterone and estrogen, cessation of the corpus luteum activity means a withdrawal of both of these hormones. As a result, the endometrium degenerates. This is associated with rupture of countless small blood vessels in the endometrium with innumerable minute hemorrhages. The disintegrated endometrium and blood and glandular secretions escape into the uterine cavity, pass through the cervix, and flow out through the vagina, carrying the tiny unfertilized ovum with them. In other words, menstruation represents the abrupt termination of a process designed to prepare lodging for a fertilized ovum. It forecasts the breakdown of a bed that is not needed because fertilization did not occur. Thus, its purpose is to clear away the old bed so that a new and fresh one may be created the next month. This phase of the cycle (from approximately the first to the fifth days) is called the *menstrual phase*.

Hormonal Control of the Cycles

The menstrual cycle is regulated primarily through the highly coordinated function of the brain, the hypothalamus, the pituitary, the ovaries, and the uterus. If it were possible to inspect the ovaries from day to day during the menstrual cycle, it would be noted that the uterine alterations are directly related to certain changes that take place in the ovary. If it were possible to look further, it might be seen that the alterations that occur regularly in the ovarian cycle are directly related to certain phenomena that take place in the anterior pituitary gland and the hypothalamus, a portion of the brain that lies above the pituitary. Thus, the whole sequence represents the harmonious, integrated reactions of several processes within the human organism, all of which are necessary to maintain proper relationships in the menstrual cycle.

ROLE OF THE PITUITARY GLAND

The pituitary gland is essential in the function of the reproductive system.* The anterior lobe of the pituitary, the "master clock," releases the gonadotropins, to stimulate the ovary, as well as other hormones. These hormones produce the ovarian alterations associated with ovulation. There are two principal gonadotropins. One is *follicle-stimulating hormone*; as its name implies, FSH stimulates the development of the follicle. The other is LH, which is principally active during ovulation and the luteal phase of the cycle.

The release of the gonadotropic hormones by the pituitary is regulated by the *hypothalamus*, a specialized structure within the brain located just above the pituitary. The hypothalamus has a vascular connection to the pituitary gland, as well as nerve connections to the central nervous system. Its function can be modified by influences within the central nervous system. Thus, the function of the pituitary gland may be affected by the brain. The cyclic release of gonadotropin by the pituitary

gland is controlled by a hormonal agent released by the hypothalamus. This is called *gonadotropin-releasing hormone* or LH/FSH-releasing hormone (GnRH or LH/FSH-RH), because it triggers the release of both FSH and LH from the pituitary gland.

CYCLIC PATTERN

Sensitive laboratory methods now allow accurate measurement of day-to-day changes in circulating pituitary and ovarian hormones (Fig. 8-15). The interplay between the pituitary and the ovary, influenced in turn by the central nervous system through the hypothalamus, brings about orderly development of the follicle and ovulation.

At the end of a given cycle and at the beginning of the subsequent cycle (see Fig. 8-15), the pituitary gland releases increased amounts of FSH. With the help of small amounts of LH, FSH stimulates maturation of several ovarian follicles. Together, LH and FSH produce modest amounts of the estrogen estradiol. The levels of estradiol in the bloodstream begin to rise, and estradiol in turn acts negatively on the central nervous system at the hypothalamic-pituitary level by inhibiting the release of additional amounts of FSH. Consequently, the level of FSH in the circulating blood begins to fall. FSH also acts on the follicle to make it more sensitive to LH.

About 2 days before ovulation, all but the one follicle that is destined to ovulate begin to regress in a process called *atresia*. That one follicle undergoes rapid growth, and estrogen production rises sharply. The increased amount of estrogen produced at this point then acts positively at the central nervous–hypothalamic level, stimulating a rapid increase in GnRH levels, In turn, GnRH causes large amounts of LH, as well as additional FSH, to be released from the pituitary gland. This dramatic rise in LH stimulates the completion of maturation of the follicle and, within 24 hours after the LH surge, ovulation takes place.

The increased levels of preovulatory estrogen prepare the genital tract for sperm migration. The secretions of the cervix, scanty and viscous early in the cycle, become thin and watery and more receptive to spermatozoa. The vaginal wall also reflects the effects of estrogen. A vaginal smear taken at this time reveals a large percentage of mature, or "cornified," cells. The endometrium displays maximal proliferation (see Fig. 8-14).

Following ovulation, the cyclic pattern continues. The ruptured follicle is transformed into a corpus luteum. The second function of LH is to maintain the corpus luteum. These endocrine events are associated with further modifications in the cervical mucus, vagina, and endometrium. The mucus becomes thick, "tacky," and viscous and is no longer as receptive to spermatozoa. The vaginal smear reflects the influence of progesterone with a decreasing "maturation index." The

---

* The posterior lobe of the pituitary gland produces oxytocin, a hormone that plays an important role in obstetrics but one that differs altogether from the purpose of the present discussion.

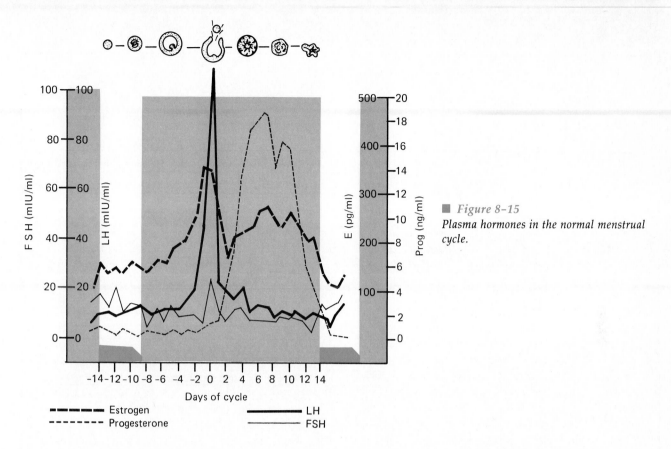

■ *Figure 8–15*
Plasma hormones in the normal menstrual cycle.

Days of cycle

- - - - - Estrogen   ——— LH
- - - - - - Progesterone   ——— FSH

endometrium takes on secretory changes preparatory to implantation.

Progesterone secretion by the corpus luteum reaches its maximum about 5 to 7 days after ovulation (see Fig. 8-15). This is the time when the fertilized egg, now a *blastocyst*, is ready to implant. If pregnancy has occurred, another hormone, *human chorionic gonadotropin (hCG)*, appears within 2 to 3 days of implantation. This hormone, which is produced by the conceptus, acts on the corpus luteum, maintaining its progesterone-providing function, and transforms it into a corpus luteum of pregnancy. If pregnancy has not intervened, the corpus luteum begins its demise at this time. Approximately 10 to 11 days after ovulation, progesterone levels decline precipitously, and on about the 14th postovulatory day, no longer receiving hormones, the endometrium begins to shed in the process of menstruation.

OTHER FUNCTIONS OF ESTROGEN AND PROGESTERONE

In addition to their role in controlling menstruation, estrogen and progesterone serve other important functions. Estrogen is responsible for the development of the secondary sex characteristics, that is, all those distinctive sex manifestations that are not directly concerned with the process of reproduction. Thus, the growth of the breasts at puberty, the distribution of body fat, the size of the larynx and its resulting influence

on the quality of the voice, as well as mating instincts, are all the results of estrogenic action.

Aside from its action on the endometrium, progesterone also helps to relax the uterine muscle. Thus, it plays an important role in preserving the life of the embryo in early pregnancy by preventing its expulsion from the uterus and by preparing the endometrium to receive and nourish it.

Variations in Cycles

Although the interval of the menstrual cycle, counting from the beginning of one period to the onset of the next, averages 28 days, there are wide variations even in the same woman. Indeed, it is rare for a woman to menstruate exactly every 28 or 30 days. This has been the subject of several studies on normal young women. These investigations show that the majority of women (almost 60%) experience variations of at least 5 days in the length of their menstrual cycles; differences in the same woman of even 10 days are not uncommon and may occur without explanation or apparent detriment to health.[7]

The degree and intensity of the outward manifestations of the ovulatory cycle vary from one woman to the next. Some women consistently experience pelvic discomfort during ovulation, or *mittelschmerz*, so named because it typically appears in the middle of a 28-day

Assessment Tool

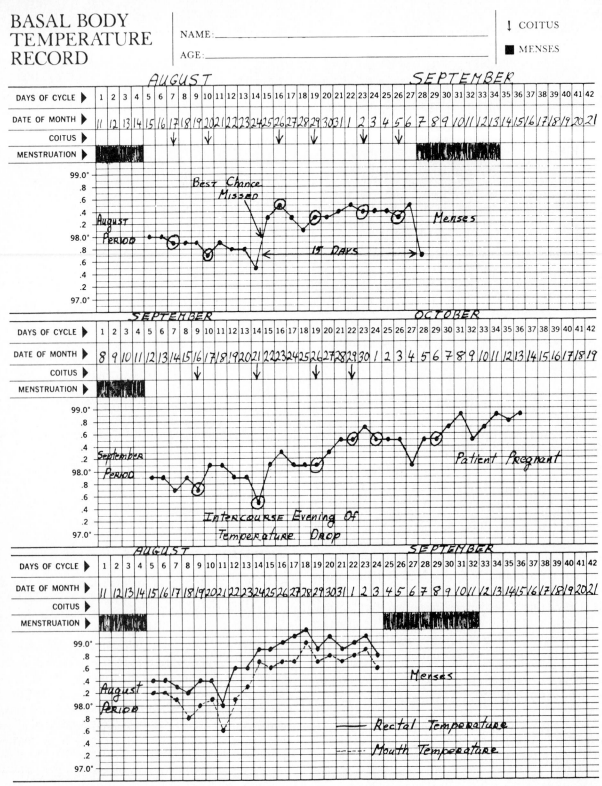

Samples of basal temperature charts indicating menstrual cycles and daily temperature readings. Temperature drops are clearly indicated on all charts, with optimal time for fertilization. Phases of the cycles are determined by these charts. Charts may be used in family planning or in management of infertility. The bottom chart contrasts oral and rectal temperatures. Directions for using this chart are given on the facing page.

(Published by Merrill-National Laboratories, Div. of Richardson-Merrill Inc., Cincinnati, Ohio 45215.)

Assessment Tool

Directions for Using the Basal Temperature Graph

1. The first day of menses is considered to be the first day of the menstrual cycle. The duration of menstrual flow is recorded, beginning on cycle day 1 (see graph). The date of onset of flow is recorded, and each subsequent date is recorded in the spaces provided. Following cessation of flow, the morning temperature is taken. Oral temperatures are as satisfactory as rectal recordings and are certainly more convenient. The temperature should be taken immediately after waking and before getting out of bed, talking, eating, drinking, or smoking. Ideally, it should be taken at about the same time every morning.
2. The thermometer is read to within 0.1 of a degree, and the reading is recorded on the chart.
3. Any known cause for temperature variation should be noted on the chart, for example, interrupted or shortened sleep, a cold, indigestion, or emotional disturbance. If intercourse has occured, that fact should be recorded with a circle around the recording the following morning.
4. Some women can recognize ovulation by mittelschmerz; others have vaginal bleeding or clear preovulatory vaginal discharge. Such manifestations should also be recorded on the chart.

menstrual cycle. Slight staining or occasional bleeding may occur in association with ovulation. In the post-ovulatory interval, there may be breast tenderness and fullness, which typically reaches a peak just before menstruation.

A variety of clinical syndromes may cause women to experience tension and other affective and somatic symptoms premenstrually. Chief among these is *premenstrual syndrome* (PMS), which involves symptoms that occur in repetitive fashion prior to menses (e.g., irritability, depression, and somatic complaints). A detailed discussion of PMS and other clinical variations in the menstrual cycle, such as dysmenorrhea and amenorrhea, is found in Chapter 48.

Determinants of Phases of Cycles

Not all menstrual cycles are of 28-day length, and ovulation cannot be determined by counting 14 days from the last menstrual period. Therefore, other means of establishing phases of ovulation have been determined. Two useful means of determining ovulation are observing daily variations in cervical mucus and checking basal body temperature. Both are used in infertility clinics and natural methods of contraception (see Chaps. 11 and 13).

VARIATIONS IN CERVICAL MUCUS

Under the influence of rapidly rising preovulatory levels of estrogen (see Fig. 8-15), the cervical mucus, scant and tacky early in the cycle, becomes copious and clear. It is most abundant on the day preceding ovulation and, not surprisingly, is most receptive to spermatozoa at that time. Following ovulation, under the influence of

progesterone, the mucus becomes scanty, thick, and sticky once again.

These cyclic changes in the quality of the cervical mucus are often easily detected by the normally menstruating woman once she is made aware of them. In some cases, a clear translucent mucus appears at the labia or may be wiped from the cervix to provide suggestive evidence of impending ovulation. In the postovulatory phase of the cycle, the sticky and less abundant mucus is not as easily detected. Daily observations of cervical mucus changes have been suggested as a useful parameter in using the rhythm method of contraception, also referred to as the *symtothermal approach*.

BASAL BODY TEMPERATURE

Beginning about the first year of life, slight daily variations in body temperature normally occur in all human beings. These temperature variations are relative to the time of the day and the nature of the circumstances surrounding the person. For example, the body temperature is lowest in the morning before breakfast, after a good night's rest, and before activity. After a day of normal activity, the body temperature is usually highest toward afternoon and early evening. The fact that physiological variations in basal body temperature also occur in relation to the menstrual cycle is important here because it can be useful in estimating the time of ovulation. Such an index becomes extremely important in studies of fertility and sterility.

In the woman who is ovulating, there is normally a rhythmic variation in the basal body temperature curve during the course of the menstrual cycle (see Basal Body Temperature Graph and Directions for Using). The basal temperature is lower during the first part of the menstrual cycle, the proliferative phase. It rises in association with ovulation and remains relatively higher during the luteal phase of the cycle. The rise in the basal temperature occurs as a result of the influence of progesterone, produced by the corpus luteum following ovulation. Progesterone causes this thermogenic effect through its influence on the central nervous system. The basal temperature rises as much as 0.5°, and a relatively higher temperature is sustained until just before the onset of the menstrual period. This interval occupies the 14 ± 2 terminal days in the cycle.

If pregnancy occurs, the progesterone level is maintained, and under its influence the basal temperature remains high past the expected time of the period. In the absence of pregnancy, the basal temperature usually drops a day or so before the menstrual period.

The Use of the Basal Temperature Graph. The basal body temperature is one of the most practical means of diagnosing ovulation. The relative difference in basal body temperature during the course of the cycle is the important diagnostic criterion for ovulation. It is only useful in the timing of ovulation retrospectively. Thus, when there is infertility, efforts to time intercourse to coincide with changes in the temperature chart may not prove helpful. In fact, such regulation of coital habits is often not recommended. However, for the diagnosis of ovulation, the temperature chart has proved valuable. The temperature chart may also be useful as an adjunct to the rhythm method of family planning (see Chap. 11).

■ MENOPAUSE

Menopause means the cessation of menstruation. In about 50% of women, this occurs between the ages of 45 and 50. About 25% will reach menopause before the age of 45, and 25% after the age of 50.[6] In common use, *menopause* generally means cessation of regular menstruation. Ovulation may occur sporadically or may cease abruptly. Hence, periods may end suddenly, may become scanty or irregular, or may be intermittently heavy before ceasing altogether. Markedly diminished ovarian activity, that is, significantly decreased estrogen production and cessation of ovulation, causes menopause. Often the terms *menopause* and *climacteric* are used synonymously, but the use is not accurate. *Climacteric* encompasses the total syndrome of endocrine, somatic, and psychic changes occurring at the termination of the reproductive period in the female. It is derived from the Greek word meaning *rung of the ladder*, or critical point in human life. The termination of cyclic estrogen production associated with greatly decreased

ovarian function causes the ovary, the uterus, and the breasts to decrease in size. The external genitals become flattened, and the vaginal walls lose their folds, elasticity, and lubrication, becoming shiny and smooth. The decrease in estrogen levels may also produce intermittent "hot flashes" and some emotional instability; for example, irritability and sudden outbursts of tears much like the emotional liability associated with PMS. Hot flashes are a result of vasomotor instability. This instability also results in sweating and brief sensations of being cold "all over." There may be redness and perspiration that are visible, or the sensations may be equally intense but with no visible signs. Their daily frequency may vary, and there can be long intervals, sometimes weeks, with no symptoms at all.

Each woman reacts somewhat differently to this withdrawal of estrogen. These reactions are unpredictable, vary from woman to woman, and depend to some extent on her previous emotional history and her present support systems within the family, and to a very real extent on the fact that the menopausal reproductive–endocrine system may be quite labile during this interval, which may last as long as 8 or 9 years.[8,9]

Artificial Menopause

Menopause may result from other than the natural physiological alterations of the climacteric. The term *artificial menopause* describes the cessation of menstruation produced by some artificial means, such as an irradiation of the ovaries or surgical operation for the removal of the ovaries (oophorectomy) or the uterus (hysterectomy). As a result of either surgery, the woman will no longer menstruate, but beyond this the manifestations in the client are not identical.

Certain misunderstandings based on incorrect interpretation of terminology are rather widespread and should be clarified. The fact that a woman has had a hysterectomy and ceases to menstruate does not mean that her healthy ovaries will not function. Hysterectomy involves only the removal of the uterus. On the other hand, if the ovaries are also removed surgically or are treated by irradiation, the source of estrogen is withdrawn abruptly and thus the symptoms caused by the sudden withdrawal of this hormone will occur. Because there is much misinformation among the public on this point, sometimes intensive preoperative and postoperative counseling is required. Abrupt interruption of ovarian function in a woman who is still having regular periods may create more withdrawal symptoms than in a woman who is in her menopausal years. The younger woman may need estrogen replacement to alleviate signs and symptoms of estrogen withdrawal. The need for estrogen replacement in the older woman after surgical removal of ovaries will vary from client to client.

Physiology of the Menopause

The endocrine and metabolic changes associated with menopause are still not completely understood. This lack of information is due, in part, to difficulties associated with long-term, longitudinal studies spanning many years. In addition, the sensitive endocrine assays that would allow study of the endocrinological events associated with menopause have only recently become available. Because of this, estrogen replacement therapy with its possible short-term or long-term effects has created much controversy in both lay and scientific literature.

It is now known that several years before menopause there is an increase in circulating levels of both FSH and LH. The actual levels of estrogen and progesterone produced by the ovaries are decreased. These are only slight changes, and in spite of them, ovulation and menstruation continue to occur. The decreasing production of estradiol and progesterone undoubtedly allows release of increased amounts of gonadotropins from the pituitary, resulting in higher circulating levels of FSH and LH.

In normal postmenopausal women, FSH and LH levels are consistently high. The ratio of FSH and LH is always greater than one. Both of the gonadotropins are released in a pulsating fashion, similar to that seen in younger women but much more pronounced, with bursts occurring every 10 to 20 minutes. There is also periodic fluctuation in gonadotropin levels that occurs about every 2 hours. After removal of the ovaries in regularly menstruating women, gonadotropin levels begin to rise within 2 days. The rise in the FSH is more dramatic than that of LH.

Estrogen production by the postmenopausal ovary is minuscule. Surgical removal of the ovaries after menopause does not affect circulating estrogens in any significant way. However, the postmenopausal ovary does continue to produce androgens and in increased amounts. The appearance of dark hair on the upper lip and chin is seen in some women. Because varying amounts of circulating estrogen are found in postmenopausal women, it has been suggested that estrogen may be produced elsewhere in the body and also that other tissues are able to convert the circulating androgens to estrogen. Fat, the liver, and some areas of the hypothalamus are capable of this conversion. Such estrogen production varies from one postmenopausal woman to the next, and this variability may account for some of the variations in menopausal symptoms.

The mechanism responsible for *vasomotor symptoms* is only partially understood. Obviously, neuroendocrinological factors are at work. It has been suggested that *catecholamines* that act as neurotransmitters in the brain—they transfer information from one neuron to another—may respond to fluctuating gonadotropin or ovarian hormone levels. Catecholamines are responsible for modulating behavior and motor activity as well as the function of the hypothalamus and pituitary. Disturbance in catecholamine activity produces vasodilatation in the brain that could bring about hot flashes.[10,11] Many other environmental influences operate in the life of a postmenopausal woman, and it is difficult to separate these from the physiological events associated with decreased ovarian function. Although it is clear that emotional and physical stress can be related to increased frequency of vasomotor symptoms and signs, this relationship does not always occur in a predictable fashion. Hot flashes are the result of vasomotor instability and are clearly related to the estrogen deficiency associated with the cessation of ovarian function.

Changes in the vaginal mucosa also vary among menopausal women. Even minimal changes may result in painful intercourse (dyspareunia). Thinning of the vaginal lining and the decrease in lubrication can be corrected with estrogen administered orally or locally with vaginal suppositories or cream. Dyspareunia is a common symptom that should not be overlooked in the management of the postmenopausal woman.

■ REFERENCES

1. Wasserman E, Gromisch D: Survey of Clinical Pediatrics, 7th ed. New York, McGraw-Hill: 1981
2. Oski FA, Feigin RD, Warshaw JB (eds): Principles and Practice of Pediatrics. Philadelphia, JB Lippincott, 1990
3. Haas A, Haas K: Understanding Sexuality. St. Louis, Times Mirror/Mosby College Publishing, 1990
4. Schwartz MW, Charney EB, Curry TA, Ludwig S: Principles and Practice of Clinical Pediatrics. Chicago, Year Book Medical Publishers, 1987
5. Scott JR, DiSaia PJ, Hammond CB, Spellacy WN (eds): Danforth's Obstetrics and Gynecology. Philadelphia, JB Lippincott, 1990
6. Cunningham FG, MacDonald PC, Gant NF: Williams Obstetrics, 18th ed. Norwalk, CT, Appleton & Lange, 1989
7. Barlow D, McPherson A: Menstrual problems. In McPherson A (ed): Women's Problems in General Practice, pp 14–42. Oxford, Oxford University Press, 1988
8. Ravnikar V: Physiology and treatment of hot flushes. Obstet Gynecol 75 (4 Suppl):3S–8S, April 1990
9. Ferguson KJ, Hoegh C, Johnson S: Estrogen replacement therapy: A survey of women's knowledge and attitudes. Arch Intern Med 149(1):133–136, January 1989
10. Bider D, Mashiach S, Serr DM, Ben-Rafael Z: Endocrinological basis of hot flushes. Obstet Gynecol Survey 44(7):495–499, July 1988
11. Rebar RW, Spitzer IB: The physiology and measurement of hot flushes. Am J Obstet Gynecol 156(5):1284–1288, May 1987

■ SUGGESTED READING

Chaffee EE, Lytle IM: Basic Physiology and Anatomy, 4th ed. Philadelphia, JB Lippincott, 1980

Cutler W, Garcia CR: Medical Management of Menopause and Premenopause. Philadelphia, JB Lippincott, 1984

Flint M, Kronenberg F, Utian W (eds): Multidisciplinary Perspectives on Menopause, Vol 592. New York, New York Academy of Sciences, 1990

Goss CM (ed): Gray's Anatomy of the Human Body, 30th ed. Philadelphia, Lea & Febiger, 1984

Greep RO (ed): Reproductive Physiology, Vol 22. Baltimore, University Park Press, 1980

Greep RO, Koblinsky MA: Frontiers in Reproduction and Fertility Control. Cambridge, MIT Press, 1977

Greep RO, Koblinsky MA, Jaffe FS: Reproduction and Human Welfare: A Challenge to Research. Cambridge, MIT Press, 1977

Hammond CB, Haseltine FP, Schiff I (eds): Progress in Clinical and Biological Research, Vol 320, Menopause: Evaluation, Treatment and Health Concerns. New York, Alan R Liss, 1989

Marshall WA, Tanner JM: Variations in pattern of pubertal changes in girls. *Arch Dis Child* 44:291–303.

Mastroianni L, Coutifaris C: Reproductive Physiology (new ed). Park Ridge, NJ, Parthenon Pub Group, 1990

Mastroianni L, Paulsen CA (eds): Aging, Reproduction, and the Climacteric. New York, Plenum Press, 1986

Speroff L, Glass RH, Kase NG (eds): Clinical Gynecologic Endocrinology and Infertility, 4th ed. Baltimore, Williams & Wilkins, 1989

Tanner JM: Growth at Adolescence, 2nd ed. Oxford, Blackwell Scientific Publications, 1962

Tanner JM, Preece NA (eds): The Physiology of Human Growth, Society for the Study of Human Biology Symposium Series 29. New York, Cambridge Press, 1989

Williams PL, Warwick R, Dyson M, Bannister LH (eds): Gray's Anatomy of the Human Body, 37th ed. New York, Churchill Livingstone, 1989

Yen SS, Jaffe RB: Reproductive Endocrinology: Physiology, Pathophysiology and Clinical Management, 2nd ed. Philadelphia, WB Saunders, 1986

9

Human Sexual Response

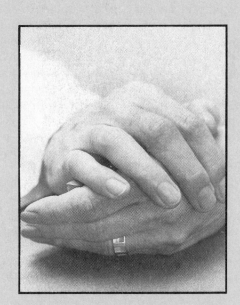

Human sexuality encompasses multiple dimensions that include physiological development, self-identity, sexual expression, reproduction, and the need for love and personal fulfillment. All people are sexual beings, with awareness of and reaction to their own femaleness or maleness. Sexuality is holistic, integrating biologic, psychological, and cultural factors into a whole that is greater than the sum of its parts. Each person has a unique style of sexuality, even those who limit sexual expression in celibacy. Human sexuality extends from before birth in early embryonic development, throughout life, and until death. It is a fundamental and pervasive characteristic of human activity and interaction.

Sexual response in men and women is a complex process with both psychological and physiological components. Sex can be considered one of the basic human drives, but it is much more malleable in expression than food and sleep, for example. Although a nearly universal behavior among humans, sex can be postponed for long periods or, in some instances, never activated, without adverse effects. Although cultural expression leads to a wide variety of sex-related behaviors, the biologic foundations of sexual interaction lead to more underlying similarities than differences among peoples.

Research on human sexuality has found that male and female sexual responses and behavior are more alike than different. The woman's sex drive is considered to be as powerful as the man's, and such behaviors as premarital and extramarital sex are becoming more similar among both sexes. While women's sexual behaviors have become less constrained, men's behaviors are becoming less promiscuous and their premarital sexual relations tend to involve one partner. The common stereotype that women need affection and intimacy to respond sexually whereas men respond regardless of the relationship has been found to have numerous exceptions. However, gender differences in attitude remain, with women more disapproving of casual sex than men. Patterns of sexual behavior continue to be most related to dominance in men and to love and affection in women.[1]

The basic similarities of physiological sexual responses between both sexes have been stressed by such researchers as Kinsey and Masters and Johnson. Aside from the obvious anatomical differences, men and women are homogeneous in their physiological responses to sexual stimuli. There are direct parallels in male and female anatomical responses to effective sexual stimulation, and the same underlying physiological mechanisms are involved: vasocongestion and myotonia. For example, vaginal lubrication in the woman is parallel to penile erection in the man, and both responses occur as a result of vasocongestion. Increases in muscle tension (*myotonia*) and changes in heart rate,

blood pressure, and respiration are common to both men and women during sexual excitement. The reflexive contractions of orgasm are virtually identical in both sexes, although there are variations in the results that these contractions produce. And, there is a considerable overlap in the subjective experience of orgasm. In a study comparing women and men's written descriptions of orgasms, in which the sex of the person writing the description could not be identified, professional judges could not distinguish the writer's sex by how orgasms were described. The study concluded that the experience of orgasm, as described by this college-age population, was essentially the same.[2]

Differences have been identified between male and female sexuality across the lifespan, which may be culturally based. Men seem to have an intense, genitally focused sexuality as teenagers. Approaching age 30, men are still highly interested in sex but without such urgency and are satisfied with fewer orgasms. With increasing age, men's sex becomes a more sensuously diffuse experience and has a greater emotional component. In contrast, women have an early awareness of the sensuous and emotional aspects of sex, but their orgasmic response is slow and inconsistent while in their teens and early 20s. By age 30 to 35, women's sexual response becomes quicker and more intense, with more consistent orgasms. Many women do not masturbate until this age, whereas most men begin masturbation in early adolescence. Sexuality for the adolescent female is person centered, emphasizing the relationships and emotions between two people. It becomes more body centered, emphasizing physical pleasure, later in midadulthood. Adolescent male sexuality is body centered and then becomes more person centered in adulthood with increasing age.[1]

The psychological and physiological components of human sexual response cannot really be separated because these are intricately interrelated and create numerous feedback loops that can enhance or inhibit sexual response. The changes in bodily function and the perceptions and emotions that precede or accompany these are closely related to physiological processes.

■ CULTURAL PERSPECTIVES ON SEXUALITY

All cultures regulate sexual behavior in some way, although there is great variation in which aspects of sexuality are regulated. This serves important functions for society and communicates social values. Cross-cultural data on human sexuality demonstrate that enormous variations exist and allow us to place the particular sexual mores of a given society in perspective. Culture and learning play an extremely important role in sexual expression and in shaping the characteristic sexuality of a society.

With its heritage of Judeo-Christianity and Victorianism, the United States has been considered a relatively sexually restrictive society up to the middle of this century. Sexual behavior and attitudes of Americans have changed substantially since then, and a more eroticized culture has emerged as the century draws to a close. Many other societies are far more permissive than the United States, however, and a few are much more restrictive.

Virtually every society regulates sex in at least two ways: prohibiting intercourse between relatives (incest) and condemning forced intercourse, such as rape. Beyond this, regulations differ greatly, as the following examples will demonstrate. Premarital sex is accepted as normal social behavior in 90% of Pacific Island, 88% of African, and 82% of Eurasian societies but is prohibited by 73% of Mediterranean societies. Homosexual behavior is strongly disapproved by some societies; it is tolerated among children but forbidden in adults in others; and it is openly accepted and even forced as part of puberty rites by still other societies. There is wide variation in socially accepted sexual techniques. Although kissing is very common, there is widespread variation in kissing methods and a few societies have no knowledge of kissing at all. Oral sex is quite common in Western and South Pacific societies, and grooming and delousing serve as foreplay behaviors in many primitive and aboriginal cultures. Most societies forbid intercourse at particular times, such as during the postpartum period.[1]

In the United States, there are large social class differences in contraceptive use and pregnancy. Women in their 20s with higher educational levels are less sexually active than those with high school or less educational levels, but they use contraceptives substantially more when they are sexually active. Among this group, women with the lowest educational levels had four times as many pregnancies as women with the highest levels.[3] In contrast, there are very few social class differences in sexual techniques, probably due to exposure to mass media. Studies have found some differences in sexual behavior between African-Americans and white Americans. African-American and white males begin masturbating at about the same age, but African-American females masturbate earlier than white females. African-American teenage females tend to have more premarital sex and have sex earlier than white teenage females. Among those who are sexually active in both these groups, about 25% do not use contraceptives. African-American female teenage girls are less knowledgeable than white teenage girls about reproductive facts, such as when during the menstrual cycle

the female is most fertile. However, such differences may be related to social class, because sexual behavior of middle class African-Americans is more similar to that of middle class whites than of lower class African-Americans.[1]

Attitudes toward premarital sex, extramarital sex, gender roles, masturbation, homosexuality, and sexual techniques differ considerably from one society to another. Sexual practices of individuals generally follow the attitudes and values predominant in the society. This underscores the importance of cultural perspectives in shaping sexual expression and the key role played by learned behaviors in human sexuality.

■ COMPONENTS OF SEXUALITY

A person's sexuality may be thought of as a complex of emotions, attitudes, preferences, and behaviors that are related to erotic expression. Among the many components of sexuality are a person's genetic (chromosomal) sex, gonadal sex, hormonal sex, morphological sex, gender identity, behavioral sex (sex role), and sexual partner preference. Usually there is congruence among these components, but this is not necessarily true. *Homosexuality* is an example of genetic, gonadal, and hormonal sex being incongruent with behavioral sex and sexual partner preference, at least by the dominant social definitions. *Transsexualism* (desiring to have the body, sexual organs, and sex role of the opposite sex) is an example of conflict between gender identity and genetic, gonadal, hormonal, and morphological sex.

In the more common case, in which there is congruence among the components of sexuality, it appears that the person's biologic equipment provides a framework through which sociocultural definitions of sexuality can be expressed. There is considerable evidence that the expression of sexuality is largely learned, although it is mediated by gonadal hormones and anatomical structures. Among humans, there are very few imperative, or unalterable, sexual behaviors; these include ejaculation in the male and menstruation, pregnancy, and childbirth in the female. These behaviors are necessary to carry out reproductive functions. All other sexual behaviors are, in a sense, optional. They are subject to environmental influences and comprise a very large sociocultural expression of sexual behavior. The following are key components of sexual expression that are largely shaped by culture rather than biology.

Gender Identity

Gender identity is the personal and private sense of being male or female, the personal experience of one's sex role. The sense of being male or female begins by the time a child is 3½ years of age. This is also the age at which a child develops conceptual language, which is involved in establishing a gender-differentiated self-concept. Information about the development of gender identity was gained from studies of children born with ambiguous genitalia, in whom it was impossible to distinguish the baby clearly as male or female. Sometimes a child is initially assigned the wrong sex according to its chromosomal sex. If during the first 12 to 18 months of life an error is discovered through chromosomal analysis, the child's identity may be changed to the opposite sex. With each subsequent month, however, changing gender identity becomes increasingly difficult.[4] Once established, gender identity is very difficult to change.[5] Although the range of behavioral expression is extremely wide, this basic sense of maleness or femaleness persists throughout life (Fig. 9-1).

Sex Role

Sex role is the public expression of gender identity. A person's sense of what are appropriate behaviors, attitudes, beliefs, and emotions for a female or male constitutes sex-role identification. In most Western societies, masculine (male sex role) behavior has been considered to be more aggressive, independent, and logical, whereas feminine (female sex role) behavior is seen as more submissive, dependent, and emotional. However, expressions of masculinity of femininity vary widely among cultures, and there are some societies in which what is considered male and female is exactly opposite of the Western stereotype.

Although most cultures place the women in the role of caretaker to children, and men in the role of breadwinner, there is no necessity that roles be assigned in

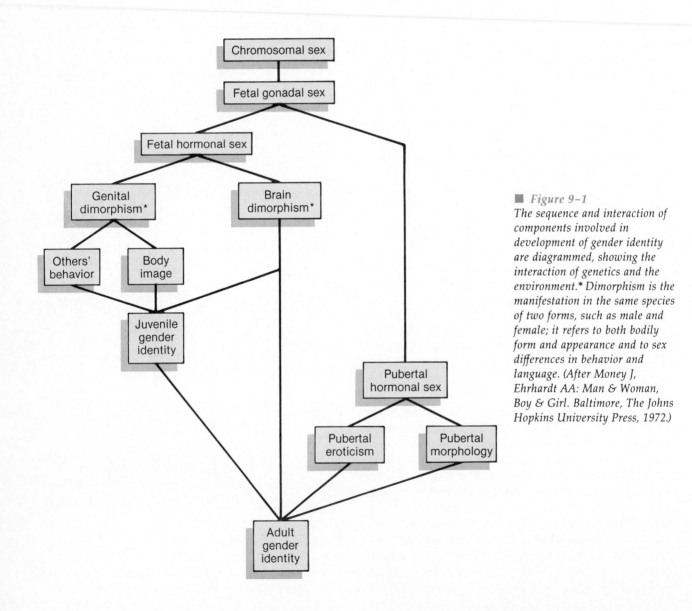

■ *Figure 9-1*
The sequence and interaction of components involved in development of gender identity are diagrammed, showing the interaction of genetics and the environment. Dimorphism is the manifestation in the same species of two forms, such as male and female; it refers to both bodily form and appearance and to sex differences in behavior and language. (After Money J, Ehrhardt AA: Man & Woman, Boy & Girl. Baltimore, The Johns Hopkins University Press, 1972.)*

this manner. Sex roles and definitions of masculinity and femininity are based on arbitrary criteria rather than on anatomical and physiological differences. Femininity and masculinity are not absolute conditions, and they can have overlapping behaviors. All humans are a mixture of maleness and femaleness and have the same types of impulses, wishes, attitudes, and basic emotional and physiological equipment (except those imperative parts of sexual function and behavior and the obvious anatomical differences). The different expressions of sex role observed in various cultures is a result of society's selective development of behavioral potentials. Sex roles are developed through family interactions, the effects of peers, social codes of dress and manners, all forms of media communication, and numerous social structures that encourage certain behaviors and inhibit others for males and females.

There is a wide expression of sex roles in the United States, but traditional gender distinctions still exert important effects. The most powerful female sex role norm is the mandate for marriage and motherhood. Male sex role norms include being competitive and successful, aggressive, sexual initiators, self-reliant, and never acting in a feminine way. These traditional norms tend to restrict women to a narrow life with limited opportunity for self-expression. Men are required to set impossibly high and demanding goals that create anxiety, frustration, and stress.[5]

Increasingly, people in the United States are expressing concern that strict gender role distinctions artificially limit the potential for finding personal fulfillment or self-actualization. More families are encouraging children to choose from the entire range of human behaviors, to express those that best suit their individual personalities. People raised in this way will be able to combine independence and other traditional male characteristics with sensitivity, emotional expressiveness, and other traditional female characteristics.[6]

Sexual Partner Preference

Preference for a sexual partner may be heterosexual, homosexual, or bisexual, and this preference may change during one's lifetime. Despite considerable research, it is far from clear how preferences for a sexual partner develop, even among heterosexuals. Sexual partner preference also appears to be on a continuum rather than an all-or-none basis, and it probably varies with the circumstances for some people. There is a difference between actual sexual experiences and sexual responsiveness in regard to partner preference. For example, a person may be exclusively heterosexual in actual experience but feel somewhat sexually attracted to people of the same sex.

There is enormous variety in sexual partner preference and associated sex-role behavior. A homosexual man may appear very masculine, carry out the role of a typical man, and have a strong gender identity as male, yet prefer a person of the same sex as an erotic partner. An effeminate-appearing male working at an occupation dominated by women may have a clear sense of male gender identity and opposite-sex erotic preference. A woman who appears and acts very masculine may have male gender identity and prefer women as sexual partners.

Many studies have examined social, psychological, and biologic factors as possible causes of homosexuality, but none are conclusive. It is well established that many people have sexual experiences with persons of the same sex, usually during childhood and adolescence. Homosexual preferences often develop before any actual sexual experience, however. Most people who have same-sex encounters do not develop homosexual partner preferences. Biologic research suggests that there may be a sex center in the fetal brain that is influenced by prenatal hormones and affects later sex-role behavior and choice of sexual partners. The mothers of some homosexuals were found to have atypical hormonal events during the critical period of sex center development during pregnancy, and it has been found that emotional stress during pregnancy causes reduced maternal androgen output, which might have contributed to feminization of male infants.[4]

The biologic linkage of sex-role and sexual partner preference in humans is far from established. "Tomboy" girls and "sissy" boys do not necessarily, or even usually, become homosexuals. The development of sexual partner preference is probably shaped by such diverse and complex factors as the prenatal hormonal environment, early mother-infant interactions, imitation by the child of the most valued parent, family dynamics and interstructure that selectively fosters and inhibits behavior, the privileges and drawbacks of social sex roles affecting value formation, and society's tolerance of variation in sexual expression.[7,8]

■ SEXUAL PSYCHOPHYSIOLOGY

Psychophysiology is a term that describes the interaction between psychological and physiological processes, between higher mental processes and the responses of muscles, glands, and organs. Two important fundamental psychophysiological principles are that a physiological response to a stimulus is influenced by past experiences and that current experiences and emotions are influenced by the body's responses. For example, a

Female and Male Sex Differences

Well-Established Differences

Size	Males are taller and heavier at birth and through life.
Musculature	Males have a greater percentage of body weight in muscles than females.
Hardiness	More males are conceived and born, but males have higher miscarriage and infant mortality rates and are more susceptible to disease, hereditary disorders, and malnutrition at all ages.
Sensorimotor	Females are more developed physically and neurologically at birth, walk earlier, and have greater pain sensitivity.
Developmental	Male children are more aggressive in social play; females comply more. Males have more reading disabilities, speech defects, school and emotional problems

Contradictory Evidence

Activity level	Male infants are reported as being more active. Many studies found no differences.
Dependency	Both sexes are equally dependent in early childhood. Females rate themselves as more dependent in later childhood and as adults. There are strong cultural influences.
Recognition of faces	Female infants recognize different faces at an earlier age found by some studies.
Confidence	Both sexes seem equally timid as young children. Older females report themselves as being more fearful than males. There are strong cultural influences.
Cognitive ability	Females appear superior in verbal abilities; they talk earlier, excel at vocabulary, reading, comprehensive and verbal creativity. Males appear superior in visual–spatial ability, such as manipulating objects in three-dimensional space. Males are found superior in mathematics by some authorities but not others.
Stress response	Males may be more vulnerable to stresses resulting from family disharmony and interpersonal conflicts. Data are preliminary.

Myths Refuted by Data or Not Documented

Task abilities	Females are better at simple, repetitive tasks, whereas males are better at complex tasks. Not true.
Preferred sensory modes	Females are more responsive to auditory stimuli, males to visual stimuli. No data to support.
Self-esteem	Females have lower self-esteem than males. Actually, self-esteem is about equal in both sexes.
Sociability	Males are less sociable than females. Actually, both sexes spend equal time with others and are equally responsive to others.
Suggestibility	Females are more suggestible than males. Actually, females are no more likely than males to conform to peer group standards or imitate others.

(Adapted from Byer Co, Shainberg LW, Jones KL: Dimensions of Human Sexuality. Dubuque, IO, WC Brown, 1985)

woman whose past experiences include frequent, intense orgasm may respond rapidly to sexual stimulation, whereas a woman who has learned not to expect to reach orgasm may have little response to the same type of stimuli. Also, awareness of the body's responses, such as vaginal congestion and lubrication in women and erection in men, can heighten pleasure and sexual feelings.

Human sexual response is determined by a delicate interaction between psychology and physiology. The nervous system has a central role in mediating sexual response by processing sexual signals of both cognitive and somatic origin. The causes of sexual arousal may be found in the interplay between the mind (conscious awareness), the brain, and the sexual organs. This framework provides an understanding of the characteristics of sexual stimuli and the wide individual variation found.

Reflexogenic and Psychogenic Stimuli

Direct stimulation of erogenous areas, usually genitals and breasts, causes sexual arousal in a reflexive, or automatic, manner. When the penis or clitoris is stroked, the peripheral nerves send a signal to a relay center in the lower part of the spinal cord, which in turn sends a signal back to the penis for erection and to the clitoris and vagina for congestion and lubrication. The cerebral cortex and higher brain centers are not involved in this transmission of signals; it is a reflexogenic response that is mediated in the same way as the knee-jerk response. This is the mechanism through which some men with spinal cord injuries are able to have erections even though they have no sensation in the pelvic area.

Psychogenic stimuli are processed through the higher brain centers and can include sensory input such as sights, sounds, tastes, smells, and touches, as well as cognitive events such as thoughts, fantasies, memories, and images. Without direct stimulation of the genitals, it is possible to become sexually aroused through any one of these types of psychogenic stimuli. Watching an erotic movie, having the earlobe stroked, listening to a song with provocative lyrics, fantasizing a favorite sexual drama, or remembering a sexual encounter can all produce sexual arousal.

Most often, a combination of reflexogenic and psychogenic stimuli is used to produce sexual arousal, and they work in a synergistic way to enhance the level of excitement. Many men have found women more rapidly responsive sexually after an evening of candlelight, soft music, and romantic interaction. After seeing an erotic picture or movie, a man will often need considerably less (maybe no) direct stimulation to have an erection. On the other hand, feelings such as anger, guilt, or anxiety inhibit sexual response when direct stimulation is being used (Fig. 9-2).

Neurological Pathways

The neurological pathways of reflexogenic stimuli are easier to trace than those of psychogenic stimuli, which involve complex mental processes and functions, such as learning, emotions, and memory. The past experiences of a person are very important in determining which types of psychogenic stimuli are perceived as arousing. Early childhood experiences of pleasurable genital touching occurring in an environment with certain smells, sights, or sounds may lead to later associ-

ation of these sensations with sexual arousal. The process continues during adolescence and adulthood as sexual experience widens and different stimuli are associated with negative or positive sexual consequences. Being interrupted during sex by parents can lead to associations of anxiety or guilt with future sexual encounters. Circumstances in which a man has difficulty with erection can result in future erection problems under similar conditions. Situations in which intense sexual pleasure was felt tend to be sought again.

The central nervous system plays a key role in processing psychogenic stimuli and in mediating the interplay between these and the activity of the peripheral nervous system. Central nervous system output travels through either the somatic or autonomic branch of the peripheral nervous system (Fig. 9-3). Generally speaking, the somatic nerves connect the central nervous system with the striated muscles. The muscle tension (myotonia) during sexual arousal is caused by stimulation of the somatic nerves. The autonomic nervous system, however, is responsible for most of the physiological changes during sexual arousal. In general, the autonomic nervous system controls the smooth muscles of the heart, internal organs, and glands whose functions are largely involuntary, or not under conscious control. Thus, sexual response has a large involuntary component, with conscious inhibition generally more effective than conscious activation.

The sympathetic and parasympathetic branches of the autonomic nervous system, with their different anatomical pathways and chemical activators of the smooth muscles and glands, are the immediate mediators of sexual response. The parasympathetic branch is also called *cholinergic* because its nerve endings release acetylcholine to transmit their messages, and the sympathetic branch is called *adrenergic* because it releases adrenaline and noradrenaline. These two branches serve different functions, with the sympathetic nervous system usually responding during times of stress, when there is a need for vigorous activity (thus the release of adrenaline), and the parasympathetic system dominating during periods of relaxation.

The sexual organs receive messages from both the sympathetic and parasympathetic systems, as do most other body organs. Penile erection and vaginal lubrication are caused by the effects of the parasympathetic system, which produce vasodilatation. As arousal progresses, the sympathetic system plays a larger role, causing increases in heart rate and blood pressure. The sympathetic system may take over completely at orgasm, with ejaculation and vaginal spasms set off by a sudden discharge of adrenaline. The autonomic imbalance produced by this sudden release of adrenaline is quickly compensated for by a release of acetylcholine that comes from the parasympathetic system. This parasympathetic rebound phenomenon, with its vaso-

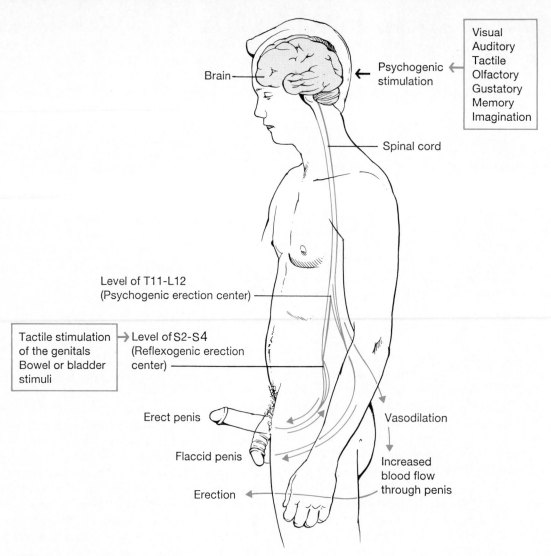

Visual
Auditory
Tactile
Olfactory
Gustatory
Memory
Imagination

Brain

Psychogenic
stimulation

Spinal cord

Level of T11-L12
(Psychogenic erection center)

Tactile stimulation
of the genitals
Bowel or bladder
stimuli

Level of S2-S4
(Reflexogenic erection
center)

Erect penis

Flaccid penis

Erection

Vasodilation

Increased
blood flow
through penis

■ *Figure 9–2*
Reflexogenic and psychogenic pathways for sexual response.

dilatation, contributes to the subjective feelings of warmth and relaxation that many people feel after orgasm.

■ PSYCHOLOGICAL MEDIATORS OF SEXUAL RESPONSE

The psychogenic stimuli that affect sexual response work largely through the relatively simple process of conditioning by association, or conditioned response. However, sexual meanings can be attached to stimuli through more complex psychological processes. The mental state in which people are likely to initiate or respond to sexual advances is created by a complex in-

terplay of many factors. Sometimes a person can identify why he or she is "in the mood" for sex or why he or she is not, but at other times the sources of reaction to sexual stimuli are elusive. Sexual feelings can be spontaneous and uncomplicated at times, but in other instances there may be conflicts, uncertainty, resistance, or hesitation. Human emotions and thoughts are very complex, so it is not surprising that sexual responsiveness varies greatly among different people and in the same person at different times.

Major psychological mediators of responses to sexual stimulation have been identified as informational responses, emotional reactions, imaginative capacity, attention, and love. These factors interact with each other and exert a direct influence on experiences in one area or another or create conflicts in responses to stimuli when there is disagreement among them. There is also a feedback loop between physiological response and the erotic stimulus: on becoming aware of physical

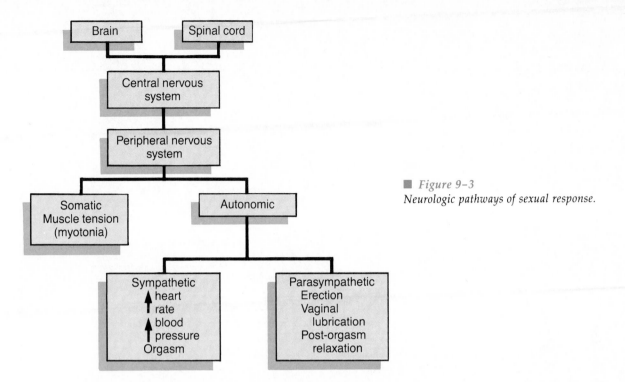

arousal, the stimulus causing arousal will be perceived as increasingly arousing (Fig. 9-4).

Informational Responses

The informational component that acts as a psychological mediator of sexual response consists of beliefs, knowledge, and labels concerning various aspects of sexuality. If a certain sexual practice is considered a perversion, such as oral–genital stimulation, then a person is unlikely to engage in this behavior and the idea of doing it would be repulsive, acting as a sexual "turn-off." If a sexual partner suggests or initiates oral–genital sex, this would effectively decrease sexual arousal and probably generate a number of negative feelings or expressions.

A person without this belief, however, who sees oral–genital sex as healthy and desirable, and who has had pleasurable past experiences, would respond with increased arousal to the idea, suggestion, or initiation of this activity. The expectations that are built on beliefs, experiences (experiential knowledge), and the labeling–categorizing process exert powerful influences on sexual responsiveness. These can either effectively shut down the physiological response or greatly enhance it.

Emotional Reactions

The emotional components in psychological mediation consist of subjective feelings and perceptions about a sexual stimulus. These follow beliefs and expectations very closely; emotions are the affective expression of values and beliefs. Feelings about sexual stimuli can range from the very positive, such as joy, happiness, and excitement, to the very negative, such as guilt, anxiety, repulsion, anger, and fear. A man exhibiting very "macho" behavior with the flavor of male superiority would probably evoke anger and repulsion in a feminist woman; therefore, he would be an ineffective visual and auditory sexual stimulus.

Many people report heightened arousal and increased intensity and rapidity of sexual response when there are deep, powerful feelings of love and commitment between partners. The boredom and diminished intensity of sexual experiences that are common among long-time married couples probably derive, at least in part, from a flattening of emotional response to each other. The sense of knowing someone too completely so there is no excitement of the unknown and unpredictable, and the little resentments that build up over years of unexpressed or unresolved conflicts so there is a smoldering anger just under the surface, constitute emotions that detract from sexual response. The directness, honesty, and humility necessary to grow out of such traps require conscious cultivation by both partners.

As previously mentioned, guilt is one of the most effective inhibitors of sexual response. Many men and women with sexual problems find early inculcation of guilty feelings about themselves as sexual beings and sex-related activities at the base of their difficulties. Making judgments about oneself or one's partner,

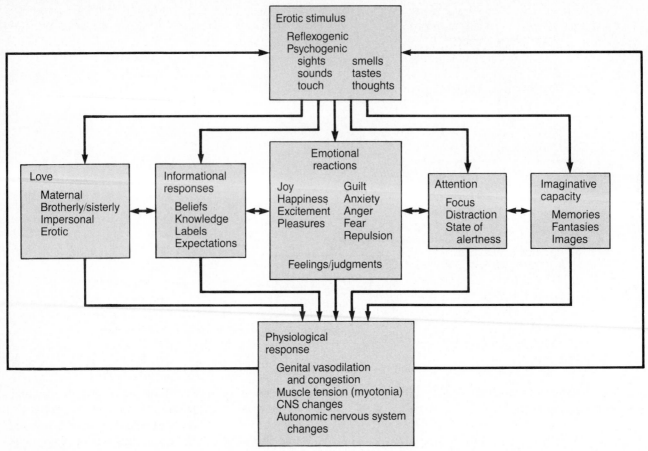

■ *Figure 9–4*
Psychological mediators of sexual response and the processing of erotic stimuli. (After Rosen R,
Rosen LR: Human Sexuality. New York, Alfred A Knopf, Inc., 1981.)

whether related to appearance or behaviors, sets up an acceptable or not acceptable dichotomy that may screen out many sexual stimuli. Judging something as ''good'' or ''bad'' is a way of expressing values and beliefs and lays the foundation for associated feelings.

Imaginative Capacity

The imaginative component in psychological mediation of sexual response includes the memories, images, and fantasies that are invoked by sexual stimuli. Almost everyone has sexual fantasies. Some people can create or enhance arousal by just thinking about them. Because some fantasies are bizarre, there is often guilt associated with them, producing a conflict in psychological input. Sexologists state that any fantasy that increases arousal is acceptable as long as it is not acted out in a way that will harm others, physically or emotionally.

Mental images have been found by sex researchers to be very important in determining sexual response. Arousal tends to be greatest with evocation of memories of the person's own past sexual acts, when what was personally experienced produced significant pleasure in sexual encounters. Imagery is so powerful that people can quickly learn to arouse themselves sexually or turn off sexual response, just by using appropriate fantasies and images.

Attention

The importance of attention in mediating sexual response is so direct and obvious that it is often overlooked. If a person is not paying attention to a sexual stimulus, then it will have very little effect, if any. Sexual response will be limited, or may not occur at all, if a person is inattentive or distracted. This was well demonstrated in a laboratory experiment in which subjects listened to an erotic tape recording through one side of an earphone headset while simple mental arithmetic problems were played through the other earphone. Using instruments to measure the subjects' penile erections, it was found that the distraction of the math problems definitely reduced the amount of erection produced in response to the erotic tape.

The effects of distraction have been felt by most people at some time. People do not respond as readily to sexual stimuli when also aware of the noises of their children in a nearby room, when thoughts of housework or office work to be done arise, when hungry and smelling food cooking, or when dissatisfied with something about their appearance or the circumstances of sex. When no environmental distractions are present, the ability to focus on the sexual encounter becomes an important part of attention processes. For no apparent reason, a person may find his or her mind wandering to totally unrelated subjects. Although the body is physically going through the motions, the level of arousal may be quite low, delaying or inhibiting orgasm when a person is not focused on the sexual experience. The state of alertness is also important; if a person is drowsy and drifting off into sleep, sexual responses will also be sluggish. This applies to the effects of certain drugs, such as alcohol, which decreases mental alertness as well as depresses physiological responses.

Sex and Love

Another important psychological mediator in sexual response is love. Similar to sexuality, love is a complex phenomenon and is variously defined and understood. There appear to be many types of love that can affect sexual development and expression. Maternal love is uncritical caring for the weak and helpless or, specifically, for one's own child. It provides a crucial foundation for developing security and self-esteem. Brotherly (sisterly) love is affection between friends or relatives, usually one's peers and close companions. It supports the sense of identity and belonging. Love of humanity is caring for all people. This love is selfless and nonsexual; it is impersonal love (because it encompasses all people and not individuals). Such love is the basis for altruism and self-transcendence.

Erotic love is most clearly expressed in sexual relationships. The feelings of affection, caring, and intimacy shared between sexual partners are often inseparable from their sexual behaviors. Some believe that sexual "freedom" means separating sex from love, something that men have long been accused of, but which now seems frequent among women also. Subordination of sex needs to love needs and expression of sexuality only in a loving (or socially approved) relationship were traditionally expected of women. Pursuit of sexual liberation through separating sex and love may prove to be unsatisfying or anxiety producing, however. More sexual activity and less emotional involvement creates an emptiness for many people. The fusion of sex with feelings of love and intimacy creates one of life's most intense experiences.

Love has developmental aspects with sexual components. Generally, a person's ability to love progresses throughout life. Some elements of sexual pleasure or sex-role expression occur in almost all types of love. When love relationships are inadequate or interrupted, sexual problems can develop. Love is essential for growth, human development, and being. In its impersonal form, it is the path to self-transcendence.

■ PRENATAL SEXUAL DIFFERENTIATION

In the process of sexual reproduction, the gametes (sex cells) of the female and male unite, combining their genetic information and producing a new member of the species. The gametes, which are the sperm of the male and the ovum of the female, are special cells because they contain only half of the genetic information of all other body cells. Each gamete has 23 chromosomes resulting from the process of meiosis, a type of cell division unique to gonadal organs, the testes in the male and ovaries in the female. In humans, meiosis results in the formation of four cells, each with 23 chromosomes. These four cells develop into four sperm in the male; in the female, they develop onto one ovum and three polar bodies that die and dissolve (see Chap. 10).

The sperm and ovum contain only one of each type of chromosome, in contrast to all other body cells that have two of each chromosome type. The chromosomes are rodlike structures containing genes composed of deoxyribonucleic acid (DNA) molecules in which genetic information is carried. When the sperm and ovum unite, the 23 chromosomes in each merge into the full complement of 46 chromosomes, and a zygote is formed. From this point on, cell division proceeds by mitosis, producing new 46-chromosome cells with the unique genetic characteristics of the new individual, half contributed by each parent.

The gametes contain 22 autosomes and one sex chromosome. In the female, before meiosis, the ovarian cells (as well as all other body cells) contain two large X chromosomes. In the male, before meiosis, the testicular cells (and all others) contain one large X chromosome and one smaller Y chromosome. Meiosis ensures that each gamete has only one sex chromosome; the ovum contains one X chromosome, whereas the sperm can contain either an X chromosome or a Y chromosome. The union of sperm and ovum produces a combination of the sex chromosomes of the parents. If each contributes an X chromosome, the result is an XX combination producing a female. If the male contributes a Y chromosome, the result is an XY combination (because the female can only contribute an X), which produces a male.

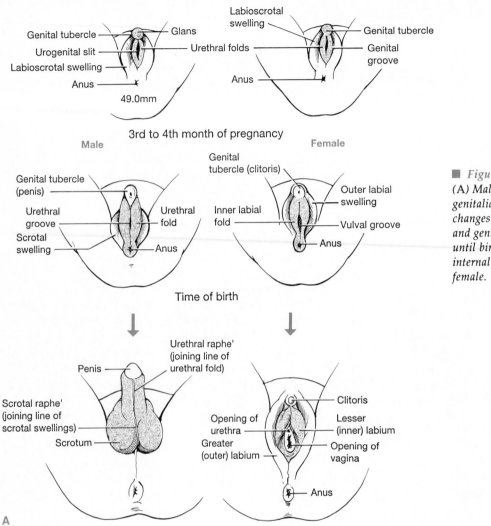

Male and Female External Genitalia
(identical at 7 weeks)

Genital tubercle — Glans
Urogenital slit — Urethral folds
Labioscrotal swelling
Anus
49.0mm

Labioscrotal swelling
Genital tubercle
Genital groove
Anus

3rd to 4th month of pregnancy

Male   Female

Genital tubercle (penis)
Urethral groove — Urethral fold
Scrotal swelling — Anus

Genital tubercle (clitoris)
Inner labial fold
Outer labial swelling
Vulval groove
Anus

Time of birth

Urethral raphe' (joining line of urethral fold)
Penis
Scrotal raphe' (joining line of scrotal swellings)
Scrotum

Clitoris
Opening of urethra
Greater (outer) labium
Lesser (inner) labium
Opening of vagina
Anus

A

■ *Figure 9–5*
(A) *Male and female external genitalia are identical at 7 weeks, but changes occur after the 3rd month and genital differentiation continues until birth. (B) Differentiation of internal sex organs of the male and female.*

The XX or XY combination of sex chromosomes passes the sexual program to the primordial gonad of the embryo. The primitive genital ducts of the embryo are identical until about 6 weeks' gestation. In the seventh week, the sex chromosomes direct the gonads to begin differentiation. A recently discovered gene, located on the Y chromosome, directs male sexual development. This sex gene, or testis-determining factor, must be present for male sexual differentiation to occur.[9,10] If it is not present because of a genetic abnormality of the Y chromosome, then testes will not develop and instead ovaries differentiate and female development follows. The individuals who result are morphologically female, with an XY sex chromosome complement, and are infertile.

In the embryo with normal XY chromosomes, testes begin to organize and grow at about 7 weeks' gestation. Cells organize into the seminiferous cords, which become the seminiferous (sperm-producing) tubules. Other cells lying between the seminiferous cords develop into the interstitial (Leydig) cells, which produce hormones, and into the tissues that form and hold the testes. The interstitial cells secrete testosterone, which induces the wolffian ducts to develop from the primitive genital ducts. The wolffian ducts develop into several internal male sex organs: the epididymis, vas deferens, and seminal vesicles. Another testicular hormone, müllerian inhibiting hormone, secreted by the Sertoli cells, causes the müllerian ducts (which would develop into female sex organs) to regress and disappear.

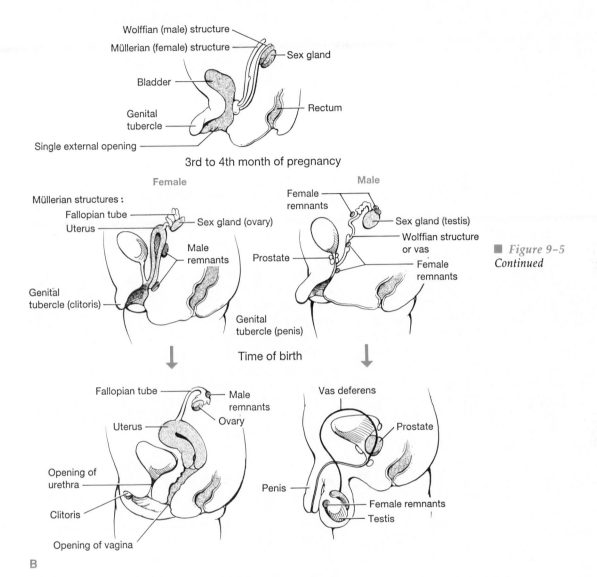

Male and Female Internal Sexual Organs
(identical at 2nd to 3rd month of pregnancy)

3rd to 4th month of pregnancy

■ *Figure 9–5*
Continued

B

In the embryo with normal XX chromosomes, the process is somewhat slower, with ovaries beginning to develop at about 11 to 12 weeks' gestation. Cells form small clusters and become follicles of the ovaries, giving rise to oocytes (immature ova) later in development. Other cells develop in the follicles that produce hormones, and still others form tissues around the follicles that become ovaries. Although the initial formation of ovaries requires the absence of a Y chromosome, continued development depends on the presence of two X chromosomes. If only one X chromosome is present, ovaries do not fully develop and the woman is infertile.

Hormones from the ovaries (estrogens) are not necessary for internal female reproductive structures to develop, although these are secreted. The lack of both testosterone and müllerian inhibiting hormone cause

the wolffian ducts to regress and disappear in the female embryo. The müllerian ducts continue to develop in the female and give rise to the fallopian tubes, uterus, cervix, and possibly the upper vagina. There seems a built-in propensity for primitive genital structures to develop in the female pattern. Androgens must be present to produce male sexual differentiation, whereas their absence leads to female differentiation. If embryonic gonads do not secrete hormones (either testosterone or estrogens), and even if embryonic reproductive tracts (without gonads) are removed in experiments and kept alive, the genital structures continue to develop the female pattern.[11,12]

The external genitals of both females and males develop from the same embryonic tissues. These folds and swellings of embryonic tissue develop into the homologous, or corresponding, structures of the male and female, as well as structures common to both, such as the bladder and urethra. The embryonic glands and genital tubercle develop into the clitoral system in the female and the penis in the male. The labioscrotal swelling becomes the female labia or male scrotum, and the urogenital slit and urethral folds form the different urethral systems in males and females. The other homologous sex organs are (male and female, respectively) (1) the prostate gland and Skene's glands; and (2) Cowper's glands and Bartholin's glands (Fig. 9-5).

■ THE SEXUAL RESPONSE CYCLE

The systems of sexual anatomy and physiology that are organized around the clitoris in women and the penis in men are exact homologues of each other. Each part in one sex has its counterpart in the other. These counterparts may be structurally the same in both women and men, may be modified to perform the same function in a different way, or may perform a different function. The sexual response cycle, with its two basic physiological mechanisms of vasocongestion and myotonia, progresses through identical phases with corresponding changes in genital and other body organs in both women and men. There are certain differences in timing and patterns characteristic of each of the sexes within this common physiological process.

Anatomy and Physiology of Sexual Response

Male and female sexual and reproductive anatomy and physiology have been presented in Chapter 8. A brief review of the most pertinent structures is included in this section, with a more detailed discussion of sexual physiology.

FEMALE SEXUAL RESPONSE

The *labia majora*, which are well endowed with fat, hair, sweat glands, blood vessels, lymphatic vessels, and nerves, respond to vasocongestion with sexual excitation by spreading apart, becoming more flattened and elongating anteroposteriorly. The *labia minora*, which are continuous with the prepuce (clitoral hood), are well supplied with blood vessels, nerves, and lymphatics. The labial skin has a pink pigmentation that deepens in color with arousal, becoming bright red or purplish red with high levels of sexual excitement. The labia minora increase in size and extend outward with vasocongestion, protruding past the labia majora and functionally elongating the vagina. Often called the "sex skin," the labia minora are highly sensitive to touch and play a major role in arousal and orgasm through their draping over the clitoris, providing continual clitoral stimulation as tension is increased and decreased with penile thrusting.

The *clitoris* is a complex anatomical structure with both external and cryptic, or hidden, parts. Its role in arousal and orgasm is central, and it appears that the sole purpose of the clitoral structure is to enhance female sexual pleasure. There are four parts to the clitoris: the glans, shaft, crus, and vestibular bulbs. The glans and shaft are the most external and smallest portions and are largely hidden under the prepuce. Comprising only one tenth of the volume of the clitoris in its resting state, the glans and shaft represent even a smaller proportion during sexual arousal when the cryptic structures may increase in size up to three times. The clitoral shaft contains two small erectile cavernous bodies enclosed in a dense fibrous membrane, similar to the male penis. The length of the shaft is about ¼ to ¾ in, although there are marked variations. The glans is on average 4 to 5 mm in diameter, although normal range encompasses 2 to 10 mm.

The clitoral glans is the most sensitive female erogenous area, with its mucous membrane so densely packed with nerve endings that there is little room for blood vessels. The entire female sexual cycle can be initiated and maintained to orgasm by stimulation of only the glans. At rest, the shaft is sharply retroflexed posteriorly. With sexual stimulation, it becomes congested, leading to erection, moving the tip through a 180-degree arc in a forward elliptical curve. As arousal proceeds, it is retracted under the prepuce and appears shorter because of the actions of muscles and the cryptic structures pulling it inward.

The cryptic structures of the clitoris include the crus and vestibular bulbs. At the end of the shaft, the clitoris

---

Homologous Sex Organs

Female Sex Organs	Male Sex Organs
Glans of the clitoris	Glans of the penis
Shaft of the clitoris	Shaft of the penis
Hood of the clitoris	Foreskin of the penis
Labia majora	Scrotal sac
Labia minora	Underside of penis
Skene's glands	Prostate gland
Bartholin's glands	Cowper's glands
Ovaries	Testes

bifurcates and branches into two crura, which extend inward bilaterally following the inferior rami of the symphysis pubis downward. The crura lie below the ischiocavernous muscles and bodies, with a tough, tendinous lower portion that anchors the clitoris to the inner surface of the ischium. The clitoral crus is homologous to the corpus cavernosum in the male, which becomes the crus of the penis. The crura play a lesser role in distention during arousal in the female than the vestibular bulbs because of their tendinous nature (Fig. 9-6).

The vestibular bulbs also divide and descend into the pelvis from the clitoral shaft. Extending outward bilaterally, they wrap fully three fourths of the way around the lower portion of the vagina. Each bulb presses closely against the lower third of the vagina, just above the vaginal opening. The vestibular bulbs are erectile and highly distensible and are covered with a mass of coiled blood vessels (*commissure of the bulbs*). These blood vessels also become distended during arousal and convey blood between the bulbs and the clitoral shaft. The greater vestibular glands (Bartholin's glands) are located at the bottom of the bulbs. The vestibular bulbs become greatly distended during arousal, contributing to the build-up of the orgasmic platform in the lower third of the vagina. The homologous structure in the male is the corpus spongiosum, which becomes the bulb of the penis.

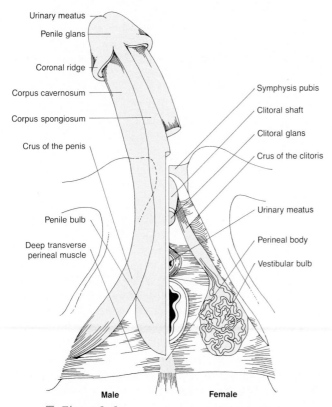

Labels (left, Male):
Urinary meatus
Penile glans
Coronal ridge
Corpus cavernosum
Corpus spongiosum
Crus of the penis
Penile bulb
Deep transverse perineal muscle

Labels (right, Female):
Symphysis pubis
Clitoral shaft
Clitoral glans
Crus of the clitoris
Urinary meatus
Perineal body
Vestibular bulb

Male　　　**Female**

■ *Figure 9-6*
Comparison of female and male cryptic structures.

The female *pelvic muscles* participate in engorgement during sexual arousal and have an important function in orgasm. The *ischiocavernous muscles* envelop the clitoral crura, and the *bulbocavernous muscles* surround the vestibular bulbs and the lower third of the vagina. Ascending from the vagina, the bulbocavernous muscles terminate in fibrous tissue dorsal of the clitoris and overlie the crura, and join the ischiocavernous to form the striated sphincter of the urethra. The *transverse perineal muscles* and *levator ani muscles* converge on the lateral walls of the lower third of the vagina and unite behind the vaginal opening to form the perineal body. These pelvic muscles become congested during arousal, and many women are aware that voluntary contractions of perineal muscles can heighten arousal. The muscles press on distended clitoral and vaginal structures, and when a critical point is reached in this distention, a reflex stretch mechanism is set off in the muscles and the contractions pressing on the distended clitoral crura, vestibular bulbs, and lower vaginal area cause orgasm.

The *vagina* is a muscular tube that is lined with mucous membranes and is richly supplied with blood vessels, glands, and lymphatics. The lower third of the vagina has many nerve endings, but the upper portion is not as well endowed and may be distended considerably laterally and posteriorly without discomfort. The circumvaginal venous plexus is a dense grouping of blood vessels surrounding the lower third of the vagina, and these vessels provide the blood supply for the massive congestion that produces vaginal lubrication during sexual arousal. They also contribute to building the orgasmic platform in later stages of excitement.

With effective sexual stimulation, pelvic venous dilatation and congestion occur quickly, and fluid from these venous networks passes into tissue spaces and causes edema. Within 10 to 30 seconds, droplets of clear fluid called *transudate* appear on the vaginal walls, coalesce, and produce vaginal lubrication. Concurrently, the upper two thirds of the vagina begins to lengthen and distend. As excitement progresses, the upper vagina balloons outward as the uterus and cervix are pulled upward into the false pelvis. In the lower pelvis, a broad platform of distended tissues forms as pelvic congestion and edema reach a peak. The vestibular bulbs and labia minora are also highly distended and congested at peak excitement. The thickened area of congested tissue surrounding the lower vagina and vaginal opening is called the *orgasmic platform* (Fig. 9-7).

When this vasocongestive distention reaches a critical point, orgasm is triggered in a mechanism involving the clitoral shaft and glans, clitoral cryptic structures, vaginal platform, and pelvic muscles. The muscles contract vigorously at intervals of 0.8 second, expelling the blood and fluid trapped in the tissues and venous plexi, and create the sensations of orgasm. Orgasm usually consists of 8 to 15 contractions; the first 5 or 6 are the

Excitement Stage

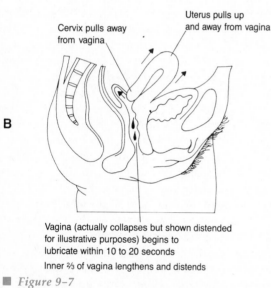

Plateau Stage

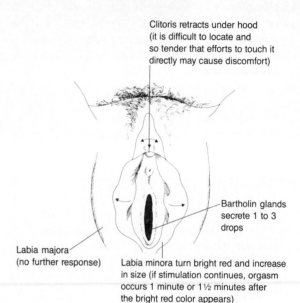

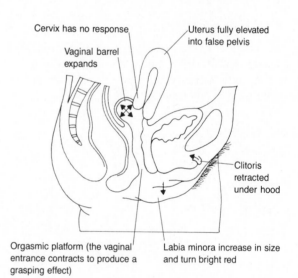

■ *Figure 9–7*

Female sexual response cycle. (A) Changes in external genitalia. (B) Changes in internal genitalia.

most intense. Mild orgasms may only have three to five contractions. Because of the extent of pelvic congestion and the capacity for distention of pelvic structures, much of the blood and edema cannot be removed and may flow back into the distended structures. As a result of this, many women are capable of restimulation seconds after orgasm and may have repeated orgasms.

The *cervix* and *uterus* have less dramatic roles in female sexual response. The uterus enlarges owing to vascular engorgement and rises gradually with increasing excitement until it is out of the true pelvis. It also pulls the upper vagina upward. Uterine contractions occur during orgasm; they are usually pleasurable, but sometimes they are not consciously perceived. For some women, however, these contractions may be painful because of prolonged spasm; most often this occurs during menopause or pregnancy, with dysmenorrhea, or when an intrauterine device is used.[13] The cervix may undergo some congestion, but there is no significant response until the cervical os opens slightly after orgasm. During the final resolution phase of the sexual cycle, the uterus drops back down into its usual position. The

Orgasm Stage

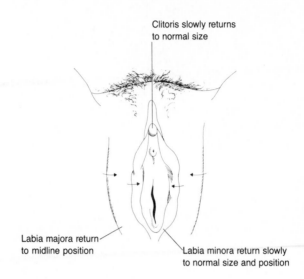

Clitoris retracted under hood

Urinary meatus dilates in some women

Labia majora (no specific response)

Labia minora (no specific response)

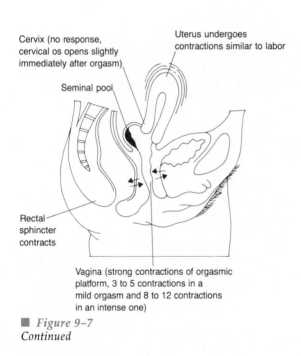

Cervix (no response, cervical os opens slightly immediately after orgasm)

Uterus undergoes contractions similar to labor

Seminal pool

Rectal sphincter contracts

Vagina (strong contractions of orgasmic platform, 3 to 5 contractions in a mild orgasm and 8 to 12 contractions in an intense one)

■ *Figure 9–7*
Continued

Resolution Stage

Clitoris slowly returns to normal size

Labia majora return to midline position

Labia minora return slowly to normal size and position

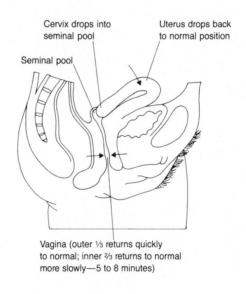

Cervix drops into seminal pool

Uterus drops back to normal position

Seminal pool

Vagina (outer ⅓ returns quickly to normal; inner ⅔ returns to normal more slowly—5 to 8 minutes)

cervical os opens more widely during this time and is positioned in the seminal pool in the upper vagina; this is believed to be an aid to sperm entry into the cervix and ultimately to conception (see Fig. 9-7).

The breasts and other nongenital areas are also involved in sexual response. During sexual excitement, the *breasts* become enlarged and the nipple becomes erect due to congestion. Both of these are erotic areas for women. Some women are able to reach orgasm by breast stimulation alone. The *skin* in some women may shown the "sex flush," a mottled pinkish discoloration that is most prominent on the chest and trunk. Spasms of the abdomen, buttocks, and thighs may also occur with high levels of excitement.

Female ejaculation, the expulsion of fluid during orgasm by women, has been reported in between 5% and 54% of women.[14-16] Researchers propose the existence of a rudimentary female prostate gland in the urethral wall near the bladder, which produces a gush of fluid from the urethra during orgasm. This has been associated with the *G spot* (for its discoverer, German gynecologist Ernest Grafenberg), a sensitive area on the anterior wall of the vagina between the symphysis pubis and the cervix. Some women find that this area is very erotic and promotes orgasm. However, the G spot has not been substantiated anatomically. The paraurethral (Skene's) glands are another possible source of female orgasmic fluid. Located on either side of the urethra,

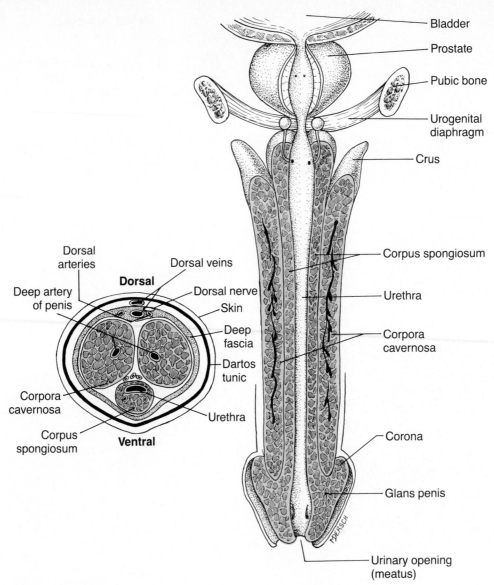

■ *Figure 9–8*
Internal structures of erect penis.

these glands develop from the same primitive tissue as the prostate gland. Studies have found that some women who ejaculate during orgasm expel a fluid that could not be distinguished from urine.[17]

MALE SEXUAL RESPONSE

The *penis* consists of three long cylinders of erectile tissue that are surrounded by an elastic sheath. Each cylinder contains blood vessels and spaces that fill up with blood during sexual arousal. The two upper cylinders, the corpora cavernosa, are responsible for the rigidity and the increase in length and width of the penis with erection (Fig. 9-8). At the base of the penile shaft, where it joins the body, the corpora cavernosa diverge into

the crura, which become tough tendinous fibers that attach to the pelvic bones. These are homologous to the clitoral crura in the female. On the underside of the penis is the third cylinder, the corpus spongiosum. On the external end it terminates in the glans, and on the internal end it terminates in the bulb. The urethra runs through the corpus spongiosum. During erection, the spongy body remains softer than the corpora cavernosa. The glans enlarges when it is excited to almost twice its quiescent size and provides a soft protective cushion for the rigid corpora cavernosa (Fig. 9-9). The glans is highly endowed with nerve endings, and it is the male's area of maximum erotic sensation.

The penile bulb becomes very rigid and distended during sexual arousal, lengthens, and increases mark-

Excitement Stage

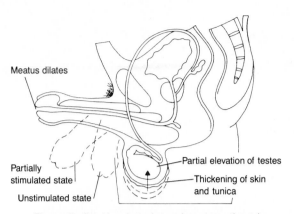

The smaller flaccid penis tends to enlarge proportionately
more in erection, thus decreasing the difference between
the larger and the smaller flaccid penis.

Plateau Stage

As seminal fluid collects in prostatic urethra,
there is a feeling of ejaculatory inevitability.
Larger fluid volume is experienced as more pleasurable.

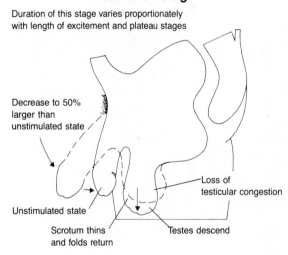

Testes fully elevated (orgasm never occurs without
elevated testes, though they may be less elevated
in men over 50 years of age.)

Orgasmic Stage

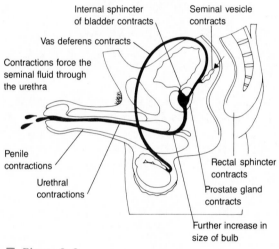

■ *Figure 9–9*
Male sexual response cycle.

Resolution Stage

Duration of this stage varies proportionately
with length of excitement and plateau stages

edly in diameter. It nearly fills the space between the
pubic rami and presses downward on the testicles. The
bulb of the penis is homologous to the female vestibular
bulbs but is not as large. The penile structures continue
to distend and enlarge until the peak of excitement is
reached. Clear mucoid fluid is secreted from the urethra,
probably from Cowper's glands or the prostate. At the
critical point of vasocongestive distention, the reflex
stretch mechanism is set off in the muscles and orgasm
occurs. The same muscles are involved in the male as
in the female, primarily the bulbocavernous, the ischiocavernous, the levator ani, and the transverse
perineum.

As muscle contractions beginning around the seminal vesicles and prostate cause emission of the semen
into the upper urethra, the man feels the sensation of

"ejaculatory inevitability," immediately followed by the
propulsive orgasmic contractions. Semen spurts out of
the urethra at 0.8-second intervals in three to seven
ejaculatory spurts. Contractions of the penis and urethra
are felt with each spurt of semen.

The skin of the *scrotum* begins to thicken and wrinkle with sexual excitement, and the *testes* begin to elevate closer to the perineum. The cremaster muscle elevates the testes and also helps to heat and to cool the
testes by bringing them closer to or farther away from
the body, maintaining an even temperature for effective
sperm production. As excitement progresses, the scrotum thickens more and the testes increase up to 50%
in size and rotate anteriorly. Vasocongestion causes increase in testicular size. At the time of orgasm, the testes
are elevated closely against the perineum and are max-

imally engorged. Following orgasm, the testes descend and decrease in size, and the scrotal skin thins and returns to its former texture (see Fig. 9-9).

The *prostate* is located just below the bladder and surrounds the urethra, and it contains an intricate series of ducts that secrete prostatic fluid. This fluid contains prostaglandins, hormonal substances that cause contractions of the uterus and are thought to aid fertilization, and other biochemical substances, including fibrinogenase, which causes temporary coagulation of semen in the vagina to prevent its dripping out. Prostatic fluid is alkaline and buffers the acidity of the vagina, allowing sperm to survive longer. It provides a vehicle for sperm transportation through the urethra and is secreted during orgasm to make up the largest part of the semen.

The *seminal vesicles* are coiled tubal structures that join the vas deferens with the ejaculatory ducts that enter the prostate. Sperm from the vas deferens mix with secretions, which are triggered by orgasm, from the seminal vesicles and pass through the prostate by way of the ejaculatory ducts. These secretions are high in fructose, a natural sugar that aids sperm motility.

The two *Cowper's glands* are the size of a pea and are located between the prostate and the urethra. They produce an alkaline secretion that neutralizes the acidity of the urethra, which is caused by transporting urine. It is important to neutralize this acidity before sperm are transported through the urethra because the acidity can damage sperm. The Cowper's glands usually secrete a drop or two of fluid, but the amount varies considerably. This fluid appears as preejaculate, and it is possible that sperm secreted into the urethra from the ejaculatory ducts might be carried along in the Cowper's gland fluid prior to orgasm. This accounts for the risk in using withdrawal for contraception, as sperm may be present in the fluid secreted before orgasm. The secretions from Cowper's glands usually appear during the plateau phase of sexual arousal, just before orgasm.

Men also experience nipple erection during sexual arousal, and they may have the sex flush, as well as spasm of the buttocks and thighs. Although no muscles play an important role in initial erection of the penile shaft, pelvic muscles are the key to the final surge to orgasm in the male. The penile bulb and corpora cavernosa are enclosed in a muscular coat, which, along with almost all other muscles in the area, is responsible for complete erection and ejaculation. Contracting in a coordinated, downward rhythm, these muscles compress the prostate, seminal vesicles, and the internal structures (penile bulb and corpora cavernosa), which in turn compress the urethra and force semen forward with considerable pressure. Blood also is forced out of the distended cavernous spaces, leading to detumescence of the penis. The penis gradually becomes flaccid

and returns to its original size after orgasm; the length of time varies for different occasions in the same man.

Patterns of Sexual Response

The sexual response cycle in men and women can be divided into several stages. The most popular model was introduced by Masters and Johnson in *Human Sexual Response*.[18] An orderly sequence of psychophysiologic events takes place and brings about marked changes in the shape and function of the genital organs, as described in the preceding section. Regardless of whether sexual stimulation is reflexogenic or psychogenic, reactions in the neurological, vascular, muscular, and hormonal systems occur that affect many parts of the body.

THE FOUR-STAGE MODEL

Masters and Johnson developed a four-stage model, which progresses from excitement to plateau, to orgasm, and finally to resolution. The *excitement stage* begins with the onset of erotic feelings and sensations. This produces an immediate and intense vasocongestion and increased myotonia if stimulation is effective. Excitement in the man is signaled by erection, with scrotal thickening and elevation of the testes. In the woman, vaginal lubrication occurs rapidly, the clitoris enlarges and becomes erect, the uterus enlarges and begins to rise, and the vagina begins to enlarge and balloon in the upper portion.

As excitement progresses, the *plateau stage* is reached; this is the stage immediately preceding orgasm. In men, the penis is fully distended and erect at its maximum size; the testes are enlarged and elevated closely against the perineum; and drops of fluid from the Cowper's glands appear at the urethral meatus. In women, pelvic congestion and edema are at a peak with maximum distention of the vestibular bulbs, labia minora, lower third of the vagina, and uterus. The orgasmic platform builds up in the lower vagina, and the uterus ascends from the true pelvis while the upper vagina widely balloons. The clitoris is completely retracted under the prepuce, is enlarged, and has completed its upward arc.

The *stage of orgasm* is reached when vasocongestion passes a critical point and a reflex stretch mechanism is set off in the pelvic muscles of both sexes. The muscles contract vigorously, pressing on distended structures and expelling blood that is trapped in tissues and vessels, which then creates the sensation of orgasm. Ejaculation occurs in the man, with spurts of semen from the urethral meatus and contractions of the penis and urethra. In the woman, contractions occur at the same time interval (0.8 second) as blood and fluid move out of distended pelvic tissues and veins. The main sites of orgasmic sensation involve the clitoris and lower part of the vagina.

Resolution is the final stage of the sexual response cycle. The changes in genitals and other organs and structures are reversed. The testes decrease in size and descend immediately, and the scrotum relaxes and returns to its usual position. The penis becomes flaccid, usually in two stages. It reduces to half the erect size soon after orgasm and completes detumescence in 30 minutes or less. In the woman, the clitoris returns to its original position rapidly and the orgasmic platform undergoes detumescence. The vagina returns to a relaxed state in about 15 minutes, the uterus descends, and the cervical os gaps for about 30 minutes. The labia minora lose their deep coloration rapidly, but the edema takes longer to resolve. Genital swelling persists in most women for variable periods of time.

Some men and women perspire heavily and have a thin film of sweat over much of the body. There is often a feeling of calm and relaxation as muscle tension ceases; laughing or crying also happens frequently. Some people feel exhausted after orgasm and rapidly fall asleep, whereas others feel invigorated and refreshed. Some may feel mildly depressed or have a sense of letdown; others feel elated or euphoric. There do not seem to be any consistent differences in postorgasmic responses between men and women.

If orgasm does not occur, resolution follows the same physiological processes but takes considerably longer. Muscle tension and vasocongestion recede more gradually, and the pelvic area may remain congested for several hours. Response to sexual experiences without orgasm vary by occasion and individual. In some instances, it may be desirable to avoid orgasmic release, and even if not deliberate, nonorgasm on occasion is usually accepted. Consistent absence of orgasm, however, often leads to frustration, resentment, feelings of inadequacy, and unhappiness. There are cultural differences between the male and female responses to nonorgasm: a man generally is not satisfied with sex unless he has ejaculated, whereas women do not find it unusual to have some percentage of nonorgasmic sexual encounters. However, a long-term, high proportion of encounters without orgasm in women gradually can lead to less interest in sex.[19]

OTHER MODELS OF SEXUAL RESPONSE PATTERNS

Based on her work as a sex therapist, Helen Kaplan has described a *triphasic model* of sexual response.[19,20] Instead of the four sequential stages of Masters and Johnson's four-stage model, she conceptualizes three rela-

tively independent phases; two are physiological (vasocongestion, reflex muscular contractions) and one is psychological (desire). The phase of vasocongestion is comparable to the excitement and plateau phases of Masters and Johnson and is controlled by the parasympathetic nervous system. The phase of reflex muscular contractions compares to orgasm in Masters and Johnson's model and is controlled by the sympathetic nervous system. The phase of sexual desire involves psychological and cognitive factors. Because different systems are involved (perceptive, neuromuscular, and vascular), difficulties can develop in one phase relatively independently of another.

A *five-component model* has been proposed by Zilbergeld and Ellison[21] that takes psychological and subjective aspects of human sexual response into account. These five components are related to each other but are also independent. The components are (1) interest or desire: (2) arousal: (3) physiological readiness, including vasocongestion of reproductive structures, erection, and vaginal lubrication: (4) orgasm: and (5) satisfaction, the subjective feeling of the sexual experience. This model includes more focus on cognitive and subjective aspects, stressing the importance of perception and evaluation of sexual events.

MALE SEXUAL PATTERN

There appears to be less variability in the man's pattern of sexual response than the woman's. Generally, excitement progresses continuously in the man unless prolonged by deliberate use of delaying tactics, until the plateau stage is reached. Plateau lasts for a relatively short period of time, then peaks in one definitive, usually strong orgasm. Resolution occurs rather rapidly, with a supposed refractory period during which restimulation of the penis is not possible. This refractory period is much shorter in younger men, who may have another erection in a few minutes, and is longer in older men. Some have questioned the concept of a time during which the man cannot respond to sexual stimuli (Fig. 9-10). Men report experiencing orgasms of different intensity.

FEMALE SEXUAL PATTERNS

There are three basic types of sexual response patterns in women. One pattern resembles the male pattern, in that excitement builds rapidly to plateau, with some peaks and dips along the way, leading to one intense orgasm and a rapid resolution stage (see Pattern C, Fig. 9-10). A second pattern among women involves a slower progression of excitement and a longer plateau stage. An intense and definite orgasm is then experienced, followed by a slower resolution stage. Or, after

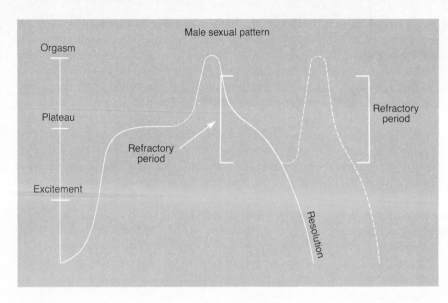

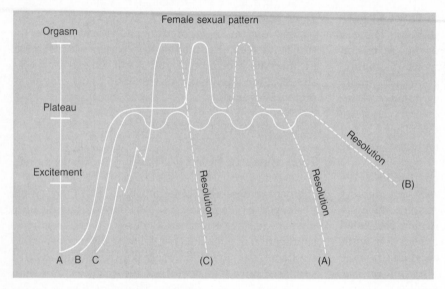

■ *Figure 9–10*

Male and female sexual response patterns. Female Sexual Patterns—(A) Steady progression to plateau stage is followed by intense orgasm; subsequent orgasms may occur; resolution is slower. (B) Slower progression to plateau stage is followed by minor surges toward orgasm causing prolonged pleasurable feelings without definitive orgasm; resolution is slowest. (C) Rapid progression to plateau stage with some peaks and dips; one intense orgasm follows with rapid resolution. This most closely resembles the male pattern.

orgasm, the woman may return to plateau for a while, then have another orgasm that may be either more or less intense. Some women can have multiple orgasms while rising and falling into plateau levels of arousal, followed by slower resolution (see Pattern A, Fig. 9-10). In the third pattern, excitement progresses more slowly until plateau is reached, then there are minor surges toward orgasm causing repeated and prolonged pleasurable and tingly sensations without a definite orgasm. Resolution tends to be longest with this pattern (see Pattern B, Fig. 9-10).[18]

There are a few other differences between the male and female sexual response that warrant discussion. Erection is attained within 3 to 5 seconds, while vaginal lubrication takes about 30 seconds. It takes longer for the woman to fill the much larger structures in her pelvic area, and greater amounts of vasocongestion and edema are required. The man has three erectile bodies to fill (two corpora cavernosa and one corpus spongiosum with its bulb), while the woman has five bodies to fill (two corpora cavernosa, two vestibular bulbs, and a large circumvaginal plexus). With all the bulbs and venous plexi maximally distended, the blood volume that a woman has to remove during orgasm is considerably greater than that of a man. Women need longer pelvic muscles to do this because the female pelvic outlet is greater in diameter. In the man, the greatest strength of muscle contractions occurs in the first three to four orgasmic contractions. This strong, concentrated muscular activity assures deposition of semen deep within the vaginal barrel. This results in a short, intense orgasm that enhances conception. The woman's orgasmic contractions generally last twice as long as the man's, and their strength is not as markedly concentrated in the first few contractions. These types of contractions remove a greater amount of the woman's more wide-

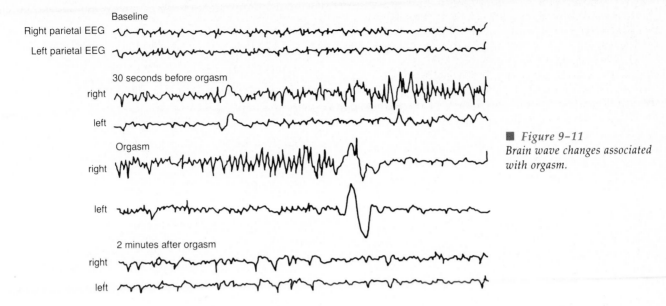

Baseline
Right parietal EEG
Left parietal EEG

30 seconds before orgasm
right
left

Orgasm
right
left

2 minutes after orgasm
right
left

■ *Figure 9–11*
Brain wave changes associated with orgasm.

spread pelvic congestion. However, as discussed previously, there is wide variation in a woman's orgasmic response with a generally greater range in intensity and duration than a man's.

Orgasm and Changes in Brain Waves

Because sexual response and orgasm are both a physical and a mental experience, it is not surprising that some striking changes in brain function have been found to parallel the physiological changes. A unique pattern in brain waves occurred in both men and women who participated in an experiment using an electroencephalogram (EEG) and physiological measures to check for changes during sexual response. The data revealed a typical pattern of brain waves through EEG recording before, during, and after orgasm. These patterns were the same for men and women (Fig. 9-11). There was a clear distinction between the left and right hemispheres of the brain just before and during orgasm. Frequency decreased in the right hemisphere to about four cycles per second, whereas in the left hemisphere it remained at about ten cycles per second. The amplitude response was also found much greater in the right hemisphere than in the left hemisphere.

The two hemispheres have been connected with different types of mental functions and cognitive activities. The left hemisphere is associated with verbal, logical, and rational thought processes. The right hemisphere has a larger role in spatial, intuitive, and emotional thought processes; it is considered the source of artistic and creative abilities. The slowing of brain wave cycles and increases in amplitude that occur in the right hemisphere with orgasm indicate its emotional–intuitive character. These brain wave patterns are unique to orgasm and do not occur with other types of activities studied in laboratories. It seems likely that the experience of orgasm is a unique state of consciousness. This may be one reason why people find the orgasmic experience difficult to describe.[22]

■ REFERENCES

1. Hyde JS: Human Sexuality, 4th ed. New York, McGraw-Hill, 1990
2. Denny NW, Quadagno D: Human Sexuality. St. Louis, Times Mirror/CV Mosby, 1988
3. Koray T, Horn MC: Contraceptive use, pregnancy and fertility patterns among single American women in their 20s. Family Plann Perspect 17:10–19, January/February 1985
4. Nass GD, Libby RW, Fisher MP: Sexual Choices. Monterey, CA, Wadsworth Health Sciences Division, 1981
5. Byer CO, Shainberg LW, Jones KL: Dimensions of Human Sexuality. Dubuque, IO, WC Brown, 1988
6. Olds L: Fully Human. Englewood Cliffs, NJ, Prentice-Hall, 1981
7. Green R: Sexual Identity Conflict in Children and Adults. New York, Basic Books, 1974
8. Money J, Ehrhardt AA: Man and Woman, Boy and Girl. Baltimore, Johns Hopkins University Press, 1972
9. Kolata G: Maleness pinpointed on Y chromosome. Science 234:1076–1077, 1986
10. Page DC, et al: The sex-determining region of the human Y chromosome encodes a finger protein. Cell 51:1091–1104, 1987
11. Johnson MH, Everett BJ: Essential Reproduction. Boston, Blackwell Scientific Publications, 1980

12. Sherfey MJ: The Nature and Evolution of Female Sexuality. New York, Random House, 1972

13. Bragonier JR: Uterine spasms elicited by orgasm. Med Aspects Human Sex 14(11):99–103, 1980

14. Ladas A, Whipple B, Perry J: The G Spot and Other Recent Discoveries About Human Sexuality. New York, Holt Rinehart & Winston, 1982

15. Masters W, Johnson V, Kolodny R: Human Sexuality, 2nd ed. Boston, Little, Brown, 1985

16. Bullough B, David M, Whipple B, et al: Subjective reports of female orgasmic expulsion of fluid. Nurse Pract 9(3):55–59, March 1984

17. Goldberg DC, et al: The Gräfenberg spot and female ejaculation: A review of initial hypothesis. J Sex Marital Therapy 9: 27–37, 1983

18. Masters W, Johnson VE: Human Sexual Response. Boston, Little, Brown, 1966

19. Kaplan HS: The New Sex Therapy. New York, Brunner/Mazel, 1974

20. Kaplan HS: Disorders of Sexual Desire. New York, Simon & Schuster, 1979

21. Zilbergeld B, Ellison CR: Desire discrepancies and arousal problems in sex therapy. In Leiblum SR, Pervin LA (eds): Principles and Practice of Sex Therapy. New York, Guilford Press, 1980

22. Cohen H, Rosen RC, Goldstein L: Electroencephalographic laterality changes during human sexual orgasm. Arch Sex Behav 5:189–199, 1976

10

Conception and Development of the Embryo and Fetus

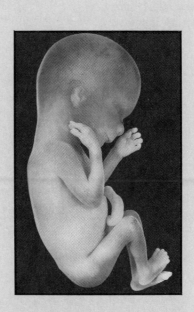

I n all of nature's wide universe, there is no process more wondrous and no mechanism more fantastic than the one by which a tiny speck of tissue, the human egg, develops into a 7-lb baby. Primitive peoples considered this phenomenon so miraculous that they frequently ascribed it to superhuman intervention and overlooked the fact that sexual intercourse was a necessary precursor. Throughout unremembered ages, our own primitive ancestors doubtless held similar beliefs, but we know that pregnancy comes about in only one way: from the union of a female germ cell, the egg, or ovum, with a male germ cell, the spermatozoon. These two germ cells, or *gametes*, become fused into one cell, or *zygote*, which contains the characteristics of both the female and the male.

■ GENETICS

Chromosomes and Genes

In all human cells, with the exception of the mature sex cells, there are normally 46 chromosomes (*chroma*, color; *soma*, body). The individual chromosomes differ in form and size, ranging from small, spheric masses to long rods (see Fig. 17-4). Normally, the chromosomes within each somatic cell are paired. Each cell contains 22 pairs of autosomes (*auto*, self) and one pair of sex chromosomes. The chromosomes are composed of strands of deoxyribonucleic acid (DNA) and protein. Genes are minute particles located in linear order on the DNA of cell nuclei. The biological and behavioral characteristics of each person are determined by genes. Pairs of autosomes that carry similar genes are referred to as *homologous*; those with dissimilar genes are referred to as *heterozygous*. It is estimated that there are as many as 100,000 genes in each cell nucleus, and these are tightly intertwined in the DNA of the 23 pairs of chromosomes.[1]

Chromosomes contain two longitudinal halves called *chromatids,* which are visible under a microscope. The chromatids are united at a point called the *centromere*. Chromosomes are classified according to their length and position on their centromere.

Female cells normally contain two X chromosomes, and male cells normally contain one X and one Y chromosome. The Y chromosomes predominantly contain genes for maleness, whereas X chromosomes carry several genes, in addition to those for sexual traits. The sex chromosome of the mature ovum is always of the X type. The mature spermatozoon may have either an X chromosome or a Y chromosome (Fig. 10-1). When fertilization occurs with a spermatozoon containing the X chromosome, a female is produced. When an ovum is

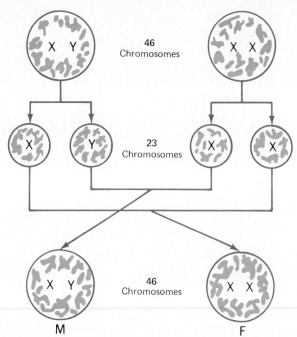

■ *Figure 10–1*

The sex of the offspring is determined at the time of fertilization by the combination of the sex chromosomes of the spermatozoon (either X or Y) and the ovum (X). The ovum fertilized by a sperm cell containing the X chromosome produces a female (44 regular chromosomes + 2 X chromosomes). If it is fertilized by a spermatozoon containing the Y chromosome, the union produces a male (44 regular chromosomes + X + Y). Note that the structures depicted as chromosomes are diagrammatic only. In this illustration it was not possible to include the total correct number.

fertilized by a spermatozoon containing a Y chromosome, a male is produced. Thus, the sex is determined at the time of fertilization by the spermatozoon, not by the ovum.

Cell reproduction is achieved by either the process of mitosis or meiosis. Mitosis is responsible for growth and development of all humans through the division, replacement, and addition of somatic cells. Meiosis is involved in *gametogenesis*, which is the process of formation and development of the specialized male (spermatozoon) and female (ovum) germ cells (gametes) for fertilization. This maturation process is called *spermatogenesis* in males and *oogenesis* in females (Fig. 10-2).

Maturation of Ovum and Sperm Cells

The oogonia enlarge to form primary oocytes during early fetal life. No primary oocytes form after birth. Although the first meiotic division of primary oocytes

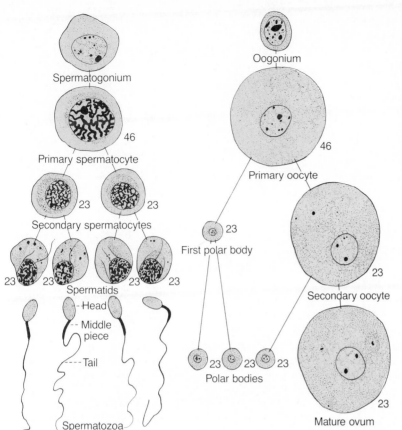

■ *Figure 10–2*
Diagram of gametogenesis. The various stages of spermatogenesis are indicated on the left; one spermatogonium gives rise to four spermatozoa. On the right, oogenesis is indicated; from each oogonium, one mature ovum and three abortive cells are produced. The chromosomes are reduced to one half the number characteristic for the general body cells of the species. In humans, the number in the body cells is 46, and that in the mature spermatozoon and secondary oocyte is 23.

begins before birth, the completion of prophase does not occur until after puberty. The ovum remains in a resting stage of development until about 2 days before ovulation. Its nucleus is large and round and has been described as vesicular because it resembles a bleb or vesicle. The ovum completes the first *meiotic division* while still in the follicle. Through meiosis, the ovum matures and its genetic material prepares for fertilization. The second meiotic division begins at ovulation; however, it is arrested until a sperm penetrates the secondary oocyte (see Fig. 10-2).

The cells that eventually produce mature spermatozoa within the seminiferous tubules of the testes are called spermatogonia. These are located at the periphery of the seminiferous tubules (see Fig. 8-3). The spermatogonia begin to increase in number at puberty. After several mitotic divisions, the spermatogonia grow and undergo gradual changes that transform them into primary spermatocytes. The primary spermatocytes subsequently undergo meiotic processes producing spermatozoa in preparation for fertilization before they leave the testis.

The spermatozoon is fully matured when it is discharged in the ejaculate.

The primary oocyte and primary spermatocyte replicate their DNA just before the first meiotic division.

Thus, at the beginning of the maturation divisions, the germ cells (primary spermatocyte and primary oocyte) contain double the normal amount of DNA and each of the 46 chromosomes is a double structure. During this reduction process, the cytoplasm divides but the chromosomes do not split; they are divided between two new cells. The daughter cell (secondary spermatocytes and secondary oocyte) contains one member of each chromosome pair (22 regular chromosomes, or *autosomes*, and an X chromosome) and thus has 23 double-structured chromosomes. The amount of DNA in each secondary cell equals that of a normal somatic cell.

Immediately after the first meiotic division, the cell begins its second maturation division in which each gamete normally receives only one chromosome of each pair and half the amount of DNA of a normal somatic cell. Thus, each mature spermatozoon has 23 chromosomes in its nucleus, and each mature ovum also contains 23 chromosomes, the haploid number.

As a result of the meiotic division, one primary oocyte produces four daughter cells, each with 22 + 1 X chromosomes. Only one of these daughter cells develops into a mature gamete, the oocyte; the other three, known as *polar bodies,* have little cytoplasm and eventually degenerate. The primary spermatocyte also gives rise to four *spermatids:* two with 22 + 1 X chromosomes and two with 22 + 1 Y chromosomes. Each spermatid develops a tail and eventually becomes a mature spermatozoon.

The importance of meiosis is that it provides for constancy of the chromosome number from generation to generation by producing haploid germ cells, and it allows independent arrangement of maternal and paternal chromosomes among the gametes.[2]

OVUM

As described in Chapter 8, one ovum per month is normally discharged from the human ovary. Under the influence of the gonadotropins, the graafian follicle, which is destined to release an ovum, has matured. The ovum has been pushed to one side of the fluid-filled cavity of the follicle. It is surrounded by a translucent coat, the *zona pellucida*. Immediately adjacent to and connected to the zona pellucida is a layer of follicular cells, the *corona radiata*, which are arranged in a radial pattern. The *cumulus oophorus* is a more loosely structured layer of cells peripheral to the corona radiata. The ovum, surrounded by this entourage of cells, having matured through release of its first polar body, is released through the process of ovulation. The ovum, within its sticky cumulus mass, rapidly and efficiently is transported into the fallopian tube, the site of fertilization. The ovum is about 0.2 mm (¹/₂₅ of an inch) in diameter and is barely visible to the naked eye.

SPERMATOZOA

Spermatozoa resemble microscopic tadpoles, with oval heads and long, lashing tails about ten times the length of the head. They are much smaller than ova; their overall length measures about one quarter the diameter of the egg, and it has been estimated that the heads of 2 billion of them—enough to regenerate most of the population of the world—could be placed, with room to spare, in the hull of a grain of rice.

The human spermatozoon consists of three parts: the head, the middle piece (neck), and the tail (Fig. 10-3). The head of the spermatozoon is covered by the acrosome. This acrosomal cap is an envelope in which enzymes that play an important role in sperm penetration are contained. The nucleus, and consequently the chromatin material, is in the head; the tail serves as a propeller.

The wriggling motions of the tails allow spermatozoa to swim with a quick vibratory motion, as fast as 3 mm/min. To ascend the uterus and the fallopian tube, they must swim against the same currents that waft the ovum downward; they are assisted by the muscular action of the uterus, which propels them upward in the direction of the tube. Spermatozoa have been observed in the fallopian tube within minutes of insemination.

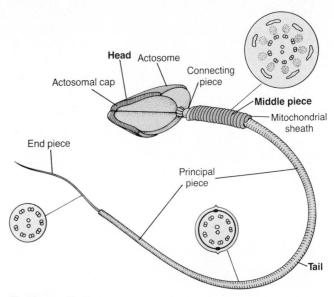

■ *Figure 10-3*

Drawing of a mammalian spermatozoon with the cell membrane removed to show the arrangement of the underlying structural components. The appearance of cross sections as seen in electron micrographs at various levels is also depicted.

The most amazing feature of spermatozoa is the huge number of them. At each ejaculation during intercourse, approximately 300 million are discharged into the vagina. If each of these could be united with an ovum, the babies that would be created would exceed the total number born in the United States during the past 100 years.

Of the millions of spermatozoa deposited in the vagina during coitus, many are expelled immediately and some remain in the vagina for an interval and are later extruded. Those retained in the vagina lose their motility in about an hour because of the acidic environment provided by the vagina.

Some spermatozoa reach the cervix almost immediately after ejaculation. Those transferred into the secretions of the cervix find a more favorable environment and may remain motile for as long as several days, especially in the preovulatory phase of the cycle.

Thousands of spermatozoa find their way into the cavity of the uterus; fewer reach the lumen of the fallopian tube. Only one is afforded the privilege of continued biological life through fertilization and, at that, only occasionally. The spermatozoa in the female reproductive tract may retain their motility for hours or days; however, few spermatozoa are capable of fertilization after more than 24 hours. It is likely that the optimum time for fertilization is substantially shorter, perhaps no more than 1 to 2 hours.[1] Spermatozoa are disposed of in the reproductive tract or in the peritoneal cavity, and, as they degenerate, they are phagocytized by white blood cells.

Spermatozoa are conditioned to fertilize an ovum after they are exposed to the female reproductive tract, a process called *capacitation* (i.e., they attain the capacity to penetrate the ovum). This mechanism involves the removal of a protein layer that coats the head of the spermatozoon as it traverses the male reproductive tract. The removal of this protein is accomplished in the fluids of the female reproductive tract and is an essential requisite to fertilization.

■ FERTILIZATION AND IMPLANTATION

Transport Through the Fallopian Tubes

The fallopian tube is an important structure that serves a number of functions in reproduction (Fig. 10-4). It is responsible for transferring the ovum into its lumen from the rupturing follicle and for providing a temporary environment for the ovum and the spermatozoon. It is also where fertilization occurs and where the ovum passes through several cell divisions during the early stages of human life. Finally, this tube is responsible for transporting the fertilized, cleaving ovum into the uterus.

The tube is uniquely designed anatomically for its various functions, containing *fimbriae* and *cilia*, which facilitate ovum transport (see Fig. 8-9 and Fig. 10-5). The structure of the fimbriated end of the tube is important in ovum pickup mechanisms. A separate strand of fimbriae, the *fimbria ovarica*, extends from the tube to the ovary to which it is attached. This contains a separate bundle of smooth muscle. During ovulation, this muscle contracts and pulls the ovary in the direction of the tubal opening. The remainder of the fimbriae are thought to embrace the ovary near or over the point of ovulation. They exercise muscular movement that

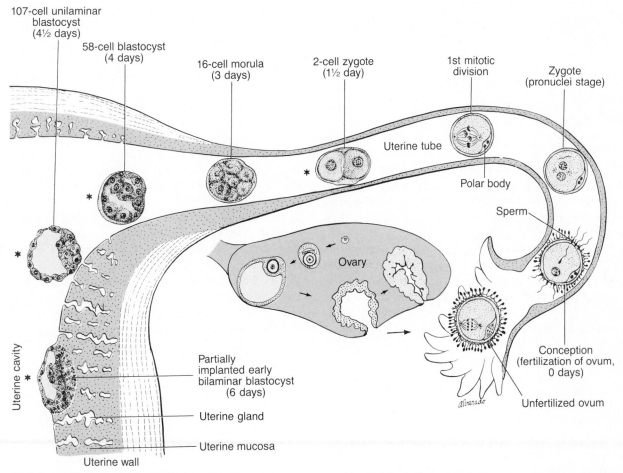

■ Figure 10–4

Transport of the ovum into the fallopian tube, and fertilization within the tube followed by cleavage (cell division) to the 8- to 16-cell stage. The product, now referred to as a morula, is delivered into the uterus where it develops into a blastocyst and implants in the endometrium on the sixth to seventh postfertilization day. (Modified from Gasser RF: Atlas of Human Embryos. Hagerstown, Harper & Row, 1975.)

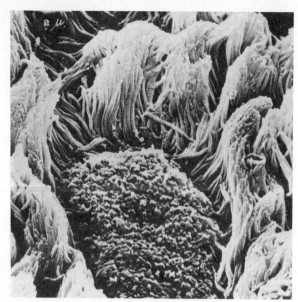

■ *Figure 10–5*
Scanning electron micrograph of the human fallopian tube showing ciliated cells surrounding a nonciliated cell in the midproliferative phase of the menstrual cycle. (Patek E, Nilsson L, Johannisson E: Scanning electron microscopic study of the human fallopian tube: The proliferative and secretory stages. Fertil Steril 23:459, 1972.)

moves them to and fro over the rupturing follicle. Thus, the cilia lining the fimbriae soon come into contact with the cumulus oophorus surrounding the ovum, and as they beat in the direction of the tubal lumen, they carry the sticky cumulus mass past the tubal ostium to a point well within the fallopian tube. An efficient process of ovum transfer is arranged through these mechanisms, and ovum pickup is practically ensured, despite the fact that the ovum is minuscule.

Once the ovum is safely past the tubal ostium, it is rapidly transported to a point well within the fallopian tube where fertilization occurs. After fertilization, the ovum passes through several cell divisions, during which it is retained in the fallopian tube for approximately 3 days. The mechanism by which the human ovum is retained in the tube is not, as yet, clear. However, the importance of the 3-day residence within the tube can be extrapolated from experiments in other mammals. In the rabbit, for example, if the fertilized ovum is removed from the tube and placed in the uterus prematurely, it degenerates and fails to implant. Although for obvious reasons this experiment has not been carried out on humans, it is generally accepted that the 3-day residence within the human tube is important. Premature expulsion of the ovum from the tube could result in failure of implantation. Prolonged retention could result in ectopic pregnancy, causing tubal rupture and hemorrhage (see Chap. 33).

Fertilization and Changes After Fertilization

After the ovum is well within the fallopian tube, the cumulus oophorus disperses. These cells begin to separate, partly as a result of the influence of the enzyme hyaluronidase contained in the acrosome surrounding the head of the spermatozoon. The spermatozoon makes its way through this peripheral layer of cells; meanwhile, the densely packed corona radiata has undergone certain changes. These cells become looser under the influence of tubal fluid, and the spermatozoon finds its way through this layer to the zona pellucida. It is thought that the zona pellucida is penetrated by the spermatozoon because of a trypsinlike enzyme present in the sperm acrosome. Before penetration, openings are created in the outer membrane of the acrosome through which the enzyme-rich contents of the acrosome escape. This process, called the *acrosome reaction*, leads to a loss of the membrane over the anterior half of the sperm head. The spermatozoon makes a channel through the zona pellucida as the trypsinlike enzyme, referred to as acrosin, dissolves the protein-containing zona with which it comes into contact. After the spermatozoon traverses the zona pellucida, it is in a position to penetrate the membrane of the ovum. As the spermatozoon penetrates the ovum, it brings its tail with it.

Once penetration is complete, a physiological barrier occurs and penetration of the ovum by other spermatozoa is prevented. Soon after penetration, the nucleus of the spermatozoon and the nucleus of the ovum undergo characteristic changes. They become pronuclei: distinct, clearly identifiable bodies of chromatin, each contained in a membrane. The male pronucleus and the female pronucleus fuse. The new cell presents the full complement, or *diploid number*, of chromosomes, one half from the spermatozoon and one half from the ovum. Soon thereafter, the first cell division occurs. In this process, the male and female chromosomes and their genes are mingled and finally split, forming two sets of 46 chromosomes, one set of 46 going to each of the two new cells. This process is repeated again and again until masses containing 8, 16, 32, and 64 cells are produced successively. These early cell divisions produce a *morula*.

At the 8- to 16-cell stage, the dividing ovum is delivered into the uterus. The fertilized ovum spends about 4 days in the uterine cavity developing further into a blastocyst before actual embedding takes place. Thus, a total interval of about 7 days elapses between ovulation and implantation. During the period when the ovum lies unattached in the uterine cavity, it lies in a lake of endometrial secretion that is rich in glycogen and provides nourishment.

Meanwhile, several important changes are occurring

in the internal structure of the fertilized ovum. Fluid appears in the center of the mulberry mass that pushes cells to the periphery of the sphere. At the same time, it becomes apparent that this external envelope of cells is actually made up of two different layers, an inner and an outer layer. The inner solid mass of cells is called the blastocyst and develops into the embryo and an embryonic membrane (the *amnion*). The outer layer is a sort of foraging unit called the *trophoblast*, which means feeding layer; it is the principal function of these cells to secure food for the embryo (Fig. 10-6). The trophoblast eventually develops into one of the embryonic membranes known as the *chorion*.

While the ovum is undergoing these changes, the lining of the uterus is preparing for its reception. Considering that ovulation took place on the 14th day of the menstrual cycle and that the tubal journey and the uterine sojourn required 7 days, 21 days of the cycle have passed before the ovum develops its trophoblastic layer of cells. This is the period when the lining of the uterus reaches its greatest thickness and succulence.

Implantation of the Ovum

The *trophoblast* is responsible for embedding the ovum. This process is carried out by means of enzymes. These cells not only burrow into the endometrium and eat out a nest for the ovum, but they can also digest the walls of the many small blood vessels that they encounter beneath the surface. The mother's bloodstream is tapped, and the ovum is deeply sunk in the lining epithelium of the uterus, with tiny pools of blood around it. Fingerlike projections, or chorionic villi, develop out of the trophoblastic layer and extend into the blood-filled spaces. Another name for the trophoblast, and one more commonly used as pregnancy progresses, is

the *chorion*. These chorionic villi contain blood vessels that are connected to the fetus and are extremely important because they are the sole means by which oxygen and nourishment are received from the mother. The entire ovum becomes covered with villi, which grow out radially and convert the chorion into a shaggy sac.

The cells of the chorionic villi begin to secrete human chorionic gonadotropin (HCG), the hormone that maintains progesterone production by the corpus luteum. In turn, progesterone stimulates and supports endometrial growth by providing a suitable environment for continued development of the conceptus. Thus, the newly formed pregnancy is essentially self-sufficient and is in control of its own environment.

Throughout the 2-week interval after fertilization, there is a substantial incidence of pregnancy loss, associated with abnormal development of the fertilized ova. Such a pregnancy loss is not surprising considering the complicated series of events that culminate in a successfully implanted pregnancy. For surviving ova, the second week of gestation marks the beginning of the embryo stage of prenatal development, in which development occurs relatively rapidly.

Multiple Pregnancies

Multiple pregnancies have become increasingly common as a consequence of infertility therapies that involve administration of human gonadotropins to women with ovulatory failure. Twinning is the most frequent type of multiple pregnancy, with an incidence of approximately 1 in 90 births.[2] There are two types of twins: dizygotic or fraternal twins originate from two zygotes; monozygotic or identical twins develop from one zygote. About two thirds of twins are dizygotic, and there is a tendency for dizygotic twins to repeat in

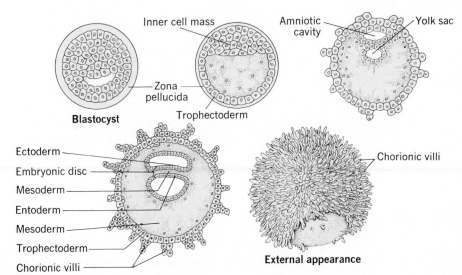

Blastocyst

Inner cell mass

Zona pellucida

Trophectoderm

Amniotic cavity

Yolk sac

Ectoderm

Embryonic disc

Mesoderm

Entoderm

Mesoderm

Trophectoderm

Chorionic villi

Chorionic villi

External appearance

■ *Figure 10–6*
Early stages of development. (Top, left and center) The cells are separated into a peripheral layer and an inner cell mass. The peripheral layer is called the trophoblast, or trophectoderm; the entire structure is called a blastodermic vesicle. (Top, right) The formation of the amniotic cavity and yolk sac is indicated. The former is lined with ectoderm, the latter with entoderm. (Bottom, left) The location of the embryonic disc and the three germ layers is shown, together with the beginning of the chorionic villi. (Bottom, right) The external appearance of the developing mass is shown; the chorionic villi are abundant.

families. Because they develop from the fertilization of two separate ova by two different sperms, dizygotic twins are genetically distinct and may be of the same sex or different sexes. In contrast, monozygotic twins are genetically identical and are of the same sex. Monozygotic twinning usually begins in the blastocyst stage as a result of the division of the inner cell mass into two embryonic primordia. A further discussion of multiple pregnancies is found in Chapter 38.

■ STAGES AND DURATION OF PREGNANCY

Development Stages: Ovum, Embryo, and Fetus

Fertilization initiates the process of human development. Prenatal development is divided into three periods, which are displayed in the box below.

Although each of the these stages is important, the embryonic period is most critical because all the main organ systems are differentiating and are vulnerable to environmental influences (e.g., teratogens such as drugs, viruses, radiation, infection). The adequacy of the mother's diet is important to the developing embryo and fetus. Nutritional deficiencies during pregnancy may contribute to smaller intrauterine growth because the needs of the rapidly growing fetus are not being met.

Duration of Pregnancy

The length of pregnancy varies greatly; it may range between 240 and 300 days and yet be entirely normal in every respect. The average duration from the time of conception is 9½ lunar months (i.e., 38 weeks or 266

days). From the first day of the last menstrual period, its average length is 10 lunar months (i.e., 40 weeks or 280 days). However, scarcely one pregnancy in ten terminates exactly 280 days after the beginning of the last period. Less than one half terminate within 1 week of day 280. In 10% of all pregnancies, birth occurs a week or more before the theoretical end of pregnancy, and in another 10%, it takes place more than 2 weeks later than expected.[3] Indeed, it appears that some fetuses require a longer time and others require a shorter time in the uterus for full development.

Viability

The length of gestation is important because it affects the unborn child's chances of survival after birth. Viability refers to the capability of the fetus to live outside the uterus at the earliest gestational age. It was formerly believed that a fetus was viable at a weight of 1000 g (about 28 weeks' gestation). The age at which a fetus reaches viability has declined in recent years as a result of improvements in maternal and neonatal care. Fetal viability has been reported as early as 22 weeks, but the chances of survival are poor until several weeks later, mainly because the respiratory system and the central nervous system are not completely differentiated.[2]

■ PHYSIOLOGY OF THE EMBRYO

Decidua

The *decidua* is the structure of thickened endometrium that develops after conception. It is a direct continuation, in exaggerated form, of the already modified premenstrual endometrium. For descriptive purposes, the decidua is divided into three portions. The part lying directly under the embedded ovum that forms the maternal component of the placenta is the *decidua basalis* (Fig. 10-7). The portion that is superficial and pushed out by the ovum is the *decidua capsularis*. The remaining portion, which is not in immediate contact with the ovum, is the *decidua vera*. As pregnancy advances, the decidua capsularis expands rapidly over the growing embryo and, at about the fourth month, lies in intimate contact with the decidua vera.

The Amnion

Even before the previously noted structures become evident, a fluid-filled space develops around the embryo.

Periods of Prenatal Development

Ovum. Fertilization through the first 2 weeks of prenatal life (includes formation of the morula, blastocyst, primary villi, and implantation)

Embryo. From the second to the eighth week of gestation during which all essential structures are developing and a definite form is being assumed

Fetus. From the eighth week to the time of birth, a period of growth and maturation of existing structures

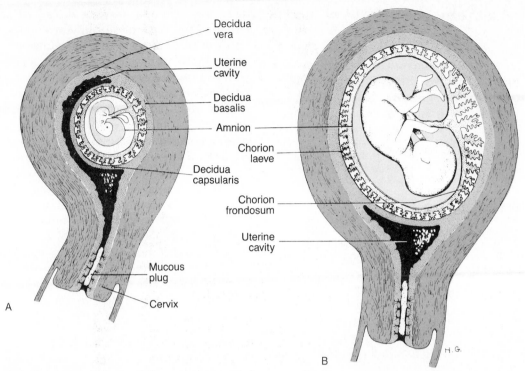

■ *Figure 10-7*
Diagrams illustrating enlargement of the chorionic vesicle and progressive obliteration of the uterine cavity. (A) At 6 weeks after fertilization. (B) At 16 weeks after fertilization. (Modified from Cunningham FG, MacDonald PC, Gant NF: Williams Obstetrics, 18th ed. Norwalk, CT, Appleton & Lange, 1989.)

This space, the amniotic cavity, is lined with a smooth, slippery, glistening membrane, the *amnion* (see Fig. 10-7). The amnion originates from the ectoderm, a primary germ layer. It has an important role in prostaglandin (PGE$_2$) formation, particularly after labor commences.

Because the amniotic cavity is filled with fluid, it is often called the bag of waters; the fetus floats and moves in the amniotic cavity. The amniotic fluid is composed of water (98%) and organic and inorganic solids (1%–2%). It serves a number of important functions for the embryo/fetus (e.g., helping maintain even body temperature, providing a cushion against possible injury, permitting symmetric external growth, preventing adherence of the amnion, and providing space for free movement).

The amniotic cavity enlarges throughout gestation; at the end of the fourth month of pregnancy, it is the size of a large orange and, with the fetus, occupies the entire interior of the uterus. By full term, this cavity normally contains from 500 ml to 1000 ml of liquor amnii, or the "waters."

Chorion

The shaggy chorionic villi that originally cover the ovum and invade the decidua basalis, enlarge and multiply rapidly to form the *chorion frondosum* (leafy chorion). This structure becomes the fetal component of the placenta. The chorionic villi covering the decidua capsularis degenerate and almost disappear, leaving only a slightly roughened membrane, the *chorion laeve* (bald chorion). The chorion laeve lies separated from the amnion by the exocoelomic cavity until near the end of the third month, after which they establish close contact. The chorion laeve and amnion form an avascular *amniochorion*, an important site of transfer and metabolic activity.[1] The fetus is thus surrounded by two membranes, the amnion and the chorion.

YOLK SAC

The small yolk sac develops as a cavity in the blastocyst about 8 or 9 days after fertilization. It serves many functions in embryonic development, such as helping to transfer nutrients to the embryo during the second and third weeks, while uteroplacental circulation is being established; and forming early blood cells until hematopoietic activity begins in the liver during the sixth week. The dorsal section of the yolk sac becomes part of the primitive gut. The yolk sac detaches from the midgut loop by the end of the sixth week and shrinks as gestation advances.

Three Germ Layers

The three germ layers that arise from the inner mass of blastocyst cells during the third week grow rapidly with adequate nutrition and give rise to all the tissues and organs of the embryo. At first. they all look alike, but soon after embedding, certain groups of cells assume distinctive characteristics and differentiate into three main groups: an outer covering layer (ectoderm), a middle layer (mesoderm), and an internal layer (endoderm).

Sex Differentiation

In the first section of this chapter, the determination of chromosomal and genetic sex is described. This is established at the time of fertilization based on whether an X-bearing sperm or a Y-bearing sperm fertilizes the X-bearing ovum. The early embryo is bipotential, with the ability to differentiate sexually (phenotypic sexual differentiation) into either male or female, at least in terms of the internal and external genitalia. The default genital phenotype is female.[3]

The two sexes have gonads identical in appearance before the seventh week; these are known as *indifferent gonads*. In the process of gonadal differentiation, the Y chromosome is of prime importance because it has a strong testis-determining effect on the medulla of the indifferent gonad.[2] It regulates the release of the testis-organizing factor (H-Y antigen), which is responsible for testicular differentiation. The primary sex cords differentiate into seminiferous tubules under the influence of the Y chromosome. A proteinaceous substance known as müllerian-inhibiting factor (MIF) is produced by Sertoli's cells of the seminiferous tubules. MIF acts locally to cause regression of the müllerian duct (i.e., it causes failure of development of the uterus, fallopian tube, and upper vagina).

Differentiation proceeds from the gonad to the internal reproductive structures and is completed with the differentiation of the external genitals as male or female.[4] Testosterone induces the development (or persistence) of the internal genital structures developed from the wolffian ducts, whereas dihydrotestosterone (peripherally metabolized from testosterone) produces normal masculinization of the external genitalia.[3] Female sexual differentiation in the fetus does not depend on hormones; it happens even if the ovaries are absent.[5]

The development of ambiguous genitalia is attributed to abnormal androgenic representation in utero.[1] In other words, an embryo that was destined to be female received too much androgen, or an embryo that was destined to be male received too little androgen.

■ SIZE AND DEVELOPMENT OF THE FETUS

Size of the Fetus at Various Months

Length is generally considered a more accurate criterion of the age of the fetus than weight. Hasse's rule suggests that for clinical purposes, the length of the embryo in centimeters may be approximated during the first 5 months by squaring the number of the month of pregnancy; in the second half of pregnancy, the month may be multiplied by five to estimate the length of the fetus. Conversely, the approximate age of the fetus may be obtained by taking the square root of its length in centimeters during the first 5 months and thereafter by dividing its length in centimeters by five. For example, a fetus that is 16 cm long is about 4 months old; a fetus that is 35 cm long is about 7 months old.

Development of the Fetus from Month to Month

Conception does not take place until ovulation, 14 days after the onset of menstruation in a 28-day cycle, and an embryo does not attain the age of 1 month until about a fortnight after the first missed period (assuming a 28-day cycle). Its "birthday" by months regularly falls 2 weeks or so after any numerically specified missed period (Fig. 10-8). If the cycle is longer than 28 days, or if ovulation was delayed in the conceptive cycle, the

---

> ### *Three Germ Layers*
>
> **Ectoderm.** The epithelium of the skin, hair, nails, sebaceous glands, sweat glands, and nasal and oral passages; the salivary glands and mucous membranes of the mouth and nose; the enamel of the teeth; the mammary glands; the central nervous system (brain and spinal cord) and the peripheral nervous system
>
> **Mesoderm.** Muscles, bone, cartilage, the dentin of the teeth, ligaments, tendons, areolar tissue, striated and smooth muscles, kidneys, spleen, ureters, ovaries, testes, the heart, blood, lymph and blood vessels, and the lining of the pericardial, pleural, and peritoneal cavities
>
> **Endoderm.** Epithelium of the digestive tract and the respiratory tract (except the nose), thymus, liver, pancreas, bladder, the urethra, the thyroid, and the tympanic antrum and auditory tube

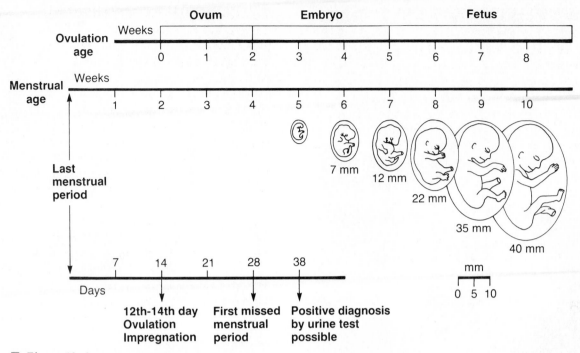

■ *Figure 10–8*
Growth of the ovum, embryo, and fetus during the early weeks of pregnancy.

duration of actual pregnancy, relative to the last menstrual period, is shorter. This should be remembered in evaluating the month-by-month development of the fetus.

Calculations of pregnancy length in lunar months refer to 4-week periods, which correspond to the usual length of the menstrual cycle (see Fig. 10-8).

END OF FIRST LUNAR MONTH

The embryo is about 4 mm to 5 mm long if measured in a straight line from crown to rump, and recognizable traces of all organs are differentiated. The backbone is apparent but is so bent upon itself that the head almost touches the tip of the tail. The head is extremely prominent, representing almost one third of the entire embryo. The head is large in proportion to the body throughout intrauterine life. This is still true at birth, but to a lesser degree.

The rudiments of the eyes, the ears, and the nose make their appearance (Fig. 10-9). The tube that eventually forms the heart has been formed, producing a large, rounded bulge on the body wall; even at this early age, this structure is pulsating regularly and propelling blood through microscopic arteries. The rudiments of the future digestive tract are also discernible. A long, slender tube leading from the mouth to an expansion becomes the stomach; connected with the latter, the beginnings of the intestines may be seen. The incipient arms and legs resemble buds.

END OF SECOND LUNAR MONTH

The fetus begins to assume human form (Fig. 10-10). As the brain develops, the head becomes disproportionately large so that the nose, the mouth, and the ears become relatively less prominent. It has an unmistakably human face, as well as arms and legs, with fingers, toes, elbows, and knees (Fig. 10-11). During the past 4 weeks, it has quadrupled in length and measures about 27 mm to 31 mm from head to buttocks. During this period the external genitalia become apparent, but it is difficult to distinguish between male and female. In the seventh week, a fetal heartbeat can be detected with real-time sonography.

END OF THIRD LUNAR MONTH

The fetus is often over 7.5 cm long and weighs almost 45 g. The sex can be distinguished because the external genitalia are beginning to show definite signs of sex. Centers of ossification have appeared in most bones; the fingers and the toes have become differentiated; and fingernails and toenails appear as fine membranes. Early in this month, buds for all the temporary "baby" teeth are present, and sockets for these develop in the jawbone. Rudimentary kidneys have developed and secrete small amounts of urine into the bladder, which escape later into the amniotic fluid. Movements of the fetus are known to occur at this time, but they are too weak to be felt by the mother.

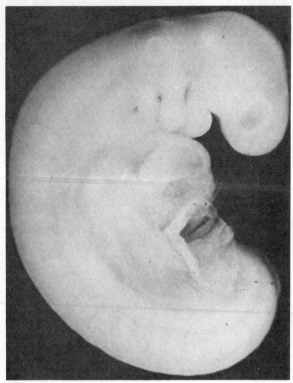

■ *Figure 10–9*
Human embryo in the first lunar month of development.
(Carnegie Institution, Washington, DC.)

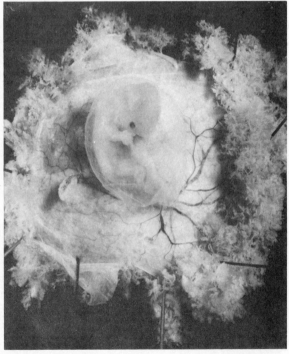

■ *Figure 10–10*
Human embryo photographed by Chester F. Reather. This
specimen represents about 40 days of development and is
shown in the opened chorion. Original magnification ×1.7.
(Carnegie Institution, Washington, DC.)

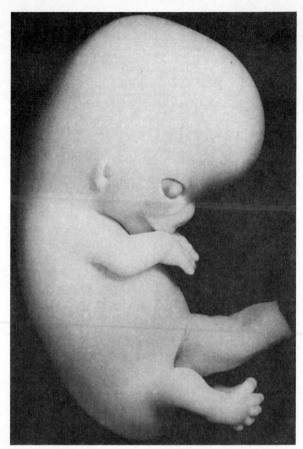

■ *Figure 10–11*
Human fetus at about 8 weeks of development. Note the
prominence of the head and the continuing development of the
extremities. (Carnegie Institution, Washington, DC.)

END OF FOURTH LUNAR MONTH

The fetus is 12 cm long from head to toe and weighs about 110 g (Fig. 10-12). The sex, as evidenced by the external genital organs, is obvious.

END OF FIFTH LUNAR MONTH

The crown to rump length of the fetus approximates 19 cm, and it weighs about 300 g. A fine, downy growth of hair, *lanugo*, appears on the skin over the entire body. Usually, the mother becomes conscious of slight fluttering movements in her abdomen as a result of fetal movement. Their first appearance is called *quickening*, or the perception of life. Fetal heart tones can easily be detected by auscultation at the end of the fifth lunar month. If a fetus is born now, it may make a few efforts to breathe, but its lungs are insufficiently developed to cope with conditions outside the uterus, and it invariably dies within a few hours at most.

*Fetal Development**

1st Lunar Month

The embryo is 4 to 5mm in length.

Trophoblasts embed in decidua.

Chorionic villi form.

Foundations for nervous system, genitourinary system, skin, bones, and lungs are formed.

Buds of arms and legs begin to form.

Rudiments of eyes, ears, and nose appear.

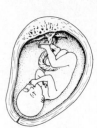

4 weeks

2nd Lunar Month

The fetus is 27 to 31 mm in length and weighs 2 to 4g.

Fetus is markedly bent.

Head is disproportionately large as a result of brain development.

Sex differentiation begins.

Centers of bone begin to ossify.

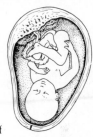

8 weeks

3rd Lunar Month

The fetus average length is 6 to 9 cm, and weight is 45 g.

Fingers and toes are distinct

Placenta is complete.

Fetal circulation is complete.

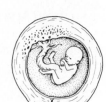

3 months

4th Lunar Month

The fetus is 12 cm in length and weighs 110 g.

Sex is differentiated.

Rudimentary kidneys secrete urine.

Heartbeat is present.

Nasal septum and palate close.

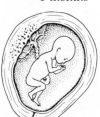

4 months

5th Lunar Month

The fetus is 19 cm in length and weighs approximately 300 g.

Lanugo covers entire body.

Fetal movements are felt by mother.

Heart sounds are perceptible by auscultation.

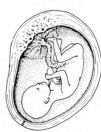
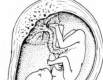

5 months

* All lengths given are crown to rump.

6th Lunar Month

The fetus is about 23 cm in length and weighs 630 g.

Skin appears wrinkled.

Vernix caseosa appears.

Eyebrows and fingernails develop.

6 months

7th Lunar Month

The fetus is 27 cm in length and weighs about 1100 g.

Skin is red.

Pupillary membrane disappears from eyes.

The fetus has an excellent chance of survival.

7 months

8th Lunar Month

The fetus is 28 to 30 cm in length and weighs 1.8 kg.

Fetus is viable.

Eyelids open.

Fingerprints are set.

Vigorous fetal movement occurs.

8 months

9th Lunar Month

The fetus' average length is 32 cm; weight is about 2500 g.

Face and body have a loose wrinkled appearance because of subcutaneous fat deposit.

Lanugo disappears.

Amniotic fluid decreases.

9 months

10th Lunar Month

The average fetus is 36 cm in length and weighs 3000 to 3600 g.

Skin is smooth.

Eyes are uniformly slate colored.

Bones of skull are ossified and nearly together at sutures.

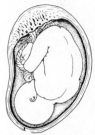
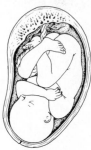

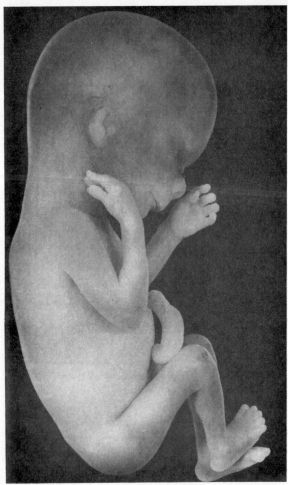

■ *Figure 10–12*
At about 4 months, external features are easily identified. Most organ systems have been formed and continue to grow and mature. (Carnegie Institution, Washington, DC.)

In Utero Fetal Behavior

As pregnancy progresses, the fetus becomes capable of increasingly complex behaviors, which may be detected in utero by sonographic techniques. By the eighth week, movements of the trunk can be observed; the limbs begin to move a week later. Hiccuping is a common occurrence that may be perceived by the mother beginning around the ninth week. By the 11th week, there is movement of the fetal chest, and soon thereafter the fetus becomes capable of moving amniotic fluid in and out of the respiratory tract—intrauterine fetal "breathing." The fetus actually swallows amniotic fluid and, because the taste buds are already developed, can actually react to substances injected into the amniotic fluid, which are swallowed by the seventh month. The internal and middle ear are well developed by mid-pregnancy, and the fetus is capable of reacting to sudden noise with active movement at about the 24th week.

END OF SIXTH LUNAR MONTH

The length of the fetus from crown to rump is 23 cm, and its weight is 630 g. It resembles a miniature baby, with the exception of the skin, which is wrinkled and red with practically no fat beneath it. At this time, however, the skin begins to develop a protective covering, *vernix caseosa*, which means "cheesy varnish." This fatty, cheesy substance adheres to the skin of the fetus and at term may be 0.3 cm thick. Increasing numbers of fetuses of this size survive in intensive-care nurseries.

END OF SEVENTH LUNAR MONTH

The fetus measures about 27 cm in length from crown to rump and weighs approximately 1.1 kg. The pupillary membrane has just disappeared from the eyes. If the fetus is born at this time, it has an excellent chance of survival.

END OF EIGHTH LUNAR MONTH

The fetus measures about 28 to 30 cm from crown to rump and weighs approximately 1.8 kg. Its skin is still red and wrinkled, and vernix caseosa and lanugo are still present. The fetus resembles a little old man. With proper incubator and good nursing care, infants born at the end of the eighth month have a better than 90% chance of survival in many nurseries in the United States.

END OF NINTH LUNAR MONTH

For all practical purposes, the fetus is a mature infant. It measures about 32 cm from crown to rump and weighs approximately 2.5 kg. Because of the deposition of subcutaneous fat, the body has become more rotund and the skin is less wrinkled and red. The fetus devotes the last 2 months in the uterus to putting on weight; during this period, it gains 220 g a week. Its chances of survival are as good as though it were born at full term.

MIDDLE OF TENTH LUNAR MONTH

Full term has been reached, and the fetus weighs, on an average, 3 kg if a girl or 3.4 kg if a boy, and it is about 36 cm long from crown to rump. Its skin is white or pink (Caucasian fetus) and thickly coated with the cheesy vernix. The fine, downy hair that previously covered its body has largely disappeared. The fingernails are firm and protrude beyond the end of the fingers.

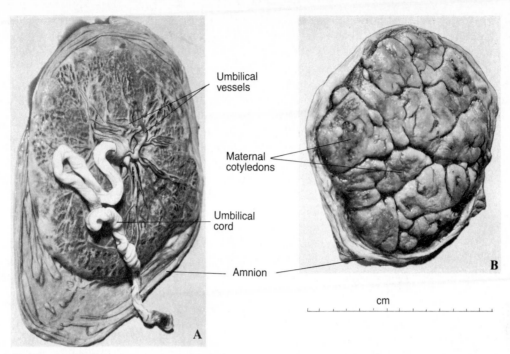

■ *Figure 10–13*
Full-term placenta. (A) Fetal surface. (B) Maternal surface. (Fitzgerald MJT: Human
Embryology: A Regional Approach. Hagerstown, Harper & Row, 1978.)

■ PHYSIOLOGY OF THE FETUS AND PLACENTA

Early in pregnancy, by the third or the fourth week, the chorionic villi develop blood vessels within them (connected with the fetal bloodstream). The trophoblast cells of the chorionic villi form spaces in the decidua basalis, which fill with maternal blood to supply nourishment to the fetus. Differentiation of the chorionic villi continues, and by the third month the placenta has formed through the union of the chorionic villi (fetal portion) and the decidua basalis (maternal portion; see Fig. 10-7).

The placenta is a fleshy, disklike organ that grows to about 20 cm in diameter and 2 cm in thickness late in pregnancy. During the course of pregnancy, its weight and mass increase in proportion with that of the fetus. The normal fetal:placental weight ratio at term is 6:1. At term, the placenta weighs about 500 g and covers about one quarter of the uterine wall.

The fetal surface of the placenta is smooth and glistening and is covered by amnion. Beneath this membrane, a number of large blood vessels may be seen. The maternal surface is red and fleshlike and is divided into 15 to 20 segments, or *cotyledons*, about 2.5 cm in diameter (Fig. 10-13).

The placenta is connected to the fetus by the *umbilical cord*, which is usually about 55 cm in length and about 1 to 2.5 cm in diameter. The cord usually leaves the placenta near the center and enters the abdominal wall of the fetus at the umbilicus, just below the middle of the median line in front. It contains two arteries and one large vein, which are twisted on each other and are protected from pressure by a transparent, bluish white, gelatinous substance called *Wharton's jelly.*

Overview of Placental Function

The human placenta is a truly versatile organ. It functions as a lung in the transfer of gases, as a gastrointestinal tract in the transport of nutrients, as a kidney in the excretion of wastes, as skin in the transfer of heat, much like a liver in its conjugation of drugs and hormones, and as an endocrine gland through production

---

Functions of Placenta

Transfer of gases

Transport of nutrients

Excretion of wastes

Transfer of heat

Hormone production

of various protein and steroid hormones. These important activities are able to be accomplished because of the unique human type of placentation (i.e., hemochorio-endothelial). The "heme" refers to maternal blood, which bathes the syncytiotrophoblasts (chorio) directly and is separated from the fetal blood by the endothelium of the fetal capillaries in the intravillous space.[1] The maternal blood entering the intervillous space from the spiral arterioles is rich in nutrients and is well oxygenated. The fetal blood contained within fingerlike villi extending into the intervillous space is deoxygenated and depleted of nutrients (Fig. 10-14); it is delivered there from the umbilical arteries. Transfer of oxygen and a great variety of nutrients from the mother to the fetus and, conversely, the transfer of carbon dioxide and other metabolic wastes from fetus to mother occur across the chorionic membrane (chorial), which constitutes the outer surface of the villi. The newly restored blood is returned to the fetus along the veins contained within the villi, which converge into the umbilical vein. The inflowing maternal arterial blood drives venous blood into the endometrial veins, which are located over the surface of the decidua basalis.

Fetoplacental Oxygen Exchange

The partial pressure of oxygen (PO_2) in the intervillous space is approximately 35 to 40 mm Hg. This is the highest oxygen tension that the fetal circulation is exposed to. At any given time, the oxygen that is contained in the intervillous space is capable of satisfying fetal oxygen consumption for approximately 1½ minutes. On their way to the intervillous space, the spiral arteries traverse the muscular wall of the myometrium. The spiral arteries are compressed by the myometrium, and blood flow through these vessels is interrupted with each uterine contraction. Thus, delivery of oxygen to the intervillous space is interrupted. The normal fetus can tolerate this brief period of oxygen deprivation without damage. In certain cases of abnormal labor, when the contractions are usually prolonged, the resulting anoxia could cause fetal damage.

The umbilical cord is the other vulnerable link in the system for maternal–fetal exchange of oxygen. Under certain conditions of labor, the umbilical cord can be compressed, for example, between the fetal head and the pelvis, or entangled above the fetus. Prolonged interference with cord circulation can seriously affect fetal oxygenation.

Gross examination of the maternal side of the placenta reveals approximately 20 cotyledons or lobes. These are further divided into approximately 200 lobules, each of which is a circulatory unit containing a single spiral artery. When a spiral artery becomes obstructed, as when there has been a thrombosis or development of a clot within its lumen, the blood supply to that circulatory unit is interfered with, resulting in tissue destruction or infarction of the area. Many term placentas contain an area of infarction. Fortunately, the placenta is endowed with a substantial reserve. It can withstand loss of an estimated 30% of the functioning villous tissue surface by fibrin deposition or 50% due to thrombotic obliterations of fetal stem vessels without fetal compromise.[3]

At the microscopic level, three layers of tissue separate the fetal circulation from the maternal blood. A molecule passing from the fetus to the mother must traverse these tissues. The outermost layer is the fetal trophoblast, which contains an outer syncytiotrophob-

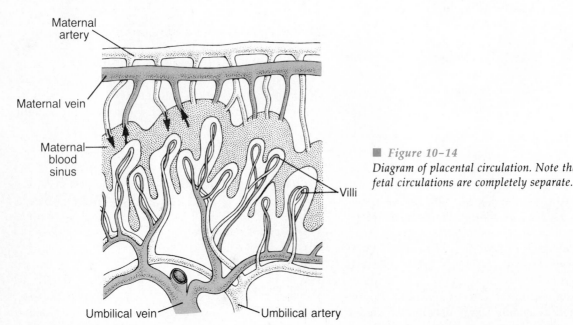

■ *Figure 10–14*
Diagram of placental circulation. Note that maternal and fetal circulations are completely separate.

Maternal artery

Maternal vein

Maternal blood sinus

Villi

Umbilical vein

Umbilical artery

last and inner cytotrophoblast. Immediately beneath the trophoblast is a connective tissue layer. The innermost layer is the endothelial layer of the fetal capillary. As pregnancy progresses, the fetal capillaries are brought closer and closer to the surface of the villi and exchange is facilitated. The diffusion distance for a molecule is approximately 3 to 6 μm.[1]

Placental Transmission of Nutrition

The six mechanisms for the transport of nutrients from the mother to the fetus are diffusion, facilitated diffusion, active transport, bulk flow, pinocytosis, and defects in placental membrane.

1. *Diffusion* is the passage of a substance from one area to another on the basis of its concentration gradient. Materials that are transported by diffusion include the respiratory gases, oxygen and carbon dioxide; the electrolytes, sodium and chloride; and some lipid-soluble vitamins. The transport of gases depends on their partial pressures.
2. *Facilitated diffusion* involves passage along a concentration gradient that occurs when the concentration of material on the maternal side is greater than that on the fetal side. This kind of transfer occurs without the use of energy, but at a faster rate than can be explained on the basis of the concentration gradient alone. This mechanism is carrier mediated (i.e., it is transferred by cellular elements that carry it into and through the membrane). Glucose, a most important fetal fuel, is transported by facilitated diffusion.
3. *Active transport* requires the passage of substances from one area to another against a concentration gradient, and it is energy dependent. This mecha-

nism requires the expenditure of energy by the cells. Amino acids are transported against a 2:1 concentration gradient from mother to fetus. Iron, calcium, iodine, and water-soluble vitamins are transported by the mechanism of active transport.
4. *Bulk flow* involves the transfer of substances by hydrostatic or osmotic gradients through micropores in the membrane. This mechanism is important in maintaining maternal–fetal exchange of water and dissolved electrolytes.
5. *Pinocytosis* involves the transfer across a cell of materials contained in small vessels located at or near the cell membrane. Microdrops of plasma are taken up by the trophoblasts, which transport immunoglobulins to the fetus.
6. *Defects in the placental membrane* can allow the transfer of large materials, such as red blood cells, from mother to fetus. This process is responsible for sensitization of the Rh-negative woman carrying an Rh-positive fetus. Rh-positive fetal red blood cells are carried into the maternal circulation and produce antibodies. This most frequently occurs at delivery when the incidence of breaks in the placental membrane is greatest.

Placental Permeability

Diffusion is the most important mechanism regulating the transfer of substances between mother and fetus. Thus, impaired diffusion is often the cause of clinically evident placental dysfunction. Diffusion depends on the characteristics of the placental membrane. It is purely a physical process and requires no energy. The process is governed by certain principles, which, in combination, are described in *Fick's law*. Fick's law states that the rate of transfer of materials is directly proportional to the thickness of the membrane. This means that the more permeable the membrane and the greater the area presented by the membrane, the greater the rate of transfer. Conversely, the thicker the membrane, the slower the rate of transfer.

Other determinants of permeability for any molecule include the size of the molecule, as well as its molecular charge and lipid-solubility properties. In general, molecules with a molecular weight greater than 1000 do not cross the placental membrane. For example, the anticoagulant heparin is a large molecule that, because of its size, does not traverse the placental membrane; hence, heparin treatment can be used safely in pregnancy. In contrast, the anticoagulant dicumarol is a much smaller molecule that readily crosses the placenta and, when used in pregnancy, may affect the fetus. Other more common drugs, such as caffeine, alcohol, and nicotine, as well as many viruses (e.g., rubella,

---

Placental Transport

Mechanism	Key Substances Exchanged
Simple diffusion	O_2, CO_2, sodium, chloride, lipid-soluble vitamins
Facilitated diffusion	Glucose
Active transport	Amino acids, iron, calcium, iodine, water-soluble vitamins
Bulk flow	Water
Pinocytosis	Immunoglobulins
Membrane breaks	Red blood cells

chickenpox, measles, cytomegalovirus), may cross the placenta and adversely influence the fetus.

Lipid solubility is an extremely important characteristic in the transport of drugs from mother to fetus, as is the electrostatic charge on the molecules. Many of the narcotic agents and analgesics used in labor and delivery are designed to reach the maternal brain quickly to provide rapid pain relief. The characteristics that allow this rapid transport to the brain also allow them to cross the placental membrane rapidly, and they can equally quickly affect the fetal central nervous system.

Factors Influencing Placental Exchange

BLOOD FLOW TO UTEROPLACENTAL CIRCULATION

In general, impaired exchange of carbon dioxide and oxygen is not usually related to problems of diffusion. There is little, if any, resistance to the diffusion of these molecules. Their transfer is most often affected by interference with blood flow into the intervillous space and back to the fetus. Oxygen is brought to the intervillous space by the maternal uterine circulation. Uterine blood flow is approximately 600 to 700 ml/min, representing 10% of the total maternal cardiac output at term. Almost 90% of the total uterine blood flow goes into the intervillous space; 10% supplies the myometrium. The amount of blood that flows into the intervillous space is directly affected by the perfusion pressure within the uterine arteries. Uteroplacental circulation is widely dilated at rest and therefore has little capacity to expand further. This circulation is, however, capable of marked vasoconstriction, which occurs through hormonal or neural mechanisms. Hence, uterine blood flow during pregnancy can be increased significantly by only one mechanism, maternal bedrest. At rest, blood flow to other organs and tissues, such as muscle and fat, is diminished and the supply of blood to the placenta and fetus is enhanced.

Many mechanisms exist by which blood flow to the uteroplacental circulation may be diminished. Each uterine contraction interrupts the supply of blood into the intervillous space. A contraction that lasts 45 seconds stops the blood flow for approximately 30 seconds. During this interval, the fetus must exist on stored nutrients or on those present in the stagnant blood of the intervillous space. This stress is well tolerated by the normal fetus. Abnormally prolonged uterine contractions or a decrease in maternal blood pressure can diminish blood flow to the uteroplacental circulation. For example, the large term uterus may compress the inferior vena cava, interfering with the return of blood to the right heart. Cardiac output and, therefore, delivery of blood to the uteroplacental unit are decreased. Diminished uterine blood flow can also result from chronic hypertension and pregnancy-induced hypertension caused by vasoconstriction. Various pharmacological agents, such as vasopressors, may also cause constriction of these vessels. Finally, vigorous maternal exercise increases blood flow to the muscles and may divert blood from the uteroplacental circulation.

FETAL BLOOD, FETAL HEMOGLOBIN, BOHR EFFECT

Several other important determinants of oxygen transfer from mother to fetus should be considered. These include the actual affinity of fetal blood for oxygen, the concentration of fetal hemoglobin within the fetal blood, and the Bohr effect. *Fetal hemoglobin*, because of its special characteristics, has a greater affinity for oxygen than does maternal blood. By virtue of certain biochemical constituents, maternal hemoglobin has a greater capacity to unload oxygen, whereas fetal hemoglobin is endowed with a greater ability to accept oxygen. The actual concentration of hemoglobin in fetal blood is also greater than in maternal blood. At 35 weeks, fetal blood contains 15 g of hemoglobin/dl and adult blood contains approximately 12 g/dl.[1] Because hemoglobin is the agent that actually carries the oxygen and because the fetus has more hemoglobin, a given unit of fetal blood can carry much more oxygen than can maternal blood.

The *Bohr effect* is the effect of pH on the ability of hemoglobin to accept or unload oxygen. A more acidic pH is associated with an increased ability of hemoglobin to unload oxygen; a more alkaline pH increases the ability to accept oxygen. Blood returning from the fetal circulation in the umbilical artery is more acidic and has a greater capacity to unload oxygen. It reaches the intervillous space, where it gives up its hydrogen ions and carbon dioxide, and its pH rises. Concomitantly, these hydrogen ions and carbon dioxide are accepted by the maternal circulation, and the pH of the maternal blood decreases. The increased fetal pH results in a greater capacity to accept oxygen, and the decreased maternal blood pH results in a greater capacity to deliver oxygen.

ADJUSTMENTS IN FETAL BLOOD FLOW

Fetal blood flow is redistributed during periods of oxygen deprivation. Increased amounts of blood are supplied to the fetal brain and heart; blood flow to the fetal gastrointestinal tract is diminished. This helps to ensure survival of the most vital fetal organs during a time of temporary oxygen lack. Nature has endowed the fetoplacental unit with a unique system of checks and balances to preserve the fetal well-being throughout pregnancy.

The Placenta as an Endocrine Organ

From early pregnancy, the cells that eventually form the placenta are hormonally active. Even before the skipped menstrual period, the trophoblastic cells that have been responsible for allowing the embryo to invade into the endometrium have begun to secrete HCG.

HUMAN CHORIONIC GONADOTROPIN

HCG, produced by the syncytial cells of the trophoblast, is a glycoprotein with a large molecular weight of 36,000 to 40,000. HCG is similar to pituitary luteinizing hormone in both structure and activity, but it differs physiologically in that its levels are maintained in the circulation for longer periods of time. It is composed of two subunits, an alpha subunit, which is similar to the alpha subunit of pituitary glycoprotein hormones, and a beta subunit, which is specific and unique to HCG. The beta subunit is used to make antibodies for a pregnancy test, which is specific for HCG levels.

HCG appears in maternal blood by the eighth day after ovulation in the fertile cycle. Its levels increase steadily in early pregnancy, reaching a maximum in 60 to 90 days, and then the levels in the blood begin to fall. Very little HCG is secreted into the fetal compartment in comparison with the large quantities that are released in the maternal circulation. Circulating HCG has served as the basis for all of the commonly used pregnancy tests.

HUMAN PLACENTAL LACTOGEN OR HUMAN CHORIONIC SOMATOMAMMOTROPIN

The placenta produces a second protein hormone, human placental lactogen (HPL), also called human chorionic somatomammotropin (HCS). This hormone is also formed in syncytial cells within the trophoblast of the placenta. Its production increases progressively during pregnancy, with a marked increase after the 20th week. Very little HPL reaches fetal circulation. There is a distinct correlation between HPL levels and placental weight. For example, maternal HPL levels are higher in multiple gestations. This hormone has an action similar to human growth hormone, and its purpose is to regulate maternal metabolism to maintain a supply of nutrients for the fetus. Specifically, HPL facilitates transport of glucose across the placenta by the process of facilitated diffusion. As its name implies, HPL also has a mammotropic effect.

PROGESTERONE AND ESTROGEN

The placenta also produces the steroid hormones progesterone and estrogen. Throughout pregnancy, there is a steady increase in *progesterone* levels, which reach a maximum just before delivery. This progesterone maintains the endometrium and endometrial blood supply, brings about uterine growth, inhibits the activity of the uterine muscle, and stimulates alveolar development in the maternal breast. It also has significant effects on the mother's metabolism.

The *estrogens*, estriol 17[beta]-estradiol, and estrone, are products of the placenta. Estriol is biologically the weakest of the three major estrogens, but it is produced in greatest quantity. Its production by the placenta involves a unique interplay among the fetal adrenals, fetal liver, and placenta. Estriol is produced by a weak androgen, dehydroepiandrosterone (DHA) sulfate, which comes from the fetal adrenal gland. Ninety percent of all the estriol seen in pregnancy is derived from fetal adrenal DHA-sulfate. The fetal liver further modifies DHA-sulfate and converts it to a hormone the placenta can use in estriol production. Thus, the requisites for the placenta to produce significant quantities of estriol are an intact fetal adrenal gland and a normally functioning fetal liver.

The placenta converts the modified DHA-sulfate into estriol. The estriol levels in the blood rise steadily during pregnancy as the fetus gains weight and the placenta increases in size. The levels of the other two hormones, estradiol and estrone, parallel the estriol levels in maternal blood.

The physiological functions of the estrogens during pregnancy are multifold. They stimulate the growth of the uterus and uterine placental blood flow, and they stimulate contractile activity of the myometrium and growth of mammary tissue. The estrogens also have significant effects on maternal metabolism.

In the past, measurement of estriol level was considered useful corroborative evidence of fetal death; however, the critical value of these tests is being questioned because of the lack of clearly established therapeutic regimens predicated on the results of estriol measurements.[1] A wide range of variation exists in the amount of urinary estriol excreted in the plasma or urine among different normal pregnant women. Factors unrelated to the fetoplacental unit may be associated with decreased urinary estriol levels (e.g., administration of potent glucocorticosteroids or certain antibiotics to the mother, or maternal pyelonephritis). Therefore, the interpretation of "abnormal" levels of urinary or plasma estriol associated with certain deficiencies in the fetoplacental unit must be made with caution. Cunningham, MacDonald, and Gant recommend verification of a single measurement falling considerably outside the "normal range."[1]

Effects on the Newborn. Maternal estrogen is transmitted to the fetus and produces striking effects on the newborn. First, as the result of the action of this hormone, the breasts of both boy and girl babies may become markedly enlarged during the first few days of life and even secrete milk—so-called witch's milk (see Chap. 29). Second, estrogen causes hypertrophy of the endometrium of the female fetus as it does in an adult woman. When this hormone is suddenly withdrawn after birth, the endometrium breaks down and bleeding sometimes occurs. For this reason, perhaps one girl baby in every 15 manifests a little spotting on the diaper during the first week of life. This is entirely normal and clears up within a few days.

■ FETAL CIRCULATION

Fetal circulation differs from extrauterine blood flow in several ways. The fetus receives oxygen through the placenta because its lungs do not function as organs of respiration in the uterus. The fetal circulation contains certain special vessels ("bypasses" or "detours") that shunt the blood around the lungs, with only a small amount circulating through them for nutrition.

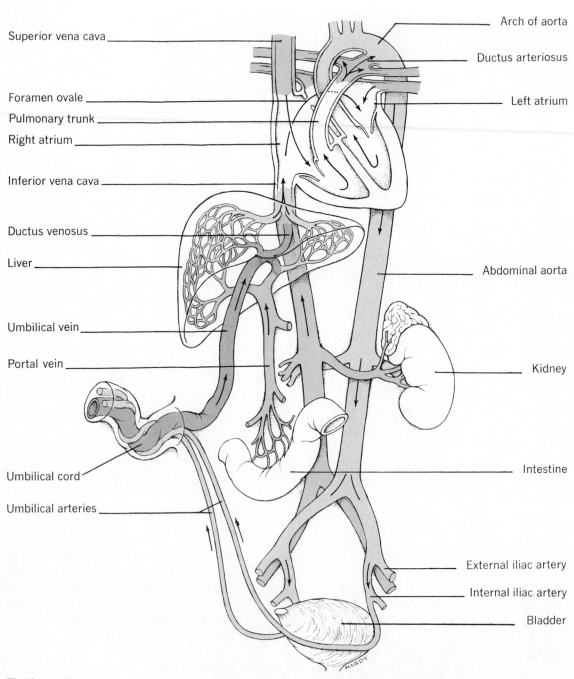

■ *Figure 10–15*
Diagram of the fetal circulation shortly before birth. The course of blood is indicated by arrows.

The oxygenated blood flows up the cord through the umbilical vein and passes into the inferior vena cava; on the way to the inferior vena cava, part of the oxygenated blood goes through the liver, but most of it passes through a special fetal structure, the *ductus venosus,* which connects the umbilical vein and the inferior vena cava. The liver is proportionately large in a newborn because it receives a considerable supply of freshly vitalized blood directly from the umbilical vein. Blood flow in the umbilical circulation has been estimated at approximately 125 ml/kg of body weight or approximately 500 ml/min in the average fetus at term.[3]

From the inferior vena cava, the current flows into the right auricle and goes directly on to the left auricle through a special fetal structure, the *foramen ovale.* It flows into the left ventricle and out through the aorta. The blood that circulates up the arms and the head returns through the superior vena cava to the right auricle again, but instead of passing through the foramen ovale as before, the current is deflected downward into the right ventricle and through the pulmonary arteries. Part of it goes to the lungs (for purposes of nutrition only), but most of it goes into the aorta through the *ductus arteriosus.*

The blood in the aorta, with the exception of that which goes to the head and the upper extremities (this blood has been accounted for), passes downward to supply the trunk and the lower extremities (Fig. 10-15). Most of this blood finds its way through the internal iliac, or hypogastric, arteries and back through the cord to the placenta, where it is again oxygenated, but a small amount passes back into the ascending vena cava to mingle with fresh blood from the umbilical vein and again makes the circuit of the entire body.

Circulation Change at Birth

The fetal circulation is so arranged that the passage of blood to the placenta through the umbilical arteries and back through the umbilical vein is possible up to the time of birth, but it ceases entirely the moment the baby breathes and begins to take oxygen directly from its own lungs. During intrauterine life, the circulation of blood through the lungs is for the nourishment of the lungs and not for the purpose of securing oxygen.

To understand, even in a general way, the course of the blood current and how it differs from the circulation after birth, it must be remembered that in infants after birth, as in the adult, the venous blood passes from the two venae cavae into the right auricle of the heart, to the right ventricle, and through the pulmonary arteries to the lungs, where it gives up its waste products and takes up a fresh supply of oxygen. After oxygenation, the arterial blood flows from the lungs, through the pulmonary veins to the left auricle, to the left ventricle, and out through the aorta, to be distributed through the capillaries to all parts of the body and eventually collected, as venous blood, in the venae cavae and discharged again into the right auricle.

Circulation Path After Birth

As soon as the baby is born and breathes, the lungs begin to function and the placental circulation ceases. This change not only alters the character of the blood in many vessels, but it also makes many of these vessels useless. The umbilical arteries within the baby's body become filled with clotted blood and are ultimately

TABLE 10-1. CHANGES IN FETAL CIRCULATION AFTER BIRTH

Structure	Before Birth	After Birth
Umbilical vein	Brings arterial blood to liver and heart	Obliterated; becomes round ligament of liver
Umbilical arteries	Brings arteriovenous blood to placenta	Obliterated; become vesicle ligaments on anterior abdominal wall
Ductus venosus	Shunts arterial blood into inferior vena cava	Obliterated; becomes ligamentum venosum
Ductus arteriosus	Shunts arterial and some venous blood from pulmonary artery to aorta	Obliterated; becomes ligamentum arteriosum
Foramen ovale	Connects right and left auricles (atria)	Obliterated usually; at times open
Lungs	Contain no air and very little blood	Filled with air and well supplied with blood
Pulmonary arteries	Bring little blood to lungs	Bring much blood to lungs
Aorta	Receives blood from both ventricles	Receives blood only from left ventricle
Inferior vena cava	Brings venous blood from body and arterial blood from placenta	Brings venous blood only to right auricle

(Guyton AC: Medical Physiology, 7th ed. Philadelphia, WB Saunders, 1986.)

converted into fibrous cords, and after occlusion of the vessel, the umbilical vein within the body becomes the round ligament of the liver. After the umbilical cord is tied and separated, the large amount of blood returned to the heart and the lungs, which are functioning, causes equal pressure in both of the auricles. This pressure causes the foramen ovale to close. The foramen ovale remains closed and eventually disappears, and the ductus arteriosus and the ductus venosus finally shrivel up and are converted into fibrous cords or ligaments in the course of 2 or 3 months. The instantaneous closure of the foramen ovale changes the entire course of the blood current and converts the fetal circulation into the adult type. The changes in the fetal circulation after birth are shown in Table 10-1.

■ REFERENCES

1. Cunningham FG, MacDonald PC, Gant NF: Williams Obstetrics, 18th ed. Norwalk, CT, Appleton & Lange, 1989
2. Moore KL: The Developing Human: Clinically Oriented Embryology, 4th ed. Philadelphia, WB Saunders, 1988
3. Scott JR, DiSaia PJ, Hammond CB et al (eds): Danforth's Obstetrics and Gynecology, 16th ed. Philadelphia, JB Lippincott, 1990
4. Money J, Tucker P: Sexual Signatures: On Being a Man or a Woman. Boston, Little, Brown & Co, 1975
5. Money J, Ehrhardt AA: Man & Woman: Boy & Girl. Baltimore, Johns Hopkins University Press, 1973.

■ SUGGESTED READING

de Vries JI, Visser GH, Mulder EJ et al: Diurnal and other variations in fetal movement and heart rate patterns at 20–22 weeks. Early Hum Dev 15(6):333–348, November 1987

de Vries JI, Visser GH, Prechtl HF: The emergence of fetal behaviour. III. Individual differences and consistencies. Early Hum Dev 16(1):85–103, January 1988

England MA: Color Atlas of Life Before Birth: Normal Fetal Development. Chicago, Year Book Medical Publishers, 1983

Havez ESE (ed): Human Reproduction: Conception and Contraception, 2nd ed. Hagerstown, Harper & Row, 1980

Klopper A, Genazzani A, Grosignori PG (eds): The Human Placenta: Serano Symposium No. 35. New York, Academic Press, 1982

Mastroianni L, Biggers J, Sadley W: Fertilization and Embryonic Development in Vitro. New York, Plenum Press, 1981

Prechtl HF: Fetal behaviour. Eur J Obstet Gynecol Reprod Biol 32(1):32, July 1988

Satler TW (ed): Langman's Medical Embryology, 6th ed. Baltimore, Williams & Wilkins, 1990

Simpson ER, MacDonald PC: Endocrine physiology of the placenta. Annu Rev Physiol 43:163, 1981

Yen SS, Jaffe, RB: Reproductive Endocrinology: Physiology, Pathophysiology and Clinical Management, 2nd ed. Philadelphia, WB Saunders, 1985

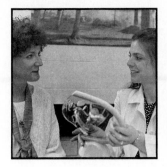

Unit II
Biophysical Aspects of Human Reproduction

CONFERENCE MATERIAL

1. Discuss the internal and external parts of the clitoral system in women and the penile system in men, and their significance in the sexual response cycle. In the discussion include their role in initiating sexual arousal, in developing vasocongestion, and in producing orgasm. Describe how the male and female systems are homologues of each other, and their homologous origins in embryonic development. Include a discussion of the critical factors for male and female embryologic sexual differentiation.

2. Describe the various patterns of male and female sexual response cycles according to the four-stage model of Masters and Johnson. What are the main differences between the male and female patterns? What are the main similarities? What anatomic and physiologic explanation can you find for the differences in male and female patterns?

3. Describe the development of the fetus from the end of the first lunar month through the tenth lunar month. Consider the significance of each period in relation to the fetus's weight, length, physiological adaptation, and behavioral development.

MULTIPLE CHOICE

Read through the entire question and place your answer on the line to the right.

1. A client who was in the later part of her pregnancy reported to the nurse that she was suffering from backache and wanted to know the cause. What is the most likely reason that the nurse could give her?
   A. The larger size of the fetus tires her more easily.
   B. Increased mobility of joints places greater weight on surrounding muscles.
   C. Some abnormality in the pelvic structures is present.
   D. The descent of the presenting part into the pelvic cavity prior to labor increases pressure against the sacrum. ____

2. The epithelium of the skin, hair, nails, sebaceous glands, and sweat glands is derived from which of the following three germ layers?

   A. The mesoderm
   B. The endoderm
   C. The ectoderm ____

3. To give adequate care to the client during and after delivery, the nurse should fully understand the structure and composition of the uterus. Which of the following statements are true of the uterus?
   A. Its muscular tissue is
      1. Predominantly striated
      2. Predominantly nonstriated
      3. Entirely striated
      4. Entirely nonstriated ____

   B. Its muscle fibers are arranged to run
      1. Circularly
      2. Longitudinally
      3. In three layers, the inner and the outer circularly, the other longitudinally
      4. In all directions ____

   C. Its blood is supplied directly from
      1. Ovarian and uterine arteries
      2. Abdominal aorta and uterine arteries
      3. Internal iliac and ovarian arteries
      4. Internal iliac and uterine arteries ____

   D. Normally, the uterus is
      1. Attached anteriorly to the bladder wall
      2. Suspended and freely movable in the pelvic cavity
      3. Suspended between the bladder and the rectum
      4. Attached posteriorly to the anterior wall of the sacrum ____

4. The perineum is a structure lying between the vagina and the rectum that is composed of
   A. A single, strong elastic muscle
   B. A strong elastic tendon
   C. A tendon to which muscles are attached
   D. Two strong muscles, the anal and the transverse perineal ____

5. A client with small breasts in her first pregnancy is worried about her ability to breast-feed her baby.

A. Which of the following responses by the nurse to the client is most correct?
1. She probably will be unable to feed her baby.
2. The size of the breasts will not influence the amount of lactation possible.
3. Mothers with small breasts usually have less difficulty feeding their babies.
4. Her baby would be fed better by means of a formula. ____

B. Which structure is most directly involved in milk production?
1. Papillae
2. Glands of Montgomery
3. Acini cells
4. Areola
5. Lactiferous ducts ____

6. The structures in the testes that are responsible for spermatogenesis are
A. The Sertoli cells
B. The seminiferous tubules
C. The interstitial cells of Leydig
D. The tunica albuginea ____

7. Seminal plasma is made up of secretions derived from
A. The seminal vesicles
B. The prostate gland
C. The bulbourethral glands
D. All of the above ____

8. The time sequence of changes that occur at puberty in the female is
A. Appearance of axillary and pubic hair, breast development, and menarche
B. Menarche, breast development, and appearance of axillary and pubic hair
C. Breast development, menarche, and appearance of axillary and pubic hair
D. Breast development, appearance of axillary and pubic hair, and menarche ____

9. The interval between ovulation and menstruation is normally
A. 31 ± 2 days
B. 14 ± 2 days
C. 28 ± 2 days
D. 21 ± 2 days ____

10. What are the ovarian hormones produced by the graafian follicle and the cells of the corpus luteum?
A. Progesterone and gonadotropin
B. Estrogen and progesterone
C. Gonadotropin and FSH
D. FSH and estrogen ____

11. The release of gonadotropins from the pituitary gland is directly regulated by
A. GNRH
B. HGH
C. Insulin
D. Androgens ____

12. Which hormone brings about the postovulatory increase in basal body temperature?
A. Gonadotropins
B. Estrogen
C. Progesterone
D. GNRH ____

13. Spermatozoa are delivered into the lumen of the seminiferous tubules by
A. Action of the Sertoli cells
B. Their own motility
C. Contraction of Leydig cells
D. Effect of testosterone ____

14. A young mother-to-be told a nurse that she was sure that she would have a boy because her husband was such a strong, physically well-developed man. The nurse could respond correctly by saying
A. "It is the female cell that determines the sex of the child."
B. "It is unlikely because there are more girls born than boys."
C. "Physical strength does not influence the sex of the child."
D. "You are probably right." ____

15. Fertilization normally occurs in
A. The uterus
B. The ovarian follicle
C. The fallopian tube
D. The vagina ____

16. Following fertilization, the ovum is
A. Transported into the uterus immediately
B. Retained in the tube for three days and then transferred to the uterus
C. Retained at the uterotubal junction for 6 days
D. Transferred to the uterus within 24 to 48 hours ____

17. Human chorionic gonadotropin (hCG) is produced by which structure?
A. The pituitary gland
B. The ovarian follicle
C. The trophoblastic cells of the embryo
D. The uterine decidua ____

18. A patient expelled a 16-cm fetus prematurely. What would be the approximate age of the fetus?
A. 2 months
B. 3 months
C. 4 months
D. 5 months ____

19. Although the exact date of delivery cannot be predetermined, if a pregnant woman's last menstrual period began on September 10, the estimated due date would be nearest

A. May 6
B. May 10
C. June 10
D. June 17 ____

20. The only direct connection between the fetus and any other structure is through the umbilical cord. The umbilical cord contains which of these important structures?
A. Umbilical artery
B. Umbilical arteries
C. Umbilical vein
D. Umbilical veins
E. Umbilical nerves
F. Wharton's jelly

Select the number corresponding to the correct letters.
1. A, D, and F
2. B, C, and F
3. C, E, and F
4. All of the above ____

21. The placenta is formed by the union of
A. The chorion frondosum and the decidua basalis
B. The chorion laeve and the decidua capsularis
C. The amnion and the chorionic cavity
D. The decidua basalis and the chorion laeve ____

22. During a uterine contraction the blood flow to the uteroplacental circulation is
A. Unchanged
B. Increased
C. Decreased
D. Completely obstructed ____

23. When genetic, gonadal, and hormonal components of sexuality are incongruent with behavioral sex and sexual partner preference, yet the person has appropriate gender identity, the condition is
A. Transvestism
B. Homosexuality
C. Transsexualism ____

24. Core gender identity has been established by age
A. 1½ years
B. 2½ years
C. 3½ years
D. 4½ years ____

25. Sexual partner preference is believed to be influenced by all but which of the following?
A. Early sexual experiences
B. Prenatal hormonal environment
C. Early mother–infant interactions
D. Values assigned to social sex roles ____

26. Stimuli leading to sexual arousal that include thoughts, fantasies, sights, or sounds are classified as
A. Reflexogenic stimuli
B. Psychogenic stimuli ____

27. Which branch of the nervous system is most immediately responsible for the sexual responses of erection in the man and vaginal lubrication in the woman?
A. Parasympathetic nervous system
B. Sympathetic nervous system ____

28. Which biochemical substance triggers orgasm?
A. Noradrenaline
B. Acetylcholine
C. Androgen
D. Adrenaline ____

29. Which psychological mediator of sexual response invokes erotic images and fantasies?
A. Informational responses
B. Emotional reactions
C. Imaginative capacity
D. Attention ____

30. In order for an embryo to differentiate as male, what hormonal event must occur?
A. Maternal estrogen secretion must decrease.
B. The fetal gonad must secrete androgen.
C. The fetal gonad must secrete estrogen.
D. Maternal androgen secretion must increase. ____

31. The process by which proteins in the uterine wall are broken down during involution is called
A. Hemostasis
B. Catabolysis
C. Autolysis
D. Regeneration ____

32. Involution is complete by 8 weeks after birth at all sites except
A. Fallopian tubes
B. Placental site
C. Cervix
D. Vagina ____

33. Lochia serosa usually begins on which postpartum day?
A. Third
B. Fourth
C. Fifth
D. Tenth ____

34. The shape of the cervical os in nulliparas is
A. Round
B. Transverse
C. Oblong
D. Truncated ____

35. Muscular–fascial relaxation of the vagina after birth may cause
A. Cystocele
B. Rectocele
C. Gaping introitus
D. Cervical erosion
E. Increased vaginal infections ____

Select the number corresponding to the correct letters.
1. A, B, and C
2. A, B, C, and D
3. A, B, C, and E
4. All of the above   ____

36. Hemodynamic changes in the postpartal period include
   A. Up to 30% increase in blood volume the first 2 to 3 days
   B. Hemodilution leading to a fall in the hematocrit
   C. Up to 35% increase in cardiac output
   D. Transient bradycardia in the first 24 to 48 hours
   E. Leukocytosis for several days

Select the number corresponding to the correct letters.
1. A, B, and C
2. B, C, and D
3. A, B, C, and D
4. All of the above   ____

37. The average time for first menstruation after delivery in nonlactating women is
   A. 6 to 7 weeks
   B. 7 to 9 weeks
   C. 9 to 12 weeks
   D. 12 to 14 weeks   ____

38. The average weight loss after delivery is
   A. 5 to 10 lb
   B. 10 to 15 lb
   C. 15 to 25 lb
   D. 25 to 30 lb   ____

39. What is the cause of postpartal afterpains?
   A. Tonic uterine contraction
   B. Intermittent uterine contractions
   C. Irritation at the placental site
   D. Inflammation of the uterine cavity   ____

UNIT III

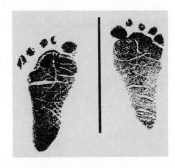

Assessment and Management in Sexuality and Reproduction

11

Sexual Health and Management of Family Planning

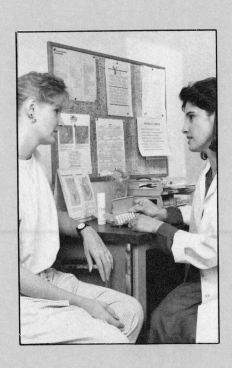

Sexual health is an integral component of each person's state of complete well-being. Attitudes toward the sexual self and beliefs about various forms of sexual expression develop gradually through childhood and into adolescence. Acceptance of sexuality begins in infancy and early childhood, with positive parental responses to genital exploration and the naming of body parts. Responses of parents and other family members to childhood sexual expression, such as sexual play, questions about sex and reproduction, nudity, explicit sexual language, masturbation, and dress continue to shape developing sexual attitudes and expression. Preparation for puberty and sex education further aid the development of the sexual self. In adolescence, the important work of identity formation takes place. Included in this task is incorporation of one's sexual identity, preferred forms of sexual expression and partner choice, and the acceptance of reproductive capacity. (Sexuality in adolescence is discussed further in Chap. 37.)

In early adulthood, the major developmental task is forming intimate relationships with others. Intimacy can occur only after identity is established and people feel comfortable enough to risk revealing their identity and sharing it with another person. Intimacy is freely chosen by consenting, equal persons who have worked out their adolescent identity processes. These relationships are characterized by mutuality, mature sharing of sexual pleasures, responsible sex, trust, and respect. A deep emotional sharing occurs between partners, with concern for one's own and the partner's well-being and sexual responses. Responsible sex includes using effective contraception unless pregnancy is sought, and taking precautions against infectious diseases. Healthy adult sexuality and the capacity for intimacy provide the foundation for pregnancy and parenthood.

Sexual health can be broadly defined as having these components:

1. Accurate information about the physical, emotional and social aspects of sexuality.
2. A well-developed identity, which includes the sexual self, and awareness of one's attitudes and values surrounding sexuality.
3. The capacity for intimacy in relationships with others.
4. The self-esteem to make choices about sexual activities congruent with one's value system and beliefs.
5. The use of effective contraception when pregnancy is not sought.
6. Taking precautions against sexually transmitted diseases (STD), including safer sex practices and selection of sexual relations.
7. Awareness of factors that may enhance or detract from the state of sexual well-being.[1]

The World Health Organization (WHO) defines a state of well-being as freedom from fear, shame, guilt, false beliefs, and other factors that might inhibit sexual responses.[2] Many people would not be enjoying a state of sexual well-being by the WHO definition, or the definition of sexual health given above. The foundation for guilt, false beliefs, shame, and fear around sexuality is established in early childhood, and these can be either reinforced by further negative experiences in later childhood and adolescence, or positively countermanded by health-promoting experiences.

Maternity nurses have an important responsibility in promoting sexual health. The integration of sexuality into the practice of nursing, assessment of sexual health and concerns of clients, and nursing intervention to promote health or alleviate problems are all part of this nursing responsibility. Assembling a database by taking a sexual history and planning interventions have become integrated into the nursing role.

The nurse is an ideal member of the health-care team to assume responsibility for counseling clients about sexuality because of a background in the social, behavioral, and physical sciences as well as knowledge of counseling techniques. Comprehensive nursing care

---

Developing Comfort with Sexuality

The nurse must be personally comfortable with the topic of sexuality to counsel effectively. Some approaches to developing this comfort include the following:

Information and Knowledge	*Attitudes and Values*
Read books and articles.	Join discussion groups (as part of classes, workshops, community activities) that cover topics such as human sexuality or values clarification.
View educational films.	
Attend workshops.	
Enroll in classes.	
Join discussion groups.	
Read popular books (source of public's information).	Take self-administered questionnaires, inventories, or tests related to sexual values and attitudes found in textbooks and journals.*

* Examples of these are found in the journal *Medical Aspects of Human Sexuality*, and in textbooks, such as "Inventory for Self-Evaluation," Appendix A, in Nass G, Libby RW, Fisher MP: Sexual Choices: An Introduction to Human Sexuality. Monterey, CA, Wadsworth Health Sciences Division, 1981. Also see chapter endings in Byer CO, Shaimberg LW, Jones KJ: Dimensions of Human Sexuality. Dubuque, IA, Brown Publishing, 1988.

Research Highlight

Contraceptive Failure Rates Higher Than Previously Found

Previous major reviews of contraceptive failure in the United States found that between 0.1% and 10% of couples who use a contraceptive method perfectly (both consistently and correctly) experience an accidental pregnancy in the first year of use. The lowest failure rates were for combined oral contraceptives (0.1%) and sterilization (0.1%–0.2%); other rates were progestin-only pills 0.5%, IUD 1% to 2%, condom 2%, diaphragm 3%, spermicides 3% to 8% and rhythm 2% to 10%. However, the underreporting of abortions, which is common in national surveys, results in serious underestimation of contraceptive failure rates.

This study undertook a different approach to obtain reliable national estimates of contraceptive failure rates, corrected for the underreporting of abortions. Data from the National Survey of Family Growth (1982, National Center for Health Statistics; used for above estimates) were combined with corrected counts of failures leading to abortions from the 1987 Alan Guttmacher Institute survey. Sophisticated statistical analysis techniques were used (log-linear hazards modeling) to derive the proportions of women using each contraceptive method and experiencing failure during the first 12 months of use.

Results of this analysis point to standardized failure rates among actual users averaging more than 30% above those previously reported. New estimates of the failure rates for the first year are 6% for oral contraceptives (all types), condom 14%, diaphragm 16%, rhythm 16%, spermicides 25%. Sterilization and the IUD were excluded from the study.

Variations in failure rates found in population subgroups were consistent with earlier analyses. The rate of contraceptive failure declines with increasing age, especially between the teenage years and ages 20 to 24. Marital status particularly affects Hispanic women, with far fewer failures in all methods among those married compared to unmarried. Nonwhites tend to have failure more often than whites. Poor women are much more prone to failure than higher income women. The most narrow range of failures was among pill users, with 2% to 18% failures; the widest was among diaphragm users with 10% to 57% failures. These variations are likely related to characteristics that affect consistency and correctness of contraceptive use, such as type of sexual relationship, attitudes about pregnancy or the contraceptive method, degree of motivation to avoid pregnancy, and amount of knowledge about how to use the method.

(Jones EF, Forrest JD: Contraceptive failure in the United States: Revised estimates from the 1982 National Survey of Family Growth. Fam Plann Perspect 21:103–109, May/June 1989)

---

requires nurses to understand the relationship of sexuality to the particular client's health needs or illness and the context of current living situations and sexual-affectional relationships to access and use support systems. Clients need adequate sex information whether they are seeking contraception, undergoing pregnancy, coping with an illness, or striving to attain a higher level of health.

Although it is always important for the nurse to be aware of his or her own feelings and attitudes toward a particular area of practice, human sexuality requires a level of self-understanding beyond that of most other areas. Nurses bring their personal experiences, values, and attitudes to the professional relationship, which may either facilitate or obstruct the process of caring for clients with sexual concerns and problems. A nurse who plans to provide sexual teaching and counseling must become comfortable with sexuality both generally and personally. Approaches to developing comfort with sexuality are summarized on the previous page.

■ SEXUAL HEALTH DURING PREGNANCY AND POSTPARTUM

Nursing Assessment

SEXUAL HISTORY

Taking a sexual history provides a base for identifying present or potential sexual problems, from which therapeutic or preventive nursing intervention can be planned. Additionally, gathering information about the couple's sexual experiences and attitudes demonstrates that the nurse is comfortable talking about sex. By taking the initiative in bringing up the subject, the nurse implicitly gives them permission to discuss sexual concerns. This legitimizes sexuality as an important component of health and an integral part of care for reproductive families and indicates that sexual counseling is an appropriate part of care they can expect to receive from health-care providers.[3]

Varying degrees of formality may be used in taking a sexual history, although it is generally best to have a flexible structure so the discussion can go in the direction the client wants it to go. If forms are used, they should be relatively short and simple to keep writing at a minimum and allow the nurse to focus attention on the interaction. A sexual history should proceed from more general to specific areas, from common to unusual, from simple to complex. Conditional statements that assume a range of behavior should be used.

The sexual history generally begins with a conditional or universal statement about why sexual health is included in the health history. The nurse might use a statement such as the following: "Sexual health is an important part of people's lives. A person's physical health sometimes affects sexual experiences, and sexual health can have effects on physical well-being. As part of your health history, I'd like to ask some questions about your sexual health that will help me to better understand your health status."

It is important to have a quiet, private place to talk and enough time for discussion and client education to conduct a history. Confidentiality must be stressed. The client should be assured that all questions are optional, and the nurse must continually assess the client's readiness as the history taking progresses. The acceptability of declining to answer must be clearly communicated.

The guidelines for taking a sexual history for a specific sexual problem include the following:

1. Description of current problem
2. Onset and course of problem
   a. Onset (age, gradual or sudden, precipitating events, contingencies)
   b. Course (change over time—increase, decrease, or fluctuation in severity, frequency, or intensity; any functional relationships)
3. Client's concept of cause and maintenance of problem
4. Past treatment and outcome
   a. Medical evaluation (specialty, date, form of treatment, results, medication taken)
   b. Professional help (type and results)
   c. Self-treatment (type and results)
5. Current expectancies and goals of treatment (concrete or ideal)[4]

SEXUAL HISTORY DURING PREGNANCY AND POSTPARTUM

Sexual expression during pregnancy is influenced by the physical and emotional changes that happen at this time, as well as attitudes and beliefs about sex during pregnancy. Difficulties can arise as a result of myths, misconceptions, and a lack of understanding of the

Assessment Tool

Taking an Adult Sexual History

These questions about sexual experiences and concerns can be included as part of the general health history.
1. When you were a child, how were your questions about sex answered (where did your sexual information come from)?
2. When you were a teenager, how were your questions about sex answered?
3. How did you first find out about sexual intercourse (how babies are made)?
4. How would you describe your current sexual activity?
5. What, if anything, would you change about your current sexual activity?
6. At this time in your life, how important is a sexual relationship to you?
7. Do you have any concerns about birth control?
8. Do you have any health problems that, in your opinion, affect your sexual health or happiness?
9. Are you taking any medicines that, in your opinion, affect your sexual health or happiness?
10. Is there anything about these questions that you would like clarified or explained?

(Mims FH, Swenson M: Sexuality: A Nursing Perspective. New York, McGraw-Hill, 1980)

Assessment Tool

Sexual History During Pregnancy

These questions about sexual experiences and concerns can be included as part of the prenatal health history. Most questions are appropriate for both partners, and a joint history-taking session is recommended.
1. How does the pregnancy make you feel?
2. How do you feel about changes in appearance and emotions?
3. How do you feel about each other's experience of the pregnancy?
4. What are your feelings about sex during pregnancy?
5. Has the pregnancy made many changes in your life? In your sexual relationship?
6. How do you think having a baby will change your life? How do you plan to manage these changes?
7. What have you heard about what you should or should not do sexually during pregnancy?
8. Do you feel any different physically now than before you were pregnant? In what ways? What medications do you take? Have you had any recent changes in your health?
9. Are there any concerns or worries about your sexual relationship during pregnancy or afterward?

physiology and emotional dynamics of couples during pregnancy.

Even if there are not significant sexual problems associated with the pregnancy, most couples have many questions about sexual activities and their sexual responses during this time and appreciate the opportunity to discuss them. Openly discussing the many changes during pregnancy with implications for sexuality can prepare the couple for potential reactions and prevent the development of conflicts and tensions in their relationship stemming from misunderstandings of physiological changes and psychodynamics.

The first few months postpartum is a time of significant change and adaptation for both partners. Partners often experience self-doubt and decreased self-esteem during the postpartum period, feeling tired, overwhelmed, ignorant, and depressed. Marital difficulties often begin around sexuality during the early months after the birth of the first child. The nurse can assist couples to prevent or deal with potential conflicts in their sexual relationship by openly discussing the changes during the postpartum period. Understanding and accepting the physiological and neurohormonal bases for many of the changes in the woman's sexuality may enable the couple to adapt successfully and find satisfying sexual expressions during the postpartum phase.

Nursing Diagnosis

Analysis of data obtained from the sexual history and from physiological and psychosocial factors may lead to the identification of problems related to sexuality.

Alterations in sexual patterns can result from pathophysiological problems, such as endocrine, genitourinary, cardiovascular, and neuromuscular diseases. Psychological factors such as anxiety, guilt, depression, fear of failure, and fear of pregnancy can also contribute to sexual difficulties. Many situational factors can be involved in sexual dysfunctions. The sexual partner may be unavailable (divorce, separation), abusive, uninformed, or unwilling to participate in satisfactory sexual relations. The environment may not be conducive, such as being in the hospital or having no privacy. Financial worries, work problems, religious proscriptions, or value conflicts may be stressors that affect sexual expression. Alcoholism, medications, chronic pain, obesity, and fatigue are other factors that affect sexuality. Lack of knowledge is a common cause of minor sexual dysfunctions.

Maturational factors can contribute to sexual problems. Absent or negative sexual teaching often leads to problems related to lack of knowledge, as well as anxiety and guilt. Ineffective role models, such as parents with sexual dysfunctions or negative attitudes toward sexuality, can lead to problems. The aging process may be a factor through loss of sexual partner, separation (e.g., through hospitalization), or declining physiological functioning.

During pregnancy and the postpartum period, sexual dysfunctions are often related to lack of knowledge, fatigue, anxiety (e.g., possibly harming the fetus), discomfort, and pathophysiological genitourinary problems. Alterations in the self-concept of both the mother and the father can contribute to ineffective sexual expression. In addition, couples during pregnancy and the postpartum period are subject to many of the other causes of sexual dysfunction mentioned above.

The North American Nursing Diagnosis Association (NANDA) has developed several diagnostic categories encompassing sexual identity, sexuality, and sexual function.[5] Altered sexuality patterns are states in which the person experiences or is at risk for experiencing a change in sexual health. These changes can be related to ineffective coping, the difficulty or inability to adapt to stressors or changes in life-style that have a negative influence on sexual functions. Changes of a body part, such as alterations in pelvic and breast structures during pregnancy and decreased postpartum vaginal lubrication, can contribute to altered sexuality patterns. Prenatal and postpartum changes also cause altered sexuality patterns, usually involving altered sexual function, feelings of undesirability, and the partner's change in usual sexual and social responses. Sexual dysfunction is a diagnostic category describing dissatisfaction with sexual response. This is a state in which people experience or may be at risk for changes in sexual function that are viewed as unrewarding or inadequate. Other diagnostic categories that may be related to sexual problems in pregnancy and the postpartum period include self-concept disturbances such as low self-esteem and body image disturbances.[5]

Nursing Planning and Intervention

Maternity nurses can provide sexual teaching and counseling as they work in prenatal, postnatal, and family-planning clinics; physician's offices; hospital maternity units; and public-health agencies. Nurses frequently conduct classes for expectant parents and classes in parenting and contraception. In any of these areas, concerns related to sexuality are likely to surface if the atmosphere is comfortable and accepting. The nurse who is prepared to deal with both information and feelings about sex has much opportunity to assist clients in a wide variety of settings.

Although intensive therapy for clients with sexual dysfunctions is usually not within the maternity nurse's role, all nurses caring for the reproductive family can contribute to their clients' sexual health by integrating some sexual teaching and counseling into their nursing care. Sexual health can be promoted by creating a climate conducive to discussing sexuality and sexual concerns, validating the normalcy of sexual practices, providing anticipatory guidance for times of altered sexuality patterns, education about various aspects of sexuality, counseling about adapting to changes in usual sexual function, and consultation and referral for more intensive sex therapy.[6]

FRAMEWORK FOR SEXUAL CARE

Sexual care occurs at various levels of depth and complexity and may involve problems of differing severity and character. The role of the maternity nurse in providing sexual care is determined by the individual nurse's background and expertise, as well as the origin and severity of the sexual problem of the client. Sexual problems range from those involving gender identity, such as hermaphroditism and transsexualism, to those resulting from misinformation, confusion about the normal sexual response cycle, and minor sexual dysfunctions.

Knowledge Problems. Lack of knowledge and misinformation are the most common and simple types of sexual problems during pregnancy and the postpartum period. Couples may be unaware of altered sexual functions, have the idea that sex during pregnancy might injure or mark the baby, think that oral sex causes an infection, or worry that orgasm may cause labor.

Fears created by minor unpleasant symptoms may lead to avoidance of sex. The common symptom of painful intercourse during pregnancy can be due to vaginitis causing perineal or vulval irritation, insufficient vaginal lubrication, normal uterine contractions during orgasm setting off Braxton Hicks contractions, or increased pelvic pressure due to the presenting part deep in the pelvis. These can be alleviated with proper medical treatment, explanation of physiological causes of the pain, and teaching of techniques to increase comfort.

Couples need specific information about sex and pregnancy. In the absence of complications, they need not avoid sex during late pregnancy or in the postpartum period once lochia has ceased. The couple's own comfort and desires are their best guide when there is no physical problem or contraindication.

Relationship Problems. Communication problems between the partners are the most common types of relationship problems. The sending and receiving of messages between people is a highly complex symbolic process, and consequently people often experience garbled messages and lack of communication.

Good communication regarding sexual needs and preferences is even more difficult than in most interpersonal situations. Some people find it hard to talk about their own sexual feelings or to accept criticism or suggestions regarding sexual performance.

Open and candid discussion of sexual preferences between partners can often dramatically improve satisfaction, but fears about propriety, hurting the other's feelings, not knowing how to say it, or being embarrassed prevent this communication from occurring.

A first step that the maternity nurse could take in dealing with common sexual problems is to encourage the couple to talk with each other about what they like and do not like in sex. If they can settle on practices that are comfortable and enjoyable to both of them, often the problem is resolved.

Many other factors can complicate communication around sexual experiences, however. Sex often has a hidden agenda that might involve a struggle for power, using sex for manipulation, expressing anger through sexual behaviors, or ways of validating or invalidating male and female sexual roles. Such feelings, whether conscious or subconscious, can interfere with giving oneself freely to the sexual experience and can lead to sexual dysfunctions.

Problems in the couple's relationship must be worked out before the sexual problem can be resolved. If the maternity nurse is skilled in family or marital counseling, she or he is able to deal with these relationship problems. Because sexual difficulties are part of the symptomatology, it is frequently necessary for the nurse–counselor to have an understanding of sexual physiology and to be familiar with basic sex therapy techniques to provide effective care.

Attitude Problems. Attitudes toward sexuality and the sexual self are established through internalized beliefs and values, originating from earliest childhood and often rooted in the unconscious levels of the psyche.

The underlying mechanism in the great majority of sexual dysfunctions is fear. Whether this fear has its origins in sociocultural values, religious inhibitions and guilt, negative early experiences, familial patterns of dominance and discipline, or temporary functional failures of performance, it is the catalyst that sets into motion the psychodynamics that produce the sexual problem. This fear of inadequacy in sexual performance is the most significant deterrent to effective sexual functioning because it completely distracts the person from natural responsiveness by blocking reception of sexual stimuli. Both partners may become self-conscious, worrying about their own and each other's sexual performance.

Specific therapeutic approaches have been developed to help people with sexual problems. These range from intensive residential sexual therapy to short-term behavior modification. Frequently, a process of reeducation is used to modify negative attitudes and counteract inhibitive beliefs. These approaches combined with teaching effective techniques for sexual stimulation have a reasonably good success rate.

When deep anxieties, unresolved guilt or conflict, or other psychopathology are present, the person usually receives psychotherapy aimed at the specific problem. Many sex therapists prefer not to explore old conflicts, but focus on changing the problematic behavior with a variety of sexual and behavioral techniques. Removal of the symptom often brings immediate relief and may result in satisfactory long-term functioning without the need for extensive insight therapy.

Nurses have become involved in this type of sex therapy after undergoing additional education in human sexuality and training in specific techniques for treating sexual problems. This level of sexual counseling is specialty practice and is often provided by a team, using the cotherapist approach (one therapist of each sex) in an extensive program involving education, attitude change, setting a permissive environment for sexual experiencing, marital counseling or psychotherapy, and application of appropriate techniques of sex therapy. The scope of maternity nursing practice usually does not include this kind of sexual therapy, unless the nurse has been specially trained and works in a setting that provides these services.

Evaluation

Progress is assessed during return visits. It is often necessary to alter approaches, try new approaches, or examine what factors are interfering with satisfactory resolution of the problem, which is frequently therapeutic. Simple sexual problems may resolve surprisingly rapidly through the reassurance of accurate information and by altering the context in which sexual activity occurs. However, there may be more deep-seated difficulty, and dealing with an apparently simple problem may reveal conflicts that require specialty referral.

In evaluating the results of nursing intervention for particular alterations in sexual patterns, the nurse can use expected outcomes to assess effectiveness. For example, if the nursing diagnosis was *altered sexual patterns related to ineffective coping with fatigue,* successful intervention can be assessed by determining if the client has identified causes of fatigue, has found constructive ways of coping with or alleviating fatigue, and has resumed satisfying sexual activity. If the diagnosis was *altered sexual patterns related to body changes of enlarged abdomen,* evaluation should include whether the following outcomes were achieved by the couple: sharing of concerns and experiences between partners, finding acceptable variations in sexual practices, and expressing satisfaction with different sexual patterns. If the diagnosis was sexual dysfunction related to decreased postpartum vaginal secretions, intervention is evaluated by ascertaining that the couple has identified practices to improve vaginal lubrication, can describe the causes of the problem and rationale for new practices, and report satisfying sexual activity.

Framework for Sexual Care

	Knowledge Problems	Relationship Problems	Attitude Problems
Occurrence	Most common	Quite common	Quite common
	Most simple	Intermediate complexity	Most complex
Origins	Misinformation	Communication patterns	Internalized beliefs and values
	Ignorance	Goals or intent in relationships and interactions	Psychological conflicts
Typical Problems	Concern over normalcy of sexual practices	Painful intercourse	Male erectile dysfunction
	Labeling activities as abnormal or dangerous	Lack of interest in sex	Premature ejaculation
	Worry over changes in sexual response patterns (i.e., during pregnancy)	Early ejaculation	Nonorgasm in women
		Nonorgasm in women	Vaginismus
	Fears about effects of birth control	Ineffective arousal	Lack of arousal
	Ineffective arousal due to lack of proper stimulation	Unsatisfying sex	
	Unsatisfying sex due to mistiming of arousal or orgasm		
Type of Teaching and Counseling	Information, clarification	Encourage discussion between partners	Sex therapy
	Reassurance of normalcy	Information, clarification	Psychotherapy
	Discussion of feelings	Family or marital counseling	
		Sex therapy	
Levels of Nurse's Involvement	Major responsibility	Initial identification and discussion; marital or family therapy if nurse is a trained therapist	Initial identification
	Provide entire counseling		Must be trained sex therapist or psychologist to undertake therapy

■ COMMON SEXUAL CONCERNS DURING PREGNANCY AND POSTPARTUM

A wide range of sexual issues may confront couples during pregnancy. Sexual problems of a dysfunctional nature include dyspareunia (painful intercourse), changing and conflicting sexual drives, and male erectile dysfunction.[3]

Other issues may relate to lack of sexual desire, breast-feeding and erotic response, and lack of arousal or dyspareunia during the postpartum period.

Lack of Sexual Desire and Avoidance of Sex

Sexual desire, or the interest in and frequency of sex, varies greatly among people. When sexual desire is persistently low or inhibited, such that it interferes with the sexual relationship, it becomes a sexual dysfunction.[7,8] People with low sexual desire usually avoid situations that evoke sexual feelings. When in a sexually arousing situation, they often feel little sexual response or may have negative, unpleasant feelings. Low sexual desire is an increasingly frequent disorder and may be the most common sexual dysfunction. A survey of normal couples (not in treatment) found disinterest in sex among 35% of the women and 16% of the men.[9]

(*Text continues on page 181*)

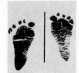

Nursing Care Plan

The Couple With Sexual Problems in Pregnancy and Postpartum

Nursing Goals

1. The pregnant couple obtains accurate information about sexuality during pregnancy and postpartum period.
2. The pregnant couple expresses concerns about sexual needs and functions related to the effects of pregnancy and the puerperium.
3. The pregnant couple indicates improvement or resolution of sexual problems and concerns during pregnancy and postpartum period.
4. The pregnant couple obtains referrals for sexual, family, or psychological counseling appropriate to their needs.

Assessment	Potential Nursing Diagnosis	Intervention	Evaluation
Changes in Sex Drive			
Stage of pregnancy and associated physical and emotional symptoms	Altered sexuality patterns related to physical and emotional changes of pregnancy, knowledge deficit, anxiety, or guilt, conflicting values	Reinforce accurate knowledge	Couple feels comfortable with changing sex drives
Level of couple's understanding of psychophysiology of pregnancy		Teach correct information, clear misconceptions	
Attitudes toward sex in pregnancy		Reassure about normality of fluctuating sex drives	
Communication patterns		Support clear communication	
Dyspareunia in Pregnancy			
Associated factors, symptoms, patterns	Altered sexuality patterns related to physical changes of pregnancy, knowledge deficits, alteration in comfort: pain	Instruct on alternate techniques and positions	Couple attains comfortable intercourse or finds acceptable alternative
Techniques of intercourse		Discuss arousal patterns	
Adequacy of stimulation		Refer for treatment of vaginitis	
Perineal irritation due to vaginitis		Teach normal variations of pregnancy (Braxton Hicks contractions with orgasm, backache)	
Avoidance of Sex			
Reasons why sex is avoided (fears, misconceptions, told by physician)	Altered sexuality pattern related to knowledge deficits, anxiety, value conflicts, fatigue, discomfort	Correct misinformation and teach normal fetal–maternal development	Couple clarifies that fears and misinformation have been cleared
Difficulties this poses for the couple		Inform when sex should be avoided and reasons why	Couple no longer avoids sex when not medically necessary
Attitudes toward sex in pregnancy		Discuss alternatives to intercourse	Couple uses acceptable alternatives if indicated

(continued)

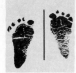

Nursing Care Plan (continued)

Assessment	Potential Nursing Diagnosis	Intervention	Evaluation
Male Erectile Dysfunction			
Extent of the problem, how often this occurs	Altered sexuality patterns related to stress, fears, anxiety or guilt, knowledge deficits, conflicting values	Teach about normal male reactions and psychological processes	Couple indicates concern decreased
Level of couple's concern		Reassure normality of occasional inability to maintain or attain erection	Able to have intercourse often enough to satisfy both partners
Level of understanding of the man's psychophysiology in pregnancy		Refer to specialist if problem is extensive	
Breast-Feeding and Erotic Response			
Loss of milk with arousal or orgasm	Altered sexuality pattern related to physical changes of postpartum period, knowledge, deficit, anxiety, guilt	Advise regarding normality of milk loss	Client indicates comfort with methods to prevent milk loss from interfering with sex
Extent to which this poses problem to the couple		Suggest wearing bra with absorbent pads if a problem	
Arousal or orgasm with nursing, level of concern about this		Avoid pressure or stimulation of breasts	Able to accept erotic feelings and continue nursing
		Advise of normality of arousal during nursing	
		Discuss discomfort and concern, and meaning of this to woman	
Postpartum Dyspareunia and Lack of Arousal			
When symptoms occur, how often, associated with what factors	Altered sexuality patterns related to physical changes of postpartum period, knowledge deficits, fatigue, value conflicts, altered self-concept, pain, lack of privacy, depression	Teach normal postpartal physiology and hormonal effects	Client indicates concern decreased
Weeks or months postpartum and stage of involution		Reinforce that arousal levels are often lower at this time	Comfortable with level of sexual arousal
Contraceptive use		Discuss techniques of arousal, advise use of lubricants if needed	Comfortable intercourse attained or acceptable alternative found
Techniques of arousal and intercourse		Refer for treatment of vaginitis	
Level of understanding of postpartum physiology		Discuss approaches to managing home and family demands to provide the couple with private time	
Perineal irritation due to vaginitis			

Most people with lack of sexual desire are able to function sexually but rarely initiate sex. Causes of this condition include restrictive religious upbringing, aversion to certain sex acts or the genitals, sexual trauma (incest or rape), depression, drug abuse, illness, aftereffects of some surgical procedures, and birth of a child.[10] In some instances, the actual level of sexual desire may not be the problem, but a discrepancy between the partners' desire levels causes conflicts.[11]

Treatment focuses on identifying the cause of low sexual desire and alleviating it when possible. This may involve short-term sex therapy, counseling, or psychotherapy. When discrepancy of sexual desire occurs, treatment includes recognition and acceptance of differences, adapting sexual practices to meet each partner's needs, and counseling for relational problems.

Fears about harming the fetus or mother may cause some couples to avoid intercourse during pregnancy. Birth of a previous abnormal baby may underlie these fears. Sexual desire may be diminished in either partner by physical and emotional changes of pregnancy and the postpartum period. For couples accustomed to regular intercourse, prolonged abstinence can cause conflicts or emotional distress.

Nursing intervention includes correcting misinformation about dangers to the fetus or mother, education about changes of pregnancy and the postpartum period, encouraging discussion of sexual needs, and assisting the couple to find sexual practices that are satisfying to both. Intercourse poses no problems even in late pregnancy if there are no complications. Once membranes have ruptured or labor has begun, or if there is vaginal bleeding, intercourse should be avoided. If premature labor threatens, intercourse should be avoided to prevent any possibility that orgasm could initiate uterine contractions. These couples should also be counseled to avoid oral or manual stimulation that can also produce orgasm and initiate premature contractions.

Changes in Sex Drive

Alterations in the woman's sexual responsiveness are common during pregnancy and are vastly different from woman to woman. In early pregnancy, some women experience a heightened sexuality, enjoy sex more, and seek it frequently. Their general level of sensuousness may increase with heightened awareness and responsiveness to stimuli. Other women have decreased sex drive during the first 2 to 3 months of gestation, often because of nausea, bloating, breast soreness, fatigue, and the many other physical changes that occur during pregnancy.

As pregnancy reaches its midpoint, heightened sexuality becomes more common. Many women report an increase in erotic feelings, more interest in sex and some even report experiencing the first orgasm. Some of this could be explained by the physiological changes of pregnancy including increased pelvic vascularity and vasocongestion which promote building an effective orgasmic platform.[12]

Expectant fathers undergo psychological processes in pregnancy resembling those of the mother and may have symptoms and alternating periods of emotional stability and well-being and times of anxiety, unexplained fears, and compulsions.[13]

As pregnancy progresses, couples experience changes in body image and self-concept. Most couples find pleasure in these changes and enjoy an expanded sense of self. Sometimes these physical changes of pregnancy can contribute to a negative self-concept or negative body image, which can lead to altered sexual responses or dysfunctions. The woman's emotional lability and fluctuating sexual responses during this time may be confusing to her and her partner.

During the first trimester, several physiological changes in the woman may generate fears and anxieties regarding intercourse: the feelings of pelvic fullness and the twinges of round ligaments that sometimes cause discomfort during intercourse; the occasional spotting, which is common; and the different sensations experienced in response to deep penile penetration due to the enlarging soft uterus. Preoccupation with these discomforts, fear, and different sensations may lead to unpredictable changes in sexual desire and decreased orgasmic response. If there are too many changes from what is usual, both partners may become concerned.

Interventions include educating couples about these normal physiological changes and anticipated alterations in sexual response, that intercourse poses no threat to pregnancy under normal circumstances, and that there is no reason to curtail their usual sexual activity if they had no unusual pathophysiological problems and were comfortable with their sexuality before the pregnancy. Variations of sexual stimulation and orgasmic release for either the man or the woman can be used during early pregnancy. Sexual techniques may need modification because of increased sensitivity of the woman's breasts and genitals. As the woman's secretions increase and change in character, she should be instructed that maintaining daily hygiene can avoid unpleasant accompanying odors. Vaginal infections, which are common during pregnancy, can also cause irritation and odor. The nurse can provide information about the prevention and treatment of vaginal infections as prescribed by the physician or midwife.

In the second trimester, early in the fourth month, the uterus enlarges rather rapidly and becomes an abdominal organ rather than a pelvic organ. As the abdomen rapidly enlarges, some concerns often arise about crushing the fetus during intercourse. There is no danger that this will happen because the fetus is well protected by the uterus and the abdominal wall. The enlarging uterus can get in the way about the fifth month if the partners assume face-to-face, prone, and supine positions for intercourse. Modifications in positioning may be needed. Intercourse using the side position may be preferred as the uterus enlarges. From a purely mechanical point of view, it is necessarily gentle. As the uterus grows larger, the expectant mother is usually much more comfortable lying on her side, with her uterus supported by a pillow. If she is on her back for any length of time, with the enlarged uterus pressing on the abdominal aorta and the vena cava, there may be problems with hypotension and lightheadedness. Using a pillow under the hips during intercourse can be helpful in avoiding hypotension.

Stress incontinence of urine (losing urine with coughing, sneezing, or orgasm) may occur because the uterus is pressing on the bladder. Some women might confuse this with loss of amniotic fluid and become frightened during intercourse.

Vaginal spotting after intercourse may be related to cervicitis or cervical friability. Although some spotting during pregnancy is normal, spotting and bleeding *can* signal spontaneous abortion and should be evaluated.

During the third trimester, the uterus is distended and there is increasing pelvic and perineal pressure. Backaches, leg cramps, and shortness of breath may increase the woman's discomfort. Vaginal secretions are increased, and some discharge of colostrum from the nipples may occur. Many couples find intercourse difficult and uncomfortable toward the end of pregnancy. They may substitute other forms of sexual expression, such as oral or manual sex, caressing and holding.

Dyspareunia During Pregnancy

Painful intercourse during pregnancy can be caused by a number of factors. Pressure on the pregnant abdomen may cause a generalized discomfort. Deep penile thrusting may be painful when there is pelvic congestion, when the presenting part is deep in the pelvis, or when certain positions are assumed that exaggerate pressure. Although vaginal secretions are increased during pregnancy, in some instances there may be a relative lack of lubrication because of inadequate stimulation, which leads to discomfort with intercourse. Irritation of the perineum or introitus, secondary to vaginitis, causes burning or pain on penetration and during intercourse. Cramps and backache may occur after coitus as the result of increased vasocongestion of sexual arousal combined with that of pregnancy. Orgasm may initiate Braxton Hicks contractions, which may continue and cause considerable pain. Aching postcoital pain may result from lack of orgasm to assist removal of the pelvic congestion associated with plateau levels of sexual arousal. If the woman experiences conflicts about having intercourse while pregnant, there may be a psychological overlay with the dyspareunia.

Male Erectile Dysfunction During Pregnancy

Almost all men, at one time or another, fail to have an erection during a sexual encounter. This does not indicate significant dysfunction and is usually connected with being upset, tired, or preoccupied or having too much alcohol. Occasionally, men are unable to attain or maintain an erection during their partner's pregnancy. This is a type of secondary erectile dysfunction; it may be a situational phenomenon with no long-term repercussions, or it may indicate a more significant psychological problem with sexual dysfunction. As men experience emotional upheavals during pregnancy, they may at certain times be disinterested in sex because of psychological processes. For some men, a reawakening of maternal relationships and the projection of this relationship onto their pregnant wife create conflicts interfering with erotic response. If the woman's body is perceived as unattractive, sexual arousal may be blocked. This may also occur when the man fears injuring the mother or fetus, or if he is feeling a close identification with his partner in vicariously experiencing the pregnancy.

Inability to attain erection on occasion during pregnancy does not indicate a significant sexual problem. Expectations of male performance create enormous pressures on men and often exaggerate fears of inadequacy, which further interfere with sexual arousal, perpetuating the difficulty in having or maintaining erections. A man is considered to have significant erectile dysfunction when he cannot achieve penile erection in 25% of his sexual attempts.[14]

Breast-Feeding and Erotic Response

The sexual response involving the breasts has effects during lactation that may cause problems for some couples. The contractile tissues that surround the milk ducts are stimulated during orgasm. Sexual stimulation leading to tissue contraction may produce a "let down" reflex, causing milk to leak or spurt. If this is a concern to the couple, the woman can wear a bra with absorbent pads and avoid pressure on the breasts. Breast tenderness can also present a problem during the postpartum period, but this is a temporary condition and the couple can avoid breast stimulation until the soreness subsides.

Another relatively common occurrence is sexual arousal in response to the baby's sucking. This may range from pleasant, mild excitation to orgasm. If women are aware that this is a normal response, they may become comfortable with this experience. Some women discontinue breast-feeding, however, because they do not feel comfortable with these responses. Women who breast-feed also tend to resume intercourse sooner postpartum than those who do not, presumably because of the increased eroticism associated with breast-feeding.

Postpartum Dyspareunia or Lack of Arousal

During the first 6 months after delivery, the vagina does not lubricate well because of relatively low levels of steroid hormones, which inhibit the vasocongestive response to sexual stimulation. Also, 3 to 6 weeks are needed for healing to occur after childbirth, including the episiotomy; cervical, vaginal, or perineal lacerations; and the site of placental attachment. Couples are usually advised to resume intercourse by the third or fourth postpartum week, if the bleeding has stopped and if the episiotomy is not painful. Their own comfort and sexual desires are used as the guide for resumption of intercourse if there are no contraindications.

However, women are at times concerned with their lack of sexual response in the months after childbirth. Taking their mothering responsibilities into consideration, with the lack of sleep, fatigue, and juggling of activities this usually requires, it is not surprising that their sexual interest might be low even without the additional factor contributed by their sexual physiology after delivery. Understanding this may alleviate fears and enable women to await full restoration of their hormonal and physical status. Residual tenderness of the perineum or vagina can also contribute to painful intercourse as well as to a lack of interest in sex. Vaginitis can result from low estrogen levels, further creating problems with dyspareunia. Fears that intercourse may be permanently affected by pregnancy, labor, and delivery grow out of the belief that these cause damage to the woman's genitalia. Painful intercourse and lack of arousal during the postpartum period can be taken as evidence that these fears have been realized unless the couple can be assisted in understanding the physiological processes of childbirth and of the postpartum period and their temporary effects on sexual functioning.

■ FAMILY PLANNING

Assisting the couple to select and use an effective contraceptive method is an important part of the maternity nursing role. Nurses providing postpartum care, both in the hospital and in the ambulatory setting, must be able to counsel couples about appropriate contraceptives. Understanding one's own philosophy is important to avoid presenting biased information. During the last trimester of pregnancy, it is helpful to initiate discussion about family planning needs and goals. The couple can begin to consider spacing children, or avoiding future pregnancies, well before they must decide and implement contraceptive methods.

Although highly effective contraceptive methods are available, their effectiveness is often lowered by inappropriate use. In addition, their safety has not yet reached levels at which risk is truly minimal. The ideal contraceptive would be a method that is 100% safe and 100% effective, inexpensive, simple to use and understand, not directly connected to intercourse, totally reversible at any time, and readily available. No available contraceptive method meets all these criteria. Despite the risks involved, people desire the benefits of reproductive choice and must therefore make decisions about methods based on personal values and a full understanding of the risks and benefits involved.

The majority of American women, regardless of religious affiliation, approve of and use contraception. Having fewer children puts less strain on the family's resources and enhances the family's opportunities for economic and personal advancement. A well-informed public, supported by changing social values that encourage individual choice and smaller family sizes, expects access to professional advice and contraceptive techniques as an integral part of health-care services.

Motives for contraceptive use are unique, and the choice of method and its meaning are highly individual. Therefore, differences must be respected by the nurse, without presumption based on external characteristics, and the full range of contraceptive possibilities needs to be discussed with each person or couple so a fully informed and satisfactory choice can be made.

Nursing Assessment

Because family planning deals with people's sexuality, a private setting should be arranged whenever possible. Feelings about contraception must be explored in a nonjudgmental way and the variety of choices must be summarized to allow selection of a method that fits the unique circumstances of the person or couple. There is no "best method" of contraception, but there is always a method that can work best in the circumstances at hand.

The choice of a suitable contraceptive depends on factors that can vary even from year to year in any couple's contraceptive life span. These factors include expense, bathroom facilities, frequency of intercourse, sexual practices, number of children, the risk of pregnancy the couple wishes to accept, illness, and physical problems.

Assessment covers the client's knowledge, understanding, and experience using various birth-control methods. Historical data include general health, menstrual and reproductive histories, sexual patterns, family structures and relationships, and other significant demographic or socioeconomic information. Certain minimal laboratory work is indicated when the method of choice is sterilization, IUD, or an oral contraceptive.

Pregnancy prevention ideally involves the participation of both male and female partners. Family planning generally encourages participation of the man and provides an opportunity for him to share responsibility for fertility control. A discussion of some methods which require the man to assume primary responsibility such as a vasectomy, using condoms, or even the rhythm method, should be included.

HISTORY

The contraceptive database includes a history of the immediate family for diabetes, bleeding, or clotting problems, heart problems or high blood pressure, migraine headaches or seizure disorders, kidney or liver disease, anemia, tuberculosis, stroke, cancer, or mental problems. This information provides a baseline on diseases for which the client may be at risk and helps identify contraindications, especially when oral contraceptives are being considered. The woman's own past medical history is elicited, covering the above problems in addition to previous hospitalizations, operations, and other major illness. Menstrual and obstetric histories are of particular importance, with any complications or abnormalities carefully noted. Previous use of and experience with contraceptives also are included. Nutritional status is assessed. Allergies and the current use of medications alert the practitioner to potential problems.* Key points in the client's history include the following:

- *When did menarche occur, and have menses been irregular or skipped?* Late menarche and irregular menses indicate a possible endocrine abnormality, and the woman may be having anovulatory cycles. In this case, oral contraceptives should not be used until her endocrine status has been investigated. Otherwise, permanent anovulation with subsequent infertility could result.
- *Are menstrual periods heavy with clotting and cramping?* The IUD causes these problems to become worse, and often oral contraceptives improve them. However, extremely heavy flow, particularly in the woman over 30, needs investigation before the pill is prescribed. The diaphragm may be a better choice in this situation.
- *Is there a history of pelvic inflammatory disease (PID)?* This is a contraindication for the IUD.
- *Is there a history of severe migraine, cerebral arterial insufficiency, cardiovascular disease, liver disease, severe diabetes, genital or breast cancer, thrombotic problems, high blood pressure, or a family history of stroke?* These are contraindications for oral contraceptives.
- *What type of contraceptive was used before? Was it effective or did a pregnancy occur?* Information is gained here about the probability of the successful use of certain contraceptive methods, and some idea is provided about the client's level of knowledge and understanding of these methods.
- *What are the most important reasons for contraceptive use?* This question helps the nurse assess the presence of realistic or unrealistic expectations that should be cleared up in discussion, and the client should be helped to understand the practical benefits of contraception. Goals and priorities can also be identified. If the woman feels strongly that pregnancy must be prevented, a highly effective method is indicated. If delay or spacing of pregnancy is actually the goal and if the woman is concerned about any alterations in her body physiology and functions, a method with somewhat greater pregnancy risk but no systemic or local alterations would be more appropriate.

Any positive responses in the history must be fully explored and considered in making decisions about the appropriateness of any particular method.

PHYSICAL EXAMINATION

The extent of the physical examination performed depends on policies and practices in the particular setting, positive responses from the history, and the type of contraceptive method desired. At the very least, it should include a breast examination, pelvic examination, a Pap smear, and blood pressure check.

A more thorough physical examination is necessary when oral contraceptives, other hormonal methods, an IUD, cervical cap or diaphragm, or sterilization are considered as methods of contraception. The areas covered in physical examination include:

Vital signs: Blood pressure, pulse
Appearance: Weight, age
Head and neck: Eyes, thyroid gland
Chest: Lung fields, heart, breasts
Abdomen: Organs, masses, large vessels

---

* Parts of the sections entitled "History," "Physical Examination," and "Laboratory Tests" are adapted from Martin LL: Health Care of Women. Philadelphia, JB Lippincott, 1978.

Pelvic: Vulva, vagina, cervix, uterus, tubes, ovaries
Rectal: Sphincter tone, masses
Extremities: Varicosities, pulses, circulation
Skin: Lesions, color, pigmentation

Findings and abnormalities in the physical examination that contraindicate or affect use of particular types of contraceptives are described in the Nursing Guidelines.

LABORATORY TESTS

A Pap smear should be performed during the pelvic examination, and chlamydia and gonorrhea cultures should be obtained when indicated. Urinalysis is simple and inexpensive and provides screening for diabetes, urinary tract infections (UTI), and kidney function. A complete blood count rules out anemia or systemic infection in most cases and gives an indication of the con-

---

Nursing Guidelines:
Abnormalities Found During Physical Examination That Affect Use of Particular Types of Contraceptives*

- *Eyes.* Check for signs of glaucoma such as narrow anterior chamber and cupping of discs or increased cup:disc ratio; conditions of veins and arteries, particularly arteriolar narrowing or venous nicking; and condition of retina.
- *Thyroid.* Examine for nodules and diffuse enlargement. Oral contraceptives alter thyroid function tests, although there is no evidence at present that they cause either hypothyroidism or hyperthyroidism.
- *Chest.* Examine lung fields, heart, and great vessels. Any heart murmurs, bruits, or adventitious lung sounds indicate the need for consultation.
- *Breasts.* Any masses, nodules, or discharge from the nipples contraindicates oral contraceptives, at least initially, and calls for consultation. There is some evidence that the pill may be helpful in certain types of benign breast disease, but it is recommended that the pill not be used in cases of suspected or proved breast cancer.
- *Abdomen.* Examine for bruits, masses, and hepatosplenomegaly.
- *Skin.* Signs of chloasma (mask of pregnancy) or history of this is a relative contraindication for oral contraceptives. Acne may be improved.
- *Extremities.* Varicose veins are a relative contraindication for oral contraceptives. Peripheral pulses that are weak or absent indicate circulatory or arteriosclerotic problems, and further investigation is necessary with avoidance of oral contraceptives until the safety of their use is determined.
- *Pelvic examination.* Significant pelvic relaxation with prolapse, cystocele, or rectocele makes effective use of the diaphragm impossible. Anatomical anomalies such as a small cervix or short anterior vaginal wall also dictate against this method. An infantile cervix and uterus suggest endocrine problems, and oral contraceptives or an IUD should not be used until this possibility has been ruled out. Pelvic inflammatory disease and extensive cervicitis contraindicate the use of IUDs. Biopsies should be taken of suspicious cervical lesions before any contraceptive method is instituted. Uterine myomas make IUD placement difficult and may be stimulated to increase with the use of oral contraceptives; therefore, foam, a condom, or a diaphragm would be the method of choice. Ovarian or tubal masses should be referred at once for consultation, and no contraceptive should be given until their nature has been ascertained and the problem has been treated. Vaginitis is not a contraindication to either the IUD or an oral contraceptive, although it may influence the type of pill used and should, of course, be treated. Severe retroversion or anteversion of the uterus contraindicates use of the IUD.
- *Weight.* Obesity must be viewed as a serious problem when oral contraceptives are desired. Some consider it a contraindication because of the pill's effects on carbohydrate and lipid metabolism. It definitely puts the client at increased risk for several complications. The obese woman also presents difficulties in fitting a diaphragm and inserting an IUD. It is difficult to find anatomical landmarks and determine the size and position of the uterus. Foam or condoms seem to be the contraceptives of choice until weight is lost.
- *Age.* Oral contraceptives carry a greater risk for the very young woman, whose endocrine system is immature, and for the woman over 35, who is increasingly susceptible to thromoembolic problems and hypertension.
- *Blood Pressure.* Elevation of the blood pressure contraindicates the use of combined oral contraceptives. There is a direct relation between the estrogen in the pill and hypertension, and a certain percentage of normotensive women develop high blood pressure under the influence of these drugs. When there is marginal or established hypertension, the risk of serious complications is increased. The minipill or another method of contraception is indicated.

* Positive findings and abnormalities indicate further consultation or referral.

dition of the platelets. If there are any questions about liver function, liver enzymes should be obtained because impaired liver function is an absolute contraindication to oral contraceptives. A VDRL or other serological test for syphilis is frequently obtained.

Other laboratory tests less frequently ordered might include a lipid profile if there is cardiovascular risk, hemoglobin electrophoresis if there is risk of hemoglobinopathies, glucose screening to test for diabetes, rubella screen (if not obtained for prenatal work-up), and herpes smear if indicated.

Nursing Diagnosis

The nursing diagnosis is made based on historical and physical examination data obtained from nursing assessments.

Health-seeking behaviors related to family planning is a common nursing diagnosis. The clients are actively seeking ways to alter health practices to move toward higher wellness, in this instance, to prevent unwanted pregnancy that might have untoward emotional and physical consequences. *Knowledge deficit* is a frequent contributing factor and has the potential for altering the client's health status. Deficits may occur in cognitive knowledge or psychomotor skills necessary for effective contraceptive use. *Potential for infection or injury* could result from improper use of contraceptive methods, lack of knowledge about dangers and risks, inadequate personal hygiene, and increased physiological susceptibility during the postpartum period.

Decisional conflict is common when selecting a contraceptive. Clients are often uncertain about the best choice, are aware of the undesired consequences of each contraceptive alternative, may vacillate between alternatives, and delay decision making placing them at risk for pregnancy. For some, considerable distress is experienced and personal values and beliefs are called into question as they attempt to make a decision. There is a high risk for *altered sexual patterns*, depending on the requirements of a given contraceptive method that may interfere with the couple's usual sexual practices. Contraceptive methods that are *not* reliable enough for the client's needs or that pose health risks beyond the client's level of comfort can cause anxiety and inhibit sexual response.

Nursing Planning and Intervention

The nursing plan is based on the diagnoses. Interventions are designed and carried out to promote behavior that helps improve or maintain the client's health. The nurse may carry out interventions directly or may facilitate or arrange for others to provide the necessary services.

Intervention focuses on assisting the client or couple through the decision-making process in selecting an appropriate contraceptive method. Knowledge deficits are remedied through teaching about various contraceptives, correcting misinformation as needed. Decision conflict is reduced by thorough discussion of the risks and benefits of each potential contraceptive choice. Fears need to be expressed, uncertainties clarified, and personal preferences identified. The effectiveness of a contraceptive method is of primary concern to both clients and professionals. When counseling clients on effectiveness, nurses must be familiar with different effectiveness rates.

Maximal effectiveness is the method's effectiveness in preventing pregnancy under ideal conditions (i.e., when it is completely understood and used perfectly). This is the method's lowest failure rate; if a pregnancy occurs, it is due to a failure of the method, not how it is being used. *Typical effectiveness* takes into consideration the method's effectiveness under actual use, in which some people use the method correctly and others use it carelessly or incorrectly. Typical effectiveness rates are lower, naturally, because the human error factor is included.

In answering questions about effectiveness, the nurse may show bias by quoting maximal effectiveness figures for preferred contraceptive methods and typical effectiveness figures for those methods not favored. This provides misleading data to the client and may be an attempt to influence choice. Ethical counseling requires consistency in presenting effectiveness data. Some nurses present both sets of figures, so the potential for error in use can be clearly assessed. Figures for maximal and typical effectiveness of common contraceptive methods are shown in Table 11-1.

When assisting clients select a contraceptive method, it is good to keep in mind that the "best method" of contraception is one that a couple will use most consistently and correctly, and this is often the one that feels most natural and comfortable. The assessment tool entitled "Questions Regarding Contraceptive Effectiveness" provides a guide to factors that might lower effectiveness in contraceptive use for couples. Any "yes" response indicates potential problems, and most people have several "yes" answers for any contraceptive method. The one with the fewest "yes" responses would be best for that couple.

There is a certain amount of risk in every contraceptive method, from either the method or the risk of pregnancy due to contraceptive failure or misuse. The mortality associated with pregnancy is greater than that of any commonly used contraceptive method. Often

TABLE 11-1. EFFECTIVENESS AND RISKS OF CONTRACEPTIVES AND PREGNANCIES PER 100 WOMEN PER YEAR

Method	Maximal Effectiveness	Typical Effectiveness	Continuing Pregnancies	Deaths due to Pregnancy	Deaths due to Contraception	Major Morbidity (%)	Minor Morbidity
No contraception			89–90	0.016	0		
Oral contraceptives (combined)	0.1–0.5	2–4	0.5	0	0.003	1	40
Low-dose oral progestin	1–1.5	5–10					
IUD	1–2	5	3	0.001	0.001	1	40
Diaphragm	2–3	13–19	12	0.002	0		
Rhythm (calendar)	10–14	21	25	0.005	0		
BBT only	7	21					
Cervical mucus only	2	25					
Early abortion*	0	0	0	0	0.003	1	8
Laparoscopic tubal ligation	0–0.2	0.4	0.4	0	0.03	0.6	1
Vasectomy	0–0.1	0.15	0.15	0	0	1	5
Condom†	2–3	10–15					
Spermicides†	3	13–22					
Condom + spermicide	<1	5					
Withdrawal†	3–16	15–25					
Cervical cap†‡	5–8	16–18					
Vaginal sponge†‡	5–8	16–28					
Injected progestogen	0.3	0.3					
Hormone implants	0.2	0.2					

 * Abortion is not a method of contraception, but is included here for comparison.

 † Data on continuing pregnancies and deaths due to pregnancy are not available, but typical effectiveness figures indicate these would be in the range found for the diaphragm.

 ‡ Data are inadequate for accurate comparisons.

 (After Hatcher RA, Stewart F, Trussell J et al: Contraceptive Technology 1990–1992, 15th rev ed. New York, Irvington Publishers, 1990; and Romney SL et al: Gynecology and Obstetrics: The Health Care of Women. New York, McGraw-Hill, Blakiston, 1975)

the risk a given method poses for the person cannot be completely determined in advance, although in many instances contraindications can be identified for known health problems or personal characteristics. Still, an apparently healthy woman with no major contraindications to a given method can develop serious complications, some of which are life threatening. Although the incidence of such complications is low, it is the client's right to be well informed about the risks, benefits, and effectiveness of all contraceptive methods.

When the client has experienced prior difficulties with certain methods, intervention focuses on the meanings attached and perceived reasons for problems. The nurse can assist in values clarification, so the client

may better understand the psychodynamics of unsuccessful contraceptive use. The client's health beliefs, values, fears related to physical or psychoemotional harm, and personal reactions to contraceptive experiences are explored. This process assists the client in clarifying values, understanding behaviors, and making personal choices that work better in achieving goals.

Informed Consent

The nurse often is responsible for obtaining informed consent for contraceptive methods or procedures (see Chap. 7). The important components in providing suf-

Assessment Tool

Questions Regarding Contraceptive Effectiveness

Answer "yes or "no."
1. Am I afraid of using this method of birth control? _____
2. Would I really rather not use this method? _____
3. Will I have trouble remembering to use this method? _____
4. Have I ever become pregnant while using this method? _____
5. Are there reasons why I will be unable to use this method as prescribed? _____
6. Do I still have unanswered questions about this method? _____
7. Has my mother, father, sister, brother, or a close friend strongly discouraged me from using this method? _____
8. Will this method make my periods longer or more painful? _____
9. Will prolonged use of this method cost me more than I can afford? _____
10. Is this method known to have serious complications? _____
11. Am I opposed to this method because of my religious beliefs? _____
12. Have I already experienced complications from this method? _____
13. Has a nurse or doctor already told me not to use this method? _____
14. Is my partner opposed to using this method? _____
15. Am I using this method without my partner's knowledge? _____
16. Will the use of this method embarrass me? _____
17. Will the use of this method embarrass my partner? _____
18. Will my partner or I enjoy sexual activity less because of this method? _____
19. Will this method interrupt lovemaking? _____

Every "yes" response indicates a potential problem with this method of contraception. You will probably be most comfortable with the method getting the fewest "yes" responses.

---

ficient information for contraceptive choices include discussing the benefits and risks of each method, discussing alternatives including abstinence and no method, supporting the client's rights and responsibility to ask questions about methods, explaining the use and results of each method, and assuring the client that she (or the couple) may choose to leave or not use any method without jeopardizing their right to care. The nurse obtains the client's signature on a consent form, which contains an outline of these components and the information provided. This form must be witnessed by the person obtaining consent and another person of the client's choice.

Further nursing interventions related to choice and utilization of specific contraceptive methods are discussed in the section entitled "Contraceptive Methods."

Evaluation

Evaluation of the contraceptive plan involves observing for desired changes in knowledge, understanding, or behavior in the client. Often evaluation leads to another round of assessment, diagnosis, and planning as problems are refined and better understood.

The most basic level of evaluation is whether or not the client uses the selected method of contraception effectively. Prevention of pregnancy is the basic outcome criterion. Other levels of evaluation consider the client's satisfaction with the method, ease in use, compatibility with life-style, acceptability in relation to values and cost, response of sexual partner, and concern with side-effects. If difficulties are experienced in any of these areas, the nurse reassesses the situation in partnership with the client or couple. A new diagnosis is made, and appropriate intervention is planned and evaluated.

Legally, the nurse must enter a record of the information covered in the client's chart and make some notation to document client understanding. Often, clients are asked to sign a statement at the end of the record of information, such as, "I have read and discussed the above information about contraception (or the specific method) and I fully understand these points." The importance of a voluntary decision by the client, without coercion or professional bias, is evident.

Informed choice is both a safeguard for the client
(*Text continues on page 192*)

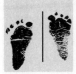

Nursing Care Plan

Couples Seeking Contraceptive Methods

Nursing Goals

1. Couple receives accurate information about modes of action, methods for use, risks, and benefits of all contraceptives.
2. Couple clarifies misunderstandings and knowledge deficits regarding particular contraceptive methods.
3. Couple selects appropriate contraceptive method for their particular needs, considering effectiveness, safety, and acceptability.
4. Couple understands use of selected contraceptive method and has opportunity for questions to be answered.
5. Couple understands and accepts potential side-effects and complications of their selected contraceptive method and can identify problems that need immediate attention.

Assessment	Potential Nursing Diagnosis	Intervention	Evaluation
All Types			
Understanding of sexuality, characteristics of sexual activity (i.e., regular or occasional intercourse, one or several partners)	Knowledge deficit related to sexual and reproductive functions, contraceptive methods (use, effectiveness, risks, mechanisms of action)	Reinforce accurate knowledge	Affirms understanding, no further questions
Knowledge of contraceptives and understanding of their use		Teach correct information, clear misconceptions	Able to select method and feel comfortable with it
Satisfaction and dissatisfaction with previous contraceptive practices	Noncompliance related to health beliefs and values, prior unsuccessful experience with method, increased symptoms with method, or disturbed self-concept (not taking responsibility for self-care)	Provide information about methods not well understood	Effective contraceptive use (i.e., no unwanted pregnancies)
Menstrual and pregnancy history		Provide feedback about effectiveness rates, reasons why method not effective	
General health history		Provide feedback about risks and contraindications of various methods	
Expectations of benefits from contraceptive method	Decisional conflict related to use or type of birth control	Reinforce accurate expectations, clear misconceptions	
Concerns about various methods related to religious affiliation, life-style, and values such as naturalism		Discuss various methods, mechanisms of action, and implications	
		Encourage discussion of decisional conflicts, advantages and disadvantages of choices	
Oral Contraceptives			
Determine if contraindications are present from history and physical examination	Knowledge deficit related to contraindications, monitoring needs, use, side-effects and complications,	Advise if contraindicated	Finds method suitable and uses effectively
		Discuss regular use of medication, need for periodic checkup, blood pressure, and Pap smears	Comfortable with decision not to use

(continued)

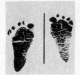

Nursing Care Plan (continued)

Assessment	Potential Nursing Diagnosis	Intervention	Evaluation
Explore understanding of requirements for this method to be effective (i.e., regularity of pill taking)	risks and benefits of oral contraceptives Knowledge deficit related to learning that impairs ability to follow regimen Decisional conflict related to health beliefs and values inconsistent with oral contraceptive use	Explain how to begin and discontinue pills Discuss side-effects, serious complications, when to seek medical care, what to do if one or more pills are forgotten Discuss advantages and disadvantages	Satisfied with experience using method
IUD			
Determine if contraindications are present from history and physical examination Explore understanding of requirements for this method to be effective (i.e., checking IUD strings)	Knowledge deficit related to contraindications, insertion and removal techniques, monitoring needs, side-effects and complications, risks and benefits of IUDS Decisional conflict related to health beliefs and values inconsistent with IUD use Disturbance in self-concept with inability to touch body part (genital)	Advise if contraindicated Discuss techniques and experience of IUD insertion and removal, need for periodic checkup and Pap smears Explain method, discuss side-effects, serious complications, and when to seek medical care Note when IUD must be replaced if it contains copper or hormone Discuss advantages and disadvantages	Finds methods suitable and uses effectively Comfortable with decision not to use Satisfied with experience using method
Diaphragm or sponge			
Determine if contraindications are present from history and physical examination Explore understanding of requirements for this method to be effective (i.e., insertion and removal techniques, checking for tears, using with every act of intercourse)	Knowledge deficit related to contraindications, requirements for effective use, risks and benefits of sponge or diaphragm Disturbance in self-concept with inability to touch body part (genital) Noncompliance related to inappropriate environment and life-style for use requirements Noncompliance related to deficit in psychomotor	Advise if contraindicated Discuss insertion and removal techniques, instruct and have client practice until correctly done Explain method and necessity for constant use, applying more spermicide with additional acts of intercourse, and for leaving in 6–8 hours (diaphragm); wet sponge before insertion, remove within 30 hours	Finds method suitable and uses effectively Comfortable with decision not to use Satisfied with experience using method

(continued)

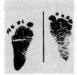

Nursing Care Plan (continued)

Assessment	Potential Nursing Diagnosis	Intervention	Evaluation
	skills that impairs ability to follow regimen	Advise that diaphragm must be refitted after each delivery and if substantial amount of weight is lost or gained Discuss advantages and disadvantages	
Fertility awareness Explore understanding of requirements for this method to be effective (i.e., long periods of abstinence, regular menstrual periods, ancillary techniques to increase effectiveness)	Knowledge deficit related to requirements for effective use, risks and benefits of fertility awareness Knowledge deficit related to learning ability that impairs ability to follow regimen Alteration in family processes related to goal conflicts with sexual partern	Discuss methods to establish baseline menstrual patterns and identify ovulation Instruct on calculating fertile period Discuss advantages and disadvantages	Finds method suitable and uses effectively Comfortable with decision not to use Satisfied with experience using method
Spermicides and Condom Explore understanding of requirements for this method to be effective (i.e., timing of applications, regular use, precautions to avoid leakage or decreasing spermicide effectiveness)	Knowledge deficit related to requirements for effective use, risks and benefits of spermicides and condom Noncompliance related to inappropriate environment and life-style for use requirements Noncompliance related to lack of motivation for regular and consistent use	Instruct on proper insertion of spermicides and application of condom Advise on repeated acts of intercourse and reapplications, care in condom removal, no douching for 6–8 hours when spermicides are used Discuss advantages and disadvantages	Finds method suitable and uses effectively Comfortable with decision not to use Satisfied with experience using method
Sterilization Determine understanding of procedure as ending fertility and irreversible Obtain childbearing history, ages and health of children, marital situation, and values assigned to reproductive role	Knowledge deficit related to indications for sterilization, types of procedures, permanence of procedures, risks and benefits Decisional conflict related to health beliefs and values inconsistent with sterilization Disturbance in self-concept due to loss of body function	Discuss permanence of sterilization Explore meanings to couple Explain various procedures and required follow-up	Affirms understanding of performance, desire to end childbearing; accepts requirements of procedure; satisfied with outcome

and a way of increasing proper contraceptive use. When the woman or couple fully understand the technique, have weighed the possible adverse effects against the convenience and acceptability of the method for them, and have made a choice based on which method best meets their needs, the likelihood of discontinuation and misuse is reduced.

■ CONTRACEPTIVE METHODS

Oral Contraception

Oral contraceptives ("the pill") are hormonal agents consisting of a combination of estrogen and a synthetic progestational agent or only progestin. They act principally at the central nervous system level to inhibit ovulation through suppression of follicle-stimulating hormone (FSH) and luteinizing hormone (LH). There are secondary effects on endometrial development, tubal motility, and cervical mucus. Under the influence of the progestational agent, the cervical mucus becomes thick, viscous, and unreceptive to spermatozoa. However, the most important effect of standard-dose combination pills is the inhibition of ovulation.

About 10 million women in the United States and 56 million women worldwide use oral contraceptives. The lowest failure rate with consistent and accurate usage of pills is 0.1%. More typical failure rates of average users range from an overall 0.34% to 4.7% for users less than 22 years old. An important factor decreasing use-effectiveness is the high attrition rate among pill users. Only 50% to 75% of women starting on the pill are still using them after 1 year. Most women discontinue the pill for nonmedical reasons, and many pregnancies occur after discontinuing the pill because women fail to start other contraception. Because of high discontinuation rates, women starting the pill should be provided with a second method of contraception and encouraged to become familiar with it.[15]

Oral contraceptives do not provide protection against human immunosuppressive virus (HIV) infections or other STD. The pill may contribute to higher STD rates because barrier methods are not used and women may have increased sexual activity when protected from unwanted pregnancy. Although lower rates of gonococcal PID have been found among pill users, evidence indicates that lower genital tract infections are more common, especially due to *Chlamydia trachomatis*.

COMBINATION ORAL CONTRACEPTIVES

Combination oral contraceptives, containing continuous doses of both estrogen and progestin, are available in 21- and 28-day packages. In the 21-day packs, a pill is taken each day for 3 weeks, followed by a week without any pills. In the 28-day pack, a pill is taken every day for 4 weeks, but only those taken during the first 3 weeks have active hormonal ingredients; those pills taken during the last week consist of lactose or ferrous sulfate, but no hormones. The purpose of a week of nonhormonal pills is to keep the woman in the habit of taking a pill a day and, in some instances, to provide an iron supplement for prevention of anemia. Two or 3 days after the last pill containing hormone is taken there is usually a "withdrawal" menstrual flow.

A large number of oral contraceptives are available, with differing combinations of estrogen or progestin doses (Table 11-2). There are three types: combination pills, which contain estrogen and progestin and are available at the standard or low (micro) dosage levels; triphasics, which contain three different combinations of estrogen and progestin; and the progestin-only type (minipills). Because the majority of serious side-effects are due to estrogen, the trend has been toward reducing this hormonal agent from the original dosage of 80 to 100 μg to doses ranging from 40 to 20 μg. However, use of 20- or 30-μg pills is associated with higher rates of breakthrough bleeding and unpredictable menses, making them less acceptable to some women.

TABLE 11–2. MOST CURRENTLY AVAILABLE COMBINATION, MICRODOSE, AND PROGESTIN ORAL CONTRACEPTIVES

Product/Manufacturer	Type	Estrogen	Progestin
Enovid-E/Searle	Combination	100 μg mestranol	2.5 mg norethynodrel
Ortho-Novum/Ortho	Combination	100 μg mestranol	2 mg norethindrone
Norinyl/Syntex	Combination	100 μg mestranol	2 mg norethindrone
Ovulen/Searle	Combination	100 μg mestranol	1 mg ethynodiol diacetate
Ortho-Novum1/80/Ortho	Combination	80 μg mestranol	1 mg norethindrone
Norinyl 1 + 80/Syntex	Combination	80 μg mestranol	1 mg norethindrone
Norlestrin/Parke-Davis	Combination	50 μg ethinyl estradiol	2.5 mg norethindrone acetate
Norinyl 1 + 50/Syntex	Combination	50 μg mestranol	1 mg norethindrone
Ortho-Novum 1/50/Ortho	Combination	50 μg mestranol	1 mg norethindrone
Norlestrin/Parke-Davis	Combination	50 μg ethinyl estradiol	1 mg norethindrone acetate
Ovral/Wyeth	Combination	50 μg ethinyl estradiol	0.5 mg norgestrel
Demulen/Searle	Combination	50 μg ethinyl estradiol	1 mg ethynodiol diacetate
Ovcon-50/Mead Johnson	Combination	50 μg ethinyl estradiol	1 mg norethindrone
Brevicon/Syntex	Combination	35 μg ethinyl estradiol	0.5 mg norethindrone
Ovcon-35/Mead Johnson	Combination	35 μg ethinyl estradiol	0.4 mg norethindrone
Modicon/Ortho	Combination	35 μg ethinyl estradiol	0.5 mg norethindrone
Norinyl 1 + 35/Syntex	Combination	35 μg ethinyl estradiol	1 mg norethindrone
Ortho Novum 1/35/Ortho	Combination	35 μg ethinyl estradiol	1 mg norethindrone
Demulen 1/35/Searle	Combination	35 μg ethinyl estradiol	1 mg ethynodiol diacetate
Ortho-Novum 10/11/Ortho	Combination-Biphasic	35 μg ethinyl estradiol	0.5 mg norethinhdrone (days 1–10) 1 mg norethindrone (days 11–21)
Nordette/Wyeth	Combination	30 μg ethinyl estradiol	0.15 mg levonorgestrel
Loestrin 1.5/30/Parke-Davis	Combination	30 μg ethinyl estradiol	1.5 mg norethindrone acetate
Lo/Ovral/Wyeth	Combination	30 μg ethinyl estradiol	0.3 mg norgestrel
Loestrin 1/20/Parke-Davis	Combination	20 μg ethinyl estradiol	1 mg norethindrone acetate
Micronor/Ortho	Progestin		0.35 mg norethindrone
Nor-QD/Syntex	Progestin		0.35 mg norethindrone
Ovrette/Wyeth	Progestin		0.075 mg norgestrel
Ortho-Novum 7/7/7/Ortho	Triphasic	35 μg ethinyl estradiol	0.5 mg norethindrone (1–7) 0.75 mg norethindrone (8–14) 1.0 mg norethindrone (15–21)
Tri-Norinyl/Syntex	Triphasic	35 μg ethinyl estradiol	0.5 mg norethindrone (1–7) 1.0 mg norethindrone (8–16) 0.5 mg norethindrone (17–21)
Triphasil/Wyeth Tri-Levlen/Berlex	Triphasic	30 μg ethinyl estradiol 40 μg ethinyl estradiol 30 μg ethinyl estradiol	0.05 mg levonorgestrel (1–6) 0.075 mg levonogestrel (7–11) 0.125 mg levonorgestrel (12–21)

For these reasons, the trend among family planning providers is to prescribe pills containing less than 50 μg of estrogen, mainly those containing ethinyl estradiol. The wide variety of combination pills available allows the provider to select according to individual client needs and responses. Among the considerations are relative estrogen potency, estrogenic effects of progestin, and androgenic effects of progestin. Adjustments can be made for side-effects clients experience, such as fluid retention, spotting, and headaches.

Side-Effects and Contraindications. Common estrogen-related side-effects of the combination pill include accentuation of such premenstrual symptoms as breast tenderness, irritability, edema, nausea, headaches, spotting, cyclic weight gain, missed periods, and increased vaginal yeast infections. The major life-threatening estrogen effects include blood clots in the legs, pelvis, lungs, heart, or brain and hepatocellular adenomas or cancer. The risk of heart attack is increased in women over 40, especially if they smoke. Gallbladder disease and hypertension also are serious complications.

Progestin-related side-effects of combination pills include increased appetite and weight gain, depression, fatigue, decreased libido, acne, oily skin, increased breast size, diabetogenic effect, headaches, pruritus, increased low-density lipoprotein cholesterol levels (LDL), and decreased high-density lipoprotein cholesterol levels (HDL). Hypertension, myocardial infarction, and cervical dysplasia are more serious effects attributable to both estrogenic and progestogenic components.

Generally accepted absolute contraindications to combined oral contraceptives include a history of thrombophlebitis, thromboembolic disorders, cerebro-vascular accident, ischemic heart disease, coronary artery disease, hepatic adenoma, or malignancy of the breast or of the reproductive tract, the presence of marked impairment of liver function, and pregnancy. Strong relative contraindications include migraine, hypertension, diabetes, gallbladder disease, sickle cell disease, undiagnosed vaginal bleeding, age over 35 and currently a heavy smoker, age over 40 and cardiovascular risk factor, fibrocystic breast disease, and less than 2 weeks postpartum.

TRIPHASIC ORAL CONTRACEPTIVES

Pills containing three different combinations of estrogen and progestins have been available in the United States since 1984. These pills usually increase progestin in three phases during the cycle, and some alter estrogen dosage as well. Triphasic oral contraceptives are available in 21- and 28-day regimens. Failure rates have been reported as somewhat higher than for low-dose combination pills.[15] Advantages of triphasics include less progestin than in low-dose combination pills; fewer metabolic effects on lipids, blood pressure and carbohydrate metabolism related to progestins; fewer progestin side-effects; and increased patient or provider acceptance. Triphasics are promoted as "more natural" than combination pills, because they more closely approximate the natural hormonal pattern of women. However, the effect produced, a state of anovulation, is certainly unnatural in women unless they are pregnant or lactating.

Disadvantages of triphasic pills include confusion because of three or four different colored pills per cycle, making it difficult for clients and providers to quickly determine the phase of the cycle. More spotting and breakthrough bleeding have been reported with triphasics than the most commonly used low-dose combination pills. There is less flexibility to delay menses by taking a few additional pills, to begin taking pills on a day other than that recommended on the package insert, or to double up on pills to control spotting.

PROGESTIN-ONLY PILLS (MINIPILLS)

Oral contraceptives containing only progestins have been available in the United States since 1973. Minipills use the same progestins as those in combination pills, but in smaller doses. The absence of estrogen in minipills is the basis for both the advantages and disadvantages. The advantage is that they do not carry the risks of complication and side-effects of increased estrogen, but the disadvantages include less predictable menstrual patterns and increased irregular bleeding.

Minipills prevent ovulation in only 15% to 40% of cycles, thus their contraceptive effect depends on other factors such as unfavorable cervical mucus, inhibited sperm migration, disturbed endometrial development, and an inadequate luteal phase. Women for whom the minipill may be the oral contraceptive of choice include those who are over 35, women with a history of headaches or mild hypertension, women who are lactating and those experiencing estrogen-related side-effects such as headaches, hypertension, leg pain, chloasma, weight gain, and nausea. Continuation rates of minipills are probably lower than with combined pills and are reported as less than 50% after 1 year of use. Because the progestin dose is low, excellent compliance in taking pills is necessary. Missing one or two tablets leads to a much higher risk of accidental pregnancy than with combination pills. Even with perfect compliance, failure rates are higher than those of combination pills. Pregnancies per 100 woman-years are reported at 0.5 to 3.7 in the United States, with higher rates in the first 6 months of use.[15]

Side-Effects and Contraindications. Because of increased spotting and breakthrough bleeding, undiagnosed abnormal vaginal bleeding is an important contraindication to minipill use. Other contraindications include acute mononucleosis or liver disease. Minipills do not protect against ectopic pregnancy as well as against intrauterine pregnancy, so the risk of an ectopic pregnancy is greater when conception occurs. Because minipills contain no estrogen, theoretically they should not cause serious estrogen-related complications such as thromboembolic disease and hypertension. However, data are not available to document this advantage.[15]

Side-effects include variations in cycle length (both shorter and longer), headaches, weight gain, breast discomfort, nausea, and vomiting. Less hypertension, dysmenorrhea, and premenstrual syndrome are reported. Progestins have no measurable effect on carbohydrate metabolism, lipid metabolism, and blood pressure. The side-effects of oral contraceptives, according to the excess or deficiency of hormone responsible for the symptoms or condition, are shown in Table 11-3.

NORPLANT IMPLANTS

Norplant is a long-acting subdermal hormonal contraceptive approved by the FDA for use in the United States in 1991. The Norplant System consists of six Silastic membrane capsules, each containing 35 μg of levonorgestrel, a type of progestin. All six capsules are inserted subdermally in the woman's upper arm and provide effective contraception for up to 5 years. Levonorgestrel slowly diffuses through the slender, flexible capsules, providing a constant low dose of hormone. About 50 to 80 μg are released daily for the first few weeks, decreasing to 30 to 35 μg daily over the next 2 to 6 months, and gradually reducing to 25 μg/day after 5 years.[16] The capsules are removed after 5 years, or at any time the woman desires to reverse the contraceptive. Fertility returns to preinsertion levels shortly after the capsules are removed.

The Norplant System is highly effective in preventing pregnancy. The pregnancy rate for the first year is about 0.2%, with an annual rate of 0.8 per 100 users during 5 years of use. This rate is better than the low-dose oral contraceptive rate and approaches the rate of tubal sterilization, but Norplant is reversible. Pregnancy rates with Norplant gradually increase over 5 years to 2.5 to 3 pregnancies per 100 users. Women who weigh over 154 lb are more likely to experience pregnancy; their annual pregnancy rate is 1.7 per 100 users over 5 years.[17]

This method is particularly suitable for women who desire long-term but reversible contraception. Good candidates include women who have had children but are not prepared to undergo tubal sterilization, who have had side-effects from combined oral contraceptives, who have experienced contraceptive failure with

TABLE 11-3. HORMONAL BASIS OF SIDE-EFFECTS OF ORAL CONTRACEPTIVES

Estrogen		Progestin		Androgen
Excess	*Deficiency*	*Excess*	*Deficiency*	*Excess*
Nausea, vomiting	Amenorrhea	Acne, oily scalp	Hypermenorrhea with clotting	Acne
Fluid retention (premenstrual tension, irritability, breast tenderness, corneal swelling, cramping, edema)	Oligomenorrhea	Increased appetite	Late-cycle spotting	Oily skin
	Early-cycle or midcycle spotting	Weight gain	Delayed onset of menses	Rashes
	Loss of pelvic tone	Fatigue	Dysmenorrhea	Increased hair growth in male pattern
	Hot flashes	Depression	Weight loss	Increased interest in sex
Increased vaginal discharge	Nervousness, irritability	Hair loss		Cholestatic jaundice
Chloasma	Decreased interest in sex	Headahces when not taking pills		Increased appetite
Headaches		Increased breast size		Pruritus
Increased breast size		Increased muscle mass		
Weight gain		Increased monilial vaginitis (*Candida*)		
Increased cervical ectropion		Breast tenderness not related to fluid retention		
Increased size of fibroids		Short menses		
Telangiectasia		Relative endometrial atrophy		
Thromboembolic disorders		Decreased interest in sex		
Reduction of lactation		Cholestatic jaundice		
Possible hypertension		Decreased carbohydrate tolerance		
Hepatic adenoma		Dilated leg veins		

other methods, or who are late in their reproductive years and prefer not to use an estrogen-containing method. Norplant's advantages include being long-lasting, easily reversible, not related to intercourse, no estrogen side-effects, high effectiveness, and not user dependent. Its disadvantages include the necessity of insertion and removal, visibility under the skin, and menstrual irregularity.

As a progestin-only contraceptive, Norplant's modes of action include suppression of ovulation, thickening of cervical mucus, changes in the endometrium making it unreceptive to implantation, and more rapid tubal transport of the ovum. Over time, about 50% of women using Norplant will have some ovulatory cycles, but this does not increase their risk of pregnancy because of the additional modes of action.

Insertion Procedure. The Norplant capsules are 34 mm long and 2.4 mm wide, about the size of lead in a pencil. The inner surface of the woman's upper arm is used as the insertion site. Local anesthetic is injected into the skin and insertion areas, which include six lines in a fanlike position. A small (2 mm) incision is made in the skin with a scalpel, then a trochar is inserted just under the skin. The first capsule is inserted through the trochar, which is withdrawn, leaving the capsule in place. This procedure is repeated until all six capsules are inserted in the fanlike position under the skin (Fig. 11-1). The incision is closed with a butterfly; suturing is not necessary. The insertion area is covered with a dry compress and gauze for hemostasis; the bandage is removed in 3 days. The procedure takes about 10 minutes. For removal, a 4-mm incision is made near the end of the implants, which are pushed downward toward the incision until the end can be grasped with a mosquito forceps. The tissue capsule that has formed around the implant is opened with the scalpel, and the tip of the implant is grasped with another forceps and gently

pulled out. If the woman wishes to continue using Norplant, new implants can be inserted through the same incision, but fanning in the other direction.[15]

Side-Effects and Contraindications. Contraindications include undiagnosed vaginal bleeding, active thrombophlebitis or thromboembolic disorders, pregnancy, liver disease, coronary artery or cerebrovascular disease, and breast cancer. Norplant can be used by lactating women and must be inserted at least 6 weeks after delivery.

The most common side-effect is menstrual cycle irregularities, which may include prolonged menstrual flow during the first months of use, bleeding or spotting between periods, or amenorrhea. These usually subside in 3 to 6 months, and a pattern of light and infrequent periods develops. About half of the women using Norplant have changes in their menstrual pattern during the first year, and 10% stop using the method because of this. Women continuing to use Norplant have, on average, 5 days of bleeding per month with less blood loss, but the bleeding pattern is more irregular.

Some women experience pain or discomfort with insertion and removal. Infection may occur at the insertion site, with expulsion of capsules, but this is uncommon and usually associated with improper asepsis. Local reactions, including itching and pain, usually resolve within a month but may persist longer. Pregnancy is infrequent, but the capsules must be removed immediately if it does occur. There is no increase in ectopic pregnancies. No excess cardiovascular complications have been identified with Norplant.

SYSTEMIC EFFECTS OF SYNTHETIC HORMONES

The estrogens and progestins used in oral contraceptives have widespread effects in many body systems, in addition to their effects on the reproduction system.

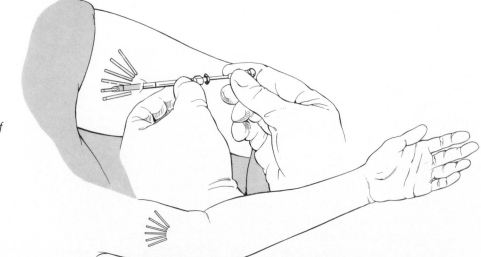

■ *Figure 11-1*
The insertion and placement of Norplant under the skin.

Cardiovascular Effects. The most serious complications of pill use are cardiovascular problems. Several studies have found heart attacks and strokes to occur more frequently in women who use the pill than in women who do not.[18] Other life-threatening cardiovascular complications of oral contraceptives include hypertension and blood clots in the legs, pelvis, lungs, heart, or brain. The hormones in the pill, particularly estrogen, cause more rapid fibrin formation with increased clot firmness, increase in coagulation factors, increased platelet counts with changes in electrophoretic mobility of platelets, and increase in vascular lesions and venous stasis.[19] The risk of death from clotting disorders is reduced among women taking pills with less than 50 μg estrogen and among women under age 35.

Cardiovascular complications occur primarily in a small subgroup of women using oral contraceptives. Characteristics of women in this subgroup include smoking; over age 35; health problems such as hypertension, diabetes, or cardiovascular disease; and family history of diabetes or heart attacks under age 50. The more of these characteristics a woman has, the greater her risk. Young women in good health, who do not smoke, can use the pill with little risk of developing a serious cardiovascular complication.[20]

Effects of Cigarette Smoking. Oral contraceptives have a synergistic effect with cigarette smoke that significantly increases a woman's risk of myocardial infarction, stroke, and thromboembolic disorders. These effects are particularly found among women over age 35. All women seen for reproductive care should be discouraged from smoking and warned about the dangers of secondary smoke. Oral contraceptives can be used by young women with no additional health risks. A survey of family planning providers found that 95% would give combination oral contraceptives to a 20-year-old woman with no contraindications to pill use other than smoking one pack of cigarettes per day.[21]

Hypertensive Effects. Blood pressure increases in some women who take oral contraceptives. Usually this is rapidly reversible once the pill is discontinued, but it can lead to permanent complications if the blood pressure elevation is high enough or persists for some time. In normotensive women, it is difficult to predict who will develop hypertension, so blood pressure monitoring is essential for all pill users.

Lipid Effects. Estrogens tend to have a beneficial effect by increasing HDL and reducing LDL. Progestins have the opposite effect and reduce HDL while increasing LDL. Progestins also modify the composition of total HDL by changing the relative amounts of HDL_2 and HDL_3. HDL_2 provides a protective effect against cardiovascular disease. Some progestins (e.g., in Triphasil) reduce HDL_2 while not changing the total HDL profile.[22]

Effects on Carbohydrate Metabolism. Higher-dose combination oral contraceptives cause an increase in glucose levels, plasma insulin levels, and decreased glucose tolerance. These changes are affected by both the estrogen and progestin in combined pills. Progestins alone may produce an increase in tissue resistance to insulin by decreasing the number of insulin receptors.[23] Recent studies of low-dose combined pills showed minimal or no change in glucose tolerance and plasma insulin. These pills apparently may be used with some gestational diabetics and women with a family history of diabetes, although there is conflicting opinion and such clients must be monitored closely.[24]

Neoplastic Effects. More than a dozen studies have failed to demonstrate an increased risk of breast cancer among women using oral contraceptives. Increased risk has been suggested in young, nulliparous women taking pills with high progestin activity. Other subgroups whose risk needs more study include women with a family history of breast cancer and women with benign breast disease.[25,26]

A decreased relative risk of ovarian cancer among pill users has been demonstrated by nine epidemiological studies. Pills also protect women from endometrial cancer. Both of these decreased risks persist for at least 10 years after women have discontinued oral contraceptive use.[25]

There is mixed evidence about the relationship between oral contraceptives and cervical cancer. Some studies have found a significantly increased risk of cervical neoplasia in pill users, whereas others found no statistically increased risk.[25] Confounding factors in the relationship between oral contraceptives and cervical cancer include the frequency of Pap smears obtained by women using the pill, leading to early diagnosis and treatment of dysplasia, and the increased number of sexual partners of pill users.

Long-term oral contraceptives have increased incidence of hepatocellular adenomas. These benign tumors can lead to rupture of the liver capsule with extensive bleeding and death. Pills with high hormonal potency, used by women over age 30, further increase the risk of liver adenomas. Although the relationship of pills to hepatocellular carcinoma is less clear, studies have suggested there is an increased risk, especially with long-term pill use (over 8 years).[27]

Fetal Abnormalities. There appears to be no increase in fetal abnormalities among women who have used oral contraceptives but discontinued them before conception. Women who take oral contraceptives in early pregnancy have been found by some researchers at slightly increased risk for having babies with limb and heart defects. This increased risk of birth defects from pill use increases the incidence from about 30 per 1000 (average population risk) to 31 per 1000. Other researchers have found no association between pill use and birth defects.[28]

Safer Sex Practices

The basic principle in prevention of AIDS is to avoid exchanging body fluids that contain the human immunosuppressive virus (HIV). The transmission of HIV occurs primarily through exchange of infected blood, semen, or vaginal secretions. Barriers that prevent the exchange of body fluids (condoms) are the best line of defense. Condoms used with spermicides are even safer.

Safe Sexual Activities

Sexual fantasies and sex talk

Hugging and holding

Massage and body rubbing

Social (dry) kissing

Masturbation

Hand–genital stimulation

Possibly Safe Sexual Activities

French (wet) kissing

Vaginal intercourse using latex condom (spermicide increases safety)

Oral sex on man using latex condom

Oral sex on woman using vaginal condom, or when no vaginal discharge is present

Anal intercourse using latex condom

Unsafe Sexual Activities

Vaginal intercourse without latex condom (unless in mutually monogamous relationship)

Anal intercourse without latex condom

Oral sex on man without using latex condom

Oral sex on woman with vaginal discharge

Unprotected oral–anal contact

Blood contact, including sharing needles and contact with menstrual blood

(McIlvenna T (ed): The Complete Guide to Safe Sex. The Institute for Advanced Study of Human Sexuality. Beverly Hills, Specific Press, 1987; and Planned Parenthood Guidelines, 1987)

NURSING INTERVENTION FOR ORAL CONTRACEPTIVES

When oral contraceptives have been selected, and a specific type of pill prescribed, nursing care focuses on providing information and education about effective use. Education includes how to start taking the pills, how to develop a reliable routine for taking pills, what to do if pills are forgotten, how to assess spotting and when this becomes a problem that needs evaluation,

Client Education

"ACHES" System: Pill Danger Signs

A   Abdominal pain (severe)

C   Chest pain (severe) or shortness of breath

H   Headaches (severe)

E   Eye problems (blurred vision, loss of vision)

S   Severe leg pain (calf or thigh)

common side-effects, and more serious dangers that require immediate medical attention. Women are advised to select and keep handy a backup method of birth control, such as condoms or foam. Women should be reminded that pills provide no protection against HIV and other STD, and safe sex practices should be discussed. Written information, package inserts, and visual aids enhance the teaching–learning process.

Teaching clients the "ACHES" system of remembering early danger signs is an effective method. Some women may experience these symptoms for weeks or months before seeking help. Women should call the clinic or physician right away if any of these danger signals develop.

A follow-up visit is usually scheduled for 4 to 6 months after pills have been used. At this time, side-effects are reviewed with special attention to headaches, blurred vision, chest pain, and leg pain. The client's experiences and practices using the pills are discussed, and questions are elicited and answered by the nurse. Physical examination includes blood pressure and weight checks. If no difficulties are encountered, another 6-month visit is scheduled, then visits become annual with repeat of the pelvic examination, Pap smear, and breast examination.

Women using oral contraceptives who want to stop taking them to become pregnant should be instructed on how to do this safely. They should be instructed to use another reliable birth control method after stopping the pills until experiencing two or three normal menstrual cycles. There may be a 1- to 2-month delay in the resumption of menses and ovulation after discontinuing oral contraceptives. If pregnancy occurs before normal cycles have been established, it is difficult to calculate an accurate delivery date.

Intrauterine Device

The intrauterine device (IUD) is a small, usually flexible appliance that is inserted by a health-care professional into the uterine cavity. The use of foreign objects placed inside the uterus to prevent pregnancy is an ancient practice.

Intensive research and development of IUDs in the 1950s and 1960s produced a number of devices that were widely used in the United States and worldwide. About 85 million women throughout the world use IUDs, most of whom are in China (70%). In the early 1980s, 2.2 million women in the United States were using IUDS, which constituted about 10% of the reversible contraceptives then in use. Since then, IUD use has dropped markedly and was estimated at 1.4 million in 1985.[15]

Public and professional concern about the serious consequences of pelvic infections associated with IUD use led to withdrawal of many IUDs from the market. The IUD linked with the largest proportion of pelvic infections, subsequent infertility, and lawsuits is the Dalcon Shield. All women with Dalcon Shields have been advised by their producer, AH Robbins, to have these devices removed. Robbins declared bankruptcy in 1985 as a result of Dalcon Shield lawsuits. Pharmaceutical companies gradually discontinued production and sales of their IUDs because of numerous lawsuits, declining market shares, liability insurance costs, and the economic unprofitability of IUDs. Only two IUDs are produced and distributed in the United States, the Progestasert and the Copper-T380A (Fig. 11-2). Some family planning clinics and physician offices still have older devices, such as the Lippes Loop, CU-7, and CU-T200. Many clients have these types of devices in place.

IUDs prevent pregnancy by way of several mechanisms: by inducing a local inflammatory response causing blastocyst or sperm lysis or preventing implantation; increasing local production of prostaglandins that inhibit implantation; interfering with enzymatic and hormonal activity on the endometrium; disrupting the blastocyst from the endometrium; increasing motility of the ovum in the fallopian tube; and immobilizing sperm as they pass through the uterine cavity. In progestin-containing IUDs, the proliferative, secretory maturation process of the endometrium is disrupted, causing endometrial suppression and impairing implantation; and thick cervical mucus is produced that discourages sperm transport.

The effectiveness of IUDs is slightly less than that of oral contraceptives. The lowest reported pregnancy rate with medicated IUDs (copper, progestin) is about 1%, whereas with unmedicated IUDs this rate is 2% to 3%. The first-year failure rate of IUDs in typical users is 6%. Use effectiveness depends on several factors, including clinician experience in insertion, likelihood of expulsion, ability of the client to detect expulsion, type of device, frequency of intercourse, and the client's access to medical services.

The IUD offers certain advantages to women who have no contraindications to insertion. Continuous protection against pregnancy is provided without the need to remember taking pills, inserting a diaphragm, or applying condoms or foam. The contraceptive is separated from intercourse, a distinct advantage to some women. IUDs can be inserted at any time during the menstrual cycle, when pregnancy has been excluded, and they may be inserted immediately after an abortion. Contraceptive effects of the IUD are readily reversible once the device is removed. Because IUDs have no systemic hormonal effects such as those created by oral contra-

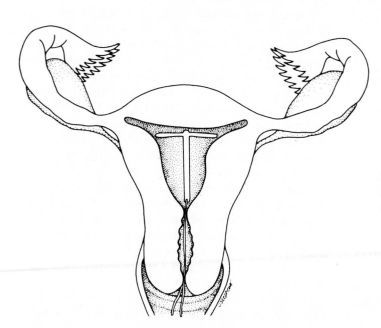

Progestasert

■ *Figure 11–2*
Progestasert-T IUD in place in the uterine cavity.
(Childbirth Graphics, Rochester, NY)

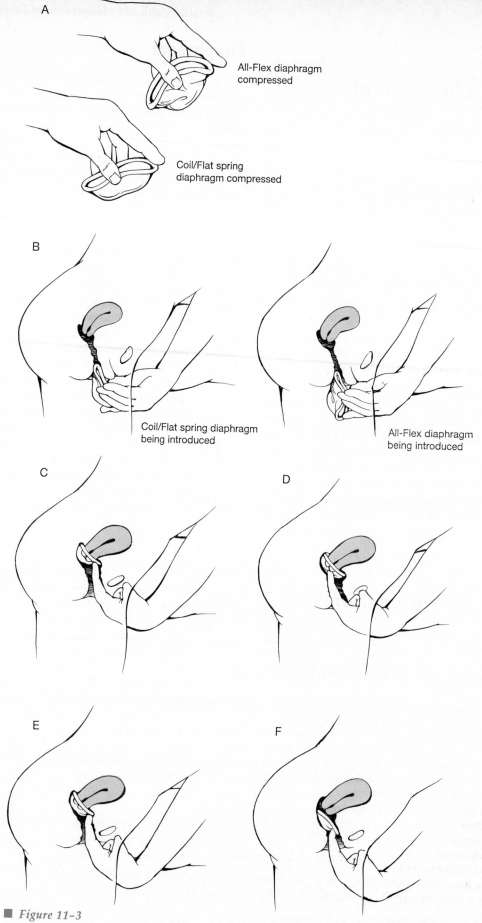

A

All-Flex diaphragm
compressed

Coil/Flat spring
diaphragm compressed

B

Coil/Flat spring diaphragm
being introduced

All-Flex diaphragm
being introduced

C

D

E

F

■ *Figure 11–3*
Diaphragm insertion, placement, and removal.

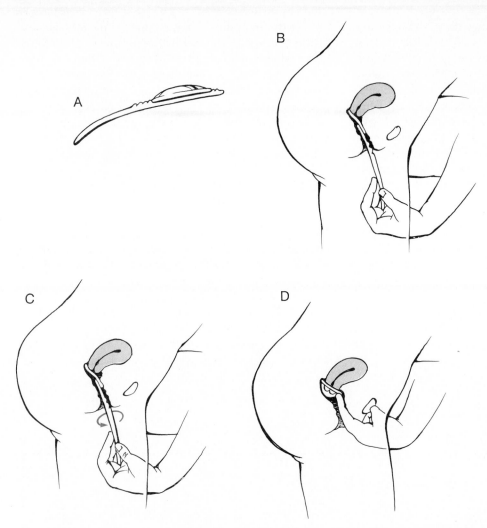

■ *Figure 11–4*
Use of an inserter to position the diaphragm minimizes genital touching and may be easier for some women. (A) The inserter with diaphragm (flat or coil spring) in place. (B) The inserter with diaphragm is positioned deep in the posterior fornix. (C) The inserter is twisted to release the diaphragm. (D) The diaphragm is pushed behind the symphysis pubis with a finger; here it is correctly positioned over the cervix. (Whitley N: A Manual of Clinical Obstetrics. Philadelphia, JB Lippincott, 1985)

The diaphragm appears to be an excellent contraceptive for younger, nulliparous women who do not have intercourse with great regularity. In a study at the Sanger Bureau in New York, involving 2175 women over 2 years, an actual failure rate of two pregnancies per 100 users per year was documented. Most of the women in the study were under 30 (80%) and were unmarried (70%).[30]

Diaphragms are available in a range of sizes and in four styles, which include the flat spring, coil spring, arcing spring, and wide seal rim. Each has particular uses depending on vaginal tone and pelvic anatomy. The newest version, the wide seal rim, has a flange on the inner rim that creates a better seal between the diaphragm and vaginal wall. The flat spring is useful with firm vaginal tone, and the coil spring is useful with average vaginal tone. Both can be used with an inserter (Fig. 11-4). The arcing spring is easier to insert manually and is useful with lax vaginal tone, cystocele, or rectocele.

The goal in fitting a diaphragm is to select the largest rim size that is comfortable for the client, taking the above factors into consideration. Sizes that are too small may fail to maintain position covering the cervix, whereas those that are too large may cause vaginal pressure, abdominal pain or cramping, vaginal ulceration, or recurrent UTI. Fitting rings or whole diaphragms with a cut-out center can be used for fitting. Rings are not helpful for patient practice because the woman needs to feel the cervix through the rubber dome of the inserted diaphragm.

Diaphragms with spermicide provide protection against STD. Spermicidal ingredients have been found lethal to organisms causing gonorrhea, herpes, PID, and trichomoniasis. Although in-vitro activity of spermicides against HIV has been demonstrated, it is not known whether any significant protection is provided. Protection against chlamydial diseases and hepatitis is also not known. There is lower risk of cervical dysplasia and cancer among women using diaphragms more than 5 years. Research on diaphragm and spermicide inhibition of *Staphylococcus aureus*, which causes toxic shock syndrome (TSS), has been contradictory.[15]

COMPLICATIONS AND SIDE-EFFECTS

Although there are few serious complications with use of the diaphragm, studies have reported several cases of TSS occurring in association with diaphragm use. These cases occurred on days when the women were not menstruating, and data provide no reliable way to estimate the background incidence of TSS on nonmenstrual days. Cases of TSS are infrequent, and the risk of death is low (0.3 deaths per 100,000 women using barrier contraceptives). No increase in relative risk with diaphragm use has been suggested.[31] However, women using the diaphragm should know the danger signs of TSS and should be instructed in taking TSS precautions.

Contraindications to diaphragm use include history of TSS, allergy to latex or spermicide, recurrent UTI, and abnormalities of vaginal anatomy that prevent satisfactory fit or stable placement (such as uterine prolapse, extreme retroversion, vaginal septum). Severe pelvic pain (due to herpes, recent episiotomy, PID, tight introitus) precludes diaphragm use, although it can be used when the condition is resolved. Women must be refitted after each pregnancy but should wait about 12 weeks postpartum before using the diaphragm. If proper insertion technique cannot be learned, diaphragm use is contraindicated.

Recurrent cystitis can occur due to upward pressure of the diaphragm rim against the urethra, and cramps or rectal pressure might also be felt. Often the diaphragm is too large when these occur. Some women or their partners have allergic reactions to rubber or spermicides. Vaginitis or foul vaginal discharge may be caused by spermicide or leaving the diaphragm in the vagina too long. Vaginal trauma or ulceration can result from excessive rim pressure or prolonged wear.

NURSING INTERVENTION FOR THE DIAPHRAGM

Nursing care for the clients using the diaphragm focuses on education about effective use, safety, and prevention of side-effects. After the client has been fitted with an appropriate size and type of diaphragm, the nurse provides teaching about insertion and removal. Although this can be time-consuming, the importance of feeling comfortable with these techniques must be emphasized. Proper placement is critical to effective pregnancy prevention, and correct removal prevents damage to the

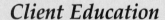

Client Education

Instructions for Inserting and Removing Diaphragm

1. When being fitted for a diaphragm, practice insertion and removal several times before leaving the office or clinic and have the provider check your placement of the diaphragm after practice. If the diaphragm feels uncomfortable, or if you think it may be too small or too large, return to the office with it in place for a reexamination.
2. Apply contraceptive jelly or cream by holding the diaphragm with the dome down, like a cup. Place about one tablespoon of cream or jelly into the dome and spread a thin layer around the rim also. The cream or jelly remains an active spermicide for up to 6 hours, so the diaphragm can be inserted well before intercourse.
3. With the dome down, insert the diaphragm by squeezing the opposite sides of the rim together. Spread the lips of the labia with one hand and insert the folded diaphragm with the other. The best positions for insertion are standing with one foot propped up, squatting, or lying down. Push the diaphragm downward into the vagina as far back as it will go, then tuck the front rim up behind the pubic bone inside the vagina. Check for proper placement by feeling for the cervix, which should be covered by the rubber dome of the diaphragm.
4. If you have intercourse more than once, you must apply more spermicidal cream or jelly with an applicator before each act of intercourse. Do not remove the diaphragm, but place the cream or jelly in front of it. You may use condoms for subsequent intercourse instead of more applications of spermicide.
5. After intercourse, the diaphragm must be left in place for 6 to 8 hours. Do not douche during this time.
6. Remove the diaphragm by placing your index finger behind the front rim and pulling down and out. If the suction is tight, insert a finger between the diaphragm and the pubic bone to break suction. If the rim is hard to reach, bear down to bring it forward. Be careful not to puncture the diaphragm with long fingernails.
7. After use, clean the diaphragm with soap and water, rinse thoroughly and dry with a towel. You may dust it with cornstarch, but do not use talcum or perfumed powder because these damage the diaphragm and may irritate the vagina and cervix. Store the diaphragm in its plastic container in a cool, dry place.
8. Inspect the diaphragm each time you use it for tears or holes. Do not use petroleum jelly because it can cause deterioration of the rubber of the diaphragm. Use K-Y Jelly or spermicidal jelly for additional lubrication. The diaphragm will become darker, mottled brown over time, but will last several years if properly cared for.
9. Have your diaphragm fitting checked if you gain or lose more than 10 to 20 lb, if you have a pregnancy or abortion, if you have pelvic surgery, if the diaphragm causes discomfort or pain, or if you think it is too large or too small.

vaginal mucosa and the diaphragm. Storage techniques to prevent diaphragm deterioration and reduce risk of infection are emphasized.

Signs and symptoms of TSS and vaginitis are reviewed with the client. The importance of seeking care without delay if the woman thinks she might have TSS is stressed. (For a more thorough discussion of TSS, see Chap. 48.) Clients are advised to return annually for health maintenance and rechecking the diaphragm fit. The need for refitting after significant weight gain (greater than 10 lb), pelvic surgery, and full-term delivery is reviewed. The nurse should be aware of those clients with higher probability of diaphragm failure, and provide particular emphasis on the need for consistent and proper use. Higher failure rates have been found in women who have had children and who have frequent intercourse (four or more times per week).

Cervical Cap

The cervical cap resembles a diaphragm that is small and has a tall dome (Fig. 11-5). It fits snugly over the cervix and is held in place by suction between its firm but flexible rim and the cervix. Cervical caps are made of soft rubber and are available in three styles. The rubber causes a strong vaginal odor after 36 to 48 hours, and these caps are not suitable for prolonged use. Approximately one third of the inside of the cap is filled with spermicide. Time rules for insertion and removal are the same as for diaphragms. When properly positioned, the cap is a barrier to sperm entering the cervix, producing the same contraceptive effect as the diaphragm. Insertion and removal of the cervical cap are somewhat more difficult than with the diaphragm.

Cervical caps have been widely used in Europe since 1930 and are used in several other countries including Canada and Australia. The Prentif Cavity-Rim cervical cap was tested in clinical research studies in the United States beginning in 1980. The device is marketed in the United States under a premarket Federal Drug Administration (FDA) approval.

The cervical cap is similar to the diaphragm in its effectiveness in preventing pregnancy. First-year failure rates range from 8 to 27 pregnancies per 100 women who begin using the method. A study comparing the Prentif cap with the diaphragm found 17.4 pregnancies per 100 woman-years during the first year with the cap, and 16.7 pregnancies with the diaphragm. The continuation rate after 12 months for the cap was 59%.[15]

The provider's goal in fitting the cervical cap is to select a size that fits well or to recommend another type of contraception if a good fit cannot be obtained. A Prentif cap that is too tight can cause cervical trauma, and if it is too loose it can be easily dislodged. Women with an acutely anteflexed uterus, with a cervix facing downward, may find that the cap dislodges with intercourse. About 6% of women cannot be satisfactorily fitted with cervical caps.

COMPLICATIONS AND SIDE-EFFECTS

Although there is limited information on safety and side-effects of the cervical cap, problems may arise due to prolonged cervical exposure to secretions, spermicide, and bacteria trapped within the cap. Trauma could result to the cervix or vagina from insertion and removal or prolonged retention of the cap. There may be interference with the normal flow of cervical mucus or menstrual blood.

Contraindications to cervical cap use include history of TSS, recurrent UTI, cervical papillomavirus (HPV) infection, full-term delivery in the past 12 weeks, acute PID or cervicitis, undiagnosed vaginal bleeding, abnormal Pap smear, recent cervical surgery, cervical neoplasia, allergy to rubber or spermicide, anatomical abnormalities or variations (extremely shallow or long cervix, severe lacerations), inability to learn insertion and removal technique, lack of privacy or facilities for washing and cleaning cap. The role the cervical cap may play in development of progressive cervical neoplasia needs further research. Women are advised to have a Pap smear before using the cap and repeat Pap smears after 3 months of use and annually thereafter.

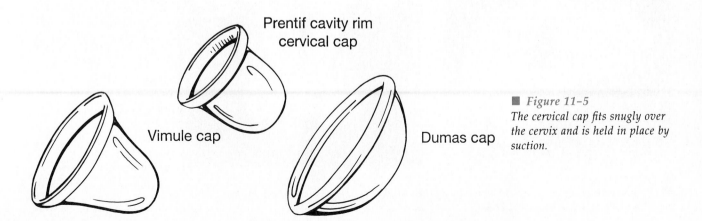

Prentif cavity rim cervical cap

Vimule cap

Dumas cap

■ *Figure 11–5*
The cervical cap fits snugly over the cervix and is held in place by suction.

Vaginal irritation and foul-smelling discharge are associated with prolonged cap use. Because of this and concerns about TSS, women are advised to leave the cap in place only 24 hours. Cervical abrasions and lacerations can occur with prolonged use and difficult removal.

NURSING INTERVENTION FOR THE CERVICAL CAP

As with the diaphragm, women must practice inserting and removing the cap after they have been fitted. The nurse instructs in this practice, using techniques similar to manual diaphragm insertion and removal. It is critical that the client can identify her cervix and check that the cap is properly attached over the cervix. The client is reminded to use spermicide with the cap and leave the cap in place at least 6 to 8 hours after intercourse up to 24 hours. The cap must not be worn during the menstrual period. Douching while the cap is in place is to be avoided, and extra spermicide should be used before additional intercourse.

Precautions to reduce risk of TSS are taught by the nurse. The cap should be cleaned with plain, mild soap and water after removal, dried, and placed in its case. Cornstarch can be used to dust the cap, but not talcum powder. The cap should be checked for tears with each use, and petroleum products should be avoided.

A return visit is scheduled in 3 months for a repeat Pap smear. If the smear is abnormal, use of the cap must be discontinued. An annual gynecological examination is scheduled, with a Pap smear, recheck of the cervical cap's fit, and review of the women's experience using the cap.

Vaginal Sponge

Since ancient times, natural sea sponges have been used for contraception. In the 1970s, natural collagen and synthetic sponges were developed incorporating spermicide, with eventual FDA approval in 1983 of vaginal contraceptive sponges made of polyurethane containing 1 g of nonoxynol 9 spermicide. The sponge is 2.5 cm thick and 5.5 cm in diameter, with a central dimple that fits over the cervix and reduces chances of dislodgment during intercourse. A braided cord is attached to the other side and is used to remove the sponge. Sponges must be soaked in water before inserting and may be left in place for 24 to 30 hours (Fig. 11-6).

The sponge exerts its contraceptive effect by providing a barrier between sperm and the cervix, by trapping sperm within the sponge, and by releasing spermicide at a steady rate while in place. After use, it is discarded. No additional spermicide is needed for repeated intercourse. Sponges are available without prescription as an over-the-counter item.

The first-year failure rates for vaginal sponges range from 17 to 24 pregnancies per 100 women who use this method. Nulliparous women were found to have half the failure rate (13 pregnancies) as parous women (28 pregnancies).[32] About 54% of women using the sponge continued this method for 12 months or more.

Vaginal sponges offer some advantages common to barrier contraceptives, such as protection from STD and possibly protection against cervical neoplasia. Risk of chlamydial disease is reduced by about one third, and gonorrhea risk is reduced by two thirds.[33] Certain complaints about diaphragms and vaginal spermicides, such as their messiness and distastefulness, are avoided with use of sponges. Some women find sponges make the vagina dry, however, by absorbing vaginal lubrication.

CONTRAINDICATIONS AND SIDE-EFFECTS

Contraindications to sponge use include history of TSS, allergy to polyurethane or nonoxynol 9, anatomical abnormalities of the vagina (uterine prolapse, cystocele, rectocele, extreme retroflexion, vaginal septum), and inability to learn correct insertion technique.

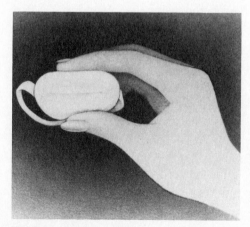
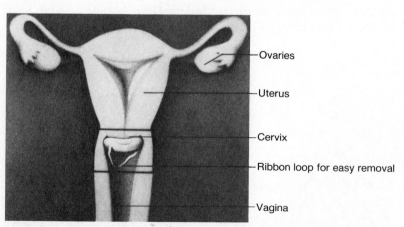

■ *Figure 11-6*
The contraceptive sponge is inserted manually by the user into the deepest part of the vagina just below the cervix. (Courtesy of Today)

Labels: Ovaries, Uterus, Cervix, Ribbon loop for easy removal, Vagina

Sensitivity to spermicide can cause vaginal irritation or allergic reactions such as vulvar erythema and edema. Sponge use may increase susceptibility to vaginal yeast infections. Difficulty removing the sponge may lead to tearing and fragmentation, which might require medical assistance for retrieving all parts and fragments from the vagina.

The risk of TSS for sponge users is similar to that for tampon users (10 per 100,000 users per year). This is the most potentially serious complication of vaginal sponge use. To reduce risk, the sponge should be removed within 24 to 30 hours and should not be used during menstruation.

Condom

Condoms ("rubbers") are thin sheaths of latex rubber or processed collagenous tissue that are placed over the penis to act as a mechanical barrier to prevent sperm from entering the vagina. Also effective in preventing venereal infections, condoms are a male method of contraception that has been used since ancient times. The condom is applied over the shaft of the penis after erection. Before withdrawal of the penis from the vagina, the condom should be held in place on the penis so that it does not slip off into the vagina.

Over 46 million couples worldwide use condoms as their contraceptive method. Condoms have been less extensively used in the United States than other countries, although this is changing with public concern about AIDS. Although in the late 1980s only 10% of married couples in the United States used condoms, their use undoubtedly is much greater among sexually active adolescents and young adults. Innovative educational and distribution programs are increasing the use of condoms throughout the world.

The first-year failure rates for typical condom users average about 12%. A much lower failure rate can be achieved among perfect users, from one to two pregnancies per 100 couples in the first year of use.[15] In British studies of older couples who were long-term condom users, having intercourse about twice per week, the failure rate was equal to only 1 in 10,000 uses.[34] Studies of condom breakage have reported an overall rate of 1 per 161 uses, with one pregnancy resulting from every 26 condom breakages. This indicates that condom breakage probably causes one pregnancy per every 4000 uses.[15]

Many brands of condoms are available, but all are approximately the same length and width in the United States. Condoms can be straight-sided or tapered, ribbed or smooth, lubricated or nonlubricated, and with or without spermicide. Some have pouches at the tip to collect semen after ejaculation. Lubricated condoms are more popular, and those with spermicides are growing in use. Spermicidal condoms are highly effective at kill-

ing sperm within the condom. About 1% of condoms are made from lamb cecum (collagenous or "skin" condoms). These condoms do not prevent passage of the hepatitis B virus (HBV) but apparently do trap larger viruses such as the retrovirus causing AIDS, cytomegalovirus, and herpes simplex virus.[35] Latex (rubber) condoms with spermicide provide the greatest protection from STD transmission. The FDA has permitted manufacturers of latex condoms to include in their labeling "for protection of sexually transmitted diseases, including AIDS."

In addition to being the major protector against STD, condoms may prevent development or cause regression of cervical neoplasia, are useful in treating premature ejaculation, and may promote conception in couples with infertility after 3 to 6 months of use by preventing the buildup of sperm antibodies in the woman. Condoms are inexpensive, widely available, and accessible without prescription. Lubricated condoms reduce vaginal friction and irritation, and condoms contain semen, which otherwise would drain from the vagina. Retail condom sales have been increasing in the United States, and about 40% of condoms are purchased by women.

Contraindications include allergy to latex, collagenous tissue, or spermicides. A small number of men cannot retain an erection when using a condom, and thus condoms are unacceptable. Some men experience greatly decreased sensation using latex condoms but may experience more satisfying sex with collagenous condoms.

SIDE-EFFECTS AND COMPLICATIONS

Allergic reactions occur in a small number of men or women; changing the type of condom may alleviate this. Psychological side-effects probably most affect condom use; these include decreased sensation for men and objection to interrupting foreplay to put on the condom. To increase sensation, collagenous, ultra-thin, or ribbed condoms can be used. Many couples have overcome the problem of interruption by having the woman put the condom on the man as part of foreplay.

NURSING INTERVENTION FOR CONDOMS

Nursing care includes education about the advantages of condoms, and instruction on effective use. The most important rule is to use condoms with every sexual activity involving exchange of body fluids or risk of pregnancy. Instructions include choices of types of condoms, and procedures for putting the condom on and removing it from the penis. Maximum protection is offered when the condom is put on before any vaginal penetration occurs. Petroleum products should not be used because they weaken the rubber. Intercourse should not

Client Education

Condom Use

Condoms can be an effective contraceptive method and can protect against the spread of sexually transmitted diseases, when these procedures are used.
- Use the condom every single time you have sex.
- Keep a supply of condoms handy, both at home and away from home.
- Put the condom on the erect penis before vaginal insertion.
- Putting the condom on as part of foreplay, done by the woman, can make it more fun and natural.
- Latex condoms with spermicide offer greater protection against both pregnancy and infections.
- Roll the condom rim all the way to the base of the penis, leaving one-half inch empty space at the end, unless the condom has a reservoir tip.
- Do not use petroleum jelly for a lubricant because this weakens the rubber.
- Wait until the vagina is well-lubricated, or use a lubricant such as K-Y jelly or spermicidal foam, before starting intercourse (this prevents condom tears).
- After ejaculation, hold the rim of the condom as the penis is removed slowly from the vagina; be careful not to spill semen near the vagina.
- Check the condom for tears after use; never use condoms more than once
- If the condom breaks or comes off in the vagina, insert spermicidal foam or gel immediately.

begin until the vagina is well-lubricated to avoid tearing the condom from friction. Condoms should be stored in a cool, dry place. Even body heat can cause the rubber to weaken.

Women who rely on condoms can be encouraged and supported to be firm about insisting on their use. Women are at much greater risk of reproductive tract damage from STD than men, and there is a high rate of transmittal of STD from infected men to their female sex partners. It is the woman's right to insist on condom use, and her right to say no to intercourse if her partner refuses to wear a condom. The nurse can discuss alternatives to intercourse that the woman can suggest to her partner if condoms will not be used. Abstinence is also a perfectly acceptable solution.

The Female Condom

A polyurethane condom for vaginal use has been developed, with flexible rims at each end connecting the condom sheath. The closed end is inserted high in the vagina with the rim surrounding the cervix; the open end fits in the introitus (Fig. 11-7). Some female condoms are lubricated. One study of married or cohabitating couples found about 66% reported the effect on sexual pleasure to be no different than with male condoms.[36] The WPC-33 female condom, made in the U.S., may provide better protection against STD and pregnancy than the male condom because it covers a larger surface area, and there seems to be less risk of exposure

to seminal fluid.[37] The WPD-33 female condom was found to perform well mechanically, with the female users reporting no severe pain and no rips over a 2-week period. Some users found the female condom less convenient and less comfortable than the male condom, had difficulty with insertion, and experienced male partner objection. Two thirds of these female users had no aversion to the female condom, whereas one third disliked it.[38]

Vaginal Spermicides

Vaginal spermicides are widely used because of their safety and simplicity. These preparations include jellies, creams, foam, suppositories, tablets, and a thin square of film. They are inserted deep into the vagina, covering the cervix, about 5 to 10 minutes before intercourse. Most remain effective for 2 hours. Tablets and suppositories take longer to dissolve, about 10 to 30 minutes. The spermicide used is usually nonoxynol 9, although some preparations use octoxynol 9.

Considerable variation in effectiveness rates has been reported for vaginal spermicides. First-year failure rates among typical users range from about 15 to 30 pregnancies per 100 woman-years, with an average of around 20. Failure rates as low as 2% to 4% in the initial year of use have been found.[15] The most common error leading to pregnancy is not using the method at all. Placing the preparation deep in the vagina and consistent use improve effectiveness (Fig. 11-8).

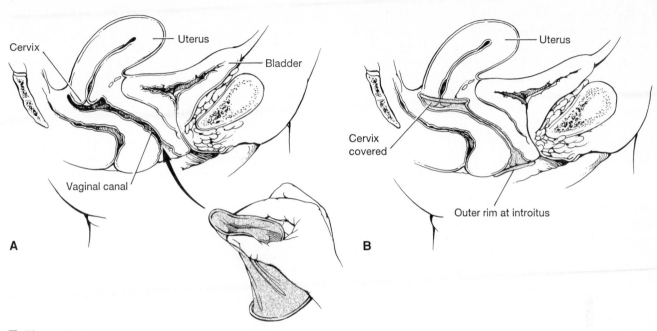

■ *Figure 11–7*
The Female Condom. (A) The flexible rim on the closed end of the condom (WPC–333) is grasped, and the condom inserted high in the vagina with the rim around the cervix. (B) When in place, the flexible rim at the open end of the condom is at the vaginal introitus.

Vaginal spermicides are readily available in drug stores and markets without prescription. Spermicides help protect against STD and have been found in vitro to kill organisms responsible for gonorrhea, trichomoniasis, herpes, and chlamydial diseases. Women using spermicides are less likely to develop PID. HIV is killed by spermicides in laboratory tests, and although they may prevent HIV transmission, spermicides should not be relied on as the sole means of prevention.

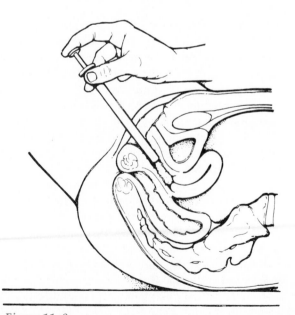

■ *Figure 11–8*
The user inserts foam or cream near the cervix.

COMPLICATIONS AND SIDE-EFFECTS

Contraindications include allergy to spermicidal foam, jelly, cream, tablets, suppositories, or film; inability to remember to use these preparations consistently at the time of intercourse; and any physical or mental disability causing problems with proper insertion and placement.

Rarely, allergies occur in either the man or woman, causing local irritation or inflammation. The tablets or suppositories may fail to melt or foam in the vagina, causing mechanical irritation and discomfort, and reducing effectiveness. Spermicides may have an unpleasant taste to couples using oral–genital sex. Studies have suggested that spermicide use around the time of conception results in a higher risk of birth defects. The incidence of birth defects found among spermicide users was 2.2%; however, the national rate of these defects is 2.1%. No single, well-defined syndrome was found among affected babies of spermicide users. It was not established that the users actually did use spermicides around the time of conception. The consensus of experts is that the evidence does not clearly support a connection between spermicides and birth defects.[39]

NURSING INTERVENTION FOR VAGINAL SPERMICIDES

Spermicide users are educated about proper use of their selected preparation. The importance of consistent use with every episode of sex is stressed. Time limits between insertion and intercourse are emphasized by the nurse. New insertions are necessary for repeated sex acts. The woman is instructed to wait 6 to 8 hours after intercourse before douching, if she chooses to douche. Spermicides can also be combined with other contraceptives to increase protection, such as with condoms or during midcycle with the IUD and fertility awareness methods.

These preparations are particularly useful as short-term contraceptives. During the postpartum period, spermicides are useful until the 4- to 6-week checkup, when a more effective method can be instituted. They are frequently recommended for 2 weeks to 1 month after insertion of an IUD or initiation of an oral contraceptive regimen, as a precaution before these methods should be relied on alone. When the pill or IUD is discontinued, spermicides can be used for a few cycles until another method is begun or pregnancy is attempted.

Fertility Awareness Methods

The rationale underlying birth control based on fertility awareness is that with regular periods ovulation occurs at approximately the same time in each cycle (i.e., 14 days before the beginning of the next cycle). The ovum is capable of being fertilized only for a period of 48 hours at the most after ovulation. Abstinence from sexual intercourse on that day and for the 2 days before and after (a total of 5 days) should forestall conception.

In actual experience, regular cycles can vary by 1 or 2 days in either direction (e.g., 28 ± 2 days). This puts the day of ovulation in the above 4-day range ± 2 days, and the period of abstinence must be at least 8 days. Due to variability of menstrual cycles, the risk of fertility often is 15 or more days, or about half of the cycle. Sperm can survive about 7 days, adding to the length of fertility risk.

Fertility awareness methods are based on calendar calculations of ovulation, changes in the basal body temperature (BBT), and changes in the condition of cervical mucus to determine ovulation. Advantages of these methods include lack of side-effects due to introduction of drugs or substances into or on the body, they are relatively inexpensive, they are acceptable to religious groups that oppose other contraceptive methods, and they are helpful in planning pregnancy due to the familiarity with signs of fertility. Disadvantages include the need to keep records for several menstrual cycles before use, the need for careful record keeping to ensure accuracy, considerable initial and ongoing counseling in their use, restriction of sexual spontaneity, and the need for abstinence or another contraceptive method for a considerable portion of the cycle. Some women are unable to recognize cervical mucus changes. Irregular cycles make calendar and BBT methods less reliable.

The first-year failure rates of fertility awareness methods among typical users is 20 to 23 pregnancies per 100 women. Sexual risk taking during fertile days accounts for most pregnancies. First-year failure rates among perfect users can be 2% to 10%.[15] Should pregnancy occur, there is increased risk that an "old" egg will be fertilized. When the ovum is fertilized late after ovulation, the deterioration of the ovum can be associated with increased risk for fetal abnormalities.[40]

CALENDAR METHOD

A menstrual calendar is kept in which the woman records the length of each menstrual cycle over 8 months. With the first day of bleeding counted as day 1, the earliest fertile day is computed by subtracting 18 days from the length of the shortest cycle. Eleven days are subtracted from the length of the longest cycle to determine the last day of fertility. These two numbers represent the beginning and end of the fertile period. During these days, intercourse must be avoided or another method of birth control must be used (Table 11-4).

This method is more effective if the woman has regular cycles and if it is used with abstinence or backup contraception through the entire first part of the menstrual cycle through the last fertile day. This method may be contraindicated among younger, postpartum, postabortion, and premenopausal women who often have irregular menstrual cycles. Use of the BBT or cervical mucus method can increase effectiveness.

BASAL BODY TEMPERATURE METHOD (BBT)

The resting temperature or BBT of a fertile woman normally rises each cycle just after ovulation. It remains higher until the next menstrual period begins. Most women can observe this temperature change if they take and record their temperature every day with a special thermometer before getting out of bed or beginning any activity, including smoking. The thermometer can be used orally or rectally and should be left in place a full 5 minutes. Temperature is recorded on a special BBT chart (see Chap. 8).

Temperature drops slightly then rises about 0.4°F to 0.8°F when ovulation has occurred. This rise is sustained until the next menstrual period. Some women have no preliminary drop before the BBT rises. Because ovulation cannot be identified until after it has happened, it is safer to abstain or use another method of contraception until the sustained rise in BBT is seen. The fertile period can be assumed to end after the BBT has remained elevated for 3 full days.

TABLE 11–4. CALCULATING THE INTERVAL OF FERTILITY

No. of Days Shortest Cycle	First Fertile Day	No. of Days Longest Cycle	Last Fertile Day
21	3rd day	21	10th day
22	4th day	22	11th day
23	5th day	23	12th day
24	6th day	24	13th day
25	7th day	25	14th day
26	8th day	26	15th day
27	9th day	27	16th day
28	10th day	28	17th day
29	11th day	29	18th day
30	12th day	30	19th day
31	13th day	31	20th day
32	14th day	32	21st day
33	15th day	33	22nd day
34	16th day	34	23rd day
35	17th day	35	24th day

Many factors such as illness, nightmares, and changes in daily schedule can influence the BBT. When the pattern of temperature rise is not clear or sustained, it is not safe to have intercourse. This method is more effective when combined with the calendar or mucus methods, which give earlier signs that ovulation is near.

CERVICAL MUCUS METHOD

Changes in the character and appearance of cervical mucus occur just before ovulation in some women. In addition, ovulatory pain may be experienced. In the ovulatory cycle, there typically is a rapid increase in the quantity of cervical mucus just before ovulation. The mucus becomes clear and stringy and may be present at the introitus or obtained from the cervix. Subsequent to ovulation, mucus becomes more viscous. When this change is associated with a rise in temperature, ovulation has probably occurred.

The woman must be careful not to confuse other substances in the vagina, such as semen, lubricants, spermicides, and discharges due to infections, with cervical mucus at midcycle. Women who douche cannot observe changes because they wash the mucus away. This method is more effective when intercourse is restricted to the postovulatory phase of the cycle and when used in combination with the calendar or the BBT method.

Women need to observe their mucus changes for several cycles before relying on this method. The peak of fertility occurs when the vagina feels wet and mucus is abundant, clear, slippery, and stretchable (can be stretched 3 to 4 in between the thumb and forefinger). After ovulation, mucus becomes thick, cloudy, and sticky or there may be no mucus. When this change is observed, the woman is no longer fertile.

SYMPTO-THERMAL METHOD

The sympto-thermal method combines approaches to fertility awareness. The most common combination is using changes in mucus (symptom) and the BBT (thermal). When using this combination, couples must wait until the fourth day after peak slippery mucus and the third day after sustained rise in BBT before resuming intercourse. If one occurs without the other, safety cannot be assumed and the couple must await the second event.

A variety of kits are available for predicting fertility. Ovulation predictor kits detect urinary LH; when a rise occurs, ovulation is expected within 24 hours. There are kits using vaginal mucus and chemical indicators to indicate fertile days. Hand-held or wrist minicomputers measure BBT or mucus to calculate fertile days. These technological aids may not be as reliable as traditional charting techniques, often do not give enough advanced warning of ovulation, are expensive, and may lead couples to defer professional counseling in fertility awareness.

NURSING INTERVENTION FOR FERTILITY AWARENESS

The nurse can play a major role in counseling and educating couples in the effective use of fertility awareness methods. Nursing care includes teaching the use of techniques to measure and charts to record menstrual cycles and changes in cervical mucus and BBT. Vagaries of individual responses are explored, and precautions are given for situations that may make measurements unreliable (e.g., infections, stress, travel). The importance of abstinence during the fertile period or use of a backup contraceptive method is emphasized.

Because fertility awareness methods require close cooperation between sex partners, the nurse can provide counseling about communication and feelings. The couple may need to clarify expectations about sex and work out mutually acceptable solutions. Couples who are reluctant to forego sexual spontaneity, or unable to keep careful records, should be advised against using fertility awareness and counseled in another contraceptive method.

Withdrawal

Withdrawal, or *coitus interruptus*, is an extensively used method of contraception in some European countries, although it is used by only 2% of U.S. couples. Couples using withdrawal have intercourse until ejaculation is impending, then the male withdraws the penis from the vagina and ejaculates completely away from the female's genitals. Withdrawal has certain advantages; it is always available at no cost and requires no devices or chemicals. It does require male awareness of and control over sexual response, and careful timing. The woman's sexual experience may be diminished unless she has orgasm before withdrawal or other techniques are used.

The first-year failure rate among typical users is about 18% to 20%. Estimate of the failure rate among perfect users is about 4% in the initial year.[15] Sperm are contained in the pre-ejaculatory fluid that seeps from Cowper's glands during intercourse. After a recent ejaculation, this fluid contains even more sperm and risk increases with multiple sex acts. Although there are no major physiological side-effects, withdrawal can diminish both partner's sexual pleasure.

Postpartum Contraception

In the absence of complications, intercourse is commonly resumed 2 to 3 weeks after delivery. The condom is a practical method to use during this period. Spermicidal foams and creams are frequently advised, either in combination with the condom or alone. If foams and creams are not used too early in the postpartum period, there does not appear to be a problem with infection.

Insertion of an IUD within the first 6 weeks postpartum is generally not recommended, because the expulsion and infection rates are higher during this time. Estrogen-containing oral contraceptives are contraindicated because of the increased incidence of thromboembolic complications associated with their use in the postpartum period. Nursing mothers are usually advised to use progestin-only oral contraceptives because lactation may be suppressed with estrogen, particularly higher-dose pills. Synthetic hormones are excreted in breast milk, but the amount that actually passes through the milk is small (approximately one fifth to one tenth of the mother's dose).

Minipills may be given immediately postpartum or at the 6-week checkup. These pills have little effect on lactation and do not pose thromboembolic risks. The American Academy of Pediatrics has approved use of combined pills in breast-feeding women, however, once lactation is well established.[41]

Sterilization

Vasectomy in the male and tubal ligation in the female are being used with increasing frequency in the United States. Approximately 61% of contraceptive users in the United States intending no additional births depended on sterilization in 1982, compared with 36% in 1973.[42] For married couples over 30, sterilization is the most common means of birth control.

VASECTOMY

Vasectomy involves surgical interruption and ligation of the vas deferens and is a relatively minor operation. It can be carried out under local anesthesia and is associated with minimal risk and only slight morbidity. It is a simple procedure that takes about 15 minutes and can be done on an outpatient basis (Fig. 11-8).

Short-term complications can include inflammation and pain, hematomas, infections, sperm granulomas, and epididymitis. No changes have been found in levels of testosterone, FSH, or LH in men with vasectomies. Prostate gland and epididymal secretions may decrease, slightly reducing semen volume. About 50% to 65% of men develop sperm antibodies, but there are apparently no pathological complications from this. Limited animal studies found that monkeys developed atherosclerotic plaques after vasectomy, and these were attributed to sperm antibodies. The reliability of these studies and their applicability to humans are questionable. Human studies have found no connection between the vasectomy and plaques.[43]

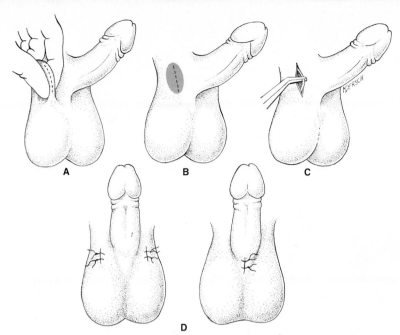

■ *Figure 11–9*
Vasectomy procedure. (A) The vas deferens is identified. (B) A small area of the skin and subcutaneous tissue is anesthetized. (C) The vas deferens is isolated from surrounding tissue and lifted through the incision. (D) Skin sutures showing one- and two-incision approaches.

The vast majority of men who have had vasectomies are satisfied with their decision and report that sexual performance is unchanged. Less than 2% report decreased sexual performance or other dissatisfaction with vasectomy.

Vasectomy failure is the result of recanalization of the ends of the ligated vas and occurs in 0.15 per 100 cases. Unprotected intercourse before the male reproductive tract is cleared of spermatozoa may result in pregnancy. Couples are advised that the first few postvasectomy ejaculates contain active spermatozoa.

Men who remarry and desire more children may request vasectomy reversal. Microsurgical procedures for reanastomosis result in the presence of sperm in almost all cases, but only 29% to 85% of men have successful impregnations.[15] The success of reanastomosis depends on the type of surgical procedure, how long since the vasectomy, and whether sperm antibodies have developed.

TUBAL LIGATION

Tubal ligation is designed to block the tubal conduit that spermatozoa and ova pass through. A number of approaches are used to interrupt the continuity of the fallopian tubes (Fig. 11-10). The procedure may be done through an abdominal incision and is commonly done along with cesarean delivery or in the first few postpartum hours.

Coagulation and interruption of the fallopian tubes can be carried out using a *laparoscopic approach* (Fig. 11-11). This procedure can be done under regional or local anesthesia, but often a general anesthetic is used. After the abdomen is distended with carbon dioxide,

the laparoscopic trocar is introduced through a small incision in the umbilicus. The laparoscope is passed into the peritoneal cavity. Visualization of the adnexa is usually complete. Forceps are used to grasp the fallopian tubes, and the tubes are occluded using a clip, ring, or band; coagulated; or cut and tied (resection).

Because the procedure is relatively simple, it can be carried out on an outpatient basis. Although it is associated with a relatively low morbidity, it is considerably higher than for vasectomy.

The *interval minilaparotomy* is a sterilization technique in which a small suprapubic incision is usually made below the pubic hair line to enter the abdominal cavity. The fallopian tubes are isolated with grasping instruments and may be crushed, ligated, embedded, clipped, or plugged as in other tubal ligation methods. Tubal ligations may also be done vaginally, but complication rates (infection, hemorrhage) are higher.

Complication rates of tubal ligation range from 0.4% to 1% and include wound infection, hematoma, uterine perforation, bladder or bowel injury, and sterilization failure. Most deaths associated with these procedures are a result of anesthesia. Other mortality risk results from sepsis, hemorrhage, and cardiovascular events. The overall case fatality rate is reported at 3 per 100,000. Put in perspective, the risk of a one-time sterilization procedure is far less for a healthy woman over 35 to 40 years than that posed by use of oral contraceptives or a term pregnancy.[15]

Studies of the effect of tubal ligation on hormonal function have found levels of LH, FSH, testosterone, and estrogen within the normal range. Contradictory evidence exists for a decrease in progesterone after sterilization. Changes in menstrual bleeding patterns have

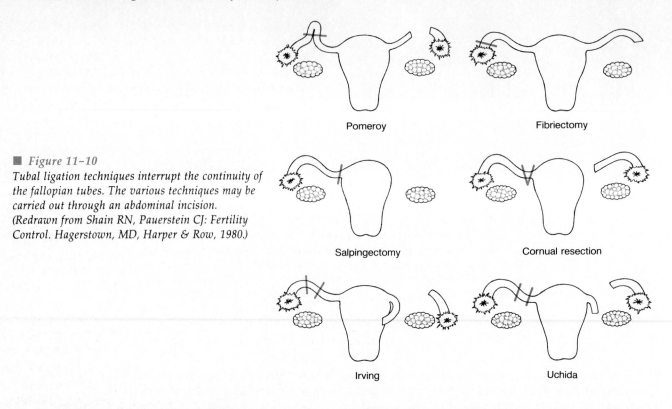

■ *Figure 11–10*
Tubal ligation techniques interrupt the continuity of the fallopian tubes. The various techniques may be carried out through an abdominal incision.
(Redrawn from Shain RN, Pauerstein CJ: Fertility Control. Hagerstown, MD, Harper & Row, 1980.)

been a concern, but data from large studies found no changes in the amount of bleeding, for six menstrual functions before and after sterilization, or significant and consistent changes in patterns even when slight increases in menstrual disorders were reported. There is also no increase in hospital admissions for gynecological procedures or hysterectomy after sterilization.[44,45]

Failure rates for tubal ligation range from 0 to 4 per 1000 procedures. Many failures occur because sterilization is done in the second half of the menstrual cycle, and an already fertilized oocyte implants. Most women are satisfied with sterilization, which is considered a permanent procedure, but a small number (04.–3%) request reversal. The client's candidacy for a reversal must be determined according to the amount of tubal damage caused by the sterilization procedure. A laparoscopy to

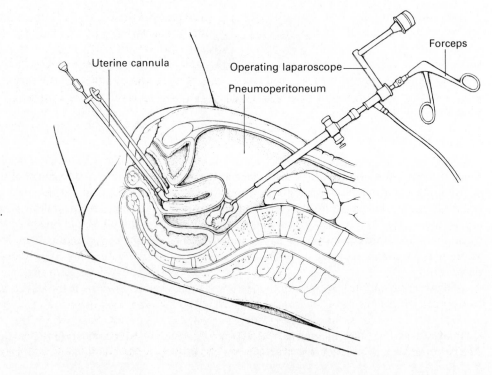

■ *Figure 11–11*
The one-incision technique for tubal ligation using the laparoscopic approach may be performed on an outpatient basis.

Counseling Clients About Sterilization: "BRAIDED" Technique

The nurse can use the BRAIDED technique to cover important components of informed consent in counseling clients who are requesting sterilization procedures for contraception.

B *Benefits:* Permanent, very effective, relatively inexpensive when years of use are considered, further contraception decisions not needed, comfortable, no chemicals or devices

R *Risks:* Surgical procedures can have complications or, rarely, death; expensive in short run; slight chance of future pregnancy (not 100% effective); considered permanent and reversal procedures are expensive and not always successful.

A *Alternatives:* Other forms of reversible contraceptives discussed, also abstinence, chance, pregnancy, and sterilization of the partner

I *Inquiries:* Client is encouraged to ask questions; information is provided to clear myths and misconceptions.

D *Decision to say no:* Client can freely decide not to have sterilization procedure, without experiencing hostility or punishment such as withdrawal of care or welfare benefits.

E *Explanation:* Sterilization procedure and possible side-effects are explained in detail, emphasizing permanence with accurate estimates of successful reversal. Explanation includes cost, where surgery can be done, and what is known about potential psychological and physiological effects (i.e., hormones, weight, menses, sexual response).

D *Documentation:* Written instructions, written risks, and written, signed and witnessed consent for the specific sterilization procedure must be done as part of the informed consent.

(Adapted from Hatcher RA, Stewart F, Trussell J et al: Contraceptive Technology 1990–1992, 15th rev ed. New York, Irvington Publishers)

evaluate tubal status is recommended. Surgery for reanastomosis can be done on about 70% of women with tubal ligations, with successful reversals resulting in pregnancy in 40% to 75%.[46]

NURSING INTERVENTION FOR STERILIZATION

Nursing care focuses on assisting the couple or client to make a sound, well-informed decision to have a va-

sectomy or tubal ligation. Because these are permanent procedures, the decision to have surgery must be carefully considered. The nurse makes certain both partners or the client understands that these methods are considered irreversible. If any doubt about sterilization exists, another contraceptive method should be advised. Family and personal circumstances that could influence the decision are reviewed in depth, including number and ages of children, stability of the marriage, likelihood of future marriage if single, age of partners, and ability to use reversible contraceptive methods.

These laws and regulations are important in counseling about sterilization:

- Strict adherence to informed consent procedures and voluntary choice are essential, both legally and practically.
- There is no legal requirement for partner or spouse consent.
- When federal and, in some instances, state funds are used, the client must be age 21 or older, mentally competent, and must wait 30 days after signing the consent before the procedure can be performed.

Postcoital Contraception

After unprotected intercourse at midcycle, women may take postcoital oral contraceptives to prevent fertilization or implantation. Diethylstilbestrol (DES) has been used, but Ovral has a similar low failure rate with fewer adverse side-effects. Two tablets of Ovral are taken within 12 to 72 hours of coitus, and two more tablets are taken 12 hours later. The failure rate is 0.16% to 1.6%. Low-dose ethinyl estradiol or high-dose estrogens can also be taken for several days after intercourse. These are effective, resulting in pregnancy rates of 0.4% and 0.9%, respectively.[15] Side-effects include nausea and vomiting. Combined estrogen–progestin oral contraceptives can also be used.

■ REFERENCES

1. Covington TP: Sex Care. New York, Pocket Books, 1987
2. World Health Organization: Education and treatment in human sexuality: The training of health professionals. Technical Report Series No 572. Geneva, WHO, 1975
3. Zalar MK: Sexual counseling for pregnant couples. MCN 1(3):176–181, May/June 1976
4. Mims FH, Swenson M: Sexuality: A Nursing Perspective. New York, McGraw-Hill, 1980

5. Carpenito LJ: Nursing Diagnosis: Application to Clinical Practice, 3rd ed. Philadelphia, JB Lippincott, 1989
6. Woods NF: Human Sexuality in Health and Illness. St Louis, CV Mosby, 1984
7. Hyde JS: Understanding Human Sexuality, 4th ed. New York, McGraw-Hill, 1990
8. Byer CO, Shainberg LW, Jones KL: Dimensions of Human Sexuality, 2nd ed. Dubuque, IA, WC Brown, 1988
9. Frank E, Anderson C, Rubenstein D: Frequency of sexual dysfunction in "normal" couples. N Engl J Med 299:111–115, March 1978
10. Rosen RC, Leiblum SR: Current approaches to the evaluation of sexual desire disorders. J Sex Res 23:141–162, 1987
11. Zilbergeld B, Ellison LR: Desire discrepancies and arousal problems in sex therapy. In Leiblum SR, Pervin LA (eds): Principles and Practice of Sex Therapy. New York, Guilford Press, 1980
12. Martin LL: Health Care of Women. Philadelphia, JB Lippincott, 1978
13. Coleman AD, Coleman LL: Pregnancy: The Psychological Experience. New York, Herder and Herder, 1971
14. Masters WH, Johnson VE: Human Sexual Inadequacy. Boston, Little, Brown & Co, 1970
15. Hatcher RA, Stewart F, Trussell J et al: Contraceptive Technology 1990–1992, 15th rev ed. New York, Irvington Publishers
16. Franklin M: Recently approved and experimental methods of contraception. J Nurse Midwifery 35(6):365–376, November/December 1990
17. Pollack A: Norplant: What you should know about the new contraceptive. Med Aspects Human Sexuality 34–38, January 1991
18. Pike MC, Henderson BE, Krailow MD et al: Breast cancer in young women and use of oral contraceptives: Possible modifying effect of formulation and age of use. Lancet 2:926–930, 1983
19. Ory HW, Rosenfield A, Landman LC: The pill at 20: An assessment. Fam Plann Perspect 12(6):278–283, November/December 1980
20. Layde PM, Beral V, Kay CR: Further analyses of mortality in oral contraceptive users. Lancet 1:542–546, 1982
21. Ortho-Novum 7/7/7 preferred for new patients by 47% of respondents. Contraceptive Technology Update 7:101–114, 1986
22. Marz W et al: Effect of oral contraceptives on serum lipoprotein patterns in healthy women. Advances in fertility control and treatment of sterility. Dublin, Proceedings of symposium, 11th World Congress, 99–109, 1984
23. Wynn V, Godsland I: Effects of oral contraceptives on carbohydrates metabolism. J Reprod Med 31(Suppl 9: 892–897, 1986
24. Skouby SO, Anderson O, Kuhl C: Oral contraceptives and insulin receptor binding in normal women and those with previous gestational diabetes. Am J Obstet Gynecol 155:802–807, 1986
25. Rubin GL, Peterson HB: Oral contraceptive use and cancer. Contraceptive Technology Update, January 1985
26. McPherson K, Neil A, Vessey MP et al: Oral contraceptives and breast cancer (letter). Lancet 2:1414–1415, 1983
27. Newberger J, Forman D, Doll R et al: Oral contraceptives and hepatocellular carcinoma. Br Med J 292:1355–1357, 1986
28. Stewart F, Guest F, Stewart G et al: Understanding Your Body. New York, Bantam, 1987
29. Alza Corporation: Progestasert intrauterine progesterone contraceptive system. Alza Product Information, 1986
30. Lane M, Arleo R, Sobrero AJ: Successful use of the diaphragm and jelly in a young population: Report of a clinical study. Fam Plann Perspect 8(2):81–86, March/April 1976
31. Pettiti D, D'Agostino RB, Oldman MJ: Nonmenstrual toxic shock syndrome: Methodological problems in estimating incidence and delineating risk factors. J Reprod Med 32:10–16, 1987
32. Edelman DA, McIntyre SL, Harper J: A comparative trial of the Today contraceptive sponge and diaphragm. Am J Obstet Gynecol 150:869–876, 1984
33. Rosenberg MJ, Rojanapithayakom W, Feldblum PJ et al: Effect of contraceptive sponge on chlamydial infection, gonorrhea, and candidiasis. JAMA 257:2308–2312, 1987
34. Gallen ME, Liskin L, Kak N: Men—new focus in family planning. Popul Rep [J] (33), 1987
35. Minuk G: Passage of viral particles through natural membrane condoms. Proceedings of conference: Condoms in prevention of sexually transmitted diseases. Atlanta, GA, February 20, 1987
36. Bounds W, Guillebaud J, Stewart L et al: A female condom (Femshield): A study of its user acceptability. Br J Fam Plann 14:83–87, 1988
37. Leeper MA, Conrady M, Henderson J: Evaluation of the WPC-33 female condom. Abstract No 6305, 5th International Congress on AIDS, Montreal, Canada, June 1989
38. Sakondhavat C: The female condom (letter). Am J Public Health 80:498, April 1990
39. Kowal D: Study raises questions of spermicide safety. Contraceptive Technology Update 2:57–61, 1981
40. Hatcher RA, Stewart GK, Guest F: Fertility awareness methods. In JW Sciarra (ed): Gynecology and Obstetrics. Philadelphia, Harper & Row, 1984
41. American Academy of Pediatrics: Breast-feeding and contraception. Pediatrics 68(1):138–140, 1981
42. Bachrach CA: Contraceptive practice among American women, 1973–1982. Fam Plann Perspect 16(6):253–259, November/December 1984
43. Association for Voluntary Sterilization: Immunologic aspects of vasectomy and atherosclerosis. Biomed Bull 1:2, 1980
44. DeStefano F, Huezo CM, Peterson HB et al: Menstrual changes after sterilization. Obstet Gynecol 62:673–681, 1983
45. Vessey M, Huggins G, Lawless M et al: Tubal sterilization: findings in a large prospective study. Br J Obstet Gynaecol 90:203–209, 1983
46. Siegler AM, Hulka J, Peretz A: Reversibility of female sterilization. Fertil Steril 43:499–510, 1985

12

Clinical Interruption of Pregnancy

PATIENTS' RIGHTS, PROFESSIONAL RESPONSIBILITY, AND ETHICS

ABORTION SERVICES AND FINANCING

CARE OF THE ABORTION PATIENT

Nursing Assessment

Nursing Diagnosis

Nursing Planning and Intervention

    Exploring Alternatives

    Education About Procedures and Experiences

    Providing Supportive Care

    Prevention of Complications

    Follow-up Care

Evaluation

LONG-TERM SEQUELAE OF ABORTION

ABORTION PROCEDURES

First-Trimester Procedures

    Vacuum (Suction) Curettage

    Dilation and Curettage (D&C)

    Menstrual Extraction

    Prostaglandins

Second-Trimester Procedures

    Dilation and Evacuation (D&E)

    Hypertonic Saline

    Hypertonic Urea

    Intra-amniotic Prostaglandin F_{2a}

    Vaginal Prostaglandin E_2

    Hysterotomy

RU 486 (MIFEPRISTONE)

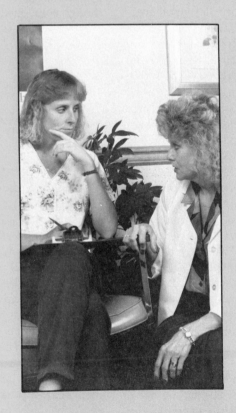

In general, attitudes toward abortion and the availability of abortion procedures are strongly influenced by prevailing societal values. Whether the society's approach is permissive or restrictive depends on several factors: culture, economy, and ecology. For example, the existence of a predominant religion in a country can affect abortion laws and practices, as can the country's economic or sociopolitical system and its population trends, level of technology, and standard of living.

Women have long sought abortion as a solution to unwanted pregnancy, regardless of whether their culture approved or disapproved of this practice. Interruption of pregnancy is sought by women for a variety of reasons, including health, economics, marital status, family stability, the circumstances of conception, personal goals, age, and many other social and psychological factors. Although accurate abortion statistics are difficult to obtain, especially in countries where the procedure is illegal, it is estimated that from 30 to 60 million pregnancies are purposefully ended each year throughout the world.[1]

The abortion rate in the United States is about 28 to 29 per 1000 women of reproductive age. Slightly over 1.5 million legal abortions are performed annually, obtained predominantly by young, white, unmarried women. The rate of abortion is about twice as high for nonwhite as for white women, although the number of abortions is smaller for nonwhites because of their smaller population proportions. About 30% of all pregnancies are terminated by legal abortion.[2]

In the United States, about half of all abortions are done within 8 weeks of the woman's last menstrual period (LMP). Ninety percent of abortions occur within 12 weeks of the LMP, with less than 1% done after 20 weeks. The performance of legal abortions early in pregnancy has reduced morbidity and mortality, which is less than that expected for term pregnancy. Nearly 90% of abortions are performed in nonhospital settings. The mortality rate from abortions is 0.6 per 100,000 legal abortions.[1]

The U.S. Supreme Court liberalized abortion laws in 1973, permitting early interruption of pregnancy (before viability) at the woman's request. Laws regulating second-trimester abortion were left to the individual states' discretion. The Hyde Amendment, passed by the U.S. Congress in 1976 and upheld as constitutional by the U.S. Supreme Court in 1980, forbids the expenditure of federal funds for abortion services except in cases in which continuation of the pregnancy threatens the woman's life.

Although abortion is legal, it is still viewed with misgivings by many because of religious and personal attitudes. Most, if not all, agree that abortion is not a happy substitute for pregnancy prevention and that the procedures necessary for bringing about termination, although generally safe, are associated with a higher morbidity than are most contraceptive methods.

Abortion remains a highly controversial issue in the United States. Since liberalization of the abortion laws in 1973, opponents have tried many strategies to restrict or prevent legal abortions. Legislative attempts to give the spouse veto power over the woman's abortion decision, or to require parental notification of abortion request by a teenager, have in general not been successful. Restricting access to abortion by limiting use of federal or state funding has had an impact on poor and minority women, who rely on governmental sources for health-care payments. Harassment of abortion providers has been increasing in an attempt to discourage both professionals and clients. Between 80% and 90% of abortion facilities have experienced some form of harassment, including picketing outside clinics, vandalizing or bombing facilities, and tracing the identity of clients. Telephone lines have been jammed, mass no-show appointments have been scheduled, and clients have been blocked from entering clinics. Occasionally, the homes of staff members have been picketed, and death threats have been made. These activities make abortion services more difficult and costly to provide, with increased expenditures for security, legal services, and insurance. Staff may be hard to recruit or retain under such conditions. The average number of abortions performed at the larger clinics has not decreased, although some facilities have closed.[3]

■ PATIENTS' RIGHTS, PROFESSIONAL RESPONSIBILITY, AND ETHICS

As professionals, nurses are committed to responding in a caring, competent manner to the needs of their patients. Women seeking abortion services have the right to expect and receive empathic, supportive, and nonjudgmental care from nurses. Nurses, as persons and as professionals, have the right to their values, beliefs, and ethical perspectives. For many nurses, moral convictions and personal ethics dictate that abortion is unacceptable and that any participation in the care of abortion patients violates these convictions. In this instance, the rights of patients and the rights of nurses are in conflict. The nurse has the right to refuse to participate in the care of abortion patients, in keeping with personal moral and ethical beliefs. Most nurses with such beliefs avoid working in facilities that provide abortions. Only in the instance when a patient's life is in immediate danger would it be necessary for nurses

Research Highlight

African-American Urban Adolescents Choosing Abortion have Better Educational, Economic, and Psychological Outcomes

About 40% of U. S. teenagers who conceive each year elect to terminate their pregnancies. Childbearing among adolescent mothers has adverse effects on subsequent schooling, economic and social status, marital stability, maternal and infant health. This study compared effects of obtaining an abortion with continuing the pregnancy among 360 black teenage women of similar socioeconomic background in an urban setting. Subjects were recruited from two family planning clinics and were of lower socioeconomic status, 17 years or younger, unmarried, and none had a baby of her own to care for.

Closed-ended questionnaires were used for data about household structure, education, jobs, economic wellbeing, health, growth, sexual and contraceptive behavior, and conception and fertility. Subjects were given psychological tests including the Rosenberg Self-Esteem Scale, Rotter Locus of Control scale, and Spielberger State-Trait Anxiety Index. The baseline data were collected before the outcome of the pregnancy was known. Two years later the same data were collected from over 90% of the baseline sample.

At baseline, the groups (abortion, continued pregnancy, negative pregnancy test) were similar for most variables. After 2 years, the young women who terminated their pregnancies were far more likely to have graduated from high school, or to still be in school at the appropriate grade level than were those who continued their pregnancies to term, or whose pregnancy test was negative. Those obtaining an abortion were better off economically with more working adults; the childbearing teenagers' families deteriorated in terms of working adults.

Analysis of psychological stress showed the women terminating pregnancies experienced no greater levels of stress or anxiety than the other teenagers at that time. Two years later, those undergoing abortion were no more likely to have psychological problems and had experienced less negative change than the other teenagers with slightly higher self-esteem and locus of control (not reaching statistical significance). They were also less likely to have experienced a subsequent pregnancy and slightly more likely to practice contraception.

Two years after their abortions, the black teenagers who had chosen to terminate their pregnancies were, on most measures, doing better than those continuing pregnancy or not pregnant.

Zabin LS, Hirsch MB, Emerson MR: When urban adolescents choose abortion: Effects on education, psychological status and subsequent pregnancy. Fam Plann Perspect 21(6):248–255, November/December 1989

to assist women undergoing abortion, even if this violates the nurse's beliefs. Other nurses may choose to present alternatives to the patient through counseling and referral services. Although nurses are entitled to their own perspectives on abortion, in general, the responsibility of the professional is to advise the client of all options and expected outcomes and to assist the client in making a personally satisfactory decision. The client's perspective should be respected, although it may differ from the nurse's perspective.

Nurses need to examine their values and beliefs carefully and decide whether to participate in the care of abortion patients. Conflicts, doubts, and confusion on the nurse's part are frequently communicated to the patient and may cause additional distress. Self-honesty and values clarification are important for the nurse; honoring the self must be done before effective, caring services can be provided to the patient.

Chapter 7 provides a more detailed discussion of ethical perspectives and legal developments related to elective abortion.

■ ABORTION SERVICES AND FINANCING

As a result of the Hyde Amendment, there has been a virtual withdrawal of federal funds to subsidize abortions for indigent women. Many states have adopted the Hyde restrictions or sought even narrower ones, instead of assuming the costs of abortions for poor women. Some of the more populous states (i.e., California, New York, Pennsylvania) have maintained more liberal standards for abortions and paid for services with state funds.

Although the restrictions on publicly funded abortions did not completely eliminate use of federal funds, they have had a major impact. The number of subsidized abortions decreased by more than one third, and in states with restrictive policies regarding use of state funds, abortions for poor women with public support were virtually eliminated. A large estimated unmet need for publicly funded abortions existed before these funding restrictions, and it has increased substantially after the institution of these restrictions.

The impact of this decrease in publicly funded abortions is felt in several ways. Indigent women who are able to raise the money to pay for their own abortions often do so at the expense of their rent or utility bills, by pawning household goods, by diverting food or clothing money, or possibly by fraudulent use of a relative's insurance policy. Some women have been driven to theft. It was found that the price Medicaid-eligible women were paying for abortions was almost the same as that paid by those not eligible; they paid the full price themselves. The distress and hardship involved in obtaining or forgoing an abortion are hardly reflected in the statistics; cases have been reported of indigent women attempting self-induced abortion or suicide after being denied publicly funded abortions.[4]

Medicaid-eligible women can obtain medically necessary abortions in those states in which public funds are approved for abortions. However, many states do not receive Medicaid funds or approve their use for abortions.

The accessibility of facilities that perform abortions is an important factor. Nearly all abortions in the United States are done in metropolitan areas (about 98%), and most nonmetropolitan counties do not have any services for women seeking abortions. This problem has intensified with the decline in the number of hospitals that offer abortion services. The unwillingness of most hospitals and physicians to perform abortions has partially been offset by an increase in the number of free standing clinics that offer abortion procedures. About two thirds of all abortions are done in such specialized clinics.[5] Abortion rates vary dramatically by state, resulting from a number of factors, including availability of abortion services, the proportion of nonwhite Hispanic population (which have above average abortion rates), degree of urbanization, and state policies, especially related to public payment for abortion services for low-income women. States with the highest abortion rates include California, New York, Hawaii, Nevada, New Jersey, Delaware, and District of Columbia. Those with the lowest abortion rates include Wyoming, South Dakota, West Virginia, Idaho, Mississippi, Arkansas, and Indiana.

Many women travel to bordering states to obtain an abortion when there are no services in their home state. The distance that women must travel can be important in determining whether they can obtain services when needed. It is more difficult to obtain information about facilities when these are distant. Travel expenses may be prohibitive for poor women, including the costs of overnight lodging and loss of pay due to absence from work. Health risks are greater, because rapid diagnosis and treatment of postabortion complications are more difficult. Privacy is jeopardized by the need to be away from home and work for a longer time. The greater the distance that a woman must travel to an abortion facility or service, the less likely she is to utilize that service successfully. Nationally, about 6% of abortions are performed on nonresidents of the state providing the service. Some states provide abortion services for a large proportion of nonresidents, however; over half of the abortions done in the District of Columbia were for nonresidents, and about 40% or more abortions were for nonresidents in Kansas, Kentucky, and North Dakota.[5]

The loss of hospital abortion services has left increasing numbers of women without any provider in their local areas. The shift of abortions from hospitals to free standing clinics is probably related to cost advantages of clinics and their ability to provide abortions later in gestation. The clinics offer many advantages to women: professional staff who understand problems faced when seeking abortion, who have extensive experience and competence in abortion procedures, and who provide emotional support and referral services.

The inequity in access to abortion services continues to worsen, however, with the shift from hospital to clinic providers. The overall effect has been to reduce abortion services in states and counties where they were already limited. Women in many parts of the country must travel long distances to obtain abortions, resulting in considerable personal hardship and often delaying the procedure until later in pregnancy, when the risks are greater.

■ CARE OF THE ABORTION PATIENT

The nurse is often a key professional in providing counseling to clients considering abortion. The need to weigh alternatives and make responsible decisions about an unwanted pregnancy may become apparent in the prenatal or family-planning clinic or other health-care setting. As part of client education and the supportive role, the nurse may offer initial discussion and assistance in problem solving to women or couples facing the problem of an undesired conception.

Nursing Assessment

Nursing assessment of the woman or couple seeking pregnancy termination includes psychological, social, and physiological data. The nurse often encounters the client at an early stage in decision making and can provide valuable assistance in considering alternatives and in arriving at a choice with which the client is comfortable. The history follows the format used with women seeking contraception (see Chap. 11), with special attention to menstrual and obstetrical history, past medical history and family history for conditions placing the woman at increased risk for a surgical procedure, contraceptive and prior abortion history.

An exploration of psychological factors is particularly important, with attention to evidence of ambivalence or conflict. The highest value placed on women in most societies is their role as mothers, and powerful systems of reinforcement operate to make motherhood central to women's lives. A decision to interrupt a pregnancy is rarely taken without some conflict because of the complex meanings and values associated with reproduction and motherhood. Even if the outcome of pregnancy (a child) is consciously unwanted, the woman may on some level desire to be pregnant as a symbol of potency, vitality, or reconnection with primal inner forces. Although pregnancy can be completely accidental, it is often used to affect relations with important people in the woman's life, such as parents, husband, or lover.

A teenage girl may become pregnant to demonstrate her maturity, prove her sexuality, or bolster her self-concept as a woman. She may become pregnant because her romantic ideals of motherhood and man–woman relations preclude the use of contraceptives, which imply premeditated sexual activity. Or pregnancy may result from sexual experimentation when neither partner takes responsibility for avoiding unwanted consequences. A woman at any age may use pregnancy as a means of alleviating feelings of inadequacy or doubts about her femininity. A woman entering menopause may conceive to reinforce her sexual self-image or to avoid facing the loss of reproductive capacity. Although pregnancy may be desired in these instances, the woman may find she cannot face the responsibilities of caring for and raising a child and so elects abortion as the most reasonable solution.

Marital status can also affect the decision to continue or interrupt a pregnancy. Many unmarried women feel incapable of raising a child outside of marriage, although there are increasing numbers of single parents and more social acceptance of this situation. A critical factor is the quality of the man–woman relation and its meaning for the woman in terms of commitment and dependability. Pregnancy has historically been used to force a man into marriage but has proven to be a poor basis on which to build a lifetime relationship. In marriages that are in trouble and facing dissolution, pregnancy may be used as an attempt to prevent a breakup. A woman may also become pregnant, even though she does not truly desire a child, to meet her partner's expectation, for example, if the man's sense of masculinity or potency requires that "his woman" become pregnant. In many of these cases, however, the pregnancy does not produce the desired result, and the woman may seek abortion when she realizes that motives for pregnancy were not appropriate for her.

Poor physical or mental health can lead a woman to interrupt her pregnancy if pregnancy poses a risk to her life or a drain on her already depleted energies. A life crisis or emotional upheaval may lead a woman to feel incapable of coping with pregnancy and motherhood until her life becomes less chaotic.

Abortion may also be chosen when a pregnancy is untimely. Education or professional goals may have higher priority at the time, or pregnancy may occur too early in a marriage or too soon after the birth of a child. Or the couple may feel emotionally or economically unable to manage parenthood. Couples frequently seek abortion for economic reasons. They prefer to strive for a higher standard of living and greater social opportunity for themselves and their children and are unwilling to be subjected to increased material hardship.

Abortion may be sought for eugenic reasons, even if pregnancy and the child are desired. Clients are becoming better informed about the hereditary genetic defects that may be of risk to their offspring. They are taking advantage of screening programs to detect such conditions as Tay-Sachs disease, hemophilia, Down's syndrome, sickle cell disease, and other genetic abnormalities. Awareness of fetal anomalies caused by rubella, exposure to radiation, and teratogenic drugs may cause some women to elect abortion if they have been exposed during the first trimester.

With the widespread availability of fetal diagnosis, women experience pressures to abort abnormal fetuses. With limited social support to families and people with disabilities, parents feel direct responsibility both emotionally and economically for the care of disabled children. To spare their families and babies the consequences of congenital diseases, many women seek all available technology to detect defects through prenatal diagnosis and feel little choice but to abort fetuses whose disabilities would be a drain on personal and societal resources.[6] Some women decide to continue the preg-

---

Psychological Factors in Pregnancy and Abortion

Purpose for Becoming Pregnant (complex meanings and values associated with reproduction and motherhood)
- Symbol of potency, vitality, or reconnection with primary inner forces
- Symbol of man's virility, potency
- Manipulation of relationships with particular people
- Maturity, sexuality, self-concept
- Elimination of feelings if inadequacy or doubts about femininity
- Avoidance of facing loss of reproduction capacity in the older woman

Purpose for Interrupting Pregnancy
- Marital status
- Quality of man–woman relationship
- Realization that motives for pregnancy were not appropriate
- Poor physical health (risk to life)
- Poor mental health (drain on energies, unable to cope)
- Educational or professional goals
- Conception too early in marriage
- Conception too soon after birth of previous child
- Emotionally unable to handle parenthood
- Financially unable to handle parenthood
- Hereditary genetic defects
- Possible fetal anomalies
- Possible reactions of peers, family, community

---

nancy even in the face of known fetal abnormalities, and they utilize the time for practical and emotional preparation. For many, the opportunity provided by fetal diagnosis offers a positive experience to relieve suffering and the burden of chronic diseases and genetic disorders.[7]

The nurse assesses the woman's or couple's decision-making processes, with particular attention to expressions of ambivalence, confusion, or conflict. This process usually begins as soon as the woman suspects she may be pregnant, although some women may have thought through their desires and choices before becoming pregnant. Because time is critical in the abortion decision, with the objective of obtaining an abortion within the first 8 weeks of gestation to minimize the risk of complications, the nurse must focus carefully on decisional conflicts. Intervention to assist the client in resolving any conflicts or confusion needs to be instituted at the earliest possible time. The woman may want her partner, or other significant persons, to be involved in the decision-making process. It is important to honor the client's wishes about involvement of important

people, because this contributes to overall satisfaction with the experience.

A focused physical examination is performed, with particular attention to signs of current illness, risk factors that might increase the potential for complications, the condition of the pelvic organs, and stage of gestation. An accurate estimation of uterine size is made, and the weeks of gestation are estimated and compared with those by dates of the LMP. The position of the uterus is important for safe execution of the uterine evacuation procedure (e.g., anteversion, retroversion). The presence of physical structures that might interfere with the abortion procedure, such as uterine fibroids or adnexal masses, is carefully assessed.

Laboratory tests are routinely performed for abortions. These include a pregnancy test (urine or serum) for positive confirmation of pregnancy, hemoglobin or hematocrit to rule out anemia, and Rh determination so that Rh-negative women can receive Rh immune globulin if they are not already sensitized. Screening is done for sexually transmitted diseases (STDs) according to clinic or office protocol; many recommend routine screening because of the increasing prevalence of STDs. Common STD tests include gonorrhea and *Chlamydia* cultures, tests for syphilis (venereal disease research laboratory [VDRL], serological test for syphilis [STS]), wet mounts for *Monilia* and *Trichomonas*, and screening tests for human immunodeficiency virus (HIV) and HBV (hepatitis B virus).

Ultrasound evaluation of the uterus is often recommended to assess the stage of gestation, to detect ectopic pregnancies, and to confirm pelvic architecture and fetal position. Routine abdominal sonography for all abortion patients has been recommended, followed by transvaginal sonography on those in whom pregnancy could not be confirmed with the abdominal procedure. This has the advantage of detecting ectopic pregnancies, molar pregnancies, women who are not pregnant, and pregnancies at a later gestational stage than clinical examination had diagnosed. The additional cost in clinics that perform over 3000 procedures annually would be only $15 per case.[8]

Nursing Diagnosis

The nursing diagnosis is based largely on psychosocial data obtained during assessment. Although several diagnoses may be made, much of nursing intervention involves providing care for the client/family with a knowledge deficit. Initially, this deficit is related to options available and procedures to be used. Later knowledge deficit is related to self-care, expected bleeding or cramping, signs and symptoms of complications, sexual activity, contraception, and community resources.

Ineffective coping and alteration in family processes

Preabortion History and Examination

History

Past medical history (major illness, surgery, hospitalization)

Family history (familial and hereditary diseases, risk factors)

Current health status:
  Recent menstrual history
  History of prior pregnancies (surgical procedures, complications, outcomes)
  Contraceptive history, plans for future contraception
  Drugs currently used (prescription and nonprescription)
  Substances used (alcohol, tobacco, illicit drugs)
  Allergies to local anesthetics, analgesics, antibiotics, and other drugs
  Current acute or chronic illness (requires further evaluation)

Psychological and social concerns

Factors affecting decision making

Examination

Vital signs

Cardiac, circulatory, and lungs

Breasts

Abdomen

Pelvic examination
  Vulva, introitus, vagina
  Cervix and uterus
  Estimation of gestation by uterine size
  Position of uterus (anteversion, retroversion)
  Presence of physical structures that might interfere with the abortion procedure (uterine fibroids, adnexal masses)

Diagnostic Tests

Pregnancy test (urine or serum)

Hemoglobin or hematocrit

Rh determination (Rh-negative women should receive Rh immune globulin)

STD screening as appropriate (gonorrhea culture, VDRL, *Chlamydia* culture, wet mount, HIV and HBV screen)

Ultrasound evaluation of the uterus (assess gestation, ectopic pregnancy, pelvic architecture, fetal position)

---

disapproval by others, inadequate problem solving, inadequate support systems, or a loss/grief reaction about the pregnancy. Fatigue, sleep disturbances, lack of appetite, and crying episodes may accompany depression and ineffective coping. Altered family processes may occur due to the stress of an unwanted pregnancy, in which the family system does not communicate openly and effectively or adapt constructively. Family members (usually the couple) may express fear or anger, may argue, and may be unable to make a decision together.

The woman may experience a self-concept disturbance related to the pregnancy and her desire for termination. She may experience negative feelings about herself or her capabilities, expressing shame or guilt, or feeling unable to deal with events and make decisions. Decisional conflict may be present, in which the women/couple feel uncertain about which course of action to take. They often express the undesired consequences of either choice (undergo abortion, continue pregnancy) and vacillate between the alternatives. This can delay decision making and lead to a later abortion with increased stress and risk of complications. Lack of information or confusion about abortion procedures may contribute to decisional conflict.

Spiritual distress may occur for women whose religious or personal ethical convictions are opposed to abortion. Conflict is experienced between religious or spiritual beliefs and other values or perceived needs (practical, economic, eugenic, self-actualizing) that would support the importance of terminating the pregnancy. There may be anxiety, guilt, grief, a sense of loss, doubt, powerlessness, depression, feeling trapped, or anger. Questions about the beliefs may arise, with doubt and confusion adding to the woman's distress.

A common nursing diagnosis is altered comfort: acute pain related to the abortion procedure. The anticipation or fear of pain can be addressed in preabortion counseling about anesthesia and analgesia. Women undergoing abortions also have potential for infection related to introduction of pathogens during the procedure, or postabortion exposure to infection, especially if precautions are not followed. Women undergoing abortions are also at risk for injury from hemorrhage and retained products.

Nursing Planning and Intervention

Nursing intervention usually covers such areas as assisting the client to consider all choices, to understand requirements for various abortion procedures, to examine supports and resources, to understand her reactions and find expression for emotional needs, to locate or take advantage of facilities or financing methods, and to provide education about the processes of abortion and contraception.

are two other potential diagnoses for this situation. Ineffective coping may be related to depression or to feelings of failure, sadness, worry and fear. Underlying this could be moral or ethical conflict, negative self-concept,

---

Nursing Diagnoses Applicable to Pregnancy Termination

Knowledge deficit
  Options available for unwanted pregnancy
  Procedures and requirements related to gestation
  Risks and dangers of abortion procedures
  Experience of undergoing abortion
  Experience after abortion
  Self-care after abortion

Ineffective coping
  Depression, grief, sadness, worry, fear
  Feelings of failure
  Moral or ethical conflict
  Negative self-concept
  Disapproval by others
  Inadequate problem solving
  Inadequate support systems

Altered family processes
  Stress of unwanted pregnancy
  Ineffective communication
  Ineffective adaptation and decision making

Self-concept disturbance
  Ambivalence over terminating pregnancy
  Negative feelings about self
  Feels incapable of dealing with events

Decisional conflict
  Ambivalence over terminating pregnancy
  Values/beliefs in conflict
  Couple with conflicting desires
  Confusion about choices and procedures
  Vacillate and delay decision making

Spiritual distress
  Conflict between religious/spiritual beliefs and felt
    need to terminate pregnancy
  Questions/doubts about religious/spiritual beliefs
  Confusion about what is right or acceptable

Altered comfort: acute pain
  Related to the abortion procedure
  Anticipation of painful procedure

Potential for infection or injury
  Introduction of pathogens during procedure
  Introduction of pathogens by not following postabortion precautions
  Increased postabortion susceptibility
  Risk of hemorrhage or retained products

EXPLORING ALTERNATIVES

Many women need help to think beyond their first reaction to the unwanted pregnancy. They need to be encouraged to consider other options available to them. Many women feel ambivalent and confused and are under pressure from family or their own social values.

It is important that the nurse encourages the woman to make the decision for herself, because there is less regret and emotional sequelae when the choice is not perceived as being forced by other people. Exploring alternatives realistically helps clarify the situation and places manageable boundaries within which the decision can be made. Thinking through what each choice means not only for present feelings and relations but also for future circumstances, goals, and needs, both from a practical and from an emotional-values standpoint, encourages a carefully weighed choice. While the counseling is in progress, tests are carried out to confirm the pregnancy and determine the length of gestation, and the type of abortion procedure indicated is discussed. These factors alone may influence the decision. Simply knowing that the pregnancy has progressed beyond the time when simple evacuation can be used and that the abortion may actually involve labor and expulsion of the fetus may cause a woman to decline abortion. In any event, understanding the nature of the procedure required is essential to informed decision making (Fig. 12-1).

EDUCATION ABOUT PROCEDURES AND EXPERIENCES

Information about the requirements of various types of abortion procedures and what women usually experience when undergoing these procedures is an important nursing intervention. The type of procedure is determined by the length of gestation and the experience of the physician as well as the medical evaluation of suitability of patient to procedure. In the United States, surgical methods are most commonly used, including vacuum curettage, dilation and evacuation (D&E), dilation and curettage (D&C), and hysterotomy or hysterectomy. Vacuum (suction) curettage is the most widely used procedure, generally done before 9 weeks' gestation. This method can be done in an office setting up through 16 weeks' gestation, when there is appropriate backup available for handling complications. D&E extends the vacuum curettage into the second trimester, using cervical dilation to accommodate removal of gestations ranging from 13 through 20 weeks' gestation. The traditional D&C uses a sharp metal curette and is infrequently used because it is more painful and causes more blood loss with greater cervical dilation. Hysterotomy and hysterectomy are used when concomitant sterilization or other gynecological surgery is necessary. These procedures are discussed in the next section.

Most women who undergo suction or vacuum curettage experience pain during and after the uterine evacuation. Abortion pain is ranked as moderately intense, but there is a wide range in women's pain experience. Preabortion depression is the principal predictor of pain intensity in abortion and is significantly correlated with other measures of emotional distress,

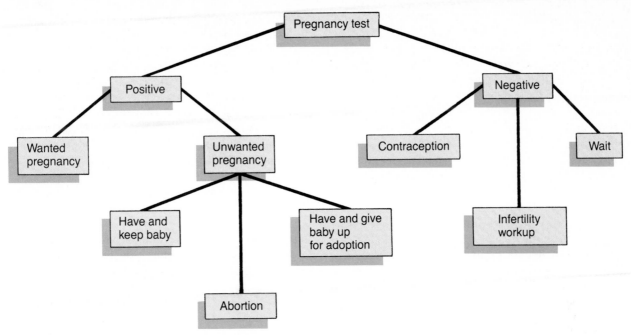

■ *Figure 12–1*
Decision tree for pregnancy alternatives.

such as anxiety, ambivalence, fear, greater pain expectancy, and tendency toward emotionality. Women who are younger and less educated report higher levels of pain, as do those with moral conflicts and concerns about others' judgment. Other factors associated with higher levels of pain include dysmenorrhea, a retroverted uterus, and early (5–7 weeks) or later gestations (more than 16 weeks) that require additional dilation and aspiration.[9]

In many clinics, a laminaria is inserted shortly before the abortion procedure. This small stick of compressed *Laminaria* seaweed or $MgSO_4$ material is highly hygroscopic and expands to dilate the cervix over a 6-hour period. This is relatively painless and effective, slowly dilating the cervix to facilitate the curettage procedure and decrease the chance of cervical laceration. Local anesthesia (paracervical block) is administered in most settings, often accompanied by mild analgesic or sedative medication.

Early abortion under local anesthesia is well-tolerated by most women, especially those who are clear about their desire to terminate pregnancy, who are more mature and well educated, and who do not have anatomical or physiological variations contributing to more intense pain experiences. Women who are ambivalent or depressed before the procedure, who are younger, who have moral and social concerns or a low pain threshold, and other anatomical or physiological factors associated with higher levels of pain may require additional pain management to ensure a comfortable and safe abortion. This might include additional narcotic analgesia or a general anesthetic.[9]

Complications from early abortions are extremely infrequent, and compared to childbirth, legal abortion is remarkably safe. Deaths due to abortion range from 0.5 per 100,000 abortions at 8 weeks or less to 7.8 per 100,000 abortions at 16 to 20 weeks' gestation. Younger women have fewer complications than older women. Problems related to abortions are lower when the pregnancy is early, the patient is healthy, and the patient is not ambivalent about having the abortion performed. The training and experience of the provider are also important in abortion outcomes. Whereas over 70% of U.S. residency programs in obstetrics and gynecology include first-trimester abortion techniques in their training programs, the number of residents receiving this training appears to have declined slightly over the past decade. Nearly all the programs teaching first-trimester abortion techniques also teach second-trimester techniques. Limited experiences in residency programs support the need for specialized focus among physicians offering abortion services.[10]

The nurse utilizes these data about procedures and women's experiences to plan client education and to assist the women to seek the approach most appropriate for her. Recognizing factors that increase risk, both physiological and psychological, enables the nurse to plan interventions that take these factors into account.

PROVIDING SUPPORTIVE CARE

A major focus of nursing intervention for the woman or couple terminating a pregnancy is to provide emotional support and a caring environment. Most nursing diagnoses applicable to pregnancy termination involve psychological factors and emotional distress. Nursing interventions include assisting the client to identify and express feelings, supporting positive self-evaluations and coping behaviors, mobilizing support systems, helping the client learn new coping skills, and assisting in exploring values conflicts and using values clarification techniques. The nurse can teach constructive problem-solving techniques and can assist the client to develop strategies that utilize her personal strengths and previous experiences. Discussing alternatives and helping with making a fully informed decision are at the core of nursing interventions.

When family processes are altered, the nurse assists the family to acknowledge feelings about the situation, to communicate openly about perceptions and feelings, to expand understanding of the other family members' experiences, and to identify and utilize family strengths. The family is helped to appraise the situation, identify choices and consequences, and find sources of additional professional or social assistance.

PREVENTION OF COMPLICATIONS

The nurse provides education to the client to facilitate recognition of and prevention of postabortion problems. The most common complications include infection, retained products of conception, intrauterine blood clots, continuing pregnancy, cervical or uterine trauma, and bleeding. Infection is the most common problem, and the nurse teaches the woman to identify the signs of infection and report these promptly to the provider or clinic. The woman is also taught how to prevent infection after the abortion.

The woman receives instruction on what to expect physiologically and emotionally after abortion. This assists the woman to recognize normal postabortion experiences and to know when to seek help for possible complications in the areas of bleeding, cramping, clots, and continuing pregnancy. Emotional responses are discussed, and parameters for normal postabortion feelings are identified.

FOLLOW-UP CARE

It is standard to have a follow-up office visit in 2 weeks, at which time contraceptives are prescribed if not already begun. The client's adjustment to termination of pregnancy, as well as her partner's or family's reactions, can be discussed, and referral can be made if needed for psychological, social, or economic reasons.

By 2 weeks after abortion, uterine size should be normal and bleeding usually should have ceased. The client is evaluated for any signs of complications or for continuing pregnancy (ongoing symptoms of pregnancy, enlarged uterus). Any concerns about long-term sequelae of abortion can be discussed.

Evaluation

The client's care has been successful when the client has been able to make a decision (whether to interrupt

---

Client Education

Signs of Postabortion Infection

- Fever over 100.4°F
- Prolonged, heavy bleeding
- Severe cramping or one-sided abdominal or pelvic pain
- Change in odor (foul) of vaginal discharge
- Passing large clots or white-gray tissue

Information to Have When You Call the Clinic

- Your temperature taken within the last hour
- Number of pads used during the last 2 hours
- Any medicine taken (aspirin, acetaminophen) and how long ago
- The telephone number of your pharmacy

Client Education

Preventing Postabortion Infections

Taking good care of yourself after your abortion can make a big difference in the way you feel. These things can bolster your general health and help to prevent infection.

- Listen to your body and keep alert to signs of infection. Take your temperature twice each day. Call the clinic if it is over 100.4°F, which could indicate infection
- Avoid inserting anything into the vagina.
- Do not use tampons until your first normal period. Use only pads.
- Do not take tub baths, use hot tubs or douches, or go swimming for at least 2 weeks.
- Do not have vaginal intercourse or oral-vaginal sex for at least 2 weeks. Other forms of lovemaking are fine.
- Eat foods that are good for you. Vegetables, protein, and whole grains help you recover more quickly.
- Get enough sleep and rest. This allows your body to use its energy to heal. Avoid putting pressure on yourself for a few weeks.
- Exercise sensibly. If your usual exercises cause increased bleeding, stop them for 1 week.

---

the pregnancy or to continue the pregnancy), feels comfortable with her decision, and follows through in an acceptable manner. The latter involves choosing an acceptable method for abortion or seeking prenatal care for herself and her baby. She has adjusted well if she expresses emotional responses openly and seeks resolution to her conflicts and problems.

Effective care also results in her returning for a follow-up visit and using a suitable contraceptive method to prevent further unwanted pregnancies.

If the woman continues to experience emotional distress, problems with self-concept, ineffective coping, or altered family processes, care is evaluated according to whether she has initiated psychological counseling either individually or for the family, as appropriate. Additional nursing intervention may be necessary for unresolved problems or when the indicated counseling assistance has not been sought.

■ LONG-TERM SEQUELAE OF ABORTION

Data on the long-term physiological complications of legal abortions show that the most common methods pose no major risks. Early first-trimester abortion using the vacuum curettage technique has little association with subsequent infertility, spontaneous abortions, premature delivery, and low-birth-weight babies. Any risk of subsequent adverse reproductive outcomes

would probably be increased for women who have undergone repeated elective abortions.[11]

Studies show that psychological problems after induced abortion are rare. Distress and depression are more commonly reported before the abortion than afterwards. Relief and happiness are much more common in the weeks after abortion of an unwanted pregnancy. When women do have negative reactions after abortion, these are mainly related to uncertainty about having the abortion, delay in decision making, lack of support from others, and need to terminate a wanted pregnancy (i.e., for fetal defects).[12]

The rates of admission to psychiatric hospitals were found to be higher among postpartum and postabortion women who were separated, divorced, and widowed than among those currently or never married. Among this latter group, the admissions after abortion were considerably higher than those after delivery. The interaction of stress, lack of social support, and reversal of original intention for a previously desired pregnancy was felt to account for the higher rates among postabortion women.[13]

In a longitudinal study of children born to women who had been denied an abortion for that pregnancy, persistent and significant differences were found between children in the study group and those in control groups. When the children were 9 years of age, the study group children had a higher incidence of illness despite the same biological start in life, had poorer grades in school despite the same levels of intelligence, and had worse integration in the peer group. At ages 14 to 16, more children in the study group did not con-

Client Education

What to Expect After Abortion

Bleeding

Bleeding similar to that of your menstrual period, lasting about a week, is the most usual pattern after abortion. Every woman is an individual, and the amount of bleeding varies. Some women have almost no bleeding; others have heavier than usual bleeding. Excessive bleeding would be soaking through several pads in 2 to 3 hours, having a very heavy flow for more than 2 days, and bleeding that lasts more than 2 weeks.

Cramping

It is not unusual to have cramping for a few days after the abortion. Aspirin, acetaminophen, or heat to the abdomen usually relieves the cramps.

Clots

Blood clots may or may not be expelled after an abortion. These are usually dark red or brown. Cramping may get worse as the uterus is trying to expel clots. It may help to massage your lower abdomen. Cramps usually stop once the clots are expelled. Severe persistent cramps and clots that are gray-white may indicate complications.

Menstruation

The next normal menstrual period usually begins in 4 to 6 weeks, although a few women have a period in 2 weeks. If birth control pills are started right after an abortion, the next period should occur 2 to 3 days after the last active pill in the pack. If menstruation has not occurred by 8 weeks, medical evaluation is indicated.

Breast Soreness

Some women may have breast tenderness for the first few days after an abortion. Occasionally there may be a little milk the second through fourth day, which stops in a few days.

Contraception

Pregnancy can occur before your next period. You should decide on a contraceptive method and be prepared to use it as soon as you resume intercourse. If you have not selected another method, you should insist that your partner use a condom and/or use foam. Using both together is most effective.

Medications

If your provider has given you medications (antibiotics are most common), be sure to take all the pills as directed. If you notice a rash or hives, call the clinic right away.

Feelings

Many women experience strong feelings after an abortion. You may feel great relief and elation that you have made a difficult decision and come to terms with yourself; or, you may feel sadness and a sense of loss. This is a normal feeling, and you may want to talk with someone close about how you feel. Sometimes women experience feelings that seem beyond their control, such as depression or anger. Discussing your feelings with friends or seeing a counselor can provide important support.

tinue into secondary education but began jobs without vocational training and found their mothers inconsistent in emotional behavior toward them. When these children were 16 to 18 years of age, the boys in the study group more often reported that they felt neglected or rejected by their mothers than did the controls; however, no difference could be found among the girls.

The study concluded that "unwantedness" during early pregnancy is a significant risk factor for the subsequent life of the child.[14]

Urban African-American adolescent women undergoing abortion were found to experience less negative change than a control group that continued their pregnancies. After 2 years, the young women who terminated their pregnancies were far more likely to have graduated from high school or still be in school at the appropriate grade level. They were also better off economically and had not experienced greater levels of stress or anxiety than the other teenagers at the time of the pregnancy test. The teenagers who obtained abortions were less likely that those continuing pregnancy to have a subsequent pregnancy, and were slightly more likely to practice contraception. The young women choosing abortion were doing well on several measures of psychological well-being.[15]

When abortion is legal and there are generally accepting social values, deciding to have an abortion does not present a traumatic experience and is usually emotionally well accepted.

Psychological sequelae are usually of short duration and reflect the circumstances surrounding abortion and attitudes conveyed by peer groups, family, and health providers.[16]

With increasing use of specialized abortion facilities, which have supportive and experienced professional staff, the negative experiences women may have related to abortion should decrease. Greater social acceptance is indicated by significant increases in support for pro choice positions shown on public opinion polls. From the late 1980s to the early 1990s, there was a 6% increase in Americans who said abortion should be legal under any circumstances, and a 5% drop in those who said it should be illegal under all circumstances. Over 85% to 90% of Americans approve of abortion for health endangerment, rape, and fetal defect.[17]

■ ABORTION PROCEDURES

The approach to pregnancy termination varies according to gestational age. Before the 12th week, abortion is generally a relatively uncomplicated vaginal procedure, employing vacuum curettage, D&E, or D&C. In the early stages of pregnancy, prostaglandins may be used in the form of vaginal suppositories, intramuscular injections, or transcervical instillation to induce abortion. Or a suctioning method for menstrual extraction or regulation may be carried out by means of a small cannula (Fig. 12-2). This procedure is occasionally used during the first 2 weeks after a missed menstrual period, frequently before pregnancy is confirmed.

Beyond the 12th week, interruption requires more complex procedures. Second-trimester abortions usually involve amniocentesis, for which 1 to 3 days of hospitalization are often necessary and the complication rate is considerably higher. D&E is the most frequently used method and the safest in the 13- to 16-week interval, but has an increased rate of morbidity and mortality over first-trimester procedures. Serial intramuscular injections of prostaglandins (15-methyl analogues) have been successful during this time but with significant effects on temperature regulation and gastrointes-

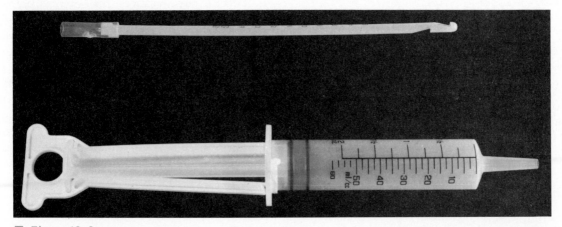

■ *Figure 12–2*
A flexible plastic Karman cannula and a self-locking syringe for menstrual extraction. (Rocket of London)

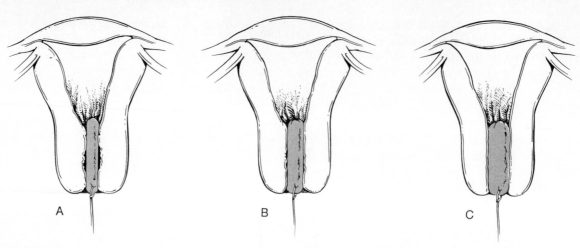

■ *Figure 12–3*
Lamineria used for cervical dilation. (A) Inserted in cervical canal beyond internal os.
(B) Hygroscopic material absorbs fluid and distends. (C) Maximum distention and cervical
dilation in 6 to 12 hours.

tinal symptoms. Intra-amniotic instillations of saline, urea, or prostaglandins are most effective after 16 weeks' gestation but with substantially increased complication rates.

Providers are performing an increasing percentage of second-trimester abortions using a combination of techniques for their dilating, fetocidal, and uterine-contracting effects. For example, *Laminaria* may be used for dilation, intrauterine instillation of urea may be used for fetocidal effects, and prostaglandin may be used for uterine-contracting effects[11] (Fig. 12-3).

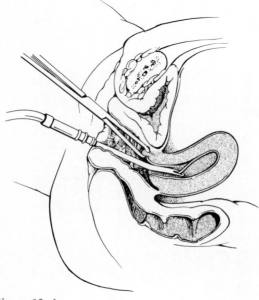

■ *Figure 12–4*
Vacuum curettage.

First-Trimester Procedures

VACUUM (SUCTION) CURETTAGE

The procedure of choice for the termination of early pregnancy is vacuum *curettage* (Figs. 12-4 and 12-5). A local anesthetic (paracervical block) or a spinal anesthetic may be used. The cervix is dilated with graduated dilators, and a suction curette is placed into the endometrial cavity to the fundus. Suction is applied, usually by an electric pump, and the products of conception are evacuated into a container. These are usually sent to the pathology laboratory for confirmation of the pregnancy and to rule out unusual conditions such as hydatidiform mole. Generally, recovery takes from 2 to 3 hours, during which time the client is observed for excessive bleeding.

In some circumstances, the cervix is prepared for the abortion by the use of *Laminaria*. These lengths of sterile hydroscopic material derived from seaweed absorb moisture at a rapid rate. When placed in the cervical canal, they expand in 3 to 6 hours and cause cervical dilatation. Insertion of a laminaria several hours before a first-trimester abortion can reduce the need for mechanical cervical dilatation. Some feel that using a laminaria decreases the incidence of cervical lacerations. The most common complications of vacuum curettage are infection, hemorrhage, and retained products or blood clots in the uterus, and cervical or uterine trauma.

DILATION AND CURETTAGE

D&C, using a surgical (sharp) curette, occasionally is used for first-trimester abortions but requires a general

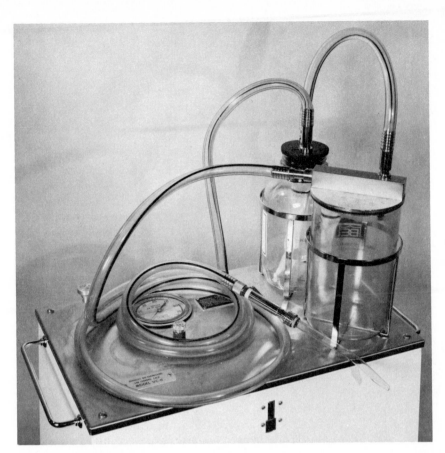

■ *Figure 12–5*
Electric suction apparatus with a swivel handle and a curette. (Model V C II by Berkeley Bio-Engineering, Inc.)

anesthetic and the usual preoperative precautions. The cervix must be dilated more than for vacuum curettage, and there is more danger of cervical laceration and blood loss. The advantage of this technique is that it is widely used and known by family physicians, general practitioners, and obstetrician–gynecologists.

MENSTRUAL EXTRACTION

Aspiration of the endometrium on an outpatient basis performed from 5 to 7 weeks after the LMP is called menstrual extraction, menstrual regulation, menstrual induction, minisuction, miniabortion, and interception. The procedure is simple and relatively atraumatic; little or no cervical dilation is required, and usually no anesthetic is given. A 4- to 6-mm flexible plastic cannula and a syringe or other low-pressure suction are used. The uterus does not need to be clinically enlarged, and often a pregnancy test is not required, because one of the advantages of the procedure is that the woman need not know for certain if she is pregnant. Although this procedure has been taught and used among women's groups as a self-administered technique, it is not safe to use it this way because of the dangers of hemorrhage, retained products, and infection.

PROSTAGLANDINS

Prostaglandins, a group of fatty acids found in the semen, are effective abortifacients at any stage of pregnancy. The exact mechanisms by which they work are not clearly understood. Oral administration is impractical because of the high incidence of side-effects, the most common being vomiting, diarrhea, fever, and shaking. Vaginal, intramuscular, and transcervical administration produce fewer side-effects, and serious complications are rare. Prostaglandins may be used more frequently as preparations are refined and side-effects are minimized.

Second-Trimester Procedures

DILATION AND EVACUATION

Over two thirds of all second-trimester abortions are done by D&E.[18] It is particularly used in the 13- to 16-week interval, when intra-amniotic procedures are often ineffective. The procedure is an extension of vacuum curettage and traditional D&C. The cervix requires greater dilation because the products of conception are larger. Usually a laminaria is inserted for gradual cervical dilation before the procedure. After administration of a paracervical block or general anesthesia, graduated metal dilators are introduced until the cervix is adequately dilated. A large suction cannula (14–16 mm) is used to remove pregnancy tissue. Forceps or crushing instruments may be needed to remove fetal tissue completely.

After the uterus has been emptied, a sharp curette is often used to explore the cavity for any remaining tissue. All fetal parts must be accounted for before administration of oxytocins. Some providers use prophylactic antibiotics (usually tetracyclines) to reduce the risk of infection. The most common complications are infections, retained products, hemorrhage, and cervical injury. D&E has about half the mortality associated with instillation methods. There is some evidence that the greater cervical dilation required for D&E in the second trimester is associated with a higher risk of delivering a subsequent low-birth-weight infant.[19]

D&E abortions are less stressful for women than instillation abortions, which involve labor and fetal expulsion. Because D&E often requires a destructive procedure, the psychological impact of second-trimester abortion may be transferred from the woman to the physician.

HYPERTONIC SALINE

When pregnancy has progressed beyond the 16th week, termination is often carried out by instilling *hypertonic saline* into the amniotic cavity. This procedure is most easily carried out when there is sufficient fluid in the amniotic cavity to be identified and aspirated. The bladder is emptied, and the client is placed in the supine position. The skin is prepped and draped with sterile towels and infiltrated with a local anesthetic over the injection site. An 18-gauge spinal needle is inserted through the uterus into the amniotic cavity. When properly placed, clear amniotic fluid flows into the syringe attached to the needle. After a small amount of fluid is removed to verify proper placement of the needle, hypertonic saline (20%–25% solution) is injected

into the amniotic cavity. Initially, a small amount is placed, and if there is no reaction, additional amniotic fluid is withdrawn and replaced with saline for approximately 15 minutes.

After a latent period of several hours, labor usually ensues and the fetus with part or all of the placenta is delivered within 24 to 72 hours. If the placenta cannot be extracted completely after delivery, a curettage must be carried out to complete the abortion. During the course of labor, the contractions can cause considerable discomfort. As the cervix dilates, the client should be medicated at intervals; generally, a substantial amount of emotional support is needed during this process. The previable fetus is usually dead at the time of delivery, but at this late stage of gestation it has human form.

Oxytocin infusion is often used as an adjunct to saline abortion to decrease the time needed for completion of the process. Oxytocin is used in a manner similar to that employed for induction of labor (see Chap. 38), except that a more concentrated solution is used. The oxytocin drip is begun 6 to 12 hours after amnioinfusion of saline. Maximum time of oxytocin use should be limited to 24 hours. If it is used longer, there is an increased incidence of water retention, which could lead to water intoxication.

In cases in which the hypertonic saline fails to induce contractions, a repeat dose must be administered. In some circumstances, such as in severe hypertension, infusion of hypertonic saline is contraindicated. Complications most often include hemorrhage, infection, and retained placenta. Occasionally, more serious complications occur as a result of the intravenous injection of saline, including hypernatremia, amniotic fluid embolism, disseminated intravascular coagulation, and necrosis of the myometrium from saline entering the uterine musculature.

HYPERTONIC UREA

A 30% solution of urea is increasingly being used to terminate second-trimester pregnancies, following the same technique described for the hypertonic saline in-

TABLE 12–1. MORTALITY RATES FOR ABORTION PROCEDURES*

Type of Procedure	Deaths	Abortions 000s	Rate	Relative Risk
Vacuum curettage/sharp curettage	46	5,786	0.8	1.0
Intra-amniotic infusions	11	222	4.9	6.1
Hysterotomy/hysterectomy	3	5	58.9	73.6
TOTAL	60	6,087†	1.0	———

* Deaths per 100,000 abortions, with relative risk based on index rate for vacuum curettage abortions.
† Total includes 4.2 million abortions with procedure unknown; rate includes these.

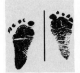

Nursing Care Plan

The Woman/Couple Interrupting a Pregnancy

Nursing Objectives

1. Woman/couple reaches acceptable decision regarding continuing or interrupting pregnancy.
2. Woman seeks early confirmation of pregnancy and first-trimester abortion to minimize risk and trauma, or seeks early prenatal care if pregnancy is to be continued.
3. Woman/couple understands procedures as indicated by gestational age and clarifies misunderstandings or fears.
4. Woman/couple obtains psychological counseling if indicated.
5. Woman/couple obtains information about effective contraception to avoid future unwanted pregnancy.

Assessment	Potential Nursing Diagnosis	Intervention	Evaluation
Menstrual history and last menstrual period, use of contraceptives	Knowledge deficit related to options available, procedures, normalcy of emotions, self-care, postprocedure care, expected bleeding or cramping, signs and symptoms of complications, resumption of sexual activity, contraception, sexuality, community resources, follow-up care	Advise of length of gestation and what type of procedure this indicates; discuss various types of abortion procedures, time in hospital or if outpatient, techniques and what the experience entails, risks, and complications	Able to reach decision about pregnancy termination with which woman/couple feels comfortable
Assist in physical examination, collection of specimens, pregnancy tests to determine length of gestation			Accepts requirements of various procedures as indicated by gestational age
Understanding of physiology of conception and contraceptive methods		Explore alternate choices (*i.e.*, have abortion or continue pregnancy and either keep baby or give baby for adoption) and meanings these have for woman, partner, and family	Affirms understanding of process of conception and effective use of contraception
Consideration of alternatives to abortion	Alteration in comfort: pain related to abortion procedure		Returns for follow-up visit and institutes contraceptive method
Pregnancy and health history to identify special needs and risks	High risk for infection related to tissue trauma	Assist during procedures; minimize tissue trauma and risk of infection; provide pain relief, support, and clarification; and keep client informed of process	Feels accepting of abortion if undertaken; no serious emotional problems
		Advise of postabortion complications, when to seek medical care, preventive measures, and when to resume activities and sex	Seeks prenatal care if abortion decided against
		Discuss contraception follow-up visits, and emotional reactions	Avoids future unwanted pregnancies
		For midtrimester abortion, monitor during labor, pro-	

(continued)

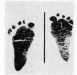

Nursing Care Plan (continued)

Assessment	Potential Nursing Diagnosis	Intervention	Evaluation
		vide pain relief and supportive care, and facilitate presence of companion if desired	
Circumstances surrounding unwanted conception Level of ambivalence or certainty about abortion decision	Ineffective individual coping leading to depression related to unresolved emotional responses (guilt, regret) Self-concept disturbance related to pregnancy	Initiate referral to psychological counseling if indicated Provide opportunity to express emotional responses, conflicts, problems	Initiates psychological counseling if emotionally distressed Expresses emotional responses openly, seeks resolution to conflicts and problems
Involvement of partner, family, parents, and sources of support Presence of crisis, need for further psycholgoical counseling	Altered family processes related to the effects of abortion on relationships (disagreements, marital and personal conflicts, adolescent identity problems) Altered sexuality patterns related to stress or conflict, pain, fear	Initiate referral to psychological or sexual counseling if indicated Provide opportunity to express emotional responses, conflicts, problems	Initiates psychological/sexual counseling if emotionally distressed Expresses emotional responses openly, seeks resolution to conflicts and problems

fusion. The major advantages of this agent are its relative safety, low cost, and fetocidal effects. Used alone, however, urea has a high failure rate for inducing successful abortions. It is usually combined with prostaglandins, which stimulate uterine contractions and induce labor. Oxytocin may also be used to stimulate and continue effective labor.

INTRA-AMNIOTIC PROSTAGLANDIN F_{2A}

Instillation of prostaglandin F_{2a} into the amniotic cavity by a similar amniocentesis technique is another method of inducing midtrimester abortions; it has a lower complication rate than saline instillation in the 16- to 20-week interval and a more rapid onset of labor with subsequent expulsion. Medication can be used to control the gastrointestinal side-effects (nausea and vomiting). Women with asthma or pulmonary disease are at increased risk because the drug can cause marked bronchospasm.

When used as the only agent, 40 to 45 mg of prostaglandin F_{2a} is instilled by intra-amniotic infusion. Labor is usually shorter than with saline solution, and

related complications are avoided. Its disadvantages include the potential for delivering a live fetus, the cost of the medication, and complications such as cervical lacerations and retained products of conception.

VAGINAL PROSTAGLANDIN E_2

Prostaglandin E_2 prepared as a vaginal suppository is used in patients to induce abortions and to assist evacuation in patients with missed abortions. The 20-mg vaginal suppositories have a high incidence of gastrointestinal side-effects and often affect the thermoregulatory mechanism, causing some patients to have a temperature elevation. Other complications are similar to those with prostaglandin F_{2a}.

HYSTEROTOMY

When other methods of midtrimester abortion fail, or if D&E, saline, or prostaglandins are contraindicated for various reasons, a hysterotomy of minicesarean section may be performed. The operation is major surgery and may be done abdominally or vaginally. This procedure requires the standard preoperative preparations and general or spinal anesthesia. The morbidity and mortality from this procedure are greater than for other techniques, and a live fetus may be delivered. Advantages of this method include the opportunity for concomitant sterilization by tubal ligation or hysterectomy, and treatment of pelvic disease. Mortality rates for the commonly used methods of pregnancy interruption are summarized in Table 12-1.

■ RU 486 (MIFEPRISTONE)

Mifepristone is a progesterone antagonist that has been investigated as an early abortifacient and a midcycle contraceptive.[20,21] The action of RU 486 prevents implantation of a fertilized ovum. Taken within 10 days of the expected onset of the missed period, up to 8 weeks after conception, it is highly effective in producing an abortion. Mifepristone decreases cervical resistance to dilation in both pregnant and nonpregnant women and, therefore, may be helpful not only for first trimester abortions, but also for gynecological procedures such as IUD insertion and removal, endometrial sampling, laser treatment of cervical lesions, and diagnostic curettage.[22]

Complete abortion after administration of RU 486 occurs in 85% to 94% of women up to the 10th week of gestation.[11,23] The medication is well-tolerated with fewer gastrointestinal side-effects than prostaglandins and less severe cramping. Severe or prolonged bleeding are the main complications. In a large British trial, 9% of women experienced severe bleeding in the 2 days after the medication.[23] When abortion does not occur, uterine evacuation by vacuum curettage is facilitated by the softening effects of RU 486 on the cervix. Prostaglandins may also be used in conjunction with mifepristone. A small number of women experience a hemorrhage that requires curettage and blood transfusion.

Mifepristone is widely used in Europe and is well accepted by French and British women. It offers a reasonable alternative to instrumental abortions by vacuum or sharp curettage, which require some form of anesthetic and often analgesia. RU 486 is not yet approved for use in the United States, and there has been some public controversy about its safety and efficacy.[24]

■ REFERENCES

1. Henshaw SK: Induced abortion: A world review, 1990. Fam Plann Perspect 22(2):76–89, March/April 1990

2. Henshaw SK: Characteristics of U.S. women having abortions, 1982–83. Fam Plann Perspect 19(1):5–9, January/February 1987

3. Forrest JD, Henshaw SK: The harassment of U.S. abortion providers. Fam Plann Perspect 19(1):9–13, January/February 1987

4. Trussel J, Menken J, Lindheim BL et al: The impact of restricting Medicaid financing for abortion. Fam Plann Perspect 12(3):120–130, May/June 1980

5. Henshaw SK, Van Vort J: Abortion services in the United States, 1987 and 1988. Fam Plann Perspect 22(3):102–108, May/June 1990

6. Rothman BK: Commentary: Women feel social and economic pressures to abort abnormal fetuses. Birth 17(2):81, June 1990

7. Jackson LG: Commentary: Prenatal diagnosis: The magnitude of dysgenic effects is small, the human benefits, great. Birth 17(2):80, June 1990

8. Kaali SG, Csakany GM, Szigetavari I et al: Updated screening protocol for abortion services. Obstet Gynecol 76(1):136–138, July 1990

9. Belanger E, Melzack R, Lauzon P: Pain of first-trimester abortion: A study of psychosocial and medical predictors. Pain 36:339–350, 1989

10. Darney PD, Landy V, MacPherson E et al: Abortion training in U.S. obstetric and gynecology residency programs. Fam Plann Perspect 19(4):158–162, July/August 1987

11. Hatcher RA, Guest R, Stewart R et al (eds): Contraceptive Technology 1988–89, 14th ed, pp 388–399. New York, Irvington, 1988

12. Adler LE et al: Psychological responses after abortion. Science 248:41, 1990

13. David HP, Rasmussen NK, Holst E: Postpartum and postabortion psychotic reactions. Fam Plann Perspect 13(2):88–91, March/April 1981

14. David HP, Matéjček Z: Children born to women denied abortion: An update. Fam Plann Perspect 13(1):32–34, January/February 1981

15. Zabin LS, Hirsch MB, Emerson MR: When urban adolescents choose abortion: Effects on education, psychological status and subsequent pregnancy. Fam Plann Perspect 21(6):248–255, November/December 1989

16. Osofsky JD, Osofsky JH: The psychological reaction of patients to legalized abortion. Am J Orthopsychiatry 42(1):48–60, 1972

17. Gallop G, Newport F: Americans shift toward pro-choice position. The Gallop Poll Monthly, April 1990, p 2

18. Grimes DA: Second-trimester abortions in the United States. Fam Plann Perspect 16(6):260–266, November/December 1984

19. Grimes DA, Schulz KF: Morbidity and mortality from second-trimester abortions. J Reprod Med 30(7):505–514, 1985

20. Couzinet B, LeStrat N, Ulmann A et al: Termination of early pregnancy by the progesterone antagonist RU 486 (Mifepristone). N Engl J Med 315(25):1665–1670, 1986

21. Nieman L, Choate TM, Chrousos GP: The progesterone antagonist RU 486: A potential new contraceptive agent. N Engl J Med 316(26):187–191, 1987

22. Gupta JK, Johnson N: Effect of mifepristone on dilata-

tion of the pregnant and nonpregnant cervix. Lancet 1: 1238, 1990

23. U.K. Multicentre Trial: The efficacy and tolerance of mifepristone and prostaglandin in first trimester termination of pregnancy. Br J Obstet Gynaecol 97:480, 1990

24. The debate: Abortion pill (RU 486). We should test this drug in the USA. Opposing view: Abortion pill. Keep this chemical killer out of the USA. USA Today, January 15, 1987, p 10A.

■ SUGGESTED READING

Atrash HK, Peterson HB, Cates W et al: The risk of death from combined abortion-sterilization procedures: Can hysterotomy or hysterectomy be justified? Am J Obstet Gynecol 142:269, 1982

Berger C, Gold D, Andrew D et al: Repeat abortion: Is it a problem? Fam Plann Perspect 16(2):70–74, 1984

Callahan S, Callahan D: Abortion: Understanding differences. Fam Plann Perspect 16(5):219–221, September/ October 1984

Cates W: Late effects of induced abortion. J Reprod Med 22: 207–212, 1979

Cates W: The Hyde Amendment in action. JAMA 246:1109, 1981

Chervenak FA, Farley MA, Walters L et al: When is termination of pregnancy during the third trimester morally justifiable? N Engl J Med 310:501, 1984

Cook RJ, Dickens BM: International developments in abortion laws: 1977–88. Am J Public Health 78:1305, 1988

Corsaro M, Korzeniowsky C: A Woman's Guide to Safe Abortion. New York, Holt, Rinehart & Winston, 1983

Frohock FM: Abortion: A Case Study in Law and Morals. Westport, CT, Greenwood Press, 1983

Henshaw SK, Binkin NJ, Blaine E et al: A portrait of American women who obtain abortions. Fam Plann Perspect 17(1):90–96, 1985

Henshaw SK, Wallisch LS: The Medicaid cutoff and abortion services for the poor. Fam Plann Perspect 16(4): 170–180, July/August 1984

Hogan R: Human Sexuality: A Nursing Perspective, Chap 20, pp 307–325. Norwalk, CT, Appleton-Century-Crofts, 1985

Hogue CJR, Cates W, Tietze C: The effects of induced abortion on subsequent reproduction. Epidemiol Rev 4:66, 1982

Merton AH: Enemies of Choice: The Right-to-Life Movement and Its Threat to Abortion. Boston, Beacon Press, 1982

Pannikar K: The Karman syringe in family practice: Techniques, safety, and usage. Int J Gynaecol Obstet (Suppl) 3:29, 1989

13

Management of Infertility

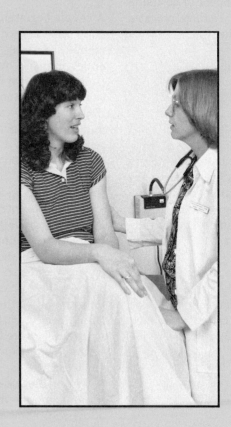

Childbearing is often considered a matter of choice. Many couples, reaching a certain point in their relationship, decide to discontinue using contraception and attempt a pregnancy. After 5 to 6 months of unprotected intercourse, most women conceive. However, for about 15% of women, pregnancy does not occur.

The number of infertile couples has risen in recent years. This can be linked to several factors. The decision to begin a career before starting a family delays childbearing. This postponement may compound further infertility problems because some disorders, such as endometriosis, tend to worsen over time. The increased incidence of sexually transmitted disease (STD) places women at greater risk of tubal damage and pelvic scarring. Men may be rendered sterile after infections such as gonorrhea.[1]

The physiological basis for reproduction discussed in previous chapters serves as the foundation for the investigation of infertility. *Primary infertility* is a condition in which a pregnancy has never occurred. *Secondary infertility* indicates that at least one prior pregnancy has occurred, but that a successful pregnancy at the current time has not been realized. *Relative infertility* refers to a set of conditions that may impede or postpone pregnancy but can often be corrected. *Sterility* indicates that a conception cannot occur, and the causative factor cannot be reversed.

■ NURSING ASSESSMENT

The inability to initiate a pregnancy is usually due to an abnormality of the anatomy or physiology of the reproductive system. Because conception requires the completion of a specific set of events within a specific time frame, the infertility investigation requires the examination of both partners as well as their ability to function as a unit.

By treating the infertile couple as a whole, neither partner needs to feel singled out. Both persons must be evaluated in a systematic, cohesive, and compassionate manner. There is no substitute for a carefully planned clinical assessment. Unless the underlying cause is discovered, treatment may be ineffectual, time-consuming, and unsuccessful.

Initiating Investigation

Because conception is the result of a complex and time-dependent process, it is not surprising that each act of unprotected intercourse does not create a pregnancy.

Under normal circumstances and without fertility disorders, a couple conceives within a 5- to 6-month period.

One year of unprotected coitus without conception was the general criterion for initiating an infertility evaluation.[2] However, because fertility declines with age, couples in their thirties who have not conceived after 6 months of exposure are being aggressively evaluated. Younger couples who demonstrate an increased risk, such as a history of STD or endometriosis, also benefit from earlier testing.

A comprehensive infertility work-up includes the examination of all factors involved in conception. The reproductive anatomy and physiology of both partners are assessed, including the hypothalamic-pituitary-ovarian axis, fallopian tube function, cervical and endometrial environments, the hypothalamic-pituitary-testicular axis, and sperm production and motility. The evaluation must also consider the frequency and methods of coitus and the emotional state of each partner. These factors and the related diagnostic tests are summarized in Table 13-1.

The Initial Interview

A couple beginning the process of an infertility evaluation often is fearful, embarrassed, and anxious. Their inability to conceive may lead them to believe that they are abnormal. They may realize that the work-up includes discussion of their intimate relationship as well as close examination of their reproductive anatomy. The initial interview can set the stage for cooperation and motivation. By creating a nonjudgmental and empathic atmosphere, the nurse can assist the couple in adjusting to the evaluation process. Acknowledgment of their frustration, fear, and anxiety helps the couple accept their situation and the offered assistance.

The initial infertility interview typically begins with a comprehensive health history of both partners. The interview may uncover factors that influence fertility and allow evaluation of lifestyle and expectations. Many agencies find that self-assessment tools, such as those found at the end of this chapter, are helpful in eliciting information pertinent to childbearing. Details of menstrual history, past pregnancies, past medical illnesses or surgical procedures, and data relating to personal habits (diet, tobacco, alcohol, or drug use) can aid the evaluation.

After the baseline medical history is established, information about the couple's sexual habits must be addressed. Some nurses are uncomfortable discussing sexual issues with clients. Nurses who are comfortable with their own sexuality and who have experience dealing with these issues have less difficulty discussing the details of a couple's sexual life. By first collecting

TABLE 13-1. SUMMARY OF PHYSIOLOGICAL FACTORS OF INFERTILITY AND METHODS OF TESTING

Factor	Test	Timing in Cycle
Male factors Sperm	Semen analysis	Anytime. Suggested as initial study
Male/female factor Mucus/sperm compatibility	Postcoital test	At time of ovulation, done 2–12 h after intercourse
Female factors Ovulation	Serum progesterone	Luteal phase, day 21–24 of 28-day cycle
Uterine environment	Endometrial biopsy	Luteal phase, day 21–24 of 28-day cycle
Tubal function	Hysterosalpingogram	Within 2–3 days of end of menstruation
	Diagnostic laparoscopy with tubal dye study	Before ovulation

data unrelated to sexuality, an atmosphere of trust can be established. Once that occurs, the interview can proceed to more sensitive areas, such as frequency and methods of coitus and sexual satisfaction.

Assessing Male Fertility Factors

Problems relating to sperm production and mortality account for 35% to 40% of all infertility cases. Evaluation of the male is simple and straightforward and should be one of the first steps in the process.

PHYSICAL EXAMINATION

Physical abnormalities of the male genitals may immediately reveal a possible cause of infertility. Undescended or hypoplastic testes are immediately evident. Postpubescent mumps orchitis can result in testicular atrophy. Blood supply can be decreased by herniorrhaphy. Decreased spermatogenesis and sperm motility can be due to a varicocele, or varicose veins within the scrotum. These are most evident when the man is in a standing position, thus allowing the veins to fill with blood. These dilated veins are thought to deliver additional heat to the testes, therefore decreasing sperm production. High ligation of these veins brings a significant improvement in semen quality in the majority of cases.

SEMEN ANALYSIS

Laboratory evaluation of semen is essential to the infertility evaluation. Careful instructions to the client will avoid erroneous results of this test. Although clinical laboratories may differ in their specific instructions,

there is a general set of guidelines to ensure obtaining the maximum information from the specimen.

The semen analysis is performed on a fresh ejaculate that is collected by masturbation after the couple abstains from intercourse for several days. The entire specimen is collected in a clean, dry container and immediately transported to the testing facility. During transport, the specimen should be kept warm by placing the container under the arm or next to the skin in some manner. Laboratory personnel need to know the time of collection because seminal fluid coagulates immediately after ejaculation and reliquefies within 20 to 30 minutes. For an accurate analysis, the ejaculate must be in the liquefied state to ensure an even distribution of spermatozoa in the counting chamber.

The specimen is analyzed for volume, density, number of mature sperm, percentage of motile sperm, quality of motility, and percentage of abnormal forms (Table 13-2). Any one or more of these factors can contribute to an abnormal semen analysis. The normal volume of a single ejaculate ranges from 2 to 5 ml. A greater volume may indicate a lower concentration of sperm; a volume less than 1 ml may indicate the inability of the semen to reach the cervix during coitus. A minimum count of 20 million sperm per milliliter is considered adequate for achieving a pregnancy, if the motility is normal. Pregnancies have been documented with counts below 20 million sperm per milliliter, although the pregnancy rate is far lower in these cases.

Because spermatogenesis is an ongoing process with sperm maturation requiring approximately 60 to 90 days, a single abnormal semen analysis should not be interpreted as a threat to the couple's fertility. Variation in the quality of semen can be influenced by prior viral infections or isolated exposure to heat in the months before collection. Normal results or information re-

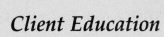

Client Education

Semen Analysis

To evaluate the quality of the semen accurately, a specimen must be collected in a specific manner. Please follow these instructions carefully.

1. Collect the specimen at approximately the same interval as your usual sexual schedule.
2. Do not use any lubricants while collecting the specimen.
3. Masturbate and ejaculate into a clean and dry plastic or glass container with a tight-fitting lid. Cap tightly. Note the time of collection.
4. Keep the specimen at body temperature by placing it under your arm or next to your chest while you are transporting it to the laboratory. Do not use artificial heating or cooling sources.
5. Transport immediately to the laboratory. The specimen must be analyzed within 1 hour of collection.

quiring further investigation may be obtained by performing repeat analyses, collected at 60- to 90-day intervals.[1]

The single most important criterion of the semen analysis is the *motility of the sperm*. The ability of sperm to move over time provides an excellent index of the possibility of insemination. Greater than 60% of the living spermatozoa should be moving for up to 2 hours after ejaculation. Living sperm that do not move do not penetrate the waiting egg.

Abnormal forms (double-headed sperm, immature forms) should be less than 40% of the total count. An increase in the number of these abnormal cells indicates a problem with spermatogenesis and should be investigated further.

Azoospermia, the absence of sperm in the ejaculate, requires additional evaluation by a urologist who specializes in male infertility. Testicular biopsy may indicate sperm production is occurring, and a blockage of the vas deferens should be considered. Blockage may be the result of a previous infection, such as tuberculosis or gonorrhea, or from prior vasectomy performed for sterilization purposes. Patency of the vas deferens may be restored by microsurgery. Genetic abnormalities must be ruled out if no sperm production is found by testicular biopsy. Total aspermia, although rare, does indicate that the man is incapable of fathering a child, and artificial insemination with donor sperm may be considered.

Excess heat to the testes, with the absence of physical abnormality, can affect semen quality. Men who habitually wear tight-fitting underwear and pants often have decreased sperm counts. The constant use of hot tubs and spas also has been found to lower sperm counts. The elimination of these habits can bring an increase of count and motility.

Exposure to pesticides, herbicides, and other toxic chemicals adversely affects the quality and quantity of sperm. Some medications, recreational drugs (especially marijuana), and cigarette smoking can also decrease the number and motility of the sperm.[1]

Another sperm factor is the *ability of sperm to penetrate the cervical mucus* and maintain motility. This is evaluated by means of the postcoital examination often referred to as the Sims-Huhner test, which analyzes the interaction between the cervical mucus and the semen.

If fewer than 15 to 20 sperm are found in the postcoital specimen, techniques of intercourse should be investigated, for the ejaculate may not be placed deep enough in the vagina for sperm movement toward the cervix. Hypospadias, a condition in which the urethra is improperly positioned on the shaft of the penis instead of at the glans, may be the cause. Other causes may include impotence or the use of positions that prohibit deep penetration during intercourse.

If a couple has a normal semen analysis and an

TABLE 13–2. NORMAL VALUES FOR SEMEN ANALYSIS

Volume	2–5 ml
Liquefaction	Complete in 20–30 minutes
Count	>20 million per ml
Motility	>60% mobile after 1 h
	>50% mobile after 2 h
Morphology	<40% of total
White blood cells	None
Bacteria	None to few

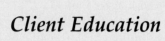

Client Education

Postcoital Examination

This examination is scheduled to coincide with the time of ovulation when the cervical mucus is clear and abundant and receptive to spermatozoa. The couple should be instructed to have unprotected intercourse 2 to 12 hours before the test; the woman should remain in bed 10 to 15 minutes after coitus. Couples should also be instructed to refrain from using lubricants or douches after coitus because some of the chemicals contained in these agents can reduce the sperm count or motility.

The procedure can be performed in the office and requires less than 10 minutes.

Patient preparation: The patient is prepared in a similar manner as for a regular gynecological examination.

Explanation of procedure: The cervix is exposed using a speculum, and a sample of cervial mucus is collected by aspirating it from the endocervical canal by way of a thin polyethylene tube. The cervical mucus is examined grossly for quality, quantity, and spinnbarkeit (ability to form a continuous, stretchy thread). Spinnbarkeit is evaluated by stretching the mucus between the tips of a forceps or gloved fingers until the mucus thread breaks. Spinnbarkeit is considered normal if the mucus stretches 8 to 10 cm. Mucus is also immediately examined under a microscope by placing a drop or two on a glass slide and covering it with a cover slip. In a normal test, 15 to 20 living motile sperm are seen in each high-powered field.

Adverse effects: None known.

The most common cause for abnormal test results is performing this examination at the wrong time of the menstrual cycle by using basal body temperature charting or urine testing for the luteinizing hormone (LH) surge.[3,4]

abnormal postcoital test, further investigation is indicated. The man may have had an isolated retrograde ejaculation, in which sperm are released into the urinary bladder instead of the ejaculate. This is often due to emotional anxiety over having to perform coitus on command and on schedule. A second postcoital test is in order and may be normal.

Cross penetration testing is available to define the causes of abnormal postcoital tests. In this test, both the man's semen and the woman's mucus are tested against donor semen and mucus, previously established as normal. Sperm motility and ability to penetrate cervical mucus are examined. Donor semen and mucus are tested against each other to ensure optimal results. This test evaluates whether the semen or the mucus is the causative factor (Table 13-3).

If sperm are found, but they are not moving or are dead, the seminal fluid and the cervical mucus may be incompatible. Antisperm antibodies, produced either by the male or female, may be found. Sophisticated immunological testing is required to document this condition. Temporary condom use or short-term oral steroid therapy or both for the man can reduce the antibody count and lead to successful insemination.[1]

The inability of the sperm to penetrate the cervical mucus can be rectified with medications or by the direct insemination of semen into the uterus. These are discussed in a later section of this chapter.

Assessing Female Fertility Factors

The woman's role in fertility is far more complex than the man's. Not only must ovulation occur, but a schedule of events must be completed for a pregnancy to implant and continue. All of these factors must be eval-

TABLE 13-3. CROSS PENETRATION STUDIES FOR CERVICAL MUCUS

Test	Result and Interpretation
Patient mucus versus donor sperm	If abnormal—mucus deficit
Patient sperm versus donor mucus	If abnormal—semen deficit
Patient sperm versus patient mucus	Previously found to be abnormal
Donor sperm versus donor mucus	Should be normal

uated in a systematic and timely fashion to determine the cause of infertility.

PHYSICAL EXAMINATION

A complete physical examination should be the starting point for any infertility evaluation. Disease processes, such as thyroid disorders and diabetes, can interfere with female reproduction. Other problems, such as hypertension, cardiovascular disease, and kidney disorders can interfere with the course of a normal pregnancy and should be evaluated.

Attention should be paid to nutritional status and body-fat ratio, because an overly lean female (such as a marathon runner, professional dancer, or a woman with an eating disorder such as anorexia) often experiences anovulation, secondary to her body habitus. A body-fat ratio of less than 10% can indicate malnutrition or overtraining. Once body fat is replaced through diet changes or reduction in exercise, ovulation usually resumes spontaneously.[3]

Pelvic examination may add evidence of reproductive failure. Ovarian masses, such as cysts, may interfere with ovulation. Thickening of the adenexa may indicate past pelvic infections and the resultant scarring. Pelvic tenderness may be a sign of a chronic subacute infection, such as *Chlamydia*. Nodularity along the uterosacral ligament or a fixed, retroflexed uterus often are linked to endometriosis. In utero exposure to diethylstilbestrol can lead to cervical anomalies.

Screening tests for *Chlamydia* and gonorrhea should be taken at the physical examination. Chronic cervical inflammation (cervicitis) or cervical dysplasia can decrease the amount and quality of cervical mucus. A Pap smear is performed, and any abnormal results are investigated within the work-up. Occasionally, correction of minor cervical problems results in a successful conception.

ASSESSING OVULATION

Ovulatory failure is one of the most common causes of infertility. Women display an amazing range of ovulatory patterns, from the expected ovulation once per cycle to ovulation only two or three times per year. Obviously, infrequent ovulation hinders fertility.

Clues to the measure and effectiveness of ovulation can be gathered by taking a careful menstrual history, by basal body temperature recording, and by examination of cervical mucus. The menstrual history may reveal irregular cycles or episodes of amenorrhea, which indicate infrequent ovulation or a dysfunction within the hypothalamic-pituitary-ovarian axis. Shifts of the basal body temperature, without the ovulatory peak, point to ovulatory problems. Cervical mucus that does

---

Client Education

Endometrial Biopsy

The endometrial biopsy can easily be performed as an office procedure and takes less than 5 minutes to perform. It is scheduled during the woman's luteal phase, approximately 7 days before expected onset of menses or between days 21 and 24 of a 28-day menstrual cycle.

Patient preparation for the procedure is the same as for a regular pelvic examination. Some physicians premedicate women with a nonsteroidal anti-inflammatory medication (ibuprofen, naprosyn sodium) about 1 hour before the procedure to help reduce cramping.

Explanation of procedure: After the position of the uterus is determined, a slender curette (4 mm or less) is introduced through the cervix to the uterine cavity (see Fig. 13-1). This indicates the depth or size of the uterus. The curette is pulled along the walls of the uterus in several places, and samples of the uterus are obtained by gentle suction. These collected samples are subsequently evaluated by a pathologist to determine the depth of the secretory glandular structure and linked to the exact day of the cycle. The biopsy also helps rule out chronic inflammation and the presence of fibroid tumors.

Adverse effects: Mild to moderate uterine cramping may occur during the procedure but usually subsides within 5 to 10 minutes. The patient is able to drive home and can return to work or normal activities immediately.

Clients should be instructed to avoid strenuous activities or lifting for 24 hours and not to douche or have intercourse for 72 hours after the test.

If the client experiences excessive bleeding (more than one pad saturated per hour) or fever or significant pain, she should notify her physician.

not change to the clear, stringing consistency that hallmarks ovulation also can indicate ovulatory disorders.[4]

Two diagnostic tests specifically help evaluate the ovulatory function: (1) serum progesterone levels and (2) endometrial biopsy. Serum progesterone levels are determined from blood tests conducted during the luteal phase, which is approximately 7 days before the expected onset of menses or between day 21 and 24 of a 28-day cycle. Ovulation is indirectly indicated by serum progesterone levels greater than 4 ng/ml. Endometrial biopsy helps indicate ovulation by the demonstration of predictable and progressive changes that normally occur to the uterine lining (endometrium) after ovulation (Fig. 13-1).

If the phasing of the endometrial stroma does not properly link to the day of the menstrual cycle or if it reflects a lagging maturation of 2 or more days behind the menstrual day, the fertilized egg may not properly implant in the uterus lining and the possibility of spontaneous abortion is likely. This is called *luteal phase defect* and is discussed later.

Recent advances in monoclonal antibody technology have resulted in the development of simple home testing kits for *urinary luteinizing hormone (LH) levels,* which is yet another indication of ovulation. LH is known to peak shortly before ovulation, and testing levels can assist in the prediction of the day of ovulation for appropriately timed coitus or insemination.[5] Urine is tested daily beginning shortly before the expected day of ovulation. A color change of the kit's reagents indicate the concentration of urinary LH.

ASSESSING UTERINE FACTORS

Closely allied with the ovulatory function is the uterine environment. As mentioned, the endometrium must be in harmony with the hormonal patterns. The uterine structure must be such that implantation and embryonic growth are possible.

Chronic inflammation of the uterus can result in adhesions that restrict the muscular growth associated with pregnancy. Adhesive disease, called *Asherman's syndrome,* often is associated with chronic and habitual abortion. Patients with this disorder often have a history of dilation and curettage (D&C) for therapeutic abortion or diagnostic evaluation followed by a postoperative infection. Repeated instrumentation of the uterus, such as repeated abortions, may contribute to this problem.[2]

Benign fibroid tumors also can contribute to repeated spontaneous abortion. The growth of these masses distort the uterine cavity and restrict implantation and growth of a pregnancy. Depending on the location of these fibroids, surgical removal is sometimes possible. Myomectomy is best accomplished when the fibroids are within the endometrial cavity or no deeper than the myometrium. Congenital malformations of the uterus also reduce fertility. Some of these are surgically

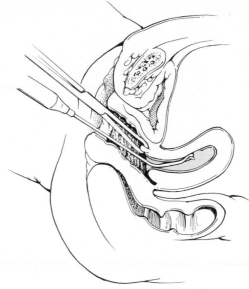

■ *Figure 13–1*
Endometrial biopsy samples the lining of the uterus to determine hormonal levels of the endometrial tissue.

correctable. Endometrial biopsy, as described previously, can assist in the diagnosis of these uterine problems.

ASSESSING TUBAL FACTORS

The fallopian tube is more than just a conduit between ovary and uterus. The tubes are involved in the retrieval of the ovum from the ovarian follicle, provide an environment in which fertilization can occur, and are the means by which the fertilized egg is transferred to the uterine environment. Any insult to the tubal structures can diminish fertility by impeding the transport of the ovum.[4]

Although congenital defects that block the tubal structures can occur, the most common cause for tubal occlusion is infection. Any anaerobic bacterial infection (acute gonorrheal salpingitis, *Chlamydia,* nonspecific pelvic inflammatory disease, etc.) can leave residual scarring, which can block the tubal lumen or damage the fimbria. The intrauterine device (IUD) is thought to cause a chronic subclinical inflammatory state and also can contribute to tubal scarring. Peritonitis from a ruptured appendix also can cause pelvic adhesions.[4]

Endometriosis, a condition in which the endometrial tissue has been displaced into the peritoneal cavity, also can cause scarring and adhesions. Each month, in response to cyclical hormonal levels, this displaced tissue bleeds into the peritoneum. Because the bleeding causes irritation to the surrounding tissues, the body responds by surrounding the irritation with scar tissue. The pelvic architecture ultimately becomes distorted with adhesions, and tubal function is compromised. Conservative therapy aims to restore fertility. This includes surgery to remove the adhesions and return the pelvic anatomy

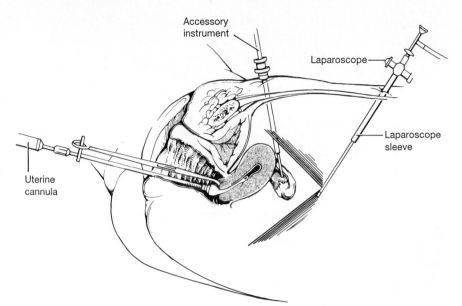

■ *Figure 13–2*
Diagnostic laparoscopy permits the direct visualization of pelvic organs. Tubal patency can also be evaluated during this procedure.

to as normal a state as possible. Drug therapy, which provides a pseudomenopause, encourages the endometrial tissue to diminish and prevents further scarring.[2]

Evaluation of tubal function requires visualization of the structures, either by direct vision or x-ray fluoroscopy by way of a surgical procedure, *diagnostic laparoscopy* (Fig. 13-2).

If an endometrial biopsy is needed in addition to the laparoscopy, the surgeon may elect to precede the laparoscopy with a D&C under the same general anesthetic.

Advances in fiberoptic technology allow the physician to see inside the uterus with a *hysteroscope.* Direct

visualization can assist with the diagnosis of intrauterine adhesions, fibroid tumors, and other uterine anomalies. Both hysteroscopes and laparoscopes have video capabilities. A video system allows better visualization and magnification of the surgical field for close examination.

If tubal blockage is diagnosed by laparoscopy, a *hysterosalpingogram* (HSG) is necessary to determine the exact location of the obstruction (Fig. 13-3).

The hysterosalpingogram may be curative. Passage of the dye through the tubes can remove minor adhesions. It is also thought to stimulate the ciliary action within the tubes.

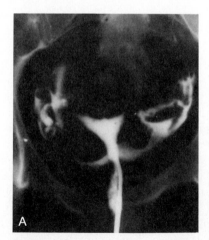
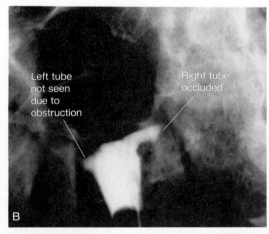

■ *Figure 13–3*
Hysterosalpingogram. (A) In a normal hysterosalpingogram, dye passes easily through the entire length of the tube and into the pelvic cavity. (Willson JR, Carrington ER: Obstetrics and Gynecology, 8th ed. St. Louis, CV Mosby, 1987.) (B) This abnormal hysterosalpingogram shows tubal blockage near the cornua. (B Courtesy of Diagnostic Imaging Department, North Bay Medical Center, Fairfield, CA.)

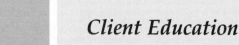

Client Education

Diagnostic Laparoscopy

This surgical procedure is performed under general anesthesia in the outpatient surgery unit. The procedure takes less than 30 minutes.

Patient preparation for the procedure is the same as any general anesthesia procedure, and the patient is required not to eat or drink anything for 6 to 8 hours before the surgery. Shaving or enema is not required for most patients.

Explanation of procedure: The surgeon is able to inspect the reproductive organs and surrounding tissue by inserting a laparoscope (fiberoptic telescope) through a small incision made near the umbilicus. Carbon dioxide is introduced into the abdominal cavity, which causes the abdomen to balloon, enhancing the field of vision. A second small incision is made above the pubic hairline through which a calibrated wand is passed. This wand can be fitted with microsurgical instruments that allow the surgeon to manipulate the organs, cut adhesions, or take selected biopsies as needed. Tubal patency can be evaluated by injecting dye through the cervix while the surgeon observes the dye passing through the fimbriated ends of the tubes. No spillage of dye into the tubes indicates the tubes are blocked. The patient is generally kept in the hospital for 4 to 6 hours after the surgery and is discharged when she is awake and able to tolerate oral fluids, demonstrates no significant bleeding from the incisions, and is able to urinate. The patient should not drive for 24 hours after receiving the general anesthesia and should arrange for someone to drive her home after discharge. The patient should be able to return to work within 2 to 3 days.

Adverse effects: The patient may experience tenderness at the incision sites and bloating of the abdomen, often manifesting as pain to one or both shoulders. The gas insufflation often allows residual gas to become trapped beneath the diaphragm, causing shoulder pain. Discomfort may last for 1 to 2 days after surgery. Codeine and codeine analogues are effective in controlling pain.

TIMING OF TESTING PROCEDURES

Infertility can place a physical, emotional, and financial burden on a couple who desires a child. By the time evaluation is sought, they have probably attempted pregnancy for many cycles and have felt profound dis-appointment with each menstrual cycle. When testing procedures are outlined, the infertile couple usually wants to proceed in the safest and fastest manner to find an answer to their dilemma.

As previously discussed, many of the baseline testing procedures are done at a specific point in the men-

Client Education

Hysterosalpingogram

This procedure is usually performed in the radiology department and requires about 20 to 30 minutes.

Patient preparation: Ibuprofen or naprosyn are administered 1 hour before the procedure. Once in the radiology suite, the patient is prepared the same as for a pelvic examination.

Explanation of procedure: Radiopaque dye is infused through the cervix and observed by fluoroscopy to enter the uterus and tubes. Patency of tubes is confirmed when the dye is seen entering the peritoneal cavity. If one or both tubes are blocked, the point of occlusion can be observed when the dye ceases to progress further. X-rays are taken at appropriate intervals for a permanent record and to assist the surgeon if tubal reconstruction is attempted.

Adverse effects: Cramping may last for 1 to 2 hours after the procedure. Most women can return to work the same day or the next day without any significant pain or discomfort.

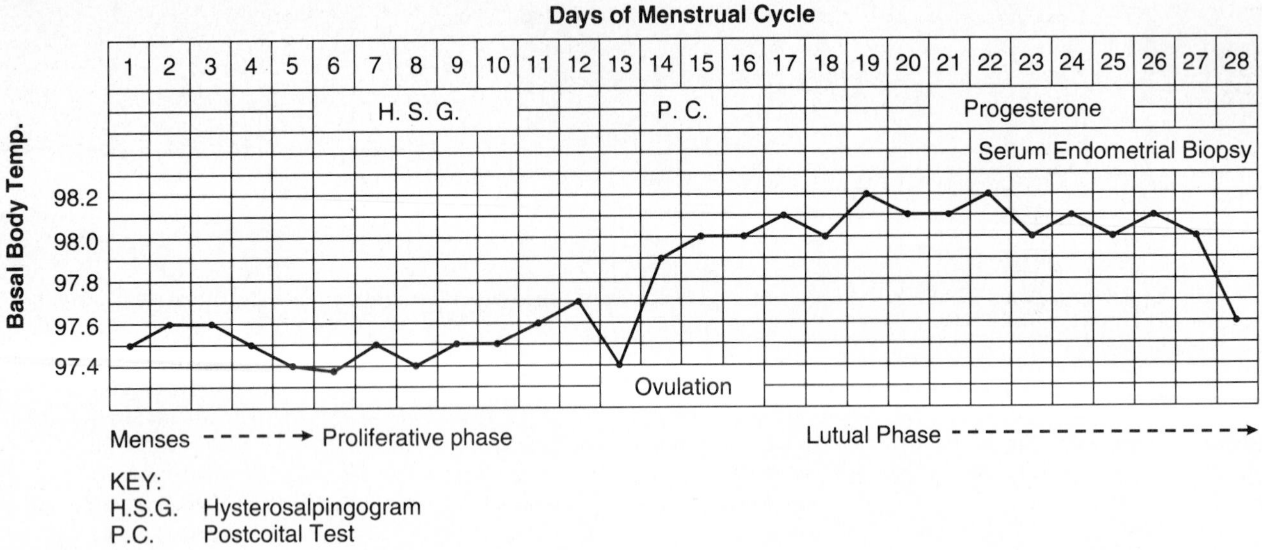

Days of Menstrual Cycle

■ *Figure 13–4*
Timing of baseline infertility studies within one menstrual cycle.

strual cycle. With proper planning, these studies can be accomplished in one cycle, removing the possible delay in reaching a diagnostic conclusion. Figure 13-4 shows the schedule of baseline testing within one cycle, using a basal body temperature chart. At the end of this cycle, all of the diagnostic data can be evaluated to plan for further testing or treatment.

■ NURSING DIAGNOSIS AND INTERVENTION

Infertility can lead to a life crisis. Childbearing often is seen as one of the most basic of life's achievements. For those who cannot achieve a pregnancy, feelings of failure, depression, isolation, guilt, and anger accompany their desire for a child. Acknowledgment of these intense feelings aids the couple in their quest for solutions and acceptance of the testing procedures.

The nurse can easily set a stage for a healthy provider/patient relationship through an attitude of acceptance. In many fertility clinics and agencies, it is the nurse who gathers the initial history and may even order baseline tests. By providing clear explanations, the nurse can assist the couple in their creation of realistic expectations and can encourage acceptance of the information gathered. Nursing diagnoses are related to the investigation of fertility disorders and may be seen at any point in this process.

The goal of an infertility evaluation is not solely that of a completed pregnancy. Equally important is the establishment of a treatment plan acceptable to the

couple and a realistic prognosis. If a couple is unable to conceive and carry their own biological child, options are presented to aid them in fulfilling their desire for a family. These options may include assisted reproductive technology (ART), such as in vitro fertilization, gamete intrafallopian transfer (GIFT) procedures, artificial insemination, surrogate parenting, and adoption.

Infertility evaluation and treatment can be a time- and resource-consuming process. This process should proceed on a schedule that meets the needs of the couple, and if at any point, they elect to stop, they must be allowed to do so. They should be advised of the consequences of their decision, but the decision must be theirs. Many couples have reached a point where they elect to remain a family of two. This is their option.[2]

Potential Nursing Diagnoses

Knowledge deficit related to sexual anatomy and/or physiology

Knowledge deficit related to sexual functioning

Anxiety or fear related to the unknown or to the outcome

Alterations in comfort (pain) related to tests or treatment

Ineffective individual or family coping, powerlessness related to reproductive processes

Disturbances in self-concept

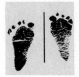

Nursing Care Plan

The Infertile Couple

Nursing Objectives:

1. Obtain a complete assessment through history taking, records, and behavioral observation.
2. Provide thorough explanation as necessary of infertility conditions and options for remedial help.
3. Allay anxiety through information and emotional support.

Assessment	Potential Nursing Diagnosis	Intervention	Evaluation
Couple's knowledge about the reproductive process	Knowledge deficit related to sexual anatomy or physiology	Take complete history regarding this area Provide accurate information as needed Allow time for feedback and questions	Couple demonstrates that they have accurate information
Couple's knowledge and technique regarding sexual behavior	Knowledge deficit related to foreplay or coital techniques	Same as above	Same as above
Couple's family coping styles (e.g., cohesiveness, blaming, sharing responsibility)	Ineffective coping styles	Take complete history in this area Observe family interaction Clarify observations Feedback behavior when appropriate	Couple demonstrates realistic appraisal of the situation
Couple's general life-style including substance use, nutrition	Knowledge deficit related to impact of life-style on fertility	Take complete history (use self-assessment form as necessary) Clarify misinformation Feedback negative aspects of life-style if appropriate	Couple can verbalize accurate information and make positive changes as indicated
Feelings of self-esteem	Lowered self-esteem related to inability to conceive	Clarify misinformation Support positive feelings	Couple demonstrates more positive attitude
Degree of anxiety or fear regarding conditions and treatment options	Anxiety or fear related to the unknown and treatment procedures and outcomes	Provide adequate time for questions Provide accurate information and clarification of treatment procedures as indicated Provide opportunity to verbalize concerns Provide referrals as necessary Schedule tests and procedures carefully with the clients' interests in mind	Couple indicates that their fear and anxiety have lessened Couple follows through with regimen

Couples may decide to continue the evaluation and treatment. Whereas most of the baseline testing can be accomplished in a short period of time, treatment may be a long process. The financial, emotional, and physical drain may influence couples to proceed slowly or to stop completely for a period of time. Reproductive technology is changing rapidly, and new doors are constantly opening for those who may have been considered irreversibly sterile.

Nursing intervention is aimed at providing factual information to assist the couple in their decision-making process and to enable them to establish realistic expectations at each point. Emotional support is critical to the successful completion of evaluation and treatment, regardless of the final outcome.

Patient education often becomes the nurse's responsibility. To inform clients of needed testing procedures, their purposes, and possible outcomes requires that the nurse understand the process as a whole. From this framework, the nurse can provide factual information, which allows the couple to make informed decisions that reflect their desires, resources, and acceptance of the situation.

It is not unusual for infertile couples to suggest and request treatment that is totally inappropriate for them. They bring stories of what worked for their friends, neighbors, or families. The nurse's knowledge and empathic understanding can assist the couple in letting go of hopes that may not be appropriate for their situation.

The nurse can aid the couple in their ongoing acceptance of their fertility dilemma. Many couples experience a grief reaction to the news that childbearing may be difficult or impossible for them. The common themes of denial, anger, guilt, bargaining, and, finally, resolution often are displayed by the infertile couple. Nonjudgmental acceptance of their emotional state can provide the best atmosphere in which the couple can grow and move toward final acceptance.

Isolation is a common feeling of infertile couples. They may find it difficult to share their feelings and emotions with their peers, who seem to conceive and carry pregnancies without problem. Isolation is a result of the couple's sense of personal failure, inadequacy, and decreased self-image. Again, the nurse can be of greatest value by encouraging open communication between partners and with the health-care team.

Support groups have made important inroads in the area of psychological care for infertile couples. Resolve, Inc., a national support group for infertile couples, has chapters around the country in which couples can find support and guidance as they seek answers to their reproductive predicaments. Resolve also serves as a national resource center, gathering and disseminating information about the latest developments in infertility treatment.

Nonmedical Factors Inhibiting Fertility

Not all cases of infertility are related to medical problems. Sometimes a couple may engage in sexual habits and preferences that are inadvertently detrimental to conception. It is extremely important for the nurse to gather as much information regarding these practices from the couple during the interview and evaluation so they can alter them.

The use of lubricants, such as petroleum jelly and water-soluble lubricant jelly, during coitus may inhibit sperm motility or actually serve as a spermicide.[6]

The use of postcoital douches or the act of the woman rising immediately after intercourse can remove the semen pool from the vagina. Women should be advised to remain supine for approximately 30 minutes after intercourse to allow the semen pool to reach the cervix.

Premature ejaculation can inhibit fertility because the semen is not correctly placed within the vagina to reach the cervix. This disorder may be embarrassing and frustrating for the man, but it is important to discover this information, so that he may be referred for counseling from a qualified sex therapist. This condition can be reversed with specific exercises and alternative positions for coitus.

Psychological factors, such as job or financial stress, family illness, depression, and fatigue, may influence infertility. The stress and frustration of being unable to conceive may further inhibit the couple's chances to conceive. The stress and anxiety surrounding intercourse and the rigorous time schedules imposed by some infertility treatments may create tension and emotional distress between couples. Cases have been seen when couples who have been infertile conceive after just one or two visits to the doctor. It is believed that the act of seeking medical assistance may relieve emotional stress for some couples. Although research does not confirm this correlation, this also has been observed in couples who decide to adopt a child. It is presumed that once the stress of scheduled intercourse is relieved, sexual activity can proceed in a more relaxed atmosphere and on the couple's own schedule, therefore enhancing the chances for conception.[1,6]

Lack of knowledge about sexuality or reproductive anatomy and physiology also can play a role in infertility. It is important that the nurse or health provider educates the couple about how to enhance the possibilities of conception naturally (e.g., basal body temperature, assess for mucus quality, positions for optimum semen pool). Some couples may be infertile because they are unable to complete intercourse because of female anatomical malformations that prevent full

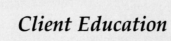

Client Education

Increasing Fertility

There are several simple things you can do to increase your chances of becoming pregnant.
1. Stay healthy. Maintain good nutrition, reduce stress, get regular exercise. Avoid alcohol, tobacco, and recreational drugs.
2. Encourage communication with your partner. "Trying" to get pregnant can become a chore and increases stress. Relax. Talk about your expectations and desires.
3. Do not stress conception as the end product of sexual relations. Enjoy being with your partner.
4. Do not use lubricants or douches before, during, or after intercourse. They can have an adverse affect on the sperm and the cervical mucus.
5. Do not rise to urinate immediately after intercourse. Remain flat in bed or elevate your hips slightly to allow the sperm to reach the cervix. You may rise after 20 to 30 minutes.
6. Maximize your chances of pregnancy by timing intercourse around the time of ovulation. Have coitus at intervals of 36 to 48 hours during the midpoint of your cycle. There are several methods to help you identify your fertile time. Your health-care provider can assist you in learning about these methods.

---

penetration, such as a tight hymenal ring, a rigid perineal body, or vaginismus.

■ MEDICAL INTERVENTIONS

Reduced Sperm Count or Motility

There are several treatments for reduced sperm count or decreased sperm motility including surgical treatment of varicoceles, reduction of heat to the scrotum, hormonal treatments with clomiphene citrate to increase sperm count, and artificial insemination.

In cases of decreased count or motility that are not reversible, direct insemination with the male partner's sperm is performed. Artificial insemination with husband's sperm (AIH) is indicated when count and motility are slightly below normal ranges. In cases of aspermia, artificial insemination with donor sperm (AID) can be used. In both AIH and AID, the semen is directly delivered to the cervix by means of a cup device, similar to a diaphragm or cervical cap (Fig. 13-5A). This is left in place for several hours and allows the cervix to rest in the seminal pool. If cervical mucus is suspect, the semen can be injected directly into the uterine cavity by means of a slender flexible plastic catheter (see Fig. 13-5B). This procedure is called intrauterine insemination (IUI). With both procedures, the semen is processed with an albumin solution to concentrate the sperm, remove bacteria, and enhance motility.[1]

Timing of insemination is greatly dependent on ovulation. With the use of basal body temperature charts or home ovulation predictor kits, inseminations are scheduled to precede ovulation immediately and are repeated on alternate days until ovulation occurs.

Donor insemination has decreased in the past years due to the possibility of transmitting the *human immunodeficiency virus* (HIV). Donors are carefully screened for HIV, and sperm banks test every semen specimen for the presence of this virus. This testing has raised the price of donor sperm significantly. Both fresh and frozen sperm are available, although success rates with frozen sperm are somewhat less.[1]

Cervical Problems

Although artificial insemination with husband's sperm and artificial insemination with donor sperm often are employed to bypass the cervical mucus, some cervical problems can be treated. Chronic inflammation, cervicitis, and cellular abnormalities can be treated with cryosurgery (freezing). When the cervix heals, the epithelium should return to its normal mucus-producing patterns. Medications are available to change vaginal and cervical pH to normal levels.

Medications may be tried to improve the characteristics of cervical mucus. These include guaifenesin (to increase the mucus flow), doxycycline (to reduce bacterial contamination), and sodium bicarbonate douches (to decrease the acidity). In women who pro-

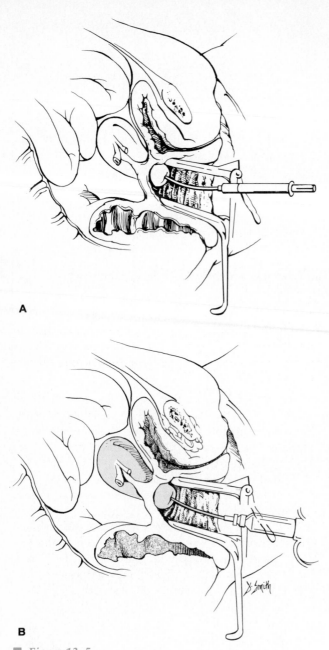

A

B

■ *Figure 13–5*
Artificial insemination. (A) Semen is placed in direct contact with the cervix by means of a cervical capping device. (B) Prepared semen is injected directly into the uterine cavity.

duce scanty amounts of cervical mucus, oral hormonal supplementation may increase the volume and make the mucus more hospitable to sperm. These treatments have limited success.[2]

Ovulation failure is not always the result of ovarian pathology. The cause may be at any point in the hypothalamic-pituitary-ovarian axis or may be a disorder of the thyroid or adrenal glands. Patients suspected of having ovarian-related infertility must be screened for deficiencies of these endocrine glands.

A serum prolactin is ordered if a patient exhibits *galactorrhea,* a spontaneous breast milk discharge. The cause may be a pituitary adenoma, a space-occupying tumor of the anterior pituitary. An elevated serum prolactin, without evidence of pituitary enlargement, may indicate hyperprolactinemia, which is often successfully treated with *bromocriptine,* a dopamine receptor agonist. This drug lowers prolactin levels, allowing the resumption of ovulation.

Clomiphene citrate (Clomid, Serophene), an estrogen antagonist, is the drug of choice for women with decreased serum progesterone levels and evidence of continuing estrogen production. This medication enhances follicular development and induces ovulation. To titrate clomiphene to the individual's needs, clients should have serum progesterone levels measured after the first cycle. If no increase is shown, the dosage is increased for the next cycle, and the serum progesterone measurement is repeated. This procedure is followed until ovulatory progesterone levels are reached. Clients also should be examined each cycle for the presence of ovarian cysts. If a cyst develops, the drug should be discontinued for one cycle. Cysts that do not spontaneously resolve may require surgical drainage. Twins result from clomiphene therapy in about 10% of cases.

Human menopausal gonadotropin (hMG; Pergonal) is used for ovulatory failure at the hypothalamic-pituitary level. Unfortunately, this drug often overstimulates the ovaries, creating multiple follicles, which result in a high rate of multiple gestations. Because of the high infant mortality with gestations of three or more fetuses, hMG is reserved for women attempting in vitro fertilization.

Uterine Problems

As previously stated, congenital anomalies of the uterus, fibroid tumors, and intrauterine scarring may contribute to habitual abortion more than to infertility. These problems often are surgically correctable. Use of the hysteroscope has enhanced the ability to correct uterine anatomy without incising the body of the organ.

Habitual abortion may be caused by asynchronous hormone levels. During the luteal phase, inadequate amounts of progesterone are secreted and the endometrium cannot support a gestation. This problem, luteal phase defect, can be treated by the administration of progesterone by injection or vaginal suppository, beginning as soon as pregnancy is confirmed. Therapy is continued at least until the 16th week, when the placenta is mature enough to support the pregnancy with its hormone production. Early detection of pregnancy is essential to preserve the gestation.

Tubal Problems

Success in correcting tubal occlusion depends greatly on the extent of damage to the adenexa. Severe endometriosis, extensive scarring from repeated infections, or recurrent ectopic pregnancy make correction of defects unlikely. However, if at the time of laparoscopy and HSG, the tubal structures are found to be minimally compromised, or if minor adhesions impede the fimbria, microsurgery may be successful.

Advances in microsurgery, plastic surgery, and laser procedures have increased the success rate of tubal reconstruction. Tubes can withstand reanastomosis and reimplantation, depending on the location of the occlusion. However, due to the structure and size of the tube, greater than 50% of these procedures fail to correct the problem.

Tubal ligation or fulguration, done as sterilization procedures, can be reversed but these procedures have the same dismal failure rate. Women undergoing any tubal surgery must be advised of their increased risk for ectopic pregnancy. Postoperative damage to the tube, although patent, may decrease the lumen to such an extent that the fertilized egg is too large to pass through to the uterus. Women should be advised of the signs and symptoms of ectopic pregnancy and should seek pregnancy verification as soon as a menses is missed.

Assisted Reproductive Technology

No longer are all children conceived within the body of their biological mothers. Several techniques have been developed that employ the mixing of ovum and sperm outside of the body with the subsequent transfer to the woman's body. Significant controversy has arisen over these techniques. Opponents state that in vitro conception is inappropriate. However, the American Fertility Society regards these procedures as an acceptable treatment for couples who would otherwise be hopelessly infertile.

The first technique developed was in vitro fertilization with embryo transfer (IVF-ET). In 1978, the birth of Louise Brown in England heralded the beginning of this new era in reproductive medicine.[7] IVF-ET involves the overstimulation of the ovaries with clomiphene or hMG so that multiple follicles are developed. When mature (determined by ultrasonography), they are harvested by way of laparoscopy or needle aspiration and fertilized in vitro with washed sperm. When the oocytes reach the four- to eight-cell stage, they are transferred to the uterus (Fig. 13-6).

GIFT produced its first success in 1984. This procedure is far more simple than IVF-ET, although it too requires laparoscopy. With GIFT, multiple follicles are produced and harvested. They are mixed with the

(*Text continues on page 256*)

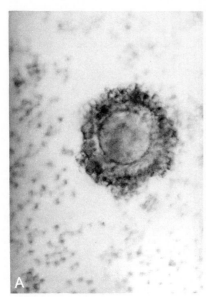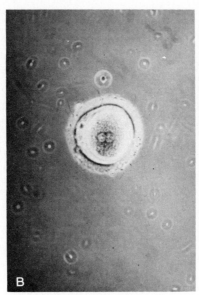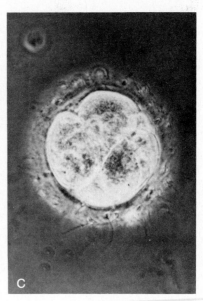

■ *Figure 13–6*
In vitro fertilization involves obtaining an oocyte, fertilizing it, and then transferring it to the uterus. (A) Mature egg just aspirated. (B) Fertilized egg (two pronuclei seen) 16 hours after insemination. (C) Four-cell embryo shortly before embryo transfer. (Pace-Owens S: In vitro fertilization and embryo transfer. JOGN Nurs Supplement 14:44s–48s, November/December 1985.)

Husband's Medical History Form, Infertility Clinic

Name: Date:
Address: Tel.:
Occupation: Age: Religion:
Employer: Ins.:
Bus. Tel.:   Cert. No.:
Referred by: Gr. No.:
Birth Place: Name Rel./Friend:
Birth Date: Address:

All previous occupations:	List all states or countries in which you have lived:

Education: Please encircle the last   Grade   5   High School   1 2 3 4   Post Grad. _____ yrs.
              grade you completed   6 7 8   College   1 2 3 4   Degrees

CHIEF COMPLAINTS
Please list all symptoms you have NOW.
1. _____
2. _____
3. _____
Routine checkup—no symptoms [ ]

P. I. Please do not write in this space.

FAMILY HISTORY	Age	If Living Health	Age at death	If Deceased Cause	Please Encircle — Has any blood relative had		Who
Father					Cancer	no	yes
Mother					Tuberculosis	no	yes
Brother or sister 1.					Diabetes	no	yes
2.					Heart trouble	no	yes
3.					High blood pressure	no	yes
4.					Stroke	no	yes
5.					Epilepsy	no	yes
Husband or wife					Mental illness	no	yes
Son or daughter 1.					Suicide	no	yes
2.					Congenital deformities	no	yes
3.							
4.							
5.							
6.							
7.							

NOTE:

This is a confidential record of your medical history and will be kept in this office. Information contained here will not be released to any person except when you have authorized us to do so.

PERSONAL HISTORY
ILLNESS: Have you had
(Please Encircle all Answers no or yes)

Measles or German measles	no	yes
Chickenpox or mumps	no	yes
Whooping cough	no	yes
Scarlet fever or scarlatina	no	yes
Pneumonia or pleurisy	no	yes
Diphtheria or smallpox	no	yes
Influenza	no	yes
Rheumatic fever or heart disease	no	yes
Arthritis or rheumatism	no	yes
Any bone or joint disease	no	yes
Neuritis or neuralgia	no	yes
Bursitis, sciatica or lumbago	no	yes
Polio or meningitis	no	yes
Bright's disease or kidney infection	no	yes

Gonorrhea or syphilis	no	yes
Anemia or jaundice	no	yes
Epilepsy	no	yes
Migraine headaches	no	yes
Tuberculosis	no	yes
Diabetes or cancer	no	yes
High or low blood pressure	no	yes
Nervous breakdown	no	yes
Food, chemical or drug poisoning	no	yes
Hay fever or asthma	no	yes
Hives or eczema	no	yes
Frequent colds or sore throat	no	yes
Frequent infections or boils	no	yes
Any other disease	no	yes

ALLERGIES: Are you allergic to

Penicillin or sulfa	no	yes
Aspirin, codeine or morphine	no	yes

Mycins or other antibiotics	no	yes
Merthiolate or mercurochrome	no	yes
Any other drug	no	yes
Any foods	no	yes
Adhesive tape	no	yes
Nail polish or other cosmetics	no	yes
Tetanus antitoxin or serums	no	yes

INJURIES: Have you had any

Broken bones	no	yes
Sprains or dislocations	no	yes
Lacerations (extensive)	no	yes
Concussion or head injury	no	yes
Ever been knocked out	no	yes

TRANSFUSIONS: Have you ever had

Blood or plasma transfusion	no	yes

Weight: now _____ one year ago _____
Max _____ when _____ Height _____

Please review the section you have just completed and wherever you answered "yes" fill in the year (guess if necessary) and also where there is more than one illness to a line encircle the ones you have had. Example: Chickenpox or mumps .... 1961 .... no (yes)

(continued)

SURGERY: Have you had

Tonsillectomy	no	yes
Appendectomy	no	yes
Any other operation (give details)	no	yes

Give DETAILS below of all hospitalizations for surgery or illness including name and address of Doctor and Hospital . . . .

Have you ever been advised to have any surgical operation which has not been done? [1] no   [2] yes   what ....

Systems: Please check those you have had.

Eye disease [ ], Eye injury [ ], Impaired sight [ ], Ear disease [ ], Ear injury [ ], Impaired hearing [ ],

Trouble with: Nose [ ], Sinuses [ ], Mouth [ ], Throat [ ], Have you checked any in this group? .... no   yes

Fainting spells [ ], Loss of consciousness [ ], Convulsions [ ], Paralysis [ ], Frequent or severe headaches [ ], Dizziness [ ], Depression or anxiety [ ], Hallucinations [ ], Have you checked any in this group? .... no   yes

Enlarged glands [ ], Goiter or enlarged thyroid [ ], Skin disease [ ], Have you checked any in this group? .... no   yes

Chronic or frequent cough [ ], Chest pain or angina pectoris [ ], Spitting up of blood [ ], Night sweats [ ], Shortness of breath [ ], Palpitation or fluttering heart [ ], Swelling of hands, feet, or ankles [ ], Varicose veins [ ], Extreme tiredness or weakness [ ], Have you checked any in this group? .... no   yes

Kidney disease or stones [ ], Bladder disease [ ], Albumin, sugar, pus, etc. in urine [ ], Difficulty in urinating [ ], Awake to urinate nightly [ ], Have you checked any in this group? .... no   yes

Stomach trouble or ulcers [ ], Indigestion [ ], Liver or gallbladder disease [ ], Colitis or other bowel disease [ ] Appendicitis [ ], Hemorrhoids or rectal bleeding [ ], Constipation or diarrhea [ ], Recent change in bowel action or stools [ ], Recent change in appetite or eating habits [ ], Have you checked any in this group? .... no   yes

HABITS: Do you

Sleep well?	no	yes
Use alcoholic beverages	no	yes
Every day?	no	yes
Smoke?	no	yes
How much?		
Exercise enough	no	yes
Is your diet well balanced?	no	yes

List any drugs or medications you take regularly or frequently:

_____
_____
_____
_____
_____
_____
_____
_____

MARITAL HISTORY

Prior marriage? ....   When? (Dates) ....

Was pregnancy achieved? ....   Any other proof of fertility? ....
....
....
....

Is sex entirely satisfactory? ....   Estimated frequency of coitus (intercourse) per month: ....

Reaction of wife: ....   Remarks: ....
....
....
....
....
....

INFERTILITY STUDIES

	Result	Date	Where Done
Semen analysis			
Thyroid tests:			
Hormone tests:			
Medicines given:			
Other tests:			

(Courtesy of Division of Human Reproduction, Hospital of the University of Pennsylvania, Philadelphia, PA)

Wife's Medical History Form, Infertility Clinic

Name:	Date:	Unit No.:
(Nee):	Tel.:	Husb.:
Address: Age:	Ins.:	Occupation: Age:
Occupation:	Cert. No.:	Employer
Employer:	Gr. No.:	Bus. Address:
Bus. Tel.:	Name Rel./Friend:	Bus. Tel.:
Referred by:	Address:	Religion: Husb. Wife:
Birth Place:		[ ] Single [ ] Divorced
Birth Date:		[ ] Married [ ] Widow (er)

All previous occupations: List all states or countries in which you have lived:

Education: Please encircle the last   Grade   5   High School   1 2 3 4   Post Grad. _____ yrs.
              grade you completed   6   7   8   College   1 2 3 4   Degrees

Date of last physical exam.

Chief Complaints: Please list all symptoms you have NOW.

1. _____
2. _____
3. _____

Routine checkup—no symptoms [ ]

P. I. Please do not write in this space.

FAMILY HISTORY

FAMILY HISTORY	Age	If Living Health	Age at death	If Deceased Cause
Father				
Mother				
Brother or sister 1.				
2.				
3.				
4.				
5.				
Husband or wife				
Son or daughter 1.				
2.				
3.				
4.				
5.				
6.				

Please Encircle

Has any blood relative had			Who
Cancer	no	yes	
Tuberculosis	no	yes	
Diabetes	no	yes	
Heart trouble	no	yes	
High blood pressure	no	yes	
Stroke	no	yes	
Epilepsy	no	yes	
Mental illness	no	yes	
Suicide	no	yes	
Congenital deformities	no	yes	

NOTE: This is a confidential record of your medical history and will be kept in this office. Information contained here will not be released to any person except when you have authorized us to do so.

PERSONAL HISTORY

ILLNESS: Have you had
(Please Encircle all Answers no or yes)

Measles or German measles	no	yes
Chickenpox or mumps	no	yes
Whooping cough	no	yes
Scarlet fever or scarlatina	no	yes
Pneumonia or pleurisy	no	yes
Diphtheria or smallpox	no	yes
Influenza	no	yes
Rheumatic fever or heart disease	no	yes
Arthritis or rheumatism	no	yes
Any bone or joint disease	no	yes
Neuritis or neuralgia	no	yes
Bursitis, sciatica or lumbago	no	yes
Polio or meningitis	no	yes
Bright's disease or kidney infection	no	yes

Gonorrhea or syphilis	no	yes
Anemia or jaundice	no	yes
Epilepsy	no	yes
Migraine headaches	no	yes
Tuberculosis	no	yes
Diabetes or cancer	no	yes
High or low blood pressure	no	yes
Nervous breakdown	no	yes
Food, chemical or drug poisoning	no	yes
Hay fever or asthma	no	yes
Hives or eczema	no	yes
Frequent colds or sore throat	no	yes
Frequent infections or boils	no	yes
Any other disease	no	yes

ALLERGIES: Are you allergic to

Penicillin or sulfa	no	yes
Aspirin, codeine or morphine	no	yes
Mycins or other antibiotics	no	yes
Merthiolate or mercurochrome	no	yes
Any other drug	no	yes
Any foods	no	yes
Adhesive tape	no	yes
Nail polish or other cosmetics	no	yes
Tetanus antitoxin or serums	no	yes

INJURIES: Have you had any

Broken bones	no	yes
Sprains or dislocations	no	yes
Lacerations (extensive)	no	yes
Concussion or head injury	no	yes
Ever been knocked out	no	yes

TRANSFUSIONS: Have you ever had

Blood or plasma transfusion   no   yes
Weight: now _____ one year ago _____
Max _____ when _____ Height _____

Please review the section you have just completed and wherever you answered "yes" fill in the year (guess if necessary) and also where there is more than one illness to a line encircle the ones you have had. Example: Chickenpox or mumps ....1961 ....no (yes)

(continued)

SURGERY: Have you had   no   yes   Give DETAILS below of all hospitalizations for surgery or illness including name and address of
Tonsillectomy ....   Doctor and Hospital . . . .
Appendectomy .... no   yes
Any other operation (give details)   no   yes

Have you ever been advised to have any surgical operation which has not been done? [1] no [2] yes what ....

Systems: Please check those you have had.

Eye disease [ ], Eye injury [ ], Impaired sight [ ], Ear disease [ ], Ear injury [ ], Impaired hearing [ ],

Trouble with: Nose [ ], Sinuses [ ], Mouth [ ], Throat [ ], Have you checked any in this group? .... no   yes

Fainting spells [ ], Loss of consciousness [ ], Convulsions [ ], Paralysis [ ], Frequent or severe headaches [ ], Dizziness [ ], Depression or anxiety [ ], Hallucinations [ ], Have you checked any in this group? .... no   yes

Enlarged glands [ ], Goiter or enlarged thyroid [ ], Skin disease [ ], Have you checked any in this group? .... no   yes

Chronic or frequent cough [ ], Chest pain or angina pectoris [ ], Spitting up of blood [ ], Night sweats [ ], Shortness of breath [ ], Palpitation or fluttering heart [ ], Swelling of hands, feet, or ankles [ ], Varicose veins [ ], Extreme tiredness or weakness [ ], Have you checked any in this group? .... no   yes

Kidney disease or stones [ ], Bladder disease [ ], Albumin, sugar, pus, etc. in urine [ ], Difficulty in urinating [ ], Awake to urinate nightly [ ], Have you checked any in this group? .... no   yes

Stomach trouble or ulcers [ ], Indigestion [ ], Liver or gallbladder disease [ ], Colitis or other bowel disease [ ], Appendicitis [ ], Hemorrhoids or rectal bleeding [ ], Constipation or diarrhea [ ], Recent change in bowel action or stools [ ], Recent change in appetite or eating habits [ ], Have you checked any in this group? .... no   yes

HABITS: Do you

Sleep well? .... no   yes
Use alcoholic beverages ...... no   yes
    Every day? .... no   yes
Smoke? .... no   yes
    How much? ....
Exercise enough .... no   yes
Is your diet well balanced? no   yes

List any drugs or medications you take regularly or frequently:

_____
_____
_____
_____
_____
_____

OBSTETRICAL-GYNECOLOGICAL REVIEW

Age at first menstruation _____ Age at first coital experience ____ Number of living children (at present) _____
Number of pregnancies _____
Number of live births _____ Number of multiple pregnancies _____
Number of stillbirths (more than 20 weeks) _____
Number of abortions, miscarriages (20 weeks or less) _____
Number of children dead _____ Age of oldest child _____
Number of births with deformities _____

GYNECOLOGICAL HISTORY

Are menstrual cycles regular? .... Are your periods similar? ....
Interval between periods ....
Length of flow .... Date of last menstrual cycle ....
Amount of flow ....[1] Light [2] Moderate [3] Heavy
Was the quality, quantity, and duration of flow for this last cycle similar in comparison with previous cycles? ....
   [1] No (specify how it differed) ....
   .... [2] Yes
Has there been any bleeding in between periods? ....
   [1] No   [2] Yes (specify) ....

Were any medications taken during cycle? ....
   [1] No   [2] Yes (specify)
Dysmenorrhea (menstrual discomfort) ....
   [1] None   [2] Intermittent   [3] Constant
Type of menstrual discomfort experienced
   [1] None   [3] Dull   [5] Cramp
   [2] Sharp   [4] Ache   [6] Backache

PREMENSTRUAL SYMPTOMS

Bloating .... no   yes
Breast tenderness .... no   yes
Pelvic pain .... no   yes
Backache .... no   yes
Headache .... no   yes
Irritability .... no   yes
Edema .... no   yes
Acne .... no   yes

INTERMENSTRUAL DISCHARGE

Type [1] None   [3] Yellow [5] White
      [2] Tan   [4] Bloody [6] Other (specify)
Amount .... Scant Heavy
Itching .... no   yes
Odorless .... no   yes
Frequent .... no   yes
Regular pattern .... no   yes

MARITAL HISTORY

Prior marriage? .... when? (Dates) ....
Is sex entirely satisfactory? ....
Estimate frequency of coitus (sexual intercourse) per month: ....
Reaction of husband: ....
Remarks: ....

Was pregnancy achieved? ....
Dyspareunia (discomfort during coitus): no .... yes ....
Does coitus occur during menses? Yes .... No ....
On which days of flow? ....
Is this consistent? ....

....
....

Assessment Tool   (continued)

INDICATE THE INFORMATION FOR ANY OF THE FOLLOWING STUDIES WHICH YOU HAVE HAD.

	Date	Result	Doctor
Basal body temperature record:			
Biopsy test:			
Thyroid test:			
Gas (Rubin) test:			
X-ray of uterus and tubes:			
Postcoital test: (survival of seed in your secretions)			
Cautery of cervix:			
Hormone test:			
Inseminations:			
Medicines given:			
Other:			

(Courtesy of Division of Human Reproduction, Hospital of the University of Pennsylvania, Philadelphia, PA)

treated sperm and immediately introduced into a tubal segment known to be patent. Fertilization is said to occur in the tube, and the embryo then moves to the uterus. Some tubal function is required for GIFT. It is most appropriate for women who have marginal tubal function, endometriosis, or damaged fimbria.

Ovum transfer or surrogate embryo transfer (SET) is a more complicated procedure. With this process, a donor ovum is used. The donor and recipient are matched genetically, medically, and psychologically. Their menstrual cycles are synchronized using oral hormones. After synchronization, and at the time of ovulation, the donor is inseminated with the biological father's sperm. Five days later, the donor's uterus is lavaged and the fertilized ovum is retrieved. It is then transferred to the recipient's uterus.

With all three techniques, success rates vary from institution to institution, as does cost. Generally, less than 20% of all attempts result in normal pregnancies. Attempts may range over many cycles, each costing several thousand dollars; therefore, the financial investment is enormous. Despite enthusiastic claims from proponents of ART, these procedures are costly both in terms of resources and human input. When a pregnancy is not achieved, the sense of failure is shared by both the fertility team and the couple, and the level of disappointment can be significant.[1,6,8] Ethical and legal considerations must be addressed as technology advances in this field (see Chap. 7).

■ UNEXPLAINED INFERTILITY

Occasionally, in spite of normal results in every diagnostic testing procedure and one or many corrective surgical procedures, a couple fails to conceive. Unexplained infertility occurs in a small number of couples, but it is perhaps more devastating than infertility that can be linked to a physical cause. In this case, the couple appear to be functioning normally but do not conceive. The health-care team can feel defeat as acutely as the couple. It is difficult to give up, but many couples reach a point where they voluntarily end testing and trying. Providers must accept that decision.

■ ALTERNATIVES TO CHILDBEARING

After years of testing and trying, many couples find that their solution lies outside of biological parenting. Adoption is a viable alternative. Although the numbers of infants available for adoption has decreased, adoption remains a satisfactory solution for some couples.[2]

Unlike in the past, adoption can be an open agreement between biological and adoptive families. A birth mother can work with an attorney or physician to select a family for her child. Communication between the two parties can be as limited or as open as desired. Agencies specializing in open adoption can provide psychological counseling for the birth mother to assist her adaptation to the adoption.

Closed adoptions are also available, should the birth mother wish no contact with the adoptive family. Most government and church agencies function with this model and encourage the birth mother to have no contact with her child after its birth.

Childlessness is another alternative. Couples who have explored various alternatives to their own satisfaction may finally decide to abandon their quest for offspring. Some find that their sense of self-worth can be fulfilled in other ways through career orientation or altruistic activities. Others may turn to foster parenting. Whatever their decision, the health-care team must support their conclusions.

■ REFERENCES

1. Speroff L, Glass RH, Kase NG: Clinical Gynecologic Endocrinology and Infertility, 4th ed. Baltimore, Williams & Wilkins, 1989
2. Cefalo RC: Clinical Decisions in Obstetrics and Gynecology. Rockville, MD, Aspen, 1990
3. Green BB, Weiss NS, Daling JR: Risk of ovulatory infertility in relation to body weight. Fertil Steril 50:721, 1988
4. Cunningham FG, MacDonald PC, Gant NF: Williams Obstetrics, 18th ed. Norwalk CT, Appleton & Lange, 1989
5. Vermes M, Kletzky OA, Davajan V et al: Monitoring techniques to predict and detect ovulation. Fertil Steril 47:259, 1987
6. Hatcher RA, Stewart F, Trussell J et al: Contraceptive Technology 1990–1992, 15th ed. New York, Irvington Publishers, 1990
7. Navot D, Laufer N: Assisted reproductive technology: A clinical appraisal. J Reprod Med 34:3, 1989
8. American College of Obstetrics and Gynecologists: Precis IV, An Update in Obstetrics and Gynecology. Washington, DC, American College of Obstetrics and Gynecologists, 1990

■ RESOURCES

American College of Obstetricians and Gynecologists
409 12th Street SW
Washington, DC 20024-2188

American Fertility Foundation
2131 Magnolia Avenue
Suite 201
Birmingham, AL 35256
205-251-9764

RESOLVE, Inc
5 Water Street
Arlington, MA 02174
617-643-2424

TABLE 14–2. AUTOSOMAL RECESSIVE TRAITS

Principal Characteristics

- Each parent of an affected person must carry at least one mutant allele (normal parents are carriers).
- Every affected person is homozygous for the given allele.
- People processing a single mutant allele do not show the trait.
- Either sex may be affected.
- There is a 25% risk of involvement of the siblings of an affected person.
- The disease tends to be rare and more severe than dominantly inherited conditions.

Examples of Autosomal Recessive Disorders

Albinism

α-Thalassemia

β-Thalassemia

Congenital adrenal hyperplasia

Cystic fibrosis

Deafness

Familial Mediterranean fever

Friedreich's ataxia

Galactosemia

Hemochromatosis

Hereditary emphysema

Homocystinuria

Microcephaly

Phenylketonuria

Sickle cell anemia

Tay-Sachs disease

Wilson's disease

(Adapted from Waechter EW, Phillips J, Holaday B: Nursing Care of Children, 10th ed. Philadelphia, JB Lippincott, 1985 and Cunningham FC, MacDonald PC, Gant NF: Williams Obstetrics, 18th ed. Norwalk, CT, Appleton & Lange, 1989.)

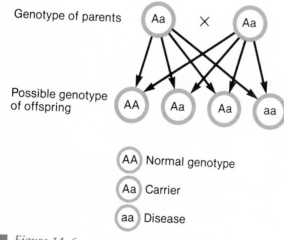

■ *Figure 14–6*

Recessive inheritance (A, normal gene; a, abnormal gene; AA, normal genotype; Aa, carrier; aa, disease). Note that the frequency of aa children when both parents are Aa carriers is 1:4, or 25%.

outpatient setting, the nurse often has brief, sporadic contact with the expectant couple. However, the value of these visits can be maximized by application of the nursing process at each appropriate point in the genetic testing schedule.

As the nursing role expands, nurses are electing to further their education and become specialists in the field of genetics. The genetic nurse–counselor also utilizes the nursing process to enhance the care provided. The nurse–counselor often integrates aspects of the medical and nursing disciplines and can employ the nursing process to design information-gathering techniques, teaching plans, and appropriate emotional support. The nursing process also enables the nurse–counselor to evaluate accurately the patient outcome.

Nursing Assessment

The nurse providing prenatal care is often involved in initial client contact and assessment. Within the early

TABLE 14-3. X-LINKED RECESSIVE TRAITS

Principal Characteristics

- Affected people are nearly always male.
- The mother is usually a carrier, and she transmits the disease to 50% of her sons.
- One half of carrier mothers' daughters will be carriers.
- Affected men transmit their mutant allele to each of their daughters and none of their sons.
- The uninvolved sons do not transmit the disease.

Examples of X-Linked Disorders

Chronic granulomatous disease

Color blindness

Fabry's disease

Glucose 6-phosphate dehydrogenase deficiency

Hemophilia A and B

Hypophosphatemic rickets

Kinky-hair syndrome

Ocular albinism

Testicular feminization

(Adapted from Waechter EW, Phillips J, Holaday B: Nursing Care of Children, 10th ed. Philadelphia, JB Lippincott, 1985 and Cunningham FC, MacDonald PC, Gant NF: Williams Obstetrics, 18th ed. Norwalk, CT, Appleton & Lange, 1989.)

phases of prenatal care, factors of potential impact on the pregnancy are identified. The nurse must not only be aware of predisposing conditions but knowledgeable about the procedures and resources available for prenatal diagnosis. Ideally, factors affecting the genetics of an unborn child should be identified before conception. However, it cannot be assumed that potential parents are aware of specific risks, and it is often only after

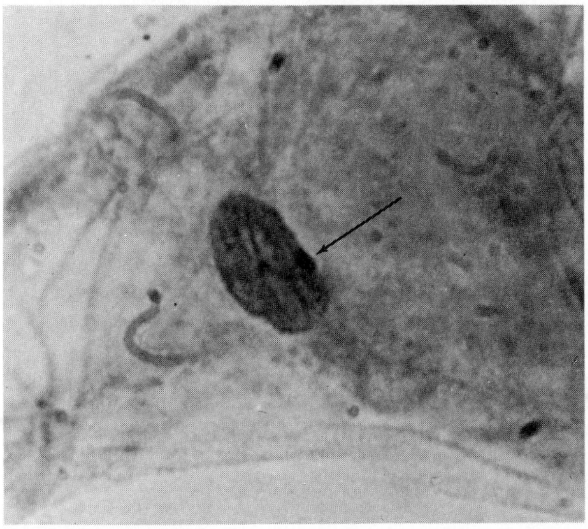

■ *Figure 14-7*
Cell from buccal mucosa. Arrow points to Barr body.

pregnancy occurs that care is sought. Timely diagnosis and intervention are of the utmost importance.

The nurse is often the primary liaison between the couple and the geneticist. In this role, it is the nurse's responsibility to assess the couple's level of understanding and to identify any emotional factors (e.g., fear and anxiety) that may affect the process.

Several factors may alter the course of genetic counseling. First, *more and more families have a higher awareness of genetic problems and testing* as genetic information enters the public domain. Families are often self-referred. This increase of knowledge affects the client's perception of and response to testing. The nurse–counselor ascertains what information the family has gathered and what sources were used. This allows for clarification and for the correction of misinformation.

Second, *the nurse encourages exploration of the family's feelings about the pregnancy.* It should be determined if the pregnancy was planned or if there is some ambivalence surrounding the event. If these feelings are not addressed, the focus of the client during counseling may be diverted and clouded by denial and anxiety.

Third, *the nurse determines how the family will use the information gathered in the testing process.* Would they elect to continue or terminate the pregnancy? A diagnosis of a fetus with Down syndrome or other major anomaly leads some families to choose to terminate the pregnancy in the first 20 weeks. However, the alternative of abortion is not acceptable to certain cultural, political, or religious segments of the population. It is important to clarify that prenatal diagnosis serves as more than a means to justify abortion. When testing procedures yield normal results, the family is reassured and their anxiety over the pregnancy decreases. When an abnormality is detected, the health-care team and family can begin to plan specialized prenatal care and delivery of the infant under specific circumstances. This can facilitate decision making surrounding interventions. Most importantly, the foreknowledge of a problem provides the family with time to adjust to the potential disability and prepare themselves for the birth and the events that follow.[2]

IDENTIFICATION OF THE COUPLE AT RISK

Most pregnancies have a positive process and outcome (i.e., a normal gestation followed by the birth of a healthy and intact neonate). However, certain genetic predispositions, familial health problems, environmental factors, and maternal influences can alter the chances of a positive outcome.

The initial prenatal interview can identify patients at risk for genetic disorders. A brief screening questionnaire (e.g., the American College of Obstetricians and Gynecologists' Sample Prenatal Genetic Screen) can be used to discover some risk factors. Using this information as a baseline, the nurse can ask for specific in-

formation related to the couple's history. In addition, the following information should be reviewed with the couple:

Maternal Age. The risk of having a child with chromosomal abnormalities (especially Down syndrome) increases with maternal age, particularly if the woman is 35 or older at the time of the birth.

Ethnic Background. Certain genetic diseases are found within the population from specific ethnic backgrounds. For example, Tay-Sachs disease is found in offspring of Middle European Jews, Mediterraneans have a greater chance of thalassemia, and African-Americans have an increased chance of carrying the sickle cell trait. Should a history of such disorders exist, a genogram is helpful in analyzing the familial pattern (Fig. 14-8).

Family History. The occurrence of certain diseases (hemophilia, Huntington's chorea, Parkinson's disease, and so forth), birth defects (neural tube defects, abdominal wall defects, congenital heart disease, and so forth), and mental retardation may increase the chance that future children will have these problems. Consanguinity can also be determined through the genogram.

Reproductive History. A history of previous stillbirths, numerous spontaneous abortions, and children with birth defects or genetic diseases may indicate an in-

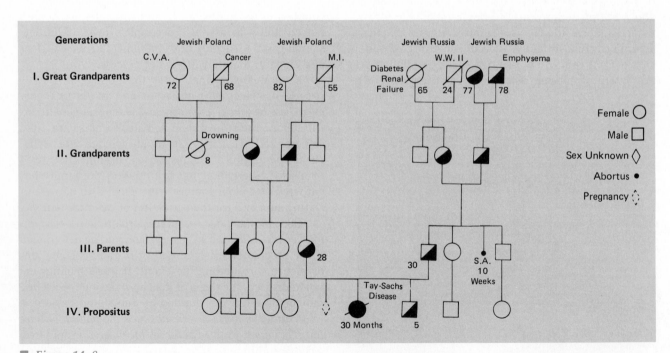

■ *Figure 14-8*
Sample pedigree demonstrating recessive inheritance of Tay-Sachs disease and the carrier state.
Slanted line (/) through symbol represents deceased individual. Carriers are depicted by
partially blackened symbol. Affected individual is depicted by totally blackened symbol.

Sample Prenatal Genetic Screen*

Name _____ Patient # _____ Date _____

1. Will you be 35 years or older when the baby is due?   Yes _____ No _____
2. Have you, the baby's father, or anyone in either of your families ever had any of the   Yes _____ No _____
    following disorders?
    *   Down's syndrome (mongolism)   Yes _____ No _____
    *   Other chromosomal abnormality   Yes _____ No _____
    *   Neural tube defect (i.e., spina bifida [meningomyelocele or open spine], anenceph-
        aly)   Yes _____ No _____
    *   Hemophilia   Yes _____ No _____
    *   Muscular dystrophy   Yes _____ No _____
    *   Cystic fibrosis   Yes _____ No _____
    If yes, indicate the relationship of the affected person to you or to the baby's father: _____
3. Do you or the baby's father have a birth defect?   Yes _____ No _____
    If yes, who has the defect and what is it? _____
4. In any previous marriages, have you or the baby's father had a child, born dead or
    alive, with a birth defect not listed in question 2 above?   Yes _____ No _____
    If yes, what was the defect and who had it? _____
5. Do you or the baby's father have any close relatives with mental retardation? Yes _____ No _____
    If yes, indicate the relationship of the affected person to you or to the baby's father: _____
    Indicate the cause, if known: _____
6. Do you, the baby's father, or a close relative in either of your families have a birth
    defect, any familial disorder, or a chromosomal abnormality not listed above? Yes _____ No _____
    If yes, indicate the condition and the relationship of the affected person to you or to the baby's father: _____
    _____
7. In any previous marriages, have you or the baby's father had a stillborn child or three
    or more first-trimester spontaneous pregnancy losses?   Yes _____ No _____
    Have either of you had a chromosomal study?   Yes _____ No _____
    If yes, indicate who and the results: _____
    _____
8. If you or the baby's father are of Jewish ancestry, have either of you been screened
    for Tay-Sachs disease?   Yes _____ No _____
    If yes, indicate who and the results: _____
    _____
9. If you or the baby's father are African-American, have either of you been screened
    for sickle cell trait?   Yes _____ No _____
    If yes, indicate who and the results: _____
    _____
10. If you or the baby's father are of Italian, Greek, or Mediterranean background, have
    either of you been tested for β-thalassemia?   Yes _____ No _____
    If yes, indicate who and the results: _____
    _____
11. If you or the baby's father are of Philippine or Southeast Asian ancestry, have either
    of you been tested for α-thalassemia?   Yes _____ No _____
    If yes, indicate who and the results: _____
    _____
12. Excluding iron and vitamins, have you taken any medications or recreational drugs
    since being pregnant or since your last menstrual period (including nonprescription
    drugs)?   Yes _____ No _____
    If yes, give name of medication and time taken during pregnancy: _____
    _____

* Any patient replying "YES" to questions should be offered appropriate counseling. If the patient declines further counseling or testing, this should be noted in the chart. Given that genetics is a field in a state of flux, alterations or updates to this form will be required periodically.

(Reprinted with permission from the American College of Obstetricians and Gynecologists: Antenatal diagnosis of genetic disorders. ACOG Technical Bulletin 108:3, 1987.)

creased risk for the unborn child. Medical records should be reviewed when available.

Maternal Disease. Mothers with diabetes, thyroid disease, heart disease, or seizure disorders may have an increased chance of bearing children with similar defects or may expose their children to the teratogenic effect of necessary medications.

Environmental Hazards. Exposure to harmful chemicals or radiation, use of certain medications, use of recreational drugs, frequent use of hot tubs and spas, and a history of poor nutrition before pregnancy can increase the chance of genetic problems.

When specific indications are identified, the family should be advised of the availability of genetic testing and diagnosis. Although most people are aware of the reasons for genetic testing, many do not know what to expect in the process. The nurse–counselor must maintain a reassuring, nonjudgmental attitude while providing factual information. Although the final decision to test rests with the family, the nurse must be able to support them throughout the decision-making and testing processes.

Once baseline information obtained by the assessment process is analyzed, the family can be referred for appropriate testing. Timely contact with the family can also minimize anxiety and maximize options dependent on gestational age. The assessment process includes information regarding normal genetic reproduction and the mechanisms involved in genetic disease. Testing procedures are outlined, and the rationales are explained. Risks, benefits, limitations, and accuracy of each of the tests are explained. Explanations should be tailored to the needs and educational level of the client. Information about post-testing evaluation and counseling also is included in the process.

Nursing Diagnosis

The stress of pregnancy is often increased when the need for genetic testing is identified. Although the final decision to proceed with testing is the couple's choice, this decision-making process is a time of increased anxiety and concern.

Appropriate nursing diagnoses allow the nurse to plan suitable intervention to support the couple at this critical time.

Nursing Planning and Intervention

Nursing care planning should emphasize interventions that gather the needed information (such as completing the intake history), increase the couples' knowledge and

---

Potential Nursing Diagnoses

Knowledge deficit related to pregnancy and genetic disorders

Fear and anxiety related to the testing process and final outcome

Powerless

Disturbance in self-concept and family process

Grieving related to the possible outcome and/or perceived loss.

Associated Diagnoses May Include:

Situational low self-esteem

Disturbance in body image

Compromised family coping

Spiritual distress related to conflicting beliefs

---

understanding of the testing process (such as providing information and answering questions), minimize the effects of fear and anxiety while supporting the couple, and normalizing their reactions to various steps in the process.

Providing factual information in clear and concise terms, answering questions, and providing support are interventions that assist the couple in coming to terms with their individual situation. The nurse should also have the information necessary to make referrals to other agencies.

The nurse must, in every situation, allow the couple to make their own decisions and support whatever decision they make.

Nursing Evaluation

Nursing care can be evaluated by assessing the couple's willingness to participate in the testing process and ability to make the necessary decisions at each juncture. The couple's increasing openness, rapport, and participation are measures of their adaptation to the genetic testing process.

■ PRENATAL GENETIC DIAGNOSTIC TESTING

Tremendous advances have been made in the field of genetic testing over the past 20 years. Progress in the fields of molecular genetics, DNA testing, and fetal

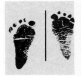

Nursing Care Plan

Families Involved in Genetic Counseling

Client Goals:

1. Client indicates understanding of the need for and the process of indicated genetic testing procedures.
2. Client demonstrates appropriate physical, emotional, and psychological responses to testing outcome.

Assessment	Potential Nursing Diagnosis	Planning/Intervention	Evaluation
Past history of pregnancy and so forth	Anxiety related to actual or perceived threat to biological integrity	Take general health and obstetrical history	Couple indicates feeling of rapport with nurse
		Obtain attitudes toward pregnancy, nuclear-family composition, initiation of referral, general knowledge and attitude toward prenatal diagnosis	Couple discusses health problems
			Couple indicates readiness for referral and counseling
Genetic history of extended family	Alteration in family processes related to birth history of previous pregnancy or of other family members	Obtain multigeneration family pedigree (when necessary, request medical records, arrange appropriate consultations, and perform laboratory studies)	Couple understands implications of high-risk factors
Psychological status of pregnancy			Couple understands vocabulary used by nurse-counselor
			Couple freely discusses genetic history of family
			Couple weighs advantages and risks for their situation
Need for counseling related to prenatal diagnosis and amniocentesis	Knowledge deficit related to purpose of tests and procedures of examinations	Provide precise, detailed information (e.g., ultrasonography and its purposes, length of time for procedures and results) in objective, nonjudgmental manner	Couple asks additional questions to clarify details
Knowledge related to ultrasound and amniocentesis			Mother is comfortable and at ease. Father feels included in procedure
		Brief overview of initial counseling (by nurse-counselor and physician)	Parents continue to develop rapport with nurse-counselor
		Assist client to examination table; position and drape client; direct father to best position to observe ultrasound	
Understanding of outcome of tests	Knowledge deficit related to outcome of tests	Review possible after-effects and complications; provide couple with phone number for an-	Couple expresses reduced anxiety
			Couple exercises control in receiving information

(continued)

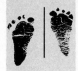

Nursing Care Plan *(continued)*

Assessment	Potential Nursing Diagnosis	Planning/Intervention	Evaluation
		swering service (24-hour availability)	Couple indicates that they feel diagnosis is accurate
		Arrange per couple's preference (call directly, referring physician call with results, or arrange return visit to review results with nurse-counselor or physician)	Couple evaluates options and makes decisions
		Arrange appointment with couple to return for detailed objective discussion of findings; be prepared to answer any questions regarding diagnosis, prognosis, and pregnancy termination	
		Suggest referral to appropriate parent support groups	

medicine has allowed the diagnosis of many more conditions than before. Testing procedures can be safely conducted earlier in the gestation and are demonstrating increased accuracy. Availability has increased. Basic screening procedures are often performed in the obstetrician's office and are part of primary care.[3]

Testing procedures fall into two categories: those that describe the phenotype of the fetus (observable characteristics), and those that identify the genotype. Although the latter is preferable in many cases, the former is usually more accessible and more widely used. Other tests include the analysis of maternal blood for fetal information.

Maternal Serum α-Fetoprotein Testing

Used as a screening test, the maternal serum α-fetoprotein (MS-AFP) test analyzes maternal blood for the presence and volume of circulating α-fetoprotein (AFP). This substance is a normal by-product of pregnancy, produced first by the yolk sac and then by the fetal liver. It is excreted by the fetal kidneys as urine and circulates with the amniotic fluid. Some crosses the placenta into the maternal bloodstream and is detectable through a simple blood test. Predictable levels are found in the first two trimesters.[3]

The blood sample for the MS-AFP must be drawn between the 15th and 20th weeks of gestation. Coupled with a precise gestational age, the patient's level of AFP can be compared with the predicted level for that week of pregnancy. An elevation of the AFP level in maternal serum can be attributed to many factors: underestimated gestational age, twins, correctable defects (omphalocele, gastroschisis), or open neural tube defects (spina bifida, meningocele). It may also be predictive of preterm labor, intrauterine growth retardation, impending intrauterine fetal demise, or premature rupture of membranes. A decreased level of AFP is predictive of trisomies in a large percentage of cases.[2-5]

In 1986, the American College of Obstetricians and Gynecologists recommended that screening programs for MS-AFP should be established with a integrated system of referral, quality control, genetic counseling, appropriate follow-up, and sonographic facilities with specific capabilities.[3] The State of California instituted such a program in 1986 and requires all prenatal-care providers to offer this test to their clients between the 15th and 20th weeks of gestation. Follow-up, including counseling, ultrasonography, and amniocentesis, is available.

It must be emphasized that MS-AFP is only a screening test. It is not diagnostic of neural tube defects or chromosomal abnormalities. An abnormal level indicates the need for further testing (ultrasonography and amniocentesis, with measurement of amniotic fluid, AFP, and chromosomal analysis). False positives and negatives of MS-AFP testing have been reported, but with appropriate follow-up testing, defects can be detected with a high degree of accuracy.[6]

Ultrasonography

Previously, roentgenograms (x-rays) performed at about 20 weeks were the only tool for diagnosing fetal deformities. Soft tissue masses and skeletal deformities were detected but only late in the pregnancy when management options were few. X-rays could not delineate fetal heart deformities, outline specific organs, or detect subtle problems. Advancements in ultrasound have made fetal x-rays obsolete while allowing earlier and more specific diagnosis.

An ultrasound (or sonogram) utilizes high-frequency sound waves to detect differences in the density of the tissues (Fig. 14-9). Structure and form of the fetus are visible as a two-dimensional image. Early in pregnancy, ultrasound can be used to determine fetal viability, because the fetal heart beat is visible at approximately 6 weeks' gestation. It can also be used to guide amniocentesis or other procedures. But one of its greatest merits is in assessing the fetus for visible anomalies.

A comprehensive ultrasound examination of the fetus includes measurements of the head, abdomen, and long bones (for estimation of gestational age and fetal weight), inspection of the thorax, heart, and abdomen (to evaluate stomach, bladder, kidneys, liver, and circulation), survey of the bony skeleton, including the head (to determine the structural integrity), evaluation of the placenta (for size and location), and estimation of the amniotic fluid volume (to determine the presence of oligohydramnios or hydramnios).[6]

With increasing frequently, physician's offices offer on-site ultrasonography screening for their pregnant clients. Many genetic problems can be detected with routine ultrasound. However, anomalies can be missed with routine scanning, and referral to perinatal centers with higher level scanning capabilities must be available for confirmation of suspicious findings.[6–8]

Within genetic testing, ultrasonography offers the advantage of viewing the image of the fetus and determining the presence or absence of suspected anom-

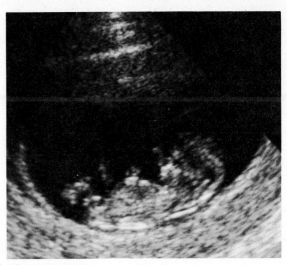

■ *Figure 14–9*
Ultrasound of fetal profile at 11 weeks. (Benson CB, Jones TB, Lavery MJ et al: Atlas of Obstetrical Ultrasound. Philadelphia, J.B. Lippincott, 1988.)

alies. Obvious deformities (e.g., hydrocephalus, spina bifida, and omphalocele) as well as subtle defects (e.g., Down syndrome, heart defects) can be detected and evaluated using sonography. When coupled with amniocentesis, the majority of genetic defects can be discerned.[6,8–10]

Amniocentesis

Analysis of the components of amniotic fluid has long been the traditional approach to perinatal diagnosis. Amniocentesis, the aspiration of fluid from the amniotic sac, is a relatively safe and simple outpatient procedure and is optimally performed between 14 and 18 weeks of gestation. Amniotic fluid contains desquamated cells from the fetus that can be cultured and analyzed for karyotype, metabolic evaluation, DNA patterns, AFP level, and a variety of other components. Cells found in the amniotic fluid are all fetal in origin and contain genetic information identical to that of the fetus.[3,6]

The list of diagnoses possible with amniocentesis has increased dramatically over the years and will continue to do so. The list includes chromosomal abnormalities (including translocation, aneuploidy, Down syndrome, autosomal disorders, and X-linked disorders), metabolic diseases, enzyme defects, hematopoietic diseases, and immunodeficiencies. Specialized tests have been developed to diagnose many of these conditions.

Indications for amniocentesis include:

1. Maternal age of 35 or older at the time of the birth
2. Previous child diagnosed with a chromosomal abnormality or major multiple birth defects

3. Parent with a diagnosed chromosomal abnormality, especially translocation errors or autosomal recessive disease
4. Mother diagnosed with an X-linked disorder
5. Familial history of neural tube defects
6. Abnormal MS-AFP level in the current pregnancy
7. Fetal abnormalities identified by ultrasonography[3,6,11]

PROCEDURE FOR AMNIOCENTESIS

After the decision to perform amniocentesis is reached, the obstetrician or geneticist counsels the client and her family (if present). Questions and concerns about the procedure should be addressed before the procedure. The client is asked to sign an informed consent outlining the procedure, including risks, benefits, and limitations of the procedure. Fetal loss is possible after amniocentesis, and the client must be aware of the chance of this event (approximately 1%–2%).[3] The procedure is explained in detail to reduce the client's anxiety.

Before the procedure, the client empties her bladder and is instructed to rest on an examining table in the supine position with legs extended. An ultrasound is performed to locate the fetus, placenta, and an adequate pocket of amniotic fluid. The skin over the selected site is prepared with an antiseptic solution, and the abdomen is prepped as a sterile field. Local anesthesia is used to prevent pain during the procedure. After the anesthesia takes effect, ultrasound surveillance is continued. With this direct and uninterrupted guidance, a 20- to 22-gauge spinal needle with trochar is inserted through the skin and into the amniotic sac. The client may experience significant pressure during the procedure (Fig. 14-10).

Once the amniotic sac is entered, the trochar is removed and fluid often spills from the needle. The first 1 or 2 ml are discarded to prevent contamination from maternal skin and tissues. Generally 10 to 30 ml of amniotic fluid are aspirated in one or two sterile syringes. These fluid specimens are labeled and transported to the laboratory.

The needle is withdrawn, and direct pressure is applied to the site. The wound is dressed, and the client is asked to rest for a brief period. Ultrasound or fetal monitoring is continued for a short time to ensure fetal well-being and to reassure the mother.

Before discharge, the client is advised to observe for complications of the procedure, including bleeding, leakage from the puncture site, fever, and decreased fetal movement. She should also be advised concerning when test results will be available (usually 2–4 weeks) and how she will be contacted. The client should be advised that the success of the cell culture can be determined in 7 to 10 days and, should a repeat amniocentesis be required, she will be notified promptly.

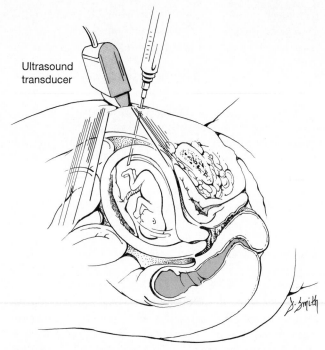

Ultrasound transducer

■ *Figure 14–10*
Amniocentesis. Amniotic fluid is withdrawn for analysis by transabdominal needle aspiration. Continuous ultrasound monitors fluid sac and fetus.

NURSING CONSIDERATIONS FOR COUNSELING AFTER AMNIOCENTESIS

After a successful amniocentesis, the client's anxiety shifts from the procedure to the results. Cell cultures require a minimum of 2 weeks for incubation, processing, and evaluation (Fig. 14-11). Three weeks are often required for a full assessment. This lengthy period can be difficult for the client and her family. Fears of an abnormal result can intensify during this time, and emotional support from the nurse–counselor and genetics team is crucial. Couples may elect not to share the news of the pregnancy with their families until the results of the amniocentesis are received. They may experience denial and increased anxiety during the waiting time. The couple should be advised that telephone communication with the nurse–counselor is available whenever they need to discuss their fears or apprehensions. Some genetics teams plan weekly calls to their clients awaiting results to reduce the predictable anxiety.

An appointment with the client's obstetrician is often planned for the time when results are available. Whether the result is positive or negative, information of this sensitive nature is best conveyed personally, not by telephone, Immediate support is available.

The news of a normal baby brings great relief and joy to most couples. They feel reassured about the preg-

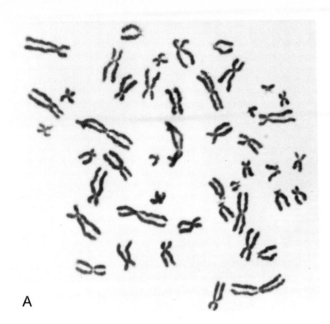

A

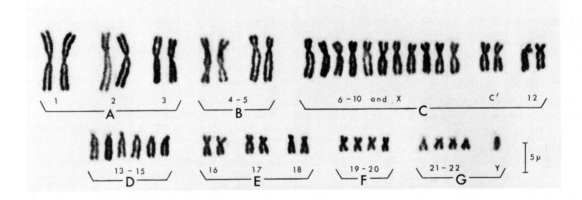

B

■ *Figure 14–11*
(A) *Chromosomes of normal human female.* (B) *Karyotype of normal human male.*

nancy and the immediate future. This is an appropriate time to plan continued prenatal care and inform the family of the need for the follow-up, because genetic diagnosis is not confirmed until the baby is born and examined.

When amniocentesis yields a positive result (the presence of an abnormality), the couple must decide the fate of the pregnancy. If termination is desired, the couple often request that it be performed immediately. The method of termination must be selected with the mother's safety in mind. The nurse–counselor remains available for emotional support during this difficult time.

It is often advisable to confirm the diagnosis with pathological examination of the fetus. Couples are often unaware of this procedure. It should be explained with sensitivity and tact. Couples should be advised that the information gathered will assist them in planning future pregnancies or aid in counseling their immediate families and their children as they reach childbearing age.

Parents who select to terminate an abnormal preg-

nancy undergo a grieving process. The nurse–counselor can assist these families by advising them of possible physical and emotional sequelae. Depression and marital discord often follow termination. Close continuing contact with the couple can minimize these problems and facilitate their resolution. Appropriate referrals for psychological counseling should be available if indicated.

Chorionic Villus Sampling

Although amniocentesis has been proven a safe and precise method of collecting fetal cells for analysis, there are circumstances when earlier diagnosis is preferred. Amniocentesis before the 12th week is not advised, due to the relatively small size of the gestational sac. Chorionic villus sampling (CVS) is an alternative method of collecting fetal genetic information.

CVS was developed in the early 1970s and became

more widely used in the 1980s. β-Thalassemia was first diagnosed by CVS in 1982, and Down's syndrome was first diagnosed by CVS in 1983. Today, most major medical centers with genetic specialty units offer this technique as an alternative to amniocentesis. CVS offers earlier diagnosis, faster reporting of results, and increased privacy for the client. Because CVS is performed in the first trimester, it analyzes cells that grow faster than those found in amniotic fluid, and it is usually performed before the pregnancy becomes physically visible, Earlier diagnosis of genetic problems provides more decision-making time for the client and allows for first-trimester therapeutic abortion if necessary.

CVS is accomplished by aspirating chorionic tissue from the placenta site. This is usually done vaginally but can be performed abdominally when necessary. A polyethylene catheter is placed, using direct ultrasound guidance, and a small amount of placental and chorionic tissue is collected (Fig. 14-12).[3,6] The tissue is processed and evaluated in a manner similar to that of amniocentesis.

There appears to be a slightly increased risk to the pregnancy with CVS. Fetal loss after amniocentesis is often quoted at 1% to 2%; data suggest that loss after CVS ranges from 2% to 4%. The risk increases dramatically when more than three attempts to retrieve chorionic villi are required.[12]

The accuracy of diagnosis by CVS has been found to equal that of amniocentesis. Although there is an increased risk of contamination by maternal cells, the analysis of a CVS specimen yields similar information about fetal karyotype and genetic structure. A common problem encountered with CVS is lack of cell growth in the culture medium, requiring an additional CVS attempt or later amniocentesis. This procedure for early genetic diagnosis continues to be tested.[13]

■ DIAGNOSIS OF GENETIC DISORDERS

A considerable number of disorders can be attributed to genetic processes. It is beyond the scope of this text to address them all. It is suggested that a current text on genetic disease be consulted for complete information. The following discussion is representative of possibilities of diagnosis encountered.

Chromosomal Abnormalities

Occurring once in every 200 births, chromosomal abnormalities account for a significant number of children affected with mental retardation, congenital anomalies, or both. These defects can be minor, major, or life-threatening.

Trisomies account for the majority of numerical genetic disorders. Trisomy 21, the presence of an extra chromosome in the 21st pair, results in a child affected with *Down syndrome* (Fig. 14-13). Mothers over the age of 35 have an increased risk for this anomaly (Table 14-4). Children affected with Down syndrome have characteristic physical features, including low-set small ears, a single transverse palmar crease (simian crease), increased epicanthal folds, cardiac defects, and poor muscle tone. Mental impairment can range from moderate to severe. *Mosaic Down syndrome* results when two cell lines are affected, one normal and one with trisomy 21. Children with this disorder may have the physical stigmata of trisomy 21 but can have normal intelligence.[1,3,11]

Trisomies 13 and 18 are severe chromosomal problems resulting in profound mental retardation and distinctive physical characteristics, including facial deformities, low birth weight, and cardiac abnormalities. These children often fail to thrive and rarely survive the first year of life.[3]

Turner's syndrome (karyotype 45 X) and *Klinefelter's syndrome* (karyotype 47 XXY) are nondisjunctive disorders that result in delayed or absent sexual maturity, skeletal anomalies, mild retardation, or behavior abnormalities. The affected child is usually diagnosed with

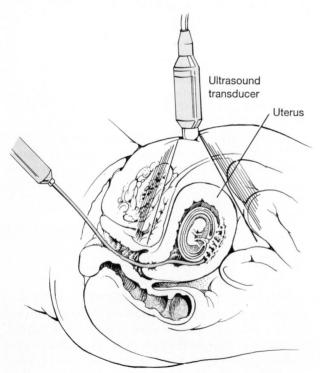

Ultrasound transducer

Uterus

■ *Figure 14–12*

Chorionic villus sampling (CVS) of placental and chorionic material with transvaginal catheter and with direct ultrasound guidance.

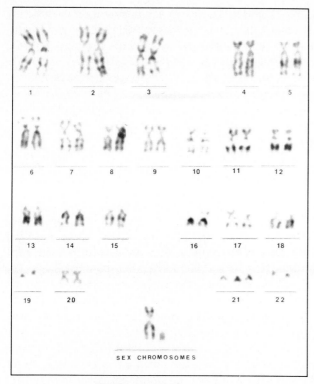

■ *Figure 14–13*
Karotype, Down syndrome.

TABLE 14–4. AGE-RELATED RISK OF DOWN SYNDROME AND CHROMOSOME ABNORMALITIES

Maternal Age	Risk of Down Syndrome	Total Risk for Chromosomal Abnormalities*
20	1/1667	1/526*
21	1/1667	1/526*
22	1/1429	1/500*
23	1/1429	1/500*
24	1/1250	1/476*
25	1/1250	1/476*
26	1/1176	1/476*
27	1/1111	1/455*
28	1/1053	1/435*
29	1/1000	1/417*
30	1/952	1/384*
31	1/909	1/384*
32	1/769	1/323*
33	1/625	1/286
34	1/500	1/238
35	1/385	1/192
36	1/294	1/156
37	1/227	1/127
38	1/175	1/102
39	1/137	1/83
40	1/106	1/66
41	1/82	1/53
42	1/64	1/42
43	1/50	1/33
44	1/38	1/26
45	1/30	1/21
46	1/23	1/16
47	1/18	1/13
48	1/14	1/10
49	1/11	1/8

* 47,XXX excluded for ages 20–32 (data not available).
(Reprinted with permission from Cefalo RC [ed]: Clinical Decisions in Obstetrics and Gynecology p 158. Rockville, MD, Aspen Publishers, Inc. ©, 1990)

karyotyping or examination of cells taken from buccal epithelium.[1,3,14]

Mendelian Disorders

Single-gene defects account for a considerable number of genetic problems. Careful history taking and appropriate genetic testing can identify pregnancies affected with these disorders.

Osteogenesis imperfecta tarda is a single-gene, autosomal dominant defect, manifesting with dental defects, increased susceptibility to long bone fractures, and otosclerosis. It is often detected after infancy. Life expectancy and intelligence are normal. With comprehensive care, the prognosis for affected people is usually good. *Congenital osteogenesis imperfecta*, an autosomal recessive disorder, results in poor mineralization of the bones, frequent fractures, blue sclerae, and short-limb dwarfism. Infants with this disease are often stillborn or do not survive the first year of life.[14]

Marfan's syndrome, an autosomal dominant defect, affects the skeletal, ocular, and cardiac systems. Affected people are usually tall with long extremities and are prone to detachment of the retina and myopia, and aortic aneurysms. Life expectancy is normal with optimal medical or surgical intervention.

Cystic fibrosis (CF) is a severe multisystem disease, hallmarked by a deficiency in pancreatic enzymes, chronic obstructive and infective pulmonary disease, and increased sweat concentrations of sodium and potassium. An autosomal recessive disease, CF is usually fatal, in spite of increasing treatment modalities. The marker gene for CF has not been identified, and prenatal diagnosis is not possible.[14]

For many years, all newborns have been tested for *phenylketonuria* (PKU), an autosomal recessive disease that affects enzyme metabolism. Dietary treatment, utilizing foods low in phenylalanine, has been found to prevent the characteristic mental retardation.

Sickle cell disease is a hemoglobinopathy primarily affecting African-Americans. An autosomal recessive condition, sickle cell disease can manifest in a wide range of clinical symptoms, from mild to life-threatening. *Sickle cell trait* is a dominant carrier state found in less than 10% of African-Americans. It is advised that all African-American women be screened for this trait during prenatal care.

Hemophilia, a bleeding disorder that prevents adequate clotting, is an X-linked recessive disease. Only males are affected. Carrier testing is advised. Hemophiliac children can be monitored and treated with prophylactic administration of the missing blood factor. Life expectancy is increasing.

A severe, debilitating, and fatal disease, *Duchenne's muscular dystrophy* is also an X-linked disease. Male children affected suffer muscle hypertrophy as a result of a defect in creatinine phosphokinase metabolism.[1,14]

Multifactoral Defects

Although most congenital malformations are multifactoral in origin, it is difficult to describe the full range of defects, due to the high number of possible genetic combinations possible. It is also thought that genetic interplay can have a cumulative effect, adding factors such as family history, chance of mutations, and adverse affects of certain environmental factors.

Neural tube defects (NTD), such as anacephaly, spina bifida, and minor vertebral defects, are thought to occur between days 26 and 28 of gestation when the neural tube normally closes. Although the exact cause is unknown, it is hypothesized that folic acid metabolism, genetic mutations, and environmental factors are involved. NTD are classified by the affected skeletal location. *Ancephaly* is the failure of the development of the skull and brain. It is the most severe NTD and is incompatible with life. *Myelomeningocele* indicates a defect in the spinal vertebra with the protrusion of meninges or spinal cord. The degree of disability depends on the size of the defect, its location, and contents. The introduction of MS-AFP testing has increased the chances of perinatal diagnosis of affected pregnancies. With prompt neurosurgical intervention and aggressive management, the prognosis for affected children is improving, but the likelihood of serious and permanent handicaps continues.[3,6,14]

Facial deformities, including *cleft lip or palate*, may be genetic in origin or the result of exposure to certain chemicals during gestation. Several medications have been identified in connection with these problems.

Extremely high-resolution ultrasound may detect these anomalies antenatally. The presence of cleft lip or palate should be viewed as a marker for the possibility of other syndromes and associated defects, and a complete examination should be conducted. When occurring as an isolated event, cleft lip and palate are surgically correctable with a high degree of cosmetic success.[3,6,14]

■ NURSING INTERVENTIONS AFTER DIAGNOSIS

Once a genetic diagnosis has been made, appropriate interventions must be planned by the couple, with the assistance of the genetic team. Obviously, the need for and the type of intervention are based on the diagnosis, its potential for life-changing consequences, and its overall prognosis. The need for this decision-making process has increased as genetic diagnosis becomes more prevalent and more accurate.

The genetic counseling process fosters an intimate relationship between the client and the genetic team. The nurse–counselor is often the primary contact throughout the process. By creating an open, honest atmosphere and relationship between patient and provider, the nurse–counselor can provide the maximum amount of information and emotional support for the expectant couple. It must be repeated that most pregnancies are normal, and, therefore, intervention is limited to the continuance of prenatal care.[15]

In the event of a positive genetic diagnosis, the genetic team must have the necessary information to facilitate the couple's decision concerning the fate of the pregnancy. If the defect is found that is incompatible with life, the couple often select to terminate the pregnancy. Termination should be accomplished as soon as desired by the couple and by the safest means. This depends on the age of the gestation.

However, couples may elect to continue the pregnancy and learn to deal with a potentially handicapped child. The nurse–counselor can provide referral to support groups and specialized medical care. For example, a family expecting a child with spina bifida may be referred to a tertiary care center for prenatal care and planned cesarean delivery, followed by immediate neurosurgery for the neonate. Referral to NTD support groups is also appropriate because they provide the practical information necessary to care for an affected child. The parent-to-parent approach is especially beneficial.

At the time of the birth of a genetically defective child, the family goes through a grief process. Even though the diagnosis was known before delivery, families often experience the same reactions of shock, denial, and anger at the time of birth. The nurse–counselor can be of tremendous assistance during this process, providing emotional support on a continuing basis.

Prenatal diagnosis is not confirmed until the child is born or the pregnancy is terminated. Careful physical examination of the infant or fetus aids in the identification of defects and their cause. Laboratory analysis of karyotype, enzyme, hematological, and metabolic factors may be necessary. The parents should be advised of the results of testing, as well as the implications for future childbearing. The nurse–counselor is often the link between the geneticist and the couple at this time and can provide empathic support as well as information.

■ REFERENCES

1. Miller WA: Medical genetics. In Ryan KJ, Berkowitz R, Barbieri RL (eds): Kistner's Gynecology, 5th ed. Chicago, Year Book Medical Publishers, 1990
2. Clark SL, DeVore GR: Prenatal diagnosis for couples who would not consider abortion. Obstet Gynecol 73:1035–1036, 1989
3. Cunningham FG, MacDonald PC, Gant NF: Williams Obstetrics, 18th ed. Norwalk, CT, Appleton & Lange, 1989
4. Drugan A, Dvorin E, Koppitch RD et al: Counseling for low maternal serum alpha-fetoprotein should emphasize all chromosome anomalies, not just Down syndrome. Obstet Gynecol 73:271–274, 1989
5. Robinson L, Grau P, Crandall BF: Pregnancy outcomes after increasing maternal serum alpha-fetoprotein levels. Obstet Gynecol 74:17–19, 1989
6. Callen PW (ed): Ultrasonography in obstetrics and gynecology. Philadelphia, WB Saunders, 1988
7. Horger EO, Tsai CC: Ultrasound and the prenatal diagnosis of congenital anomalies: A medicolegal perspective. Obstet Gynecol 74:617–619, 1989
8. Rosendahl H, Kivinen S: Prenatal detection of congenital malformations by routine ultrasonography. Obstet Gynecol 73:947–951, 1989
9. Hill LM, Guzick D, Belfar HL et al: The current role of sonography in the detection of Down syndrome. Obstet Gynecol 74:620–622, 1989
10. Hogge WA, Thiagarajah S, Ferguson JE et al: The role of ultrasonography and amniocentesis in the evaluation of pregnancies at risk for neural tube defects. Am J Obstet Gynecol 161:520–524, 1989
11. Cefalo RC: Clinical Decisions in Obstetrics and Gynecology. Rockville, MD, Aspen, 1990
12. Wade RV, Young SR: Analysis of fetal loss after transcervical chorionic villus sampling—A review of 719 patients. Am J Obstet Gynecol 161:513–519, 1989
13. Wright DJ, Brindley BA, Foppitch FC et al: Interpretation of chorionic villus sampling laboratory results is just as reliable as amniocentesis. Obstet Gynecol 74:739–743, 1989
14. Hoekelman RA: Primary Pediatric Care. St Louis, CV Mosby, 1987
15. Jennings JC: Prenatal tests: Helping the patient decide. OBG Management 61–71, March 1990

■ SUGGESTED READING

Dicke JM, Gray DL, Songster GS et al: Fetal biometry as a screening tool for the detection of chromosomally abnormal pregnancies. Obstet Gynecol 74:726–729, 1989
Hegge FN, Franklin RW, Watson PT et al: An evaluation of the time of discovery of fetal malformations by an indication-based system for ordering obstetric ultrasound. Obstet Gynecol 74:21–24, 1989
Lynch L, Berkowitz GS, Chitkara U et al: Ultrasound detection of Down syndrome: Is it really possible? Obstet Gynecol 73:267–270, 1989
Meyers CM, Elias S: Genetic screening for mendelian disorders. Contemporary OB/GYN, 35(8):56–82, 1990

Study Aids

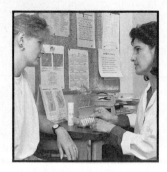

Unit III
Assessment and Management in Sexuality and Reproduction

CONFERENCE MATERIAL

1. Ruth W. is 24 years old, pregnant for the first time, and in the eighth month of pregnancy. She and her husband Tom report a generally satisfying sexual relationship during pregnancy. For the last week, however, intercourse has been quite painful on deep thrusting, and she notices continued uncomfortable contractions for one half hour after sex. Because of this, Ruth has been avoiding sex, which is creating tension in their relationship. What additional information would you need, and how would you assist this couple in understanding what is happening and finding approaches to alleviate this problem?

2. Sally and Bill S. are having their second child, and in early pregnancy they seek counseling about the changes in sex drive and responsiveness during pregnancy. They were worried and confused about these changes during the first pregnancy, and did not enjoy their childbearing experience as much as they wanted. Both usually have an intense, enjoyable sexual experience, and this is an important part of their lives. To counsel this couple effectively, what information do you need, and what specific knowledge about sexuality in pregnancy can you draw from?

3. Louise H. is a 34-year-old mother of three who has used oral contraceptives successfully for a total of 7 years. Her weight and blood pressure are normal, and there is no history of thromboembolic disease in her family. She smokes a half pack of cigarettes per day and has smoked for 15 years. She is currently taking a combination pill with 50 mcg estrogen. Louise has a stable marriage, her husband is 38 years old, and they feel their family is complete. On this visit for her biannual examination, how would you counsel Louise concerning continuation of oral contraceptives and alternative methods of birth control?

4. Aurora and Saadi are in their early 20s, unmarried and have been living together for 2 years. She had an IUD in place, but became concerned about complications and had the IUD removed last week. They are now interested in a natural method of birth control, which would be more compatible with their life-style and philosophy (includes avoiding the introduction of unnatural substances into the body). In discussing their options, what information do you need to know about Aurora's menstrual cycles, the pattern of their sexual relations, and their feelings about an acci-

dental conception? Outline the benefits and risks of using one or a combination of natural contraceptive methods.

5. Vikki is 16, a high school sophomore who is active in student government, and has a part-time job. She and her boyfriend Chris have been going steady for 3 months. Vikki has come to the family planning clinic requesting birth control pills, because she and Chris want to begin having sex but strongly want to avoid pregnancy. In counseling Vikki about contraception, what information about teenage sexuality will you draw on? How would you present their options regarding intercourse and contraception to her? What would be the main considerations in their using the following contraceptive methods: the pill, the IUD, condom, spermicidal cream or foam, diaphragm, and withdrawal?

6. A 44-year-old woman has just been evaluated for a first-trimester abortion. She has four children, ages 6 to 17, and had two miscarriages. Presently she is divorced and receiving both state welfare assistance and Aid to Dependent Children, and she has no job. The pregnancy is 10 weeks' gestation, and she is definite about wanting an abortion. She desires no further children, and had been using foam and condom as contraception. Although receiving Medicaid, she lives in a state that does not provide funds for abortions. What factors will you take into consideration in discussing the patient's options with her? Since she feels strongly about wanting to have the abortion, what types of assistance can you provide her in carrying out this decision? (Her state of health is good.)

7. Marianne is 17, unmarried, and 12 weeks pregnant. No one but her boyfriend knows that she has come to the clinic for pregnancy evaluation. She is from a middle-class family, her parents have been divorced for 5 years, and she is the oldest of three children. A junior in high school, she is not very interested in her studies and has no clear career plans. Marianne and her boyfriend Jeff have talked about getting married, but he is reluctant because he wants to go to college. She is unhappy with her home situation because she feels she has too much responsibility for her younger siblings because her mother works. She has mixed feelings about the pregnancy, is confused about what she wants to do, and has little understanding about what her choices entail. How would you counsel Marianne and Jeff about their decision making and implementing their choice?

8. Ms. T. is a 29-year-old nulligravida. She has not used any contraception in the past year. She and her partner are now interested in pursuing an infertility workup. Outline the intake interview, and discuss the preliminary testing procedures for this evaluation.

9. A 32-year-old woman presents for her first prenatal visit. During the intake interview, she states that her only son has hemophilia. She has three healthy daughters. Outline the genetic counseling for this patient, and suggest possible testing procedures. Include appropriate patient teaching strategies.

10. A 35-year-old primigravida presents for her second prenatal visit. Her family history is negative for birth defects and chromosomal abnormalities. Discuss amniocentesis for this patient, including appropriate patient education.

MULTIPLE CHOICE

Read through the entire question and place your answer on the line to the right.

1. Cervical mucus is not receptive to spermatozoa when it is
   A. Clear, abundant, and acellular
   B. Turbid and thick
   C. Under the influence of progesterone
   D. Under the influence of estrogen
   Select the number corresponding to the correct letters.
   1. A and C
   2. A and D
   3. B and C
   4. B and D   ____

2. A pituitary tumor should be suspected and ruled out in the patient with amenorrhea who exhibits
   A. Elevated levels of FSH and LH
   B. Elevated prolactin levels
   C. Low estrogen levels
   D. Pregnanediol in the urine   ____

3. A 35-year-old nulligravida has had unprotected intercourse for 10 months. She and her husband both want a pregnancy. She should be told
   A. Not to worry; it will happen in time
   B. To consider having a fertility investigation if pregnancy does not ensue soon
   C. That patients over 35 years of age have a higher incidence of children affected by Down's syndrome, and that therefore, pregnancy is unwise   ____

4. The maternity nurse without training in sex therapy can most effectively intervene in which type of sexual problem?
   A. Knowledge problems
   B. Relationship problems
   C. Attitudinal problems   ____

5. Sexual responsiveness might decrease during early to mid pregnancy because of
   A. Physiological changes (e.g., nausea, fatigue)
   B. Increased pelvic vascularity and vasocongestion
   C. Heightened sensual responsiveness   ____

6. Intercourse should be avoided during pregnancy
   A. After the seventh month
   B. When the uterus is large enough to press on the vena cava
   C. If vaginal bleeding or loss of amniotic fluid occurs
   D. If cramping occurs   ____

7. Intercourse should be resumed after delivery
   A. Following the 6-week check-up
   B. When bleeding has ceased and intercourse is comfortable
   C. When the physician permits it   ____

8. Couples who fear harming the fetus by pressure or crushing during intercourse in later pregnancy can be advised
   A. To avoid intercourse after 6 to 7 months' gestation
   B. To use the side position for intercourse
   C. To use noncoital methods   ____

9. Physiologic causes of postpartal dyspareunia or lack of arousal include all but which of the following?
   A. Low levels of steroid hormones
   B. Perineal tenderness due to episiotomy or lacerations
   C. Fatigue and lack of sleep
   D. Postpartal diuresis   ____

10. In discussing contraceptive effectiveness, the method's lowest observed failure rate, when used perfectly and understood completely, is called
    A. Maximal (theoretical) effectiveness
    B. Typical (use) effectiveness   ____

11. Ethical contraceptive counseling requires the nurse to
    A. Quote effectiveness data for all methods using only one type of failure rate
    B. Quote maximal rates for the more effective methods and typical rates for the less effective methods
    C. Avoid quoting any type of failure rates and letting the client follow her or his own inclinations   ____

12. Which of these statements is not a component of informed consent?
    A. Discussing benefits and risks of the methods being considered
    B. Discussing alternative methods
    C. Encouraging the client to ask questions
    D. Assuring that the client may stop using a method at any time without penalty

E. Explaining how to use the method
F. Discussing results expected by using the method
G. Written documentation in the chart
H. Written, signed client consent form
I. All of these are components of informed consent ____

13. Which of these statements is accurate regarding contraceptives for minors?
A. It is illegal to provide contraceptives to minors.
B. Minors may receive contraceptives only after pregnancy or abortion.
C. Minors have a constitutional right to contraception. ____

14. Absolute contraindications to use of oral contraceptives include all but which of the following?
A. Thromboembolic disorders
B. Migraine headaches
C. Pregnancy
D. Malignancy of breast or reproductive tract ____

15. Life-threatening side-effects of oral contraceptives include
A. Edema, headaches, weight gain
B. Vaginal spotting and amenorrhea
C. Thrombosis or embolus
D. Liver adenomas ____

16. The risk of cardiovascular complications, particularly fatal heart attacks and strokes, is substantially increased in women using oral contraceptives who
A. Use alcohol moderately (two drinks per day)
B. Are over age 30 to 35
C. Smoke heavily (15 or more cigarettes daily)
D. Do not exercise regularly
E. Are hypertensive
Select the number corresponding to the correct letters.
1. A, B, and C
2. B, C, and D
3. B, C, and E
4. B, C, D, and E
5. All of the above ____

17. Major contraindications to IUD insertion include all but which of the following?
A. Small uterus (sounds less than 6 cm)
B. Acute or chronic pelvic infection
C. Pregnancy
D. Uterine myomas ____

18. The most common life-threatening complication of IUDs is
A. Increased bleeding
B. Pelvic infection
C. Uterine perforation
D. Thrombosis ____

19. The contraceptive of choice for short-term use during the first 6 weeks postpartum or for 2 to 4 weeks after IUD insertion or beginning oral contraceptives is

A. Abstinence
B. Withdrawal
C. Jellies, creams, or foams
D. Fertility awareness methods ____

20. The rationale underlying natural methods of birth control based on fertility awareness includes which of the following?
A. With regular menses, ovulation occurs at approximately the same time in each cycle.
B. The ovum remains fertile for about 48 hours and sperm are viable for about 3 to 5 days.
C. Abstinence can occur during a calculated fertile period to prevent pregnancy.
D. Intercourse is safe during the prefertile and postfertile phases.
E. Intercourse is safe only during the postfertile phase.
Select the number corresponding to the correct letters.
1. A, B, C, and D
2. A, B, C, and E ____

21. The occurrence of ovulation is documented by
A. An elevated serum progesterone during the luteal phase
B. A decreased serum progesterone during the secretory phase
C. Thick cloudy cervical mucus
D. Thin clear cervical mucus
Select the number corresponding to the correct letters.
1. A and C
2. A and D
3. B and C
4. B and D ____

22. Tubal occlusion may result from
A. Prior pelvic infections
B. Endometriosis
C. Prior pelvic surgery
D. Congenital abnormalities
Select the number corresponding to the correct letters.
1. A and B
2. B and C
3. A, C, and D
4. All of the above ____

23. Maternal serum alpha-fetoprotein
A. Can diagnose neural tube defects
B. Can diagnose chromosomal abnormalities
C. Is dependent on accurate pregnancy dating
D. Can only be performed during a specific time period
Select the number corresponding to the correct letters.
1. A and C
2. B and D
3. C and D
4. B and C ____

24. Some of the indications for amniocentesis are
A. Maternal age of 35 or older at the time of the birth

B. Parents' need or desire to know the sex of the unborn child
C. Previous birth of a child with a chromosomal abnormality or major multiple birth defects
D. Mother with a history of gestational diabetes
E. Parent with a diagnosed chromosomal abnormality, especially translocation errors or autosomal recessive disease
F. Mother diagnosed with an x-linked disorder
G. Abnormal MS–AFP level in the current pregnancy
H. Fetal abnormalities identified by ultrasonography

Select the number corresponding to the correct letters.
1. A, B, C, D, E, F
2. A, C, E, F, G, H
3. B, C, D, E, F, G
4. A, D, E, F, G, H   ____

DISCUSSION

21. What preparation is necessary for the maternity nurse to provide basic sexual counseling to pregnant families?

22. What areas should be covered in taking a sexual history? What areas should be covered in taking a sexual history during pregnancy?

23. What are the common dysfunctional sexual problems during pregnancy?

24. What general principles would you discuss with parents who are concerned about how to respond to their children's questions about sex?

25. Discuss four reasons why a woman might want to terminate her pregnancy.

26. What have been three findings of studies on the psychological sequela of abortions?

UNIT IV

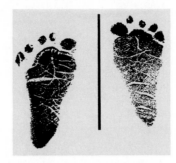

Assessment and Management in the Antepartum Period

15

Biophysical Aspects of Normal Pregnancy

SIGNS AND SYMPTOMS OF PREGNANCY

PHYSIOLOGICAL CHANGES OF PREGNANCY

16

Psychosocial Aspects of Pregnancy

CULTURAL INFLUENCES ON PERCEPTIONS OF PREGNANCY

PREGNANCY IN THE AMERICAN CULTURE

THE MEANING AND EFFECT OF PREGNANCY ON THE COUPLE

APPLYING THE NURSING PROCESS TO THE PSYCHOSOCIAL ASPECTS OF NORMAL PREGNANCY

17

Education for Pregnancy and Parenthood

FACTORS IN PARENT EDUCATION

TYPES OF EDUCATION FOR PREGNANCY, LABOR, AND POSTPARTUM

COMFORT DURING PREGNANCY

EXERCISE DURING PREGNANCY

PREPARATION FOR LABOR AND BIRTH

POSTPARTUM TEACHING

18

Nutritional Care in Pregnancy

IMPORTANCE OF NUTRITION DURING PREGNANCY

ASSESSMENT

NURSING DIAGNOSIS

PLANNING AND INTERVENTION: DIETARY COUNSELING

EVALUATION

19

Nursing Care in the Antepartal Period

INITIAL PRENATAL VISIT

RETURN VISITS

GENERAL HEALTH MAINTENANCE IN PREGNANCY

NURSING MANAGEMENT OF MINOR DISCOMFORTS

DRUG USE DURING PREGNANCY

PREPARATIONS FOR THE BABY

15

Biophysical Aspects of Normal Pregnancy

SIGNS AND SYMPTOMS OF PREGNANCY
Presumptive Signs
  Menstrual Suppression
  Nausea and Vomiting
  Frequent Urination
  Breast Changes
  "Quickening"
  Vaginal Changes
  Skin Changes

Probable Signs
  Abdominal Changes
  Changes in the Uterus
  Fetal Outline
  Cervical Changes
  Braxton Hicks Contractions
  Pregnancy Tests
Positive Signs
  Fetal Heart Sounds

Fetal Movements Felt by Examiner
  Roentgenogram
  Sonography
PHYSIOLOGICAL CHANGES OF PREGNANCY
Bodily Changes Associated with Uterine Growth
  Effects on Posture

Changes in the Body Systems
  Metabolic Changes
  Circulatory Changes
  Respiratory Changes
  Gastrointestinal Changes
  Urinary and Renal Changes
  Endocrine Changes
Immunological Response in Pregnancy

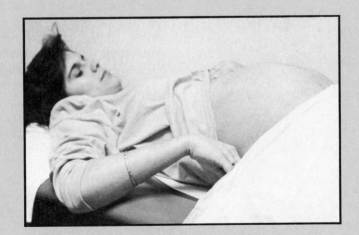

From a biological point of view, pregnancy and labor represent the primary function of the female reproductive system and should be considered a normal process. Knowledge of human reproduction, which was presented in the previous unit, is essential to the understanding of this phase of the reproductive process.

The length of human pregnancy varies greatly, but the average duration, counted from the time of conception, is approximately 267 days or 38 weeks (see Chap. 10).

Many changes in maternal physiology occur during pregnancy. These adaptations to pregnancy, although most apparent in the reproductive organs, involve other body systems as well. In addition to these physical changes, the expectant mother usually has many emotional adjustments to make; these are discussed Chapter 16.

■ SIGNS AND SYMPTOMS OF PREGNANCY

The expectant mother's first visit to a physician is usually prompted by the query, "Am I really pregnant?" Oddly

---

Important Definitions

Gravida. A women who is or has been pregnant

Primigravida. A woman pregnant for the first time

Primipara. A woman who has given birth once to a fetus that has reached the stage of viability

Multipara. A woman who has had two or more pregnancies to the stage of viability

Para I. A primipara

Para II. A woman who has had two children of viable age (and so on up numerically; para III, para IV, and so forth)

The term *gravida* refers to a pregnant woman, regardless of the duration of pregnancy. In reference it includes the present pregnancy. The term *para* refers to past pregnancies that have produced an infant of viable age, whether or not the infant is dead or alive at birth. The terms *gravida* and *para* refer to pregnancies, not to fetuses.

In many centers, it is customary to describe the past obstetrical history with a series of digits connected by dashes. The first digit refers to the number of term infants delivered, the second to the number of premature infants delivered, the third to the number of abortions, and the fourth to the number of children currently alive.

Signs and Symptoms in Pregnancy

A. Presumptive signs
   1. Menstrual suppression
   2. Nausea, vomiting, and "morning sickness"
   3. Frequency of micturition
   4. Tenderness and fullness of the breasts, breast pigmentation, and discharge
   5. "Quickening"
   6. Dark blue discoloration of the vaginal mucous membrane (Chadwick's sign)
   7. Pigmentation of the skin and abdominal striae
B. Probable signs
   1. Enlargement of the abdomen
   2. Changes in the size, shape, and consistency of the uterus (Hegar's sign)
   3. Fetal outline, distinguished by abdominal palpation and detection of a fetal part vaginally by ballottement
   4. Changes in the cervix
   5. Braxton Hicks contractions
   6. Positive pregnancy test
C. Positive signs
   1. Fetal heart sounds
   2. Fetal movements felt by examiner
   3. Roentgenogram—outline of fetal skeleton
   4. Ultrasonographic demonstration of the presence of a conceptus

---

enough, this is one question that is difficult to answer. The initial pelvic examination rarely reveals clear-cut evidence of pregnancy until two menstrual periods have been missed. However, the availability of rapid, accurate, and easy-to-perform pregnancy tests has markedly improved the ability to substantiate the diagnosis.

Certain signs are absolutely indicative of pregnancy, but even these may be absent if the fetus has died in the uterus. Some so-called positive signs are not present until the middle of gestation, and by that time the diagnosis of pregnancy can be made without them by the "circumstantial evidence" of a combination of earlier and less significant symptoms. The signs of pregnancy are usually divided into three groups: presumptive, probable, and positive.

Presumptive Signs

MENSTRUAL SUPPRESSION

In a healthy woman who has previously menstruated regularly, cessation of menstruation strongly suggests pregnancy. However, not until the date of the expected period has been passed by 10 days or more can any reliance be put on this symptom. When the second period is also missed, the probability becomes stronger.

Although cessation of menstruation is the earliest and one of the most important symptoms of pregnancy, it should be noted that pregnancy may occur without prior menstruation and that, occasionally, menstrual periods may continue after conception. An example of the former circumstance is noted in certain cultures in which girls marry at an early age; here pregnancy may occur before the menstrual periods are established. Nursing mothers, who usually do not menstruate during the period of lactation, may conceive at this time from the first postpartum ovulation. More rarely, women who think they have passed the menopause are startled to find themselves pregnant.

Conversely, it is not uncommon for a woman to have one or two periods after conception, but almost without exception these are brief and scant. In such cases, the first period ordinarily lasts 2 days instead of the usual 5 days, and the next lasts only a few hours.

Although some women claim that they menstruated every month throughout pregnancy, these claims are of questionable authenticity and can probably be ascribed to some abnormality of the reproductive organs. Vaginal bleeding at any time during pregnancy should be regarded as abnormal and should be reported at once.

Absence of menstruation may result from a number of conditions other than pregnancy. Any condition that affects the function of the central nervous system (CNS)-hypothalamic-pituitary-ovarian-endocrine axis may cause amenorrhea. Probably one of the most common causes of delay in the onset of the period is due to psychological influence. In addition, certain chronic systemic diseases, such as tuberculosis, advanced thyroid disease, chronic malnutrition, and neoplasms, may be associated with amenorrhea. Amenorrhea may also occur as a result of sustained strenuous exertion and is often seen among female athletes such as marathon runners, ballerinas, and competition swimmers. Women with eating disorders such as anorexia or bulimia not infrequently experience amenorrhea.[1]

NAUSEA AND VOMITING

Approximately half of pregnant women suffer no nausea during the early part of pregnancy; the other half do experience varying degrees of nausea. Of these, perhaps one third experience some vomiting. *Morning sickness* usually occurs in the early part of the day and subsides in a few hours, although it may persist longer or may occur at other times. When morning sickness occurs, it usually begins about 2 weeks after the first missed menstrual period and subsides spontaneously 6 or 8 weeks later.

Because this symptom is present in many other conditions, such as ordinary indigestion, it is of no diagnostic value unless it is associated with other evidence of pregnancy. When the vomiting is excessive, lasts beyond the fourth month, begins in the later months, or affects the general health, it must be regarded as pathological. Such conditions, termed *hyperemesis gravidarum* or pernicious vomiting, are discussed in Chapter 38.

FREQUENT URINATION

The sensation of bladder irritability with frequency of urination may be one of the earliest symptoms of pregnancy. Early effects of hormonal changes cause increased sensitivity in the lower bladder and trigone. The growing uterus, which stretches the base of the bladder, and the hormonal effects result in a sensation that resembles the one felt when the bladder wall is distended with urine. As pregnancy progresses, these hormonal effects are less noticeable and the uterus rises out of the pelvis, and the frequent desire to urinate subsides. Later on, however, the symptom is likely to return, because during the last weeks of pregnancy the head of the fetus may press against the bladder and give rise to similar sensations of bladder fullness and irritability.

Although frequency of urination may be bothersome or inconvenient, pregnant women need to drink substantial amounts of fluids and to void often enough to keep the bladder from becoming overdistended. Dehydration and urinary stasis from infrequent voiding predispose pregnant women to urinary tract infections.

BREAST CHANGES

Temporary enlargement of the breasts, with sensations of weight, tenderness, and fullness, are noted by most women before their menstrual periods. The earliest breast changes of pregnancy are exaggerations of these changes. After the second month, the breasts begin to become larger, firmer, and more tender (Fig. 15-1). Sensations of stretching and fullness, accompanied by tingling in the breasts and in the nipples, often develop. Many women also experience a throbbing sensation in the breasts. As pregnancy progresses, the nipple and the elevated, pigmented area immediately around it, the *areola*, become darker. The areola tends to become puffy, and its diameter, which in the nulligravida rarely exceeds 3 cm (1½ in), gradually widens to reach 5 or 6 cm (2–3 in). Small sebaceous glands embedded in the areola enlarge during pregnancy and appear as slight protuberances or follicles.

In a few women, patches of brownish discoloration appear on the normal skin immediately surrounding the areola. This discoloration is known as the secondary areola and is a sign of pregnancy, provided the woman has never nursed an infant.

With the increasing growth and activity of the breasts, a richer blood supply is needed; consequently,

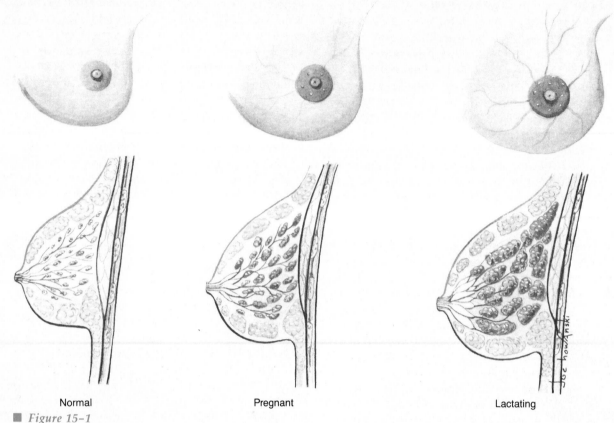

Normal · Pregnant · Lactating

■ *Figure 15–1*
Breast changes during pregnancy. (Whitley N: A Manual of Clinical Obstetrics. Philadelphia, JB Lippincott, 1985.)

the blood vessels supplying the area enlarge. As a result, the veins beneath the skin of the breasts, which previously may have been scarcely visible, become more prominent and occasionally exhibit intertwining patterns over the whole chest wall.

The alterations in the breasts during pregnancy are directed ultimately to the preparation for breast-feeding the baby. After the first few months, a thin, viscous, yellowish fluid may be expressed by gentle massage or may appear spontaneously from the nipples. This is a watery precursor of breast milk, *colostrum*. Composed mostly of protein, fat, and minerals, colostrum is important for the neonate's immunological defense because it contains secretory IgA. This immunoglobulin is not produced by the fetus or neonate; its presence in colostrum provides necessary protection in the gastrointestinal system by preventing attachment of bacteria to the mucosal surface.[2]

In the primigravida, breast changes are helpful adjuncts in the diagnosis of pregnancy, but in women who have already borne children, particularly if they have nursed an infant within the past year, these changes are much less significant.

"QUICKENING"

Quickening is an old term derived from an idea prevalent many years ago that at some particular moment of pregnancy, life is suddenly infused into the infant. At the time this notion was in vogue, the first tangible evidence of intrauterine life lay in the mother's feeling the baby move, and the conclusion was only natural that the infant "became alive" at the moment these movements were first felt. Quickening is still used in obstetrical terminology to refer to the active movements of the fetus as first perceived by the mother. Most women refer to feeling movement or feeling life.

Quickening is usually felt as a tremulous fluttering low in the abdomen toward the end of the fifth month. The first impulses caused by the stirring of the fetus may be faint; later on, however, they grow stronger and become clearly perceptible.

Many fetuses, although alive and healthy, seem to move about very little in the uterus, and not infrequently, a day or so may pass early in pregnancy without a movement being felt. Inability to feel the baby move for brief periods of time does not mean that it is dead or compromised, but, in all probability, that it has assumed a position in which its movements are not felt so readily by the mother. If a few days pass without movements, the nurse or physician should check for fetal heartbeat and movements by ultrasound or auscultation. If fetal heartbeat and movements are present, the mother can be reassured that the fetus is alive. In pregnancy near term, it is important for the mother to stay aware of fetal movement and to report significantly decreased or absent movement of more than 1 day, because this could indicate that the fetus is compromised.

Fetal movement is not a positive sign of pregnancy, because women occasionally misinterpret movements of gas in the intestines as motions of a baby and, on this basis, think that they are pregnant. Therefore, the woman's statement that she feels the baby move cannot be regarded as absolute proof of pregnancy.

VAGINAL CHANGES

During pelvic examination after about 8 to 10 weeks of pregnancy, discoloration of the vaginal mucous membrane due to the influence of elevated hormones can be observed. The vaginal mucosa frequently becomes thickened and has a dark bluish or purplish congested appearance because of increased vascularity. This dark violet-blue hue to the tissues is called *Chadwick's sign.* When contrasted with the ordinary pink color of the nonpregnancy vagina, it is considered a valuable sign of pregnancy. As a result of the rich blood supply, vaginal secretions become considerably increased, particularly toward the end of gestation. This increased vascularity extends to the other pelvic structures and tissues in the perineal region, skin, and muscles, contributing to changes in preparation for labor.

Chadwick's sign is not as predictive of pregnancy in women who have borne children. Because a bluish discoloration of the vagina may be due to any condition leading to congestion of the pelvic organs, it can be considered only a presumptive sign of pregnancy.

SKIN CHANGES

Striae Gravidarum. The abdomen gradually enlarges to accommodate the increase in size of the uterus. The distention of the abdominal wall, usually in the later months of pregnancy, causes certain pink or slightly reddish streaks, or *striations*, to form in the skin covering the sides of the abdomen and the anterior and the outer aspects of the thighs. These streaks, or *striae gravidarum*, are caused by the stretching, rupture, and atrophy of the deep connective tissue of the skin. They grow lighter after labor has taken place and finally take on the silvery whiteness of scar or cicatricial tissue. In subsequent pregnancies, new pink or reddish lines may be found mingled with old silvery-white striae. The number, size, and distribution of striae gravidarum vary, and some clients have no such markings whatever, even after repeated pregnancies.

Striae are not peculiar to pregnancy but may be found in other conditions that cause marked skin stretching, especially if the condition develops rapidly. Sudden weight gain with accumulation of subcutaneous fat or the development of large tumors of rapid growth that distend the skin can cause striae.

Striae gravidarum often develop in the breasts, the buttocks, and the thighs, probably as the result of deposition of fat in those areas with consequent stretching of the skin.

Pigment Changes. Certain pigmentary changes are also common, particularly the development of a black line running from the umbilicus to the mons veneris, called the *linea nigra.*

The external genitalia and pigmented nevi also darken. In certain women, irregular spots or blotches of a muddy brown color appear on the face. This condition is called *chloasma,* or the "mask of pregnancy." Oral contraceptives may also cause chloasma in some women. These facial deposits of pigment may cause the woman emotional distress. Although chloasma becomes lighter after delivery and often disappears after a few months, some women retain increased facial pigment. The increased pigmentation of the breasts and the abdomen never disappears entirely, although it usually becomes much less pronounced.

All these pigmentary deposits vary in size, shape, and distribution and usually are more marked in brunettes than in blonds.

Spider Hemangiomas. These vascular phenomena are minute, fiery-red blemishes on the skin with branching legs coming out from a central body. They develop more often in light-skinned women. Spiders have no clinical significance in pregnancy and are a result of hormonal effects on vasculature. Usually spiders disappear after delivery, but some may persist.

Variations in Skin Changes. The changes in the skin that may accompany pregnancy (i.e., striae gravidarum, linea nigra, chloasma, and pigmentation of the breasts, spider hemangiomas) vary greatly in different women; often they are entirely absent. The pigmentation changes are frequently absent in blonds and exceptionally well marked in pronounced brunettes. This pigmentation may remain from former pregnancies and cannot be depended on as a diagnostic sign of pregnancy in women who have borne children previously.

Sweat Glands. There is a great increase in the activity of the sebaceous glands, the sweat glands, and the hair follicles. The augmented activity of the sweat glands produces an increase in perspiration, an alteration that is helpful in the elimination of waste material.

Probable Signs

ABDOMINAL CHANGES

The size of the abdomen during pregnancy corresponds to the gradual increase in the size of the uterus, which at the end of the third month is at the level of the symphysis pubis. At the end of the fifth month, it is at the level of the umbilicus, and toward the end of the ninth month, it is at the ensiform cartilage. Abdominal enlargement may be due to a number of causes, such as accumulation of fat in the abdominal wall, edema, or uterine or ovarian tumors. However, if the uterus can be distinctly felt to have enlarged progressively in the proportions stated above, pregnancy is probable.

CHANGES IN THE UTERUS

Changes in shape, size, and consistency of the uterus that take place during the first 3 months of pregnancy are important indications. These are noted in the bimanual examination, which shows the uterus to be more anteflexed than normal, enlarged, and of a soft, spongy consistency. About the sixth week, Hegar's sign is perceptible (Fig. 15-2). At this time, the lower uterine seg-

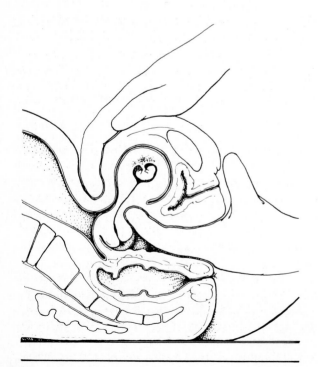

■ *Figure 15–2*
Hegar's sign.

ment, or lower part of the body of the uterus, becomes much softer than the cervix. It is so soft that it can be compressed almost to the thinness of paper. This is one of the most valuable signs in early pregnancy.

The uterus increases in size to make room for the growing fetus. It increases from approximately 6.5 cm long, 4 cm wide, and 2.5 cm deep to about 32 cm long, 24 cm wide, and 22 cm deep. The uterine wall thickens during the first few months of pregnancy from about 1 cm to almost 2 cm, but thereafter it thins to about 0.5 cm or less. By the end of pregnancy, the uterus becomes a soft-walled muscular sac that yields to the movements of the fetal extremities and permits the examiner to palpate the fetus easily. Its weight increases from 50 g to 1000 g. The small, almost solid organ that has a capacity of about 2 ml increases to become a thin-walled muscular sac capable of containing the fetus, the placenta, and over 1000 ml of amniotic fluid.

The tremendous growth is due partly to the formation of new muscle fibers during the early months of pregnancy. The major source of growth is the enlargement of preexistent muscle fibers that are 7 to 11 times longer and 2 to 7 times wider than those observed in the nonpregnant uterus. Simultaneously, fibroelastic tissue develops between the muscle bands and forms a network around the various muscle bundles. This is of great importance in pregnancy and labor because it strengthens the uterine walls. During early pregnancy, the hypertrophy of the uterus is probably due to the stimulating action of estrogen on muscle fibers.

The muscle fibers are arranged in three layers: the external hoodlike layer, which arches over the fundus; the internal layer of circular fibers around the orifices of the fallopian tubes and the internal os; and the figure-eight fibers in the middle layer, which make an interlacing network through which the blood vessels pass.

FETAL OUTLINE

After the sixth month, the outline of the fetus (head, back, knees, and elbow) can usually be identified by abdominal palpation, and this supports the diagnosis of pregnancy. As pregnancy progresses, the outline of the fetus becomes more and more clearly defined. The ability to outline the fetus makes pregnancy extremely probable. In rare instances, however, tumors of the uterus may mimic the fetal outline.

Ballottement. Another valuable sign suggesting the presence of a fetus is ballottement (from the French *balloter*, to toss up like a ball). During the fourth and the fifth months of pregnancy, the fetus is small in relation to the amount of amniotic fluid present. During vaginal examination, a sudden tap on the presenting part makes it rise in the amniotic fluid and rebound to its original position and, in turn, tap the examining finger. When elicited by an experienced examiner, this response is the most certain of the probable signs.

CERVICAL CHANGES

Softening of the cervix usually occurs about the time of the second missed menstrual period. In comparison with the usual firmness of the nonpregnant cervix (which has a consistency approximate to that of the cartilaginous tip of the nose), the pregnant cervix becomes softened, and on digital examination the external os feels like the lips or like the lobe of the ear (Goodell's sign).

Softening of the cervix may be apparent as early as a month after conception. The softening of the cervix in pregnancy is due to increased vascularity, edema, and hyperplasia of the cervical glands.

As shown in Figure 15-3, the glands of the cervical mucosa undergo marked proliferation and distend with mucus. As a result, they form a structure resembling a honeycomb and make up about one half of the entire structure of the cervix. This creates a mucous plug that seals the uterus from contamination by bacteria in the vagina. The mucous plug is expelled at the onset of labor along with a small amount of blood. This discharge of blood-stained mucus is called the bloody *show*. Frequently, the onset of labor is heralded by the appearance of bloody show.

BRAXTON HICKS CONTRACTIONS

Uterine contractions begin during the early weeks of pregnancy and occur at intervals of from 5 to 10 minutes throughout pregnancy. These contractions are painless, and the client may or may not be conscious of them. Contractions may be palpated during the later months by placing the hand on the abdomen and during the

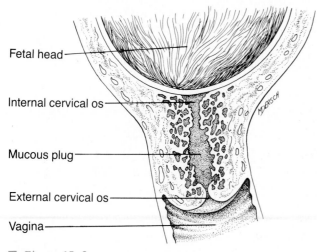

■ *Figure 15–3*
Cervix with mucous plug.

bimanual examination. These contractions cause the uterine muscles to contract and relax, thereby enlarging to accommodate the growing fetus. Braxton Hicks contractions are named after a famous London obstetrician of the last century who first described them. They are the cause of false labor.

PREGNANCY TESTS

Pregnancy tests are based on the fact that the early chorionic villi of the implanted ovum secrete human chorionic gonadotropin (hCG), which appears in the maternal blood and is excreted in the urine. This hormone is detected in maternal serum or urine by tests using immunological methods.

The level of hCG increases rapidly after implantation. When sensitive assays are employed, hCG can be detected in the maternal blood at about 8 to 9 days after ovulation and fertilization. Highly sensitive and selective assays can also detect hCG in the maternal urine before the first missed menses, or within 2 weeks of conception. There are α and β subunits of hCG; the α subunit is common to the pituitary gonadotropic hormones, including luteinizing hormone (LH) and follicle-stimulating hormone (FSH). The β subunit has molecular characteristics that are specific for hCG. Antibodies that are specific for the β subunit of hCG are utilized in many immunoassay tests, the most sensitive of which can detect minute quantities of β-hCG. The β-hCG specific tests also do not cross-react with α subunits in LH and FSH.

Radioreceptor Assay. Radioreceptor assay (RRA) is a sensitive test that identifies hCG in the blood within 1 hour. LH also produces a positive reaction in this test, so the sensitivity is usually set at above the levels of LH. Sophisticated equipment is needed to interpret the RRA, and it is available in hospital and medical center laboratories.

Radioimmunoassay for hCG. The RIA β-subunit hCG is a highly specific and sensitive serum assay that avoids cross-reaction with LH and other α unit gonadotropins. In most laboratories, as little as 5 mIU of hCG/ml of serum can be identified. This test can detect pregnancy in the first week after conception (about 6 days) with nearly 100% accuracy in 1 to 3 hours.[3]

Enzyme Immunoassay. The enzyme-based assay detects β-hCG in the urine, utilizing a matched combination of antibodies. It is highly sensitive and takes less than 4 minutes to perform in an office or outpatient setting. Elevated levels of hCG at concentrations of 50 mIU/ml urine can be detected before the first missed menses. The test does not cross-react with LH, FSH, or thyroid-stimulating hormone (TSH).[4]

Positive Signs

Although some of the signs mentioned above, particularly the immunoassay tests, ballottement, and palpating the fetal outline, are nearly positive evidences of pregnancy, they are not 100% certain. Errors in technique occasionally invalidate the tests, and on rare occasions the other signs may be simulated by nonpregnant pathological states. If the term *positive* is used in the strict sense, there are only four positive means of detecting pregnancy: the presence of fetal heart sounds, fetal movements felt by the examiner, the roentgenogram outline of the fetal skeleton, and delineation of a pregnancy by ultrasonography.

FETAL HEART SOUNDS

When fetal heart sounds are heard distinctly by an experienced examiner, there is no longer any doubt about the existence of pregnancy. Ordinarily, they become audible by stethoscope at about the middle of pregnancy, or at approximately the 20th week. If the abdominal wall is thin and conditions are favorable, they may become audible as early as the 18th week, but obesity or an excessive quantity of amniotic fluid may render them inaudible until a much later date.

Although the usual rate of the fetal heart is approximately 140 beats per minute, it may vary under normal conditions between 120 beats per minute and 160 beats per minute. The head stethoscope is used because the listener receives bone conduction of sound through the headpiece in addition to that transmitted to the eardrum (Fig. 15-4). Contractions of the fetal heart can also be detected by use of the Doppler principle with ultrasound. Using this approach, fetal heartbeats can almost always be detected by the 8th to the 10th week.

Office electronic fetal heart monitors that detect fetal heartbeat by ultrasound are widely used (see Fig. 15-4). The heartbeat is transmitted to a monitor and amplified so that it can be heard by both the examiner and the client. The use of this instrument provides an exciting experience and can be appreciated by all, including the client's partner when present.

Funic and Uterine Souffles. Two additional sounds may be heard when listening over the pregnant uterus: the funic souffle and the uterine souffle. *Souffle* means a blowing murmur or whizzing sound, and the nature of these two sounds is similar, but their timing and causation are different.

The word *funis* is Latin for umbilical cord; the term *funic souffle* refers to a soft blowing murmur caused by blood rushing through the umbilical cord. Because this blood is propelled by the fetal heart, the rate of funic souffle is synchronous to that of the fetal heart. It is heard only occasionally, perhaps in one case of every six.

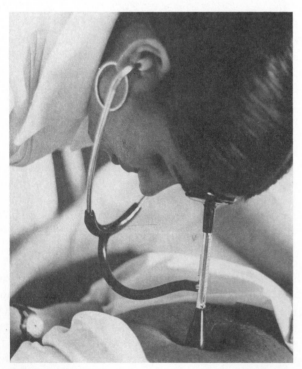
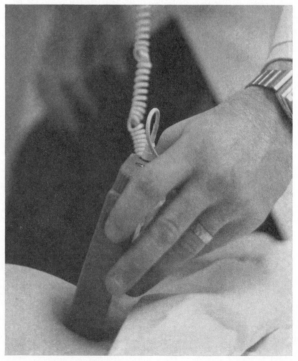

■ *Figure 15–4*
Auscultation of fetal heartbeat by means of a head stethoscope (left) and by ultrasound (right).

The funic souffle is a positive sign of pregnancy, but it is not usually so listed, because it is almost always heard in close association with the fetal heart sounds.

The *uterine souffle* is produced by blood rushing through the large vessels of the uterus. Because this is maternal blood, propelled by the maternal heart, it is synchronous to the rate of her heartbeat. The rate of the funic souffle is ordinarily approximately 140 beats per minute (or the same as that of the fetal heart rate); the rate of the uterine souffle is near 80 beats per minute (that of the maternal heart rate).

FETAL MOVEMENTS FELT BY EXAMINER

Fetal movements reported by the client may be misleading in the diagnosis of pregnancy. However, when an experienced examiner feels the characteristic thrust or kick of the fetus against the hand, this is positive evidence of pregnancy. Often this can be felt after the end of the fifth month.

ROENTGENOGRAM

A roentgenogram (x-ray) showing the outline of the fetal skeleton is proof of pregnancy. How early the fetal skeleton shows in the x-ray depends on the thickness of the abdominal wall, the x-ray equipment, and other factors. It has been demonstrated as early as the 14th week and is easily demonstrated as a rule after the 20th week. Because of the potential hazards of ionizing radiation and because the fetus can be outlined sonographically, this approach is rarely used today.

SONOGRAPHY

The presence of an early embryo can be detected by the use of ultrasound techniques. This test is useful in the diagnosis of intrauterine versus extrauterine pregnancy and in detection of fetal abnormalities. A fetal sac within the uterus usually manifests in a characteristic pattern on the sonogram. Ultrasound used for dating of pregnancy and for detecting gross fetal abnormalities is becoming a routine part of early prenatal care. Patients tend to like the ultrasound procedure because it allows them to see a moving image of the fetus. Examination at 16 to 18 weeks yields optimal information for dating pregnancy. This is especially useful when dates of the last menstrual period are uncertain. Routine office ultrasound is usually done transabdominally; however, transvaginal ultrasound is most effective in detecting ectopic and other extrauterine pregnancies.[5] There is widespread support for use of ultrasound both for antepartal diagnostic procedures and for general improvement of maternal and fetal health.[6] (The use of ultrasound is discussed in detail in Chap. 42.)

■ PHYSIOLOGICAL CHANGES OF PREGNANCY

The physiological changes of pregnancy are both local and general alterations in the woman's bodily structures and functions. Most of these changes resolve during the postpartum period.

Bodily Changes Associated with Uterine Growth

Between the third month and the fourth month of pregnancy, the growing uterus rises out of the pelvis and can be palpated above the symphysis pubis. It rises progressively to reach the umbilicus at approximately the sixth month and almost impinges on the xiphoid process at the ninth month (Fig. 15-5).

In the majority of pregnancies, the uterus is rotated to the right as it rises out of the pelvis. This dextrorotation is probably caused by the presence of the rectosigmoid on the left. As the uterus becomes larger, it comes in contact with the anterior abdominal wall and displaces the intestines to the sides of the abdomen.

Coincident with the uterine and abdominal enlargement, the umbilicus is pushed outward until about the seventh month, when its depression is completely obliterated and it forms merely a darkened area in the smooth and tense abdominal wall. Later, it is raised above the surrounding integument and may project slightly outward.

When the abdominal wall is unable to withstand the tension created by the enlarging uterus, the recti muscles become separated in the median line, termed *diastasis recti.*

About 2 weeks before labor, in most primigravidae, the fetal head descends into the pelvic cavity. As a result, the uterus sinks to a lower level and at the same time falls forward. Because this relieves the upward pressure on the diaphragm and makes breathing easier, this phenomenon of the descent of the head has been called *lightening.* These changes usually do not occur in multiparas until the onset of labor. By measuring the height of the fundus, experienced examiners can determine the approximate length of gestation.

EFFECTS ON POSTURE

Because the full-term pregnant uterus and its contents weigh about 6000 g (12 lb), pregnant women often lean backward to maintain equilibrium. This backward tilt of the torso is characteristic of pregnancy. This posture imposes increased strain on the muscles and the ligaments of the back and the thighs. This causes many of

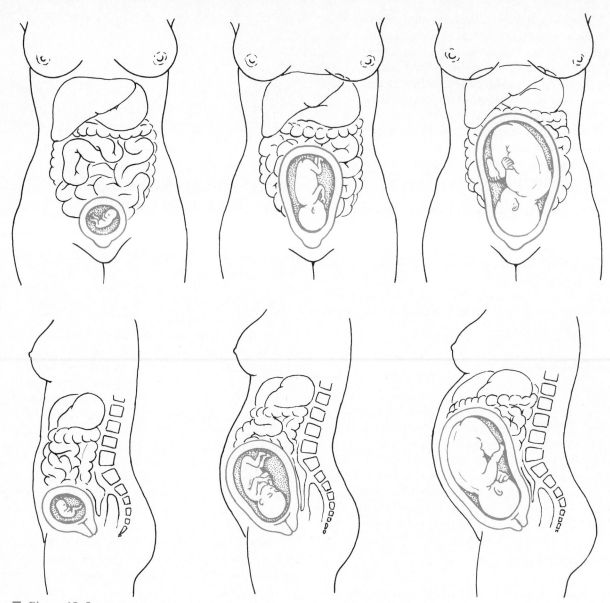

■ *Figure 15–5*

Front (top) and lateral (bottom) views of the relative size of the growing uterus, showing the fetus at 4, 6, and 9 months of gestation. The fundus reaches a height between the symphysis pubis and the umbilicus by the fourth month, is about the level of the umbilicus at the sixth month, and almost impinges on the xiphoid process at about the ninth month of gestation.

the skeletomuscular aches and cramps so often experienced in late pregnancy.

An additional contributing factor is a relaxation of the ligaments that support the joints of the spinal column and pelvis. This feature is increasingly prominent as pregnancy progresses. Relaxation of the sacroiliac joints and the pubic symphysis creates a certain amount of pelvic instability, producing additional strain on the back muscles and thighs. These changes account for the waddling gait often observed in late pregnancy and in the early postpartum period.

Changes in the Body Systems

METABOLIC CHANGES

The presence of a rapidly growing fetus and placenta and the demands of these structures bring about a number of significant metabolic changes. Although there is significant weight gain, only a small portion of this increase occurs as a result of metabolic alteration. Most weight gain is associated with the presence of the growing fetus, placenta, fetal membranes, and amniotic fluid.

Pregnancy has a marked influence on carbohydrate metabolism. In general, levels of fasting blood sugar are lower, and it has been suggested, but not proved, that secretion of insulin by the pancreas is increased. The stress of pregnancy may actually bring to light subclinical diabetes, which may be detected for the first time during the course of prenatal care (see Chap. 34).[4]

The uterus, maternal blood, and products of conception contain more protein than fat or carbohydrate. There are significant alterations in several plasma proteins. During pregnancy, albumin concentration decreases and fibrinogen levels increase, whereas immunoglobulin levels fall somewhat. In the latter half of pregnancy, there is an appreciable increase in plasma lipid, including total lipids, cholesterol, phospholipids, free fatty acids, and lipoproteins. Table 15-1 lists the

TABLE 15-1. COMMON LABORATORY VALUES IN PREGNANCY

Test	Normal Range (Nonpregnant)	Change in Pregnancy	Timing
Serum Chemistries			
Albumin	3.5–4.8 g/dl	↓ 1 g/dl	Most by 20 weeks then gradual
Calcium (total)	9–10.3 mg/dl	↓ 10%	Gradual fall
Chloride	95–105 mEq/L	No significant change	Gradual rise
Creatinine (female)	0.6–1.1 mg/dl	↓ 0.3 mg/dl	Most by 20 weeks
Fibrinogen	1.5–3.6 g/L	↑ 1–2 g/L	Progressive
Glucose, fasting (plasma)	65–105 mg/dl	↓ 10%	Gradual fall
Potassium (plasma)	3.5–4.5 mEq/L	↓ 0.2–0.3 mEq/L	By 20 weeks
Protein (total)	6.5–8.5 g/dl	↓ 1 g/dl	By 20 weeks then stable
Sodium	135–145 mEq/L	↓ 2–4 mEq/L	By 20 weeks then stable
Urea nitrogen	12–30 mg/dl	↓ 50%	First trimester
Uric acid	3.5–8 mg/dl	↓ 33%	First trimester, rise at term
Urinary Chemistries			
Creatinine	15–25 mg/kg/day (1–1.4 g/day)	No significant change	
Protein	Up to 150 mg/day	Up to 250–300 mg/day	By 20 weeks
Creatinine clearance	90–130 ml/min per 1.73 m²	↑ 40%–50%	By 16 weeks
Serum Enzymatic Activities			
Amylase	23–84 IU/L	↑ 50%–100%	Controversial
Transaminase			
Glutamic pyruvic (SGPT)	5–35 mU/ml	No significant change	
Glutamic oxaloacetic (SGOT)	5–40 mU/ml	No significant change	
Hematocrit (female)	36%–46%	↓ 4%–7%	Bottoms at 30–34 weeks
Hemoglobin (female)	12–16 g/dl	↓ 1.5–2 g/dl	Bottoms at 30–34 weeks
Leukocyte count	4.8–10.8 × 10³/mm³	↑ 3.5 × 10³/mm³	Gradual
Platelet count	150–400 × 10³/mm³	Slight decrease	
Erythrocyte count	4.0–5.0 × 10⁶/mm³	↑ 25%–30%	Begins 6–8 weeks
Serum Hormone Values			
Coritsol (plasma)	8–21 μg/dl	↑ 20 μg/dl	Peaks 28–32 weeks then constant to term
Prolactin (female)	25 ng/ml	↑ 50–400 ng/ml	Gradual, peaks at term
Thyroxine, total (T₄)	5–11 g/dl	↑ 5 mg/dl	Early sustained
Triiodothyronine, total (T₃)	125–245 ng/dl	↑ 50%	Early sustained

common laboratory values and cardiovascular changes in pregnancy.

CIRCULATORY CHANGES

Blood. The total volume of blood in the body increases approximately 30% during pregnancy. The minimal hematological values for both nonpregnant women and pregnant women are 12 g of hemoglobin, 3.75 million erythrocytes, and 35% hematocrit. If there are adequate iron reserves in the body, or if sufficient iron is supplied from the diet, the hemoglobin, the erythrocyte count, and the hematocrit values remain within normal limits during pregnancy.

During pregnancy, there is an increased production of red blood cells by the bone marrow. At the same time, the maternal blood volume, the total amount of fluid circulating in the vessels, increases. Thus, the actual concentration of red blood cells is more or less the same as under normal conditions.

IRON NEEDS. The marked increase in production of red blood cells places an inordinate demand on bodily iron stores. Iron stores in the female are often marginal anyway because of the normal loss at menstruation. Iron deficiency anemia is often present before pregnancy, especially when there has been inadequate dietary intake of iron, frequently the case among clients in poor socioeconomic circumstances. Iron deficiency is markedly aggravated by pregnancy because of the heavy demand for iron by the growing fetus, especially late in gestation. The increased demand for iron as a result of the changes associated with pregnancy should be kept in mind during the course of prenatal care, and the use of supplementary iron should be provided as indicated.

Heart. An important aspect of this increase in blood volume relates to its effect on the heart (Table 15-2). During pregnancy, the heart has about 50% more blood to pump through the aorta per minute. This augmented cardiac output attains a peak at the end of the second trimester and declines to the nonpregnant level during the last weeks of gestation. Immediately after delivery, there is a sharp rise again. In women with normal hearts, this is of no particular concern. However, in women with heart disease, this increase in cardiac workload may add to the seriousness of the complication (see Chap. 34).

Palpitation of the heart is not uncommon. In the early months of pregnancy, this is due to sympathetic nervous disturbance; toward the end of gestation, it is due to the intra-abdominal pressure of the enlarged uterus.

Blood Pressure. The arterial blood pressure of the pregnant woman is affected by her posture. Pressure in the brachial artery is highest when she is sitting and is lowest when she is in the lateral recumbent position. Ordinarily, arterial blood pressure falls during the second or early third trimester of pregnancy and rises slowly thereafter.

Systolic pressure falls slightly during pregnancy, whereas diastolic pressure decreases more markedly. These changes are due to the increased cardiac output and reduced peripheral resistance typical of pregnancy. Toward the end of pregnancy, vasoconstrictor tone usually increases, resulting in a normal rise of blood pressure toward prepregnant levels. This must be taken into account in caring for preeclamptic women who are experiencing already elevated blood pressures.[7]

Mechanical Circulatory Effects of the Enlarging Uterus. As pregnancy progresses, the enlarging uterus displaces and compresses the iliac veins, inferior vena cava, and probably the aorta. When the woman is supine, this venous compression is accentuated, producing a fall in venous return and decreased cardiac output. In some women, this results in a significant fall in blood

TABLE 15–2. CARDIOVASCULAR CHANGES IN PREGNANCY

Parameter	Amount of Change	Timing
Arterial blood pressures		
Systolic	↓ 4–6 mm Hg	All bottom at 20–24 weeks, then rise
Diastolic	↓ 8–15 mm Hg	gradually to prepregnancy values at
Mean	↓ 6–10 mm Hg	term
Heart rate	↑ 12–18 beats/min	Early 2nd trimester, then stable
Stroke volume	↑ 10%–30%	Early 2nd trimester, then stable
Cardiac output	↑ 33%–45%	Peaks in early 2nd trimester, then stable until term

pressure (hypotensive syndrome) producing nausea, dizziness, and occasionally syncope. Hypotension is relieved by changing position and lying on the side. Heart rate during these hypotensive episodes usually does not increase; actually, it may become slower (bradycardia).

Venous compression by the pregnant uterus elevates the pressure in veins draining the legs and pelvic organs. This can lead to development or exacerbation of varicose veins in the legs and vulva and to hemorrhoids, which often first appear during pregnancy. Subsequent pregnancies usually increase hemorrhoidal swelling. The rise in venous pressure is a major cause of edema in the lower extremities that often occurs in later pregnancy. Decreases in plasma oncotic pressure also contribute to edema. The hypoalbuminemia associated with pregnancy shifts the balance of the colloid osmotic pressure in favor of fluid transfer from the intravascular to the extravascular space. This mechanism of edema may be more important than venous compression.[8]

Because of venous compression, the rate of blood flow in the lower veins is markedly reduced, predisposing pregnant women to thrombosis. The effects of compression of the vena cava are partially offset by development of paravertebral collateral circulation that permits blood from the lower extremities to bypass the partly occluded vena cava.

During late pregnancy, the uterus partially compresses the aorta and its branches, which may account for lower pressure in the femoral artery compared with the brachial artery. Aortic compression is accentuated during uterine contractions and may cause fetal distress when the woman is in the supine position.

Regional Blood Flow. Blood flow to most regions of the body increases during pregnancy, reaching a plateau relatively early. In the uterus, kidneys, and skin, the blood flow increases with gestational age. This enables the kidneys and skin to eliminate waste materials better and the skin to regulate heat production. Both of these processes require large amounts of plasma, which is one reason for the disproportionate increase of plasma over red blood cells in the expansion of blood volume during pregnancy.

RESPIRATORY CHANGES

The major respiratory changes in pregnancy are caused by the mechanical effects of the enlarging uterus, the increased total body oxygen consumption, and the respiratory stimulant effects of progesterone (Table 15-3). As pregnancy progresses, the enlarging uterus places pressure upward toward the lungs and elevates the position of the diaphragm. This results in lower intrathoracic pressure and decreased resting lung volume, creating a decreased functional residual capacity (FRC) in the lungs. Reductions in the expiratory reserve volume and the residual volume of the lungs contribute to the reduced FRC. The movement of the diaphragm and the thoracic muscles is not impaired by the enlarging uterus, thus the vital capacity (VC) of the lungs is unchanged.

Oxygen Consumption and Ventilation. There is an increased need for oxygen during pregnancy, mainly by the uterus and its contents. More oxygen is required for increased renal and cardiac work, with small increments needed for work of the respiratory muscles and the breasts. Total body oxygen consumption increases about 15% to 20%. During pregnancy, the increases in both cardiac output and alveolar ventilation are greater than those needed to meet increased oxygen consumption. Therefore, despite the rise in total oxygen con-

TABLE 15-3. CHANGES IN LUNG VOLUME AND CAPACITY DURING PREGNANCY

Test	Description	Change in Pregnancy
Respiratory rate	Breaths per minute	Unchanged
Inspiratory capacity	Maximum volume air inspired from resting level	Increased about 5%
Tidal volume	Volume air inspired and expired each breath	Rises through pregnancy 40% increase (0.1–0.2 L)
Functional residual capacity	Volume air in lungs at resting expiratory level	Decreased about 18%
Vital capacity	Maximum volume air forcibly inspired	Unchanged, may be small decrease at term
Minute ventilation	Volume air inspired or expired in 1 min	Increased about 40%
Expiratory reserve volume	Maximum volume air expired after normal expiration	Decreased about 15%
Residual volume	Volume air remaining after maximum expiration	Decreases considerably

sumption, the arteriovenous oxygen difference and arterial P_{CO_2} both fall, indicating hyperventilation. Progesterone increases ventilation, making the respiratory center more sensitive to CO_2. This probably accounts for the hyperventilation of pregnancy.

In the hyperventilation of pregnancy, the P_{CO_2} falls to a level of 27 to 32 mm Hg, producing respiratory alkalosis. There is a corresponding rise in arterial P_{O_2} to about 106 to 108 mm Hg in the first trimester, with a slight downward trend as pregnancy progresses. To compensate for the alkalosis, there is increased renal bicarbonate excretion leading to a final pH between 7.40 and 7.45.

Dyspnea in Pregnancy. Respiratory rate does not change during pregnancy, but there is a rise in minute ventilation, reflecting about a 40% increase in tidal volume at term. Airway resistance is generally unchanged. Despite these effects, dyspnea is a common symptom during pregnancy. It may be related to greater differences between nonpregnant and pregnant P_{CO_2} levels in susceptible women. There are no differences in pulmonary function tests between pregnant women with dyspnea and those who do not experience this symptom.

GASTROINTESTINAL CHANGES

The intestines and stomach are displaced upward by the enlarging uterus. These positional changes may alter the physical findings in certain diseases such as appendicitis. The appendix is usually displaced somewhat laterally and upward and at times may be located as high as the right flank. The motility in the gastrointestinal tract is decreased during the course of pregnancy. These changes result in a prolonged gastric emptying time and a longer intestinal transit time. A generalized relaxation of the smooth musculature of the gastrointestinal tract occurs under the influence of progesterone. Gastric emptying time is especially prolonged during the course of active labor. The altered position of the stomach contributes to the increased frequency of heartburn in pregnancy, most likely caused by reflux of acidic secretions into the lower esophagus. Muscular tone about the stomach and esophagus is altered, resulting in lower intraesophageal pressures and higher intragastric pressures, and slower esophageal peristalsis. All of these changes contribute to gastroesophageal reflux.

There is often a vascular swelling of the gums, referred to as epulis of pregnancy. The gums become hyperemic and softened, with an increased tendency toward bleeding after brushing the teeth. These changes *per se* do not lead to an increased incidence of tooth decay and regress spontaneously after delivery.

Digestion. The function of the digestive organs may be somewhat altered during pregnancy. During the early months, the appetite may be diminished, particularly if nausea exists. Because the nutritional requirements to meet the needs of the mother's body and the growing fetus demand quality of the diet rather than an appreciable increase in the quantity of food ingested, this temporary manifestation should not produce injurious effects. As pregnancy advances and the digestive system becomes accustomed to its new conditions, the appetite is increased. Heartburn and flatulence may occur at this time. Also upward pressure from the diaphragm and the diminished tone may delay the emptying time of the stomach.

Constipation is exceedingly common in pregnancy; at least one half of all gravid women suffer from this disorder. The entire gastrointestinal tract is affected by diminished tone and pressure of the growing uterus during gestation.

Liver and Gallbladder. Although no characteristic changes in liver morphology occur during the course of normal pregnancy, there are alterations in some of the laboratory tests for hepatic function. The total alkaline phosphatase activity in serum doubles, reaching levels that would be abnormal in the nonpregnant state. This is caused not by intrinsic changes in the liver, but rather by the effect of alkaline phosphatase isoenzymes produced by the placenta. Serum cholinesterase activity normally falls during pregnancy, a change seen in certain liver diseases, and leucine aminopeptidase activity as measured in serum is markedly elevated. Palmar erythema and vascular spiders, lesions in the skin that are characteristically seen in clients with liver disease, are commonly found in normal pregnant women. These are thought to be caused by the dramatic increase in circulating estrogens; they usually disappear shortly after delivery. Gallbladder function is also altered, with a tendency toward decreased tone and distention. Gallbladder contents are thickened, and these changes could account for the increased predisposition to gallstones during pregnancy.

URINARY AND RENAL CHANGES

The urine in pregnancy usually is increased in amount and has a lower specific gravity. Pregnant women show a tendency to excrete dextrose in the urine. Although a reduction in the renal threshold for sugar is often associated with pregnancy, the presence of any sugar in the urine should always be reported to the physician. Lactosuria may be observed at times, especially during the latter part of pregnancy and the puerperium. Lactosuria is associated with the presence of milk sugar, which is from the mammary glands.

Some of the commonly used tests for renal function may be altered during gestation. Plasma creatinine and urea concentrations decrease. Urine concentration tests may be altered, and in the normal pregnant woman there may be failure to concentrate urine after withholding fluids. The kidney simply mobilizes extracellular fluid.

The *ureters* become markedly dilated in pregnancy, particularly the right ureter. This change apparently is due in part to the pressure of the gravid uterus on the ureters as they cross the pelvic brim and in part to a certain softening that the ureteral walls undergo as the result of endocrine influences.

This pregnancy-related dilatation does not appear to be accompanied by decreased ureteral peristalsis, as was previously thought. Ureteral dilatation begins in the first trimester and is present in 90% of women at term. It usually resolves within 4 to 6 weeks after delivery, although it may persist until the 12th to 16th postpartum week.

Renal Blood Flow, Fluid Volume, and Glomerular Filtration Rate. Renal plasma flow and the glomerular filtration rate (GFR) begin to increase in early pregnancy, reaching a plateau by midpregnancy at about 40% above nonpregnant levels. This persists unchanged until term. The exact mechanism of these changes is unclear; although partially related to the increased plasma volume in pregnancy, the renal changes reach a peak relatively early in pregnancy, before the maximum increase in plasma volume occurs.

The intravascular volume during pregnancy, consisting of plasma and red cell components, increases by about 50%. The plasma component increases by about twice as much as the red cell mass, leading to a fall in hematocrit beginning early in pregnancy. Extracellular volume, consisting in intravascular and interstitial components, increases throughout pregnancy, creating a physiological extracellular hypervolemia. Maternal interstitial volume has its greatest increase during the last trimester, contributing to edema.

Renin-Angiotensin Changes. Plasma concentrations of renin, renin substrate, angiotensin I and II are increased during pregnancy. Renin levels remain elevated throughout pregnancy; some of this elevated renin may represent a different, high-molecular-weight form or inactive form of the enzyme. The uterus as well as the kidneys can produce renin, and high concentrations of renin are found in the amniotic fluid. The role of renin in amniotic fluid is not fully understood.

The *bladder* usually functions efficiently during pregnancy. The urinary frequency experienced in the first few months of pregnancy is caused by hormonal effects and pressure exerted on the bladder by the enlarging uterus. Mechanical frequency is observed again when lightening occurs before the onset of labor. Urinary tract infections, especially cystitis, are not uncommon during pregnancy and may be related to urinary stasis and inadequate emptying of the bladder.

ENDOCRINE CHANGES

Placenta. The early chorionic villi of the implanted ovum secrete hCG, which prolongs the life of the corpus luteum. The result is the continued production of estrogen and progesterone, which are necessary for the maintenance of the endometrium. During pregnancy, hCG appears in maternal blood and is excreted in the mother's urine, allowing diagnosis of pregnancy by tests previously discussed.

The chorionic cells of the placenta produce another unique hormone, human chorionic somatomammotropin (hCS), which is also known as human placental lactogen (hPL). This hormone is detectable in placental cells as early as the third week after ovulation and is found in maternal serum by the sixth week. Its name suggests its actions. It influences somatic cell growth of the fetus and facilitates preparation of the breasts for lactation.

In addition to its function in the formation of hCG and hCS, the placenta takes over the production of estrogen and progesterone from the ovaries and, after the first 2 months of gestation, becomes the major source of these two hormones. The increase in these hormones in the maternal organism is thought to be responsible for many important changes that take place during pregnancy, such as the growth of the uterus and the development of the breasts. In the breasts, the development of the duct system is promoted by estrogen and the development of the lobule-alveolar system is promoted by progesterone.

Pituitary Body. The pituitary gland enlarges somewhat during pregnancy but, as such, is not essential for the maintenance of pregnancy.

ANTERIOR LOBE. The *anterior lobe* of this small gland, located at the base of the brain, is referred to as the "master clock," which, under the influence of the hypothalamus, controls the menstrual cycle. In addition to gonadotropins, the anterior lobe secretes hormones that act on the thyroid and adrenal glands and another hormone that influences the growth process. Production of these hormones continues during the course of pregnancy. Gonadotropins, on the other hand, are no longer released cyclically. The estrogen and progesterone produced by the placenta inhibit their release from the pituitary gland.

POSTERIOR LOBE. The *posterior lobe* of the pituitary secretes an oxytocic hormone, *oxytocin*, which has a strong stimulating effect on the uterine muscle. Extracts of the pituitary gland that contains oxytocin are widely used in obstetrics to cause the uterus to contract after delivery, thereby diminishing postpartum hemorrhage, and to initiate labor and to stimulate contractions during labor when they are of poor quality. Oxytocin also has an influence on the breasts. It causes *milk let-down*, or ejection of milk from the nipples. This effect is of clinical use in the care of the nursing mother. Oxytocin is available as Pitocin and Syntocinon (a synthetic product) and is usually administered parenterally.

Other Endocrine Glands. The placenta is the major endocrine gland in pregnancy. Other endocrine glands display alterations during normal pregnancy.

THYROID. During the course of pregnancy, there is slight to moderate enlargement of the thyroid. This hypertrophy of thyroid tissue is not associated with increased thyroid activity, although there is an elevation in the basal metabolic rate that increases throughout the course of pregnancy. This is a reflection of the increased oxygen consumption as a result of the metabolic activity of the products of conception.

Other parameters for the measurement of thyroid function also display changes. The serum protein-bound iodine (PBI), butyl extractable iodine (BEI), and thyroxine (T_4) levels increase, and the elevated levels are maintained until shortly after delivery. The increase is due not to increased thyroid activity as such, but rather to an elevation in the level of thyroid-binding protein normally present in the blood. Thus, although there is an increase in the amount of circulating thyroid hormones and, therefore, the total concentration of hormone is elevated, the actual amount of unbound or available hormone remains within normal limits.

The triiodothyronine (T_3) uptake test displays decreased values in pregnancy, which indicates an increase in the binding of circulating triiodothyronine. A similar increase in the level of thyroid-binding proteins is seen in the nonpregnant client after the administration of estrogen, and it is likely that in pregnancy the increase is a reflection of the high level of circulating estrogen.

ADRENALS. The *adrenal cortex* hypertrophies during pregnancy, and probably its activity increases. The actual secretion of cortisol by the adrenals is unchanged, although there are alterations in the metabolism of cortisol as a result of the influence of estrogen. There is an increase in the production by the adrenal glands of aldosterone, the hormone responsible for the retention of sodium by the kidneys. This increase begins early in pregnancy and continues throughout. The net result of the increase is a decreased ability of the kidneys to handle salt during pregnancy. In the absence of proper dietary control of salt intake, there is often fluid retention and either occult or overt edema.

OVARY. The *ovary*, except for the activity of the cor-

pus luteum of pregnancy, remains relatively quiescent. Gonadotropin levels are low, because their release is inhibited by the estrogen and progesterone produced by the placenta. Thus, follicular activity in the ovary is suppressed, and there is no further ovulation until after delivery.

Immunological Response in Pregnancy

The immunological defense system of the mother remains intact during pregnancy, protecting her and the fetus from infection and invasion by foreign substances. Of great importance is the tolerance by the mother of the antigenically different fetus during pregnancy. The presence of the fetus in the uterus can be compared to an organ transplant, in which organs of two different people are grafted together. Problems with immunological rejection of grafted tissue from another person often occur. In pregnancy, several mechanisms permit tolerance of the fetal "graft" and successful continuation of the gestation (Table 15-4).

The primary sites where maternal immunological defenses are modulated in response to the fetus are the uterus, regional lymphatics, and the placental surface. The uterus has decreased or altered afferent lymphatic systems that allow it to modify the host response to tissue grafts. The T cells, whose role is to mediate the cellular response to foreign tissue by acting to either help or suppress the immune response, are altered locally in the uterus during pregnancy. Pregnancy-related suppressor T cells, which decrease the maternal lymphocyte response, have been found. These T cells, in conjunction with actions by the placenta, can create an altered local immunological environment.

The placenta acts as an interface between the maternal and fetal systems. The separate vascular compartments of the placenta effectively remove the fetus from direct contact with the maternal immunological defense system. Tight trophoblastic intercellular junctions and a fibrinous covering of the trophoblast allow control of cellular and molecular exchange between mother and fetus. Also, the placenta does not have the major histocompatibility (HLA) antigens that are needed for maternal lymphocytes to initiate an effective immunological response.

Several plasma proteins and steroids produced by the placenta may alter maternal immune response, including pregnancy-specific β_1 glycoprotein, human placental lactogen (hPL), and hCG. These have been shown to suppress nonspecifically local immune response in pregnancy. The placenta functions as an immunoabsorbent, decreasing the response against the fetus by trapping maternal immune components.

Although tolerating the existence of the fetal

TABLE 15–4. MECHANISMS OF MATERNAL IMMUNOLOGICAL TOLERANCE OF FETAL "GRAFT"

Maternal		Fetal	
Systemic	*Uterus and Local Lymphatic Systems*	*Placenta*	*Systemic*
None (normal cell mediated immunity)	Privileged immunological site	Separation of the maternal-fetal circulations, including tight local barriers	Unidentified humoral and cellular immunosuppressive elements
	Localized, nonspecific suppression induces tolerance and generates suppressor T cells	Lack of expression of the major histocompatibility antigen (HLA) at the maternal-fetal interface	
		Nonspecific local immunosuppression through placental proteins and hormones	
		Immunoabsorbent effect of placental proteins and hormones	
		Production of masking and blocking antibodies	
		Generation of immune cell blockage	

"graft," the maternal immune system provides the usual protective responses. Nonspecific mechanisms such as phagocytosis and the inflammatory response are not affected by pregnancy. Specific immune responses, both humoral and cellular, are also not significantly affected. The leukocyte count does not change much, and the percentage and performance of B or T lymphocytes are not altered.

Maternal immunoglobulin levels do not change during pregnancy. Maternal IgG antibodies are able to cross the placenta and provide the major component of the fetal immunoglobulin in utero and during the early neonatal period. IgG is the only maternal immunoglobulin that can be transported across the placenta, providing significant passive immunity to the fetus and neonate. IgM, IgA, IgD, and IgE do not cross the placenta and do not provide any direct harm or benefit to the fetus. IgA is secreted in maternal colostrum and provides additional gastrointestinal immunity to the breast-fed newborn infant.[9,10]

The fetal immune system begins to develop early, with lymphocytes present by the 7th week and antigen recognition occurring by the 12th week. The fetus produces all types of immunoglobulins except IgA by the 12th week of gestation. Production of these immunoglobulins is progressive throughout gestation, so the newborn at term has developed a sufficient defense system to combat both bacterial and viral infections.

■ REFERENCES

1. Marshall J: Amenorrhea and abnormal uterine bleeding. In Hacker NK, Moore JG (eds): Essentials of Obstetrics and Gynecology, pp 410–417. Philadelphia, WB Saunders, 1986
2. Ross MG, Hobel CJ, Murad SH: Normal labor, delivery, and the puerperium. In Hacker NK, Moore JG (eds): Essentials of Obstetrics and Gynecology, pp 88–100. Philadelphia, WB Saunders, 1986
3. Neeson JD: Procedures and medical tests. In Clinical Manual of Maternity Nursing, pp 470–471. Philadelphia, JB Lippincott, 1987
4. Tyrey L: Human chorionic gonadotropin assays and their uses. Obstet Gynecol Clin North Am 15:467–475, 1988
5. Schurz B, Wenzl R, Eppel W, et al: Early detection of ectopic pregnancy by transvaginal ultrasound. Arch Gynecol Obstet 248:25–29, 1990
6. Ringa V, Blondel B, Breart G: Ultrasound in obstetrics: Do the published evaluative studies justify its routine use? Int J Epidemiol 18:489, 1989
7. Villar J, Rapke J, Markush L, et al: The measuring of blood pressure during pregnancy. Am J Obstet Gynecol 161(4):1019–1024, 1989
8. Valenzuela GJ: Is a decrease in plasma oncotic pressure enough to explain the edema of pregnancy? Am J Obstet Gynecol 161(6):1624–1627, 1989
9. Medearis AL: Immunology of pregnancy. In Hacker

NF, Moore JG (eds): Essentials of Obstetrics and Gynecology, pp 47–83. Philadelphia, WB Saunders, 1986
10. Adelsberg BR: Immunology of pregnancy. Mt Sinai J
Med 52:5, 1985

■ SUGGESTED READING

Bernales R, Bellanti J: Fetal and neonatal immunology. In
Quilligan EJ, Kretchmer N (eds): Fetal and Maternal
Medicine. New York, J Wiley & Sons, 1980

Cauchi M: Obstetric and Perinatal Immunology. London,
Edward Arnold, 1981

Elkayam R, Gleicher N: Cardiovascular physiology of pregnancy. In Elkayam R, Gleicher N (eds): Cardiac Problems in Pregnancy: Diagnosis and Management of Maternal and Fetal Disease. New York, Alan R Liss, 1982

Pritchard JA, MacDonald PC, Gant NF: Williams' Obstetrics, 17th ed. New York, Appleton-Century-Crofts,
1985

Quilligan EJ: Prenatal care. In Romney SL, Gray M, Little
AB (eds): Gynecology and Obstetrics: The Health Care
of Women, pp 579–594. New York, McGraw-Hill, 1980

Simpson ER, MacDonald PC: Endocrine physiology of the
placenta. Annu Rev Physiol 43:163, 1981

16

Psychosocial Aspects of Pregnancy

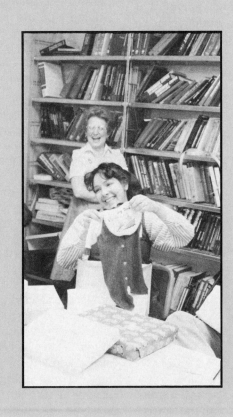

■ CULTURAL INFLUENCES ON PERCEPTIONS OF PREGNANCY

The family is society's most basic unit, surviving through the centuries as it has because it serves vital human needs. There may be different styles of family living and different ways of relating the family to the larger society. However, whatever the form, the family will no doubt continue to exist as long as humans continue to populate this planet.

Each member of the family assumes roles for which the culture dictates overt and covert behavioral expectations. Each member's perceptions of these roles also vary according to the manner of socialization and the kind of interaction he or she has had with others. As the society evolves and changes, so do the various role expectations. Each successive generation may hold different expectations as they adapt to changing times and needs, although there are always socially imposed limitations.

So it has been with childbearing. Pregnancy and birth are important events in most cultures. However, attitudes toward these processes vary considerably among different cultures and even within one society. In some cultures, birth is a social event, with open attendance by all friends and family; in other cultures, it is conducted in secrecy. Similarly, pregnancy may be seen as a normal uneventful preparatory phase to a desired change in status connoting achievement; conversely, it may be viewed as mysterious, the harbinger of possible disaster, or an atonement for simply being a lowly female.[1,2]

■ PREGNANCY IN THE AMERICAN CULTURE

There have been two competing views of pregnancy in our culture. One conceptualizes pregnancy and childbirth as a "crisis" situation; the other regards it as a normal role transition experience. Each of these attitudes has different assumptions that if carried to their logical conclusions have different implications for the delivery of health care. Unfortunately, assumptions and terminology have not always been clearly articulated, and when the rhetoric has been uncritically accepted and applied to the health-care scene, some peculiar innovations and traditions have been incorporated into the delivery of care. This chapter examines both the "crisis" and the "normal" orientations to pregnancy and their impact on the delivery of maternity and perinatal care in our culture.

Pregnancy as Crisis Versus Stress

A couple's first pregnancy, in particular, is a critical period in the evolution of a family. Beginning in the 1940s, a variety of disciplines became interested in pregnancy and the subsequent changes brought about by parenthood. Psychologists and psychiatrists, notably Bibring, Hass, Larsen, Menninger, Caplan, and Coleman and Coleman, have written about the critical nature of these events and have at least alluded to the *assumed* crisis implications.[3-8] Shainess, in fact, refers to pregnancy as a "crucible tempering the self" and suggests the possibility that the tempering process may go wrong, resulting in damage to the person and to the person's relationships with others.[9] Chertok speaks of pregnancy as a progressively developing crisis with the labor and delivery as the peak of the crisis because parturition results in separation of the mother and child and isolation from significant others.[10]

These early writings were based largely on experiential or clinical impressions of people who experienced difficulty with no comparison studies including control groups. Moreover, samples were small and skewed to the pathological end of a normal–abnormal continuum. There were problems in analysis also, because small skewed samples do not lend themselves to multivariate analysis, which is more appropriate when dealing with the multiple variables involved in family research.[1,2,11,12]

Other research led to the formulation of the concept of "normal crisis of parenthood," a contradiction in terms to say the least. Although the original focus of this crisis research was parenthood, often pregnancy became intermingled with the general research in this area with little empirical basis. The early work of Le Masters, Dyer, and Hobbs laid the foundation for this unfortunate extrapolation.[13-15]

PREGNANCY AS A STRESSOR

In many of the early conceptual formulations, both psychological and sociological, a "crisis" was considered to be a critical event but one that was not necessarily totally psychologically or interpersonally disruptive. However, the authors' true meaning was often subverted because they did not precisely define their terms.

In the original stress research on the family as exemplified by Hill and Hansen,[16,17] the term *crisis* connoted a sharp, decisive change in experience for which old patterns of behavior became inadequate.[17] Thus, there was an interruption in the family's routine, and new patterns of interaction had to be developed. There was also the implication that resolution and reintegration were not only possible (i.e., "normal") but expected and well within the family's capabilities without outside intervention.

Research Highlights

Past studies of couvade syndrome found that fathers frequently mimic symptoms of pregnancy. Strickland explored (1) the occurrence of symptoms during early, middle, and late pregnancy; (2) the association of social class, race, planning of pregnancy, and fathering experience; and (3) the relationship of symptoms expressed to the father's emotional state in expectant fathers. Excluding expectant fathers who had been diagnosed with physical and psychological illnesses or who were single, 91 expectant fathers completed and returned questionnaires at three designated stages of pregnancy.

Eighty-seven percent of the general sample reported experiencing one or more symptoms. No significant differences were found in the number of symptoms reported and the experience of the father. Significantly higher somatic symptoms were reported from the unplanned pregnancy group than the planned pregnancy group, although no significant difference was found in psychological symptoms. Data from all three stages suggested that working-class expectant fathers had significantly higher somatic and psychological symptoms than the middle-class group. African-Americans reported significantly more total symptoms than white expectant fathers in all stages of pregnancy, although differences decreased over the time of the pregnancy. Anxiety appeared to be the significant predictor of total symptoms, showing that symptom manifestation is related to emotional stress.

Evaluation of the emotional stress of the expectant father should be integrated into the nursing assessment of the expectant family. Consideration of social class, race, and whether this pregnancy is planned or unplanned would cue the nurse to watch for reports of symptoms from the father. Education of the family regarding couvade syndrome and reducing anxiety of the father may reduce symptoms.

Strickland OL: The occurrence of symptoms in expectant fathers. Nurs Res 36(3): 184–189, May/June 1987

In the 1980s and 1990s, researchers have done much to clarify and refine concepts, definitions, and measurement of family stress, the conceptualization of stressors, crisis, role transition and where pregnancy fits into the total process.[11,18–21] The topic of role transition to parenthood is addressed more fully in Chapter 27. In the newer, more refined conceptualizations, pregnancy is thought of as a potential stressor (something that can produce stress) that gives input into the entire equation of the role transition from nonparent to parent, and its impact depends on a variety of factors.

In summary, there has been some confusion, both semantically and conceptually, over the way the term *crisis* has been applied to the events of pregnancy, childbirth, and parenthood. This has sometimes led to pregnancy being viewed as disruptive and potentially damaging emotionally or psychologically. Recent research indicates that pregnancy is a time of transition but is not necessarily disruptive.

Pregnancy as a Role Transition

In a classic paper, Rossi suggested that the term *normal crisis* was a misnomer as applied to parenthood because the concepts of "normal" and "crisis" are basically incompatible—one implies natural successful resolution

and the other indicates the possibility of nonresolution.[22] She suggested that parenthood be viewed as a role transition and be based on a stage-task conceptual framework such as was found in the work of Erickson, Benedek, and Hill.[17,23,24] This type of orientation puts parenthood and other phases of the reproductive cycle, including pregnancy, into a development task formulation and allows these phenomena to be seen as essentially normal or usual, but also respects the fact that deviation, stress, or disruption can occur, depending on a variety of circumstances. It is also the orientation that is most commonly accepted and used by current researchers.[1,2,11,18,19,21,22,25,26] Chapter 27 discusses this concept as applied to the postpartum period, when parenthood becomes tangible. In this chapter, the discussion is limited to pregnancy.

LIFE SPAN CYCLES AND ROLE TRANSITION IN PREGNANCY

By viewing the total life span in terms of a developmental task interaction, we can view people's life spans as having cycles composed of stages or phases, each with its unique tasks. As the various cycles occur, social roles develop out of interaction with others in our social network. By analogy, social roles may be said to have cycles and each stage in the cycle has its set of tasks and adjustments. Rossi has outlined four broad stages in a role cycle that have implications for pregnancy as well as parenthood.[22]

1. *Anticipatory stage.* Almost all social roles have some kind of formal or informal training, either through formal schooling, role modeling, or watching others. This stage serves to socialize or train the potential actor for the role that he or she is to assume. As its name implies, this stage precedes the assumption of the role and may take place years ahead of the actual role assumption.

2. *Honeymoon stage.* This is the time immediately after the full assumption of the role. Here, intimacy and exploration occur as the person tries to adjust the "fit" of his or her personality to the role demands. Reality testing takes place rather than the fantasizing that often accompanies the anticipatory phase.

3. *Plateau stage.* This is the protracted middle period of a role cycle during which the role is fully exercised. In this phase, people validate themselves as adequate or inadequate depending on how well they and others see themselves performing in the role.

4. *Disengagement-termination stage.* This period immediately precedes and includes the actual termination of the role. For some roles, this stage is tangible. The marital role, for instance, can end abruptly with death or divorce. Similarly, pregnancy ends with labor or the termination of the pregnancy. For other roles, such as parenthood, the distinction is much less clear because there is little cultural prescription about when the authority and obligations end.[22]

Stages in the Role Cycle

Anticipatory stage—Formal/informal training for the role; socializes the incumbent-to-be. May take place years before. No role modeling for the "pregnant" role.

Honeymoon stage—Immediately follows the assumption of the role. Exploration and adjustment to the "fit" of the role to the incumbent. Reality testing.

Plateau stage—Role is fully exercised; incumbent validates his or her role-adequacy.

Disengagement-termination stage—Immediately precedes and includes role termination; sometimes tangible (pregnancy); sometimes less distinct (parenthood).

PREGNANCY AS A SOCIAL ROLE

Although there have been positive attempts to describe the various stages of pregnancy, the emotional reactions, and the developmental tasks that need to be accomplished, there are no definite boundaries, expectations, and prescriptions for the pregnant role. How are pregnant women supposed to act? What kinds of behaviors are really expected? Does one act "ill," or is pregnancy essentially a well state? Is it "business as usual," or are there special restrictions or exemptions that may be claimed? There are several interesting explanations of the many and varied behaviors that we see in parents-to-be.

Anticipatory Stage. If we examine the stages we outlined in a role cycle transition, we find that being pregnant is an anticipatory stage in a role transition to parenthood. This can cause confusion at the outset. As she enters the anticipatory stage of the pregnant role, the woman attempts to learn the role by observing others, both family and friends, and she recalls how other significant people in her life acted when they were pregnant. She also takes cues from her physician, who may overtly or covertly influence her thinking, even to the extent of regarding pregnancy as a "sick" or "well" state.[27] It is interesting that, in our culture, we do not have any socialization or role modeling for the pregnant role; little girls play at being mothers, but not at being pregnant. Thus, although certain behaviors directly relate to women and their fetuses during pregnancy and are essential for the collective well-being of the entire family (to say nothing of the happiness), the prescriptions for these activities are amorphous and vary considerably in different social classes. These include such behaviors as assuming positive personal health habits, cutting down on activities (or, conversely, exercising to maintain fitness), prompt and consistent attendance to prenatal care, and adequate nutrition practices.

Honeymoon and Plateau Stages. The honeymoon and plateau stages of the role cycle come quickly after the anticipatory stage. The showers, coffee klatches, and conversations with mother and pregnant friends or new mothers help the woman adjust the "fit" of the pregnant state to her personality. Some women find that they adore being pregnant. They feel at one with the earth and sky and see themselves at the center of the universe. They find that they seem to bloom physically and emotionally. Others find the condition almost unbearable. They feel unwell, ugly, and put upon and cannot wait to be "unpregnant." By far the more usual are those women who come to accept this condition, enjoy the positive aspects, and tolerate the discomforts and inconveniences. They see it as a necessary stepping stone to another larger role change.

Disengagement Stage. With the infant's birth comes a relatively sudden disengagement stage. There are few cultural norms concerning when the duties and privileges of pregnancy end and parenting begins, although in the space of a few short hours the mother is obviously "unpregnant." This role ambiguity can make this transition from pregnancy to actual parenthood difficult for some. (The student is referred to the list of Suggested Readings for articles that examine this issue in depth.)

■ THE MEANING AND EFFECT OF PREGNANCY ON THE COUPLE

As we discuss the impact of pregnancy on the potential father and mother, we relate some of the psychosocial aspects to the stages of the role cycle. Pregnancy is a unique experience in which a sexual union between a male and female leads to the creation of a new life. This new life, in turn, results in the creation of many new and unprecedented relationships.

Mother

Although the normal female may love her partner greatly and desire a child very much, there still are major developmental changes that she must make to become a mother. In the process of childbearing, she is creating from the union of herself and her mate another individual inside herself who must ultimately grow to become a separate person outside herself. Hence, the coming child represents the synthesis of three distinct entities: the mother's relationship to her partner, the relationship of the mother to the child as a representative of herself, and the relationship to the unique individual, which is the unborn child (Fig. 16-1). As with puberty when the person can never again be a child, or with menopause when the person can never again reproduce, with pregnancy the person can never become a completely single unit again. As long as the child lives, it never ceases to exist as a representative of the woman, her mate, and itself.

PSYCHODYNAMICS OF PREGNANCY

The pregnant woman must accomplish several psychological and cognitive tasks in pregnancy in addition to

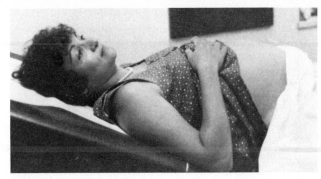

■ *Figure 16–1*
The mother can never again be a single unit. Her baby represents her relationship to her partner, her relationship to her baby as a representative of herself, and her relationship to the unique individual who will soon become a separate person outside herself. (Courtesy of Booth Maternity Center, Los Angeles, CA.)

the physiological restructuring that takes place. As her body adapts to the physiological demands of the fetus, she must adapt to the idea of being a mother of one or more children and to the incorporation of another person into her family and social sphere[26,28] (Fig. 16-2).

Psychological and Cognitive Tasks of Pregnancy. One of the first tasks the woman must accomplish is to believe she is pregnant and incorporate the fetus into her body image. Although she may be ambivalent initially about whether this is the "right time" for the pregnancy, she usually gradually resolves this cognitive dissonance and becomes enthused about the coming child. The ex-

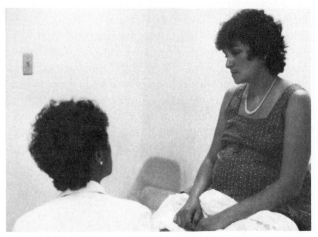

■ *Figure 16–2*
The third trimester is marked by heightened introversion as the woman looks back to her own childhood and forward to her child's future. (Courtesy of Booth Maternity Center, Los Angeles, CA.)

perience of fetal movement generally dispels doubts about the readiness or desire for a child at this time in her life. It is also a reality marker for her that she is, indeed, carrying a child. She may have had a sonogram, which also serves as a reality marker.[20,26] As the mother feels the fetus move and her body change in both subtle and apparent ways, she begins to realize that the fetus inside her is a real and separate being complete with its own boundaries and identity. This is not to say there is no turmoil; there is a great range of behavioral displays: mood swings, introspection, and physical and psychological weariness. Hence, we have many descriptions of the emotional lability of pregnancy. We must note, however, that there is evidence that the physiological and hormonal changes play an additional role in this lability.[26]

The mother's second task is to prepare for the physical separation, the birth of the infant. As with all aspects of pregnancy, there are various responses. Many women are eager to have the baby; they are "tired" of being pregnant. Some even state they are frightened to have this intrusive "invader" within them. However, others do not want to let the fetus go; they anticipate delivery as a loss of a loved object, and this anticipation may actually cause depression. Nevertheless, the task must ultimately be resolved, because every fetus lost is, in a moment, a baby gained.[26,28,29]

A third task is to resolve the identity confusions that accompany role transition and prepare for the smooth functioning of the family after birth. Researchers studying the period of pregnancy suggest that as the woman progresses in pregnancy, she becomes one with "mother," the primitive memory of the omnipotent being who nurtured her. Moreover, she becomes increasingly likely to evaluate her partner with respect to his appropriateness as a father. She may criticize his current behavior patterns to bring them more into line with her idea of what constitutes an ideal father.[26,28,29] Fishbein found that concordance between the partners about the expectations of the father role was important in reducing the father's anxiety during pregnancy.[30] Similarly, the pregnant father watches his partner become transformed into "mother" as her body changes, her behavior becomes more nesting, and so on. He is

simultaneously confronting his own feelings and aspirations as he metamorphoses into father. Pregnancy may be the first occasion in the relationship when the partners realize the extent to which they are interdependent psychologically, socially, and economically. On the one hand, this represents a physiological union that can be mystical; on the other hand, however, the merger may be experienced as a trap.[26,29] No wonder this resolution of identity confusions requires energy, commitment, and work.

Cognitive and Emotional Reactions in Pregnancy. In addition to the psychological tasks of pregnancy, the mother has certain cognitive and emotional reactions during the different trimesters of her pregnancy. Although not every woman has every reaction, research has shown that a certain pattern occurs with fair regularity.[20,21,26] Table 16-1 summarizes these reactions. (The student is referred to the list of Suggested Readings for further in-depth reading on this topic.)

Father

Men undergo far less social preparation than women do for parenthood, and there is little to prepare them for pregnancy except for the childbirth education classes that they may attend with their mates. Experience with fathers who have actively involved themselves in pregnancy indicates that men, like women, go through various phases during the pregnancy although they may not be as definitive and pronounced. As more attention is given to the father and more research efforts are directed toward his experiences, we are beginning to find out and redefine what the pregnancy experience means for him. For instance, some of the earlier research relating to body image change in fathers has been modified.[28,31]

EXPERIENCING PREGNANCY

The First Trimester. The introduction comes with the confirmation of the diagnosis of pregnancy. This places fathers almost immediately into a honeymoon stage. The reactions are as many and varied as with women. There may be unclear feelings because the intellectual focus is on the impending fatherhood, rather than the immediate state of pregnancy. Like his partner, he must assimilate the fact that the baby is his. He does not have the gross physiological changes to help him in this as the woman does, although we have seen some men who do experience some of the same physical symptoms of early pregnancy. How men accomplish this psychological task is still unclear and has been the topic of some fascinating research.[1,28,32–35]

The Mother's Psychological Tasks of Pregnancy

1. Incorporation of the fetus into her own body image
2. Perception of the fetus as a separate object
3. Readiness to assume the caretaking relationship with the baby

TABLE 16-1. MATERNAL COGNITIVE AND EMOTIONAL REACTIONS TO PREGNANCY[26,28,29,30]

First Trimester

Ambivalence

- Initial uncertainty about the timing of the pregnancy
- Physical discomforts: frequency, nausea, fatigue, restlessness and sleeplessness at night
- Uncertainty about herself and partner's role-adequacy as parents
- Uncertainty about material considerations

Fears and Fantasies

- Speculation and anticipation about new role assisted by fantasies: imagines and role-plays what her infant will be like, how she and her partner will cope, what her new life will be like
- Concerns about the future may be enhanced by fear and anxiety; if severe and unremitting, can be physically debilitating (rise in catecholamine levels)

Second Trimester

Feeling of Well-Being

- Physical symptoms and unwellness abate
- Fear and anxiety lessen and are forgotten as baby moves (if pregnancy progresses normally)

Introversion, Self-Engrossment, Introspection

- Concentration of mother on her own needs and those of her fetus
- Fascination with pregnancy and birth process; conscious of children's behavior
- Examination of her relationship with her own mother as she develops her own sense of maternal identity

- Appears egocentric, daydreams frequently
- Begins to exhibit "nesting" behavior: getting things ready for the baby and herself in anticipation of the birth

Mood Swings and Emotional Lability

- Preoccupation and mood swings may be troublesome to those around her; needs extra love, attention, and understanding

Third Trimester

Physical Discomfort Returns

- Fatigue, heaviness, frequency, sleeplessness, clumsiness

Psychosocial Dimensions Expand

- Self-image changes most in this trimester; feelings of awkwardness and clumsiness

Heightened introversion

Heightened concerns

- Fears for her own well-being and "performance" during labor
- Fears for the well-being of the infant

Contemplation of her Assumption of the Maternal Role

- Fantasizing of hypothetical situations involving parenthood
- Obsession with labor and delivery, desire for pregnancy to be over
- Increases nesting behavior: puts finishing touches on efforts

We do know that there may be guilt reactions about getting the partner pregnant or causing her to be sick and uncomfortable. On a more positive note, there may be feelings of pride at his virility or mutual pride that "We did it!" There may also be feelings of distance between him and his partner as she continues through her introverted first trimester. Jealousy, worry about the change in sexual relationships, and concern about his own competence as a man and provider may occur.[36–39]

The Second Trimester. The first perceptible movement of the fetus generally creates a profound feeling that the fetus is real; most men, when questioned, recall the time when "I first felt the baby move" or when he viewed the fetus through ultrasound. In the second trimester, more thought is given to what it means to be a father, and the plateau stage is entered. Men observe children and pregnant women more intently and become more acutely aware of their partners' growing uterus. A myriad of thoughts and concerns may sweep

over the father just as with the mother. Often these center on his ability to provide for the expanding family. However, there is also concern and thought about how well he will be able to "father" the new progeny and meet the newly evolving expectations of the mother.[1,2,39]

The Third Trimester. As with pregnancy for the woman, there is a good deal of literature that describes this period as a crisis time for fathers. Yet there is evidence to indicate that psychologically healthy men cope without major problems.[1,2] What is clear, however, is that pregnancy requires as much adjustment for the father as it does for the mother.

As is true for the mother, labor and delivery mark the disengagement-termination stage of the role transition of pregnancy for the father. How these proceed can have a profound effect on the father. Most health providers who have had experience with pregnant couples believe that men who take an active part in the pregnancy by attending childbirth and parent education classes, participating in preparations for the infant, and so on are more likely to participate in the birthing with positive psychological outcomes, and this, in turn, strengthens the parental bond (Fig. 16-3).

Laboring for Relevance. In a recent study using grounded theory, Jordan found the essence of the experience of expectant and new fatherhood is *laboring for relevance*, which has both intrapersonal and interpersonal aspects. The man labors to perceive the paternal role as relevant to his sense of self and his repertoire of roles. He labors to incorporate the paternal role into his self-identity as a salient and integrated component of his personhood and to be seen as relevant to childbearing and childrearing by others. Jordan suggests that laboring for relevance is a process consisting of three subprocesses.

1. Grappling with the reality of the pregnancy and child
2. Struggling for recognition as a parent from mate, coworkers, friends, family, baby, and society
3. "Plugging away" at the role of involved fatherhood

Each subprocess is developmental in nature, and the focal trajectory is the man's movement toward becoming an involved father. The driving force is the unfolding reality of the child. As with any process, the laboring for relevance processes occur within the larger contextual environment of interpersonal interactions and the larger society. People within the father's environment, the recognition providers, act to promote or impede his development (Fig. 16-4).

Jordan also found that, in general, men tend not to be recognized as parents but as helpmates or breadwinners, which interfered with validation of the reality of the pregnancy and later the child. They felt somewhat excluded from the childbearing experience by their mates, health-care providers, and society. Moreover, they found themselves without models to assist them in taking on the role of active and involved parent.[36] This type of study is helpful for shedding insight into the male experience of pregnancy and fatherhood and into designing interventions and supports to promote involved paternal behavior. It will fall to subsequent, replicative research to confirm these initial findings.

Body Image and the Couvade Syndrome. Body image refers to the way one pictures his or her own body. It is a composite of attitudes, feelings, and perceptions that each person has regarding how his or her body appears. In the 1960s and 1970s, researchers examined this topic to provide explanations for the appearance of pregnancy symptoms in spouses and partners of pregnant women. Early studies examined changes in body image in both the father and the mother and found similarities. Fawcett's early work suggested that it was not only the mother who experienced a change in body image perception as she literally grew during pregnancy, but her mate as well. These early data also showed that the couple's ability to identify with one another played a mediating role in the process.[33] Subsequently, more tightly designed, longitudinal studies by the same researcher and others found that, although the mother definitely experienced changes in perceived body space and global body attitude, her partner lacked significant identification with her on these dimensions and did not experience these changes.[34,35] Thus, although there is some identification on other dimensions of the pregnant state, there is no significant evidence that there are

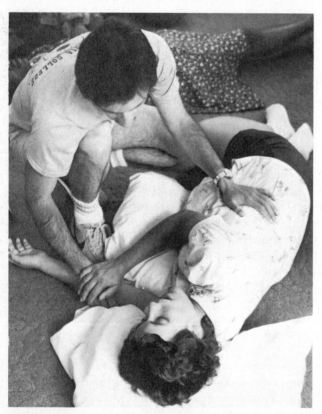

■ *Figure 16–3*
It is believed that men who take an active part in the pregnancy are more likely to have positive psychological outcomes to the birth, thus strengthening the parental bond. (Courtesy of Booth Maternity Center, Los Angeles, CA.)

Becoming a Father: Laboring for Relevance

Grappling with the reality of the pregnancy and child

Struggling for recognition as a parent from mate, family, friends, health-care providers, and society

"Plugging away" at the role of involved fatherhood without role models or support from networks

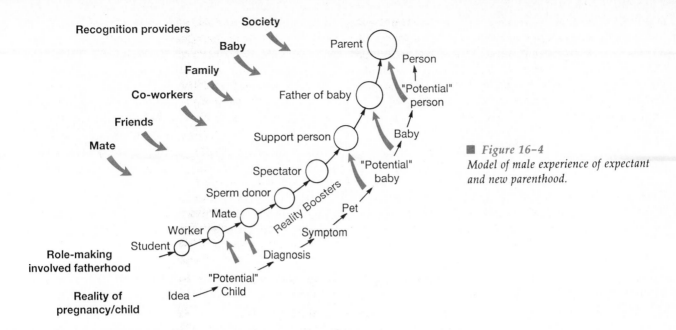

■ *Figure 16–4*
Model of male experience of expectant and new parenthood.

changes in perceptions of body image on the part of husbands and partners.

In the 1960s and 1970s, research was directed to the study of fathers who were afflicted with pregnancy-related symptoms. This phenomenon was dubbed the *couvade syndrome* because of its resemblance to some aspects of the primitive ritual couvade. In primitive cultures, couvade consists of the lying-in and simulation by the male of his mate's labor and delivery and the observation of certain proscribed dietary rituals postnatally.[37]

The most frequently exhibited couvade symptoms are alimentary and mimic symptoms common in pregnancy such as nausea, vomiting, alterations in appetite, weight gain, abdominal pain, backache, leg cramps, elusive toothaches, and other aches and pains in different parts of the body.[37,38] A variety of studies beginning in 1960s have consistently documented that husbands have a variety of these signs and symptoms.[32,37–40] The British researchers, Trethowen and Conlon, for instance, found that the men in their study experienced symptoms of physical illness during their wives' pregnancies. These include increased and decreased appetite, gastrointestinal disorders, toothache, and backache. It was noted that these men did not ordinarily experience these conditions at other times.[41] Similarly, studies of American men found that they expressed concerns about body intactness and tended to demonstrate "sympathetic" pregnancy symptoms. These included nausea and vomiting, dizziness, fainting, weight gain, backache, and leg cramps.[32,40] More recently in a longitudinal study of 91 expectant fathers, Strickland found that men who were working-class or African-American, or who reported that pregnancy was

not planned, experienced more pregnancy-related symptoms during pregnancy. White expectant fathers reported an increase in somatic symptoms as pregnancy progressed; African-American expectant fathers, on the other hand, indicated a decrease. However, African-American expectant fathers consistently reported more symptoms than white expectant fathers. Moreover, symptom manifestation in expectant fathers was positively associated with anxiety.[38]

The observation has been made and documented that the father's close proximity to the mother influences his response to the pregnancy. It is also postulated that the more closely the man identifies with his mate, the more intensely he experiences changes in his own body during pregnancy.[32,39] The importance of these findings lies in the fact that they have withstood the test of multiple studies and replication over several decades. Unlike the findings about changes in body image, which have not stood the test of time, these findings remain fairly constant. Thus, we can see what a momentous physiological, psychological, and emotional milestone pregnancy can be for both the woman and her mate.

■ APPLYING THE NURSING PROCESS TO THE PSYCHOSOCIAL ASPECTS OF NORMAL PREGNANCY

The nurse can function in collaboration with other members of the health team by providing emotional support, counseling, and teaching to the pregnant couple. Regarding pregnancy as a role transition rather than a crisis helps emphasize the normality of the condition. Care is structured to support the resources of the couple rather than looking for problems that may not exist. The key to appropriate intervention in this instance is family assessment.

Family Assessment

Certain extrafamilial stressors, both developmental and situational, must be taken into account when assessing the pregnant family's psychosocial needs. Pregnancy, parenthood, and other family life cycle changes are examples of developmental or normative stressors.[2,11] Major illness, loss of a job, destruction of property through natural catastrophes, divorce, and separation of families because of war are examples of situational stressors (Fig. 16-5). These extrafamilial stressors work in conjunction with the intrafamilial stressors (e.g., inadequate communication, personal disorganization, inadequate role relationships) to affect the role relationships within the family by producing varying amounts of difficulty in role transition. The amount of difficulty produced is related to how well the family roles are organized, how good their resources are, and how flexible they can be in defining positively the discomfort produced by the stressor.[11]

The way the family is organized (their role structure) depends on each member's values, goals, and ability to perceive and put meaning on events (definitions of the situation). On the basis of these goals and definitions, roles are given to the members and certain behaviors become associated with each role (role allocation and differentiation). Strength is gathered from the family

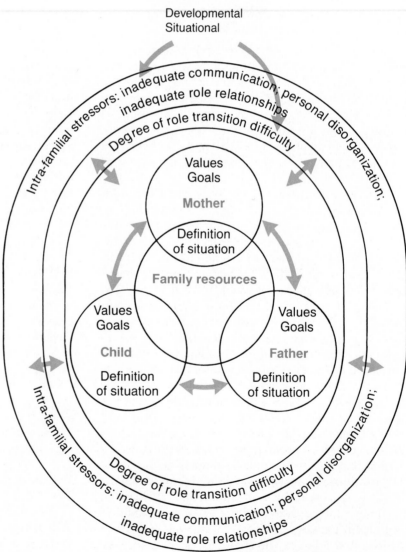

■ *Figure 16–5*
Model of family interaction during role transition and components of assessment.

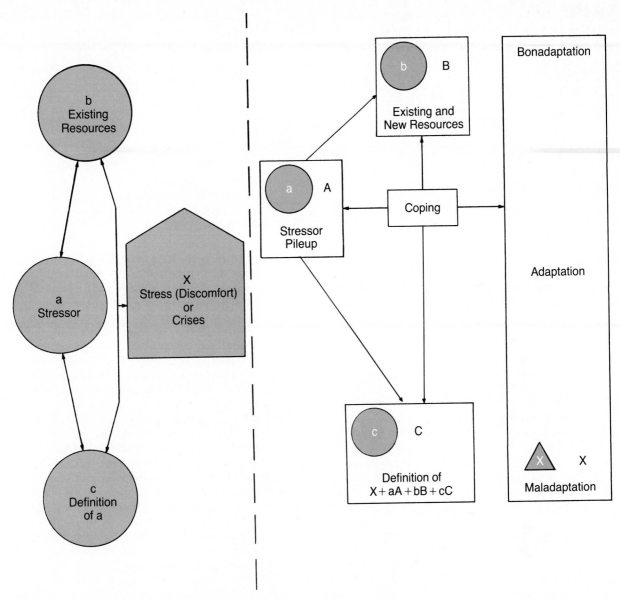

■ *Figure 16–6*
Modification of the McCubbin model for the family stress process (double ABCX). (McCubbin HI, Sussman JM, Patterson M [eds]: Social Stress and the Family, p 12. New York, Haworth Press, 1983.)

resources, which can be material (e.g., finances, material support from relatives) or interpersonal (integration, cohesiveness, good communication). Appropriately structured roles and a reservoir of family resources serve to buffer the family from the impact of the various stressors and make role transition easier.

McCubbin has pointed out that, in reality, it is infrequent that the family copes with only one stressor at a time.[11] There can be preexisting stressors or new stressors that accrue, often because of the immediate stressor, causing what McCubbin calls a "pile up" of stressors. This calls for the garnering of new resources to consolidate with the old and the redefinition of the current emerging situation. According to McCubbin's

formulation, this results in the adaptation of the family along a continuum of "good" adaptation (*bonadaptation*) through "poor" adaptation (*maladaptation*).[11] A schematic rendering of McCubbin's model can be seen in Figure 16-6.

The assessment tool shown here includes the type of questions the nurse would ask during an assessment aimed at developing a family-care plan.

Nursing Diagnosis

Assessment helps the nurse determine if members of the family are fulfilling their expected role behaviors

Assessment Tool

Assessment of Psychosocial Aspects of Pregnancy

Family Composition

1. Who are the family members? (Inlcude the extended family.)
   a. What are their ages? What are their relationships to one another?
   b. Where do they live? Do they interact frequently?
   c. Are they "close" emotionally if not physically?
   d. What is the family's relationship to the larger educational community? Is the family involved in community affairs and religious activities? What is its community support structure?

Family Functioning

1. How are the roles allocated and differentiated?
   a. Who does what in the house? Is this mutually satisfactory?
   b. Who makes decisions? How are they made? Is there mutual discussion?
   c. What are the changes that members would like?
   d. How do the parents see their roles being changed with the new infant?
2. How do members usually define situations that happen?
   a. Does the family generally consolidate in time of trouble?
   b. Do they tend to be optimistic, pessimistic, or do attitudes vary with situations?
   c. What are the communication patterns? Who talks to whom? Do problems usually get solved with discussion?
3. What are the family's material and emotional resources?
   a. Is the family's environment safe and healthful? Is housing safe and adequate? Is the house in

good repair and is there appropriate room for the expected infant? If not, what plans are being made to remedy the situation? Is the housing environment structured to prevent accidents? If not, what plans are being made to remedy this?

What is the general health status of the family? Have there been or are there now illnesses? If so, has appropriate medical (or dental) care been sought? Is there a regular source of medical and dental care for the family? Does the mother use maternity services appropriately? If not, why not? How does the family usually pay for health services? Is health insurance or health maintenance organization (HMO) service available? What are the usual health habits of the family members (exercise, rest, nutrition, smoking, substance abuse)?

   b. Are finances adequate? Who contributes? Will the pregnancy make a difference?
   c. Who turns to whom for emotional support? Who is the mother's main support at this time? Who is the father's main support at this time?
4. Are there interpersonal or intrapersonal difficulties?
   a. Are there long-term problems? What are the attempts to resolve them?
   b. Are there problems specific to this pregnancy?
   c. What alternatives for solution for the existing problems do the parents see?
5. What are the specific plans for the baby and for themselves during pregnancy?
   a. What are their plans for themselves as parents?
   b. What are their plans for the infant?
   c. Are siblings anticipated (if this is the first child)?
   d. What are plans for siblings?

appropriately. If they are at this time, the nurse can anticipate what the potential problems for the remainder of pregnancy or postpartum might be. If they are not fulfilling roles, she would ascertain how the intrafamilial and extrafamilial stressors determined by the assessment could be affecting the couple and how they perceive and are managing their resources.

Diagnoses, in this case, deal with psychosocial problems: alteration in family processes, alteration in personal and social integration, inefficient individual coping, and knowledge deficit. Both the client and the family should be considered in making diagnoses.

Planning and Intervention

The nurse who is planning interventions should keep in mind that intervention is aimed at helping the parents define possible stressors and resources within their family unit and developing strategies for coping with manifest or possible disruptive elements. By helping parents become aware of their resources and supporting them in their decision making, the nurse can minimize a great deal of stress associated with this role transition. Parents need to validate their impressions of what is

(*Text continues on page 317*)

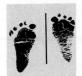

Nursing Care Plan

The Family With Pyschosocial Needs

Nursing Goals:

1. Family identifies stressors and resources.
2. Family defines their situation and coming role transition realistically.
3. Family demonstrates integration and utilizes and develops support systems.
4. Family demonstrates adaptation to the situation.

Assessment	Potential Nursing Diagnosis	Planning/Intervention	Evaluation
Family Composition Ages; relationships to one another Where they live; frequency of interaction Emotional closeness Family's relationship to larger community; family's involvement in community affairs and religious activities; community support structure Additional members in its social network; other relatives or friends available for support	Alteration in personal and social integration related to lack of support in the family and social network	Identify potential stressors and sources of support within family and between family and community Support family in their decision making Allow family to validate their impressions of what is happening to them Encourage family to use identified support systems	Family verbalizes understanding of stressors or potential stressors Family uses support systems appropriately

Family Functioning
 	
Role allocation and differentiation
  Who does what; mutually satisfactory?
  Decision maker; how made
  Any changes members would like
  Parents' views of role changes with new infant
Member definitions of situations that happen
  Family consolidation in times of trouble
  Tone of attitude: optimistic, pessimistic, or varying
  Communication patterns; who talks to whom; problem solving with discussions
	Alteration in family processes related to pregnancy
	
	Alteration in family processes related to disturbance in communication patterns
		Identify potential stressors and sources of support within familial roles or in decision making
		
		Encourage family to use identified support systems
		
		Identify family's realistic views of role changes
		
		Identify potential stressors and sources of support within family communication patterns
		
		Share with the family any nurses' perceptions of healthy communication patterns
			Family verbalizes understanding of stressors or potential stressors
			
			Family uses support systems appropriately
			
			Family has realistic perception that infant will change their lives and adjustment is possible
			
			Family verbalizes understanding of stressors or potential stressors
			
			Family uses support systems appropriately
			
			Family is perceived as drawing together by family and nurse

(continued)

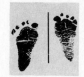

Nursing Care Plan (continued)

Assessment	Potential Nursing Diagnosis	Planning/Intervention	Evaluation

Family's material and emotional resources
  Is the general and health status of the family and environment safe and healthful?
 	
  Is housing safe and adequate with appropriate room for expected infant?
  What is the health status of the family? Recent illness? Appropriate medical and dental care sought? Regular source of medical and dental care? Clinic, insurance, HMO available?
  Maternity services appropriately used? General health habits of family healthful?
  Adequate finances; who contributes; differences with pregnancy
  Who turns to whom for emotional support; mother's support; father's support
	Ineffective individual coping related to inadequate resources
	Alteration in health maintenance related to inadequate resources
		Identify stressors in systems: environmental, emotional, and financial
		Identify alternative support systems
		Refer family to financial services as necessary
			Family shows adequate emotional and financial support systems
			Family uses support systems appropriately

Interpersonal or intrapersonal difficulties
  Long-term problems; resolution attempts
  Problems specific to this pregnancy
  Alternative solutions for existing problems
	Social isolation related to demands of pregnancy	Identify any long-term problems or problems specific to this pregnancy
		Determine best support systems and solutions for this family
			Family's long-term problems are resolved
			Family's problems specific to this pregnancy are resolved

Specific plans for baby and selves during pregnancy
  Plans for themselves as parents
  Plans for infants
  Siblings anticipated
  Plans for siblings
	Knowledge deficit related to pregnancy and inadequate resources	Identify whether plans are realistic or not
		Identify potential sibling rivalry situations
		Offer individualized family solutions
			Family has realistic plans for the pregnancy
			Parents have realistic expectations of selves as parents
			Minimal sibling rivalry experienced

happening to them, both physically and emotionally, with an outside person. Family, friends, and healthcare professionals can be useful in this way. The nurse should encourage the parents to use their network of family and friends if it is determined that this network can supply material and emotional support.

Evaluation

Intervention can be evaluated as effective if the family unit is perceived by the nurse and the family as drawing together, if there is open discussion of problems and experiences, if concrete plans are made for the infant's arrival, and if the parents have a realistic perception that the infant will change their lives and that adjustment is possible for this momentous new role.

A care plan for the psychosocial aspects of the pregnant family appears.

■ REFERENCES

1. La Rossa R, La Rossa MM: Transition to Parenthood: How Infants Change Families. Beverly Hills, Sage Publications, 1981
2. Getty C, Humphreys W: Understanding the Family: Stress and Change in American Family Life. New York, Appleton-Century-Crofts, 1981
3. Bibring GL et al: A study of the psychological processes in pregnancy and of the earliest mother–child relationship. In Psychoanalytic Study of the Child, 16:9–72. New York, International Universities Press, 1955
4. Hass S: Psychiatric implications in gynecology and obstetrics. In Ballak LC (ed): Psychology of Physical Illness. New York, Grune & Stratton, 1952
5. Larsen VL: Stresses of the childbearing years. Am J Public Health 56:32–36, 1966
6. Menninger WC: The emotional factors in pregnancy. Bull Menninger Clin 7:15–24, 1943
7. Caplan G: Patterns of parental response to the crisis of premature birth: A preliminary approach to modifying the mental health outcome. Psychiatry 23:365–374, 1960
8. Coleman AP, Coleman L: Pregnancy: The Psychological Experience. New York, Herder and Herder, 1971
9. Shainess N: The structure of the mothering encounter. J Nerv Ment Dis 136:146–161, 1963
10. Chertok L: Motherhood and Personality. London, Tavistock, 1969
11. McCubbin HI, Sussman MB, Patterson JM (eds): Social Stress and the Family: Advances and Developments in Family Stress Theory and Research. New York, Haworth Press, 1983
12. Kitson GC, Danson A, Foster RV et al: Sampling issues in family research. J Marr Fam 44:965–981, November 1982

13. Le Masters EE: Parenthood as crisis. Marr Fam Living 19:352–355, 1957
14. Dyer ED: Parenthood as crisis: A restudy. Marr Fam Living 25:196–201, 1963
15. Hobbs DJ Jr: Parenthood as crisis, a third study. J Marr Fam 27:367–372, 1963
16. Hill R, Hansen DA: The identification of a conceptual framework utilized in family study. Marr Fam Living 22:299–311, 1960
17. Hill R: Generic features of families under stress. Soc Casework 39(2–3):32–54, 1958
18. Belsky J, Rovine M: Social network contact, family support, and the transition to parenthood. J Marr Fam 46:455–462, May 1984
19. Steffenmeier RH: A role model of the transition to parenthood. J Marr Fam 44:319–347, May 1982
20. Gay JT, Douglas AB: Reva Rubin revisited. JOGN Nursing 17:394–399, November/December 1988
21. Gilliss CL, Highly BL, Roberts BM et al: Toward a Science of Family Nursing. New York, Addison Wesley, 1989
22. Rossi AS: Transition to parenthood. J Marr Fam 30:26–39, February 1968
23. Erickson E: Identity and the life cycle: Selected papers. Psychol Issues 1:1–171, 1959
24. Benedek T: Parenthood as a developmental phase. J Am Psychoanal Assoc 7(8):389–417, 1959
25. Duvall EM, Miller BC: Marriage and Family Development. New York, Harper & Row, 1986
26. Mercer RT: First-Time Motherhood: Experience from Teens to Forties. New York, Springer, 1986
27. Rosengren W: The sick role in pregnancy: A note on research in progress. J Health Hum Behav 3(3):213–218, Fall 1962
28. Stainton MC: The fetus: A growing member of the family. Family Relations 34:321–326, July 1985
29. Coleman AD, Coleman L: Pregnancy as an altered state of consciousness. Birth Fam J 1(1):7–11, 1974
30. Fishbein EG: Expectant fathers' stress—due to the mothers' expectations. JOGN Nursing 13:325–328, September/October 1984
31. Taubenheim AM, Silbernagel T: Meeting the needs of expectant parents. MCN 13:110–113, March/April 1988
32. Lamb GS, Lipkin M Jr: Somatic symptoms of expectant fathers. MCN 7:110–115, March/April 1982
33. Fawcett J: Body image and the pregnant couple. MCN 3:227–233, July/August 1978
34. Fawcett J, Bliss Holtz V, Hass J et al: Spouses' body image changes during and after pregnancy. Nurs Res 35:220–223, 1986
35. Drake ML, Verhulst D, Fawcett J et al: Spouse's body image changes during and after pregnancy. A replication in Canada. Image 20:88–95, Summer 1988
36. Jordan PL: Laboring for relevance: Expectant and new fatherhood. Nurs Res 39(1):11–16, January/February, 1990
37. Treathowan WH: The couvade syndrome. In Howell JG (ed): Modern Perspectives in Psycho-obstetrics, pp 66–93. New York, Brunner/Mazel, 1972
38. Strickland O: The occurrence of symptoms in expectant fathers. Nurs Res 36:184–189, May/June, 1987

39. May KA: Active involvement of expectant fathers in pregnancy: Some further considerations. JOGN Nursing 7:7–12, March/April 1978
40. Munroe RL, Munroe RH: Male pregnancy symptoms and cross-sex identity in three societies. J Soc Psychol 89:147–158, February 1973
41. Trethowen WH, Conlon MF: The couvade syndrome. Br J Psychiatry 11 1:57–66, January 1965

■ SUGGESTED READINGS

Clinton JF: Expectant fathers at risk for couvade. Nurs Res 35:290–295, 1986
Gaffney KF: Prenatal maternal attachment. Image 20(2): 106–109, 1988

Lerum CW, LoBiondo-Wood G: The relationship of maternal age quicking, and physical symptoms of pregnancy to the development of maternal–fetal attachment. Birth 16:13–17, March 1989
Maloni JA, McIndoe JE, Rubenstein G: Expectant grandparents class. JOGN Nursing 16:26–29, 1987
Stainton MC: Parents' awareness of their unborn infant in the third trimester. Birth 17:92–96, June 1990
Steinberg MC: The relationship between anticipated life change and nausea and vomiting during pregnancy. J Perinatol 4:24–31, Summer 1984
Tilden VP: The relation of life stress and social support to emotional disequilibrium during pregnancy. Res Nurs Health 6:167, 1983
Tilden VP: The relation of selected psychosocial variables to single status of adult women during pregnancy. Nurs Res 33:102–103, 1984

17

Education for Pregnancy and Parenthood

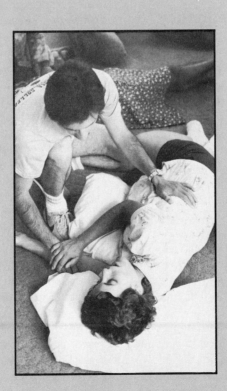

Pregnant women and their families not only are interested in learning about maternity care but also have come to view such knowledge as their right. They expect the nurse to be both willing and prepared to assist them in acquiring knowledge and to take their individual wants and needs into consideration.

The increased involvement of childbearing couples in all phases of the reproductive cycle benefits not only the parents, as receivers of care, but also nurses, as givers of care. A concerned and knowledgeable woman follows a more healthful regimen during pregnancy. A prepared woman and an involved partner can cope positively with the stresses of labor, enriching their relationship and promoting psychological maturation. Parents who are informed and who actively seek understanding of their child's numerous needs for comfort, security, and stimulation during the early formative years can attain a happier, more satisfying parent–child relationship and foster optimal growth and development of the child.

The cornerstone of client education is recognition and respect of the learning needs of clients. The nurse may design content, but if it does not meet the family's learning needs, it is pointless and ineffective. The nurse is responsible for developing the skill to assess these learning needs accurately.

■ FACTORS IN PARENT EDUCATION

Psychological Tasks of Pregnancy and Women's Interests

Nurses have long observed that pregnant women ask different kinds of questions and express different concerns in early pregnancy than in later periods of gestation.

Professional interest in the many behavior changes characteristic of pregnant women led to identification of the specific and unique psychological tasks that appear to be a universal phenomenon of pregnancy. These tasks are necessary to cope with the numerous changes, and they seem to occur at specific times during gestation (see Chap. 16).

During early pregnancy, when the woman is working through the idea of being pregnant, informational needs center on validating the pregnancy, understanding physical changes, and recognizing normal emotions and feelings. In midpregnancy, a woman begins to identify the baby as a unique person and is receptive to information about fetal growth and development and about maintaining her own health and the baby's health. As pregnancy draws to an end, the woman be-

comes concerned about preparing for the baby's arrival and becomes interested in preparation for childbirth, infant behavior, and caretaking activities including feeding, handling, bathing, and so on. By tailoring the information presented to the different interests of each group and providing women with the opportunity to express their own learning needs, nurses can conduct meaningful antepartal educational programs.

Table 17-1 lists learning needs by trimesters.[1]

Importance of Labor and Postpartum Processes

Although the experience of labor is undoubtedly significant for the woman's self-concept, maternal–infant bonding, and possibly the couple's relationship, few data are available to substantiate what impact nursing intervention during labor might have on these perceptions. Advocates of prepared childbirth believe that women move more rapidly into the caretaking role when they are awake and actively participating in their labor. There is some empirical evidence that fathers who act as labor coaches develop stronger and more recognizable paternal feelings toward the babies of these labors than toward their other children.

Effective client teaching must take into account what is known about the processes occurring during labor and the puerperium, as well as individual variation and specific need. If the labor experience is as important as we suspect, health professionals have an obligation to assist parents in preparing for it and supporting them during this stressful time. When labor has started, a certain amount of teaching is possible, and sensitive care can be helpful, but this is not as effective as antenatal preparation.

Other physiological and psychological changes that occur during the puerperium are part of the process undergone by the mother and must be taken into consideration when planning postpartum education. For further details of these physiological and psychological changes and their relation to teaching, refer to Chapters 26 and 27.

Socioeconomic and Cultural Factors

The learning process varies according to culture and the socioeconomic situation. Mothering practices in lower-income groups are influenced by economic circumstances that limit equipment, supplies, and mobility; by the organization of the family group and the authority structure; and by the accumulated folk knowledge that establishes specific practices for many common activities and problems of childrearing. Standard educational

Research Highlight

An interesting study performed by Geden in 1985 attempted to determine which of the three segments of the core content of Lamaze classes is the most effective in reducing pain: (1) informational content, (2) relaxation training, or (3) breathing exercises. In this study, 80 nulliparous college women were randomly divided into one of eight of the following treatment groups: (a) relaxation training, breathing exercises, and informational lectures, (b) relaxation and breathing, (c) relaxation and information, (d) breathing and information, (e) relaxation, (f) breathing, (g) information, and (h) no treatment.

Using standardized measurements, the researchers rated individual's heart rate, blood pressure respirations, EMG, and self-reported pain (a previously researched instrument). An examination of the overall pattern of results indicated that two of eight groups manifested significant reductions in self-reported pain, five groups manifested significant reduuctions in frontalis EMG, and all eight groups manifested significant reductions in heart rate.

Of the 15 significant findings, 9 involved treatment groups containing the relaxation component. In addition, relaxation training when delivered in isolation was the sole principle component to show significant reductions in self-reported pain, EMG activity, and heart rate. The authors concluded that "relaxation training comprised the most therapeutically active component of the current Lamaze treatment regimen." The authors did hasten to point out the limitations of their research and indicated that further clinical recommendations could not be made until further study was conducted comparing newly packaged treatment formats versus the standard labor class format.

This study seems to indicate that it would be worthwhile for nurse educators to spend more time on relaxation training with pregnant clients and to emphasize its importance in coping with labor. Many certified childbirth educators already follow these guidelines.

Geden E, Beck N, Brouder G, et al: Self-report and psychophysiological effects of Lamaze preparation: An analogue of labor pain. Res Nurs Health 8:155–165, 1985.

(A previous study of 30 postpartum women was conducted to determine which pain stimulus was most like the transition phase of labor. See Geden E, Beck N, Brouder G et al: Identifying procedural components for analogue research of labor pain, Nurs Res 32:2, March/April, 1983.)

programs about breast-feeding or formula preparation, clothing and supplies for the baby, integration of the baby into the family, and the mother's nutritional and rest needs are often meaningless to low-income mothers because of a lack of resources and a different value system. Family and friends are generally viewed as more reliable consultants for health concerns than professionals, whose assistance is sought only when community knowledge cannot solve the problem. Sometimes the use of language precludes useful exchange of information. In lower socioeconomic levels, the grandmother's word about baby care is often law, and she may be the major caretaker of the baby. Teaching given solely to the mother may be of little consequence to the actual care given to the baby. Different cultural groups also have unique approaches to childrearing and patterns of assistance to new mothers.

The nurse must come to understand different cultural and income lifestyles if effective antepartum and postpartum teaching is to occur. The approach to teaching used with these groups probably needs to shift from the giving of information to assessing present practices, supplementing these practices when necessary with information presented in a form that can be understood and accepted.

Characteristics of Adult Learners

According to Knowles,[2] adult learners differ from other learners. Because the majority of expectant and new parents the nurse comes in contact with are adults, it is important to take these differences into consideration.

The Adult Learner[3]

1. *Is independent and self-directed in learning.* The nurse serves, therefore, as a facilitator, resource person, and encourager in the learning situation as opposed to being the total director of learning.

2. *Has previous experiences that serve as rich resources for learning.* Students learn faster and better when the teacher relates new class material to their past experiences and builds on previous knowledge. Learners can also serve as resources for others in the classroom situation. The teacher is not, therefore, the source of all knowledge in the classroom.

3. *Has a readiness to learn that is based on current social roles and tasks.* Life situations influence the adult's readiness to learn. For example, a stressful life situation because of inadequate money can

TABLE 17–1. LEARNING NEEDS OF EXPECTANT PARENTS: PREGNANCY AND CHILDBIRTH*

First Trimester	Second Trimester	Third Trimester
• Physical changes of pregnancy	• Physical changes of second trimester	• Physical changes of third trimester
• Emotional changes of pregnancy	• Emotional changes of second trimester	• Emotional changes of third trimester and postpartum period

• Sexuality
  Changing relationships
  Sexual concerns
	• Sexuality
	  Changing needs
	  Sexual concerns
		• Sexuality
		  Changing needs
		  Sexual expression (different methods)
		  Sexual concerns
		  Problem solving

• Minor discomforts of pregnancy
  Frequent urination
  Nausea
  Cramps
  Vaginal discharge
  Fatigue
	• Minor discomforts of pregnancy
	  Backache
	  Varicose veins
	  Braxton Hicks contractions
	  Leg cramps
	  Vaginal discharge
	  Constipation
	  Round ligament pain
		• Minor discomforts of pregnancy
		  Frequent urination
		  Backache
		  Dyspnea
		  Varicose veins
		  Braxton Hicks contractions
		  Leg cramps
		  Vaginal discharge
		  Constipation
		  Round ligament pain
		  Fatigue

• Danger signs
  Vaginal bleeding
  Persistent vomiting
	• Danger signs
	  Vaginal bleeding
	  Abdominal pain
	  Edema of face, hands, feet
	  Severe headache
	  Visual disturbances
	  Rupture of membranes
		• Danger signs
		  Vaginal bleeding
		  Abdominal pain
		  Edema of face, hands, feet
		  Severe headache
		  Visual disturbances
		  Rupture of membranes (before 38 weeks)

• Nutrition	• Nutrition	• Nutrition

• General hygiene
  Rest and sleep
  Exercise
	• General hygiene
	  Rest and sleep
	  Exercise
		• General hygiene
		  Rest and sleep
		  Exercise

• Use of drugs
  Smoking
  Alcohol
  Over-the-counter (OTC) drugs
  Prescription drugs
	• Use of drugs
	  Smoking
	  Alcohol
	  OTC drugs
	  Prescription drugs
		• Use of drugs
		  Smoking
		  Alcohol
		  OTC drugs
		  Prescription drugs

• Fetal development	• Fetal growth	• Fetal growth

• Financial considerations	• Preparation for newborn
	  Feeding methods
	  Physical arrangements
	  Selection of pediatrician
	  Infant care
		• Preparation for breast-feeding

• How to use the health care system		• Support systems

• Resources for pregnancy and childbirth		• Preparation for childbirth
		  Common fears and anxieties
		  Father involvement in childbirth
		  The issue of choice
		  Anatomy and physiology of childbirth
		  Comfort measures
		  Pain management strategies
		  Variations in childbirth

• Myths about pregnancy and childbirth		

(continued)

TABLE 17-1   LEARNING NEEDS OF EXPECTANT PARENTS: PREGNANCY AND CHILDBIRTH *(continued)*

First Trimester	Second Trimester	Third Trimester
		Hospital routines
		Obstetrical interventions
		Special needs of multi-paras
		• Parenting
		Life-style changes
		Role changes
		Role conflict
		Balancing family demands
		Maternal role acquisition
		Maternal development tasks
		• Preparation for newborn
		• Family planning

*Adapted from Roberts J: Prenatal teaching guide. JOGN Nursing 5:18, 1976. While there is strong research support for some of these learning needs, others are based on health-care professionals' beliefs of what expectant parents need to know. The most appropriate time for the introduction of these topic areas in childbirth education classes is as yet undetermined from a scientific perspective. There is a need for the systematic documentation of the learning needs of expectant parents and the best time during pregnancy to discuss them from the parents' perspective as well as from that of health professionals.

This Table is from: Nichols Francine: The Content. In Nichols F Humenick S (eds): Childbirth Education: Practice Research, and Theory. Philadelphia: WR Saunders, 1988.

hinder readiness to learn, whereas other life situations such as pregnancy can increase the adult's eagerness to learn. The nurse needs to be sensitive to the life situations of learners and work with the adult to overcome any barriers to learning.

4. *Wants to learn things that have immediate application.* Adults often are motivated to attend classes because of a particular need. If the class can be structured so that the learner can immediately use some of the information in life situations, this enhances the learning process. Information presented on the first night of class on coping with the discomforts of pregnancy and how to develop basic relaxation skills are examples of information that the adult learner can use immediately.

5. *Prefers a problem-oriented learning approach as opposed to a subject-oriented learning approach.* Adults want to learn how to solve real-life problems; thus, they are often less interested in information presented in a subject-oriented format. When a nurse teaches fetal development by describing the anatomy and physiology of conception and subsequent development, the nurse is using a subject-centered approach. When the nurse teaches about pregnancy from the perspective of expectant parents' tasks and sensations of pregnancy while weaving in a description of the developing fetus, he or she is using a problem-centered approach to teaching fetal development. In this approach, learners can more readily apply the information to their own situation.

Time also is important to adults. Classes should start and end on time. Adults need to feel they are getting something of value out of their learning experience. Classes should be organized so that early in the first class, each learner feels his or her presence in class is important because of the material that was discussed. Ideally, each learner should come away from each class thinking it is a good thing he or she did not miss this class because important things were learned and each minute of class time was well spent.

The Cone of Learning

In addition to all the other factors just discussed, the nurse–educator must take the "learning cone" into consideration before planning content (Fig. 17-1). If learning is to occur, the nurse must do more than merely present the content and hope the patient remembers.

■ TYPES OF EDUCATION FOR PREGNANCY, LABOR, AND POSTPARTUM

Preparation for parenthood is influenced by an accumulation of experiences through infancy, childhood, adolescence, and maturity. Schools are increasingly incorporating information about childbearing and par-

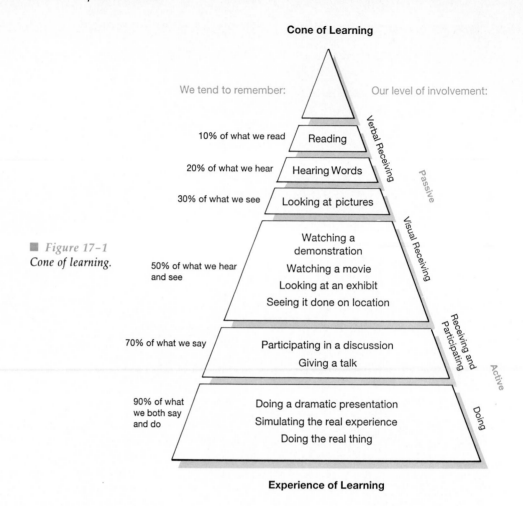

Cone of Learning

We tend to remember:

Our level of involvement:

10% of what we read	Reading
20% of what we hear	Hearing Words
30% of what we see	Looking at pictures
50% of what we hear and see	Watching a demonstration / Watching a movie / Looking at an exhibit / Seeing it done on location
70% of what we say	Participating in a discussion / Giving a talk
90% of what we both say and do	Doing a dramatic presentation / Simulating the real experience / Doing the real thing

Verbal Receiving

Visual Receiving

Passive

Receiving and Participating

Active

Doing

Experience of Learning

■ *Figure 17–1*
Cone of learning.

enthood into "health education" and "family life" courses. Classes about pregnancy, sexuality, and parenthood are becoming more common in high school and university curricula, as well as more widely available in continuing education and private adult educational programs. Couples bring a wealth of previous learning to their experience of childbearing, some of it useful and positive and some frightening and inaccurate. With the advent of pregnancy, preparation for parenthood begins in earnest.

Individual Teaching and Counseling

One-to-one teaching is widely used in all nursing settings and is frequently effective in assisting clients to understand and adapt to a variety of health problems. In most nurse–client contacts, some individual teaching occurs. Numerous opportunities are present during pregnancy for nurses to enhance the effectiveness of medical care through explanations of treatments and procedures, interpretations of what the physician tells parents, and specific instructions for carrying out the regimen of care. When the client asks questions about

symptoms or feelings or seeks general information, an on-the-spot response by the nurse meets that particular learning need.

Some clinics and offices have pamphlets or audio-visual material intended to provide individualized instruction to parents during the antepartal period. The amount of structure necessary to ensure that these materials are actually used varies widely. The effectiveness of written or media information without reinforcement through discussion is limited (see Fig. 17-1).

Counseling, an interchange of opinions or giving of advice to help direct the judgment or conduct of others, is often hard to separate from teaching. Although counseling is more personal and feeling oriented, its use in combination with presentation of facts usually results in enhanced learning. Appropriate use of counseling takes into consideration the client's viewpoint and works within an acceptable framework to bring about increased understanding, which leads to a change in behavior in the desired direction through the client's internalization of the new goals.

Individualized nursing care in which the woman is assisted to recognize her feelings and fears, is reassured that such feelings are normal, and is given certain facts to dispel myths or anticipate and prepare for coming events is an example of combined teaching and counseling in antepartal care.

Group Education

Although individual teaching and counseling continue to be a major mode of nursing intervention, concerns for more efficient use of the health professional's time have led to increased use of groups for antepartal and postpartum education. Groups are also beneficial because the exchange of experiences among parents with common concerns provides support and encouragement.

Groups also can provide increased motivation, sharing of resources, and socialization with others who share common interests.

Most institutions providing maternity care also offer some type of antepartal group instruction, but the goals and purposes as well as quality of the groups vary widely.

Classes also may be affiliated with continuing education programs in colleges and universities, adult education programs in local communities and high schools, health professionals in private practice, or national health-care organizations such as the Red Cross.

The following are examples of group classes that may be available. Some communities have a wide range available, whereas others have few.

1. *Early pregnancy classes* usually are given for women in the first trimester and include content about fetal growth and development, nutrition, early physical and emotional changes in pregnancy, drugs and toxins, exercises, and selecting a health-care provider and place of birth that shares the women's goals for the birth.
2. *Breast-feeding classes* for antepartum clients are becoming extremely popular. These classes usually consist of 8 to 10 women in their last trimester. Husbands, grandmothers, or other support people are welcome in some classes. Emphasis is placed on knowledge of the lactation process, nutrition, how to prevent and overcome the common minor problems of breast-feeding, myths and misconceptions, and information about the working mother and breast-feeding. Often, a mother and infant from a previous class return to demonstrate proper positioning, manual expression, and how to use breast pumps. These classes are often taught by certified lactation educators or certified lactation consultants, who are either hired by a hospital to teach or are in private practice.
3. *Baby care classes* usually include the father and cover safety, crying, parenting tips, car seats, buy-

ing clothes, circumcision, handling baby, and feeding. Some classes actually have each of the participants bathe, diaper, and dress a life-size and weight doll. This hands-on experience is valuable.
4. *Sibling preparation classes.* These fun classes help prepare the sibling for the new baby by discussing pregnancy, birth and newborns, and the sibling's role as a big brother or sister.
5. *Prenatal and postpartum exercise classes*
6. *Yoga classes*
7. *Childbirth education classes*
8. *VBAC (vaginal birth after cesarean) classes.* Some areas have specialized classes for women who have had a previous cesarean who are attempting a vaginal birth with the current pregnancy. In most areas, however, this group takes standard childbirth education with supplemental reading and individual discussion with the teacher.
9. *Mothers' groups*
10. *Parenting groups*
11. *Breast-feeding and returning to work*
12. *Infant and child CPR.* Because most parents do not know how to perform CPR on infants or children these classes can be valuable for parents of young children.
13. *Emergency situations classes for your child-care provider.* Relatively new in some areas, these innovative classes cover infant and child CPR, the Heimlich maneuver, how to call 911, basic first aid, poison control, common childhood illnesses, home safety, what to do in case of fire or earthquake, and kidnapping awareness.

These educational programs can enhance, strengthen, and broaden the care and services provided by the physician and maternity nurse.

■ COMFORT DURING PREGNANCY

The Nursing Process

During the many weeks of prenatal care, the nurse has a golden opportunity to help the woman be more comfortable during her pregnancy. Aches and pains are so common during pregnancy that many women are unaware there are remedies that may help (see Chap. 19).

ASSESSMENT

Prenatal assessment should include observation of posture (see Posture Checklist) as well as a thorough history

Client Education

Posture Checklist

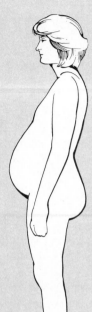

Incorrect Posture	**To Correct Posture**
Head	*Head*
Neck sags, chin pokes forward, and whole body slumps	Straighten neck and tuck chin in so body lines up
Shoulders and chest	*Shoulders and chest*
Slouching cramps the rib cage and makes breathing difficult	Lift up through rib cage and pull shoulder girdle back
Arms turn in	Roll arms out
Abdomen and buttocks	*Abdomen and buttocks*
Slack muscles cause a hollow back	Contract abdominals to flatten back
Pelvis tilts forward	Tuck buttocks under and tilt pelvis back
Knees	*Knees*
Pressed back strains joints and pushes pelvis forward	Bend to ease body weight over feet
Feet	*Feet*
Weight on inner borders strains arches	Distribute body weight through center of each foot

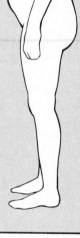

(Noble E: Essential Exercises for the Childbearing Year. Boston, Houghton-Mifflin, 1988)

of the client's discomforts and what, if anything she has found to relieve them. The nurse should also find out which sleeping positions are most comfortable for the client.

POTENTIAL NURSING DIAGNOSES

As a result of the nursing assessment, several potential nursing diagnoses may be identified that focus on the woman's comfort.

PLANNING AND INTERVENTION

Having discovered a particular woman's discomforts, the next step is to plan patient teaching strategies to help alleviate them. The nurse must first be sure that specific discomforts are not related to pathophysiology and as such need to be reported to the physician (e.g.,

---

Potential Nursing Diagnoses

Low backache related to weak abdominal muscles, poor posture, improper body mechanics

Difficulty sleeping related to knowledge deficit about pillow placement for increased relaxation and comfort

Upper backache related to poor posture

Swelling of feet and ankles related to knowledge deficit about how to minimize

Leg cramps related to pressure of uterus on nerves to lower extremities

Hemorrhoids related to constipation

Shortness of breath related to pressure on diaphragm by enlarged uterus

Client Education

Principles for ADL During Pregnancy

- Activities need to be varied (walking, standing, sitting).
- Time period should be of short duration.
- Walking back and forth is preferable to standing still.
- Standing posture should be with one leg forward so that weight can be shifted easily and efficiently from foot to foot and the body can be turned comfortably.
- Walking posture should be head erect, back upright, chin up, and pelvis tilted.
- Use a footstool when sitting.
- When climbing stairs, the entire foot should be placed on stair and leg muscles should be used to lift self up each step without leaning forward.
- Stooping and lifting should be avoided; if stooping is necessary, it is best to squat down and reach and lift, with feet wide apart and back straight. The alternate squatting position, with one foot placed forward, may also be used. The body is lowered slowly to the other knee. The front foot, which should be flat on the floor, is used for lifting. The rear foot, flexed at the toes, serves for pushing and acts as a balance.
- When carrying bulky packages (e.g., groceries), the load should be divided and carried in two hands. A cart that rolls easily should be used for heavy loads.

swelling of feet and ankles may be related to toxemia or the woman with shortness of breath may be having cardiac difficulties). Using the Posture Checklist, Principles for Activities of Daily Living (ADL) During Pregnancy, and exercises presented in Table 17-2 and in Appendix C, the nurse can plan appropriate interventions for the patient.

EVALUATION

The nurse must be realistic in the evaluation of the outcome of the nursing interventions. It is unlikely that all the woman's discomforts can be relieved, but some improvement, even temporary, should be expected. On the other hand, perhaps a reassessment can point to a misdiagnosis and lead to a more effective nursing intervention.

Posture and Body Mechanics

Maintaining correct posture and practicing good body mechanics are important in avoiding some of the more common discomforts of pregnancy. For example, a frequent cause of backache during pregnancy is poor posture. As pregnancy progresses, body proportion and weight distribution are altered. As the body's center of gravity is gradually shifted forward, the abdominal muscles often relax and the natural curvature of the

spine becomes exaggerated, shortening the muscles of the lower back. The woman often compensates for this by leaning backward slightly at the waist, which shifts her weight to her heels when walking. This results in an awkward, waddling gait and frequently contributes to backaches, particularly of the lower back.

It is important to encourage the woman to be constantly mindful of her posture and to provide her with information on correcting her body alignment (see Posture Checklist). Some exercises, such as the pelvic tilt which strengthens the muscles of the abdomen and lower back, are also helpful in correcting poor posture and relieving backaches (see Appendix C).

The importance of practicing good body mechanics should also be taught to the pregnant woman. Body mechanics involve the efficient use of the body to distribute weight and stress evenly among several muscle groups rather than overtaxing a particular muscle group with undue strain. For example, pregnant women should be instructed to avoid stooping when lifting or reaching for low objects. Bending forward or stooping may put the woman off balance and requires the muscles of the back to assume the burden of returning the trunk (and any weight that is lifted) to an erect posture. A squatting posture is much preferred when reaching for low objects. The woman should be instructed to squat with the back straight and the body properly aligned. Any weight to be lifted should be pulled close to the body, and the muscles of the thighs and legs should be used to raise the body to an erect posture.

TABLE 17-2. EXERCISES AND POSITIONS TO RELIEVE COMMON DISCOMFORTS OF PREGNANCY

Discomfort	Exercise or Position
Swelling of feet, ankles	Leg elevating
Leaking urine when coughing, laughing	Pelvic floor contraction
Heaviness in pelvis	Pelvic floor contraction
Hemorrhoids and swelling around vagina	Pelvic floor contraction
Cramps in legs	Leg elevating; calf stretching
Tired legs	Leg elevating; calf stretching
Varicose veins in legs	Leg elevating; calf stretching
Shortness of breath	Good posture; good body mechanics; rib cage lifting; shoulder circling
Low backache	Pelvic rocking; good posture; pushing position; squatting
Middle backache	Pushing position
Upper backache	Shoulder circling; good posture
Numbness in arms and fingers	Shoulder circling; lying on side
Abdominal muscle spasm (stitch)	Pelvic rocking; deep abdominal breathing

Good body mechanics relate directly to good posture. Throughout daily activities, such as household chores, walking, and climbing stairs, the woman should be encouraged to keep the back straight (but not rigid) and the body in proper alignment. Learning to maintain a correct posture and practicing good body mechanics often require a considerable amount of conscious thought and practice at first. It is not unusual for a person who has previously had poor posture to feel strange or even uncomfortable when her body is in proper alignment. However, it should be emphasized that good posture and body mechanics are beneficial throughout life, and it is hoped that the lessons learned during pregnancy carry over to a more healthful future. (See Principles for ADL During Pregnancy.)

Comfort Positions

Pregnant women often comment that they find it difficult to relax because they are unable to find a comfortable position or that heartburn, backaches, or other common discomforts interfere with their ability to relax. A variety of positions have been found effective in providing comfort and in relieving some of the discomforts of pregnancy. A comfort method for sleeping is illustrated in Figure 17-2.

It should be noted that a position that is effective for one woman may not necessarily work equally well for another. For example, some women find the squatting position relaxing and effective in relieving backaches; others find a pushing posture or some other position or exercise more effective. Women should be encouraged to try a variety of positions until they find what works best for them (see Table 17-2).

■ EXERCISE DURING PREGNANCY

Exercises performed during pregnancy increase circulation, improve muscle tone, aid in prevention of fatigue, promote physical comfort, and encourage good posture.

The Nursing Process

ASSESSMENT

Before encouraging a pregnant women to begin an exercise program, the nurse should consider several factors in the assessment. Has the woman's lifestyle been active or sedentary? Does she have any of the relative or absolute contraindications for strenuous (or any) exercise (Tables 17-3 and 17-4)? Is she already involved in an

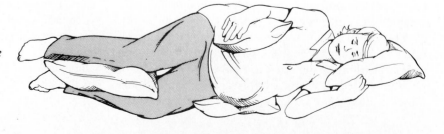

■ Figure 17-2
Comfort positions are positions in which the body is in alignment, with no body part resting on any other body part.

TABLE 17-3. CONTRAINDICATIONS THAT MAY RULE OUT VIGOROUS ACTIVITY

Hypertension
Anemia and other blood disorders
Thyroid disease
Diabetes
Cardiac arrhythmia or palpitations
History of precipitous labor
History of intrauterine growth retardation
History of bleeding during pregnancy
Breach presentation in the last trimester
Excessive obesity or extreme underweight
History of extremely sedentary life-style

(Artal R: Exercise During Pregnancy and the Postnatal Period. Washington, DC, American College of Obstetricians and Gynecologists [ACOG], 1985)

exercise program? How many times a week and for how long? How strenuous? What kinds of exercises?

PLANNING AND INTERVENTION

The nurse can either plan client education for the woman or refer her to some of the many books and videotapes available that deal specifically with exercise and pregnancy (see section entitled "Other Resources on Pregnancy and Childbirth" at the end of this chapter). Some hospitals have physical therapists who specialize in pregnancy. The community may offer pregnancy exercise classes of good quality, or community swimming pools may be available for exercising.

EVALUATION

Evaluation would include asking whether the exercises are helpful (e.g., do they decrease backache due to weak abdominal muscles? Do they increase physical stamina?). The nurse should also evaluate for any signs or symptoms that should be reported to the obstetrical care provider (see "Warning Signs and Signals During and After Exercise"). Frequency and duration of exercise periods should also be evaluated.

Potential Nursing Diagnosis

Knowledge deficit related to benefits of exercise during pregnancy, optimum frequency and length of time, most important body areas to exercise, and inappropriate types of exercises

---

Risk Factors During Pregnancy

Each woman needs to be individually evaluated regarding an exercise program. She should be instructed about the general warning signs and symptoms that should always signal her to stop exercising and contact the physician.

Warning Signs and Symptoms During or After Exercising

Pain
Bleeding
Dizziness
Shortness of breath
Palpitations
Faintness
Tachycardia
Back pain
Pubic pain
Difficulty walking

Table 17-3 lists conditions that *may* rule out vigorous activity for the pregnant client, and Table 17-4 lists *absolute* contraindications for vigorous exercise during pregnancy.[4]

General Guidelines for Exercise

The following guidelines are based on the unique physical and physiological conditions that exist during pregnancy and the postpartum period. They outline general criteria for safety to provide direction to patients in the development of home exercise programs.[4]

Pregnancy and Postpartum

1. Regular exercise (at least three times per week) is preferable to intermittent activity. Competitive activities should be discouraged.
2. Vigorous exercise should not be performed in hot, humid weather or during a period of febrile illness.

TABLE 17-4. ABSOLUTE CONTRAINDICATIONS TO VIGOROUS EXERCISE

History of more than three spontaneous abortions
Ruptured membranes
Premature labor
Diagnosed multiple gestation
Incompetent cervix
Bleeding or a diagnosis of placenta previa
Diagnosed cardiac disease

(Artal R: Exercise During Pregnancy and the Postnatal Period. Washington, DC, American College of Obstetricians and Gynecologists [ACOG], 1985)

3. Ballistic movements (jerky, bouncy motions) should be avoided. Exercise should be done on a wooden floor or a tightly carpeted surface to reduce shock and provide a sure footing.

4. Deep flexion or extension of joints should be avoided because of connective tissue laxity. Activities that require jumping, jarring motions, or rapid changes in direction should be avoided because of joint instability.

5. Vigorous exercise should be preceded by a 5-minute period of muscle warm-up. This can be accomplished by slow walking or stationary cycling with low resistance.

6. Vigorous exercise should be followed by a period of gradually declining activity that includes gentle stationary stretching. Because connective tissue laxity increases the risk of joint injury, stretches should not be taken to the point of maximum resistance.

7. Heart rate should be measured at times of peak activity. Target heart rates and limits established in consultation with the physician should not be exceeded (Table 17-5).

8. Care should be taken to rise gradually from the floor to avoid orthostatic hypotension. Some form of activity involving the legs should be continued for a brief period.

9. Liquids should be taken liberally before and after exercise to prevent dehydration. If necessary, activity should be interrupted to replenish fluids.

10. Women who have led sedentary lifestyles should begin with physical activity of low intensity and advance to higher activity levels gradually.

11. Activity should be stopped and the physician should be consulted if any unusual symptoms appear.

Pregnancy Only

1. Maternal heart rate should not exceed 140 beats per minute.
2. Strenuous activities should not exceed 15 minutes in duration.
3. No exercise should be performed in the supine position after the fourth month of gestation is completed.
4. Exercises that employ Valsalva's maneuver should be avoided.
5. Caloric intake should be adequate to meet not only the extra energy needs of pregnancy, but also of the exercise performed.
6. Maternal core temperature should not exceed 38°C.

We recognize that the exercises presented in Appendix C do not exactly follow ACOG guidelines—no exercises done on the back after the fourth month.[4] We point out, however, that all exercises except straight curl-up can be done easily in positions other than on the back. (The straight curl-up, as noted in Appendix C, is not for "late starters.")

Women should certainly be taught to watch for symptoms of dyspnea and dizziness, in which case exercise on the back is inappropriate. Women who have no symptoms may want to alternate back exercises with exercises that can be done in other positions. In any event, strenuous exercises on the back are not advisable. In Appendix C, we present some of the recommended prenatal and postpartum exercises of Elizabeth Noble.[5] For more detailed content than we can present, please refer to her book.

■ PREPARATION FOR LABOR AND BIRTH

Whether or not the maternity nurse is involved in offering classes for parents, it is important that education for childbirth be part of the professional repertoire. This information can be used for individual teaching or for reinforcing what has been learned from other sources. Including the father in this instruction helps him understand his partner's needs during the childbearing process and offer support.

The Nursing Process

During the last trimester, women become increasingly concerned about the impending labor and birth and are especially receptive to learning about that process. The

TABLE 17–5. HEART RATE GUIDELINES FOR POSTPARTUM EXERCISE

Age	Beats per Minute	
	Limit*	Maximum
20	150	200
25	146	195
30	142	190
35	138	185
40	135	180
45	131	175

*Each figure represents 75% of the maximum heart rate that would be predicted for the corresponding age group. Under proper medical supervision, more strenuous activity and higher heart rates may be appropriate.

(Artal R: Exercise During Pregnancy and the Postnatal Period. Washington, DC, American College of Obstetricians and Gynecologists [ACOG], 1985)

nurse has the responsibility of helping the woman and her labor partner prepare for that momentous event.

ASSESSMENT

Assessment concerning preparation for labor and birth covers several areas. Does the woman have someone she would like to be with her to help her during labor? If the father is unwilling or unavailable because he has to be home with the other children or at work, is there a friend or relative she could count on to be with her? What previous labor experience does the woman and the labor support person have? What have they read about the labor process? Are they planning to attend childbirth education classes? If not, why not? Has the woman (and her partner) given any thought to any of the items discussed in the section entitled "Choices in Childbirth"? This is often not given much thought, even by well-educated, well-prepared women. Many women do not know they have any choices or are not willing to do the "research" necessary to delve into this area. Others have great difficulty establishing a dialogue with their care provider that may involve assertiveness skills to obtain compromises. The nurse can be helpful as a consumer advocate by encouraging the patient to think about options and suggest reading materials.

POTENTIAL NURSING DIAGNOSES

The possible nursing diagnoses in this area are practically limitless. A few of them are listed here.

PLANNING AND INTERVENTION

Having determined a specific woman's knowledge deficits, the nurse can plan ways to assist the woman to take responsibility for her own learning. There is an abundant supply of books and audio and video materials available about labor and how to prepare for coping with labor and birth (see section entitled "Other Re-

sources on Pregnancy and Childbirth" at the end of this chapter). The nurse can be helpful in assisting the woman to choose a quality childbirth class and, in the event that the woman cannot attend, assist her in learning relaxation, imagery, breathing, and pushing techniques. In the event that the woman comes to labor not knowing how to relax and not knowing any breathing techniques, the nurse can teach her some "on-the-spot" techniques.

EVALUATION

It is unlikely that the nurse can fill all the knowledge deficits concerning preparation for labor and birth for any one patient, let alone for the many patients seen. That is why organized classes were developed and so many books have been written. However, the nurse can do a great deal for a lot of patients if he or she uses an organized approach.

Choices in Childbirth

Today, in most areas of this country, women and their partners have choices surrounding their birth experience. Although in some geographic areas choices may be few, in other areas the choices are many and varied. Some parents-to-be decide to choose their birth attendant and allow the birth attendant to make all the other choices, either because they don't want to decide or don't know about their options. Other expectant parents decide what they want in a birth experience and go out and find a birth attendant and facility they are comfortable with who can help them achieve the experience they want. "Choices in Childbirth" gives some specific labor and birth options expectant parents may want to consider. (To obtain a detailed pamphlet entitled "Planning Your Baby's Birth," see the section entitled "Other Resources on Pregnancy and Childbirth" at the end of this chapter.)

Prepared Childbirth

The late Grantly Dick-Read, a British obstetrician, emphasized certain psychological aspects of labor—that "fear is in some way the chief pain-producing agent in otherwise normal labor." The woman builds up a state of tensions because she is frightened, and these tensions create an antagonistic effect on the muscular activity of normal labor and result in more pain. The pain causes more fear, which further increases the tensions, and so on, creating a vicious circle.

Dick-Read's approach included an educational component to help women comprehend the physiological processes of labor, exercises to improve muscle tone,

(Text continues on page 334)

Potential Nursing Diagnoses

Knowledge deficits related to any special plans or choices for childbirth

Knowledge deficits related to nonattendance at childbirth education classes

Knowledge deficit related to signs and symptoms of labor and the labor process and lack of coping techniques for pain

Knowledge deficit related to what to expect in the hospital before, during, and after birth

Client Education

Choices in Childbirth

The two lists below do not represent an "either–or" situation. Most parents choose their options from both pathways. Very few doctors or midwives practice completely in accordance with either pathway. Consider and discuss each option and then decide which you prefer. Flexibility is necessary to ensure that the Birth Plan will apply in difficult or complicated labors as well as in normal and typical labors.

Medical Pathway	*Physiological Pathway*

(Which of these are routines and which are options in your hospital or birth center? Most parents choose some options from each list.)

Labor

Medical Pathway	Physiological Pathway
• Mother in wheelchair upon arrival at hospital	• Mother walks to labor and delivery
• Shave, minishave, or clipping of long hairs on perineum	• No shave or clipping of hair
• Enema	• Bowels emptied spontaneously, or enema self-administered at home
• Partner asked to leave during prep and examinations	• Partner present throughout labor and delivery
• Limit to one support person during labor and birth	• Presence of other friends, relatives, and siblings
• Confinement to bed or one position	• Freedom to walk and change position as desired

• Induction of labor
   Methods: stripping membranes, amniotomy, oxytocin
	• Spontaneous labor
	   Alternatives: making love, breast stimulation

• IV fluids for hydration and energy	• Drinking fluid or eating as desired
• Frequent vaginal examinations	• Vaginal examinations when requested by mother or for medical reasons
• Electronic fetal heart monitor	• Listening to fetal heart with fetal stethoscope
• Pain relief through medication: analgesics or anesthetics	• Relaxation, emotional support, massage, breathing

Birth

Medical Pathway	Physiological Pathway
• Lithotomy position or semisitting in labor bed for pushing	• Choice of position and freedom to move
• Prolonged breath holding and bearing down for expulsion	• Mother follows her urge to push
• Limit of 2 hours on 2nd stage, then forceps or cesarean birth	• Allow for longer 2nd stage and position variations to help progress
• Delivery table for birth	• Birth in labor bed, birth chair, or bean bag
• Lithotomy position with stirrups for birth	• Side lying, all fours, squatting, standing with leg up, semireclining with back support, no stirrups
• Mother not allowed to touch sterile field	• Mother allowed to touch baby's head as it crowns
• Catheterization in 2nd stage	• No catheterization and frequent voiding in first stage
• Episiotomy	• No episiotomy: massage, warm compresses, slower delivery, coaching to pant out baby, support to perineum Late episiotomy with no anesthetic
• Forceps or vacuum extraction	• Spontaneous delivery

(continued)

Client Education   (continued)

After Birth

- Intubation/suctioning
- Immediate care of baby done out of sight of mother (e.g., identification, Apgar, heat lamp, replace hemostat with cord clamp)

- Limit of 15–20 minutes on 3rd stage followed by manual extraction of the placenta
- Pitocin drip or injection for contraction of uterus after placenta is delivered

- Waiting to see if baby can handle own mucus
- Care done on mother's abdomen. Baby skin to skin with mother with heat lamp or blanket over them

- Delay in nonessential routines
- Allow for longer time for placenta. Allow mother to move around, nurse baby. Let cord drain
- Evaluation of uterus before using uterine stimulant routinely
- Breast-feeding

Baby

- Baby to isolette or nursery for 4–24 hours. Mother to recovery room for observation
- Eye drops–silver nitrate applied shortly after birth

- Baby's first feeding–glucose water by nurse

- Baby in nursery except for scheduled 4-hour feedings
- Circumcision
- Home in 3 or more days after delivery

- Baby held by mother or father on delivery table or in recovery
- Omit eye drops or delay administration up to 2 hours or use of other agent as alternative
- Colostrum by mother who plans to breast-feed or plain water given by mother
- Demand feeding, baby to mother when crying Twenty-four hour rooming in
- No circumcision
- Early discharge from hospital

The Unexpected

Common Medical Procedures

Cesarean Birth

- Scheduled surgery
- Mother without her support person in surgery
- General anesthesia
- Spinal or epidural
- Screen to prevent viewing surgery

- Mother not allowed to wear contacts or glasses
- Baby sent to intensive care nursery

Possible Options

- Surgery after labor begins
- Father present to support mother

- Screen lowered at time of birth or baby held up for mother and father to see
- Mother to wear contacts or glasses
- Father to hold baby and mother to see baby, if baby is not in distress
- Mother allowed to breast-feed in recovery if her and her baby's condition permits

Premature or Sick Infant

- Baby cared for by professionals

- Baby rushed to intensive care
- Baby sent to another hospital or another part of hospital

- Parents involved in care of baby, diapering, touching, talking to baby in incubator, feeding baby Mother allowed to hold and see baby, if not distressed

- Baby close to mother in same part of hospital

(continued)

Client Education (continued)

- Baby transported to hospital with intensive care unit
- Limited visits to baby from mother only
- IV and bottle feeding

- Father goes with the transport team, mother goes if she is able
- Father or extended family allowed to see baby
- Mother allowed to express her colostrum for the baby and encouraged and helped to get started at breast-feeding

(Simpkin P, Reinke C: Planning Your Baby's Birth. Seattle, The Pennypress, 1980)

and techniques to assist in relaxation and prevent the fear–tension–pain mechanism. These three components are included in most childbirth preparation programs developed after Dick-Read's work became well known.

EARLY RESISTANCE

Early in the movement in the United States, prepared childbirth earned a bad name through publicity about its more overzealous advocates. "Painless childbirth" was held up as a goal by some extremist groups, and the woman who did experience pain and resorted to pain medication during labor was made to feel a failure. This can be extremely destructive to the woman's self-concept at a time when she needs positive reinforcement in her abilities to achieve and perform competently. Fortunately, current thinking recognizes the variability in individual responses to stress and the differing character of individual labors and teaches that pain medication may at times be necessary.

In the early years, many obstetricians and labor room nurses resisted prepared childbirth. Couples who had been trained in a particular method often had to buck staff pressures in their attempt to use the relaxation and breathing techniques they had learned. Medication was at times forced on the laboring woman because the physician felt it would be best for her, even when she protested that it was not necessary. Such practices as laboring in a semiupright position instead of lying flat, having ice chips or sips of water, eliminating the perineal shave, holding and putting the baby to breast immediately after birth, and constant presence of the father throughout labor and birth caused much staff consternation and were often vetoed.

Although prepared childbirth advocates had long been reporting the increased satisfaction the couple experienced and the reduction of depressed babies when these methods were used, it took economic consumer pressure to bring about widespread acceptance of prepared childbirth. When childbearing couples began avoiding physicians and hospitals because they were not allowed to practice their method, the recalcitrants began to see the benefits of involvement and participation of the parents.

FATHER INVOLVEMENT

Prepared childbirth programs include the father as an active participant in helping the woman cope with labor. The father is made to feel involved and useful, and through learning the physiological and emotional processes of pregnancy, he may gain an appreciation of the woman's experience. He is also able to explore his feelings and role as a parent and to prepare psychologically for fatherhood.

Fathers also play another important role in labor. A study by Sosa, Kennell, and Klaus suggests that there may be major perinatal benefits of constant human support during labor.[6] The control group (no labor companion) showed a higher rate ($P < 0.001$) of subsequent perinatal problems (e.g., cesarean section and meconium staining). It was necessary to admit 103 mothers to the control group and 33 to the experimental group (supportive companions in labor) to obtain 20 in each group with uncomplicated deliveries. Also, in the final sample, the length of time from admission to delivery (primigravidas) was shorter in the experimental group (8.8 versus 19.3 hours $P < 0.001$). In another study, by Gaziano and colleagues, the women rated medication during labor of less importance than the presence of a labor companion.[7]

SELECTING A CLASS

Because prepared childbirth classes differ, it is important that couples are aware of how to shop around for a

Variables to Consider in Selecting a Childbirth Class

1. Professional credentials of instructor and type of training as a childbirth educator
2. Class size
   a. Eight couples or less—ideal for group interaction and supervised practice
   b. More than 12 couples—limited group interaction, limited supervised practice, and decreased relaxation skills mastered by couple
3. Location of class
   a. Home—usually limits class size and provides informal, relaxed atmosphere
   b. Office, school, church, or hospital—class size may escalate and atmosphere may be less than ideal
4. Total hours of class time for the fee
5. Amount of supervised practice time per session
6. Fee payment by couple
   a. Directly to instructor—instructor accountable to consumer
   b. To group or sponsoring health facility—instructor accountable to agency for content

teacher and class that suit their particular needs (see Variables to Consider in Selecting a Childbirth Class).

Lamaze or Psychoprophylactic Method

The psychoprophylactic method (PPM), or Lamaze method, is the most widely used prepared childbirth method in the United States today. It was first promoted by two Russian doctors, Nicolaiev and Velvovsky.

The rationale of the program was based on Pavlov's concept of pain perception and his theory of conditioned reflexes (i.e., the substitution of favorable conditioned reflexes for unfavorable ones).

The theory intrigued a Paris obstetrician, Ferdinand Lamaze, who studied Russian-trained mothers-to-be in a Leningrad clinic. Lamaze returned to France and began to prepare his clients in *psychoprophylaxis,* or *mental prevention* of pain in childbirth. He gradually introduced certain adaptations, the most important of which was the rapid shallow breathing that came to characterize the Lamaze method. (This breathing has since been changed.)

As the technique spread throughout Europe and Latin America, the *Lamaze method* and *psychoprophylaxis* became synonymous. The late Marjorie Karmel was perhaps the most responsible for introducing this technique to America. There are programs in psychopro-

phylaxis throughout this country. Many are under the auspices of the American Society for Psychoprophylaxis in Obstetrics, Inc. (ASPO), which was founded through joint efforts of Karmel, Elisabeth Bing, and others.

Several changes have occurred in the Lamaze method as a result of research. Class content, slower and more flexible breathing techniques, theories of learning and motivation constitute the major changes. Class content originally dealt mostly with exercises, relaxation, breathing techniques, and the normal labor and birth experience. Childbirth educators have added information on such subjects as nutrition, infant feeding, cesarean birth, medical interventions benefits and risks and other variations from usual labor, as well as discussions concerning sexuality, early parenting, and coping skills for the postpartum period.

RELAXATION

The use of relaxation as a coping skill during labor is the foundation of all the childbirth education techniques.

Many authorities regard the ability to release tension under stress as *the* most important skill being taught or learned in childbirth education classes. It is the core of all other skills, including breathing and expulsion techniques.[8] Humenick found that prenatal relaxation skill achievement was significantly related to medication used in childbirth.[9] She also found that larger childbirth class size correlated negatively with achievement of relaxation skill for expectant mothers.[10]

Tensing during labor is a natural response to the contracting uterus. Tension, however, causes exhaustion and oxygen depletion, lowers the pain threshold, and prolongs labor. Adrenaline, the hormone that accompanies the fear–tension–pain syndrome, inhibits the effects of oxytocin, which causes the uterus to contract. This interference with oxytocin actually makes the contractions of the uterus less effective and prolongs labor.[11]

Learning to relax involves an active building of awareness of the state of the muscles, either tensed or relaxed, and a conscious control by the mind of that state. It is a learned activity, a process of isolating muscle groups, differentiating between tenseness and relaxation, and a conscious letting go of or total release of muscle groups. Relaxation is an active involvement of mind over body, which requires awareness, concentration, and practice.

Constant practice or repetition of a relaxation technique is necessary to maintain a conditioned response of this nature. Continued practice establishes patterns that can be depended on if thought processes become cloudy in active labor.

The skill of relaxation is not only helpful for birth but is a lifelong skill that can be called on during the daily stresses of life.

There are many ways of teaching relaxation, including progressive relaxation, focusing, meditation, and touching.[12] Some of the methods are listed in Table 17-6.

To begin teaching relaxation it is important to start with the simple techniques and, after they are mastered, to move to the more complex. A simple general-body relaxation technique is presented to begin with (see Conditioned Relaxation), followed by Tense–Release Relaxation, and finally a neuromuscular dissociation technique. All of these Client Education charts are in Appendix C.

Many people find an audio cassette recording of a relaxation technique helpful to supplement their practice with their partner. Several are listed in the section entitled "Other Resources on Pregnancy and Childbirth" at the end of this chapter. It is also possible for a person to record her own relaxation tape by reading the exercise slowly into a tape recorder. A quick way to teach relaxation to untrained women in labor is presented in the section entitled "Jaw Relaxation" in Chapter 23..

IMAGERY

Coupled with relaxation, imagery can be a powerful coping mechanism for labor. Also called visualization, imagery is a form of daydreaming with direction and purpose. It is a conscious experience in which a person maintains a focus on one object of concentration. The physiological basis of how imagery decreases pain is not understood. However, several theories are proposed. It is known that when a person is in a highly relaxed state electroencephalographic (EEG) recordings show brain waves in the alpha state and sometimes in the theta state[13] (Table 17-7). The alpha state is most easily created in a relaxed person. This state allows a person to use the functions of the right brain more efficiently.

The brain is divided into two hemispheres with separate functions (Table 17-8). It is thought that the different hemispheres allow the brain to access the central nervous system with two different and separate methods of communication. Access to the somatic nervous system is thought to be verbal, and access to the autonomic nervous system is thought to be the language of imagery, dreams, and intuition. The autonomic nervous system prepares the body for action through the sympathetic nervous system (SNS) and prepares the body for rest through the parasympathetic nervous system (PNS). When the PNS is activated, a feeling of tranquility occurs as the breathing and heart rates slow. The person who can learn to influence those activities of the body that previously were thought to be out of one's control can benefit by stress reduction and pain control techniques.[13]

To start a learning session on imagery, the nurse must create an atmosphere in which relaxation can oc-

cur. It should be as quiet as possible, lights lowered, and everyone should be in a sitting or comfortable reclining position. Selected music often helps (see the section entitled "Music for Relaxation and Labor" at the end of this chapter for suggestions). The teacher's position in the room should be where self-consciousness or embarrassment by the person or group is minimized. Once the physical setting has been established, the next task is to orient those present to the activity. This should include explaining what sensations to expect and emphasizing the need to just "let things happen." Occasionally, as people relax, they experience new or unusual feelings, which may include a feeling of losing control. The group, however, needs to be reassured that they will always remain in control and that to gain control, they first must learn to let go. It is important to set a low achievement level and allow anyone who does not want to participate to refrain from doing so. It is important also to tell members of the group that if their minds wander, closing the eyes may help by avoiding visual distraction. If someone prefers, keeping the eyes open is fine. Once the group is oriented, the relaxation process is begun. Generally, any relaxation technique or breathing exercise can be used either in part or whole (see Conditioned Relaxation, Appendix C). When the group is relaxed, the next step is to begin the exercise in imagery (see Imagery Exercises, Appendix C). After completion of the exercise, each person needs to be directed to return slowly to the physical realities of the room and the surroundings. Afterward, the group needs to process the experience. Some people want to talk about what it was like, some find drawing or writing helpful, and others desire to be alone with their thoughts.[14]

When the nurse is working with women in labor, it is helpful to be able to assist with imagery. Whether the woman is trained or untrained, it will be beneficial. To do this effectively, the nurse must be comfortable with imagery and have a spontaneous dialogue, perhaps a loose memorization of one from a book, ready to use.

BREATHING AND PUSHING TECHNIQUES

Because the Lamaze technique is the most widely used, those techniques are presented here. The breathing techniques were modified several years ago to reflect current research, but the nurse needs to be aware that not all childbirth educators have kept pace and regional differences may be seen.

The cleansing breath is a breath taken by the woman at the beginning and at the end of each labor contraction. The cleansing breath is like a sigh—a deep, relaxed breath to enhance oxygenation and serve as a signal for relaxation. The depth of the cleansing breath should be what the woman feels is comfortable. She

(*Text continues on page 340*)

TABLE 17-6. APPROACHES TO TEACHING RELAXATION

Name and Type	Description	Feedback
Progressive relaxation (modifies muscular responses)	Systematically tensing and releasing muscles. Developed by Edmond Jacobson, modified by J. Wolpe into a 6-week approach with home practice.	Primary feedback initially described as the awareness of participant who focuses on the sensation of tensing and relaxing each muscle. Either a coach or electromyograph can provide feedback.
Neuromuscular dissociation (modifies muscular responses)	Follows progressive relaxation by asking the participant to tense some muscles and relax others simultaneously, Introduced in this country by Elisabeth Bing.	Feedback by having the coach check relaxation (see Table 17-3A) and tension was introduced by Karmel and Bing—not mentioned in books by either Fernand Lamaze or Irwin Chabon.
Autogenic training (mental control modifying muscular and autonomic systems responses)	Training through suggestions including "my right arm is heavy" or "my left arm is warm." Includes slowing of the heart and respiration as well as cooling of forehead. Developed by J. Schultz and W. Luther.	Feedback initially described as the awareness of the participant with no outside feedback. Has been used with biofeedback equipment, thermometers, and so forth.
Meditation (modifies vascular and neurotransmitter responses)	Defined by Herbert Benson as dwelling on an object (repeating a sound or gazing at an object) while emptying all thoughts and distractions in a quiet atmosphere in a comfortable position. Used in transcendental meditation and yoga.	Concentration on a focal point and on breathing patterns would be forms of meditation by Benson's definition. Participant can monitor self but also receives coach's feedback on both activities.
Visual imagery	Includes techniques such as visualizing oneself on a warm beach or as a bag of cement or going down a staircase. Often precedes introduction of other kinds of relaxation. May also be used to visualize and potentially affect specific body parts as in cancer therapy. May be used in desensitization in which one relaxes while visualizing a potentially threatening situation. Used in labor rehearsals.	
Touching and massaging	Touch has always been a way for one person to calm another. There is evidence of actual transfer of energy taking place in some forms of touching. In childbirth preparation, touching is associated with muscular relaxation (Sheila Kitzinger).	Feedback from coach include informing when muscle tension is felt, necessitating advanced coaching. Coaches may need first to discern relaxation by moving a limb.
Biofeedback	Electromyograph measures neuromuscular tension. Thermometer measures skin temperature at extremities. Galvanic skin relfex records conductivity changes because of the action of sweat glands at the surface of the skin. Electroencephalograph distinguishes alpha, beta, and theta waves in the brain.	Feedback from all these machines is in one or more of these forms: visualization of a meter, listening to a sound, or watching a set of flashing lights.

(Humenick S: Teaching relaxation. Childbirth Educator, 3(4):47, Summer 1984)

Nursing Care Plan

Couples Participating in Training for Relaxation for Pregnancy, Labor, and Birth, or Life Stress

Patient Goals

1. Woman verbalizes understanding of importance of relaxation techniques.
2. Partner is willing to assist woman to learn and practice relaxation techniques.
3. Woman practices on regular basis.
4. During practice sessions observed by the nurse, woman shows evidence of relaxation.
5. Couple appears to work together as a team.

Assessment	Potential Nursing Diagnosis	Nursing Planning and Intervention	Evaluation
1. Knowledge of benefits of relaxation in pregnancy, labor and birth, and life stress management a. ↑ O_2 to baby and uterus b. ↓ Fatigue c. ↓ Pain perception d. ↑ Feeling of competency and mastery e. Aids breathing for labor and expulsion of baby f. Facilitates labor process g. ↓ Blood pressure and stress disease h. Enhances feeling of well-being	Knowledge deficit related to relaxation skills	After finding out what woman and partner know, explain other benefits of relaxation. Include benefits for right now, labor and birth, and later life. Give other examples in everyday life that may be familiar, for example, "tension headache" (tension causes ↑ pain).	Verbalizes understanding May contribute some benefits No further question
2. Past use of relaxation techniques, meditation, or yoga in any life situation and its effectiveness		Build on what she already knows. May be able to omit more basic techniques if she is currently skilled in a technique. Encourage her to use what she knows best or what has worked in the past.	
3. Partner's or friends' willingness to help her learn and practice new skill	Noncompliance related to: a. Partner's knowledge deficit about importance of relaxation skills	Include partner in teaching when possible. Discuss health benefit for partner also. Have partner participate by doing relaxation with woman as you teach.	Woman practices three times a week
4. Motivation to practice consistently, 15–20	b. Powerlessness c. Learning deficit: inef-	Teach partner how to as-	

(continued)

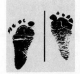

Nursing Care Plan *(continued)*

Assessment	Potential Nursing Diagnosis	Nursing Planning/ Assessment	Evaulation
min/day, three to five times per week	fective teaching	sess woman's level of relaxation and how to give positive nonjudgmental feedback to her	
		Explain it will take time and daily practice (15–20 min) to be effective in labor or stress.	
		Motivate by making sure couple understands benefits and physiological consequences resulting from unnecessary tension. Help couple plan specific home practice schedule with self-reward system to help motivate.	
		Tailor teaching to individual or with class provide multimodal approach. (see Table 17–6).	
5. Client's ability to relax during technique. 6. Client's ability to tense and release during technique. 7. Couple's ability to work together 8. Woman's ability to learn imagery 9. Woman's ability to integrate relaxation, imagery, and previously learned paced breathing techniques		1. Week 1: Start with basic whole body relaxation. (see Conditioned Relaxation—Appendix A). 2. Week 2: Progress to tense-release exercise. (see Tense Release Relaxation—Appendix A). 3. Week 3: Progress to neuromuscular disassociation exercise. (see Appendix A). 4. Week 4: Add Imagery Excercises (Appendix A). 5. Week 5: Have client integrate relaxation, breathing, and imagery during practice contractions.	Couple practices, evidenced by verbal reports and by woman's increasing ability to relax as observed by nurse during practice sessions: a. Relaxed jaw b. Slow, regular breathing c. Smoothed out facial muscles d. Legs rolled out and flexed. Arms flexed. Couple acts as team during observed practice session. Partner assists with woman's learning, practice, and evaluation; gives appropriate feedback during practice

TABLE 17-7. BRAIN WAVE STATES

Beta	Alpha	Theta
Focus attention	Pleasant feelings	Drowsiness
Visual scanning	Well-being	Daydreaming
Anxiety, worry	Tranquility	Creative processes
Concentration	Relaxation	Problem solving
Fear	Relief from attention	Uncertainty
Frustration		Future planning
Excitement	Concentration	
Hunger	Wordless images	
Surprise	Blank nothingness	

(Bressler D: Free Yourself from Pain. New York, Simon and Schuster, 1979)

should avoid a breath that is too deep that stimulates the stretch receptors in the intercostal muscles and leads to an alarm response rather than a relaxation response.[15]

The slow deep breathing pattern is called slow paced breathing. It should be at a rate that is comfortable for each woman and that provides sufficient oxygen for labor and helps the woman relax, but should be not less than one half the woman's normal rate. (The nurse needs to help the couple determine the woman's normal rate.) Clinically, one half the normal rate puts most women at six to nine breaths per minute. Whether the woman breathes in or out through her nose or mouth or in any combination is her choice. Because of the enhanced relaxation and improved oxygenation that occurs with slow paced breathing, the woman should be encouraged to use this breathing for as long as possible during labor. Throughout labor and before changing breathing patterns, women should be assessed for the need to change positions, relax more completely, uri-

TABLE 17-8. FUNCTIONS OF BRAIN HEMISPHERES

Left Hemisphere	Right Hemisphere
Speech	Images
Words	Symbols
Analytic	Impulsive
Rational	Creative
Logical	Receptive
Sequential	Intuitive
Active	Emotional
Cognitive	Spiritual
Somatic control	Autonomic control

(Bressler D: Free Yourself from Pain. New York, Simon and Schuster, 1979)

nate, and so forth to decrease pain. With time, habituation may make slow paced breathing less effective. Habituation is the decreased response to a repeated stimulus. Changing positions, walking, imagery, and changing music tapes help decrease habituation to this breathing technique, but most women eventually need to change to a breathing pattern that causes an alerting response.[15]

The second breathing technique, modified paced breathing, mediates the stress response of advancing labor by pacing the respirations at a controlled rate. Modified paced breathing is performed as an upper chest breath. It is not confined to the throat, and the chest does not move vigorously. Telling the woman to breathe at a level at which she feels comfortable may help her determine how deeply she needs to breathe to meet her own physiological needs. A delicate balance should be sought—breathing deep enough to obtain adequate ventilation, but not so shallow as to move only "dead air." Breathing should not be rapid enough to cause hyperventilation. The respiratory rate should not exceed twice the woman's normal rate. This rate has been observed empirically to be a safe upper limit. The choice of mouth or nose breathing is the woman's, however, if mouth breathing is her choice, the nurse needs to help her protect the mucous membranes by offering fluids, ice, or mouth rinses at regular intervals. Sounds (hee or haw) should be avoided because these are made by tightening the vocal cords and contracting the intercostal muscles. Relaxation is always the core on which paced breathing patterns are built.[15]

The third breathing technique is patterned paced breathing. It is performed exactly the same way as modified paced breathing with the addition of a slightly emphasized exhalation at regular intervals. A common rhythm taught is 4–1, that is, four relatively shallow upper chest breaths in and out plus one similar breath in, followed by an exhalation. This exhalation receives only minimal emphasis. Then the woman returns to the original pattern without hesitation. Patients may be taught other patterns or may make up their own variations of the patterned paced breathing. The rhythmic patterns of this breathing technique provide a mechanism for increased attention focusing by the laboring woman.[15]

Modified and patterned paced breathing are used because they provide an alerting mechanism to the brain that decreases habituation. Once this has been achieved, a return to slow paced breathing may be appropriate. Each of the three breathing techniques may be used at any time in labor without regard for any phase of dilation. The decision as to how best to use them is left up to the laboring woman.[15]

It would be helpful if the nurse would learn these techniques to assist the couple in labor, either by clarification of their use or by breathing with the woman whenever it would be helpful.

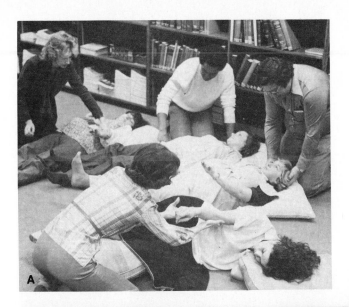

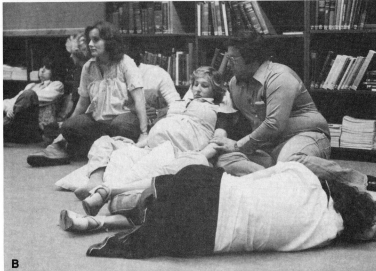

■ *Figure 17–3*
(A) *Couples practicing muscle relaxation for labor.*
(B) *Couples practicing various positions for pushing: leg holding, squatting, relaxing legs, and lying on side.*

In second-stage labor, the woman may assume any physiological position (Figs. 17-3*B* through 17-7). As the second stage proceeds, the nurse often monitors the progress of the descent of the baby. If 20 minutes pass without progress, the woman should be assisted to change positions.

Often there is a lull at the end of the first stage where women do not feel the urge to push. This pause is physiological and allows the woman to rest. The urge to push is felt only when the head is low enough to stimulate the stretch receptors in the pelvic floor. Frequently, women are urged to push before the uterus is ready instead of allowing labor to flow with its' own rhythm. Pushing with a closed glottis (Valsalva's maneuver) results in severe cardiovascular effects. This causes a high intrathoracic pressure, preventing venous return and causes a falling blood pressure, a decrease in cardiac output, and a disrupted blood flow to the uterus. Visible signs of straining include red face and tight neck muscles. When women are not directed to hold their breath, spontaneous pushing with a partially open glottis results. In spontaneous pushing, the air is audibly exhaled. Moans, grunts, and groans are the normal sounds of birth. If no sound is heard, it means the breath is being held and the body is tense.[5] Studies have found no significant difference in length of second stage with open glottis pushing.[16,17] Spontaneous pushes last only a few seconds, which is considerably shorter than when pushing is "directed" by the nurse. Caldeyro-Barcia[18] found that when women hold their breath for pushing, bearing-down efforts that last more than 5 seconds resulted in late decelerations of the fetal heart rate and marked falls in the maternal systolic and diastolic blood pressures. He suggests that if the woman is not urged to bear down long and hard, which often occurs with the "cheering section" approach to pushing, her *spontaneous* efforts are usually within physiological limits—5 to 6 seconds long—and fetal acidosis is

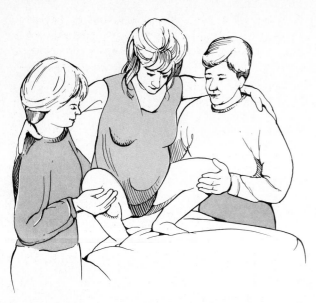

■ *Figure 17–4*
Squatting with help.

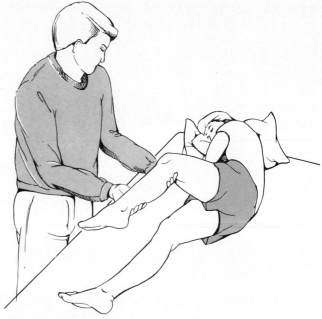

■ *Figure 17–6*
Pushing in side-lying position.

avoided. Noble[5] suggests the following for expectant women in the second stage:

- Don't strain. Let go and flow with the contraction.
- Relax the pelvic floor throughout second stage. Don't tense the muscles when you feel rectal pressure, the vagina stretching, or the gaze of many eyes! Relax *all* sphincters and the mouth, too—with your lips and jaws parted.
- Direct the push low down and in front—increase the pressure in your abdomen, not in your face! Don't strain so that you screw up your eyes—you might miss the moment of birth!

- Always take one or two deep breaths to refuel at the start and the end of a contraction. Exhale slowly as you bear down.
- Push only as long and hard as you feel the urge to do so. Avoid prolonged pushes, which affect your breathing, circulation, and also the baby's heart rate.
- When asked to refrain from pushing at any time, immediately relax the head back and pant. Keep it light and brisk. Don't blow out hard and pull in the abdominals at this time.

Breathing Techniques for Untrained Women

Nurses in some hospitals seldom see women who have not attended childbirth education classes. But nurses

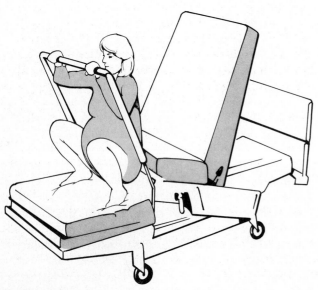

■ *Figure 17–5*
Squatting with squat-bar.

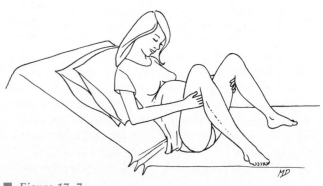

■ *Figure 17–7*
Pushing in sitting position.

occasionally come in contact with women who are in premature labor and who haven't finished or maybe even started classes. Other hospitals have only a small percentage of patients who attend classes. (Nurses from other clinical areas would do well to learn these and other pain reduction strategies to use to help any patient through a difficult procedure. Also see Chap. 23.)

If possible, before contractions become uncomfortable, teach the woman slow paced breathing. When contractions become uncomfortable, help her do the breathing. You can do the breathing with her (she focuses on your face) or verbally coach her through it.

As labor progresses, if she needs it, teach her the following simple version of modified paced breathing:

1. As the contraction begins, have the woman focus her attention on your face.
2. The woman takes a big relaxing sigh.
3. She breathes in and out through her nose or mouth at a rate of about 20 to 30 breaths per minute. You might "conduct" her breathing with rhythmic hand signals to help her pace herself.
4. The contraction ends. The woman takes another big sigh.

Other Childbirth Methods

Several other approaches to prepared childbirth are used, some of which are popular in specific geographic regions or even specific areas of a particular city.

Although these programs may derive from different theories and vary in specific techniques, they have many points in common, including the following basic beliefs:

- Fear enhances the perception of pain but may diminish or disappear when the parturient knows about the physiology of labor.
- Psychic tension enhances the perception of pain, but the parturient may relax more easily if childbirth takes place in a calm and agreeable atmosphere and if good human contacts have been established between her and the personnel attending her.
- Muscular relaxation and a specific type of breathing diminish the pain of labor.

The *Bradley method,* also called husband-coached childbirth, emphasizes slow, deep breathing along with complete deep relaxation. The Academy of Husband-Coached Childbirth is the organization that trains teachers to conduct classes in the Bradley method.

The *Wright method* is based on psychoprophylaxis but uses less active breathing than is taught in the Lamaze method. The breathing "levels" become more complex as labor progresses. This method is also referred to as the *new childbirth.*

The *psychosexual method* of Shelia Kitzinger is not based on psychoprophylaxis but on a method using sensory memory as an aid to understanding and working with the body in preparation for birth. Included also is the Stanislavsky method of acting as a basis for teaching relaxation. Kitzinger advocates chest breathing but teaches release of the abdomen at the same time. Her method is called the psychosexual method because she saw sexuality as part of the larger whole encompassing family relationships, birth, cuddling, and feeding.[19]

Yoga, although not a method of prepared childbirth, has been used by numerous women in labor, sometimes in combination with other specific methods of childbirth preparation. Yoga teachings include relaxation, concentration, and a combination of abdominal and chest breathing called "complete breathing." It is not unusual to see childbirth educators teaching different techniques from several methods in an eclectic or "holistic" preparation for childbirth.

Hypnosis is a technique that induces a state of extreme suggestibility in which the client is insensible to outside impressions, except the suggestion of her attendant. There is no particular "program" associated with the use of this technique; rather, training in achieving a hypnotic state or autohypnosis is usually given by a person who is specially trained in this area. Although there is no general regimen for learning this technique, the conditioning required is usually presented in several individual sessions, usually in the latter half of pregnancy.

The major drawback to this technique lies in the difficulty of securing adequately prepared therapists in some areas of the country.

Participants also usually enroll in childbirth education classes.

■ POSTPARTUM TEACHING

Parenthood often constitutes a stress in the developmental processes of both mothers and fathers. The postpartum period is particularly stressful because of the numerous physical changes the mother undergoes, the incomplete integration of her pregnancy and labor experiences, the changing roles that must occur within the family complex, and the uncertainty of the nature of the early mother–child relationship. Fatigue, confusion, feelings of helplessness and inadequacy, and depression often complicate this period. Isolation from the extended family, lack of community resources, economic strains, and pressures on the woman to resume her full previous role within the family as rapidly as possible create additional stresses. Factors that may influence teaching and learning in the postpartum period are outlined in Table 17-9.

The nurse working on the postpartum unit has a unique opportunity to intervene early in the developing mother–child relationship and to assist the parents to anticipate and plan for the first few critical weeks at home. If the mother can attain a level of confidence in her ability to perform caretaking tasks and begin to recognize her baby's behavioral messages, a good foundation can be laid and later difficulties can be minimized.

The needs of the hospitalized postpartum woman may conflict with the nursing staff's needs to maintain the routine or provide the teaching they believe necessary. Mothers progress at different speeds in assuming the caretaking role and have individualized concerns. Finding a way to respond to individual needs yet conduct an efficient postpartum educational program is a major challenge to postpartum nurses.

Sources for continuing care and counseling need to be available to parents during the baby's first few months at home, especially because most women leave the hospital 6 to 48 hours after birth. The postpartum nurse must know about resources in the particular community.

For specific postpartum teaching, see Chapters 26 and 28.

The Nursing Process

ASSESSMENT

As in other areas, a postpartum teaching assessment can best be accomplished using a written assessment tool. Many postpartum areas have specific checklists of items that are common to most of the unit's postpartum

TABLE 17-9. FACTORS INFLUENCING TEACHING AND LEARNING

Factor	Implications
Infant's condition	Preparation of the parents of a preterm infant or an infant with significant neonatal problems differs considerably from that of parents of the healthy, full-term infant.
Parental age	Parental age reflects development status. For example, the adolescent may need more concrete examples and be less able to assimilate written material.
Marital status	Marital status may influence the paternal role. Whether married or not, there is need to determine desired paternal involvement. Father should be included in caretaking activities when interested. Marital instability usually increases the anxiety level and makes teaching more difficult.
Parity	When there are siblings, the family usually needs more of a review of child care than actual teaching. Some teaching should be directed at interaction with the other children and meeting their needs as well as the infant's.
Socioeconomic status	Socioeconomic status influences the parent's ability to provide material things for the infant, and it usually influences childrearing practices.
Educational levels of the parents	Appropriate vocabulary should be used for verbal instruction and written material.
Experimental readiness	Previous learning transfers to the new situation. Insight enables the learner to apply older learning to a new situation.
Health beliefs and behaviors of the family	When health beliefs deviate from the usual, teaching may be difficult and more time may be required to convince the family of the need to change.
Emotional state of the learner	Some anxiety may enhance the learning process, but high anxiety militates against learning. Efforts should be made to lower high anxiety levels before proceeding with instruction. Attempts should be made to help parents work through feelings about their child's illness before attempting to teach.
Physical state of the learner	Physical discomfort may preclude or reduce learning
Parental questions	The type of questions asked indicates learning needs.
Parental motivation	Motivated parents are usually easier to teach. The nurse needs to find ways of stimulating the apparently unmotivated.
Interest in the infant	Lack of interest in the infant makes teaching very difficult. When interest appears slight there should be exploration of apparent disinterest.

(Oehler JM: Family-Centered Neonatal Nursing Care. Philadelphia, JB Lippincott, 1981)

population. This is especially helpful due to the short stay of most postpartum patients and the numbers of different staff that may be involved in the nursing process.

POTENTIAL NURSING DIAGNOSES

Potential nursing diagnosis are many and varied. A few are listed below:

Knowledge deficit related to improper breast-feeding position
Knowledge deficit related to pericare
Knowledge deficit related to handling a newborn

PLANNING AND INTERVENTION

In planning teaching strategies, the nurse must take into consideration many factors that may influence both teaching and learning in the postpartum period (see Table 17-9).

EVALUATION

The nurse's evaluation of the success of the instruction is both observable and measurable. The nurse can evaluate by asking whether there has been a change in how the mother positions the baby for breast-feeding since the nurse's instruction? Does she do pericare as frequently as prescribed? Is she progressing in her ability to handle the baby more confidently? With evaluation, the feedback loop of reassessment occurs and the nursing process begins anew.

Individual Teaching

Part of the postpartum nurse's daily responsibility is to provide individual instruction and support to mothers. This can range from information about infant sleep and activity patterns, growth and development, and how to dress the baby for different types of weather to sibling rivalry, contraception, and organizing the household to get the necessary tasks done. Mothers' concerns may be small and particular, such as getting the baby to stay awake and suck well, or they may be larger and more general, such as the changes in her own and the father's lifestyle after the birth of the baby. The nurse needs to be informed about a wide variety of topics, including contraception, sexuality, and family dynamics, as well as infant care and involutional physiology.

Individual teaching allows the nurse to respond to the personal questions and concerns of mothers and to relate information to that particular situation. Reinforcement of mothering skills is particularly effective on an individual basis, as is counseling regarding family problems or emotions. However, the nurse may not have the time to give each mother the amount of individual teaching and counseling needed. Certain types of teaching can be effectively achieved in groups, and the use of postpartum groups has increased on hospital postpartum units.

Group Education

POSTPARTUM CLASSES

The organization of classes for postpartum mothers and fathers differs considerably from one institution to another. Each unit must work out the most convenient time for both staff and parents and a method of communication to ensure maximum attendance. Sometimes a conference room on the unit is used, or a large patient room can be adapted and extra chairs brought in. The teachers may be postpartum nurses only, or they may be nursery nurses, physicians, social workers, dietitians, or physical therapists. A variety of media aids can be used, ranging from films to flip charts, books, or other printed material. Closed-channel television, which can be viewed by each mother in her room, is also used as a method of postpartum group instruction.

The content of postpartum teaching varies, but generally it includes content about the mother and her needs and information about the care of a newborn. Content about the mother should include getting enough rest, postpartum blues, family adjustment to a new baby, involutional physiology, pericare, breast care, sexuality, contraception, nutrition, and postpartum exercises. Mothers should be instructed in bathing and dressing the baby, breast-feeding or bottle-feeding, holding and handling, cord care and care of the circumcision, routine tests (e.g., the PKU test), and the normal range of newborn behaviors, including sleeping and crying. Some classes may include time for the mother to practice what she has just been taught while the nurse is available for assistance.

Some postpartum units organize special classes for mothers with particular needs (e.g., breast-feeding classes). The mothers are instructed in techniques of breast-feeding, and possible problems and their prevention are discussed. Experienced mothers can be encouraged to attend, because they are most helpful to new mothers who have never breast-fed before. Common situations that breast-feeding mothers might encounter are discussed, and group solutions are developed. Having the telephone number of the nurse for consultation if problems arise after discharge is helpful to mothers and promotes continued success with breast-feeding. Many hospitals are hiring certified lactation educators and consultants to provide specialized service and expertise to this growing population of clients.

If the hospital is large enough to have a regular census of diabetic, adolescent, or other special groups of postpartum mothers, postpartum classes to address their particular needs and concerns are helpful. Perhaps women who had a cesarean birth could make up another group, because their physiological problems often affect accomplishment of mothering tasks. If, however, the maternity service is relatively small and cannot support many different postpartum groups, the common concerns of baby care can be taught to a group of varied composition, with needs for particular information handled on an individual basis.

OUTPATIENT CLASSES

With 6- to 24-hour discharge common in some areas and 48-hour discharge the norm, the postpartum nurse has little time for postpartum teaching. In addition, the new mother can only absorb so much. For these reasons, nurses and other health professionals are increasingly aware of the need to extend services to parents after discharge from the hospital. These services may be provided through the public-health department, hospital-affiliated clinics, private physicians' offices, a community liaison nurse from the postpartum unit, or health professionals in private practice.

Postpartum nurses should be able to inform new parents about how they can contact these community resources for postpartum education. Some hospitals provide patients with lists of these classes, or the patient can contact a childbirth educator who frequently knows about these resources.

Parenting Groups. The importance of the first year of life in the child's development, both behaviorally and physically, has led to establishment of "parenting groups" in a variety of settings. Because most couples are unprepared for the realities of parenthood, there is a need to educate parents with respect to basic processes of parenting to foster more realistic expectations.

The goal is generally to promote healthy parent–child relationships by educating parents about the varied aspects of parenting and child development. The group also promotes problem-solving skills, enhances parenting skills, and facilitates growth.

The groups serve four primary functions: a source for socioemotional support, a forum to address specific problems, a setting in which the leader serves as a role model, and an arena in which to address common problems of all new parents.[20]

These groups are often under the auspices of community adult education groups, church groups, large teaching hospitals (department of psychiatry), and professionals in private practice.

Mothers' Groups. Mothers' groups provided by local facilities can also be helpful to new mothers. If mothers receive little or no instruction in the hospital before discharge, these groups can offer answers to many common concerns about care of the baby and support in mothering abilities.

The content of each group varies (e.g., La Leche League provides a mothers' group in support of breast-feeding. Distribution of information and group sharing of solutions to breast-feeding and other common questions of new mothers make this a valuable source of support for new and expectant mothers.)

Exercise Classes. These classes usually include pregnant and postpartum women. As the women give birth, they return with their infant and begin their postpartum recovery exercises. The pregnant women have a good opportunity to see the new mothers tending to their newborns and to hear about labors as well as what the early weeks and months are like with a new baby. This is a much more valuable learning experience than any pregnancy class "discussion" about the early weeks of mothering.

Working and Breast-feeding Classes. Another relatively new class available in some areas, this concept is an offshoot of the more common prenatal breast-feeding class. Most prenatal classes contain some content about working and breast-feeding, but how much is retained at that time is questionable. It is much more relevant to discuss this content just before or even during the experience.

Postpartum Exercise

POSTURAL REFLEX

The postural reflex needs to be reestablished postpartum so that the woman doesn't continue the stance she had during pregnancy. This means she must consciously contract the abdominal and pelvic floor muscles to balance the pelvis again after the sudden loss of its load. Because of the hormones of pregnancy, the joints are still at risk for a few weeks, and good body mechanics are essential to protect the joints and ligaments. The abdominal muscles are obviously in need of exercise.[5]

The goal is to achieve a flat abdomen and good posture, with the pelvis titled back to realign correctly with the spine.[5]

DIASTASIS RECTI

It is not uncommon for the longitudinal muscles (recti) of the abdomen to separate (diastasis) during pregnancy,

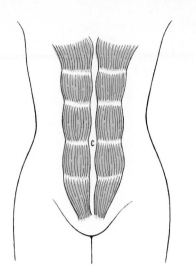

■ *Figure 17-8*
Diastasis recti. (From Noble E: Essential Exercises for the Childbearing Year. Boston, Houghton-Mifflin, 1988.)

labor, or delivery (Fig. 17-8). The gaping can be slight or severe. If these muscles are not corrected, the abdominal wall remains weakened and will not be supportive for a subsequent pregnancy. Because the recti muscles are important in controlling the tilt of the pelvis, their weakness can give rise to poor posture and pain in the lower back. A postpartum check of the recti muscles is performed about the third day after delivery. Until this time, the entire abdominal area feels so slack that the test is not reliable.[5]

The following exercise may be done to see if diastasis has occurred. Lie on back with knees bent. Press the fingers of one hand firmly into the area around the navel. Slowly raise head and shoulders until neck is about 8 inches from the bed. The bands of muscles on each side pull toward the midline, pushing the fingers out of the way. A slight gap, one or two fingers, is just tissue slackness and will tighten by itself. A gap of three, four, or more fingers between the muscles requires a special exercise to restore the integrity of this area (Fig. 17-9).[5]

If diastasis has occurred, the exercise is done by lying on the back with knees bent. Cross hands over the abdominal area to pull the muscles toward the midline as head is raised. Take a deep breath. Raise the head (and later the shoulders) to a 45° angle off the bed while exhaling, and at the same time pull the muscles together. Return slowly to the original position. Repeat exercise often and gradually work up to at least 50 times a day. Until the diastasis has closed, the woman should avoid exercises that rotate the trunk, twist the hips, or bend the trunk to one side.[5]

PELVIC FLOOR CONTRACTIONS

The purpose of the pelvic floor exercise after delivery is to enable the muscles to resume their role in sup-

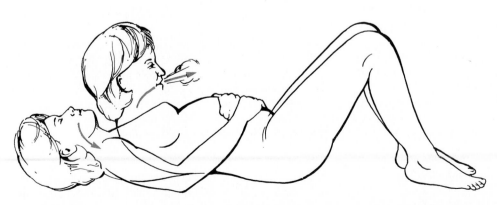

■ *Figure 17-9*
Woman supports the recti muscles as she raises her head on outward breath.

porting pelvic contents and to reestablish sphincter control. It is an excellent exercise to maintain lifelong pelvic floor tone and to enhance sexual enjoyment. It is also widely used by women with sexual dysfunction to increase their capacity for orgasm, and it is helpful for minor degrees of cystocele. (See Appendix C for specifics.)

During the puerperium, the 6 weeks after childbirth, the body undergoes major changes. Postpartum exercises are important in restoring muscle tone and the woman's figure. Often the exercises recommended during the prenatal period are also useful in the postpartum exercise program (see Appendix C). Many communities offer special exercise classes for pregnant and postpartum women. A group setting is often beneficial because motivation and learning are enhanced. In an uncomplicated birth, simple exercises should begin during the first postpartum day. If the woman had an abdominal delivery or extensive perineal repair, the beginning exercises may differ. The physician should be consulted before resuming fitness activities such as jogging. (See section entitled "General Guidelines for Exercise" and Table 17-5 earlier in this chapter.)

The nurse's role in parent education is a challenging one and one that requires much thought and preparation. The rewards for the nurse are equally great— hearing the grateful comments of parents and having participated in a special memorable event in their lives.

menick S (eds): Childbirth Education: Practice, Research, and Theory. Philadelphia, WB Saunders, 1988

9. Humenick S: Assessing the quality of childbirth education: Can teachers change? Birth Fam J 7:82–90, Summer 1980
10. Humenick S, Marchbanks P: Validation of a scale to measure relaxation in childbirth education classes. Birth Fam J 8:141, Fall 1981
11. Ewy D, Ewy R: Preparation for Childbirth. New York, New American Library, 1982
12. Humenick S: Teaching relaxation. Childbirth Educator, 3(4):47, Summer 1984
13. Bressler D: Free Yourself from Pain. New York, Simon and Schuster, 1979
14. Steffes S: Relaxation: Imagery. In Nichols F, Humenick S (eds): Childbirth Education: Practice, Research, and Theory. Philadelphia, WB Saunders, 1988
15. Rose A, Hilbers S: Relaxation: Paced breathing techniques. In Nichols F, Humenick S (eds): Childbirth Education: Practice, Research, and Theory. Philadelphia, WB Saunders, 1988
16. Barnett M, Humenick S: Infant outcomes in relation to second stage labor pushing method. Birth 9:221, 1982
17. Knauth D, Haloburo E: Effect of pushing techniques in birthing chair on length of second stage labor. Nurs Res 35:49, 1986
18. Caldeyro-Barcia R: The influence of maternal bearing-down efforts during second stage on fetal well-being. Birth Fam J 6:17, Spring 1979
19. Bean CA: Methods of Childbirth. New York, Doubleday, 1990
20. Heinicke C, Carlin E, Given K: Parent and mother–infant groups. Young Children, March 1984

■ REFERENCES

1. Nichols F: The content. In Nichols F, Humenick S (eds): Childbirth Education: Practice, Research, and Theory. Philadelphia, WB Saunders, 1988
2. Knowles M: The Modern Practice of Adult Education. Chicago, Association Press, 1980
3. AuKamp V, Humenick S, Frederick A: The Learner. In Nichols F, Humenick S (eds): Childbirth Education: Practice, Research, and Theory. Philadelphia, WB Saunders, 1988
4. Artal R: Exercise During Pregnancy and the Postnatal Period. Washington, DC, American College of Obstetricians and Gynecologists (ACOG), 1985
5. Noble E: Essential Exercises for the Childbearing Year. Boston, Houghton-Mifflin, 1988
6. Sosa R, Kennell J, Klaus M: The effect of a supportive companion on perinatal problems, length of labor, and mother–infant interaction. N Engl J Med 303:597–600, 1980
7. Gaziano E, Garvis M, Levine E: An evaluation of childbirth education for the clinic patient. Birth Fam J 6:89, Summer 1979
8. Shrock P: The basis of relaxation. In Nichols F, Hu-

■ SUGGESTED READING

Artal R: Exercise during pregnancy and the postnatal period. ACOG, May 1985
Bing E: Six Practical Lessons for an Easier Childbirth. New York, Bantam Books, 1977
Humenick S: Relaxation tapes for childbirth preparation: A review. Birth 9(4):281, Winter 1982
Karmel M: Thank You, Dr. Lamaze. Philadelphia, JB Lippincott, 1959
Nichols F, Humenick S: Childbirth Education: Practice, Research, and Theory. Philadelphia, WB Saunders, 1988
Noble E: Essential Exercises for the Childbearing Year. Boston, Houghton-Mifflin, 1988
Rozdilsky ML, Banet B: What Now? A Handbook for New Parents. New York, Charles Scribner's Sons, 1975
Simkin P, Reinke C: Planning Your Baby's Birth. Seattle, WA, The Pennypress (1100 23rd Avenue East, Seattle, 98112; 50¢), 1980
Simkin P: The Birth Partner: Everything You Need to Know to Help a Woman Through Childbirth. Boston, Harvard Common Press, 1989

Other Resources on Pregnancy and Childbirth

RELAXATION TAPES FOR CHILDBIRTH PREPARATION (AUDIOCASSETTES)

"Labor-eze" by Kenneth and Gloria Price, 2 sides, 20 minutes each. 12800 Hillcrest Road, Suite 116, Dallas, TX 75230

"Letting Go of Stress" by Emmet Miller and Steve Halpern, Halpern Sounds, 1980

"Preparing for Easier Childbirth: Home Practice Exercises" by Elizabeth Bing, 2 sides, 29 minutes each. 200 Park Avenue South, New York, NY 10003 ($9.95)

"Relaxation Tapes for Childbirth. . .and After" by Rae Grad, 6 sides, 12 to 15 minutes each. Box 6358, Alexandria, VA 22306 ($18.00 plus $1.00 shipping)

MUSIC FOR RELAXATION AND LABOR (AUDIOCASSETTES)

"Celtic Harp" by Patrick Ball, Fortuna Records, 1982

"Fairy Ring" by Mike Rowland, Sona Gaia Productions, 1982

"Pachabel Canon and Other Baroque Favorites" by Paillard Chamber Orchestra, RCA, 1983

"Pachabel's Greatest Hit, Canon in D" by Pachabel, RCA, 1984

"Seascapes" by Michael Jones, Narada Productions, 1984

"Silverwings" by Mike Rowland, Antiquity Records, 1983

"Solace" by Mike Rowland, Antiquity Records, 1985

VIDEOTAPES

"The Lamaze Method: Techniques for Childbirth Preparation," narrated by Patty Duke Astin, ASPO/Lamaze, Embassy Home Entertainment, 1983 (45 minutes, color, VHS)

"Postnatal Exercise Program," American College of Obstetricians and Gynecologists, Feeling Fine Programs, Inc., 1985 (55 minutes, color, VHS)

"Pregnancy Exercise Program," American College of Obstetricians and Gynecologists, Feeling Fine Programs, Inc., 1985 (51 minutes, color, VHS)

FOR AUDIOCASSETTES AND VIDEOTAPES CONTACT:

ASPO of Los Angeles, Inc.
2931 South Sepulveda Blvd., Suite F
Los Angeles, CA 90064
(213) 479-8669

COMPREHENSIVE MAIL-ORDER CATALOGUE OF BOOKS AND PAMPLETS:

Birth and Life Bookstore
P.O. Box 70625
Seattle, WA 98107-0625
(206) 789-4444

Research Highlight

Food beliefs of 15 African-American, 20 Puerto Rican, and 21 Haitian pregnant women, attending an urban prenatal clinic, were explored through the use of 24-hour dietary recall and interviews during the first trimester at the first prenatal visit, and at visits during the second and third trimesters. In response to questions about why each food was selected and what the subjects believed was "good" or "bad" about each food, the investigators identified food beliefs that were unique to each culture.

Food intake in five food groups (meat, milk-cheese, vegetable, fruit, and bread-cereal) was given a score and compared with food beliefs. Positive and negative correlations were found between food beliefs and food intake from the various food groups. These correlations followed unique patterns for each of the three cultures. For example, the belief that a food would be good for the mother and baby was significantly correlated with the milk-cheese and the fruit groups for the African-American women, with the bread-cereal group for the Puerto Rican women, and with the fruit group for the Haitian women.

Although the small sample size and other study limitations interfere with generalization of the findings, the study does support the importance of identifying a pregnant woman's food beliefs and related food behaviors. This information can assist the nurse in nutritional counseling that might increase the recommended nutrient and calorie intake and reduce deficiencies.

(Gulick EE, Franklin CM, Elinson M: Food beliefs and food behaviors among minority pregnant women. J Perinatol VI:197–201, 1986)

birth weights in the supplemented group when supplements of high protein density are used,[4] and other studies have shown little difference between supplemented and nonsupplemented groups regardless of type of supplement.[4,5] Most studies, however, have generally substantiated the belief that improving maternal nutrition during pregnancy is important for optimal maternal and fetal outcome.

A study at the Montreal Diet Dispensary provided supplemental foods to women who were found to be at risk nutritionally. The study demonstrated that women receiving the supplemental foods had better pregnancy outcomes for themselves, including easier deliveries with fewer cesarean sections, and had infants with a greater mean birth weight and considerably lower neonatal morbidity and mortality.[6] In the United States, evaluation of the Special Supplemental Food Program for Women, Infants and Children (WIC) has shown some improved pregnancy outcomes, such as increased mean birth weight and larger infant head circumference, after provision of supplemental foods to low-income women.[4]

Effects on Mental Development

When discussing the effects of nutrition on mental development, it is difficult to differentiate between prenatal and postnatal nutritional effects. The critical period for brain cell development begins during pregnancy and continues during the first year of life. The nutritionally deprived fetus may have decreased development of brain cells, but if optimum nutrition is provided after birth, the effects may be reversible.[7]

Inductees into the Dutch armed forces whose conception, gestation, or birth occurred during the 1944 to 1945 famine were compared with other Dutch inductees who were born in the same time period, but not living in the famine area. Although birth weights in the famine area were significantly lower than in other areas, intelligence tests failed to show significant differences between famine and nonfamine subjects.[7] A possible explanation for the good mental outcomes of the survivors of the famine in spite of their prenatal nutritional deprivation is that the Dutch were generally well nourished before and after the famine, in contrast to many other study populations who suffer from chronic malnutrition and other deprivations.[8]

On the other hand, when malnutrition during and after pregnancy is associated with other forms of environmental deprivation, mental retardation and severe, long-lasting behavioral effects, such as learning disabilities, are more frequent. The Montreal Diet Dispensary study indicates that improved nutrition during pregnancy and lactation improved the mental development of the children in the study, compared with siblings who were born before the mother received supplements.[9]

■ ASSESSMENT

Each pregnant woman has a unique nutritional background. Many factors influence her nutritional status and her daily food intake. To be able to help these women choose the best possible diets during their pregnancy, the nurse needs to be aware of the factors, their effect on each person, and ways of obtaining information about them.

Assessing Dietary Intake

To gather information about the client's food habits and actual food intake, an atmosphere and opportunity must be provided for the woman to discuss her concerns about food and diet and to give information about her current dietary patterns. Nutritional evaluation requires information on what is eaten, as well as the quantities and the method of preparation. Information regarding purchasing practices is also needed. The purchase of certain foods may be avoided because of cost, and suggestions for more economical substitutes may be needed.

The *Nutritional Questionnaire for Pregnant Women* developed by the California Department of Health Services[10] is a useful tool for assessing the client's food habits and related nutritional concerns. It should be completed by the client, either independently or with assistance, on her first prenatal visit. It is used to identify problems and as a basis for a nutritional counseling interview. Some questions may not be applicable to all client populations; some questions may require further clarification during the interview.

Obtaining information about dietary intake is another important aspect of nutritional assessment. Several methods can be used to attempt to determine actual eating patterns. For a *24-hour recall,* the woman writes down or tells the interviewer her food intake for the past 24 hours. This should include the time, place, and the type and amount of food eaten. This method is relatively simple to complete and not too time consuming.

Another method of obtaining the information is to have the woman keep a *food record* or *food diary* of everything she eats for 2 or 3 days. She should be advised to avoid holidays or days with atypical diet patterns, to record everything as soon after eating as possible, and to write down amounts of each food as accurately as she can. The Instructions for Completing a 24-Hour Diet Recall are useful here as well. Some women have difficulty remembering to write things down, but even if the diary is incomplete, it can still provide useful information.

With the *dietary history* method, an interviewer asks the woman to describe her food intake for a usual day. This method has the advantage of providing a more accurate estimate of the quantities of nutrients consumed and the balance of nutrients. The interviewer, however, must be highly skilled and trained, and the process is time consuming.[10] The *Dietary Intake* form can be used for either a 24-hour recall, a food record, or a dietary history.

Assessing Nutritional Status

Gathering information about a variety of maternal characteristics can help in assessing a woman's nutritional status.

Anthropometric evaluation includes various measurements of the body. Height and weight are the most common measurements taken. Comparing height to pregravid weight gives an estimate of body build, which is useful in determining standard weight and identifying the underweight person. Recording weight at intervals throughout the pregnancy also allows comparisons of the person's weight gain pattern with the recommended pattern (see Prenatal Weight Gain Grid on Assessment Tool entitled "Nutritional Assessment for Pregnant Women"). Measurement can also include the use of tape measures and calipers for skinfold width, but these are not usually done and are not necessary for most women.

Laboratory tests are used to determine the presence of adequate amounts of certain nutrients. Hemoglobin and hematocrit are measured routinely to evaluate the woman's iron status and need for supplements. The serum folacin level may be used as an indicator of nutritional intake.[11] Determination also might be made of serum albumin, total serum protein, and serum vitamin B_{12}. Additional hematological values may be obtained in assessing specific nutrient-related problems.[10]

The *Nutritional Assessment for Pregnant Women* provides a convenient way to record initial assessment data, plus ongoing assessment for three or more additional visits and allows the nurse to assess changes over time.

General physical assessment of the pregnant woman can provide useful information in assessing nutritional status. Alone, the signs may not be reliable indicators, but considered together, and with laboratory tests and dietary history, they can provide useful clues for further investigation (Table 18-1).

Assessing Individual Dietary Factors Involved in Food Choices

The *psychological aspects of nutrition* are important determinants of food choice but do not lend themselves to clear-cut analysis. Food is a basic need for survival, and hunger is one of the most fundamental of all sensations.

(Text continues on page 356)

Assessment Tool (continued)

15. Do you live: ☐ Alone ☐ With own family ☐ With other people

16. Check if you have the following: ☐ Stove ☐ Oven ☐ Refrigerator

17. a. Do you plan your own meals? ☐ Yes ☐ No

    b. Do you buy your own food? ☐ Yes ☐ No

    c. Do you prepare your own food? ☐ Yes ☐ No

18. How would you describe the type and amount of food in your household?

    ☐ Enough of the kind you want   ☐ Sometimes not enough

    ☐ Enough, but not always the kind you want   ☐ Often not enough

19. Are you receiving any of the following?

    ☐ Food stamps   ☐ Medi-Cal   ☐ Donated food/meals

    ☐ WIC   ☐ AFDC/welfare   ☐ Other: _____

20. a. How do you plan to feed your baby?

    ☐ Breast-feed   ☐ Both breast and formula

    ☐ Formula-feed   ☐ Other: _____

    b. Have you ever breast-fed or tried to breast-feed before? ☐ Yes ☐ No

    c. If yes, how long did you breast-feed? _____

    d. Why did you stop breast-feeding? _____

(Nutrition During Pregnancy and the Postpartum Period: A Manual for Health Care Professionals. Sacramento, Maternal and Child Health Branch, WIC Supplemental Food Branch, California Department of Health Services, 1989)

Related to hunger, but of a different origin, is appetite. Appetite is Nature's primary defense for the prevention of hunger. Based on the anticipation of eating, the impulse is determined by the person's previous experience. Only by coincidence and training does appetite become associated with health-giving foods. Factors affecting food-seeking behavior are the main determinants of eating (i.e., hunger, appetite, and custom). The great deterrents to normal appetite are worry, fear, and preoccupation with troublesome or difficult problems. These may be reflected in either an increase or a decrease in appetite. Some of the positive emotional stimulants include situations that encourage feelings of calm, contentedness, mild elation, or ego stimulation.

Food choices are a combination of heritage, superstition, custom, knowledge, and opportunity. Subtle cravings are passed along from one generation to the next by the process of training and imitation. Unique methods of food preparation as well as food selection, combinations, and prejudices are embodied in this training. Congeniality and hospitality are enhanced by the serving of good food, and it has become the custom to serve food at practically all functions, business as well as social.

From infancy onward, food and closeness are associated with love and security. Food and eating are looked on as symbolizing interpersonal acceptance, warmth, and sociability. Throughout all societies, this symbolic undertone is unmistakable; from the "breaking of bread" in antiquity to the modern banquet, the serving of food is a vehicle for expressing honor, joy, or mutual bonds. It is easy to see why food has become associated with the symbolism of motherliness. Feeding is not only kindly and warm in its emotional meaning to those who receive food, but it is also essential to growth and well-being; hence, it has become bound up with the idea of the mother, the one who originally nurtured, loved, and supported.

Women may crave or reject certain foods, due more to symbolic meanings of the food than to any physio-

Assessment Tool

Dietary Intake (24 hour recall)

Do Not Write In This Space
Intake Summary

Name		Age	Height	Weight	Animal protein	Veg. protein	Milk products	Breads/cereals/grains	Vit C frt/veg	Vit A frt/veg	Other fruits/veg	Fats/sweets/other foods
Time	Place	Amount	Foods Eaten									
Influences on Diet, Comments and Follow-up		Servings Eaten										
		Servings Needed										
		Difference										
Condition/ Diagnosis	Visit No.	Weeks Gestation	Date	Interviewer								

Sample Instructions for Completing A 24-Hour Diet Recall

1. Please write down everything, all foods and liquids, that you consumed during the last 24 hours—from the time you awakened yesterday morning until you awakened this morning.
2. Indicate the amount actually eaten, not how much was put in the dish.
3. Use measuring cups or spoons to describe the amount. For example:
   1 cup cornflakes
   ½ cup milk (whole)
   1 tsp sugar
4. For pieces of food that do not fit into a cup or spoon, write down the size. For example:
   1 tortilla (6 in across)
   1 piece cheese ($3 \times 3 \times \frac{1}{4}$ in)
5. Tell what is in a mixed food. For example:
   1 cup stew (¼ cup meat, ¼ cup potato, ¼ cup carrot, ¼ cup gravy)
6. Describe preparation method. For example:
   1 chicken drumstick (fried in shortening, no flour or batter)
7. Remember to write down the little things like butter, jelly, sugar, gravy, or salad dressing.
8. Remember to write down the snacks and drinks between meals.

(Nutrition During Pregnancy and the Postpartum Period: A Manual for Health Care Professionals. Sacramento, Maternal and Child Health Branch, WIC Supplemental Food Branch, California Department of Health Services, 1989)

logical factors. These responses may, for example, be related to the pregnant woman's close identification of food with mother, to fears that certain foods "mark" the baby, or to beliefs that specific foods give the baby strength or other desirable characteristics. It is crucial that the meaning food has for the client be explored and that her feelings and attitudes be respected.

The *stage of growth and development* of the client may also influence her food choices. For instance, foods enjoyed by adolescents are often different from those enjoyed by adults. When people marry younger and become parents, they often carry their adolescent eating patterns into marriage with them. In addition, in an

(*Text continues on page 361*)

Assessment Tool

Nutritional Assessment for Pregnant Women

Source   Date

Identification

Nutritional Risk Factors

Very overweight ☐	Hypovolemia ☐	Medical/obstet. complications ☐
Underweight ☐	Prev. obstet. complications ☐	Low income ☐
Inadequate gain ☐	Adolescence ☐	Substance abuse ☐
Excessive gain ☐	High parity ☐	Pica ☐
Anemia ☐	Short inter-preg. interval ☐	Psychological problems ☐

Prenatal Weight Gain Grid

Age (at conception) _____
Prepregnant weight: _____
Height (w/o shoes) _____
Desirable weight: _____
% Desirable weight: _____
Body mass index: _____
Term weight goal: _____

Weight Gain (lb)

Weeks Gestation

Visit 1

Date _____
Week gest. _____
Weight _____
BP _____
Comment _____
Alb _____
Glu _____
Ket _____
Edema _____

Dietary Assessment

Daily avg. from _____ days:

Food Group	Min. Amt./Serv.	Amt./Serv. Eaten	Sugg. Change
Animal protein	6 oz.	_____	_____
Vegetable protein	1	_____	_____
Milk products	3	_____	_____
Breads/cereals/grains	7	_____	_____
Vit. C-rich frt./veg.	1	_____	_____
Vit. A-rich frt./veg.	1	_____	_____
Other fruit/veg.	3	_____	_____

Excessive: ☐ Fat   ☐ Sugar   ☐ Salt
            ☐ Caffeine   ☐ Alcohol

Comments:

Laboratory Observations

TEST	Values			
	Date	Date	Date	Date
Hemoglobin (g/dl)				
Hematocrit (%)				
MCV (μ^3 or fL)				
Cervical cytology				
1-hour oral glucose load				

(continued)

Assessment Tool *(continued)*

Visit 2

Date _____
Week gest. _____
Weight _____
BP _____
Comment _____
Alb _____
Glu _____
Ket _____
Edema _____

Dietary Assessment

Daily avg. from _____ days:

Food Group	Min. Amt./ Serv.	Amt./ Serv.	Amt./ Serv. Eaten	Sugg. Change
Animal protein	6 oz.			
Vegetable protein	1			
Milk products	3			
Breads/cereals/grains	7			
Vit. C-rich frt./veg.	1			
Vit. A-rich frt./veg.	1			
Other fruit/veg.	3			

Excessive: ☐ Fat ☐ Sugar ☐ Salt ☐ Caffeine ☐ Alcohol

Comments:

Visit 3

Date _____
Week gest. _____
Weight _____
BP _____
Comment _____
Alb _____
Glu _____
Ket _____
Edema _____

Dietary Assessment

Daily avg. from _____ days:

Food Group	Min. Amt./ Serv.	Amt./ Serv.	Amt./ Serv. Eaten	Sugg. Change
Animal protein	6 oz.			
Vegetable protein	1			
Milk products	3			
Breads/cereals/grains	7			
Vit. C-rich frt./veg.	1			
Vit. A-rich frt./veg.	1			
Other fruit/veg.	3			

Excessive: ☐ Fat ☐ Sugar ☐ Salt ☐ Caffeine ☐ Alcohol

Comments:

Visit 4

Date _____
Week gest. _____
Weight _____
BP _____
Comment _____
Alb _____
Glu _____
Ket _____
Edema _____

Dietary Assessment

Daily avg. from _____ days:

Food Group	Min. Amt./ Serv.	Amt./ Serv.	Amt./ Serv. Eaten	Sugg. Change
Animal protein	6 oz.			
Vegetable protein	1			
Milk products	3			
Breads/cereals/grains	7			
Vit. C-rich frt./veg.	1			
Vit. A-rich frt./veg.	1			
Other fruit/veg.	3			

Excessive: ☐ Fat ☐ Sugar ☐ Salt ☐ Caffeine ☐ Alcohol

Comments:

(Nutrition During Pregnancy and the Postpartum Period: A Manual for Health Care Professionals. Sacramento, Maternal and Child Health Branch, WIC Supplemental Food Branch, California Department of Health Services, 1990)

TABLE 18–1. PHYSICAL INDICATORS OF NUTRITIONAL STATUS

Body Area	Normal Appearance	Signs Associated With Malnutrition
Hair	Shiny, firm, not easily plucked	Lack of natural shine; hair dull and dry; thin and sparse; fine, silky, and straight; color changes (flag sign); can be easily plucked
Face	Skin color uniform; smooth, pink, healthy appearance; not swollen	Skin color loss (depigmentation); skin dark over cheeks and under eyes (malar and supraorbital pigmentation); lumpiness or flakiness of skin of nose and mouth; swollen face; enlarged parotid glands; scaling of skin around nostrils (nasolabial seborrhea)
Eyes	Bright, clear, shiny; no scores at corners of eyelids; membranes a healthy pink and are moist; no prominent blood vessels or mound of tissue on sclera	Eye membranes are pale (pale conjunctivae); redness of membranes (conjunctival injection); Bitot's spots; redness and fissuring of eyelid corners (angular palpebritis); dryness of eye membranes (conjunctival xerosis); cornea has dull appearance (corneal xerosis); cornea is soft (keratomalacia); scar on cornea; ring of fine blood vessels around cornea (circumcorneal injection)
Lips	Smooth, not chapped or swollen	Redness and swelling of mouth or lips (cheilosis); especially at corners of mouth (angular fissures and scars)
Tongue	Deep red in appearance; not swollen or smooth	Swelling; scarlet and raw tongue; magenta (purplish color) of tongue; smooth tongue; swollen sores; hyperemic and hypertrophic, and atrophic papillae
Teeth	No cavities; no pain; bright	May be missing or erupting abnormally; gray or black spots (fluorosis); cavities (caries)
Gums	Healthy; red; do not bleed; not swollen	"Spongy" and bleed easily; recession of gums
Glands	Face not swollen	Thyroid enlargement (front of neck); parotid enlargement (cheeks become swollen)
Skin	No signs of rashes, swellings, dark or light spots	Dryness of skin (xerosis), sandpaper feel of skin (follicular hyperkeratosis); flakiness of skin; skin swollen and dark; red, swollen pigmentation of exposed areas (pellagrous dermatosis); excessive lightness or darkness of skin (dyspigmentation); black and blue marks due to skin bleeding (petechiae); lack of fat under skin
Nails	Firm, pink	Nails are spoon shaped (koilonychia); brittle, ridged nails
Muscular and skeletal systems	Good muscle tone; some fat under skin; can walk or run without pain	Muscles have "wasted" appearance; baby's skull bones are thin and soft (craniotabes); round swelling of front and side of head (frontal and parietal bossing); swelling of ends of bones (epiphyseal enlargement); small bumps on both sides of chest wall (on ribs)—beading of ribs; baby's soft spot on head does not harden at proper time (persistently open anterior fontanel); knock-knee or bowlegs; bleeding into muscle (musculoskeletal hemorrhages); person cannot get up or walk properly
Internal systems Cardiovascular	Normal heart rate and rhythm; no murmurs or abnormal rhythms; normal blood pressure for age	Rapid heart (above 100 tachycardia); enlarged heart; abnormal rhythm; elevated blood pressure
Gastrointestinal	No palpable organs or masses (in children, liver edge may be palpable)	Liver enlargement; enlargement of spleen (usually indicates other associated diseases)
Nervous	Psychological stability; normal reflexes	Mental irritability and confusion; burning and tingling of hands and feet (paresthesia); loss of position and vibratory sense; weakness and tenderness of muscles (may result in inability to walk); decrease and loss of ankle and knee reflexes

(Reprinted with permission from Nutritional Assessment in Health Programs. Am Public Health 63: November 1973 Supplement)

effort to exert their independence, they may reject many foods, such as milk, vegetables, and cereal because they are associated with "home" and a period of dependency. The desire to be free and to select the "forbidden," often non-nutritious foods, is strong.

The *religious, racial,* and *ethnic background* of the client and her family is also an important consideration in nutritional counseling. Regional or national food preferences may be different from the standard American diet usually portrayed in diet plans. Certain foods may be highly valued and others may be excluded from the diet, according to laws or customs of various religious or cultural groups. Methods of food preparation may also be different. In each group there are some differences that are beneficial and others that are detrimental. During counseling, the nurse can encourage the beneficial practices and assist in finding acceptable substitutes for those that negatively affect the health of the mother, fetus, or infant.[10] For those who have recently arrived in this country, assistance may also be needed to find sources of their accustomed foods or alternatives.

Knowing the client's ethnic background can be helpful in understanding her dietary habits (Table 18-2), but there is much variation within ethnic groups. These differences may be related to climate, growing conditions, geographic relocation, intermarriage, and individual differences. Therefore, assumptions should not be made about a client's food habits based only on surname or language spoken.

An *individual dietary pattern, vegetarianism,* has become the dietary choice of an increasing number of people. Some abstain from eating meat for religious or health reasons, whereas others choose the vegetarian way to make more efficient use of the world's resources or to economize on their food bills. Vegetarian diets vary in the extent to which they exclude animal sources of protein. Lacto-ovovegetarians exclude meat, but include eggs and dairy products and sometimes fish, poultry, and liver. Lactovegetarians exclude all animal protein sources except dairy products. A small minority of vegetarians in the United States are "pure" vegetarians, or *vegans,* who exclude *all* animal sources of protein. Besides the obvious need to make sure the pregnant vegetarian obtains enough high-quality protein, it is also important for the nurse to be aware that some vegetarians, especially the vegans, may have diets lacking in other nutrients. Their caloric intake may be low, leading to low prepregnancy weight and low pregnancy weight gain. Because they avoid dairy products, they may not get enough calcium in their diets. They also run the risk of developing a vitamin B_{12} deficiency, because this vitamin is found only in foods of animal origin.[12]

Food allergies or *intolerances* can develop to a number of different foods. Adjustments in the diet may be required to avoid these foods and still obtain adequate amounts of the essential nutrients. Intolerance to the milk sugar lactose is a particular problem during pregnancy because it is difficult to meet the pregnant woman's need for calcium, protein, and certain vitamins and minerals without using milk.

Assessing Nutritional Risk Factors

Certain factors place women "at risk" for nutritional problems related to pregnancy and require special attention to nutritional needs. These factors can be grouped into categories (Table 18-3).

AGE

A woman's age can affect her nutritional needs during pregnancy as well as her dietary habits. *Women under the age of 17* who become pregnant have their own growth needs to satisfy in addition to their pregnancy needs and those of the fetus. This increases their nutritional requirements at a time when they may be reluctant to follow dietary instructions or to gain weight. Adolescent pregnancies have been associated with low birth weight, prematurity, and increased perinatal mortality (see the section entitled "Special Nutritional Concerns of the Pregnant Adolescent" for further discussion).

Older gravidas also may be at increased nutritional risk, mostly because they have a greater chance of being in one of the other risk categories.

OBSTETRIC HISTORY

High parity or frequent conceptions can cause depletion of maternal nutrient stores, leading to pregnancy complications, unless the diet is of high quality.

Previous obstetric complications, such as inadequate weight gain, preeclampsia and eclampsia, anemia, gestational diabetes, antepartum hemorrhage, premature or small-for-gestational-age infants, and fetal or neonatal death, have nutritionally related factors and may recur in the present pregnancy. These women need good nutritional guidance.

PREGNANCY COMPLICATIONS

Complications that develop during the current pregnancy, such as anemia, gestational diabetes, or preeclampsia, may indicate the development of nutritional deficiencies due to increased nutritional needs. Continuing emphasis on a well-balanced diet is important, as well as specific help, possibly from a dietitian, to meet the individual needs related to the condition.

(*Text continues on page 365*)

TABLE 18-2. ETHNIC DIETARY CHARACTERISTICS

Ethnic Group	Protein Foods	Milk and Milk Products	Grain Products	Vegetables and Fruits	Counseling Suggestions
Mexican-American	Variety of meats; poultry, legumes, eggs	Not usual part of adult diet as beverage; small quantities of cheese in cooking	Tortillas and rice are staples	Tomatoes, chili peppers, fried potatoes, other raw or boiled vegetables, oranges, apples, bananas	Increase cheese and milk in cooking, and milk as beverage. Encourage variety of vegetables eaten raw or cooked for short time in small amount of water Decrease consumption of carbonated beverages and other empty-calorie foods Encourage use of enriched flour for tortillas
Puerto Rican	Beans, chicken, pork, beef, eggs; ham butts and sausage used for flavoring, not as a protein source	Limited use—"cafe con leche" may contain 2 to 5 oz of milk	Rice; French bread, rolls, crackers, increasing use of cereals	Pumpkins, carrots, green pepper, tomatoes, sweet potatoes, special boiled root vegetables, canned fruits and nectars	Encourage milk and cheese Suggest meat source with bean meal Urge more leafy green vegetables Increase use of citrus and other fresh fruits and use of whole grain or enriched breads, cereal, and rice
African-American / Southern	Beef, pork, chicken; legumes as accompaniment	Some milk, buttermilk, cheese, ice cream	Rice, biscuits, white and corn bread	Greens, sweet potatoes, okra, cabbage, corn, green beans, usually boiled; seasonal fruits, limited citrus	Increase milk and decrease carbonated beverages Encourage whole-grain cereals and bread Decrease water and time for cooking

(continued)

TABLE 18–2. ETHNIC DIETARY CHARACTERISTICS *(continued)*

Ethnic Group	Protein Foods	Milk and Milk Products	Grain Products	Vegetables and Fruits	Counseling Suggestions
					greens and other vegetables
					Eat some raw vegetables
					Increase vitamin C sources
Chinese	Fish, chicken, pork, legumes, eggs, nuts	Ice cream, flavored milk, some milk in cooking	Rice, millet, noodles	Variety of vegetables, often stir-fried with minimal nutrient loss; many fruits, usually fresh	Increase serving size of protein foods, or use as snacks
					Increase calories
					Encourage dairy products in cooking and use of tofu (soybean curd)
					Discourage washing rice because of nutrient loss
Southeast Asian	Legumes, fish, fish sauce, eggs, poultry, beef, organ meats, pork	Ice cream, milk (infrequently)	Rice, French bread, noodles	Variety of fresh, uncooked vegetables and fresh fruit	Describe combinations of foods in terms of meals with rice at the center
					Reinforce use of vegetable protein such as mung beans, and calcium-rich foods such as fermented fish sauce, soft shelled crabs, and small whole fish
					Increase calories
Japanese	Variety of meat and fish, eggs, nuts, legumes, tofu (soybean curd)	Milk and milk products limited	Polished rice, some wheat products	Variety of fruits and vegetables	Encourage use of dairy products to overcome major dietary problem

(continued)

TABLE 18–2. ETHNIC DIETARY CHARACTERISTICS *(continued)*

Ethnic Group	Protein Foods	Milk and Milk Products	Grain Products	Vegetables and Fruits	Counseling Suggestions
					Use of calcium and vitamin D supplements if necessary
					Avoid par-cooking of vegetables and washing of rice to avoid nutrient loss

TABLE 18–3. NUTRITIONAL RISK FACTORS

Category	Factor	Significance
Age	Adolescence	Increased nutritional needs; possible poor food habits
	Older gravidas	Possible increased incidence of other risk factors
Obstetric history	High parity or frequent conceptions	Depletion of maternal nutrient stores
	Previous obstetric complications	Possible nutritional relationship may recur
Medical history	Preexisting medical problems	May affect ingestion, utilization, or absorption of nutrients
Complications of current pregnancy	Development of complications, such as anemia, preeclampsia, or gestational diabetes	Development of nutritional deficiences due to increased nutritional needs
Maternal weight	Low prepregnancy weight	Increased incidence of pregnancy and neonatal complications
	Insufficient weight gain	Indication of poor maternal and fetal nutrition; increased number of low-birth-weight infants
	Obesity	Possible poor nutritional habits; increased incidence of pregnancy complications
	Excessive weight gain	If sudden, may indicate preeclampsia; lack of agreement on other possible risks
Dysfunctional dietary patterns	Dietary faddism	Diets often inadequate to meet fetal or maternal nutritional needs
	Pica	Displacement of nutritious foods, often related to iron deficiency anemia
	Excessive use of alcohol, drugs, or tobacco	Interference with appetite and with utilization of some nutrients
Socioeconomic status	Low income	Limited ability to buy sufficient food; possible chronic malnutrition
Cultural or ethnic group	Ethnic or language differences	Interference with ability to find usual foods; misinterpretation of dietary instructions
Psychological conditions	Depression, anorexia nervosa	Possible reduced caloric and nutrient intake

MEDICAL HISTORY

Preexisting medical problems, including anemia, cardiac disease, diabetes, hypertension, and infections, may affect the ingestion, absorption, or utilization of nutrients. These clients need nutritional guidance to meet their pregnancy needs and to incorporate any diet therapy for the particular condition.

MATERNAL WEIGHT

The pregnant woman's weight, as measured by prepregnancy weight-for-height and serial weight measurements during the pregnancy, has been found to have clinical value in assessing gestational weight gain.[13] Weight-for-height can be expressed as a percentage of a standard or as body mass index (BMI), defined as weight/height^2.

Low prepregnancy weight is defined as 10% or more under the standard weight for height or a BMI of less than 19.8. Underweight women have been shown to have more pregnancy complications, and their infants have a higher incidence of prematurity and low birth weight, lower Apgar scores, and increased neonatal morbidity. Improved nutrition with adequate weight gain during the pregnancy has been shown to improve the outcome.

Insufficient weight gain during pregnancy has been shown to be correlated with low-birth-weight infants and may indicate poor maternal and fetal nutrition. A woman's weight that falls below her prepregnant weight in the first trimester, or a gain of 2 lb or less per month, or less than 0.5 lb per week in the second and third trimesters would be considered insufficient.[10]

Obesity can be divided into two categories: overweight, which is defined as a weight 20% above the standard weight for height (BMI 26.0 to 29.0) and very overweight, defined as greater than 35% over the standard weight for height (BMI 29.0).[13] The obese maternity client is at higher risk for developing such problems as hypertension, gestational diabetes, and thrombophlebitis. The obesity may also indicate in many cases that her nutritional habits are not optimal.

Excessive weight gain during pregnancy has not been well defined, nor is there agreement on whether it should be considered a risk factor. Pitkin defines excess weight gain as a gain of 3 kg (6.6 lb) or more per month,[14] and others say 4 kg (8.8 lb) per month or 1 kg (2.2 lb) per week.[13] Some studies have shown that pregnancy outcome continues to improve as maternal weight gain increases, but others indicate that there can be problems above a certain optimal gain.[15] Those favoring unrestricted weight gain cite concern that any limitation may limit needed nutrients, whereas others are concerned high gains may result in fetal macrosomia and later maternal obesity.[13]

DYSFUNCTIONAL DIETARY PATTERNS

Dietary faddism refers to diets that are very restrictive or food habits that concentrate on certain foods or food groups to the exclusion of others. Food regimens such as the macrobiotic diet, the Atkins diet, or the Stillman diet are insufficient for even a nonpregnant woman if pursued for a prolonged period of time. For the pregnant woman, with her increased nutritional needs, they should not be used at all. Besides endangering the fetus, they sometimes induce harmful metabolic changes in the mother.

Pica is usually defined as the craving for and ingestion of nonnutritive substances such as clay, laundry starch, raw flour, or ice. In some cases, there are regional preferences for certain substances. The cause is unknown, but in many instances it appears to be related to iron deficiency anemia as either a cause or an effect. Some studies indicate that the ingested substances could lead to anemia by displacing iron-containing foods, but others have demonstrated that iron therapy can stop the cravings.[16,17] When large quantities are ingested, there is usually some displacement of nutritious foods to the detriment of the woman's nutritional status.

Excessive use of alcohol, drugs, or tobacco can interfere with appetite and with the utilization of some nutrients, sometimes resulting in congenital anomalies, low birth weight, and, in the case of alcohol and drugs, withdrawal symptoms in the infant after delivery (see Chap. 8 for further discussion).

SOCIOECONOMIC STATUS

Low income limits the amount of money available for food and may be related to an inadequate nutrient intake. Low maternal nutrient stores may also be a problem caused by chronic malnutrition. There is an increased likelihood of low-birth-weight babies and other reproductive problems in low socioeconomic groups.

ETHNIC OR LANGUAGE DIFFERENCES

Ethnic or language differences may contribute to nutritional problems in the pregnant woman. She may not be able to find the foods she is used to cooking, and substitutions may not furnish the same nutrients. Also, if English is not spoken, she may misunderstand or misinterpret dietary instructions or recipes.

PSYCHOLOGICAL CONDITIONS

Mental illness such as depression, and eating disorders such as anorexia nervosa or bulimia, may lead to a reduced caloric and nutrient intake. (See section entitled "Eating Disorders" for further discussion of this topic.)

(*Text continues on page 368*)

Client Education

Nutritional Teaching Guides

Food Group	One Serving Equals		Recommended Minimum Servings	
			Male/non-pregnant female	Pregnant*/breast-feeding
Protein Foods Excellent sources of protein, vitamin B$_6$, iron, and zinc. Animal protein supplies vitamin B$_{12}$. Vegetable protein is a good source of folic acid, magnesium, and fiber.	**Animal Protein:** 1 oz cooked lean meat, fish, poultry, or seafood 1 egg 2 hot dogs 2 slices luncheon meat 2 oz or 3 links sausage 2 fish sticks	**Vegetable Protein:** ½ cup cooked dry beans 3 oz tofu 1 oz or ¼ cup peanuts, pumpkin, or sunflower seeds 1½ oz or ⅓ cup other nuts 2 tbsp peanut butter	5	7 Have at least 1 serving from vegetable protein
Milk Products† Excellent sources of protein and calcium. In addition, milk products are good sources of vitamins A, B$_{12}$, riboflavin, and zinc. Fortified fluid milk contains 100 IU of vitamin D per cup.	1 cup milk or yogurt 1 cup milkshake 1½ cups cream soups (made with milk) 1½ oz or ⅓ cup grated brick-type cheese (like cheddar or jack)	1½ slices presliced American cheese 4 tbsp parmesan 2 cups cottage cheese 1 cup pudding or custard 1½ cups ice cream or frozen yogurt	2 (3 for teens)	3
Breads, Cereals, Grains All provide carbohydrates and some protein, as well as thiamine, riboflavin, niacin, and iron. Whole grains provide additional vitamin B$_6$, folic acid, vitamin E, magnesium, zinc, and fiber.	1 slice bread 1 dinner roll ½ bun, bagel, English muffin or pita 1 small tortilla ¾ cup dry cereal ½ cup granola	½ cup cooked cereal, noodles, or rice 4 tbsp wheat germ 1 4-in pancake or waffle 1 muffin 8 medium crackers 4 graham cracker squares	6	7 Have at least 4 servings from whole-grain products
Vitamin C-Rich Fruits and Vegetables Excellent sources of vitamin C and fiber. They also supply vitamins A, B$_6$, and folic acid	6 oz orange, grapefruit, tomato, vegetable juice cocktail, or fruit juice enriched with vitamin C 1 orange, kiwi, mango ½ grapefruit, cantaloupe ¼ papaya 2 tangerines, tomatoes	½ cup strawberries, broccoli, brussels sprouts, cabbage, cauliflower, snow peas, sweet peppers, or tomato puree 2 tbsp fresh or ½ cup cooked hot peppers	1	1

† See Nondairy Calcium-Rich Foods above.

(continued)

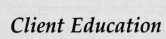

Client Education *(continued)*

Food Group	One Serving Equals		Recommended Minimum Servings	
			Male/non-pregnant female	Pregnant*/ breast-feeding
Vitamin A-Rich Fruits and Vegetables Excellent sources of beta-carotene and vitamin A. Most are good sources of fiber. The dark green vegetables also supply good amounts of vitamin B₆, folic acid, and magnesium.	6 oz apricot nectar or vegetable juice cocktail 3 raw or ¼ cup dried apricots ¼ cantaloupe or mango ½ papaya 1 small or ½ cup sliced carrots	½ cup greens (beet, chard, collards, dandelion, kale, mustard, spinach) ½ cup pumpkin, sweet potato or winter squash 2 tbsp raw or cooked hot peppers 2 tomatoes	1	1
Other Fruits and Vegetables Provide carbohydrates and fiber as well as smaller amounts of other essential vitamins and minerals	6 oz fruit juice 1 medium or ½ cup sliced fruit (apple, banana, berries, cherries, grapes, peach, pear) ½ cup pineapple or watermelon ¼ cup dried fruit	½ cup sliced vegetable (asparagus, beets, green beans, celery, corn, eggplant, mushrooms, onion, peas, potato, summer squash) ½ artichoke 1 cup lettuce	3	3

Folic Acid-Rich Foods

These foods are rich in folic acid, a B-vitamin especially important during pregnancy because of its role in growth and repair. Pregnant women should have at least four servings daily of these foods.

Protein Foods

Beans: baked, garbanzo, kidney, navy, pinto, pork'n'beans	Peanuts
Lentils	Split peas
Liver	Sunflower seeds
	Yeast, nutritional

Fruits and Vegetables

Asparagus	Lettuce: bibb, Boston, endive, romaine

Nondairy Calcium-Rich Foods

Each of the following is approximately equivalent in calcium to one serving from the milk products group (250–300 mg calcium):

Almonds	4 oz
Beans: baked, pork'n'beans	2 cups
Broccoli, fresh cooked	1½ cups
Greens: turnip, cooked	1½ cups
Greens: bok choy, collard, dandelion, cooked	2 cups
Greens: kale, mustard, cooked	3 cups
Molasses, blackstrap	2 tbsp
Oranges	5 medium
Salmon (with bones)	½ cup canned

(continued)

Client Education *(continued)*

Folic Acid-Rich Foods		*Nondairy Calcium-Rich Foods*	
Avocado	Orange	Sardines	5 medium or 2½ oz
Beets, fresh	Orange juice	Tofu (must be processed with calcium salt)	9 oz
Broccoli	Peas	Tortillas, corn	7 medium
Brussels sprouts	Pineapple juice		
Cabbage	Spinach		
Corn	Tomato juice		
Greens: collards, mustard	Vegetable juice		

* All pregnant women should have at least four servings of the foods rich in folic acid.
(California Department of Health Services, MCH/WIC: Nutrition During Pregnancy and the Postpartum Period: A Manual for Health Care Professionals, 1990)

The result may be poor maternal weight gain with the possibility of low-birth-weight infants and increased perinatal mortality.

■ NURSING DIAGNOSIS

Nutritional assessment of the pregnant woman can lead the nurse to a variety of nursing diagnoses that can be used in planning and implementing care. Most of these nursing diagnoses would involve the diagnostic category Alteration in Nutrition and would be related to different factors that might put the expectant mother or fetus at increased risk for problems. Some possible diagnostic statements include the following:

Alteration in nutrition: less than body requirements, related to inadequate caloric intake
Alteration in nutrition: less calcium than required for pregnancy, related to decreased intake of dairy products secondary to lactose intolerance
Alteration in nutrition: inadequate weight gain, related to self-imposed limitation of calories

Knowledge Deficit is another diagnostic category that might be appropriate for nutritional problems of the pregnant woman. A possible diagnostic statement would be Knowledge Deficit regarding nutritional needs during pregnancy, related to lack of information resources.

■ PLANNING AND INTERVENTION: DIETARY COUNSELING

In contacts with women during the reproductive cycle, the nurse has many opportunities to use the nursing process in assisting each woman to improve her nutritional status. Drawing from the information in the previous section on assessment, the nurse can work with individuals or groups of clients to plan and implement nutritious food choices.

The responsibility for initial and ongoing dietary evaluation and counseling varies from one prenatal setting to another. If a dietitian or nutritionist is available, he or she may see all clients at least one time, or services may be limited to seeing high-risk clients and consulting with staff concerning other clients. In the absence of a nutritionist or dietitian, the primary responsibility for nutrition counseling may rest with the nurse. Whether it is the nurse's primary responsibility or a shared responsibility with other members of the health-care team, the nurse plays an important role because he or she usually sees the client at each visit and often is the one available to answer questions. If more than one person is involved in the counseling, it is important that there be consistency in the nutritional information taught and the advice given. Nutrition counseling ideally begins at the first prenatal visit, starting during the assessment of dietary intake.

As the nurse and the woman plan together, the client's likes and dislikes are recognized, and those foods that provide the essential nutrients are encouraged. Suggestions may be given for the addition of certain foods or the modification of existing methods of selecting or preparing it. Incorporating the woman into the planning and allowing her choices whenever possible, helping her to increase her knowledge of nutrients, encouraging and reinforcing correct choices or willing adaptations, and giving firm guidance when indicated, all help the client and the nurse to achieve their respective goals.

Many women are already eating an adequate diet. They may only need reinforcement of their dietary habits and encouragement to continue what they are doing. For those women whose dietary intake is not adequate or whose history indicates one or more risk factors, consistent counseling toward optimum nutritional intake is vitally important.

The nurse must have a tolerant and nonjudgmental attitude and should respect the client's right to reject dietary information if she chooses. This attitude may be difficult for the nurse to achieve, because health-care providers traditionally expect their advice to be followed. However, more may be gained in the long run by accepting the "client's right to choose." A client is more likely to seek care from those she feels respect her views, even when these views differ from those of the provider.

Dietary counseling should be an ongoing aspect of prenatal care. It is not enough to talk about it at the first visit and hand out a suggested diet plan or food guide. There should be some discussion of nutrition at each follow-up visit, with reinforcement or additional suggestions as needed. Periodic use of diet recall or a food diary can be helpful in assessing the extent to which the suggestions are being followed. The following sections include information on specific areas that may be helpful in counseling.

Calorie Intake and Weight Gain

Calories provide the energy requirements for the body and are needed to maintain bodily processes, thermal balance, and physical activity. Caloric allowances are established to provide for adequate energy requirements and to support growth and body weight levels for the fetus and mother that are commensurate with health and well-being.

In the past, attempts were made to limit weight gain by caloric restriction, with the purpose of preventing and controlling preeclampsia. However, controlled studies have not supported the contention that caloric intake as reflected by weight gain causes pre-eclampsia. To the contrary, there is evidence that limiting weight gain decreases essential nutrient intake, which is thought to be one of the contributing factors in the development of preeclampsia.

During pregnancy, there is an increased need for calories to meet the energy requirements for building fetal and placental tissue and for maintaining the woman's tissue requirements. The recommended dietary allowance (RDA) during the second and third trimesters of pregnancy is 300 kcal/day above the woman's usual RDA. For the individual woman, actual needs could vary according to many factors, including her size and activity. Vermeersch suggests calculating individual needs by allowing approximately 40 kcal/kg of pregnant body weight or about 18 kcal/lb.[18] In a study group at the Montreal Diet Dispensary, additional calories are recommended for specific conditions such as protein deficiency, underweight, and special conditions of stress.[9]

One of the main risks to the newborn is low birth weight and the problems that accompany it. The outcome for the infant has been shown to improve as the birth weight increases. Many studies have shown the relationship between maternal weight gain and birth weight. These findings, coupled with concern over relatively high U.S. perinatal mortality, have led to the recommendation of more liberal weight gain for the mother during pregnancy.

The 1990 recommendations for weight gain during pregnancy from the Food and Nutrition Board of the National Academy of Sciences[13] suggest a total gain of 25 to 35 lb for women whose prepregnancy weight falls within the normal weight range. Although this is an increase from previous recommendations, they also emphasize more individualization of weight gain recommendations based on the woman's prepregnant weight for height and certain individual factors (Table 18-4). Higher weight gains may be appropriate for those who tend to have smaller babies such as young adolescents, African-American women, women who smoke, and those with multiple pregnancies. Very short women and women who are very overweight may do well with lower weight gains. Studies have found that the very overweight have the lowest perinatal mortality when they gain 15 to 16 lb.[15]

It is sometimes tempting for the obese client to try to lose weight during pregnancy, but this should be discouraged. When caloric intake is low enough to cause weight loss, maternal fat stores are catabolized for energy, resulting in ketonemia, which may adversely affect the fetus. Also, environmental contaminants stored in the fat may be released during the process and affect the fetus. Emphasizing nutritious foods, rather than weight reduction, may help improve dietary habits and lead to easier weight reduction after pregnancy.

TABLE 18-4. RECOMMENDED PRENATAL WEIGHT GAIN* ACCORDING TO PREGRAVID WEIGHT FOR HEIGHT

Pregravid Status	Range of Gain (lb)
Underweight (<90% of desirable weight)	28–40
Desirable weight (90%–120% of desirable weight)	25–35
Moderately overweight (121%–135% of desirable weight)	15–25
Very overweight (>135% of desirable weight)	15–20
Overall range	15–40

* For women age 18 years and older. Women 17 years or below, women carrying twins or triplets, or women who smoke may gain above these ranges irrespective of their pregravid weight.

(Nutrition During Pregnancy and the Postpartum Period: A Manual for Health Care Professionals. Sacramento, Maternal and Child Health Branch, WIC Supplemental Food Branch, California Department of Health Services, 1990)

COMPONENTS OF WEIGHT GAIN

For some time, it was taught that maternal weight gain was adequate if it consisted only of the amount necessary for the products of conception and that anything over that would just be stored by the mother as "unwanted fat." Although the exact components of weight gain and the proportions of each are not known, and probably vary from one pregnancy to another, a possible distribution of average weight gain is shown in Figure 18-1 and Table 18-5.

These figures are rough estimates only, and if actual weights could be measured, they might differ. The fat component is sometimes quoted as being closer to 2 kg,

and in some analyses, part of the maternal gain is credited to lean muscle mass.

It is apparent from Figure 18-1 that most of the gain during the second trimester is related to maternal tissues, whereas the fetus gains the most during the third trimester. The pattern of total weight gain is also illustrated in this figure. This pattern is believed to be much more important than the actual amount of weight gained. The usual pattern consists of a 1- to 2-kg (2–4 lb) weight gain during the first trimester, followed by an average, fairly steady, gain of about 0.4 kg (0.9 lb) per week during the last two trimesters.[12]

The Prenatal Weight Gain Grid on page 358 shows the recommended pattern. It can be used to plot the pattern of each person's weight gain and to detect any deviation. For example, a sudden, sharp increase in weight after the 20th week may indicate excessive water retention and the onset of preeclampsia. Inadequate weight gain or weight loss can also be noted.

PROMOTING ADEQUATE WEIGHT GAIN

Counseling in regard to weight gain varies from one client to another. Some women have been counseled to restrict weight with previous pregnancies or have heard about this practice from friends and believe it is the best way. They may need reassurance that gaining over 20 lb is beneficial for both themselves and the baby. Other women may think that they can limit the size of the baby and have an easier delivery if they eat less. They can be helped to understand that if the mother's nutritional status is poor, the labor and delivery might be difficult regardless of the size of the baby.

Some women are weight conscious and may resist gaining adequate weight because of fears that they will not be able to lose it after the baby is born. Careful explanation of the distribution of the additional weight and the importance of good nutrition to the outcome of pregnancy may help them accept the weight gain.

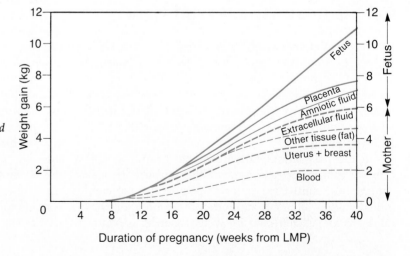

■ *Figure 18–1*
Pattern and components of cumulative gain in weight during pregnancy, assuming total gain of 11 kg. (Pitkin RM: Nutritional support in obstetrics and gynecology. Clin Obstet Gynecol 19[3]:491, September 1976.)

TABLE 18-5. COMPONENTS OF WEIGHT GAIN DURING PREGNANCY

	kg	lb
Fetal components		
Fetus	3.4	7½
Placenta	0.6	1½
Amniotic fluid	1.0	2¼
Maternal components		
Uterus and breasts	1.6	3½
Blood	2.0	4½
Extracellular fluid	1.6	3½
Other tissue (fat)	0.8	1¾

Holey states, "Knowing from her first prenatal visit that her 'temporary pounds' will influence her unborn child and prepare her for the work of motherhood is not only fascinating to the mother, but makes sense of the puzzle—'Why should I gain so much weight?'"[19]

Women who gain weight rapidly during the first two trimesters may reach what they consider to be maximum gain by the seventh month. They attempt to cut down on what they eat to try to avoid gaining any more weight. This deprives them of adequate nutrients at the time when fetal brain cells are growing the fastest and when the fetus is depositing a protective layer of fat.[20] These women need encouragement to continue eating adequately.

MAKING CALORIES COUNT

"Making calories count" is not the same as saying that pregnant women should count their calories; it is to emphasize the importance of eating only foods that contribute necessary nutrients to the diet. "Empty calories" are to be avoided, especially if the woman's appetite is poor or her food dollar is limited. The obese woman also benefits from this kind of instruction, not only during pregnancy, but also in planning a weight reduction program after pregnancy. "Eat to appetite" may be a good slogan to promote adequate weight gain during pregnancy, but it is only valid when the woman is taught which foods to eat to obtain the most nutrients.

The woman whose diet consists mainly of foods such as doughnuts, candy bars, and soda pop may satisfy her appetite, but her nutritional status suffers and she gets a poor return for her food dollar. This does not mean that desserts must be eliminated from the diet. Custard, made from eggs and milk, is an example of a nutritious dessert. The nutritive value of other desserts such as baked goods can be improved by the use of whole grain flour and the addition of wheat germ or extra eggs and milk.

Nutrient Needs

A brief review of basic nutrition may be helpful to the nurse in teaching her clients about good nutrition during pregnancy. All foods are made up of a combination of classes of nutrients: carbohydrates, proteins, fats, vitamins, minerals, and water. Carbohydrates, proteins, and fats constitute the group referred to as "energy nutrients" because they contribute energy or "calories" to the diet. Vitamins, minerals, and water do not contribute to the caloric content of food.

RECOMMENDED DIETARY ALLOWANCES

The Food and Nutrition Board of the National Research Council sets standards for the daily intake of calories and nutrients by people in the United States. RDAs are defined as "the levels of intake of essential nutrients that, on the basis of scientific knowledge, are judged by the Food and Nutrition Board to be adequate to meet the known nutrient needs of practically all healthy persons."[21] The 10th edition, published in 1989 (Table 18-6), includes some changes from the 9th (1980) edition, but overall the recommended allowances are similar for most nutrients. RDAs are based on reference individuals, using actual height and weight medians for the U.S. population of the designated age. Allowances vary according to age and during pregnancy and lactation. They are meant to be used as a basic reference and adjusted according to individual need.

CARBOHYDRATE

The main function of a carbohydrate is to produce energy. It is necessary in adequate amounts to spare protein for growth needs. The main sources of carbohydrate in the diet are fruits, vegetables, and grain products. The unrefined sources contribute valuable fiber. Sugars and sweets are also sources of carbohydrates but are often called empty calories because they do not contribute many nutrients to the diet.

FAT

Fat is a concentrated source of energy, yielding over twice as many calories per gram as carbohydrates. Besides supplying energy, fat in the diet provides essential fatty acids and supplies and carries the fat-soluble vitamins, A, D, E, and K. Also, fats, such as butter, margarine, and salad oil, add to the palatability of food.

PROTEIN

The main function of protein is to build and repair all body cells. An increased amount is needed during pregnancy for growth and maintenance of maternal and

TABLE 18–6. RECOMMENDED DIETARY ALLOWANCES* DURING PREGNANCY AND LACTATION

Recommended Energy Intake Females:

Age or Condition	Weight[†] kg	Weight[†] lb	Height[†] cm	Height[†] in	Average Energy Allowance (kcal) per kg	Average Energy Allowance (kcal) per day
11–14	46	101	157	62	47	2200
15–18	55	120	163	64	40	2200
19–24	58	128	164	65	38	2200
25–50	63	138	163	64	36	2200
Pregnant (1st trimester)						+0
Pregnant (2nd and 3rd trimester)						+300
Lactating (1st 6 months)						+500
(2nd 6 months)						+500

Recommended Protein, Vitamin and Mineral Allowances

	Pregnant	Lactating 1st 6 months	Lactating 2nd 6 months
Protein (g)	60	65	62
Fat-Soluble Vitamins			
Vitamin A (μg RE)[‡]	800	1300	1200
Vitamin D (μg)§	10	10	10
Vitamin E (mg α TE)‖	10	12	11
Vitamin K (μg)	65	65	65
Water-Soluble Vitamins			
Vitamin C (mg)	70	95	90
Thiamine (mg)	1.5	1.6	1.6
Riboflavin (mg)	1.6	1.8	1.7
Niacin (mg NE)#	17	20	20
Vitamin B_6 (mg)	2.2	2.1	2.1
Folate (μg)	400	280	260
Vitamin B_{12} (μg)	2.2	2.6	2.6
Minerals			
Calcium (mg)	1200	1200	1200
Phosphorus (mg)	1200	1200	1200
Magnesium (mg)	320	355	340
Iron (mg)	30	15	15
Zinc (mg)	15	19	16
Iodine (μg)	175	200	200
Selenium (μg)	65	75	75

* The allowances, expressed as average daily intakes over time, are intended to provide for individual variations among most normal persons as they live in the United States under usual environmental stresses. Diets should be based on a variety of common foods to provide other nutrients for which human requirements have been less well defined.

† Weights and heights of Reference individuals are actual medians for the U.S. population of the designated age. The use of these figures does not imply that the height-to-weight ratios are ideal.

‡ Retinol equivalents. 1 retinol equivalent = 1 μg retinol or 6 μg β-carotene.

§ As cholecalciferol. 10 μg cholecalciferol = 400 iu of vitamin D.

‖ α-Tocopherol equivalents. 1 mg d-α tocopherol = 1 α-TE.

1 NE (niacin equivalent) is equal to 1 mg of niacin or 60 mg of dietary tryptophan.

(Adapted from National Research Council (US) Subcommittee on the Tenth Edition of the RDAs: Recommended Dietary Allowances. Washington, DC, National Academy Press, 1989)

fetal tissues. Proteins are made up of different combinations of the more than 20 amino acids. Eight of these cannot be synthesized by the body and are referred to as *essential amino acids,* which must be supplied by the diet. All eight must be present in the correct proportion at the same meal to be used by the body.

Proteins that contain adequate amounts of all eight essential amino acids are called *complete proteins.* Most animal sources fall into this category. Most vegetable protein sources are deficient in one or more of the essential amino acids. Those amino acids that are in short supply in any given protein are called *limiting amino acids.* The body can only use the protein to the level of the limiting amino acid, and what is left over is used for energy. Two or more "incomplete" protein sources with different limiting amino acids can be combined in the same meal and are used by the body as a complete protein.[22]

VITAMINS

Vitamins are organic substances that are essential to life and must be supplied by the diet in minute amounts daily. They are directly involved in regulating the metabolism of carbohydrate, protein, and fat, and they assist in regulating reactions by which body tissues are maintained. Many reactions in the body require more than one vitamin, and the lack of any one can interfere with the function of another. Most vitamins cannot be synthesized by the body.

Fat-Soluble Vitamins. Fat-soluble vitamins are stored by the body, so large doses, especially of vitamins A and D, can be toxic. Excesses usually come from excessive supplementation, not from food sources.

Vitamin A assists in maintaining the integrity of the mucous membrane, which increases the body's resistance to infection. It is also essential for normal skeletal and tooth development and plays a role in night vision. Carotene, which is synthesized by plants and is the usual form of the vitamin in foods, is the precursor of vitamin A. Dark green and deep yellow vegetables and fruits are the best sources of vitamin A. Some foods, such as milk, are fortified with vitamin A.

Vitamin D is important for its role in the absorption and utilization of calcium and phosphorus in skeletal and tooth bud formation. Egg yolk, liver, and some fish contain small amounts of vitamin D. Cod liver oil was used as a supplement for years to prevent rickets in children. Most milk is fortified with 400 IU of vitamin D per quart. Although some vitamin D can be produced by the body from sunlight on the skin, this is not a reliable source because of the variability of exposure to the sun and interferences with the rays, such as smog or dust.

Vitamin E is primarily an antioxidant. It reduces oxidation of the polyunsaturated fatty acids, helping to maintain the integrity of the cell membranes. It is also involved in certain enzymatic and metabolic reactions. The main sources of vitamin E in the diet are vegetable fats and oils, leafy green vegetables, grains, nuts, and egg yolks.

Vitamin K is an essential factor in the formation of prothrombin and is therefore necessary for normal blood clotting. Leafy green vegetables and pork liver are excellent dietary sources of this vitamin. Vitamin K is also synthesized by bacteria of the lower intestinal tract. Dietary deficiency is not usually a problem.

Water-Soluble Vitamins. Water-soluble vitamins are not stored in any significant amount, so deficiencies develop more easily than with the fat-soluble vitamins. The *B complex* actually consists of a number of different vitamins that are essential to good nutrition. The Food and Nutrition Board lists allowances for thiamine (vitamin B_1), riboflavin (vitamin B_2), niacin (vitamin B_6), folacin (folic acid), and vitamin B_{12}. They serve as components of enzymes and coenzymes in many reactions in the body, such as cell respiration, glucose oxidation, and energy metabolism. Requirements are increased to meet the increased metabolic and growth needs of pregnancy. The B vitamins are not all found together in the same foods; however, if the diet includes milk, organ and other meats, eggs, whole grain or enriched cereals and breads, legumes, and dark green vegetables, most of them probably are present. Vitamin B_{12} is only found in foods of animal origin.

Folic acid is one of the B vitamins that has received increasing attention in recent years. It is involved in deoxyribonucleic acid (DNA) and ribonucleic acid (RNA) synthesis. If there is a lack of folic acid, cell division cannot proceed normally. Needs are increased during pregnancy for growth of the fetus and expansion of maternal blood volume. Maternal serum folate levels are often low during pregnancy, but megaloblastic anemia, a sign of folic acid deficiency, is seldom seen. Leafy green vegetables, other green vegetables, liver, yeast, legumes, nuts, and whole grains are sources of folic acid, but as much as 80% of the vitamin may be destroyed in cooking or storage, so supplementation is often advised.[23]

Vitamin C (ascorbic acid) is essential for the formation of *collagen,* which is sometimes called the "cement" that holds the body's cells and tissues together. This helps explain the importance of vitamin C in building strong bones and teeth, healing wounds, and aiding the ability of the body to withstand the stresses of injury and infection. Vitamin C is found in fresh vegetables and fruits, especially citrus fruits. Fresh strawberries, cantaloupe, pineapple, guavas, tomatoes, and the green vegetables are also good sources. Other fruits and vegetables can be important dietary sources if eaten in sufficient quantity. Vitamin C is easily destroyed by exposure to air, overcooking, or cooking in too much water. The exact amount of vitamin C needed in the diet to promote optimum health is not known, but it probably varies from person to person. Infections and stress may increase requirements. The current RDA is 60 mg for adults, with an additional 10 mg for pregnant women.[21]

MINERALS

There are 14 or more mineral elements that are essential for good nutrition. Some of these are found in fairly large amounts in the body, and others, called *trace elements or micronutrients*, are found in minute amounts. The minerals are constituents of vital body materials, and some act as regulators and activators of body functions.

Calcium is an important constituent of bone and teeth. It is also used by the body for other functions, such as normal blood clotting, promoting muscle tone, and regulating the heart beat. Although two thirds of the calcium in the fetus is deposited during the last month of pregnancy, the mother's daily requirement of calcium is increased during the entire course of pregnancy to prepare adequate storage for this demand. The principal foods from which calcium is obtained are cheese, eggs, oatmeal, vegetables, and milk. A quart of milk alone supplies 1.2 g of calcium.

Phosphorus is an essential constituent of all the cells and the tissues of the body. Milk provides an abundant source of phosphorus. Actually, because phosphorus is an almost invariable constituent of protein, a diet that includes sufficient protein-rich foods, such as eggs, meat, cheese, oatmeal, and green vegetables, provides an adequate amount of phosphorus.

Iron is one of the chief components of hemoglobin, the substance in the blood responsible for carrying oxygen to the cells. During pregnancy, iron is needed to manufacture hemoglobin for fetal red blood cells as well as for maternal red blood cells. During the first two trimesters of pregnancy, iron is transferred to the fetus in moderate amounts, but during the last trimester, when the fetus builds up its reserve, the amount transferred is accelerated about ten times. The diet should be rich in iron-containing foods (e.g., liver, wheat germ, egg yolks), but dietary sources of iron and limited maternal stores often cannot supply the amounts needed for pregnancy.

Therefore, daily iron supplementation is usually recommended, beginning about the 12th week of gestation. Foods rich in ascorbic acid appear to enhance the absorption of dietary iron, but the same effect has not been demonstrated with most iron supplements.

Iron tablets taken between meals are absorbed more completely than those taken with food.[13]

Iodine is only needed in small amounts for the health of the woman and the fetus. This mineral is obtained readily from seafood and cod liver oil. In certain localities around the Great Lakes and in parts of the Northwest, the water supply and the vegetables grown are poor in iodine. Hence, daily use of iodized salt ensures an adequate intake of iodine and prevents deficiency.

Zinc has recently been shown to be important during pregnancy. Deficiency has been linked to congenital malformations and labor and delivery complications, including prolonged labor.[24] Lack of sufficient zinc in the diet is also thought to predispose to bacterial infections of the amniotic fluid, which may lead to preterm labor and delivery.[25] Meats, fish, egg yolks, and most other protein foods have a relatively high zinc content, so a diet meeting the RDA for protein should also furnish sufficient amounts of zinc.[24]

Sodium is present in foods of animal origin and in some vegetables, but the major dietary source is salt. There is increasing recognition of the importance of adequate sodium intake during pregnancy. In the past, like calorie restriction, restriction of salt was thought to be an important factor in the prevention of toxemia. Clinical and laboratory data indicate that the sodium requirement is increased during pregnancy. Restriction, therefore, can be harmful when imposed indiscriminately. An adequate renal and placental blood flow demands an adequate circulating blood volume. When there is a stringent reduction in sodium intake, there is a reduction in circulating blood volume, which is intolerable during pregnancy and causes damage to both mother and fetus. Thus, the routine restriction of salt is no longer practiced. The use of diuretics for reduction of edema that was previously thought to be associated with sodium retention caused by excessive salt in the diet has also been discontinued.

The need for sodium during pregnancy does not mean that pregnant women, as a group, need to increase their salt intake. The recommendation is for the daily consumption of no less than 2 to 3 g of sodium.[17] The usual diet of most women in the United States easily meets this requirement.[21]

VITAMIN AND MINERAL SUPPLEMENTS

There is no universal agreement on the use of vitamin and mineral supplements during pregnancy. Ideally, the diet should supply all the nutrients needed so supplements are not necessary. Some physicians prescribe a multivitamin and mineral supplement to be "on the safe side." The Subcommittee on Dietary Intake and Nutrient Supplements During Pregnancy[13] considers supplementation during pregnancy as an intervention to be

Client Education

Sample Meal Plan for Pregnant or Lactating Female—Moderate-Calorie Diet*

Meal	Menu	Protein	Milk	Grains	Vit. C	Vit. A	Other
Breakfast	2 cups puffed wheat 8 oz low-fat milk 1 banana 1 bran muffin 1 tsp. butter**		1	1 1			1
Snack	¼ cup frozen strawberries, sweetened				½		
Lunch	2 slices whole-wheat bread 2 oz tuna, canned in oil, drained 2 tsp. mayonnaise** 1 carrot, raw 4 oz low-fat milk	2	½	2		1	
Snack	4 graham cracker squares 4 oz lowfat milk		½	1			
Dinner	4 oz ground beef ½ cup refried beans ¾ oz American cheese 2 flour tortillas ½ cup corn, frozen 1 medium tomato, sliced	4 1	½	2	½		1
Snack	½ cup peaches, canned light syrup 6 oz low-fat yogurt, fruited		1				1
TOTALS		7	3	7	1	1	3

Food Groups (spanning Protein, Milk, Grains, Vit. C, Vit. A, Other)

* 2218 Kcal in basic diet.

** This food is optional and represents extra calories added to the basic diet.

(Adapted from Nutrition during Pregnancy and the Postpartum Period: A Manual for Health Care Professionals. Sacramento, Maternal and Child Health Branch WIC Supplemental Food Branch, California Department of Health Services, 1990)

used only when specifically indicated. They point out that supplementation can create imbalances, because increasing one nutrient often changes the requirement for other nutrients and all essential nutrients may not have been identified yet.

Iron and folacin are the most frequently recommended supplements, because they are difficult to obtain by diet alone. The Subcommittee recommends a low-dose supplement of 30 mg/day of elemental iron. Folate is also recommended if there is any evidence of an inadequate intake. Because large doses of iron appear to depress plasma zinc in pregnant women, zinc supplementation may be needed when a supplement of more than 30 mg of elemental iron per day is taken. If zinc is given, the Subcommittee recommends the addition of a 2-mg copper supplement to offset zinc's depressive effect on copper absorption.[13]

Certain conditions or habits of the pregnant woman may increase requirements for certain nutrients. For example, women carrying more than one fetus, or women who smoke cigarettes, drink alcohol or use illicit drugs may require additional supplementation. Special attention also needs to be given to the adequacy of calcium and vitamin D intake for pregnant women under age 25, because their bone mineral density is still increasing.[13] Calcium supplements might be advised for women who drink little or no milk, and vitamin B_{12} might be needed by the vegan who eats no animal protein.[17] If any vitamin or mineral supplements are used, it is important for the woman to understand that these are in addition to, not instead of, her recommended dietary intake.

Megadoses of Vitamins and Minerals. The idea that if a little is good, a lot is even better is applied by some people to vitamin supplementation. As more is learned about vitamins and their uses in the body, it is becoming more apparent that doses far in excess of body requirements may cause chemical imbalances that can lead to adverse effects. Toxic effects have been seen in people consuming large amounts of certain vitamins. Evidence of detrimental effects during pregnancy is limited at present, but the embryo or fetus is thought to be particularly vulnerable to toxic effects of vitamin and mineral megadoses.[26] One reason for this is that the placental transport system concentrates some nutrients in fetal blood in an effort to make sure that the fetus has a sufficient amount, and thus excessive maternal intake exposes the fetus to unusually high levels. Another reason is that the excretory capacity of the fetus is limited. Susceptibility to damage is greatest during early pregnancy, when organ systems are developing.[27]

The fat-soluble vitamins, especially *vitamin A* and *vitamin D*, have been linked to birth defects by both human case reports and animal studies. Some infants whose mothers took large doses of vitamin A during pregnancy have been born with urinary tract malformations, and others have developed behavioral problems and learning disabilities.[26]

Retinol or preformed vitamin A has been shown to be teratogenic. Carotene, the vitamin A precursor found in foods, does not appear to be harmful, even in large amounts, primarily because it is not efficiently absorbed and converted to vitamin A.[13]

Vitamin D has the smallest margin of safety of any of the vitamins. Among the adverse conditions associated with an excess intake during pregnancy is infantile hypercalcemia, which is characterized by damage to the cardiovascular and renal systems and the brain.

Although water-soluble vitamins are not stored in the body in the same way that fat-soluble vitamins are, some of them have been shown to have adverse effects in excessive amounts. There is some evidence that the fetus may become accustomed to the high levels during pregnancy and show withdrawal symptoms after birth. Some infants of women who took large amounts of *vitamin C* during pregnancy have shown scurvylike

symptoms when their high prenatal intake was cut off at birth.[27]

To help avoid potential dangers of vitamin overdosage, questions about vitamin supplementation should be included in the initial dietary assessment of the pregnant woman. As with other aspects of dietary counseling, the nurse can assist the expectant mother in planning a diet that includes appropriate amounts of nutrients and avoids excesses.

WATER AND OTHER FLUIDS

Water is often omitted when nutrients are listed, but it is, in fact, an essential nutrient. It is an important solvent that is necessary for digestion, nutrient transport to the cells, and removal of body wastes. It is also a lubricant and helps to regulate body temperature.

Fluids should be taken freely. The woman should drink an average of six to eight glasses daily. Water and juices are good choices. Some beverages contain ingredients that should be used sparingly in the prenatal diet. For example, regular soft drinks contain many empty calories, dietetic soft drinks contain artificial sweeteners, and cola, tea, and coffee contain caffeine (see section entitled "Food Additives"). Women who drink large quantities of any of these beverages should be counseled to decrease their intake.

Although there is no definite evidence at present that tea and coffee should be eliminated from the prenatal diet, women are usually advised to at least cut down. Using decaffeinated coffee or tea and removing the teabag promptly when brewing regular tea help to decrease the amount of caffeine per cup.

Planning the Diet

The following discussion and tables are provided to assist the nurse in helping the pregnant woman plan her diet and follow basic guidelines for good nutrition during pregnancy. Planning a menu to include all the essential nutrients would seem impossible if each nutrient had to be considered individually. Fortunately, nutrients are found in foods in certain combinations, so division of foods into groups according to the major nutrients they supply, as in Table 18-7, can simplify the planning.

The four basic food groups are: protein foods, milk and milk products, breads, cereals and grains, and fruits and vegetables. The Daily Food Guide (see Table 18-7) further differentiates fruits and vegetables into three groups: vitamin C-rich, vitamin A-rich, and other.

The Daily Food Guide is meant to be used to plan nutritionally adequate diets with clients. The woman should eat the number of servings recommended from each food group every day. The Nutritional Teaching Guides (page 366) are helpful in selecting the foods. The Sample Meal Plan (page 375) illustrates how the

Client Education

Basic Guidelines for Good Nutrition During Pregnancy

1. Use the Daily Food Guide to plan each day's meals.
2. Include a wide variety of foods.
3. Gain weight gradually and steadily.
4. Use supplements if prescribed.
5. Avoid:
   - Weight reduction diets
   - Sodium restriction and diuretics
   - Harmful substances such as alcohol, drugs, and nicotine
   - Excessive fat, salt, caffeine, sugar, and sweeteners

guide can be used. Note that the Daily Food Guide serves as a framework for the menu but does not limit the foods that can be included. The nurse can assist the woman in deciding where ethnic foods fit into the plan as shown in the Sample Menus to Meet the Daily Food Requirements During Pregnancy for Ethnic Groups. Intake of specific nutrients varies depending on the foods selected, but using the Daily Food Guide leads to an average intake of adequate amounts of most of the essential nutrients. The woman should be counseled to include additional nutritious food to meet her caloric needs.[10]

PROTEIN FOODS

Seven or more 1-oz servings of protein-rich foods such as beef, pork, lamb, veal, organ meats, or vegetable protein sources are recommended daily. At least one of the servings should come from vegetable sources such as legumes (e.g., dried beans, peas, and lentils) or nuts. In addition to their main value of providing amino acids, the protein foods are also good sources of many vitamins and minerals. In keeping with current concerns about limiting the intake of fat to 30% of calories consumed, protein-rich foods can be distinguished as those that are low in fat (<5 g/serving) and those that are high in fat (>5 g/serving).

Often the family's budget restricts the quantity and the variety of protein foods, especially meat. The substitution of cheese, peanut butter, poultry, fish, or legumes may be suggested. Advice regarding the preparation and use of the organ meats that are rich in protein, vitamins, and minerals may also be helpful. Many women may avoid these foods because they are unfamiliar with them, are unaware of their nutritional value, or dislike the taste. With a little ingenuity and suggestions from a good nutrition book or cookbook, the nurse can often help the family use this valuable and inexpensive source of protein. Liver, for instance, can be lightly broiled, ground, and incorporated into a meatloaf or ground meat patties to disguise the taste and looks, and to make the meat go farther.

Women who follow a vegetarian diet, especially vegans, may also need assistance in meeting their protein needs. Vegetarian diets can be adequate in protein if the person is knowledgeable about the complemen-

(*Text continues on page 380*)

TABLE 18-7. DAILY FOOD GUIDE FOR WOMEN

Food Group	Minimum Number of Servings		
	Non-pregnant Adolescent Female	*Non-pregnant Adult Female*	*Pregnant/Lactating Adolescent/Adult Female*
Protein foods	5*	5*	7*
Milk products	3	2	3
Breads, cereal grains	7†	6†	7†
Fruits and vegetables:			
Vitamin C-rich	1	1	1
Vitamin A-rich	1	1	1
Other	3	3	3

* Each serving is equivalent to 1 oz of animal protein; at least one serving should be from the vegetable protein list (two servings during pregnancy or lactation).
† At least 4 servings should be from whole grains
(California Department of Health Services, MCH/WIC: Nutrition During Pregnancy and the Postpartum Period: Manual for Health Care Professionals, 1990)

Client Education

Sample Menus to Meet the Daily Food Requirements During Pregnancy for Ethnic Groups

			Food Groups					
Mexican	**African-American**	**Lacto-Ovovegetarian**	*Protein*	*Milk*	*Grains*	*Vit. C*	*Vit. A*	*Other*
Breakfast								
½ cup oatmeal	1 slice whole-grain toast	½ cup Wheatena			1			
1 sweet roll (pan dulce)	½ cup grits	½ cup granola cereal			1			
1 cup low-fat milk	1 cup whole milk	1 cup nonfat milk		1				
Sugar*	Margarine, bacon*	Margarine*						
Lunch								
Tostadas:	Chiliburger:	Soup and Salad:						
2 oz chicken breast	2 oz hamburger	1 ½ cups lentil soup	} 3					
½ cup refried beans	½ cup chili beans	1 egg hard boiled (in salad)						
2 corn tortillas	1 hamburger bun, white	2 whole-grain rolls			2			
Fresh chili salsa:	Cole slaw:	Salad:						
½ tomato + ½ tbsp. chili pepper	½ cup cabbage + dressing*	1 fresh tomato				½		
1 cup romaine lettuce	½ cup french fries	1 cup romaine lettuce						1
¾ oz jack cheese	½ cup vanilla milkshake	½ cup nonfat milk		½				
Dinner								
Bistec ranchero:	Pork chops:	Stuffed pita:						
3 oz chuck steak	3 oz pork chop	½ cup kidney beans	} 4					
½ cup kidney beans	½ cup baked beans	6 oz tofu						
		½ cup hummus						
½ cup red potatoes	½ cup mashed potatoes	½ cup mushrooms						1
Fresh chili salsa: ½ tomato + ½ tbsp. chili pepper	½ medium orange	¼ cup tomato purée				½		
2 corn tortillas	2 whole-grain rolls	1 pita, whole-wheat			2			
¼ fresh mango	½ cup mustard greens	½ cup carrots, raw					1	
Snacks								
Licuado:		Smoothee:						
1 cup low-fat milk	1 cup fruit yogurt	4 oz nonfat milk + ½ cup yogurt		1				
1 cup banana + sugar, vanilla*	15 small grapes	1 banana + honey*						1
¾ cup corn flakes	8 whole-wheat crackers	8 whole-wheat crackers			1			
½ cup low-fat milk	¾ oz American cheese	¾ cups frozen yogurt		½				
		TOTALS	7	3	7	1	1	3

Each menu meets the minimum number of servings for all groups in the Daily Food Guide for Women. One extra serving from the breads/cereals/grains group is included in each menu to follow customary eating habits.

* Indicates foods that provide extra calories only.

Client Education

Sample Menus to Meet the Daily Food Requirements During Pregnancy for Ethnic Groups

			Food Groups					
Chinese	*Japanese*	*Southeast Asian*	Protein	Milk	Grains	Vit. C	Vit. A	Other
Breakfast 1 egg, soft-boiled 1 cup oatmeal, cooked 1 cup low-fat milk	1 egg, hard-boiled 1 cup steamed rice 1 cup low-fat milk	1 oz pork, stir-fried 1 cup rice noodles ½ cup evaporated milk (in decaf coffee)	1	1	2			
Lunch Chicken and soup noodles: 2 oz chicken, boiled Soy sauce, ginger* 1 cup noodles, boiled ½ cup snow peas ½ cup bean sprouts, onions Jasmine tea*	Soup and Salad: 2 oz beef, boiled Miso soup broth* 1 cup buckwheat noodles (soba) ½ cup broccoli 1 cup head lettuce, white radish Seasoned rice vinegar*	BBQ beef: 2 oz beef strips, grilled Lemon grass, garlic, oil* 1 cup rice noodles 6 oz orange juice 1 cup green leaf lettuce Fish sauce, hot red pepper*	2		2	1		1
Dinner Mongolian beef: 3 oz beef strips Garlic, soy sauce, green onions* 1 cup white rice, steamed 2 medium plums ½ cup bok choy, stir-fried Soup: 3 oz tofu Parsley, chicken broth*	Teriyaki salmon: 3 oz fresh salmon fillet, broiled Shoyu marinade* 1 cup white rice, steamed ½ cup cucumber salad ½ cup carrots 3 oz tofu (in soup) 1 cup miso soup with onion*	Stir-fry chicken and cabbage: 3 oz chicken Fish sauce, chili* 1 cup white rice, steamed ½ cup bean sprouts Soup: ½ cup mustard greens 1 oz pork Broth*	3 1		2		1	1
Snacks 1 cup low-fat milk 1 medium apple 8 whole-wheat crackers	1 cup low-fat milk 15 small grapes 8 whole-wheat crackers	½ cup evaporated milk (in decaf coffee) 1 medium banana 8 whole-wheat crackers		1	1			1
		TOTALS	7	2	7	1	1	3

Each menu contains at least the minimum number of servings for each food group in the Daily Food Guide for Pregnant Women, except the milk products group. Women who are able to drink milk or who will take lactose-reduced milk can include more milk products to meet the need for calcium. Additional calcium is supplied by broccoli, greens, and tofu.

None of these menus supplies the recommended four servings from whole grains, and the Southeast Asian menu does not include the recommended two servings of vegetable protein, because the menus reflect usual cultural practices. Women should be encouraged to eat more whole-grain breads or crackers and vegetable protein to meet the recommended number of two servings each.

* Indicates foods that provide extra calories only or are used for seasonings.

(California Department of Health Services, MCH/WIC: Nutrition During Pregnancy and the Postpartum Period: A Manual for Health Care Professionals. 1990)

tarity of protein foods with different limiting amino acids to ensure the presence of complete proteins (Table 18-8). However, some of the people who adopt vegetarian diets do not have the knowledge or the resources to select or obtain the appropriate foods. They need help in finding sources of information and in planning menus.

MILK AND MILK PRODUCTS

Three 1-cup servings of fluid milk (1 qt) daily, or the equivalent, is the recommendation for the expectant mother. Milk has been called Nature's most nearly perfect food, and it is an invaluable source of nutrients during pregnancy. It contains vitamins, such as vitamin A and riboflavin, and minerals, such as calcium and phosphorus, that are needed for fetal development. Milk's high content of calcium and phosphorus is in the correct proportions and in a digestible form that permits optimum utilization by both mother and fetus. It is not only an excellent source of protein, but it is also the most readily digested and easily absorbed of all food proteins.

When a woman indicates that she does not drink milk or drinks very little, it is important to pursue the subject and find out the basis for the avoidance. She may not like milk or be able to tolerate it well. After the cause is established, a plan can be developed with her to make milk more palatable or to include adequate substitutes.

The instant nonfat and whole dry milks may be used in a quantity that provides an adequate intake. Approximately 5 tablespoons of dried skim milk equals 1 pt of fluid milk. The milk may be used dry and worked into meatloaf, mashed potatoes, cereals, sandwich spreads, baked articles, and so on. Reconstituted with less than the usual amount of water, it has a richer taste than the regular liquid skim milk. Certain condiments

TABLE 18–8. COMPLEMENTARY PLANT PROTEIN SOURCES

Food	Amino Acids Deficient	Complementary Protein
Grains	Isoleucine	Rice + legumes
	Lysine	Corn + legumes
		Wheat + legumes
		Wheat + peanuts + milk
		Wheat + sesame + soybean
		Rice + seasame
		Rice + brewer's yeast
Legumes	Tryptophan	Legumes + rice
	Methionine	Beans + wheat
		Beans + corn
		Soybeans + rice + wheat
		Soybeans + corn + milk
		Soybeans + wheat + sesame
		Soybeans + peanuts + sesame
		Soybeans + peanuts + wheat + rice
		Soybeans + sesame + wheat
Nuts and seeds	Isoleucine	Peanuts + sesame + soybeans
	Lysine	Sesame + beans
		Sesame + soybeans + wheat
		Peanuts + sunflower seeds
Vegetables	Isoleucine	Lima beans ⎫
	Methionine	Green peas ⎪ + sesame seeds or
		Brussels sprouts ⎬ Brazil nuts or
		Cauliflower ⎪ mushrooms
		Broccoli ⎭
		Greens + milet or converted rice

(After Lappé FM: Diet For a Small Planet. Ballantine, NY, 1975. By Frances Moore Lappé, Friends of the Earth/ Ballantine, New York, 1975)

and flavorings (e.g., vanilla, nutmeg, cinnamon) enhance the flavor of milk. Some clients may prefer evaporated milk, buttermilk, nonfat, or low-fat milk instead of whole milk. Milk can also be taken in some other form, such as in soups or custards.

Other dairy products, such as cottage cheese, ricotta cheese, farmer's cheese, hoop cheese, yogurt, and the hard cheeses, are also adequate substitutions. One ounce of cheese contains approximately the same amount of minerals and vitamins as a large glass of whole milk. However, the total protein and fat content varies and must be considered when making substitutions. Cream cheese has a high percentage of fat and a low calcium content so it is not a good substitute for the other cheeses. Also, products such as "cheese foods" and "cheese spreads" are diluted and therefore contain fewer nutrients per serving.

Lactose Intolerance. Many adults, especially Hispanics, African-Americans, Asians, and Native Americans, have difficulty digesting milk because of an insufficient amount of the enzyme lactase in the small intestine. Lactase is responsible for breaking down lactose (milk sugar) into glucose and galactose. If the available lactase is not sufficient to hydrolyze the amount of lactose ingested, fermentation occurs in the large intestine and causes abdominal cramps, diarrhea, bloating, and flatulence.

Not every woman who says "I don't like milk" or "Milk doesn't agree with me" is lactose intolerant. On the other hand, encouraging the truly lactose-intolerant person to "drink more milk" can be counterproductive if it causes symptoms. Aside from the discomfort caused by symptoms, the increased stool frequency and mass can lead to the increased loss of nutrients, including calcium in the feces. This, in turn, can cause a negative calcium balance.[28]

When counseling these women, special attention should be directed to meeting calcium, protein, vitamin, and mineral requirements. Certain dairy products, such as cheeses, are lower in lactose and can be used in place of fluid milk (Table 18-9). Some women may find that, due to improved efficiency of lactose absorption during pregnancy, they are able to tolerate small amounts of fluid milk at a time.[10] Also, it has been found that ingesting milk and milk products in combination with other foods may help lactase-deficient women tolerate them better. Women who consume less than the recommended number of servings of milk products can be advised to substitute foods from the nondairy calcium-rich list included in the Nutritional Teaching Guides.

BREAD, CEREAL, AND GRAINS

Seven or more servings should be included from this group daily. At least four of these should be whole-grain products, which contain vitamins and minerals not found in refined flour and not replaced by the enriching process. The germ of the grain, removed in the refining process, also contains protein of value comparable to that from animal sources. Wheat germ can be purchased separately and eaten as a cereal or added to foods, such as baked goods or meatloaf, to increase the nutritional value.

Cereal products are a primary source of energy in the diet, and they make an important contribution to every nutrient need except calcium, ascorbic acid, and vitamin A. When bread is buttered, it even contributes to the vitamin A intake. Whole-grain cereal and breads also add fiber to the diet to help counteract constipation.

VEGETABLES AND FRUITS

Five or more servings of fruits and vegetables, some raw, should be included in the diet daily. Fruits and vegetables contain variable amounts of vitamins and minerals, and most are excellent sources of fiber. Breaking the vegetable and fruit group into the subgroups of vitamin C-rich, vitamin A-rich and other, helps to ensure that vitamins A and C are adequately included in the diet.

Vegetables. Vegetables are particularly rich sources of iron, calcium, and several vitamins. The dark green vegetables are good sources of vitamin A, folacin, and iron. The deep yellow fruits and vegetables are also good sources of vitamin A. Fresh or frozen vegetables can be used interchangeably. Canned vegetables may be used if necessary, but some nutrients are lost in the cooking and canning process.

Careful preparation and cooking of vegetables helps to retain the maximum vitamin and mineral content. Presoaking should be avoided. Steaming and stir-frying are preferred methods of cooking. Steamer baskets to fit standard size pans are widely available. Some vegetables contain incomplete proteins that add to the total protein intake.

In addition to their value as nutrient agents, these vegetables deserve an important place in the diet as laxative agents because their fibrous framework increases the bulk of the intestinal content and thereby stimulates elimination.

Fruits. Citrus fruits such as oranges, lemons, and grapefruit are the best sources of vitamin C. Most of these fruits also supply vitamins A and B. Tomatoes are also an excellent source of vitamin C; the amount eaten, however, must be twice that of the citrus fruits to supply the same amount of vitamin. Other fruits, raw and cooked, such as prunes, raisins, and apricots, contain important minerals (e.g., iron and copper) as well as vitamins. Fruits may stimulate a lagging appetite and

TABLE 18-9. COMPOSITION AND COMPARISON OF DAIRY PRODUCTS

Products and Amount	Calories	Protein (g)	Lactose (g)	Lactose Ratio to Milk	Calcium (mg)	Calcium Ratio to Milk
Sandwich cheese (2 oz)						
American	210	12.6	0.96	0.09:1	364	1.4:1
Cheddar	230	14.2	1.18	0.11:1	386	1.5:1
Cream cheese	196	4.8	1.14	0.11:1	40	0.15:1
Swiss	210	15.6	0.96	0.09:1	522	2.0:1
Cottage cheese (4 oz)						
Plain, creamed	108	14.0	2.4	0.23:1	68	0.3:1
Low fat (2%)	96	15.6	3.7	0.36:1	100	0.4:1
Uncreamed	92	21.2	0.8	0.08:1	28	0.1:1
Ice Cream (4 oz)						
Vanilla (12% fat)	254	4.4	8.0	0.77:1	164	0.6:1
Ice Milk (4 oz)						
Vanilla	166	4.4	8.4	0.8:1	156	0.6:1
Milk (8 oz)						
Whole milk (3.5% fat)	141	7.3	10.4	1:1	260	1:1
Chocolate drink	136	7.3	9.6	0.9:1	247	0.95:1
Egg nog (6% fat)	304	10.4	12.8	1.2:1	343	1.3:1
Skimmed	73	7.3	10.4	1.1	266	1:1
Yogurt (8 oz)						
Blueberry	257	9.6	10.4	1:1	282	1:1
Plain	134	12.0	13.6	1.3:1	362	1.4:1
Strawberry	232	10.4	12.0	1.2:1	314	1.2:1
Vanilla	195	11.2	12.8	1.2:1	336	1.3:1
Milk (reconstituted; 8 oz)						
Nonfat dry	80	8.0	12.4	1.2:1	300	1.2:1
Evaporated whole	174	8.8	12.5	1.2:1	325	1.3:1
Evaporated skim	96	9.6	13.9	1.3:1	350	1.4:1
Liquid breakfast mix (1-serving envelope)						
Vanilla	130	7.0	12.2	1.2:1	50	0.2:1

Figures are calculated from nutritional analysis information provided by the Kraftco Corporation and the Carnation Company on their own products. (Luke B: Lactose intolerance during pregnancy: Significance and solutions. MCN 2(2)95, March/April 1977)

counteract constipation. They may be used as juices, combined in salads, as additions to cereals or plain yogurt, as in-between-meal refreshments, and in desserts, such as gelatins and puddings. Fruits contain some incomplete proteins but only supplement the other proteins.

FOOD QUALITY

Women may need to be reminded to select foods that are fresh and of good quality, because they are more appealing and safer as well. Foods that have been on the shelf a long time are more likely to begin to deteriorate or become rancid, interfering with their nutritive value. Aflatoxins and other mycotoxins are produced by fungal growths on a wide variety of foodstuffs. They can be toxic to humans and are suspected of being teratogenic and carcinogenic. Therefore, pregnant women

should be warned against eating any foods that are fermented, moldy, rotten, discolored, or malodorous because they are potentially contaminated.[29]

FOOD ADDITIVES

Food additives are substances, added either directly or indirectly to a food, that become a component of the food or affect its functional characteristics.[30] Some additives are necessary to our food supply to prevent spoilage and ensure that certain products are safe to eat. Other additives are used to improve the flavor, odor, texture, color, or the nutritional quality of foods.

The FDA monitors additives and bans those that cause cancer or other problems in animals. There is often controversy over the safety of additives. Nitrates and nitrites, for example, can be converted by the body to nitrosamines, which have been shown to be teratogenic and carcinogenic in rats, but they are still used to preserve processed meats and other foods until adequate substitutes can be found. The safety of artificial sweeteners has been questioned in recent years. The use of saccharin as an additive in commercial products has decreased markedly since it was linked with the development of bladder cancer in animal studies. There is no real evidence that other artificial sweeteners such as aspartame (Nutra-Sweet) are harmful, but most dietitians recommend that they be used with caution during pregnancy. BHA and BHT, which are used in many foods, including cereals, oils, and snack foods, are other additives whose safety has been questioned.

Although caffeine is not really an additive, it is a substance of potential concern to the pregnant woman. There have been conflicting results, but it has been shown to be teratogenic and mutagenic in some experiments on rats and mice. There is insufficient evidence to label it as a teratogen in humans, but it should be used with caution (see Chap. 19 for further information).

Teratogenicity is usually considered to be dose related, so that, although it may be impossible to eliminate additives from the diet, reducing the amount during pregnancy would lower the risks.[30] Until more is known, it is wise for the pregnant woman to read labels carefully and choose products with as few additives as possible.

Special Nutritional Concerns for the Pregnant Adolescent

If the pregnant client is in her teenage years, nutritional concerns arise that need to be highlighted in her care. Adolescents, as a group, have repeatedly been shown to have poorer pregnancy outcomes than older pregnant females. This has sometimes been attributed to a competition for nutrients between the growth requirements of the adolescent and those of the fetus. Current information, however, indicates that, except for those of low gynecological age, the adolescent's nutrient needs are not very different from those of other pregnant woman.[13,21,31] The pregnant adolescent is at higher nutritional risk, though, for a number of reasons. She is more likely to begin pregnancy in poor nutritional status as evidenced by being underweight, iron deficient, and consuming inadequate amounts of calcium and other important nutrients.

Factors leading to inadequate nutrition for the pregnant adolescent include the desire to be slim, peer food practices, and resistance to adult advice. Eating nutritionally may also be of low priority to the pregnant adolescent, who may be much more concerned with meeting her social and emotional needs. Because adolescent pregnancy is most common among the poor and socially disadvantaged, and therefore among those least likely to receive needed medical and social support, the risk for poor nutritional status is further increased. Appropriate referrals to WIC (the Special Supplemental Program for Women, Infants and Children) and other resources, such as classes and programs for pregnant adolescents, are important.[31]

FOOD SELECTION

The teenager's food choices often include many "fast foods" and non-nutritious snacks. This leads to a low intake of fresh fruits and vegetables, which in turn limits the intake of vitamins and minerals, especially vitamins A and C. If milk and milk products are also avoided, there may be a lack of certain B-complex vitamins and vitamin D, in addition to inadequate intake of calcium and protein.

WEIGHT GAIN

The levels of protein and energy intake and the pregnancy weight gain needed to promote optimal intrauterine growth for the infants of adolescent mothers are not unequivocally established.[32] Theoretically, the ideal weight gain would include the usual pregnancy recommendation plus, for the girl who is still growing, the amount she would have gained in the process of maturation during the 9-month period if she had not become pregnant. Younger adolescents (12–15 years) would therefore be expected to gain more than older adolescents (16 and over), whose growth rate would have slowed down or stopped.[33] Chronological age, however, is less important in this regard than gynecological age (number of years past the onset of menarche), the girl's individual growth pattern, her prepregnancy weight for height, and her level of activity.

Weight-conscious teenagers may resist continuous weight gain, especially if they have gained a lot in early pregnancy. They need extra help in understanding the importance of weight gain throughout the pregnancy, and the potential dangers to the fetus of dieting during this time when extra nutrients are needed.

EATING DISORDERS

Weight consciousness and equating thinness with attractiveness have led to an increased incidence of eating disorders. Anorexia nervosa and bulimia are found most frequently in the adolescent and young-adult age-groups. Fertility is usually reduced in the anorexic female, who is rarely able to conceive or carry a pregnancy. Bulimia, however, which is becoming more common among teenagers, is less likely than anorexia to affect fertility. The bulimic, through her binging and purging, is in far from an optimum nutritional state in spite of near-normal body weight. Because recognition of bulimia is relatively recent, little research is available on how best to manage the pregnant bulimic female.[17]

Some possible effects from the practice of bulimia, besides the nutritional deficits, are tooth decay and possible esophageal damage caused by the repeated vomiting, rectal bleeding, and electrolyte imbalance caused by the continual use of laxatives, and possible diabetes or hypoglycemia resulting from the stimulus of food without its nutritional effects.[34] Theoretically, the primary problem during pregnancy is the effect on the fetus of the potentially detrimental changes in its biochemical environment resulting from the maternal binging, vomiting, and purging.[17]

To provide sufficient nourishment to support the pregnancy and attempt to avoid detrimental effects on the fetus, the bulimic woman needs psychological intervention. The nurse's primary role with these people is detection of the problem and referral to an appropriate source for psychological help.

COUNSELING

The pregnant adolescent benefits most from counseling designed to meet her individual needs. Many teenagers do eat nutritionally sound diets and just need reinforcement of their good eating habits and information about additional pregnancy needs. Others need more specific assistance. Although some may respond to the appeal to eat well for a healthy baby, to many the unborn child does not seem real until late in the pregnancy or after the birth. The nurse working with these girls may find it more helpful to stress the girl's own growth and development needs.[33] When pregnant teenagers are well-nourished throughout their pregnancy, they are much less likely to develop complications and much more likely to produce a healthy infant.

Resources

The nurse should be aware of available resources for nutritional counseling, education, and support. This assists in keeping nutritional education up to date and also enables the nurse to make appropriate referrals.

When consultation with a nutritionist is advisable and one is not available on the clinic or hospital staff, it may be possible to locate one in the area through the local community-health department or a home economist's office. Publications, visual aids, charts, and so on may be secured from city, county, and state health departments. The March of Dimes Birth Defects Foundation also provides many teaching aids and reminders about nutrition during pregnancy.

The U.S. Government Printing Office is another invaluable source of publications. The Food and Nutrition Board, National Research Council, Council on Foods and Nutrition, American Medical Association, American Home Economics Association, and American Public Health Association are all professional organizations that offer additional resources. The above associations are only a few of the resources that the nurse and the physician have to assist their clients in planning for adequate nutrition.

WIC

A source of nutritional help for some pregnant women is the *Special Supplementary Food Program for Women, Infants and Children,* better known as *WIC.* This program was initiated in 1973 to provide food for low-income families at critical times of growth and development. Funds for the program come from the U.S. Department of Agriculture and are administered at the state and local levels by state health departments.[4]

At the local level, specific foods are provided for pregnant and lactating women, in addition to infants and children up to 5 years of age, who are determined to be at risk nutritionally and who otherwise would be unable to afford an adequate diet. Food vouchers or supplemental foods are distributed at designated health clinics. The WIC program seeks to do more than just provide food for needy families. Nutrition education is mandated to be an integral part of the program. The educational component of the program uses a variety of teaching modalities, including lectures, films, group or individual discussions, and written material. It is planned to take into account socioeconomic, educational, and cultural factors and the level of understanding of the recipients.

■ EVALUATION

The nurse can use the evaluation phase of the nursing process to improve the effectiveness of nutritional care for the pregnant patient. Nutritional interventions are evaluated by monitoring changes in the patient's nutritional status, absence of nutritionally related diseases, such as preeclampsia and anemia, changes she makes in her diet to follow the Daily Food Guide, appropriate weight gain, and adequate fetal growth. Ongoing evaluation occurs throughout pregnancy through use of the weight gain grid, repeated use of dietary recall, and assessments of changes in nutritional status and fetal growth. Revisions in the nursing care plan are made during pregnancy in response to the evaluation. Optimal outcomes, including a full-term pregnancy, an uncomplicated birth and an adequate size, healthy baby, would be evaluated after the baby's birth.

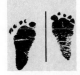

Nursing Care Plan

The Pregnant Woman and Her Nutritional Needs

Patient Goals

1. Patient is free of nutritionally related problems such as preeclampsia or anemia.
2. Patient demonstrates implementation of suggested dietary changes through use of dietary recall or food diary.
3. Patient's weight gain is adequate and follows recommended pattern.
4. Patient's fetus/neonate demonstrates adequate growth and well-being.

Assessment	**Potential Nursing Diagnosis**	**Planning and Intervention**	**Evaluation**

Nutritional status
  Physical indicators
  Prepregnant weight
  Pregnancy weight gain
  Laboratory values (hemoglobin, hematocrit)
Current dietary habits
  Daily food intake
  Individual factors in food selection
Nutritional risk factors
Client understanding of nutrition
  Importance of good nutrition during pregnancy
  Important nutrients
  Importance of weight gain
	Alteration in nutrition: less than body requirements, related to: inadequate caloric intake or inadequate financial resources or dysfunctional dietary patterns
	
	Alteration in nutrition: less calcium than pregnancy requirements, related to: lactose intolerance
	
	Knowledge deficit regarding nutritional needs during pregnancy, related to lack of information
	
	Alteration in nutrition: inadequate weight gain, related to self-imposed limitation of calories
		Use assessment tools to determine individual client needs
		
		Provide dietary counseling as needed:
		  Involve client in planning
		  Consider individual needs, preferences, attitudes, family needs, and cultural or ethnic background
		  Provide information about nutrient needs
		  Encourage and reinforce appropriate food choices and preparation
		  Plan menus with client including foods she likes and can afford, and is able to prepare
		  Give careful, thorough explanation of rationale for any suggested changes
		
		Teach importance of weight gain; use and discuss weight gain grid at each visit
		
		Refer to dietitian when appropriate
			Absence of nutritionally related problems such as preeclampsia and anemia
			
			Repeat dietary recall or food diary indicates use of Daily Food Guide and implementation of suggested changes
			
			Weight gain is adequate and follows recommended pattern
			
			Fetal growth and well-being follow optimal pattern

■ REFERENCES

1. Committee on Maternal Nutrition, Food and Nutrition Board, National Research Council: Maternal Nutrition and the Course of Pregnancy. Washington, DC, National Academy of Sciences, 1970
2. Luke B: Maternal Nutrition. Boston, Little, Brown & Co, 1979
3. Rosso P, Cramoy C: Nutrition and pregnancy. In Winick M (ed): Nutrition—Pre and Postnatal Development, p 176. New York, Plenum Press, 1979
4. Rush D: Effects of changes in protein and calorie intake during pregnancy on the growth of the human fetus. In Chalmers I, Enkin M, Keirse MJNC (eds): Effective Care in Pregnancy and Childbirth, pp 255–280. New York, Oxford University Press, 1989
5. Worthington-Roberts BS, Klerman LV: Maternal Nutrition. In Merkatz IR, Thompson JE: New Perspectives on Prenatal Care, pp 235–271. New York, Elsevier, 1990
6. Primrose T, Higgins A: A study in human antepartum nutrition. J Reprod Med 7(6):257–264, December 1971
7. Winick M: Malnutrition and mental development. In Winick M (ed): Nutrition—Pre and Postnatal Development, p 52. New York, Plenum Press, 1979
8. Stein Z (ed): Famine and Human Development: The Dutch Hunger Winter of 1944–1945. New York, Oxford University Press, 1975
9. Higgins A: Montreal diet dispensary study. In Nutritional Supplementation and the Outcome of Pregnancy, pp 93–110. Washington, DC, National Academy of Sciences, 1973
10. Nutrition During Pregnancy and the Postpartum Period: A Manual for Health Care Professionals. Sacramento, Maternal and Child Health Branch, WIC Supplemental Food Branch, California Department of Health Services, 1990
11. Kitay DZ: Dysfunctional antepartum nutrition. J Reprod Med 7(6):251–256, December 1971
12. Dwyer J: Vegetarian diets in pregnancy (proceedings of a workshop). In Committee on Nutrition of the Mother and Preschool Child, Food and Nutrition Board, Commission on Life Sciences, National Research Council: Alternative Dietary Practices and Nutritional Abuses in Pregnancy, pp 61–83. Washington, DC, National Academy Press, 1982
13. Food and Nutrition Board, Institute of Medicine, National Academy of Sciences: Nutrition During Pregnancy; Part I, Weight Gain; Part II, Nutrient Supplements. Washington, DC, National Academy Press, 1990
14. Pitkin RM: Nutritional influences during pregnancy. Med Clin North Am 61(1):3–14, January 1977
15. Naeye RL: Weight gain and the outcome of pregnancy. Am J Obstet Gynecol 135(1):3–9, September 1979
16. Luke B: Understanding pica in pregnant women. MCN 2(2):97–100, March/April 1977
17. Worthington-Roberts BS, Williams SR (eds): Nutrition in Pregnancy and Lactation, 4th ed. St Louis, CV Mosby, 1989
18. Vermeersch J: Physiological basis of nutritional needs. In Worthington B (ed): Nutrition in Pregnancy and Lactation, 3rd ed. St Louis, CV Mosby, 1985
19. Holey ES: Promoting adequate weight gain in pregnant women. MCN 2(2):86–89, March/April 1977
20. Shearer M: Malnutrition in middle-class pregnant women. Birth Fam J 7(1):27–35, Spring 1980
21. National Research Council (US) Subcommittee on the Tenth Edition of the RDAs: Recommended Dietary Allowances. Washington, DC, National Academy Press, 1989
22. Lappe FM: Diet for a Small Planet. New York, Ballantine Books, 1975
23. Williams SR: Essentials of Nutrition and Diet Therapy, 5th ed. St Louis, Times Mirror/Mosby, 1990
24. Lemasters GK: Zinc insufficiency during pregnancy. JOGN Nurs 10(2):124–125, March/April 1981
25. Naeye RL: Effects of maternal nutrition on fetal and neonatal survival. Birth 10(2):109–113, Summer 1983
26. Luke B: Megavitamins and pregnancy: A dangerous combination. MCN 10(1):18–23, January/February 1985
27. Pitkin RM: Megadose nutrients during pregnancy (proceedings of a workshop). In Committee on Nutrition of the Mother and Preschool Child, Food and Nutrition Board, Commission on Life Sciences, National Research Council: Alternative Dietary Practices and Nutritional Abuses in Pregnancy, pp 203–211. Washington, DC, National Academy Press, 1982
28. Luke B: Lactose intolerance during pregnancy: Significance and solutions. MCN 2(2):92–96, March/April 1977
29. Streitfeld PP: Congenital malformation: Teratogenic foods and additives. Birth Fam J 5:1, Spring 1978
30. Green ML, Harry J: Nutrition in Contemporary Nursing Practice, p 228. New York, John Wiley & Sons, 1981
31. Winick M: Nutrition, Pregnancy, and Early Infancy. Baltimore, Williams & Wilkins, 1989
32. Zuckerman B, Walker DK, Frank DA et al: Adolescent pregnancy and parenthood. Advances in Developmental and Behavioral Pediatrics 7:275–311, 1986
33. Ritchey SJ, Taper LJ: Maternal and Child Nutrition. New York, Harper & Row, 1983
34. Williams SR: Nutrition and Diet Therapy, 5th ed, pp 809–813. St Louis, Times Mirror/Mosby, 1985

19

Nursing Care in the Antepartal Period

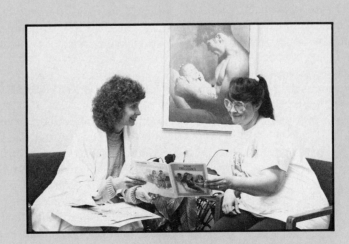

regnancy is a normal physiological process. The vast majority of births do not require active management by health professionals, because the natural reproductive process unfolds according to biological patterns. Normal pregnancy does, however, significantly alter the woman's psychophysiological systems and has the potential to affect the woman's and baby's health status. The most frequent stressors reported by women during pregnancy are related to physical symptoms, body image, welfare of the baby, changes in living patterns, emotional disturbances, and worries about problems in pregnancy, labor, and delivery.[1]

Antepartal care includes both the medical and nursing components of care given to the pregnant woman during the period between conception and the onset of labor. Adequate antepartal care is concerned with the physical, emotional, and social needs of the woman and her unborn baby, her partner, and their other children, if any. The goals are to provide the best of medical and nursing science to protect the life and health of the mother and fetus, and to ensure a satisfying and growth-promoting experience for the woman and family. Prenatal care takes into consideration the sociocultural conditions under which the family lives (i.e., its economic status, educational level, community setting, nutrition, support systems, and cultural perspectives; see Chaps. 5 and 6).

The goals of antepartal care are accomplished through the combined efforts of the expectant parents, the physician, the nurse, and various other members of the health team. Emphasis is on increasing the knowledge and expanding the abilities of the expectant parents and family, so that all members may experience pregnancy in a positive way, the health of mother and infant is promoted, and the family transition to include its new member proceeds smoothly.

Nurses provide essential care to prenatal women and their families. An ongoing relationship can be established, with regular contact and opportunity to assess client and family needs. Nursing responsibilities for prenatal care include physiological and psychosocial assessment, education, and counseling for pregnant women and their families, and identification of needs for other types of services with appropriate community and specialty referrals.

■ INITIAL PRENATAL VISIT

When a woman thinks she may be pregnant, she makes an appointment with the physician or clinic. The visit for confirmation of pregnancy may be combined with the prenatal work-up, or two visits may be required,

depending on office or clinic routines. The prenatal work-up consists of a thorough history, a physical examination, and laboratory tests. Prenatal forms are used by most facilities to summarize data and to serve as a flow sheet for continuing visits throughout pregnancy. Frequently the nurse is responsible for obtaining the history, collecting specimens, participating in or conducting the physical examination, and providing client education and orientation to the services that are offered.

Initial contact is particularly important. By greeting the client in a pleasant and professional manner the nurse can initiate a productive relationship that conveys interest and concern.

Diagnosis of Pregnancy and Estimating Date of Delivery

Early, accurate diagnosis of pregnancy has been aided by development of radioassay and immunological pregnancy tests, which can often confirm pregnancy before or shortly after the first missed menstrual period. Although highly sensitive and specific, these tests occasionally are inaccurate. The absence of menses, and the other signs and symptoms of pregnancy, are used to support the diagnosis of pregnancy (see Chap. 15).

An accurate estimation of the date of delivery (EDD) is important, because this allows the nurse and physician to assess the progress of gestation and evaluate term pregnancy more readily. A correct and definite date for the last menstrual period facilitates estimation of delivery date, but many women do not keep careful menstrual records or may have irregular periods. Various approaches are used to calculate delivery date, such as Nägele's rule based on last menstrual period (LMP), progressive measurements of the height of the funds (McDonald's rule), and ultrasonography to measure various parameters of fetal growth.

Nursing Assessment

Nursing assessment begins with the initial visit to confirm pregnancy and continues throughout the prenatal period at each contact with the pregnant woman and her family. Information about the client and her family, current health status and past medical history, pregnancy and gynecological history, and behavioral habits is gathered. Most health facilities use a prenatal form and flow sheet to organize and focus these data. A thorough physical examination is done to evaluate health condition and status of the pregnancy, and a panel of laboratory tests are obtained. From this information, a plan of continuing care for the woman and her family

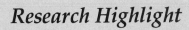

Research Highlight

Use of Immersion for Treating Edema of Pregnancy

Rest and leg elevation are standard treatment of edema during pregnancy. Both bed rest and immersion in warm water lead to mobilization of extravascular fluid and reduce edema. With rest and leg elevation, gravitational force on the long venous blood columns is reduced and capillary pressure is decreased. The shift in Starling forces leads to reabsorption of extravascular fluid into the vascular space, which reduces edema. The excess fluid is then eliminated from the body by the kidneys. During immersion, the hydrostatic force of water actively pushes extravascular fluid into the vascular space. Hydrostatic force, which acts within seconds, is proportional to the depth of the water. Profound diuresis occurs after immersion.

This study compared three treatments for edema in healthy pregnant women in the third trimester. Each subject experienced the three treatments at different sessions, with random assignment to the first treatment. One hour before the treatment, the subjects voided completely and were weighed; pulse and blood pressure were measured; and urine and blood samples were taken. The women spent 50 minutes lying in the lateral supine position in bed, in a standard bathtub with warm water at waist level, or in an immersion tub with warm water at shoulder level. After the treatment, blood was drawn within 10 minutes and the women voided and were reweighed in 1 hour.

All three treatments produced diuresis and reduced edema. The diuresis was more than twice as great after immersion as after bed rest. The bathtub treatment was as effective as bed rest in producing diuresis. The same result found in the immersion tub treatment can be obtained by static immersion in a swimming pool or in water-aerobics programs. There was no drop in plasma volume after immersion despite significant diuresis. Serum and plasma parameters remained stable despite large fluxes in fluid and electrolytes. Serum sodium, potassium, total protein, osmolarity, and serum creatinine concentrations were unchanged. There was a drop in mean arterial pressure during immersion, probably due to the large mobilization of extravascular fluid in pregnant women.

The study results provide evidence for the safety of immersion as a treatment for edema. Nurses can recommend this method to women as an alternative to bed rest and leg elevation. Deeper water, such as in swimming pools and hot tubs (warm water temperature), produces more effective diuresis.

Katz VL, Ryder RM, Cefalo RC et al: A comparison of bed rest and immersion for treating edema of pregnancy. Obstet Gynecol 75(2):147–151, February 1990.

is developed to promote a healthy, satisfying pregnancy and delivery.

The nurse often is responsible for a considerable portion of prenatal assessment. In the initial interview, a relationship of confidence, trust, and respect can be established, which facilitates care throughout pregnancy. The client often is accompanied by her partner or other family members, and the nurse establishes a therapeutic relationship with them as well. When others are included in the prenatal interview, the nurse has opportunity to assess interaction among family members and observe aspects of family coping style and support. Social support has been found exceedingly important in positive experiences and outcomes of pregnancy. Emotional disequilibrium and anxiety during pregnancy decrease with good social support systems, and psychosocial measurements demonstrate increased health among women who receive social support during pregnancy.[2,3]

HISTORY

Inquiries are made into the family history, with special reference to any condition likely to affect childbearing, such as hereditary diseases, tuberculosis, or multiple pregnancy. Then the personal history of the client is reviewed, not only with regard to previous diseases and operations, but particularly in relation to any difficulties experienced in previous pregnancies and labors, such as miscarriages, prolonged labor, death of infant, hemorrhage, and other complications.

Inquiry is made into the history of the present pregnancy, especially in relation to nausea, edema of the feet or the face, headache, visual disturbance, vaginal bleeding, constipation, breathlessness, sleeplessness, cramps, heartburn, lower abdominal pain, vaginal discharge, and varicose veins. A sample prenatal history form is given below.

Estimated Date of Delivery (EDD)

Nägele's Rule

Count back 3 months from the first day of the LMP and add 7 days. Correct for year if necessary.

$$EDD = LMP - (3\ months) + 7\ days$$

Considerations for using Nägele's rule: Assumes a 28-day menstrual cycle with conception occurring on the 14th day. Adjustments must be made for shorter or longer cycles.

McDonald's Rule for Fundal Height

Height of fundus (cm) $\times$ 2/7
= gestation in lunar months
Height of fundus (cm) $\times$ 8/7
= gestation of pregnancy in weeks

Considerations in using fundal height measurements: Such factors as hydramnios, multiple gestation, very large fetus, and obesity affect the accuracy of measurement. For women weighing over 200 lb, subtract 1 cm from the measurement obtained. Technique can vary measurements; providers need to standardize approaches when more than one person takes serial measurements.

Ultrasonography

Four methods for estimating fetal age are the following:
- Determination of gestational sac dimensions (used as early as 6–10 weeks; fetus appears in sac about 7–8 weeks after the LMP, fetal heart activity appears by 9–10 weeks, and fetal movement is seen by 11 weeks)
- Measurement of crown–rump length (between 7 and 14 weeks)
- Measurement of femur length (after 12 weeks)
- Measurement of biparietal diameter (BPD) of fetal head (after 12 weeks. BPD is frequently used for diagnosis of term pregnancy. Fetal weight and BPD are well correlated, and at 36 weeks BPD should be about 8.7 cm. At term, the BPD is usually greater than 9.8 cm.)

As time permits, the nurse can use the initial visit to expand on historical information for assessment purposes, both nursing and medical. The following areas are generally included:

1. Social and personal characteristics of the client: age, marital status, occupation, ethnicity, religion, height, weight, number of children in the home
2. Information summary of spouse (father of baby): name, address, age, height, weight, ethnicity
3. Characteristics influencing the course of pregnancy: EDD, LMP, blood type and Rh, pertinent

medical conditions or hospitalizations, current medications, usual bowel patterns, usual sleep patterns, dietary habits, substance use (tobacco, alcohol, recreational drugs)
4. Attitudes toward the pregnancy:
Was this child planned?
What are the client's goals and values regarding this pregnancy and other relevant areas?
Does she view this pregnancy positively or as an interference in her life?
What is her knowledge about health in general and pregnancy and childbearing in particular?
Does she have any previous experience with pregnancy or childbearing?
What are her expectations and concerns about this pregnancy, birth, and care of the infant?
What is her apparent willingness or disinclination to prepare herself in the areas that need attention?
5. Resources:
What appears to be her general level of intelligence or education?
What is the level of economic stability?
Is the family intact?
Is there extended family available to her?
Does she have sufficient friends from whom she can get tangible help and emotional support if necessary?
6. Antenatal classes and instruction: antenatal classes and films attended, individual and group instruction and counseling

PHYSICAL EXAMINATION

A thorough physical examination is usually performed to establish a baseline for the woman's general state of health and to evaluate the pregnancy. Vital signs including temperature, blood pressure, pulse, respiration, height, and weight are taken. The Components of the Prenatal Physical Examination assessment tool summarizes the techniques for examination and normal and abnormal findings, which are generally included in the prenatal physical examination.

The nurse who is alert to the clues and the events that transpire during the physical examination may use this information to interpret instructions or answer questions that the client may ask afterward. Often a client hesitates to discuss some matter with a physician because she considers it too trivial, but she may feel comfortable talking about it with the nurse. In turn, the nurse may consider this a problem of some importance and on reporting it to the physician may find that it has a bearing on the course of treatment that is prescribed.

Because the initial examination is thorough, the client disrobes completely and wears a gown that opens

(Text continues on page 393)

Prenatal History

Name _____   Date _____
Address _____   Phone number _____
_____   Date of birth _____

Physician _____

I. Health History

Family History

Health status of parents, siblings (if deceased, note cause of death):

_____
_____
_____
_____

Occurrence or history of the following diseases in parents, siblings, and close relatives:

diabetes mellitus _____   hypertension _____   renal disease _____   vascular disease _____
tuberculosis _____   cardiopulmonary _____   neuromuscular disease _____
complications of pregnancy or congenital anomalies (specify) _____
psychiatric disorders (specify) _____
cancer (specify) _____

Personal and Health History

Personal characteristics:

age _____   habits:
racial/ethnic background _____   smoke _____
relationships (husband, partner, children,   alcohol _____   drugs _____
support networks) _____   exercise _____
_____   relaxation _____
_____   misc. _____

Past medical history:
childhood diseases: _____
_____

immunizations (including rubella): _____
_____

hospitalizations (reasons, years): _____
_____

surgery (type, year): _____
_____

blood transfusions: _____
drug sensitivities: _____
allergies (foods, allergens): _____

diseases: vascular disease _____   endocrinopathy _____
diabetes mellitus _____   sexually transmitted disease _____   severe anemia _____
rheumatic fever _____   asthma _____   blood dyscrasias _____
cardiopulmonary _____   psychiatric disorders _____   malnutrition _____
hypertension _____   cancer _____   malignancy _____
tuberculosis _____
renal/urinary tract disease _____
injuries (especially to pelvic organs or structures): _____

(continued)

Menstrual history:
  age at menarche _____
  describe present cycle (interval between menses _____, amount of flow _____, pain _____, clots _____,
    intermenstrual bleeding) _____:
  problems and procedures (e.g., D&C _____, conization, _____, irregular bleeding _____, amenorrhea _____):
Sexual history:
  sexual learning and understanding of sexual functions: _____

_____

  sexual self-concept and identity: _____

_____

  attitudes toward sexuality, particularly as affected by pregnancy: _____

_____

  current sexual practices and satisfaction with these: _____

_____

  contraceptive history and practice: _____
    method _____ effective/satisfied with use _____ problems_____
    method _____ effective/satisfied with use _____ problems_____
    method _____ effective/satisfied with use _____ problems_____
    sexually transmitted diseases and treatment: _____
    type of STD _____ date _____ Rx _____
    type of STD _____ date _____ Rx _____
    type of STD _____ date _____ Rx _____

II. *Pregnancy History*

Past Obstetric History

Year	Length Gest	Probs During Preg	Onset Labor	Length Labor	Complications Labor

Current Pregnancy

Last menstrual period (LMP): _____ Prior menstrual period (PMP): _____
Date fetal movement first felt: _____
Symptoms: nausea _____ urinary frequency _____ headache _____ leukorrhea _____
edema _____ constipation _____ bleeding _____ abdominal pain _____
others _____

Drugs or medications taken since pregnancy began:
_____

_____

Exposure to communicable disease (especially rubella if not immune): _____

_____

Illnesses since beginning of pregnancy (colds, flu, etc): _____

Occupation: _____ Possible workplace exposure to toxins: _____

(continued)

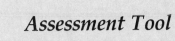

Assessment Tool

Reactions and adaptation to pregnancy (Was pregnancy planned? Is woman pleased or concerned?): _____
_____
_____

Reactions of partner and family: _____
_____

Data about father:
    age _____   height _____   weight _____
    racial/ethnic origins: _____
    health status: _____
    medical history: _____
_____

    response to pregnancy: _____
_____

    relationship with client and family: _____
_____

    occupation: _____   potential health hazards: _____
Interviewed by: _____   Date: _____
Comments:

---

easily. In addition, the expectant mother should be covered with a small sheet to prevent unnecessary exposure and chilling. The nurse instructs the woman to empty her bladder, because a full bladder is uncomfortable and may interfere with the examination. A good footstool is necessary for the woman to mount the table in safety and comfort.

During the physical examination, particular attention is paid to the teeth and throat, thyroid gland and lymph nodes, lungs, heart, breasts, skin, extremities, and abdomen (Fig. 19-1). Characteristic changes of pregnancy are noted (see Chap. 15), and signs of infection or systemic disease are identified if present.

Physical indicators of high-risk pregnancy can often be determined in initial examination, such as obesity, hypertension, severe varicosities, preeclampsia, or inappropriate uterine size for dates.

Pelvic Examination. Pelvic examination provides data relevant to confirming the pregnancy and determining the length of gestation, pelvic characteristics, and any abnormalities that might produce complications of pregnancy. At the same time, specimens are obtained to screen for potential problems. The pelvic examination includes both speculum and bimanual examinations. On speculum examination, the characteristics of the vaginal and the cervical mucosa are examined, and vaginal discharge is evaluated. Unusual lesions are identified and biopsies are taken, as well as smears for vaginitis and cultures for gonorrhea. Pap smears to screen for cervical cancer are done routinely.

The bimanual examination provides information about the consistency of the cervix; the size, shape, and consistency of the uterus; the condition of the fallopian tubes and ovaries; and the configuration of the bony pelvis. Uterine size is useful in determining length of gestation, and pelvic measurements enable a clinical appraisal of potential pelvic contractions that might lead to cephalopelvic disproportion in labor. Other abnormalities of the birth canal, such as soft-tissue masses, can also be identified.

The vaginal or pelvic examination deserves special consideration because often it is the most stressful part of the experience for the client. This examination is carried out with the woman in the dorsal recumbent position. In this position, she lies on her back with the lower extremities flexed and rotated outward. Her heels are supported in stirrups, which are level with the table,

Assessment Tool

Components of Prenatal Physical Examination

Part Examined, Examination Technique	Normal Findings	Abnormal Findings
Head and Neck		
Palpation, inspection with otoophthalmoscope, and visual inspection of mouth	Hyperemia of nasal and buccal mucous membranes, slight diffuse enlargement of thyroid	Enlarged lymph nodes, thyroid nodules or irregular enlargement, lesions of eyes or mouth, caries and abscesses of teeth, ear infections
Chest and Heart		
Auscultation with stethoscope, percussion and visual inspection	Lungs clear, heart in regular rhythm (occasionally a soft, short functional murmur due to hemodynamic changes of pregnancy)	Adventitious lung sounds (rales, wheezes, rhonchi), irregular cardiac rhythm, nonphysiological murmurs
Breasts		
Palpatation and visual inspection	Enlargement of breasts with increased vascular patterns, darkened areola with prominent tubercles, clear fluid from nipples in later pregnancy	Masses or nodules, bloody or serosanguineous nipple discharge, nipple lesions, erythema
Skin		
Visual inspection	Pigmentation changes (linea nigra, mask of pregnancy), enlargement of nevi, appearance of spider angiomas, mottled erythema of hands	Pallor, jaundice, rash, skin lesions
Extremities		
Visual inspection and palpation, percussion with reflux hammer	Mild pretibial and ankle edema in third trimester, slight edema of hands in hot weather	Limitations of motion, varicosities, more than slight pretibial, hand, or ankle edema, edema of face or sacrum, hyperreflexia and clonus

(continued)

perhaps a foot in front of her buttocks. In this position, the anxious woman, already under stress during the physical examination, is likely to tense her abdominal, pelvic, and thigh muscles, attempting to adduct her thighs. If she arches her back as her tension increases, her pelvis is tilted downward, a position that makes the pelvic examination almost impossible to achieve.

The nurse can be effective in assisting the client to relax if she encourages her to keep breathing naturally, reminds her to breathe if she holds her breath, and reminds her to press the small of her back down on the table. The nurse needs to give the client direct guidance to relax, often step by step. For example, if the client is clenching her fists, the nurse may say, "See, your wrists and hands are tense. Try to let them go limp—very limp—like a rag doll's. That's it—very limp." And a moment later, "Keep breathing naturally." Such short, explicit requests and instruction give the mother a simple

Assessment Tool (continued)

Part Examined, Examination Technique	Normal Findings	Abnormal Findings
Abdomen		
Palpation, visual inspection, auscultation, percussion	Enlarged uterus, palpation of fetal outline in later pregnancy, fetal heart sounds, contractions in last trimester	Uterus too large or too small for dates, absence of fetal heart sounds beyond 10 weeks (using Doppler), transverse lie of fetus, fetal head in fundus, tonic uterine contractions, enlarged liver or spleen
Pelvis		
Speculum exam, bimanual exam with inspection and palpation, collection of specimens	Speculum exam: Bluish discoloration of mucosa of vagina and cervix, congested cervix, ectropion in multigravidas, increased leukorrhea	Speculum exam: Yellow, purulent, frothy, cheesy white or homogeneous gray, foul-smelling discharge, friable, bleeding lesions of cervix; vaginal lesions; bleeding from cervical os, amniotic fluid
	Bimanual exam: Cervix soft, admits a finger or two (depending on gravida and length of pregnancy), uterus soft and enlarged, fetal head or parts may be felt in lower uterine segment, gynecoid pelvic configuration	Bimanual exam: Cervix dilated and effaced (unless labor has begun); cervical or vaginal masses; excessive amniotic fluid (uterus unusually enlarged); adnexal masses or fullness; rectal masses; hemorrhoids; contractions of the pelvic inlet, midpelvis, or outlet
	Pap smear: Squamous metaplasia, negative or normal, adequate or increased estrogen, endocervical cells present, hyperplasia is considered borderline	Pap smear: Inflammation, presence of *Trichomonas* or fungi, diminished or absent estrogen, atypical or suspicious cells, atypical hyperplasia, dysplasia, neoplasia, or carcinoma

task that she can do with guidance. This diverts her attention from the anticipated discomfort and promotes relaxation.

Steps in the Pelvic Examination. To see the cervix clearly, the examiner sits on a stool and focuses a good light into the vagina. Any equipment that is needed, such as vaginal speculum, swabs, cotton balls, slides, and lubricating jelly, should be within reach.

The pelvic examination begins with an examination of the external genitalia, including the urethra and Skene's and Bartholin's glands. If any unusual discharge is present, a specimen may be obtained for culture or microscopic examination.

Usually, the next step is to insert a speculum into the vagina to distend the folds to provide a clearer view of the cervix (Fig. 19-2). If a Pap smear is to be taken, no lubricating jelly is used; instead, the speculum may be rinsed under *tepid* running water to facilitate insertion. Occasionally, the dilation of the vagina by the speculum may cause an unpleasant sensation of stretching (Fig. 19-3).

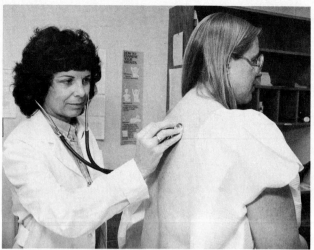

■ *Figure 19–1*
A thorough physical examination is done early in pregnancy to assess the mother's health and the status of the pregnancy. (Courtesy of Media Services, Sonoma State University, Rohnert Park, CA.)

As the examination proceeds, the cervix is visualized, and the examiner notes its color and character. Normally, the cervix of the primigravida is pink or bluish and smooth, with a dimple for the os. The cervix of a multigravida may have an irregular os owing to lacerations from previous deliveries (Fig. 19-4). Ectropion is often present around the os in multigravidas; this is a darker pinkish-red, bumpy tissue composed of columnar epithelium, which lines the endocervical canal. Unless infection is present, this tissue is considered a normal variant during the years of active estrogen secretion. Any discharge that is purulent, greenish, or frothy is considered to be abnormal, and a specimen may be secured for microscopic examination or culture.

After the cervix has been examined, the examiner withdraws the speculum and proceeds with the biman-

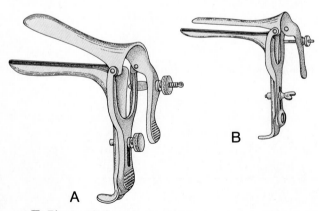

■ *Figure 19–2*
Instruments of the gynecologic examination. (A) Graves speculum. (B) Pederson speculum.

ual examination to evaluate the uterus and the adnexa (Fig. 19-5). The size, consistency, and contour of these organs, as well as the relationship of the uterus to the pelvis, are determined. Pelvic measurements are taken at the same time. The examination is usually completed with an examination of the rectum to ascertain the presence of hemorrhoids, polyps, or other abnormalities. When the examination is completed, disposable tissues should be offered the client to wipe the perineum adequately.

Pap Smear. The Pap smear is obtained during speculum examination. The cervix is cleansed with a dry cotton ball to remove excess mucus, and a cotton-tipped applicator or cytobrush is introduced into the endocervical canal. It is rotated several times, withdrawn, and rolled on a glass slide. The smear is fixed immediately with commercial fixatives or immersed in 95% ethyl alcohol to prevent the specimen from drying, which distorts the cells. Next, a wooden or plastic spatula is used to obtain the ectocervical sample. The shaped end is introduced slightly into the cervical os and turned firmly several times to scrape the tissue of the squamocolumnar junction (where the endocervical epithelium meets that of the ectocervix; Fig. 19-6.) This is the area where most malignancies arise and can be seen as a color change of cervical epithelium. This specimen is smeared on a glass slide and fixed as above. Some providers place both endocervical and ectocervical specimens on one slide. A vaginal pool sample may also be taken by introducing the rounded end of the spatula into the posterior vaginal fornix or by aspirating fluid with a vaginal pipette. The smears should be accompanied by data about the woman's age, LMP, pregnancy or postpartum status, gynecological surgery, and use of hormones.

LABORATORY TESTS

Laboratory tests are initiated early in pregnancy to provide additional data about the physiological changes in pregnancy and to identify risks or problems (Table 19-1). Urinalysis and urine culture are done, and smears or cultures are taken of cervical and vaginal secretions. Blood samples are drawn for a complete blood count, blood type, Rh factor and titer if indicated, syphilis, and rubella titer. Screening for gestational diabetes is recommended between the 24th and 28th weeks of pregnancy, with blood sugar drawn after 50 mg of oral glucose are administered. Elevated blood sugar levels indicate the need for a subsequent 3-hour glucose tolerance test (GTT). Other blood tests that might be ordered include hemoglobin electrophoresis for sickle cell anemia and thalassemias, hepatitis B antigen, and HIV (human immunodeficiency virus) antibody assay as indicated by risk characteristics (see Chap. 35).

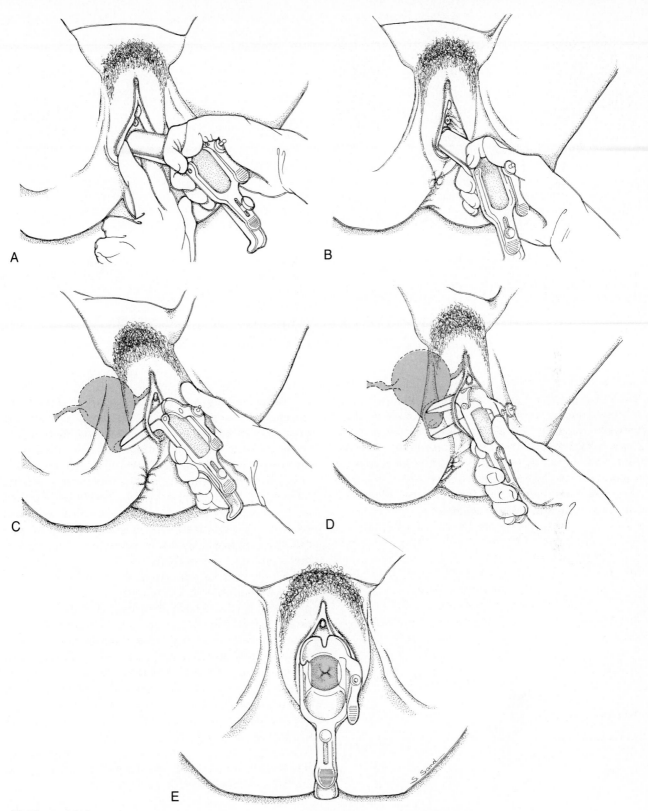

■ *Figure 19–3*
Insertion of the speculum. (A) Opening the introitus. (B) Oblique insertion of the speculum. (C) Final insertion of the speculum. (D) Opening the blades of the speculum. (E) View of the cervix through the speculum.

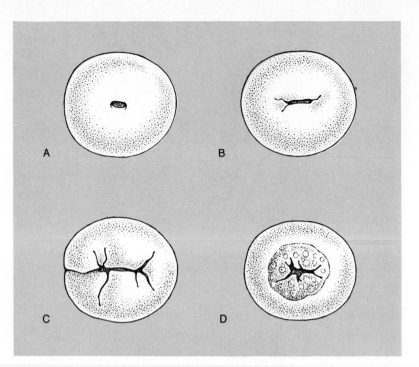

■ *Figure 19–4*
Common appearance of the cervix. (A) The nulliparous cervical os is small and either round or oval. (B) After childbirth the os presents a slitlike appearance. (C) Difficult deliveries may tear the cervix, producing permanent lacerations. (D) Ectopion, often present in multigravidas, is a pinkish-red, bumpy tissue composed of columnar epithelium. (Redrawn from Bates B: A Guide to Physical Examination, 2nd ed. Philadelphia, JB Lippincott, 1979)

Blood may be drawn for α-fetoprotein (AFP) to screen for neural tube defects. The test must be done between the 15th and 20th weeks of pregnancy. Increased levels of AFP indicate possible neural tube defects and should be followed by ultrasonography or amniocentesis. Other laboratory tests, such as electrocardiogram and kidney function tests, are ordered depending on maternal health conditions.

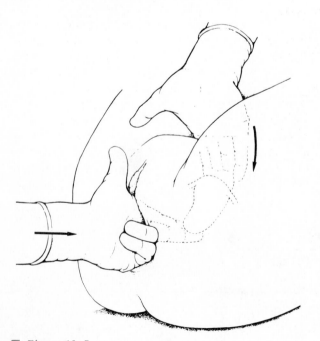

■ *Figure 19–5*
Bimanual palpation of the uterus.

Ultrasonography is used frequently to provide information about gestational age, fetal position, multiple pregnancy, placental location, growth retardation, and to detect several fetal abnormalities. Ultrasound may also identify the sex of the fetus; parents are usually asked if they wish to know this information. Studies have not found demonstrable adverse effects of pulsed or continuous ultrasound waves.[4] Amniocentesis with fetal cell culture is used when indicated to detect chromosomal disorders, neural tube defects, and certain metabolic disorders of the fetus.

Women who are over age 35 are at increased risk for fetal abnormalities. Diagnostic procedures in early pregnancy to detect such abnormalities as Down's syndrome, neural tube defect, and other chromosomal disorders are recommended. Procedures commonly done include chorionic villi sampling, which can be scheduled between 7 and 9 weeks and involves transcervical aspiration of placental samples; and amniocentesis, which is scheduled at 12 to 14 weeks and involves intraabdominal aspiration of amniotic fluid samples (see Chap. 42).

IDENTIFICATION OF INCREASED RISK DURING PREGNANCY

Prenatal nursing assessment identifies clients who are at increased risk for complications during pregnancy and who are at risk for parenting difficulties. Any condition that might adversely affect the health of the mother or fetus during pregnancy, labor, and delivery places the pregnancy in a high-risk category (see Chaps.

Indicators of High-Risk Pregnancy

Social-Behavioral Factors

Age (less than 16 or greater than 35)

Poverty, low income

Nutritional (underweight, overweight, poor diet)

Substance use (tobacco, alcohol, drugs)

High-risk sexual behavior

High risk for family or environmental violence

Work exposure to toxins

Health Conditions—Deviations in Health

Chronic illness (diabetes, cardiovascular disease, renal disease, respiratory disorders, blood dyscrasias, others)

Sexually transmitted disease (current, past history of)

Other infectious diseases (urinary tract, communicable diseases)

Pregnancy-Related Conditions

Previous pregnancy complications (preterm birth, recurrent abortions, ectopic pregnancy, operative delivery, breech delivery, prolonged labor, infection, hemorrhage, still-birth, gestational diabetes, hydatidiform mole)

Previous infants with birth defects

Previous low-birth-weight infants, macrosomia

Multiple pregnancy

Gestational diabetes

Rh or ABO sensitization

Recent previous delivery (less than 1 year)

Uterine or ovarian tumors

Bleeding problems

Reproductive tract abnormalities (contracted pelvis, vaginal septum, septate uterus)

Indicators of High-Risk Parenting

Unplanned pregnancy

Single parent, limited support systems

Adolescent pregnancy

Substance abuse by parents (alcohol, drugs)

Psychiatric history or mental retardation in parents

Ambivalence or negativity about pregnancy or parenthood

History of abuse as a child

Previous stillbirth, neonatal death

Extreme desire for child of particular sex

Severe marital discord, spousal abuse

Previous child relinquished for adoption

Previous child with anomalies, chronic illness

History of abusing and neglecting previous child

Multiple recent moves, no permanent living plan, homeless

Several small children close together in age

---

33 through 38). Various psychosocial and developmental factors can place the mother and father at high risk for parenting difficulties. The nurse needs to assess the family structure, communication, supports, and coping behaviors to identify strengths and stressors (see Chaps. 4 through 6).

Nursing Diagnosis

Data from the health and pregnancy history and the physical examination are used to formulate nursing diagnoses. Each pregnant woman and her family respond to pregnancy in a different way; these responses along with the woman's health status and physiological response to pregnancy largely determine nursing diagnoses and interventions. Probably the most common nursing diagnosis is knowledge deficit, which may be related to emotional and physiological changes of pregnancy, what to expect during the course of prenatal care, self-care during pregnancy, and family adjustments. Health-seeking behaviors is an appropriate diagnosis for most pregnant women who seek prenatal care to help achieve a successful pregnancy outcome, and desire to learn and follow practices to promote the growth, development, and delivery of a healthy baby.

During early pregnancy, the woman may experience altered nutrition: less than body requirements related to nausea and vomiting during the first trimester. Anxiety related to physical changes of pregnancy, fear of pregnancy loss, emotional reactions to being pregnant, and concerns for safety may be diagnosed. Alterations in comfort often occur related to breast tenderness, lower abdominal achiness, and the need for frequent urination in early pregnancy. Sexuality patterns may be altered related to early pregnancy discomforts, nausea and vomiting, or emotional reactions.

Altered family processes may be diagnosed, related to the family's response to the pregnancy. Pregnancy often acts as a stressor that alters the family's function, and calls for different coping strategies and role adjustments. Potential for growth in family coping may be diagnosed, as the family responds creatively through

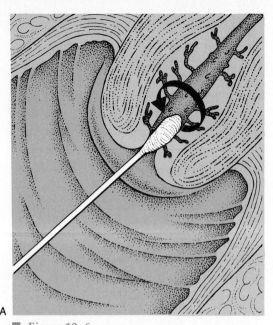
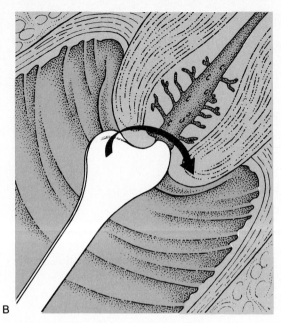

■ *Figure 19–6*
The Pap smear. (A) Obtaining the endocervical sample. (B) Obtaining the ectocervical sample.

planning and preparing for changes necessary for birth and care of the infant. When families have destructive behavior patterns, or respond ineffectively to stressors, the nursing diagnosis is ineffective family coping. Ineffective coping may be related to many factors, such as addictions, emotional disturbances, adolescent parents, physical illness, inadequate financial resources, and abusive family patterns.

Nursing Planning and Intervention

At the initial visit, counseling and education in response to knowledge deficits should be brief and focused on immediate and short-term needs. The mother's initial questions should be answered, and an overview should be given of the process of prenatal care. Explanations are given about testing and diagnostic procedures, when these are to be done, why, and what to expect. Current problems, such as alterations in comfort (nausea and vomiting, frequent urination, breast and abdominal pain) are discussed. The nurse interprets any treatments ordered by the physician and ascertains the client's understanding and ability to follow the prescribed regimen.

Problems identified by nursing assessment that exert immediate effects on maternal or fetal well-being are addressed during the first visit. If the pregnant woman is currently smoking (altered health maintenance related to tobacco use), nursing intervention focuses on encouraging and supporting her to stop smoking or reduce cigarette consumption as much as possible. Adverse effects of smoking are directly related to daily cigarette consumption, so even some decrease is beneficial. The

TABLE 19–1. LABORATORY TESTS DURING PREGNANCY

Test	Source of Specimen	Purpose
Urine		
Urinalysis Sugar Albumin Microscopic	Clean voided urine	Sugar (glycosuria)—screen for diabetes Albumin (proteinuria)—screen for preeclampsia, kidney stress, or renal problems RBCs, WBCs, epithelial cells, casts, microorganisms—screen for renal disease, urinary tract infection

(continued)

TABLE 19-1. LABORATORY TESTS DURING PREGNANCY *(continued)*

Test	Source of Specimen	Purpose
Urine culture	Clean voided urine	Diagnose urinary tract infections; often done routinely on all pregnant women; done when urinary symptoms are present to identify organism
Blood		
CBC	Venous blood	
Hematocrit and hemoglobin		Hematocrit and hemoglobin—screen for anemia
White blood cell count and differential		White blood cell count and differential—identify infectious processes; screen for blood dyscrasias, folic acid deficiency
Platelets		Platelets—assess blood-clotting mechanisms
Serologic test for syphilis	Serum	Screen for syphilis (if positive must confirm with FTA-ABS)
Rh factor and blood type	Venous blood	Determine the blood type and Rh factor (positive or negative): blood type is important in case of hemorrhage; Rh factor alerts providers to possible incompatibility disease in fetus
Rh titers	Venous blood	Done when mother is Rh negative and father is Rh positive to assay danger to fetus (signified by rising titer)
Rubella antibodies	Venous blood	Determine if mother has been exposed previously to rubella and has built up antibodies (i.e., is immune or not)
α-fetoprotein	Serum	Screen for neural tube defects between 15th and 20th weeks of gestation
Glucose (blood sugar)	Venous blood	Screen for gestational diabetes (if elevated, 3-hour glucose tolerance test is done)
Hemoglobin electrophoresis	Blood	Diagnose hemoglobinopathies (e.g., sickle cell anemia, thalassemias)
BUN, creatinine, total protein, electrolytes	Serum	Evaluate renal function and diagnose renal disease
Hepatitis B antigen	Serum	Infection by hepatitis B virus
HIV antibody assay (ELISA—enzyme-linked immunosorbent assay)	Serum	Infection by human immunodeficiency virus
Cervical/Vaginal		
Gonorrhea culture	Cervical discharge	Diagnose gonorrhea; often done routinely because gonorrhea is frequently asymptomatic in women
Pap smear	Cervix, vagina	Screen for cervical intraepithelial neoplasia; herpes simplex type 2
Chlamydia culture	Cervical discharge	Diagnose *Chlamydia* trachomatis, often done routinely because infections may be symptomatic and often co-occur with gonorrhea infections
Other		
Tuberculin skin test	Applied to skin	Screen high-risk women for tuberculosis
ECG, chest x-ray	Heart, lungs	Evaluate cardiac and pulmonary function
Ultrasonography	Uterine contents	Evaluate gestational age, fetal position, multiple pregnancy, placental location, growth retardation, fetal abnormalities
Chorionic villi sampling	Placental villi	Detect fetal chromosomal disorders, some metabolic disorders
Amniocentesis	Amniotic fluid	Detect fetal chromosomal disorders, some metabolic disorders

---

*Nursing Diagnoses Applicable
to Early Pregnancy*

Knowledge deficit related to:
 Emotional and physiological changes of pregnancy
 Course of prenatal care
 Self-care during pregnancy
 Family adjustments to pregnancy
 Tests and procedures

Health-seeking behaviors to:
 Achieve a successful pregnancy outcome
 Learn practices to promote growth, development, and delivery of a healthy baby
 Prevent complications

Altered nutrition: less than body requirements related to:
 Nausea and vomiting during first trimester

Anxiety related to:
 Physical changes of pregnancy
 Fear of pregnancy loss
 Emotional reactions to being pregnant
 Concerns for safety

Alterations in comfort related to:
 Breast tenderness
 Abdominal cramping, discomfort
 Frequent urination

Altered sexuality patterns related to:
 Early pregnancy discomforts
 Emotional reactions to pregnancy
 Fears of harming the baby

Altered family processes related to:
 Family's response to pregnancy
 Need for different coping strategies
 Need for role readjustments
 Potential for growth in family coping

Ineffective family coping related to:
 Addictive or abusive processes
 Emotional disturbances
 Adolescent parents
 Physical illness
 Inadequate financial resources

---

nurse educates the patient about health risks of tobacco use to the fetus, other children at home, herself, and others. Benefits of quitting are clearly described, and strategies to stop smoking are discussed (see Chap. 36). Many approaches are available, ranging from stopping "cold turkey" to ongoing smoking cessation groups and residential programs. Some degrees of success have been reported by various self-help smoking cessation approaches with pregnant women in health maintenance organizations and health departments,[5,6] and in WIC clinics (Special Supplemental Food Program for Women, Infants and Children).[7]

Alcohol use during pregnancy presents significant risk to the fetus of fetal alcohol syndrome and other more subtle developmental disorders. Evidence of maternal alcohol use (altered health maintenance related to alcohol use, ineffective denial related to acknowledgement of substance abuse) during the initial assessment leads to immediate nursing interventions. The objective is to assist the pregnant women to stop drinking, because no safe level of alcohol use during pregnancy has been established.[8] The use of street drugs and abuse of over-the-counter and prescription medications also call for early nursing intervention to stop or control use during pregnancy. Interventions for alcohol and drug use during pregnancy are presented in Chapter 36.

Depending on the duration of pregnancy, the nurse reviews important danger signs with the patient and when to contact the health provider. In early pregnancy, indicators of complications include vaginal bleeding, abdominal cramping, persistent and frequent nausea and vomiting, and elevated temperature.

---

*Nursing Diagnoses Applicable to
Mid-Late Pregnancy*

Knowledge deficit related to:
 Self-care to reduce minor discomforts
 Preparation for labor, delivery, and parenthood
 Signs of complications
 Safety measures

Anxiety related to:
 Increasing discomforts of late pregnancy
 Approaching labor and delivery

Alterations in comfort related to:
 Increased abdominal size
 Increased pelvic pressure
 Digestion and elimination disturbances
 Changes in body alignment (backache)

Altered sexuality patterns related to:
 Later pregnancy discomforts
 Fear of harming fetus
 Changes in body image

Potential for injury related to:
 Lack of safety measures (e.g., seatbelts)
 Mother's altered balance
 Risks of labor and delivery

Sleep pattern disturbance related to:
 Physiological changes (respiratory, urinary)
 Physical discomforts

Activity intolerance related to:
 Changes in center of gravity
 Increased weight

It is better to postpone further routine health teaching and counseling about weight gain, diet, exercise, sexuality, and other areas until a subsequent visit, when the mother is not so overloaded with new stimuli.

Evaluation

Nursing interventions are effective when the patient expresses increased understanding of areas identified as knowledge deficits, states that her questions have been adequately answered, and indicates concurrence with plans for prenatal care such as diagnostic tests and return visits. The patient is able to repeat symptoms of pregnancy complications and what to do if these occur. When alterations in health maintenance are diagnosed (smoking, alcohol or drug use), nursing intervention is effective when the patient acknowledges the risks to herself and the baby and agrees to a plan for stopping the substance use. Subsequent evaluation of the level of substance use is necessary.

■ RETURN VISITS

Regular return visits are scheduled throughout pregnancy to provide continuous monitoring of maternal and fetal status, to institute treatment and further diagnostic tests as necessary, and to offer ongoing opportunity for support and education. The usual schedule of visits is once a month until the seventh month, every 2 weeks during the seventh and eighth months, and weekly during the ninth month until delivery. Visits are scheduled more frequently if problems arise. Routine return visits consist of follow-up history, physical examination, and client education.

Assessment

Nursing assessment includes physiological data on maternal adaptations to changes of pregnancy, measures of fetal well-being, identification of signs or symptoms of complications, maternal and family psychological adaptation to pregnancy, compliance with medical regimens, and preparations for parenthood. There is also great opportunity to identify other health problems within the pregnant family, but not directly related to pregnancy. Such problems may need immediate attention or may be appropriately dealt with in the future.

Inquiry is made each visit about how the client and family are feeling and the presence of any concerns or symptoms. New signs or physical findings, such as excessive weight gain or glycosuria, are explored through

---

Schedule of Return Prenatal Visits

First through sixth month—visits once per month
Seventh and eighth months—visits every 2 weeks
Ninth month until delivery—visits once per week

Included in Visit	When Done
Weight	Each visit
Blood pressure	Each visit
Fundal height (McDonald's)	Each visit
Fetal heart rate	Each visit
Check for edema	Each visit
Pelvic examination	Middle of ninth month, then weekly as indicated
Other examination	As indicated by symptoms
Inquiry about symptoms, signs, or problems	Each visit
Prenatal education*	Each visit
Nutrition and appetite	Each visit
Family and personal adjustment	Each visit
Urinalysis for glucose and albumin	Each visit
Hematocrit and hemoglobin	At 32 to 34 weeks (more often if anemic)
Urine culture	As indicated by symptoms or signs
Rh titers	If initially negative, twice more during pregnancy; if positive, more often as indicated by titer levels
α-Fetoprotein	At 15 to 20 weeks
Glucose (blood sugar)	At 24 to 28 weeks
Ultrasonography	For fetal age, best between 8 and 16 weeks
Other tests	As indicated by symptoms or signs

* See Prenatal Teaching Checklist later in this chapter.

---

a series of questions. The woman is asked about other signs and symptoms, including edema of the fingers or face, bleeding, constipation, and headaches. During these visits, the woman is encouraged and given ample opportunity to ask any questions of concern to her.

Weight, blood pressure, fundal height, and fetal heart rate are taken during each return visit (Fig. 19-7).

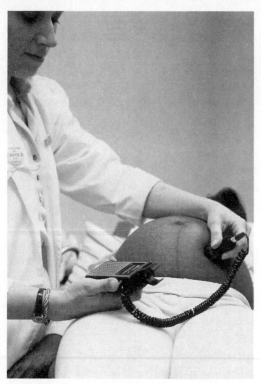

■ *Figure 19–7*
Assessment of FHR using doppler.

Weight is plotted on a graph or flow sheet, and deviations from expected progression are noted and explored.

Legs and feet are examined for edema and development of varicosities. Other aspects of the physical examination are performed if indicated by signs or symptoms.

Vaginal examinations are usually not done on return visits until the client nears term. Vaginal examinations begin about 2 or 3 weeks from EDD to assess the status of the cervix, fetal presentation, and the degree of engagement.

Abdominal Examination

Abdominal examination is useful in providing information about the position of the fetus after the 13th week of gestation (Fig. 19-8). Leopold's maneuvers help determine position and presentation of the fetus, and auscultation of the fetal heart tones can provide an indication of fetal conditions. (Leopold's maneuvers are discussed in Chap. 20. Monitoring of fetal heart tones is discussed in Chap. 42.)

Fetal activity can be assessed by asking the mother about the frequency of fetal movements. The height of the fundus can be used to approximate the length of gestation by McDonald's technique. A flexible tape measure is used to measure the distance from the upper border of the symphysis pubis to the top of the uterine fundus. Frequently the tape measure is curved over the mother's abdomen, although some providers hold it straight between the fingers with the hand at a right angle to the top of the fundus (Fig. 19-9). The distance measured in centimeters, multiplied by two and divided by seven gives the duration of pregnancy in lunar months. During the first 24 to 26 weeks, the fundal height in centimeters is roughly equal to the weeks of gestation (e.g., 20 cm fundal height equals 20 weeks' gestation). Using *McDonald's rule* increases accuracy during the second and third trimesters (see rule given earlier in this chapter).

Diagnostic Tests

Urine is tested on each return visit for glucose and protein (albumin). Multi-chemistry urine strips are frequently used, which also report leukocytes, nitrites, pH, blood, and ketones. Any abnormalities on these screening urine tests are followed with further diagnostic testing, such as urine cultures, microscopic examination of urinary sediment, or glucose challenge tests. Many offices perform routine urine screening cultures because of the prevalence of asymptomatic bacteriuria during pregnancy.

Hematocrit (and sometimes hemoglobin) is repeated at 32 to 34 weeks to detect anemia. Further serum iron studies are indicated when these levels are significantly low. α-Fetoprotein testing is frequently done between 15 and 20 weeks. Routine 50-mg glucose challenge testing is recommended at 24 to 28 weeks, followed by a 3-hour GTT if values are elevated. Ultrasonography is becoming more common as a routine screening test, used primarily for determination of fetal age; the greatest accuracy for this purpose is obtained between 8 and 16 weeks.[4,8]

Additional diagnostic tests are done as indicated during pregnancy. Tuberculin skin testing is advisable in high-risk and symptomatic clients. Renal function tests, such as blood urea nitrogen (BUN), creatinine, electrolytes, and total protein excretion, are obtained when renal complications or conditions are suspected. Problems such as cardiac disease are evaluated with electrocardiogram (ECG) and echocardiogram, pulmonary problems are evaluated with chest x-ray and pulmonary function studies, and hemoglobinopathies are evaluated with hemoglobin or protein electrophoresis (see Table 19-1).

Nursing Diagnosis

A variety of nursing diagnoses may be made during the antepartal period because pregnancy causes numerous

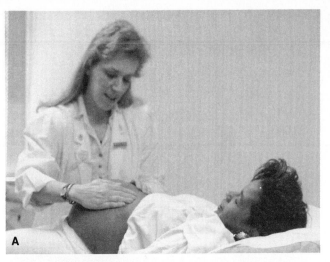

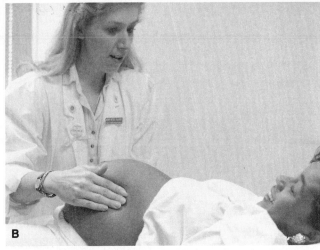

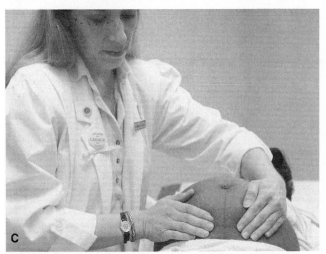

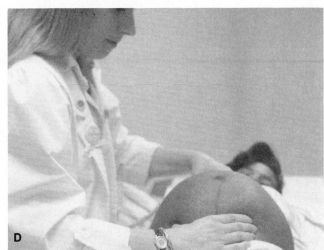

■ *Figure 19–8*
Lespold's maneuvers to assess fetal position and presentation.

physiological and psychosocial changes to which the woman and her family must adapt (see Chaps. 15 and 16). In addition to most of the nursing diagnoses discussed for early pregnancy, there may be knowledge deficits related to self-care to reduce common discomforts, and preparation for labor, delivery, and parenthood. Potential for injury related to lack of safety measures, such as proper use of seatbelts, is a common nursing diagnosis. Anxiety related to the increasing discomforts of later pregnancy and approaching labor may be present. Toward the end of pregnancy, many women experience sleep pattern disturbance related to physiological changes and physical discomforts; or may have activity intolerance related to changes in center of gravity and increased weight. Sleep pattern disturbance related to physiological and physical changes of pregnancy is common in the later third trimester. There is potential for injury or trauma to mother and fetus related to the mother's altered balance, and to the risks of labor and delivery (infection, hemorrhage, hypoxia, tissue damage).

Planning and Intervention

Nursing intervention uses techniques of teaching, support, advice, self-care preparation, direct physical care,

---

Danger Signals to Be Reported Immediately

Vaginal bleeding, no matter how slight

Swelling of the face or the fingers

Severe continuous headache

Dimness or blurring of vision

Flashes of light or dots before the eyes

Pain in the abdomen

Persistent vomiting

Chills and fever

Sudden escape of fluid from the vagina

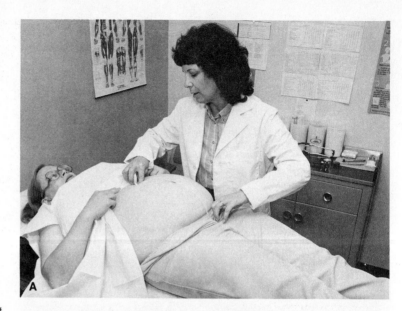

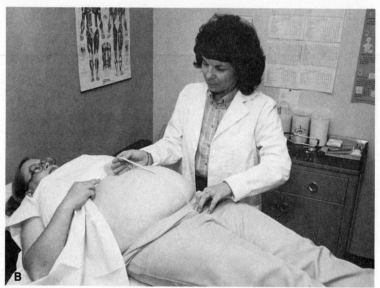

■ *Figure 19–9*
Measurement of fundal height: McDonald's technique. (A) The tape measure is curved over the mother's abdomen. (B) The tape measure is held straight between the fingers with the hand at a right angle to the top of the fundus. (Courtesy of Media Services, Sonoma State University, Rohnert Park, CA.)

and referral or coordination of services. The scope of nursing care includes helping client and family understand and adapt to physiological and emotional changes of pregnancy, deal with minor discomforts effectively, recognize and, if possible, avoid potentially serious complications, plan for parenthood and integrating the new baby into the family, understand and comply with the medical regimen, and attain optimal health status.

WEIGHT GAIN

The pregnant woman's weight is measured at each prenatal visit. During early pregnancy, the average gain in weight of the fetus is 1 g daily; nine tenths of the fetus' weight is gained after the fifth month, and one half of this weight is acquired during the last 8 weeks. Explain-

ing to the woman how pregnancy weight is distributed and the patterns in which it is gained helps her understand why increased weight is necessary for normal fetal development (see Chap. 18).

A total weight gain during pregnancy of 10 to 12 kg (22–26 lb) has been described as generally acceptable by the American College of Obstetricians and Gynecologists (ACOG).[9] Maternal weight gain is positively and significantly associated with birth weight and exerts a direct influence on pregnancy outcome. Optimal weight gain guidelines depend on maternal prepregnancy body mass and must be individualized for each client, especially those under and over average prepregnant weights. Underweight mothers have significantly lower birth weight infants, whereas for the obese mother, the impact of pregnancy weight gain on infant birth weight is diminished. The influence of maternal weight gain on birth weight occurs at all different levels of prepregnancy body mass, age, parity, and education.[10]

Weight gain in the range of 20 to 40 lb has been associated with good pregnancy outcome (full term, appropriate for gestational age infant) in women with underweight, normal, and overweight prepregnant body mass. Fewer women with pregnancy weight gain at the lower end (20–22 lb) had good pregnancy outcomes, however. The majority of women tend to gain more than the recommended upper limits, with weight gain closer to 30 lb.[11] Good outcomes have been found even at 40 to 45 lb maternal weight gain. Whereas the lower end of the ACOG range is important, a higher weight gain does appear consistent with good pregnancy outcome.[12]

INSTRUCTIONS AND ANTICIPATORY GUIDANCE

During prenatal visits, the client may be instructed regarding diet, rest and sleep, elimination, proper exercise, fresh air and sunshine, bathing, clothing, recreation, and dental care. Therefore, it is necessary for the nurse to have broad knowledge and understanding about the physiology of pregnancy and childbearing; general hygiene; nutrition; the emotional, psychological, and socioeconomic aspects of family living; and the part played by a family in the larger community.

Explanation of the changes that are taking place within her body is provided by the nurse. Exploration with the client regarding her concerns about these changes and appropriate instruction give her greater reassurance and self-confidence. An understanding and empathic attitude does much to buoy the client's morale and to diminish unnecessary anxiety.

As the client approaches full term, she can also be instructed about the signs and symptoms of oncoming labor, so that she may know when the process is beginning and when to notify the physician. At this time, she needs to report the frequency of contractions and any other pertinent symptoms. See the accompanying Prenatal Teaching Checklist for items to be discussed.

Teaching sessions are individualized for each client and should include instruction in maintaining good health habits in daily living, interpretation of the reasons these practices are important, and suggestions of ways undesirable habits may be changed or modified.

The first step toward this goal is to identify the level of knowledge and understanding of the client about the topic in question. Second, any misinformation or misconceptions must be clarified. The final step is to add to the base of knowledge and understanding through reinterpretation, clarification, reemphasis, and reinforcement.

VISUAL AIDS AND TEACHING GROUPS

In hospitals and offices where the appointment system is used, the waiting time for the client is minimized. In others, the client may have to wait longer periods. Waiting time in any setting may be used advantageously by providing reading material that contributes to the client's knowledge of her condition. Visual aids such as posters and charts may be both instructive and diverting. Some simple computerized programmed instruction or interactive computer educational programs are being used more frequently.

Offices and, increasingly, clinics are using a group approach for discussion, teaching, and guidance. These groups are usually under the leadership of the nurse and provide a maximum amount of instruction for a large number of clients in a short period of time. In addition, in the large, busy clinic, this group discussion technique provides clients with a feeling of continuity of care, because the nurse leader remains a stable figure (see Chap. 17).

HOSPITAL TOUR

Most hospitals conduct routine tours of the maternity division for the expectant parents. It is advisable to encourage parents to take advantage of this opportunity sometime during the pregnancy. Becoming familiar ahead of time with the surroundings where the mother will deliver the baby reduces the anxiety that may be experienced in going to a strange hospital for the first time after labor begins. The details of the hospital admission routine are explained, so that the parents are familiar with this procedure before admission for delivery.

REFERRALS

Emotional and social problems identified during pregnancy may interfere with the client's ability to derive full benefit from health services. Nursing care includes exploring in what ways the client needs help and making appropriate referrals when indicated (e.g., to the nurse in the community, to community services, or to other members of the extended health team). Through the use of such referrals, lines of communication can be kept open between the particular health agency, the community, and the members of the health team. This is one of the nurse's most important functions. Thus, comprehensive care for the client is ensured.

COMMUNITY RESOURCES

The nurse in the office or clinic may find actual or potential health problems that affect both the woman and her family who could benefit from a home visit by a

Assessment Tool

Prenatal Teaching Checklist

Pregnancy and Health Status

Date   Initials

Date	Initials	
————	————	Prenatal history and physical examination results discussed
————	————	Prenatal laboratory panel results discussed
————	————	Medications and teratology discussed
————	————	Nutritional counseling
————	————	Preferred weight gain ————————————
————	————	Emotions of pregnancy

The following minor problems discussed:

————	————	Constipation or hemorrhoids
————	————	Backache
————	————	Stretch marks
————	————	Difficulty sleeping
————	————	Ankle edema
————	————	Nausea and vomiting
————	————	Heartburn
————	————	Varicosities
————	————	Headache
————	————	Stuffy nose and allergies

The following danger signs discussed:

————	————	Vaginal bleeding
————	————	Swelling of face and fingers
————	————	Severe continuous headaches
————	————	Dimness or blurring of vision
————	————	Flashes of light before eyes
————	————	Severe abdominal pain
————	————	Persistent vomiting
————	————	Chills and fever
————	————	Sudden escape of fluid from vagina

Preventive Health Care

————	————	Smoking discussed
————	————	Activity, exercise, travel, working discussed
————	————	Sexual activity discussed
————	————	Accident prevention
————	————	Dental care
————	————	Alcohol discussed

(continued)

Assessment Tool (continued)

_____ _____ Community-health resources

_____ _____ Contraception discussed. Plans: _____ birth control pills, _____ IUD, _____ diaphragm, _____ foam and condom, _____ tubal ligation, _____ vasectomy, _____ rhythm or ovulation, _____ vaginal sponge, _____ none

Preparation for Labor, Delivery, and Parenthood

_____ _____ Prenatal classes discussed

_____ _____ Enrolled in class: date _____ type _____

_____ _____ Hospital arrangements discussed (visit and register)

_____ _____ Breast-feeding versus bottle-feeding discussed

_____ _____ Type selected _____ Breast care taught _____

_____ _____ Management of labor and delivery discussed

Anesthesia/analgesia _____
Prepared childbirth _____

_____ _____ Partner in delivery room discussed. Yes _____ No _____

_____ _____ Signs of labor discussed (when to go to hospital)

Instructed on what to do about the following:

_____ _____ Ruptured membranes
_____ _____ Bleeding
_____ _____ Fever

_____ _____ Fetal monitoring equipment discussed

_____ _____ Circumcision discussed

_____ _____ Special requests related to birth _____

_____ _____ Infant care

_____ _____ Rooming-in

_____ _____ Pediatrician

_____ _____ Layette

---

community-health nurse (CHN). If such a situation arises, the woman can be informed about available community-health services and what services the CHN might offer during a home visit, and how such a visit can be beneficial. A referral can be made through established agency procedures.

Community-Health Nurse. The nurse in the community may work in either an official or a voluntary agency. The official health agency may have an antepartal clinic offering complete antepartal services for families with financial need.

Home Visits. Real value may be derived from a visit in which the nurse is able to see the woman in her usual surroundings. For instance, if the woman has the problem of excessive weight gain and is not responding to clinic therapy, the CHN can visit the home and gain some insight into the basis of the problem. In her report to the clinic or the office staff, she relates information that contributes to both the medical and the nursing management of this pregnancy.

In situations in which the clinic program is limited in educational opportunities, such as parents' classes or individual guidance, the CHN's visit to the home may be necessary to supplement the health-care teaching and anticipatory guidance done in the clinic.

Assessment of the situation at each home visit includes finding out what the woman needs to know. Communication and observation skills are of paramount importance. The nurse takes cues from the mother and handles each need as it arises, focusing teaching on the mother's concerns and limiting the amount of material taught during each visit. Topics may include basic information about pregnancy, hygiene, and nutrition; specific preparations for the baby; how to handle sibling rivalry; and so on. These subjects may come up naturally in the course of the visits, or the nurse can guide conversation around to them as she explores with the mother certain areas of need. By the end of the antepartal period, all necessary counseling usually can be accomplished.

Medical Social Worker. The medical social worker, a member of the health team, works closely with the nurse in the care of pregnant woman. Most hospitals and community-health agencies have a social service department.

The function of social service workers is to help people meet and cope with problems that interfere with social functioning. These problems may include unmarried parenthood, divorce, desertion, placing older children during the mother's hospital stay, arranging for a working housekeeper, planning convalescent care for the mother, or arranging financial or material assistance.

By observation, counseling, and liaison work, the social worker combines efforts with the other members of the health team to see the client not only as an individual maternity client, but also as an important member of the family, and the family as an integral part of the community.

Summary. Comprehensive antepartal care is concerned with the total health and the well-being of the pregnant woman and her family. With this as the central objective, the combined efforts of several disciplines, in addition to those of medicine and nursing, may be required in the cooperative plan.

A positive effort on the part of the health team becomes possible if each member has a clear understanding of his or her own role, appreciates and understands the contribution of the other professions represented on the team, knows something of the processes involved in the differing approaches, recognizes commonality of interest and skill, and has the intellectual and the emotional capacity to enter into a team relationship.

■ GENERAL HEALTH MAINTENANCE IN PREGNANCY

During pregnancy, women are encouraged to continue their usual habits with little change, unless they have previously been living in ways not conducive to health and well-being. Although pregnancy creates numerous physiological and psychoemotional changes, women with basically positive attitudes and good health are able to adapt without undue stress. Many find these changes interesting and enjoyable—part of the mystery of the phenomenon of childbearing. During the months of antepartal care, the nurse has many opportunities to assist clients to attain healthier patterns of living and to reinforce health-promoting behaviors.

Rest, Relaxation, and Sleep

Because rest and sleep are so essential to health, it is important to emphasize this detail in parent teaching. Pregnant women become tired more readily. Nature has made provision for some reduction in normal energy without injury to health. Beyond this limit, the symptoms of fatigue are evidenced in irritability, apprehension, a tendency to worry, and restlessness. These symptoms are sometimes subtle and misleading. The pregnant woman should rest to prevent this fatigue.

The expectant mother ought to get as much sleep as she believes she needs. Some people need more than others. It can be beneficial to take a nap or rest for a half hour every morning and afternoon. If this is not possible, shorter rest periods, preferably taken lying down (several times a day), are beneficial.

Not all mothers are able to follow the recommended rest periods. Both the woman who works throughout her pregnancy and the mother of preschool children need special attention in planning for adequate rest. The nurse can search with the mother for minutes in her busy day that can be used for rest. Counseling the family may be necessary to maximize the mother's free moments. Resting might include lying down or sitting comfortably to rest the body, mind, abdominal muscles, legs and back, and to stretch out whenever possible so it is easier for the heart to pump the blood to the extremities.

During the last months of pregnancy, a small pillow used for support of the abdomen while the pregnant woman lies on her side does much to relieve discomfort.

Conscious relaxation can be used to advantage by the pregnant woman. Various techniques are available, including such approaches as progressive relaxation, breathing exercises, attention focusing, imagery, and forms of meditation. Practiced regularly, relaxation is refreshing, energizing, and effective in counteracting stress. If the mother does not already practice relaxation, the nurse can teach her a simple technique. Relaxation techniques are discussed in Chapter 17; exercises are given in Appendix C.

Exercise

Exercise during pregnancy is usually beneficial. However, the degree of exercise recommended depends on
(*Text continues on page 413*)

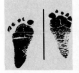

Nursing Care Plan

The Pregnant Woman

Nursing Goals

1. Women seek diagnosis of pregnancy and regular prenatal care.
2. Women and families understand the progress of pregnancy and anticipated changes.
3. Women learn self-care and health maintenance during pregnancy.
4. Women are able to alleviate minor discomforts of pregnancy.
5. Women can identify potential or actual complications and seek appropriate care.

Assessment	Potential Nursing Diagnosis	Planning/Intervention	Evaluation
Physiological status of pregnancy (vital signs, weight, urine, fundal height, fetal heart rate and activity, symptoms, test results)	Knowledge deficit of effects of pregnancy on body systems Knowledge deficit of fetal growth and development Concomitant medical conditions	Take general health history and obstetric history, physical examination, and laboratory tests as part of antepartal work-up; continue surveillance at return visits	Client repeats EDD Client understands implications of minor health problems and complications
Psychosocial status of pregnancy (responses to pregnancy, family adaptations, knowledge of psychosocial effects)	Knowledge deficit related to effects of pregnancy on psychosocial domain Knowledge deficit of effects of pregnancy on sexuality Disturbance in self-concept related to effects of pregnancy on biopsychosocial patterns	Discuss client profile, identifying data, family composition, attitudes toward pregnancy, knowledge levels, expectations related to pregnancy, family and personal resources, coping mechanisms, and economic situation	Client discusses expectations of pregnancy Client realizes who support persons are Client clarifies her understanding of (or lack of) information
Health maintenance needs (self-care, diet, rest and exercise, substance use, medications, sexuality)	Health-seeking behaviors achieve successful pregnancy outcome Knowledge deficit of nutritional requirements Knowledge deficit of hazards of smoking, alcohol, drugs Alterations in health maintenance related to increased psychophysical needs	Provide information about ways to promote health and well-being during pregnancy (i.e., rest, exercise, work, recreation, travel, medications and immunizations, skin care, breast care, clothes, teeth, bowel habits, douching, smoking, sexual relations, drug and alcohol use) Refer to appropriate health professional or agency when significant problems are identified	Client acknowledges areas needing improvement Client seeks information on changing behavior Client follows through on referrals, recommendations, and treatment plans
Minor discomforts (symptoms in specific systems: genitourinary, gastrointestinal, urinary, musculoskeletal, neurological)	Alteration in comfort: nausea or vomiting, heartburn, constipation, headaches, hemorrhoids, flatulence, backache, dyspnea, leg cramps, vaginal discharge	Provide information and instruction about occurrence and alleviation of such discomforts as urinary frequency, nausea and vomiting, heartburn, constipation, flatulence,	Client identifies discomforts Client understands remedies for symptoms Client receives comfort from remedies

Nursing Care Plan (continued)

Assessment	Potential Nursing Diagnosis	Planning/Intervention	Evaluation
	Activity intolerance related to fatigue and dyspnea	hemorrhoids, backache, dyspnea, varicosities, leg cramps, and vaginal discharge	
	High risk for vaginal infection due to hormonal changes	Refer to physician or other health professional if difficulties persist or if there is present significant interference with daily activities	Client follows through on referral
Preparation for parenthood (knowledge of effects of pregnancy, fetal development, prenatal routines, preparing for delivery and child care)	Knowledge deficit of fetal growth and development Knowledge deficit of effects of pregnancy on body systems Knowledge deficit related to effects of pregnancy on psychosocial domain Knowledge deficit of childbirth preparation resources	Provide specific information and instruction related to growth and development of the fetus, progression of pregnancy, physical and emotional changes, prenatal management routines, and preparation for childbirth or refer to sources providing these educational services (i.e., childbirth classes, nutritionist)	Couple attends childbirth classes Couple indicates understanding of fetal development, effects of pregnancy, and prenatal routines Couple makes plans for labor and delivery Couple makes plans for infant care at home
Indicators of complications of pregnancy (i.e., rising blood pressure, facial edema, bleeding, excessive weight, inappropriate fundal measurements for dates)	High risk for pregnancy complication (related to specific symptoms) Anxiety and fear related to potential complication	Notify physician, obtain additional physical data and laboratory tests as indicated, explain to client the meaning of symptoms and signs and the plan of care	Client affirms understanding of complications Client cooperates with treatment Client controls signs and symptoms of complications
Indicators of stress and psychosocial problems (i.e., missed appointments, noncompliance, affect, direct expression of concerns, acting out behavior of children, complaints)	High risk for disturbance in self-concept related to pregnancy or other life situations High risk for alteration in parenting or family processes related to psychosocial problems High risk for pregnancy complication (related to specific behaviors)	Determine sources of problems, whether economic, interpersonal, or due to emotional illness, cultural discrepancies, or conflicts with the system of health care; provide counseling according to level of skills, refer as needed for more intensive therapy; use community resources for socioeconomic, cultural disparity problems; work with agency and health team to improve client relations if this is a problem	Client keeps appointments Client follows through on referrals Client implements suggestions and recommendations Client reports recommendations have been helpful Client affirms improvement of problems

the woman, her general condition, and the stage of pregnancy.

There are differences in the amount of exercise for the early and late periods of pregnancy. When pregnancy is advanced, exercise may be limited in comparison with the amount advised previously. Exercise provides a diversion, reduces anxiety and tension, quiets the mind, promotes sleep, helps decrease constipation, and stimulates the appetite, all of which are valuable aids to the pregnant woman.

Walking is generally a preferred form of exercise during pregnancy because it stimulates the muscular activity of the entire body and is available to all women. Exercise of any kind should not be fatiguing; to secure the most beneficial results, it should be combined with periods of rest. Sitting or standing for long periods should be avoided.

Interest in active exercise has been increasing among pregnant women, as in the general population.

Most fetuses can tolerate strenuous maternal exercise when women are accustomed to this level of activity and continue exercise programs into their pregnancies. New strenuous exercise should not begin during pregnancy. In physically fit women, the ventilatory reserve and cardiovascular changes of pregnancy contribute to increased fetal tolerance of the circulatory and respiratory challenges of strenuous maternal exercise.[13]

Prenatal exercises have been standard components of childbirth education, with the intention to strengthen abdominal muscles, relax muscles of the pelvic floor, teach the pelvic tilt, stretch and adduct the thighs, and limber specific body parts (see Chap. 17 and Appendix C).

Employment

Women frequently continue work during pregnancy. The type of work, level of physical activity, environmental risks or occupational hazards, and obstetric or medical problems of the woman affect whether she should work and the length of time she should continue working during pregnancy. Avoidance of work environments that expose the pregnant woman to fetotoxic substances is a major consideration (Table 19-2).

In general, jobs requiring moderate manual labor should be avoided if they must be continued over long hours or if they require delicate balance, constant standing, or constant working on night shifts. Actually, the woman who has a "desk job" in an office often does less strenuous work than the average homemaker who does not go out to work. Positions that require the worker to sit constantly can be extremely tiring. Adequate rest periods and opportunities to stand and walk

should be provided for all pregnant women employed in such positions.

Women whose jobs require prolonged periods of standing, repeated stooping and bending, climbing ladders or stairs, and heavy lifting have been found to have more placental infarcts and lower birth weight infants. These women are advised to stop working several weeks before term.[8]

During the prenatal assessment, the nurse discusses the mother's work environment and identifies sources of possible risk. Education and counseling by the nurse help the woman make an informed decision about the risks and benefits of continuing to work in a potentially hazardous environment. Steps to minimize or avoid risky activities or fetotoxic substances can be identified. Guidelines for employment of pregnant women have been developed by the U.S. Children's Bureau (Standards for Maternity Care and Employment).

Recreation

Recreation is as necessary during pregnancy as it is at other times in life.

Activities that are diverting, healthful, and relaxing help the client and the family to keep the pregnancy in a positive perspective. The nurse can discuss with the mother types of recreation that are most relaxing and pleasing for her and her family. Family group activities can still be enjoyed, even though the mother's energy and dexterity may be somewhat curtailed.

The mother should avoid situations that are likely to cause discomfort. Amusements, exercise, rest, and recreation at proper intervals help to keep the pregnant woman well and happy in an environment conducive to her well-being.

Travel

Even though there is little restriction on travel from a medical point of view, it should be discussed with the mother to clarify concerns or misinformation. Pregnant women are generally advised to avoid any trip that will cause undue fatigue or stress. For traveling long distances, flying is safest and provides greatest comfort. If travel is by automobile, rest periods of 10 to 15 minutes ought to be planned at least every 2 hours. This not only helps to avoid fatigue but also benefits circulation by providing the chance to stretch and walk.

The pregnant woman should be advised to use seatbelts during all automobile travel. Risks of injury and death to mother and fetus are increased when seatbelts are not used.[14] Placental separation can also occur with an automobile accident, because the force of the

(*Text continues on page 416*)

TABLE 19–2. OCCUPATIONS COMMONLY HELD BY WOMEN WORKING IN INDUSTRY AND POTENTIAL OCCUPATIONAL HAZARDS

Occupation	Potential Hazard	Known or Suspected Effects on Reproduction

Hospital workers
  Nurses
  Anesthetists
  Lab technicians
  Physicians
  Dentists
  Dental assistants
	Radiation	Chromosomal aberrations, sterility, birth defects, leukemia, miscarriages, retarded fetal development, carcinogen

	Benzene	Chromosomal aberrations, aplastic anemia and leukemia, prolonged menstrual periods
	BIS (chloromethyl ether)	Known human carcinogen, possible fetal effects (BIS ether formed by combination of formaldehyde and HCl in warm, moist air)
	Toluene	Chromosomal aberrations (derivative of benzene, less toxic)
	Anesthetic gases	Birth defects, miscarriages, infertility, low-birth-weight infants
	Hexachlorophene	Cogenital malformations
	Mercury	CNS damage in humans, cerebral palsy symptoms in exposed infants, behavioral alterations in animal offspring
	Estrogens	Birth defects (teratogenic), carcinogenic in offspring (DES), heavier and more frequent menses, enlarged breasts and impotence in male workers
Clerical workers	Asbestos	Chronic lung disease (asbestosis) with reduced fetal oxygenation
	Trichloroethylene	Liver and kidney damage, suspected carcinogen
	Benzene	See above
	Toluene	See above
Laundering and dry cleaning	Perchlorethylene	Liver damage, suspected carcinogen, CNS effects (dizziness, nausea), extended exposure can cause death, fetal studies not complete
	Carbon tetrachloride	Specific toxicity to liver and kidneys, suspected carcinogen, passes placental barrier to cause fetal liver damage in animals
	Petroleum solvents	Reproductive failure in both men and women
	Trichloroethylene	See above
	Benzene	See above
Textile and apparel	Carbon disulfide	Menstrual irregularities, decreased fertility, miscarriage, decreased sex drive and sperm abnormalities in men
	Dyes, aniline	Carcinogenic
	Chloroprene	Functional disruption of spermatogenesis in men, miscarriage rate increased three times in their wives, chemically related to vinyl chloride
	Cotton dust	Chronic lung disease (byssinosis, brown lung) with reduced fetal oxygenation
	Benzene	See above
	Toluene	See above
	Asbestos	See above
	Trichloroethylene	See above

(continued)

TABLE 19–2. OCCUPATIONS COMMONLY HELD BY WOMEN WORKING IN INDUSTRY AND POTENTIAL OCCUPATIONAL HAZARDS *(continued)*

Occupation	Potential Hazard	Known or Suspected Effects on Reproduction
Electronic workers, rubber workers	Perchlorethylene	See above
	Nitrosamides	100% incidence of nervous system tumors in animal studies in offspring
	Lead	Sterility, birth defects, prematurity, mental retardation, chromosomal aberrations, menstrual disorders
	Polychlorinated biphenyls (PCB)	"Cola-colored babies" with high frequency of growth retardation, gingival hyperplasia, spotted skull calcification, stillbirths, liver cancer, and reduced fertility in animals
	Arsenic	Carcinogenic; can cause death
	Mercury	See above
	Trichloroethylene	See above
Agricultural workers	Pesticides (chlorinated hydrocarbons)	Carcinogenic, abnormalities in offspring and infertility in animals, kepone causes decreased sex drives and sterility in human males
	Dioxin (2, 4, 5T)	Miscarriages in humans; mutations, birth defects, and miscarriages in animals
	Heptachlor and chlordane	Carcinogenic in animals; possibly cause neuroblastomas and leukemia in prenatally or postnatally exposed children
	Chloroprene	See above
Outdoor work Toll booth workers Traffic controllers Airline stewardesses	Carbon monoxide	Acute exposure has caused fetal and fetal–maternal deaths; chronic exposure causes decreased birth weight and increased neonatal mortality in animals
Hairdressers and cosmetologists	Hair dyes	Mutations in bacterial lab cultures, possibly carcinogenic, chromosomal damage in women using hair dyes
	Vinyl chloride (aerosol sprays)	Documented carcinogen, linked to angiosarcoma of the liver, possible chromosomal aberrations of sperm, increased miscarriage rate and birth defects in humans
	Asbestos (hair dryers)	See above
	Benzene, toluene	See above
Arts and crafts Painters Printers Potters Silkscreen, woodwork, stained glass	Benzene, toluene	See above
	Lead	See above
	Mercury	See above
	Lithium, barium	Heavy metal poisioning
	Chromium	Suspected carcinogen
	Benzidine dyes	Suspected carcinogen
Various	Cadmium	Implicated in bronchogenic and prostatic cancer, testicular damage, sterility, teratogenic effects, low birth weight in animals, cigarette smoke high in cadmium and heavy smoking increases risk
	Manganese	Impotence and decreased sex drive in exposed males

(After Greenberg J: Implications for primary care providers of occupational health hazards on pregnant women and their infants. J Nurse Midwifery 25(4): 21–30, July/August 1980)

Standards for Maternity Care and Employment (U.S. Children's Bureau)

1. Facilities for adequate prenatal medical care should be readily availalbe for all employed pregnant women, and arrangements should be made by those responsible for providing prenatal care, so that every woman has access to such care. Local health departments should make the services of prenatal clinics available to industrial plants, and the personnel management or physicians and nurses within the plant should make available to employees information about the importance of such services and where they can be obtained.

2. Pregnant women should not be employed on a shift including the hours between 12 midnight and 6 AM. Pregnant women should not be employed more than 48 hours per week, and it is desirable that their hours of work be limited to not more than 40 hours per week.

3. Every woman, especially a pregnant women, should have at least two 10-minute rest periods during her work shift, for which adequate facilities for resting and an opportunity for securing nourishing food should be provided.

4. It is not considered desirable for pregnant women to be employed in the following types of occupations, and they should, if possible, be transferred to lighter and more sedentary work:
   a. Occupations that involve heavy lifting or other heavy work
   b. Occupations that involve continuous standing and moving about

5. Pregnant women should not be employed in the following types of work during any period of pregnancy
   a. Occupations that require a good sense of bodily balance, such as work performed on scaffolds or stepladders and occupations in which the accident risk is characterized by accidents causing severe injury, such as operation of punch presses, power-driven woodworking machines, or other machines having a point-of-operation hazard
   b. Occupations involving exposure to toxic substances considered to be extra hazardous during pregnancy, including the following:
      Aniline
      Benzene and toluene
      Carbon disulfide
      Carbon monoxide
      Chlorinated hydrocarbons
      Lead and its compounds
      Mercury and its compounds
      Nitrobenzol and other nitro compounds of benzol and its homologues
      Phosphorus
      Radioactive substances and x-rays
      Turpentine
      Other toxic substances that exert an injurious effect upon the blood-forming organs, the liver, or the kidneys

   Because these substances may exert a harmful influence upon the course of pregnancy, may lead to premature termination, or may injure the fetus, the maintenance of air concentrations within the so-called maximum permissible limits of state codes is not, in itself, sufficient assurance of a safe working condition for the pregnant woman. Pregnant women should be transferred from workrooms in which any of these substances are used or produced in any significant quantity.

6. A minimum of 6 weeks' leave *before* delivery should be granted with the presentation of a medical certificate of the expected date of confinement.

7. At any time during pregnancy, a woman should be granted a reasonable amount of additional leave with the presentation of a certificate from the attending physician to the effect that complications of pregnancy have made continuing employment prejudicial to her health or to the health of the child.

   To safeguard the mother's health she should be granted sufficient time off after delivery to return to normal and to regain her strength. The infant needs her care, especially during the first year of life. If it is essential that she return to work, the following recommendations are made:
   a. All women should be granted an extension of at least 2 months leave of absence after delivery.
   b. Should complications of delivery or of the postpartum period develop, a woman should be granted a reasonable amount of additional leave beyond 2 months following delivery with presentation of a certificate to this effect from the attending physician.

collision alters the contours of the uterine muscle and displaces placental attachment.[15] Proper placement of seatbelts during pregnancy is important. The woman should wear both shoulder and lap belts, with the lap belt worn low and under the abdomen. The shoulder belt is worn above the uterus and below the neck, with the woman sitting upright and using a headrest to minimize flexion-extension injuries (Fig. 19-10).

Less than half of pregnant women interviewed in a small study reported using seatbelts regularly. Fewer than 25% recalled having received information about seatbelt use from their physician or nurse during preg-

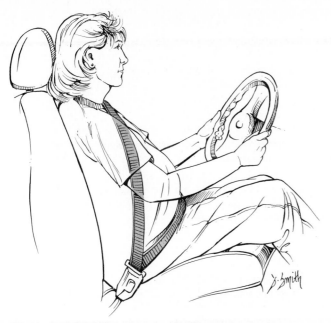

■ *Figure 19–10*
Pregnant women should wear seat belt with shoulder strap above the uterus and below the neck and lap belt low and under the abdomen.

nancy. Their major source of information was from posters and pamphlets in the waiting room.[16] This suggests that health providers need to place greater emphasis on seatbelt use during prenatal counseling.

Although traveling in general is not usually contraindicated during pregnancy, each expectant mother should seek individual consultation concerning the advisability of extensive travel at any time during the pregnancy.

Immunizations During Pregnancy

As a general rule, immunizations are best avoided during pregnancy. Several factors enter into the decision about immunizing a pregnant woman against an infectious disease, including the possibility of exposure, the effect on mother and fetus if the disease is contracted, susceptibility to the disease, and risk to the fetus from the immunization. Immune globulins, toxoids, and vaccines made from inactivated organisms are usually safe during pregnancy. Vaccines made from live organisms should not be given during pregnancy except in acute situations and emergencies, because these vaccines may infect the fetus.

Pregnant women with chronic cardiac, pulmonary, or metabolic diseases should be evaluated carefully for immunization against influenza and pneumonia. Rec-

ommendations for travel immunizations during pregnancy by the American College of Obstetricians and Gynecologists with updates are summarized in Table 19-3.

The nurse can advise the pregnant woman to plan travel during pregnancy to minimize exposure to infectious diseases. Any febrile or rash illness should be reported to the physician without delay. Education about updating immunizations after delivery is provided to reduce future risk. Delay of conception for an appropriate time period after receiving live organism vaccinations is stressed.

Skin Care

The glands of the skin may be more active during pregnancy, and there may be increased perspiration, resulting in irritation or odor. Elimination through the skin is an important method of removing body waste products. A bath or a shower should be taken daily because it is stimulating, refreshing, and relaxing. Baths should not be taken after rupture of the membranes. The only danger from tub baths during the last trimester of pregnancy is that the heavy weight of the large abdomen may put pregnant women off balance and make climbing in and out of the tub awkward. Therefore, the likelihood of slipping or falling in the bathtub is increased.

Breast Care

Special care of the breasts during pregnancy is an important preparation for breast-feeding. During the antepartal period, the breasts often have a feeling of fullness and become larger, heavier, and more pendulous. A well-fitted supporting brassiere that holds the breasts up and in may relieve these discomforts. It may also help to prevent the subsequent tissue sagging often noticeable after delivery due to the increased weight of the breast during pregnancy and lactation.

Early in pregnancy, the breasts begin to secrete colostrum. The breasts should be bathed daily with a clean washcloth and warm water. Some studies have demonstrated that the use of soap, alcohol, and other such materials during the antepartal period tends to be detrimental to the integrity of the nipple tissue because they remove the protective skin oils and leave the nipple more prone to damage. Rubbing the nipples with a bath towel or rolling them between thumb and forefinger during the last trimester of pregnancy may be helpful in attempting to toughen them.

The position of the thumb and finger should be

TABLE 19-3. IMMUNIZATIONS DURING PREGNANCY

Measles (rubeola) and mumps	Live virus vaccines, should not be given during pregnancy. Measles immune globulin given for postexposure prophylaxis.
Rubella	Live virus vaccine, should not be given during pregnancy. Virus can infect placenta and fetus.
Influenza	Evaluate risk to pregnant women with chronic cardiac, pulmonary or metabolic diseases, may be indicated
Pneumonia	Evaluate risk to pregnant women with chronic cardiac, pulmonary, or metabolic diseases; may be indicated.
Poliomyelitis	Usually not given during pregnancy; except during epidemics or travel to endemic areas.
Hepatitis A	Given during pregnancy after exposure or for travel to endemic areas; one dose given to infants born to infected mothers.
Hepatitis B	Immune globulin given to pregnant women at risk due to work or travel; immune globulin given to newborn followed by HBV vaccination.
Rabies	Antirabies series given only after exposure
Cholera	Killed bacteria, given only with travel to areas of increased risk for exposure.
Chickenpox (varicella)	Immune globulin given to pregnant women with exposure; globulin given to newborns whose mothers develop varicella perinatally.
Tetanus, diphtheria	Toxoid given if no primary series or no booster within 10 years; immune globulin and toxoid with exposure in unvaccinated woman.
Typhoid	Recommended for travel in endemic areas.
Yellow fever	Live virus vaccine, not given during pregnancy unless with travel to endemic area or exposure.
Plague	Given only if great risk of exposure.

gradually shifted around the circumference of the nipple until a complete circuit has been made.

Clothing

During pregnancy, the clothes should be comfortable and nonconstricting. Most women are able to dress in their usual manner until the enlargement of the abdomen becomes apparent. Maternity specialty shops and department stores carry a wide variety of maternity fashions.

Designers have given consideration to the pregnant mother's clothing, making it easy to dress attractively and feel self-confident about appearance. Maternity clothes are designed to be comfortable and "hang from the shoulders," thus avoiding any constriction; they are made in a variety of materials. The expectant mother can dress according to the climate and the temperature for her comfort.

Pregnant women should avoid any type of clothing or accessories that constrict movement or circulation. Tight belts, garters, knee socks, knee-high stockings, panty girdles, garter belts, stretch pants, and so forth should not be worn. Particularly dangerous are round garters, rolled stockings, and tight knee-high stockings that might restrict circulation in the lower extremities. These can aggravate varicose veins, cause edema of the lower legs and feet, and produce venous stasis.

Clothing that fits snugly in the perineal area, such as tight pantyhose and stretch pants, can contribute to vaginal infections and heat rash (miliaria). Pantyhose are preferable to hose held up by garters or tight waist garter belts, but should not be constricting and should have cotton crotches.

BREAST SUPPORT

Every pregnant woman should wear a well-fitted brassiere to support the breasts in a normal uplifted position.

Client Education

Techniques Used During Pregnancy to Prepare Nipples for Breast-feeding

Nipple Rolling. The nipple is placed between thumb and fingers and rolled gently. This helps toughen the nipple surface.

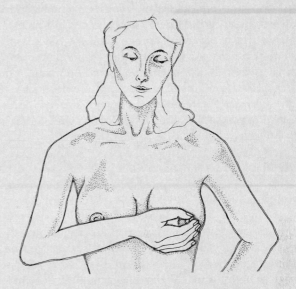

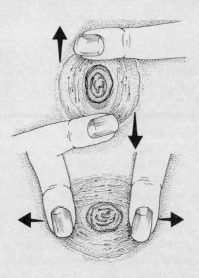

Nipple Stretching. The fingers or thumbs are placed close to the nipple and pressed firmly into the breast tissue. Gradually the fingers are pushed away from the nipple toward the edge of the areola and beyond. Stretching is done vertically and horizontally and repeated several times. This helps to evert nipples that are flat or inverted.

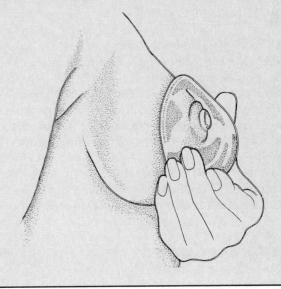

Nipple Cup. Plastic cups can be used to help correct inverted nipples. These cups apply a constant, gentle pressure around the areola and push the nipple forward through a central opening in the inner shield. They can be worn for several hours a day toward the end of pregnancy.

Proper support of the breasts is conducive to good posture and helps to prevent backache.

The selection of a brassiere is determined by individual fitting and is influenced by the size of the breasts and the need for support. It is important to see that the cup is large enough and that the underarm is built high enough to cover all the breast tissue. Wide shoulder straps afford more comfort for the woman who has large and pendulous breasts. Again, the size of the brassiere is determined by the size of the woman, but in most instances the brassiere is approximately two sizes larger than that usually worn. The mother who is planning to breast-feed finds it practical to purchase nursing brassieres with drop flaps over the nipples, which can be worn during the latter months of pregnancy, as well as during the postpartal period for as long as she is nursing her baby.

SHOES

A comfortable, well-fitted shoe is essential for the expectant mother. The postural changes that occur as the mother's abdomen enlarges may be aggravated by wearing high-heeled shoes and may cause backache and fatigue. Low-heeled shoes should be worn during working hours and for daytime activities. For more fashionable attire, a 2-in heel is acceptable if the client does not develop backache from the increased lordosis induced by the heels, and if she can maintain adequate balance.

Shoes also should provide adequate support to the arch and sides of the foot to promote comfort.

ABDOMINAL SUPPORT

If the mother's abdomen is large or if previous pregnancies have caused her abdominal musculature to become lax or pendulous, a properly made and well-fitted maternity girdle gives support and comfort. The purpose of the garment is support, not constriction of the abdomen. When putting the girdle on, the woman should lie on the bed rather than stand and should fasten it from the bottom upward, so support is provided to the uterus from below. Abdominal support provided by a maternity girdle can help relieve backache, prevent fatigue, and assist in maintaining good posture.

Care of the Teeth

Good dental care is necessary because the teeth are important for adequate mastication of food. The teeth should be brushed carefully on arising, after each meal, and before retiring at night. An alkaline mouthwash may be used if desired. It is advisable for the expectant mother to visit her dentist at the beginning of pregnancy

and follow any recommendations made. Any extensive elective work is better postponed until after the pregnancy. The most favorable period for routine, minor procedures is from the fourth to the seventh month. The mother is usually less nauseated and, in general, feeling well.

Diagnostic dental x-rays should be postponed until the latter half of pregnancy. A lead apron over the abdomen gives sufficient protection.

The old saying, "For every child a tooth," based on a belief that the fetus takes calcium from the mother's teeth, has no real scientific basis. An adequate diet during pregnancy supplies the baby with calcium and phosphorus in sufficient amounts to build bones and teeth.

Bowel Habits

The pregnant woman with regular elimination habits often experiences little or no change in the daily routine. Those who have a tendency toward constipation become noticeably more irregular during pregnancy because of decreased physical exertion, relaxation of the bowel smooth-muscle systems, and pressure of the enlarging uterus. The presenting part of the fetus exerts pressure on the lower bowel, especially during the latter part of pregnancy. Iron supplementation during pregnancy is an additional contributing factor to constipation.

Constipation may be prevented or alleviated by maintaining regular bowel elimination, drinking a large amount of fluids daily, and maintaining a diet that contains several daily servings of fresh fruit and raw vegetables, whole-grain breads and cereals, and particularly products with whole bran. If these measures are not effective, a stool softener such as dioctyl sodium sulfosuccinate or a mild laxative such as milk of magnesia may be recommended. Harsh laxatives and purgatives are contraindicated. Mineral oil should not be used because it prevents absorption of fat-soluble vitamins from the gastrointestinal tract. Lack of vitamin K can lead to hemorrhagic disease of the newborn.

HEMORRHOIDS

Pregnancy often precipitates the occurrence of hemorrhoids (anal varicosities), partially as a result of constipation. Maintaining regular bowel habits, keeping the stool soft, and avoiding straining at stool can help prevent or minimize hemorrhoids. Standing for long periods of time and wearing constricting clothing are aggravating factors. Passage of hard fecal material can injure the rectal mucosa and cause bleeding from fissures or hemorrhoids. Hemorrhoids may become thrombosed or protrude through the anus. The little bumps and nodules seen in a mass of hemorrhoids are the distended portions of the affected vessels. As with varicosities in other areas, they are caused by pressure interfering with return venous circulation and are aggravated by constipation. They often cause discomfort during pregnancy and, due to pressure at the time of delivery, may cause great distress during the postpartal period.

The prevention and the treatment of constipation can minimize the severity of hemorrhoids. When internal hemorrhoids protrude through the rectum, the mother can be instructed to replace them carefully by pushing them gently back into the rectum. Usually she can manage this after a thorough explanation or demonstration. She lubricates her finger with petrolatum or mineral oil to aid ease of insertion and to avoid trauma to the veins. If the client wishes, a finger cot can be used to cover her finger. Also, taking either the knee–chest position or elevating her buttocks on a pillow facilitates replacement through gravity.

The application of an icebag or cold compresses wet with witch hazel or Epsom salts solution provides relief. The physician may order tannic acid in suppositories, or compresses of witch hazel and glycerin. Surgery is seldom resorted to during pregnancy. Doing Kegel's exercises regularly helps prevent and control hemorrhoids.

Sexuality During Pregnancy

Although sexuality has become a more open topic in today's society, there is a wide variety of views among people of different cultural backgrounds. Nonetheless, there is a growing expectation on the part of clients that health professionals will offer counseling related to sexuality as an integral part of health care. Particularly in maternity nursing, sexual concerns are close to the surface, providing a ready situation for intervention and satisfying sexual adjustments. Being willing to explore and respond to a client's sexual concerns and having knowledge of appropriate sources of referral for sexual counseling are part of the function of the maternity nurse (see Chaps. 8, 9, and 11).

■ NURSING MANAGEMENT OF MINOR DISCOMFORTS

The minor discomforts of pregnancy are commonly experienced by most expectant mothers, to some degree, in the course of a normal pregnancy. Not all women experience these discomforts, and some go through the entire antepartal period without any. Although the discomforts are not serious, their presence detracts from the mother's feeling of comfort and well-being. In many instances, they can be avoided by preventive measures or can be reduced by healthful practices once they do occur.

Client Education

Kegel's Exercises

Tightening and relaxing the pubococcygeal muscle keeps the vagina toned, increases the strength of the perineum, and helps prevent or control hemorrhoids. This contributes to the strength of the pelvic sling in supporting the fetus, increases sexual pleasure, and enhances urinary control.

The muscle that is used to stop the flow of urine is the pubococcygeal muscle. Practice stopping urine by squeezing this muscle several times to become familiar with it. When lying down, insert one finger into the vagina and contract the pubococcygeal muscle; note the feeling of contraction around your finger.

1. Squeeze the pubococcygeal muscle for 3 seconds, relax for 3 seconds, and squeeze again. Begin with 10 three-second squeezes per day, and increase gradually until you are doing 100 twice daily.
2. Squeeze and release, then squeeze and release alternately as rapidly as you can. This is called the "flutter" exercise.
3. Bear down as during a bowel movement, but concentrate on the vagina instead of the rectum. Hold for 3 seconds.

Kegel's exercises can be done anywhere and anytime. The increased control gained over the pubococcygeal muscle is useful throughout pregnancy, during labor, during intercourse, and to prevent loss of vaginal tone with aging. This exercise, done regularly, is useful for the rest of your life.

Gastrointestinal Discomforts

NAUSEA

Nausea and vomiting to mild degree (morning sickness) constitute the most common discomfort of the first trimester of pregnancy. Symptoms usually appear about the end of the 4th or 6th week and last until about the 12th week. Nausea occurs in about one half of all pregnant women; of these, about one third experience some vomiting. Usually, it occurs in the morning only, but a small percentage of women may have nausea and vomiting throughout the entire day.

Altered hormonal status, with high levels of human chorionic gonadotropin (HCG) and progesterone, is involved in producing these symptoms through effects on gastrointestinal smooth musculature. Changes in carbohydrate metabolism and other metabolic processes may also contribute.

Manifestations. The typical sign of morning sickness starts with a feeling of nausea when the woman is getting out of bed in the morning. She is unable to retain her breakfast, but by noon she feels much better and usually has no further episodes until the next morning. The nausea may happen in the afternoon or in the evening. In a few women, the nausea and vomiting may persist throughout the day and even be worse in the afternoon. With the majority of women, this problem lasts from 1 to 3 months and then suddenly ceases. There may be slight loss of body weight but no other signs or symptoms.

Nursing Care. Often this condition can be controlled or relieved by various before-breakfast remedies. Taking a dry piece of toast, plain popcorn, or crackers a half hour before getting out of bed may produce relief. In some instances, sips of hot water (plain or with lemon juice), hot tea, clear coffee, or hot milk have been tried and found successful. However, the dry carbohydrate foods seem to be more effective. After remaining in bed for about a half hour after taking these remedies, the woman gets up and dresses slowly (sitting as much of the time as possible). After this, she is usually ready for breakfast.

Greasy foods and those known to cause disagreeable after-effects should be avoided in the diet. Other suggested remedies include eating an increased amount of carbohydrate foods during this time or eating simple and light food five or six times a day instead of three regular full meals. Sweet lemonade, about half a lemon to a pint of sweetened water is usually welcome after a bout of vomiting. Small amounts of ginger ale, cola drink, or spearmint, raspberry, or peppermint tea also may be helpful.

Once nausea and vomiting are established, they are difficult to overcome; therefore, it is especially desirable to prevent the onset, or control this condition as soon as possible after it develops. Vomiting can deplete the body of necessary nutrients at a time when daily health should be maintained. Eating high-protein meals (e.g., eggs, cheese, meat), fruit, and fruit juices may help prevent morning sickness by avoiding hypoglycemia. Taking 10 mg of vitamin B_6 at bedtime may be helpful also.

Pregnancies differ, and what may help one person may not benefit another. The trial-and-error method often is necessary to obtain results. If persistent vomiting develops, as it does with a small number of women, the condition is no longer considered a minor discomfort but a serious complication called hyperemesis gravidarum (see Chap. 33).

HEARTBURN

Heartburn is a neuromuscular phenomenon that may occur any time during pregnancy. As a result of diminished gastric motility, reverse peristaltic waves cause regurgitation of the stomach contents into the esophagus. This irritation of the esophageal mucosa causes heartburn. It may be described as a burning discomfort diffusely localized behind the lower part of the sternum, often radiating upward along the course of the esophagus. Although called heartburn, it really has nothing to do with the heart. Often it is associated with other gastrointestinal symptoms, of which acid regurgitation, belching, nausea, and epigastric pressure are most troublesome. Stress, tension and emotional disturbances, worry, fatigue, and improper diet may contribute to its intensity.

Little fat should be included in the diet, because fatty foods are especially aggravating.

Coffee and cigarettes tend to make heartburn worse because they stimulate acid secretion in the stomach and irritate the mucosa.

Eating several small meals daily instead of three large ones may help prevent heartburn. Wearing clothes that are loose around the waist may also be helpful. When heartburn occurs, it may be relieved with small sips of water, milk, or a carbonated drink. Lying down makes regurgitation worse, so it is best to sit upright. Relaxing and breathing deeply for several minutes may help. The "flying exercise" is also suggested: sitting tailor fashion, the arms are raised and lowered quickly, bringing the hands together over the head; this is repeated several times.

When antacids are used, those with an aluminum or magnesium base should be taken. Many over-the-counter remedies contain sodium, which promotes water retention and could lead to edema. Women are advised to avoid Alka-Seltzer, Fizrin, and baking soda (sodium bicarbonate), which are high in sodium ions.

Equally effective medications are aluminum compounds, such as aluminum hydroxide gel, or this medication in tablet form with magnesium trisilicate.

FLATULENCE

Flatulence is a somewhat common and often disagreeable discomfort. Usually it is due to bacterial action in the intestines, which results in the formation of gas. Eating only small amounts of food and masticating it well may prevent this feeling of distress after eating. Regular daily elimination is of prime importance, as is the avoidance of foods that form gas (e.g., beans, parsnips, corn, sweet desserts, fried foods, cake, and candy). If these measures fail to relieve the condition, the physician should be consulted.

Backache

Most pregnant women experience some degree of backache. As pregnancy advances, the woman's posture changes to compensate for the weight of the growing uterus. The shoulders are thrown back as the enlarging abdomen protrudes, and, for body balance to be maintained, the inward curve of the spine is exaggerated. The relaxation of the sacroiliac joints, in addition to the postural change, causes varying degrees of backache after excessive strain, fatigue, bending, or lifting.

The woman can be advised early in pregnancy how to prevent such strain through good posture and body mechanics, and avoidance of fatigue. Appropriate shoes worn during periods of activity and a supporting girdle may be helpful (see section entitled "Clothing").

The key to good posture is to sit, stand, walk, and lie in a way that minimizes the hollow or curvature of the lower back. To do this, the abdominal and gluteal muscles are contracted and those of the lower back are relaxed, while the pelvis is tilted slightly upward and forward. The pelvic tilt exercise brings the pelvis into this alignment (see Chap. 17). Sitting posture can be improved by using armrests, foot supports, and a pillow for the back. The tailor position or lotus position used for yoga is useful for relief of back pain. The mother should always bend from the knees rather than the back when lifting, keeping the spine straight. Avoiding forward leaning while doing chores helps prevent strain on the back. Adjusting the height of the work surface or the mother's position to maintain proper posture when standing or sitting reduces back strain.

Daily exercises such as walking, swimming, and stretching are effective ways of preventing backache. The knee–chest twist is a particularly beneficial exercise. When backache occurs, it may be relieved by applying a heating pad or hot water bottle to the lower back, by having a back rub, or by sitting in a Jacuzzi that is not too hot.

Dyspnea

Difficult breathing or shortness of breath occasionally results from pressure on the diaphragm by the enlarged uterus. Dyspnea may interfere with the client's sleep and general comfort during the last weeks of pregnancy. Dyspnea is relieved by lightening (the settling of the fetus into the pelvic cavity with relief of the upper abdominal pressure) or after the birth of the baby, when it disappears spontaneously. It is most troublesome when the client lies down, and her comfort may be greatly enhanced by propping her up in bed with pillows. In this semisitting posture, she can sleep better and longer than with her head low. The nurse demonstrates how these pillows may be arranged comfortably so that the client's back is adequately supported.

In clients with known heart disease, shortness of breath, especially of rather sudden onset, may be a sign of oncoming heart failure and should be reported at once to the physician.

Varicose Veins

Varicose veins or varices may occur in the lower extremities and, at times, may extend up as high as the external genitalia or even into the pelvis. A varicosity is an enlargement in the diameter of a vein due to a thinning and stretching of its walls. Such distended areas may occur at short intervals along the course of the blood vessel; they give it a knotted appearance. Varicosities generally are associated with hereditary tendencies and are enhanced by advancing age, multiple pregnancy, and activities that require prolonged standing.

During pregnancy, the pressure in the pelvis due to the enlarged uterus, which presses on the great abdominal veins, interferes with the return of blood from the lower extremities; the greater the pressure in the abdomen, the greater the chance of varicose veins of the lower extremities and the vulva. Therefore, any occupation that keeps a client constantly on her feet, particularly in the latter part of pregnancy, causes an increase in abdominal pressure and so acts as an exacerbating factor.

Symptoms. The first symptom of the development of varicose veins is a dull aching pain in the legs due to distention of the deep vessels. Inspection may show a fine purple network of superficial veins that cover the skin in a lacelike pattern, although this does not always appear. Later, the true varicosities appear, usually first under the bend of the knee, in a tangled mass of bluish or purplish veins, often as large as a lead pencil. As the condition advances, the varicosities extend up and down the leg along the course of the vessels, and in severe cases they may affect the veins of the labia majora, the vagina, and the uterus.

Nursing Care. Treatment for varicose veins begins by eliminating constricting garters, stockings, or other clothing that causes pressure, particularly on the legs or thighs. If varicosities persist, the client can be taught the right-angle position (lie on the floor with her legs extended straight into the air at right angles to her body, with her buttocks and heels resting against the wall; see Chap. 17). This position is taken for 2 to 5 minutes several times a day.

Late in pregnancy, this position may be too difficult to assume because of pressure against the diaphragm.

To give support to the weak-walled veins, a full-length elastic stocking (support pantyhose) often is recommended. Many women who must be on their feet a great deal and do not have the opportunity to rest frequently wear these stockings during working hours as a prophylactic measure. The nurse can be helpful in apprising mothers of the varieties of hose available to meet individual needs.

Varicosities of the vulva may be relieved by placing a pillow under the buttocks and elevating the hips for frequent rest periods or by taking the elevated Sims' position for a few moments several times a day (Fig. 19-11). Clients suffering from this condition should not stand when they can sit, and they should not sit when they can lie down.

Prevention of varicosities should be emphasized by the nurse. Every pregnant woman should be advised to sit with her legs elevated whenever possible. When the legs are elevated, care should be taken to see that there are no pressure points against the legs to interfere with the circulation, particularly in the popliteal space.

A *varicose vein in the vagina* may rupture during the antepartal or intrapartal period, but this is rare. The hemorrhage is venous and can be controlled readily by pressure. The foot of the bed can be markedly elevated.

Cramps

Cramps are painful spasmodic muscular contractions in the legs. They may occur at any time during the pregnancy but are more frequent during the later months owing to pressure of the enlarged uterus on the nerves affecting the lower extremities. Other causes have been attributed to fatigue, chilling, tense body posture, and insufficient or excessive calcium in the diet. Cramps are commonly noted after the use of diuretics.

A quart of milk in the daily diet has been recommended to meet the calcium needs during pregnancy. However, studies show that large quantities of milk or dicalcium phosphate predispose to muscular tetany and leg cramps as a result of the excessive amount of phos-

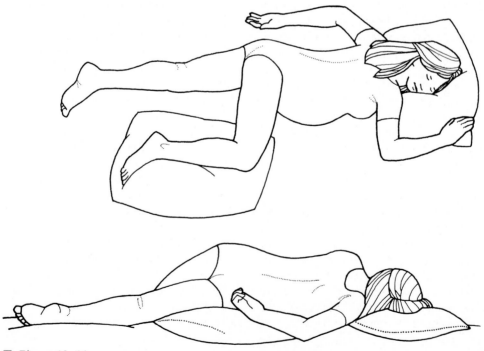

■ *Figure 19–11*
Sims' position for varicosities of the vulva and rectum.

phorous absorbed from these products. Some authorities suggest that small quantities of aluminum hydroxide gel be taken with the quart of milk because it removes some of the dietary phosphorus from the intestinal tract. Immediate relief may be obtained by forcing the toes upward and by putting pressure on the knee to straighten the leg. Elevating the feet and keeping the extremities warm are preventive measures.

Cramps, although not a serious condition, are excruciatingly painful for the duration of the muscle contraction. Regular exercise to keep circulation good in the legs helps prevent cramps. Taking a warm bath before bedtime can improve circulation at night. Cramps are often brought on by pointing the toes when stretching; the woman needs to be reminded to avoid this. Massaging the cramped muscle, soaking it in warm water, using a heating pad, and standing and walking when able relieve cramps.

Edema

Swelling of the lower legs and ankles is common during pregnancy and is sometimes uncomfortable. It is especially likely to occur in hot weather. Often it may be relieved by a proper abdominal support or by resting frequently during the day. Elevating the feet or taking the right-angle position often gives relief.

Edema may be reduced by avoiding highly salted foods, eating high-protein foods, and avoiding tight clothing. Women who work or must remain standing or sitting for long periods need to rest two to three times daily with legs raised for about 20 minutes. When edema occurs, elevating the legs as much as possible reduces swelling and discomfort.

Resting with legs elevated has been the standard treatment for edema during pregnancy. Immersion in warm water has been found to be a safe and more rapid method than rest to mobilize extravascular fluid in pregnant women. Diuresis is more than twice as great after immersion in a tank (similar to a hot tub) than after rest. In a bath tub with water at waist level, diuresis is the same as with rest. No changes in serum and plasma parameters occurred despite large fluxes in fluid and electrolytes. A simple bath seems to be as effective as an hour of rest in reducing edema during pregnancy.[17]

Although edema of the ankles, feet, and even hands is common, particularly in late pregnancy, the nurse must always be alert for possible complications. *Edema is one of the signs of preeclampsia and must not be overlooked.* Sudden weight gain of more than 2 lb/week needs careful evaluation. The nurse should look for distribution of edema on the face and sacrum as additional indices of preeclampsia. This must be brought to the

physician's attention. The prevention of various minor discomforts of pregnancy, medications to avoid, and safe natural remedies are described in Table 19-4.

Vaginal Discharge

In pregnancy, there are increased vaginal secretions so that a heavier discharge at this time usually is physiological. However, the client should call to the attention of the physician any copious, yellow or greenish foul-smelling or irritating discharge. This may indicate a possible infection with gonorrhea, *Chlamydia,* or *Trichomonas* (see Chap. 35). Urinary manifestations such as burning on urination and frequency may indicate a urinary tract infection. The microscopic result of a smear or culture indicates whether or not treatment is necessary.

■ DRUG USE DURING PREGNANCY

The use of all medication is to be avoided or minimized during pregnancy. Evidence regarding the adverse effects of many chemical substances when taken by a pregnant woman continues to accumulate. Because of the rapid formation of fetal organ systems and development of cellular functions, the first trimester is a particularly susceptible time. However, ingestion of drugs at any time during pregnancy holds potential for fetal damage. The impact of a drug on the developing fetus may range from no measurable effect to such marked toxicity that the embryo is killed (aborted). Sublethal doses of drugs may result in gross anatomical defects or a permanent subtle metabolic or functional deficit.

About half of all drugs taken during pregnancy are over-the-counter (OTC) products used to relieve symptoms of physiological changes of pregnancy. Most commonly used are preparations for nasal congestion, backache, constipation, hemorrhoids, and heartburn. Despite long-standing and continuing use, there is little information about possible harmful effects of these drugs during pregnancy.

Used occasionally in small doses, adverse effects of most OTC products on mother or fetus are unlikely. However, most studies of these drugs have been on animals and do not accurately predict damage to the human fetus.[8] There have been few human investigations.[18] The safest approach is to avoid OTC drugs and to discuss their use with the physician if symptoms cannot be relieved by natural remedies (see Chap. 36).

(Text continues on page 428)

TABLE 19–4. NATURAL REMEDIES FOR MINOR DISCOMFORTS OF PREGNANCY

Prevention	Natural Remedies	Medicines Not to Be Used*
Nausea and Vomiting		
Eat high-protein meals and fruit and drink fruit juices to avoid hypoglycemia	Eat dry bread or crackers	Antihistamines (contained in most antinausea medicines)
Eat several small meals daily	Sip soda water	
Avoid fried foods	Take a walk in fresh air	
Drink liquids between meals rather than with meals	Drink spearmint, raspberry leaf, or peppermint tea	
Get out of bed slowly, avoid sudden movements		
Eat dry bread or crackers before rising (keep by bed)		
Eat yogurt or drink milk at night or before rising		
Headache		
Get enough sleep at night and enough rest during the day	Apply a cool, wet washcloth to forehead and back of neck (some prefer warm cloth)	Narcotic analgesics
Do not go for long periods without eating	Massage neck, shoulders, face, scalp, forehead	Aspirin, Excedrin, Percogesic, Cope
Drink plenty of fluids	Take a walk in fresh air	Advil, Tylenol
Avoid things that contribute to headaches (e.g., eye strain, stuffy rooms, cigarette smoke, rushing around)	Take a warm bath	
	Find a quiet place and relax	
	Meditate or do yoga	
Difficulty Sleeping		
Exercise daily	Relax and do not worry about not sleeping; even lying in bed is restful to the body	Sleeping aids (Sleep-Eze, Nytol, Sominex, Compoz, and so forth)
Take a warm bath at bedtime	Read for a while	Sedatives
Drink hot water with lemon, or warm milk, at bedtime	Follow suggestions under prevention	Tranquilizers
Do not eat a large meal within 2–3 h of bedtime		
Decrease noise and lights		
Do relaxation exercises		
Use pillows under knees, back, or abdomen		
Avoid caffeine		
Stuffy Nose and Allergies		
Avoid allergens	Breathe steam from hot shower, pot of boiling water, or vaporizer/humidifier	Antihistamines (in most cold remedies—Contac, Coricidin, Allerest, Dristan, and so forth)
Do not smoke cigarettes, avoid smoke-filled rooms	Drink plenty of liquids	
	Use salt-water nose drops (¼ tsp salt in 1 cup warm water)	
	Use warm, moist towel on sinuses; massage sinuses	

(continued)

TABLE 19-4. NATURAL REMEDIES FOR MINOR DISCOMFORTS OF PREGNANCY *(continued)*

Prevention	Natural Remedies	Medicines Not to Be Used*
Heartburn		
Avoid foods known to cause gastric upset	Take small sips of water	Sodium base antacids (e.g., Maalox, Alka-Seltzer, Fizrin, Soda Mint, baking soda)
Avoid greasy, fried foods	Sip carbonated beverage	
Avoid highly seasoned foods	Sit upright	
Eat several small meals daily	Relax and breathe deeply for several minutes	
Avoid coffee and cigarettes	Do the "flying exercise"	
Wear loose clothes at waist	Use aluminum base antacids	
Drink 6–8 glasses water daily		
Fatigue		
Get enough sleep and rest	Take the time to rest when the body demands it	Caffeine (e.g., coffee, tea, cola drinks, stay-awake pills)
Take naps during the day	Sit with feet up whenever possible	Amphetamines
Pace daily life to provide for extra rest	Follow suggestions under Prevention	
Eat well-balanced meals		
Exercise regularly		
Leg Cramps		
Get enough calcium (milk, dark green leafy vegetables, supplements)	Sit down, straighten the leg, point or pull toes upward toward the knees	Quinine
Exercise regularly	Massage the cramped muscle	Muscle relaxants
Keep the legs warm	Walk around when able	
Take a warm bath at bedtime	Soak cramped muscle in warm water or use heating pad	
Do not point the toes when stretching		
Constipation		
Drink plenty of fluids (6–8 glasses of water daily)	Drink either hot or very cold liquid on an empty stomach	Laxatives that are other than bulk producing (best to avoid all laxatives; at least use only twice per week; taking too many laxatives causes more constipation)
Exercise regularly	Follow suggestions under Prevention	
Eat raw vegetables, cooked fruit (e.g., prune juice), 3 Tbsp bran daily, whole grain bread and cereal, oatmeal, brown rice	Use bulk-producing laxatives (e.g., Metamucil, Effersyllium)	
Caution—raw apples and coffee increase constipation		
Chew food thoroughly		
Have good bowel habits (do not force bowel movements, go when having the urge, take time for bowel movements, raise feet on stool to reduce strain)		
Varicose Veins		
Exercise regularly	Lie with feet raised several times daily	No medications
Avoid tight or binding clothes (especially garters, knee-length stockings)	Lie with feet against wall	

(continued)

TABLE 19–4. NATURAL REMEDIES FOR MINOR DISCOMFORTS OF PREGNANCY *(continued)*

Prevention	Natural Remedies	Medicines Not to Be Used*
Wear full-length support hose when standing or walking for a long time Avoid sitting or standing for a long time Wear shoes with well-padded soles to absorb shock	Wear elastic support hose (put on before rising)	
Hemorrhoids		
Prevent constipation and straining during bowel movements Follow good bowel habits Do not sit for a long time on the toilet Do Kegel's exercises regularly	Sit in warm tub for 15–20 min three to four times daily Apply dilute lemon juice or vinegar compresses, use Tucks or witch hazel compresses Use bulk-producing laxatives to keep stool soft	Local anesthetic creams (Preparation H, Americaine, Anusol)
Backache		
Maintain good posture Bend from knees when lifting Wear supportive shoes with low heels Exercise regularly Do prenatal exercises or yoga Maintain normal weight gain	Do prenatal exercises (especially the pelvic tilt and knee–chest twist) Apply heat to the lower back Have a back rub or back massage Rest the back	Analgesics Aspirin, Tylenol
Edema		
Eat high-protein foods Avoid highly salted foods Avoid standing for long periods Avoid tight clothing and constrictions of legs Rest and elevate legs two to three times daily for 20 min	Sit in warm bathtub or hot tub for 20–30 min Lie or sit with legs raised as much as possible Follow suggestions under prevention	Diuretics (prescriptions and over-the-counter water pills)

* In severe cases, the physician may prescribe a medication after weighing the benefits to the mother and risks to the fetus.

■ PREPARATIONS FOR THE BABY

As the time of delivery nears, parents become involved in planning for the baby's homecoming. The baby's layette and equipment are of special interest. The nurse should be familiar with clothing and equipment needed and should advise parents accordingly. Costs should be in keeping with the family's economic circumstances.

Layette

Baby clothing should be comfortable, lightweight, and easy to put on and launder. Any clothing that comes in contact with the infant's skin should be made of soft cotton material. Wool should be avoided because it can irritate an infant's skin. Knitted materials are preferred because they are easy to launder and can stretch sufficiently to allow more freedom in dressing the baby. Caution should be taken that the materials are fire resistant. Garments that open down the full length and fasten with ties or grippers are easier to put on. Ties or grippers are also safer than buttons.

The geographic location and climate greatly influence the selection of the infant's clothing. Size 1 shirts and gowns are recommended, because the infant grows rapidly in the first 6 months and quickly outgrows garments. It is important to remember that clothing should not inhibit the baby's normal activities.

DIAPERS

The selection of diapers should be considered from the standpoint of their comfort (soft and light in weight), absorbency, cost, and washing and drying qualities. The mother who plans to use a commercial diaper service may use either the company's diapers or her own. Disposable diapers are frequently used, but they may be more expensive in the long run than cloth diapers or a diaper service.

Nursery Equipment

In choosing the equipment, again the family's financial and social circumstances should be considered. Expense, space, and future plans all influence the selection. Furniture should be selected that will be suitable for and appeal to the child as he or she grows and develops.

Layette

Layette Necessities

Five or six shirts

Three to four dozen diapers (if diaper service is not used)

Four to six receiving blankets (These are very versatile items and can be used in various ways. For instance, they can be rolled firmly and used to support the back when the infant is on his side; in emergencies, they can used as bath towels, diaper pads, and sheets.)

Three to six nightgowns, kimonos, or sacques

Six cotton covered waterproof diaper pads (11 in × 16 in)

Two waterproof protectors for under diaper pads

Two afghans or blankets ⎱ (if climate is cold)
One bunting ⎰

Two to four soft towels (40 in × 40 in)

Two to four soft washcloths

Nursery Equipment

Basket, bassinet, or crib

Mattress (firm, flat, and smooth)

Mattress protector (waterproof)

Sheets or pillowcases for mattress

Chest or separate drawer

Cotton crib blankets

Bathtub

Diaper pail

Equipped toilet tray

Absorbent cotton or cotton balls

Baby soap (bland, white, unscented)

Rustproof safety pins

Soapdish

Bath apron (for mother)

Table for bathing or dressing

Chair (for mother)

Additional Suggestions for Layette and Equipment

Sweaters

Crib spreads

Bibs

Clothes dryer

Chest of drawers

Nursery stand

Footstool

Diaper bag (for traveling)

Disposable diapers

Nursery light

Carriage or stroller

Car seat

Study Aids

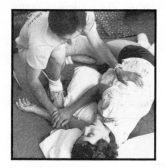

Unit IV
Assessment and Management in the Antepartum Period

CONFERENCE MATERIAL

1. A mother in her first trimester of pregnancy is undergoing a difficult divorce. She appears very anxious and upset and tells you that she sometimes feels like she is losing her mind. What do you know about the psychological and physiological effects of anxiety during pregnancy? What specific interventions would you plan to help this mother?

2. A couple comes to childbirth education classes, and the husband complains that he had symptoms of morning sickness during the first trimester and is now experiencing low back pain and aching legs. What might your counseling be for this couple?

3. A young husband complains to you that his wife's sexual desire has changed since she became pregnant. When he tells you, you note that his wife becomes flushed and tense. What would you tell this couple to reassure them about their apparent problem?

4. What childbirth education classes are available in your community? How do they compare to the "Variables to Consider in Selecting a Childbirth Class" (see display box in Chap. 17)?

5. What community resources are available for prenatal and postpartum exercise classes and parenting classes?

6. A 34-year-old woman delivered her first baby a few hours ago. She and her husband attended childbirth classes. The woman requested and received 50 mg demerol during her labor. She tells you how guilty she feels because she needed medication for pain since she and her husband had hoped to have a "natural birth." How would you respond to this patient?

7. Examine several women on their third postpartum day for diastasis recti. Depending on the results of your findings teach each woman an appropriate exercise to strengthen her abdominal muscles.

8. A 15-year-old mother from a low-income family will be going home with her baby in 2 days. She will be living with her mother and father. What specific teaching measures would you include in discharge planning for this patient?

9. Dorothea W. is a 28-year-old married mother of two, presently in the seventh month of her third pregnancy. Her husband Sam works as a printer; the children are both boys, ages 7 and 4. Dorothea quit her secretarial job last month, and plans not to work until the new baby is about 2 years of age. Her pregnancy has been progressing normally; she has experienced recent discomfort with hemorrhoids and heartburn. At her prenatal visit, you notice that she has gained 8 lb since the last visit 1 month ago, and she has moderate edema of the ankles and hands. The couple will begin childbirth classes in 2 weeks; both previous deliveries have been conscious and participative, without complications. In conducting Dorothea's prenatal visit, discuss how you would approach and manage the following areas:

- Assessment of potential occupational hazards to the fetus
- Counseling her about prevention and control of hemorrhoids and heartburn
- Evaluation of her weight gain and edema
- Assessing the family's economic situation
- Determining her educational and informational needs at this stage of pregnancy

10. Sally S. has come to the clinic for her first antepartal visit. She is 20 years old, unmarried, and is 16 weeks pregnant. She is presently unemployed and is receiving welfare assistance; she lives at home with her divorced mother and two siblings. Sally is in good general health, but is 30% overweight and smokes one and one half packs of cigarettes per day. She wants to keep the baby, and relates that her mother will help her care for it. In your antepartal assessment, what areas will receive particular attention, both psychosocial and physical? What types of problems and complications are potentially present in Sally's situation? Based on the information given, what risks can you identify for Sally, and what risks for the baby? How will you counsel Sally about weight gain during pregnancy? How will you counsel her about cigarette smoking? What types of community agency or specialist referrals might be appropriate for Sally?

11. One of the patients you have been following in the prenatal clinic, Mrs. Scott, has missed several appointments. She is a 43-year-old multipara with several moderately severe physical problems, including vulvar varicosities and gestational diabetes. Because of her missed appointments, a thorough antepartal assessment has not been done. How-

ever, the history does reveal that her last pregnancy, 3 years ago, ended in an unexplained stillbirth. Today Mrs. Scott has kept her appointment. When discussing the missed appointments, she mentions that she has been preoccupied with family troubles and difficulties with the children. She appears distracted and has a hard time keeping focused in the discussion. What specific problems will you consider as potential causes of Mrs. Scott's behavior? How will you further assess these problems? What risks are present for the fetus with each problem? What nursing intervention is appropriate, and what types of referrals might be indicated?

MULTIPLE CHOICE

Read through the entire question and place your answer on the line to the right.

1. Below are some signs, symptoms, and conditions commonly associated with pregnancy. Those that the patient might notice and describe in the first trimester of pregnancy are
    A. Amenorrhea
    B. Enlargement and tenderness of breasts
    C. Enlargement of uterus
    D. Frequent micturition
    E. Goodell's sign
Select the number corresponding to the correct letters.
    1. A and C
    2. A, B, and D
    3. B, D, and E
    4. All of the above _____

2. In pregnancy, morning sickness is most common during which of the following periods?
    A. First month
    B. First 6 weeks
    C. Sixth week to 12th week
    D. First 4 months
    E. Eighth week to 16th week _____

3. A pregnant woman seen for the first time in the antepartal clinic has a hemoglobin of 10 g. The nurse should understand that this condition is
    A. A true anemia
    B. Caused by increased blood volume
    C. Dangerous to the baby's development
    D. Predisposing to postpartal hemorrhage _____

4. Active fetal movements are usually first perceived by motion
    A. In the third month of gestation
    B. Toward the end of the fifth month
    C. Between the sixth and seventh months _____

5. Which of the following placental hormones is detected by immunologic tests for pregnancy?
    A. Estrogens
    B. Progesterone
    C. Human placental lactogen (HPL)
    D. Human chorionic gonadotropin (hCG) _____

6. During her first visit to the clinic, the mother confides to the nurse that she is afraid to have a baby. The most appropriate response of the nurse might be
    A. "Modern obstetrics makes having a baby so safe that you have absolutely nothing to fear."
    B. "Perhaps if you discussed this with a psychiatrist he would help you to overcome this feeling."
    C. "Many women feel this way, so I wouldn't be concerned about it if I were you."
    D. "I can understand that you might feel this way. What is it in particular that you are worried about?" _____

7. Pregnancy has been referred to as a critical event in the lives of parents. Which of the following descriptions best describes pregnancy?
    A. Pregnancy is always a crisis.
    B. Pregnancy is a role transition.
    C. Pregnancy is just a normal developmental stage people go through. _____

8. *Current* research on pregnancy demonstrates that
    A. Spouses or partners do not experience changes in their body image during their wives' pregnancy.
    B. Men may have the physiological symptoms of pregnancy that their mates experience.
    C. Men do not identify with their mates very well during pregnancy.
Select the number corresponding to the correct letter or letters.
    1. All of the above
    2. A and B
    3. A and C
    4. B and C
    5. C only _____

9. Several psychological tasks have to be accomplished by the mother during pregnancy. Which of the following is *not* a usual task?
    A. Preparation for physical separation from the infant
    B. Belief that she is pregnant and incorporation of the fetus into her body image
    C. Working through the anger that usually accompanies pregnancy
    D. Resolution of the identity confusions that accompany role transition _____

10. The term "laboring for relevance" refers to
    A. The mother's striving to have a relevant childbirth experience
    B. The father's attempts to perceive the paternal role as relevant to his sense of self and his repertoire of roles
    C. The couple's working together for the incorporation and integration of the fetus into their cognitive and emotional structure
    D. The partner's immersing himself in preparations for the coming labor, delivery, and parenthood _____

11. Expectant parents should consider which of the following variables when selecting a childbirth class?
   A. Class size
   B. Instructor's age
   C. Whether or not the instructor has given birth
   D. Professional credentials of instructor and type of training as a childbirth educator
   E. Amount of class hours for the fee
   Select the number corresponding to the correct letters.
   1. A, C, D, and E
   2. D and E
   3. A, D, and E
   4. A, B, D, and E
   5. All of the above _____

12. The purpose of breathing techniques for labor is to
   A. Increase pain perception
   B. Provide oxygenation
   C. Aid in relaxation
   D. Obviate the need for analgesics
   Select all that are correct. _____

13. Which exercise can help relieve low backache in pregnancy?
   A. Shoulder circling
   B. Back massage
   C. Calf stretching
   D. Pelvic rocking or pelvic tilt _____

14. Both prenatal and postpartum exercises are concerned with which of the following?
   A. Improving circulation
   B. Strengthening abdominal muscles
   C. Improving tone of pelvic floor muscles
   D. Strengthening leg muscles
   E. Improving posture
   F. Developing an awareness of relaxation of pelvic floor muscles
   Select all that are correct. _____

15. Relaxation is
   A. A learned activity
   B. A passive process
   C. An active process
   D. Requires awareness and concentration
   E. A natural reaction
   Select the number corresponding to the correct letters.
   1. A, B, D, and E
   2. A, C, D, and E
   3. A, D, and E
   4. A, C, and D
   5. A, B, and D _____

16. Which of the following statements is true regarding weight gain during pregnancy?
   A. Excessive weight gain is a cause of preeclampsia.
   B. The obese client should be advised to limit her weight gain to 10 lb or less.
   C. Inadequate weight gain during pregnancy is related to an increased incidence of low-birth-weight infants.
   D. A weight gain of 20 lb is sufficient for most women during pregnancy. _____

17. Protein needs
   A. Are decreased during pregnancy
   B. Can be met by a combination of foods from plant and animal sources
   C. Require inclusion in the diet of 20 essential amino acids
   D. Are more important than the need for other nutrients _____

18. Which of the following questions would be helpful in the dietary assessment of a pregnant woman?
   A. Where are you from?
   B. Who purchases the food for your household?
   C. Are there any foods you cannot eat?
   D. All of the above _____

19. Two physical examination procedures performed during antepartal visits that assess the condition of the fetus are
   A. Leopold's maneuvers and fetal heart beat
   B. Chadwick's sign and fundal height
   C. Fetal heart beat and fetal presentation
   D. Fundal height and fetal heart beat _____

20. Information provided by Leopold's maneuvers includes
   A. Fetal presentation
   B. Fetal position
   C. Fetal growth status
   D. Fetal heart beat
   Select the number corresponding to the correct letters.
   1. A and B
   2. B and C
   3. C and D
   4. A, B, and C _____

21. Return visits for uncomplicated pregnancies routinely include
   A. Fetal heart beat
   B. Leopold's maneuvers
   C. Measurement of fundal height
   D. Pelvic examination
   E. Examination for edema
   F. Urinalysis for glucose and protein
   Select the number corresponding to the correct letters.
   1. A, B, C, and D
   2. C, D, E, and F
   3. A, B, C, E, and F
   4. All of the above _____

22. Danger signs that should be reported immediately to the physician during pregnancy include
   A. Bleeding from vagina
   B. Loss of amniotic fluid
   C. Persistent blurred vision or light flashes

D. Severe headache
E. Abdominal pain and cramping
F. Pain and swelling of calf
Select the number corresponding to the correct letters.
1. A, B, C, and F
2. A, B, C, D, and F
3. A, B, C, E, and F
4. All of the above   _____

23. What is considered an acceptable weight gain during pregnancy for a woman at ideal body weight?
A. 20 lb
B. 30 lb
C. 40 lb
D. 50 lb   _____

24. Which statement is true regarding pregnant women who are obese?
A. Weight gain should be limited to 20 lb.
B. Weight gain should be about as much as for nonobese women.
C. Weight loss of about 10 lb should be sought.
D. Weight should be monitored carefully but no limits set.   _____

25. Hemorrhoids may be prevented or minimized during pregnancy by which measures?
A. Adequate dietary roughage to avoid constipation
B. Adequate fluids to prevent dehydration
C. Regular bowel habits to evacuate colon
D. Avoiding long periods of standing or sitting
E. Adequate exercise for muscle tone
Select the number corresponding to the correct letters.
1. A, B, and C
2. A, C, and D
3. A, B, C, and D
4. All of the above   _____

26. Risks to the fetus from maternal smoking include
A. Low birth weight
B. Premature labor and delivery
C. Hypoxia from bleeding problems (placenta previa, abruptio)
D. Congenital defects (cleft palate, heart, anencephaly)
Select the number corresponding to the correct letters.
1. A and B
2. A, B, and C
3. All of the above   _____

27. What advice should be given to pregnant women regarding alcohol consumption?
A. There is no safe level of alcohol consumption during pregnancy.
B. Less than 1 to 2 drinks per week are safe.
C. Less than 3 to 5 drinks per week are safe.
D. Less than 1 drink per day is safe.   _____

28. What is the danger of a boggy uterus?
A. Urinary retention
B. Hemorrhage
C. Severe afterpains
D. Hematomas   _____

29. Early ambulation after delivery promotes maternal health and comfort by
A. Reducing the risk of thrombophlebitis
B. Improving bladder function
C. Improving bowel elimination
D. Reducing abdominal distention
E. Reducing the incidence of postspinal headache
Select the number corresponding to the correct letters.
1. A, B, and C
2. A, B, C, and D
3. B, C, and D
4. All of the above   _____

30. How may leg cramps be prevented during pregnancy?
A. Regular exercise
B. Warm bath at bedtime
C. Not pointing toes when stretching
D. Aluminum hydroxide gel
Select the number corresponding to the correct letters.
1. A and B
2. A, B, and C
3. A and C
4. A, B, C, and D   _____

31. In evaluating edema in later pregnancy, what signs would raise your suspicion of preeclampsia?
A. Weight gain of more than 2 lb in one week
B. Edema over sacrum
C. Edema of face
D. Pretibial edema
Select the number corresponding to the correct letters.
1. A and B
2. A, B, and C
3. A, C, and D
4. A, B, C, and D   _____

32. Vaginal infection during pregnancy characterized by thick, white, curdy discharge, itching, and inflammation of the vulva is due to
A. *Candida albicans*
B. *Trichomonas vaginalis*
C. *Gardinerella*
D. *Chlamydia trachomatis*   _____

33. What general advice is given to pregnant women about use of drugs?
A. All medications are to be minimized during pregnancy.
B. The fetus is particularly susceptible to teratogenic effects during the first trimester.
C. Ingestion of drugs at any time during pregnancy has potential for fetal damage.

D. Many over-the-counter drugs have not been thoroughly investigated for their fetal effects; the safest approach is to avoid them.

E. Medications prescribed by the physician are safe during pregnancy.

Select the number corresponding to the correct letters.

1. A, B, and C
2. B, C, and D
3. A, B, C, and D
4. All of the above _____

34. Which of the following immunizations are contraindicated during pregnancy?

A. Rubeola
B. Mumps
C. Rubella
D. Tetanus toxoid

Select the number corresponding to the correct letters.

1. A and B
2. A, B, and C
3. A and C
4. A, B, C, and D _____

35. Natural remedies to prevent or control nausea during pregnancy include

A. Dry toast, plain popcorn
B. Frequent, light meals
C. Separate liquids from dry foods
D. Spearmint, raspberry, or peppermint tea
E. High-protein meals and fruit

Select the number corresponding to the correct letters.

1. A, B, and C
2. A, B, C, and D
3. A, B, C, and E
4. All of the above _____

36. Backache during pregnancy may be prevented or relieved by

A. Pelvic tilt while sitting, standing, and walking
B. Sitting in tailor or lotus positions
C. Avoiding fatigue
D. Using proper body mechanics in lifting and moving
E. Daily exercise such as walking, swimming, or stretching

Select the number corresponding to the correct letters.

1. A, B, and C
2. B, C, and D
3. C, D, and E
4. All of the above _____

37. Varicose veins during pregnancy may be treated by

A. The right angle position for 5 minutes several times per day
B. Wearing elastic support stockings daily
C. Avoiding constricting clothing
D. Sclerosing injections into the veins
E. Anticoagulants to prevent thrombosis

Select the number corresponding to the correct letters.

1. A, B, and C
2. B, C, and D
3. B, C, and E
4. All of the above _____

38. When can the postpartal mother take tub baths?

A. In 1 week
B. In 2 weeks
C. In 3 weeks
D. In 4 weeks _____

39. How can the nurse determine that the patient is adequately emptying the bladder?

A. The amount of voiding is 100 ml or more.
B. The uterus is not displaced.
C. The mother fails to report suprapubic discomfort.
D. Lochia is normal in amount.
E. The bladder is not palpable.

Select the number corresponding to the correct letters.

1. A, B, and C
2. A, B, C, and D
3. A, B, D, and E
4. All of the above _____

40. Signs and symptoms of thrombophlebitis include

A. Unilateral calf swelling
B. Unilateral erythema and tenderness of calf
C. Pain in calf on flexion of foot (Homan's sign)
D. Reduced or absent pulses in foot on affected side

Select the number corresponding to the correct letters.

1. A and B
2. A, B, and C
3. A, B, C, and D _____

41. Contraceptive counseling for nonlactating postpartal mothers includes

A. Although unlikely, ovulation can occur before 6 weeks.
B. Short-term contraception using foam or jelly and condom is preferred.
C. IUD insertion or oral contraceptives should be delayed until 6 weeks.
D. There is no reason to delay intercourse after lochia has ceased and there is no perineal discomfort.
E. There are often emotional benefits for couples by resuming intercourse early following birth.

Select the number corresponding to the correct letters.

1. A, B, and C
2. A, B, C, and D
3. All of the above _____

DISCUSSION

42. Why is regular exercise so important during pregnancy? What are some exercises the nurse could advise the mother to do?

43. Name three occupational hazards to which women are frequently exposed, and describe the dangers to the fetus or mother from these.

44. Describe preventive measures in breast care during pregnancy that help mothers avoid nipple cracking and infection later while nursing.

UNIT V

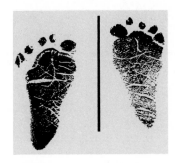

Assessment and Management in the Intrapartum Period

20

Assessment of the Passageway and Passenger

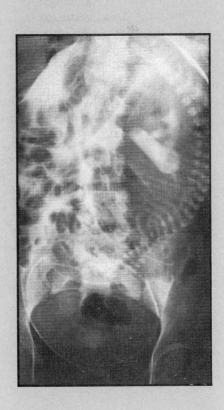

The process of labor can be divided into three components, each of which must be normal for progress to be made and birth to occur. These components may be described as the powers (forces) of labor, the passenger, and the passageway. The powers, including uterine contractions with the addition of maternal "bearing down" during the second stage, must be of adequate strength with coordination of muscle activity. These forces propel an irregular object, the infant or *passenger*, through the birth canal or *passageway*. The passenger must be of appropriate size and shape and able to undergo the necessary maneuvers to pass through the different dimensions of the birth canal. The passageway must also be of normal size and configuration, not presenting any undue obstacles to the descent, rotations, and expulsion of the baby. The passageway and passenger are discussed in this chapter, and the powers are discussed in Chapter 21. When nature tries to propel the fetus through the birth canal and fails to do so, there are problems in the powers, the passenger, or the passageway. These problems are discussed in Chapter 38.

■ THE PASSAGEWAY

The entire childbirth process centers on the safe passage of the fully developed fetus through the pelvis. Slight irregularities in the structure of the pelvis may delay the progress of labor, and any marked deformity may render delivery through natural passages impossible.

True Pelvis

True and false pelves were discussed briefly in Chapter 8. The difference between the two is illustrated in Figure 20-1. It is the true pelvis that concerns us here.

The true pelvis, or lower part, forms the bony canal through which the fetus must pass during parturition. It is divided into three parts: an inlet or brim, an outlet, and a cavity.

PELVIC INLET

Continuous from the sacral promontory and extending along the ilium on each side in circular fashion is a ridge called the *linea terminalis*, or brim (see Fig. 20-1A). This bounds an area or plane, the *inlet*, so named because it is the entryway or inlet through which the fetal head must pass to enter the true pelvis.

The pelvic inlet, sometimes called the pelvic brim or superior strait, divides the false pelvis from the true pelvis. It is heart shaped, and the promontory of the sacrum forms a slight projection into it from behind (see Fig. 20-1B). Generally, it is widest from side to side and narrowest from back to front (i.e., from the sacral promontory to the symphysis). It should be noted that the fetal head enters the inlet of the average pelvis with its longest diameter (anteroposterior) in the transverse diameter of the pelvis (Fig. 20-2A). In other words, the greatest diameter of the head accommodates itself to the greatest diameter of the inlet (Fig. 20-2B).

Because the inlet is entirely surrounded by bone, it cannot be directly measured with the examining fingers in a living woman. However, the measurements of its

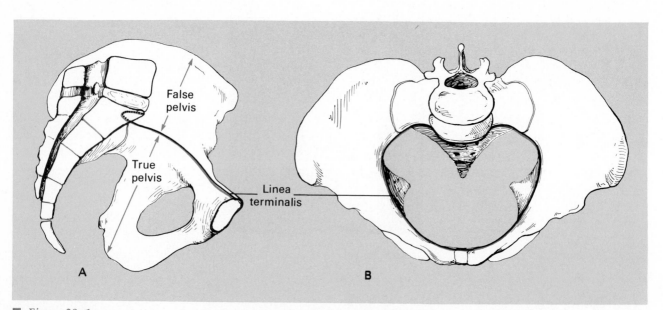

■ *Figure 20-1*
(A) Side view of true and false pelvis. (B) Front view showing linea terminalis (pelvic brim).

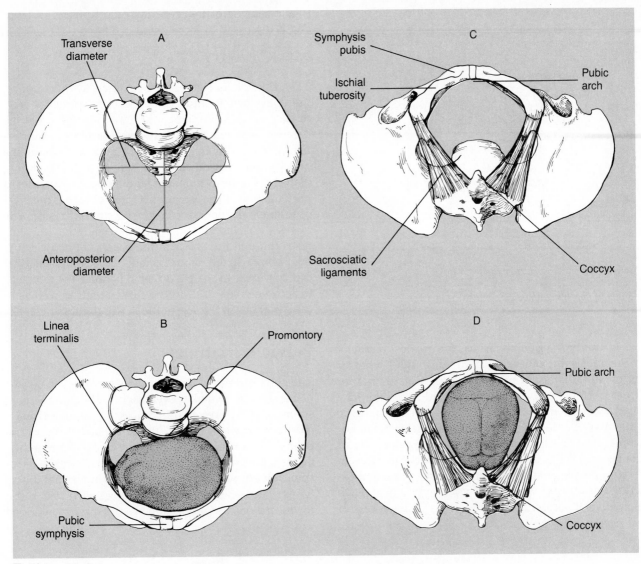

■ *Figure 20–2*
Views of pelvic inlet and outlet with fetal head in place. (A) Inlet of normal female pelvis showing transverse and anteroposterior diameters. (B) Largest diameter of the fetal head passing through the largest diameter of the inlet; therefore, it enters transversely. (C) Pelvic outlet and sacrosciatic ligaments. (D) Largest diameter of the fetal head passing through the largest diameter of the outlet; therefore, it passes through anteroposteriorly.

anteroposterior diameter can be estimated on the basis of the diagonal conjugate diameter (Fig. 20-3). The measurement of the diameters is important, because variations from the normal (e.g., smaller in size or flattened) may cause grave difficulty at the time of labor (see Chap. 25).

PELVIC OUTLET

When viewed from below, the *pelvic outlet* is a space bounded in front by the symphysis pubis and the pubic arch, at the sides by the ischial tuberosities, and behind by the coccyx and the greater sacrosciatic ligaments (see

Fig. 20-2C). The front half of the outlet resembles a triangle, the base of which is the distance between the ischial tuberosities, and the other two sides of which are represented by the pubic arch. From an obstetric point of view, this triangle is of great importance because the fetal head must use this space to exit from the pelvis and the mother's body (see Fig. 20-2D). Nature has provided a wide pubic arch in females, whereas in males it is narrow (Fig. 20-4). If the pubic arch in women were as narrow as it is in men, vaginal delivery would be extremely difficult because the fetal head, unable to traverse the narrow anterior triangle of the outlet, would be forced backward against the coccyx and the sacrum, where its progress would be impeded.

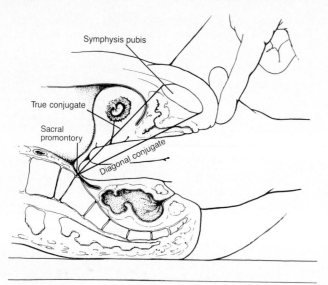

■ *Figure 20–3*
Method of obtaining diagonal conjugate diameter.

In the typical female pelvis, the greatest diameter of the inlet is the transverse (from side to side), whereas the greatest diameter of the outlet is the anteroposterior (from front to back, see Fig. 20-2*A* and *C*). As the fetal head emerges from the pelvis, it passes through the outlet in the anteroposterior position, again accommodating its greatest diameter to the greatest diameter of the passage. Because the fetal head enters the pelvis in the transverse position and emerges in the anteroposterior, it is obvious that it must rotate approximately 90 degrees as it passes through the pelvis. This process of

rotation is one of the most important phases of labor and is discussed in more detail in Chapter 21.

PELVIC CAVITY

The *pelvic cavity* is the space between the inlet above, the outlet below, and the anterior, the posterior, and the lateral walls of the pelvis. The upper portion of the pelvic canal is practically cylindrical, and the lower portion is curved. It is important to note the axis of the cavity when viewed from the side (Fig. 20-5). During delivery, the head must descend along the downward prolongation of the axis until it almost reaches the level of the ischial spines and begins to curve forward. The axis of the cavity determines the direction that the fetus takes through the pelvis in the process of delivery. As might be expected, labor is made more complicated by this curvature in the pelvic canal because the fetus has to accommodate itself to the curved path as well as to the variations in the size of the cavity at different levels.

Pelvic Variations

The pelvis presents great individual variations: no two pelves are exactly alike. Even clients with normal measurements may present differences in contour and muscular development that influence the actual size of the pelvis. These differences are due in part to heredity, disease, injury, and development. Heredity may be responsible for passing on many racial and sexual differences. Diseases such as tuberculosis and rickets cause malformations. Accidents and injuries during childhood

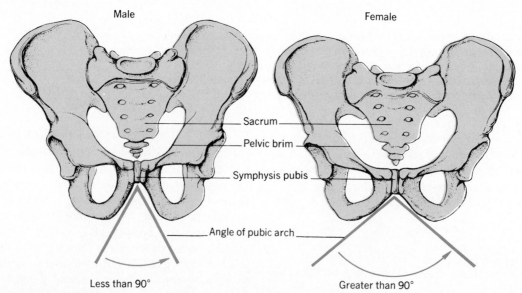

Male   Female

Sacrum
Pelvic brim
Symphysis pubis
Angle of pubic arch

Less than 90°   Greater than 90°

■ *Figure 20–4*
Comparison of the male and female pelvis. (Left) The male pelvis is narrow and compact; the pelvic arch is less than a right angle. (Right) The female pelvis is broad and capacious; the pubic arch is greater than a right angle.

There are several types of pelves. Even pelves whose measurements are normal differ greatly in the shape of the inlet, in the proximity of the greatest transverse diameter of the inlet to the sacral promontory, in the size of the sacrosciatic notch, and in their general architecture. These characteristics have been used in establishing a classification of pelves, which is useful in understanding the mechanisms of labor. The four main types according to this classification are shown in Figure 20-6. The gynecoid pelvis is most common, found in almost 50% of women, and best suited for childbearing. The anthropoid pelvis is found in nearly 50% of nonwhite women and 25% of white women. The android pelvis and platypellic pelvis are less common. The manner in which the fetus passes through the birth canal and, consequently, the type of labor vary considerably in each pelvic type.

In addition, many pelvic types result from abnormal narrowing of one or the other diameters. These contracted pelves are described in Chapter 38.

In comparing male and female pelves, several differences are observed (see Fig. 20-4). The most conspicuous difference is in the pubic arch, which has a much wider angle in women. The symphysis is shorter in women, and the border of the arch probably is more everted. Although the female pelvis is more shallow, it is more capacious, much lighter in structure, and smoother. The male pelvis is deep, compact, conical, and rough in texture, particularly at the site of muscle attachments. Both males and females start life with pelves that are identical in type; the major differences do not appear until puberty and are created by sex hormones. (For the definition and description of the sex hormones, see Chap. 8.)

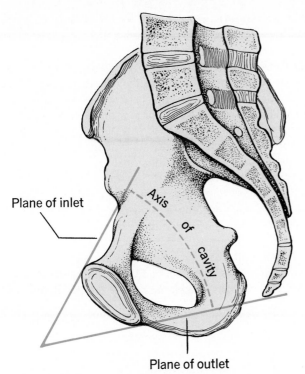

■ *Figure 20–5*
Pelvic cavity showing plane of inlet and outlet. The direction the fetus takes through the pelvis is determined by the axis of the cavity.

or at maturity result in deformities of the pelvis or other parts of the body that affect the pelvis. Adequate nutrition and well-formed posture habits and exercise have much influence on the development of the pelvis, which is completed at approximately 20 to 25 years, when ossification is concluded.

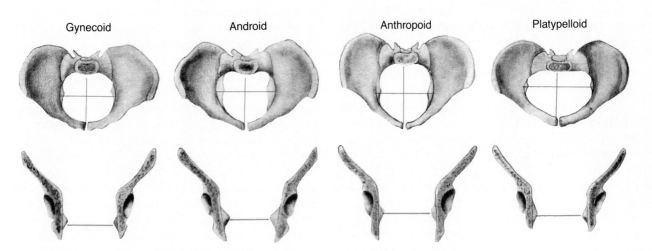

■ *Figure 20–6*
Caldwell-Maloy classification of pelvic types. (Top) The typical shape of the inlet for each type is shown. A line has been drawn through the widest transverse diameter, dividing the inlet into an anterior and posterior segment. The longitudinal line illustrates the anteroposterior diameter of the inlet. (Bottom) The typical interspinous diameter of each type is depicted.

Assessment: Pelvic Measurements

The pelvis of every pregnant woman should be measured accurately in the antepartal period to determine whether or not there is anything about the condition of the mother's pelvis that may complicate the delivery. This examination is a part of the antepartal evaluation. It is most useful to know in advance whether there are any abnormalities in the size or configuration of the pelvis, and this information is most readily and appropriately obtained well in advance of the onset of labor.

TYPES OF PELVIC MEASUREMENTS

Internal pelvic measurements, made manually, are an important means of estimating the size of the pelvis. These are optimally performed close to the 34th to 36th week of gestation when increased joint mobility and soft-tissue distensibility make the procedures easier and more comfortable for the client.[1] A number of external pelvic measurements were recorded in the past. Most of these procedures are considered of dubious value and are no longer used, with the exception of measurement of the outlet. In many abnormal pelves, the most marked deformity affects the anteroposterior diameter of the inlet.[1]

Diagonal Conjugate. Internal pelvic measurements are made to determine the actual diameters of the inlet. The chief internal measurement taken is the *diagonal conjugate*, or the distance between the sacral promontory and the lower margin of the symphysis pubis. The client should be placed on her back on the examining table, with her knees drawn up and her feet supported by stirrups. Two fingers are inserted into the vagina and, before the diagonal conjugate is measured, the contour of the pelvis is evaluated by palpation. Included in this evaluation are the height of the symphysis pubis, the shape of the pubic arch, the motility of the coccyx, the inclination of the anterior wall of the sacrum and the side walls of the pelvis, and the prominence of the ischial spines.

To obtain the length of the diagonal conjugate, the two fingers passed into the vagina are pressed inward and upward as far as possible until the middle finger rests on the sacral promontory. The point on the back of the hand just under the symphysis is marked by putting the index finger of the other hand on the exact point (see Fig. 20-3). The fingers are withdrawn and measured. The distance from the tip of the middle finger to the point marked represents the *diagonal conjugate measurement*. This distance may be measured with a rigid measuring scale attached to the wall or with a pelvimeter. If the measurement is greater than 11.5 cm,

it is justifiable to assume that the pelvic inlet is of adequate size for childbirth.

True Conjugate. An extremely important internal diameter is the *true conjugate* or the conjugata vera, which is the distance between the posterior aspect of the symphysis pubis and the promontory of the sacrum. However, direct measurement of this diameter can only be made by means of an x-ray study; consequently, it has to be estimated from the diagonal conjugate measurement. It is believed that if 1.5 to 2 cm, according to the height and the inclination of the symphysis pubis, is deducted from the length of the diagonal conjugate, the true conjugate is obtained. For example, if the diagonal conjugate measures 12.5 cm and the symphysis pubis is considered to be "average," the conjugata vera may be estimated as being about 11 cm. In this method, the problem consists of estimating the length of one side of a triangle, the conjugata vera; the other two sides, the diagonal conjugate and the height of the symphysis pubis, are known. If the symphysis pubis is high and has a marked inclination, the examiner takes this into consideration and may deduct 2 cm.

The length of the conjugata vera is of utmost importance, because it is the smallest diameter of the inlet through which the fetal head must pass. Indeed, the main purpose in measuring the diagonal conjugate is to give an estimate of the size of the conjugata vera.

Obstetric Conjugate. The term *obstetric conjugate* is used to identify a diameter that begins at the sacral promontory and terminates on the inner surface of the symphysis pubis, a few millimeters below its upper margin. The obstetric conjugate is the shortest diameter through which the fetal head must pass as it descends into the true pelvis. It normally measures 10 cm or more but may be shortened in abnormal pelves. A distinction is rarely made between the conjugata vera and the obstetric conjugate, except in pelvimetry.

Biischial Diameter. Next to the diagonal conjugate, the most important clinical dimension of the pelvis is the transverse diameter of the outlet, the diameter between the ischial tuberosities. This is sometimes called the biischial diameter or intertuberous diameter. A measurement greater than 8 cm is considered adequate. The biischial diameter is determined by placing a closed fist against the perineum between the innermost and lowermost aspect of the ischial tuberosities, on a level with the lower border of the anus (Fig. 20-7). The diameter of the closed fist, which has been previously measured, can be used as a reference; generally it is wider than 8 cm. The shape of the subpubic arch also can be evaluated by palpating the pubic rami from the subpubic

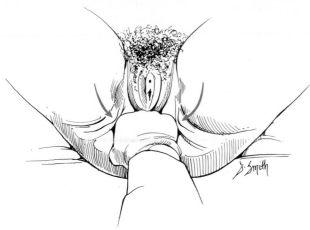

■ *Figure 20–7*

Measurement of the bi-ischial diameter. The distance across the top of a closed fist can be measured and this used as a frame of reference to estimate the distance between the ischial tuberosities, indicated by the arrows. (Cunningham FC MacDonald PC, Gant NF: Williams Obstetrics, 18th ed. Norwalk, CT, Appleton & Lange, 1989)

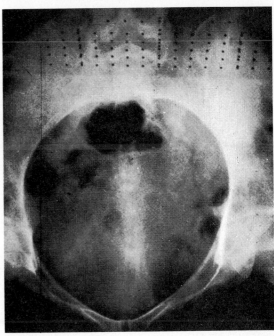

■ *Figure 20–8*

Pelvic inlet roentgenogram. The scale represents corrected centimeters for various levels of the pelvic canal. The top line is used for measuring the diameters of the inlet. The other levels are established on the lateral roentgenogram. Pelvic morphology is readily established by viewing both lateral and inlet views. This is known as Thoms' technique.

area to the ischial tuberosities. This procedure is performed with the client in the lithotomy position and the legs widely separated.

X-RAY PELVIMETRY

Although x-ray pelvimetry is used less frequently than in the past, it remains an important and accurate means of determining pelvic size in certain clinical circumstances. The method subjects the maternal ovaries and fetal gonads to a certain amount of radiation; however, the slight risk from exposure appears justifiable whenever information critical to the welfare of the fetus or mother is likely to be obtained.[2] The American College of Obstetricians and Gynecologists and the American College of Radiology have endorsed and recommended limited application of this technique.[3,4] The main reason for performing x-ray pelvimetry should be to determine the safety of vaginal deliveries for breech babies.[5] Pelvimetry also may be indicated to evaluate women with a history of previous injury or disease that could have affected the bony pelvis. X-ray pelvimetry is no longer considered necessary in the management of a labor with a cephalic fetal presentation in which the mother is suspected of having pelvic contraction.

A variety of pelvimetry techniques have been developed to provide exact mensuration of the inlet and the interischial spinous diameter of the midpelvis (Fig. 20-8), as well as the anteroposterior dimensions of the pelvis including the obstetric conjugate (Fig. 20-9). It is

also possible to gain an impression of the size of the fetal head.

OTHER TECHNIQUES: COMPUTED TOMOGRAPHY (CT SCANNING) AND MAGNETIC RESONANCE IMAGING

Digital radiographs obtained with computed tomographic (CT) scanners also are being used to measure pelvic diameters and to evaluate fetal presentation. The anteroposterior digital radiograph provides clear visualization of the attitude of the fetal head and position of the limbs, as well as measurement of the transverse diameter of the pelvic inlet. The lateral digital radiograph is used to measure the anteroposterior diameter of the pelvic inlet and the posterior sagittal diameter of the midpelvis. With the CT system, the fetus is exposed to approximately one third of the radiation used in x-ray pelvimetry.[5] Other advantages include greater accuracy of CT scanning as compared to conventional x-ray pelvimetry, increased client comfort, and simplicity in performing the procedure.[6] For digital pelvimetry the client lies supine on the CT table, which is positioned so the geometric center of the pelvis corresponds with

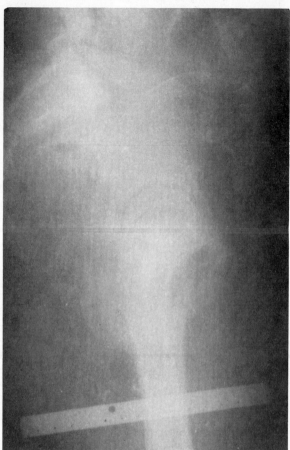

■ *Figure 20–9*
Lateral roentgenogram. The scale represents corrected centimeters in the midplane of the body. The various diameters may be measured with calipers. The lateral morphologic aspects are readily visualized.

the geometric center of the CT gantry circle. Less than 10 minutes are generally required for this procedure.

Magnetic resonance imaging (MRI) provides another method for obtaining accurate pelvic measurements and complete imaging of the fetus. Although this method benefits the client by eliminating exposure to ionizing radiation, it is expensive, time-consuming, and requires equipment that is not available in many health-care settings.

■ THE PASSENGER

Even in an adequately sized pelvic outlet, there may be difficulties in delivery of the passenger if the fetus is too large or in a difficult position. There are various means of assessing the fetal head, fetal lie, fetal attitude, fetal presentation, and fetal position.

Fetal Head

From an obstetric viewpoint, the head is the most important part of the fetus. If it can pass through the pelvic canal safely, there is usually no difficulty in delivering the rest of the body, although occasionally the shoulders may cause trouble.

The cranium, or skull, is made up of eight bones. Four of the bones—the sphenoid, the ethmoid, and the two temporal bones—lie at the base of the cranium, are closely united, and are of little obstetric interest. On the other hand, the four bones forming the upper part of the cranium—the frontal, the occipital, and the two parietal bones—are of great importance. These bones are not knit closely together at the time of birth but are separated by membranous interspaces called *sutures*. The intersections of these sutures are known as *fontanels* (Fig. 20-10).

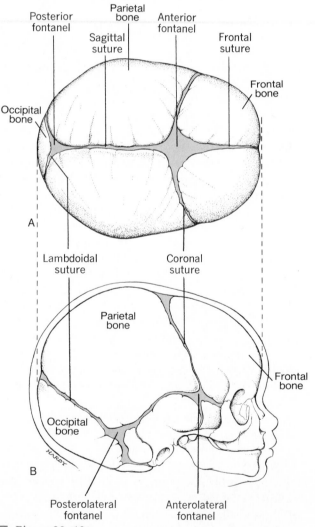

■ *Figure 20–10*
Fetal skull showing fontanels, bones, and sutures. (A) Superior aspect. (B) Lateral aspect.

By means of this formation of the fetal skull, the bones can overlap each other somewhat during labor and so diminish materially the size of the head during its passage through the pelvis. This process of overlapping is called "molding," and after a long labor with a large baby and a snug pelvis, the head often is so definitely molded that several days may elapse before it returns to its normal shape.

The most important sutures are the sagittal, between the two parietal bones; the frontal, between the two frontal bones; the coronal, between the frontal and parietal bones; and the lambdoid, between the posterior margins of the parietal bones and the upper margin of the occipital bone. The temporal sutures, which separate the parietal and the temporal bones on either side, are unimportant in obstetrics because they are covered by fat parts and cannot be felt on the living baby.

The important fontanels are the anterior and the posterior. The anterior fontanel is large and diamond shaped and is located at the intersection of the sagittal and the coronal sutures; the small triangular posterior fontanel lies at the junction of the sagittal and the lambdoid suture. The sutures and the posterior fontanel ossify shortly after birth, but the anterior fontanel remains open until the child is over a year old, constituting the familiar "soft spot" just above the forehead of an infant.

By feeling or identifying one or another of the sutures or fontanels and considering its relative position in the pelvis, one is able to determine accurately the position of the head in relation to the pelvis.

FETAL SKULL MEASUREMENT

The principal measurements of the fetal skull are shown in Figure 20-11. The most important transverse diameter is the biparietal; it is the distance between the biparietal protuberances and represents the greatest width of the head. It measures, on an average, 9.5 to 9.8 cm.

There are three important anteroposterior diameters of the fetal skull: the suboccipito-bregmatic, which extends from the undersurface of the occiput to the center of the anterior fontanel and measures about 9.5 cm; the occipitofrontal, which extends from the root of the nose to the occipital prominence and measures about 12 cm; and the occipitomental, which extends from the chin to the posterior fontanel and averages about 13.5 cm.

When the head is in complete flexion and the chin is resting on the thorax, the smallest diameter, the suboccipito-bregmatic, presents itself into the pelvis; whereas, if the fetal head is extended or bent back (flexion is absent), the greatest anteroposterior diameter presents itself to the pelvic inlet. Herein lies the great importance of flexion; the more the head is flexed, the smaller is the anteroposterior diameter that enters the

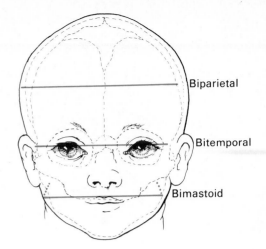

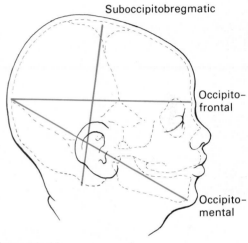

■ *Figure 20–11*
Fetal skull showing various diameters.

pelvis. This basic principle is shown in diagrammatic form in Figure 20-12.

Fetal Lie

The lie of the fetus refers to the relation of the long axis of the fetus to that of the mother. Longitudinal lies are present in over 99% of labors at term.[2] When the long axis of the fetus is approximately perpendicular to that of the mother, the condition is referred to as a transverse lie. When it forms an acute angle in relation to the axis of the mother, it becomes an oblique lie. An oblique lie is usually converted during the course of early labor to either a longitudinal or a transverse lie. The common causes of the transverse lie are abnormal relaxation of the abdominal wall due to grand multiparity, pelvic contraction, and placenta previa.

Fetal Attitude

The attitude of the fetus means the relation of the fetal parts to one another. The most striking characteristic of

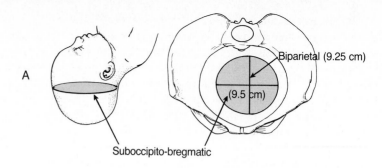

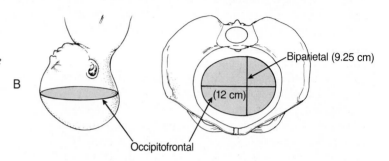

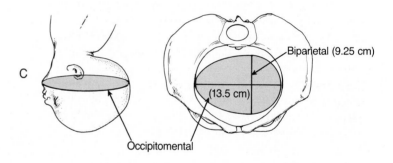

■ *Figure 20–12*
(A) Complete flexion allows the smallest diameter of the head to enter the pelvis. (B) Moderate extension causes the larger diameter to enter the pelvis. (C) Marked extension forces the largest diameter against the pelvic brim, but the head is too large to enter the pelvis.

the fetal habitus is flexion. The spinal column is bowed forward, the head is flexed with the chin against the sternum, and the arms are flexed and folded against the chest. The lower extremities also are flexed; the thighs are on the abdomen, and the calves are against the posterior aspect of the thighs. In this state of flexion the fetus assumes a roughly ovoid shape, occupies the smallest possible space, and conforms to the shape of the uterus. In this attitude it is about half as long as if it were completely stretched out. However, there are times when the fetus assumes a different position.

Fetal Presentation

The term *presentation* or *presenting part* is used to designate that portion of the infant's body that lies nearest the internal os, or in other words, that portion that is felt by the examining fingers when they are introduced into the cervix. When the presenting part is known by abdominal palpation, it is possible to determine the re-

lation between the long axis of the baby's body and that of the mother (Fig. 20-13).

Head or *cephalic presentations* are the most common; they are seen in 96% to 97% of all cases at term. Cephalic presentations are divided into groups according to the relation of the infant's head to its body. The most common is the *vertex presentation*, in which the head is sharply flexed so that the chin is in contact with the thorax; thus, the vertex is the presenting part. The *face presentation*, in which the neck is sharply extended so that the occiput and the back come in contact, is more rarely observed.

Breech presentation is the next most common; it is present in about 3% to 4% of cases at term. The incidence of breech increases in preterm fetuses, multiple gestation, and in women with a history of previous breech delivery. In breech presentation, the thighs may be flexed and the legs extended over the anterior surface of the body (*frank breech presentation*), or the thighs may be flexed on the abdomen and the legs on the thighs (*full breech presentation*), or one or both feet may be the lowest part (*foot* or *footling presentation*).

When the fetus lies crosswise in the uterus, it is in a transverse lie and the shoulder is the presenting part— *shoulder presentation.* Shoulder presentations are relatively uncommon, and, with rare exceptions, the spontaneous birth of a fully developed child is impossible in a "persistent transverse lie."

Fetal Position

In addition to knowing the presenting part of the baby, it is important to know the exact position of the presenting part in relation to the pelvis. This relationship is determined by finding the position of certain points on the presenting surface and relating these to the four imaginary divisions or regions of the pelvis. For this purpose, the pelvis is considered to be divided into quadrants: left anterior, left posterior, right anterior, and right posterior. These divisions aid in indicating whether the presenting part is directed toward the right side or the left side and toward the front or the back of the pelvis.

Certain points on the presenting surface of the baby have been arbitrarily chosen as points of direction in determining the exact relation to the presenting part of the quadrants of the pelvis. In vertex presentations, the occiput is the guiding point; in face presentations, the chin (mentum); in breech presentations, the sacrum; and in shoulder presentations, the scapula (acromion process).

Position has to do with the relation of some arbitrarily chosen portion of the fetus to the right or the left side of the mother's pelvis. Thus, in a vertex presentation, the back of the head (occiput) may point to the front or to the back of the pelvis. The occiput rarely points directly forward or backward in the median line until the second stage of labor, but usually it is directed to one side or the other.

The various positions are usually expressed by abbreviations made up of the first letter of each word that describes the position. Thus, left occipitoanterior is abbreviated L.O.A. This means that the head is presenting with the occiput directed toward the left side of the mother and toward the front part of the pelvis. If the occiput is directed straight to the left with no deviation toward front or back of the pelvis, it is termed left occipitotransverse, or L.O.T. The occiput might also be directed toward the back or posterior quadrant of the pelvis, in which case the position is left occipitoposterior, or L.O.P. There are also three corresponding positions on the right side: R.O.A., R.O.T., and R.O.P.

The occipital anterior positions are considered the most favorable for both mother and baby, and of these, the L.O.A. position is most common.

The same system of terminology is used for face and breech presentations, as illustrated in Figure 20-13.

Although it is customary to speak of all "transverse lies" of the fetus simply as shoulder presentations, the terminology sometimes used to express position in the shoulder presentation is L.A.D.A.—left acromiodorso-anterior, L.A.D.P.—left acromiodorso-posterior, R.A.D.A.—right acromiodorso-anterior, and R.A.D.P.—right acromiodorso-posterior. Left acromiodorso-anterior (L.A.D.A.) means that the acromion is to the mother's left and the back is anterior.

ASSESSMENT

Assessment of fetal position is made in five ways: abdominal palpation, vaginal examination, combined auscultation and examination, ultrasound, and, in certain doubtful cases, the roentgenogram. The first three are discussed here. Ultrasound and roentgenograms are discussed in Chapter 42.

Palpation. It is extremely helpful to palpate the abdomen before listening to the fetal heart tones. The region of the abdomen in which the fetal heart is heard varies according to the presentation and the extent to which the presenting part has descended. The location of the fetal heart sounds by itself does not give important information as to the presentation and the position of the child, but it sometimes reinforces the results obtained by palpation. To obtain satisfactory information by abdominal palpation for the determination of fetal position, the examination should be made systematically by following the four *Leopold maneuvers* (Fig. 20-14).

The client should empty her bladder before the procedure begins. This not only contributes to her comfort but also aids in gaining more accurate results in the latter part of the examination. The client's abdomen should be observed before palpation is done. The examination is performed with the client lying flat on her back, with her knees flexed to relax the abdominal muscles. The examiner should lay both hands gently and, at first, flat on the abdomen. If done in any other manner than this, or if the hands are not warm, the stimulation of the fingers causes the abdominal muscles to contract. One should become accustomed to palpating the uterus in a definite, methodical way.

FIRST MANEUVER. The examiner should ascertain what is lying at the fundus of the uterus by feeling the upper abdomen with both hands (see Fig. 20-14A). Generally, one finds that there is a mass, which is either the head or the buttocks (breech) of the fetus. The pole of the fetus can be ascertained by observing the following three points:

1. Its relative consistency. The head is harder than the breech.
2. Its shape. The head is round and hard, and the transverse groove of the neck may be felt; the

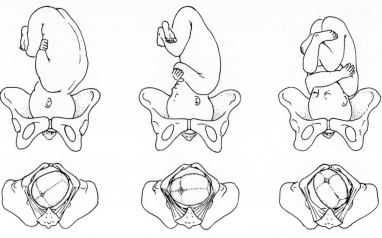

Left Occipitoanterior (LOA)   Left Occipitotransverse (LOT)   Left Occipitoposterior (LOP)

Vertex presentations

■ *Figure 20–13*
Fetal presentations. (Redrawn from Benson RC: Handbook of Obstetrics and Gynecology, 7th ed. Los Altos, CA, Lange Medical Publications, 1980.)

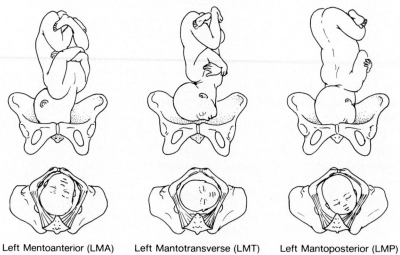

Left Mentoanterior (LMA)   Left Mantotransverse (LMT)   Left Mantoposterior (LMP)

Face Presentations

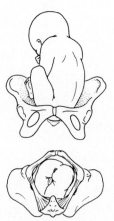
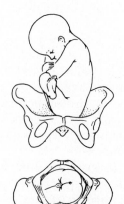
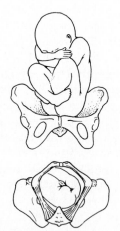

Left Sacroanterior (LSA)   Left Sacrotransverse (LST)   Left Sacroposterior (LSP)

Breach Presentations

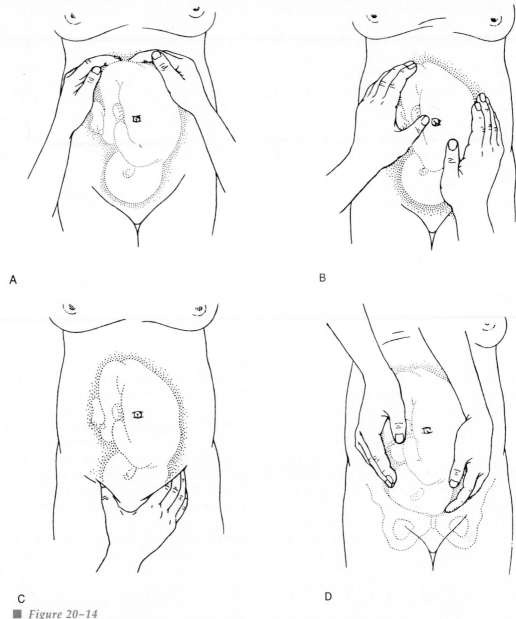

A

B

C

D

■ *Figure 20–14*
Leopold maneuvers, or palpation of fetal position. (A) First maneuver. (B) Second maneuver. (C)
Third maneuver. (D) Fourth maneuver.

breech has no groove and usually feels more angular.

3. Mobility. The head moves independently of the trunk, but the breech moves only with the trunk; the ability of head to be moved back and forth against the examining fingers is spoken of as ballottement.

SECOND MANEUVER. Having determined whether the head or the breech is in the fundus, the next step is to locate the back of the fetus in relation to the right and left sides of the mother. Still facing the client, the examiner places the palmar surfaces of both hands on either side of the abdomen and applies gentle but deep pressure (see Fig. 20-14B). If the hand on one side of the abdomen remains still to steady the uterus, a slightly circular motion with the flat surface of the fingers on the other hand can gradually palpate the opposite side from the top to the lower segment of the uterus to feel the fetal outline. To palpate the other side, the functions of the hands are reversed (i.e., the hand that was used to palpate remains steady and the other hand palpates the opposite side of the uterus).

A smooth, hard, resistant plane, the back, is felt on one side; on the other, numerous angular nodulations are palpated, the knees and the elbows of the fetus.

THIRD MANEUVER. The third maneuver is an effort to find the head at the pelvic inlet and to determine its mobility. It should be conducted by gently grasping the lower portion of the abdomen, just above the symphysis pubis, between the thumb and the fingers of one hand and pressing together (see Fig. 20-14C). If the presenting part is not engaged, a movable body is felt, which is usually the head.

FOURTH MANEUVER. The fourth maneuver is conducted while facing the client's feet. The tips of the first three fingers are placed on both sides of the midline about 2 inches above Poupart's ligament. Pressure is made downward and in the direction of the birth canal, the movable skin of the abdomen being carried downward along with the fingers (see Fig. 20-14D). The fingers of one hand meet no obstruction and can be carried downward well under Poupart's ligament; these fingers glide over the nape of the baby's neck. The other hand, however, usually meets an obstruction an inch or so above Poupart's ligament; this is the brow of the baby and is usually spoken of as the "cephalic prominence." This maneuver gives several kinds of information, such as the following:

1. If the findings are as described above, it means that the baby's head is well flexed.
2. Confirmatory information is obtained about the location of the back, as naturally the back is on the opposite side from the brow of the baby, except in the uncommon cases of face presentation, in which the cephalic prominence and the back are on the same side.
3. If the cephalic prominence is easily palpated, as if it were just under the skin, a posterior position of the occiput is suggested.
4. The location of the cephalic prominence tells how far the head has descended into the pelvis. This maneuver is of most value if the head has engaged, but may yield no information with a floating, poorly flexed head.

Vaginal Examination. During a vaginal examination, the fontanels and the suture lines of the fetal skull are identified. Before the onset of labor, the vaginal examination gives limited information concerning the position of the fetus because the cervix is closed and the landmarks on the fetal head are not palpable. However, during labor, after dilatation of the cervix, important information about the position of the fetus and the degree of flexion of its head can be obtained, by palpating and identifying the fontanels through the dilated os. When the head is well flexed, the posterior fontanel is easily identified by palpating the junction point of the

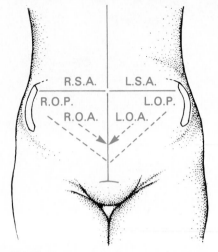

■ *Figure 20–15*
Fetal heart tone locations on the abdominal wall indicate possible corresponding fetal positions and the effects of the internal rotation of the fetus.

sagittal suture and the two lambdoid sutures. When the fetal head is well flexed, the anterior fontanel is located well within the birth canal. It is diamond shaped and has four sutures that lead to it: the sagittal posteriorly, two coronal laterally, and the frontal. One can easily develop skill at identifying these landmarks on the fetal skull by palpating the skull of the newborn after delivery, first with eyes closed and then confirming their location visually. The steps in a vaginal examination and an illustration are given in Chapter 25.

Auscultation. The location of the fetal heart sounds, as heard through the stethoscope, yields helpful information about fetal position, but it is not wholly dependable. Certainly, it never should be relied on as the sole means of diagnosing fetal position. Ordinarily, the heart sounds are transmitted through the convex portion of the fetus, which lies in intimate contact with the uterine wall, so that they are heard best through the infant's back in vertex and breech presentations and through the thorax in face presentation.

In cephalic presentations, the fetal heart sounds are heard loudest midway between the umbilicus and the anterior superior spine of the ilium (Fig. 20-15). In general, in L.O.A. and L.O.P. positions the fetal heart sounds are heard loudest in the left lower quadrant. A similar situation applies to the R.O.A. and R.O.P. positions. In posterior positions of the occiput (L.O.P. and R.O.P.) often the sounds are heard loudest well down in the flank toward the anterior superior spine. In breech presentation, the fetal heart sounds usually are heard loudest at the level of the umbilicus or above.

■ REFERENCES

1. Scott JR, DiSaia PJ, Hammond CB et al: Danforth's Obstetrics and Gynecology, 6th ed. Philadelphia, JB Lippincott, 1990
2. Cunningham FG, MacDonald PC, Gant NF: Williams Obstetrics, 18th ed. Norwalk, CT, Appleton & Lange, 1989
3. American College of Obstetricians and Gynecologists: ACOG Bull 23:10, 1979
4. American College of Radiology: ACR Bull 35:2, 1979
5. Kopelman JN, Duff P, Karl RT et al: Computed tomographic pelvimetry in the evaluation of breech presentation. Obstet Gynecol 68:455–458, 1986
6. Adam PH, Alberge AT, Castellano S et al: Pelvimetry by digital radiography. Clin Radiol 36(3):327–330, 1985

■ SUGGESTED READINGS

Creasy RK, Resnik R (eds): Maternal–Fetal Medicine: Principles and Practice, 2nd ed. Philadelphia, WB Saunders, 1989
Dickinson RL, Belskie A: Birth Atlas, 6th ed. New York, Maternity Center Association, 1968
Dunnihoo DR: Fundamentals of Gynecology and Obstetrics. Philadelphia, JB Lippincott, 1990
Friedman EA: Labor: Clinical Evaluation and Management, 2nd ed. New York: Appleton-Century-Crofts, 1978
Steer CM (ed): Moloy's Evaluation of the Pelvis in Obstetrics, 3rd ed. New York, Plenum Medical Books, 1975
Titus P: Atlas of Obstetric Technic, 2nd ed. St Louis, CV Mosby, 1949

21

Phenomenon of Labor

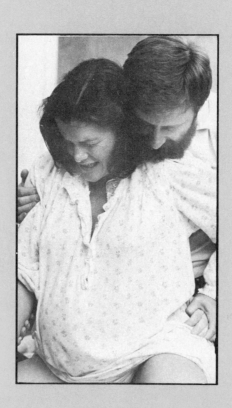

*L*abor refers to the series of processes by which the products of conception are expelled by the mother. It implies physical exertion applied to attaining a specific goal. Other terms for these processes are childbirth, parturition, accouchement, and confinement. The actual birth of the baby is called *delivery*.

The onset of labor usually occurs when the fetus is mature enough to cope with extrauterine conditions but not yet large enough to cause mechanical difficulties in labor. The actual mechanisms responsible for the initiation of this process have not yet been clearly identified.

■ CAUSES OF ONSET OF LABOR

During pregnancy, the uterus consists of a large number of greatly hypertrophied smooth muscle cells. Each cell is activated by a series of chemical reactions to begin rhythmic contractions in a highly coordinated way and with such force that the cervix is dilated and the baby is expelled. The fundamental question is what stimulates these uterine cells (at a precise time in most pregnancies) to begin labor contractions. Various theories have been advanced to explain the onset of labor. It appears that several mechanisms are involved in initiating and maintaining labor, each having varying importance depending on individual circumstances.[1]

Progesterone Deprivation Theory

This theory proposes that progesterone, the hormone essential in maintaining pregnancy that is secreted first by the corpus luteum and then by the placenta, acts to inhibit uterine contractility. The onset of labor results from the withdrawal of progesterone at a time of relative estrogen dominance. The role of a "progesterone block" in the maintenance and termination of pregnancy remains controversial. Although one investigator has reported a fall in circulating progesterone with a continuing increase of estrogen in women during the 5 weeks preceding labor, support for this theory is based largely on animal research.[2] In humans and other primates, there is a lack of substantial evidence that a demonstrable withdrawal of progesterone exists when labor commences.[3]

Oxytocin Theory

This theory suggests that oxytocin stimulates contractions of the uterus by acting directly on the myometrium and indirectly to increase the production of prostaglandin in the decidua.[4] The uterus becomes increasingly sensitive to oxytocin as pregnancy advances. Research findings provide inconsistent support for this theory. Although some studies link increasing levels of oxytocin to onset of labor, others do not indicate that levels of this hormone increase before labor or through the first stage.[5-7] The highest concentration of oxytocin-like activity in the blood has been found during the second stage of labor. Because humans and other mammals go into labor normally after removal or destruction of the hypophysis which secretes oxytocin, it is unlikely that this hormone alone is the initiator of the labor process. Oxytocin may well play a significant role in combination with other substances.

Fetal Endocrine Control Theory

At the appropriate time of fetal maturity, it is proposed that the fetal adrenals secrete cortical steroids that trigger the mechanisms leading to labor. The suggested mechanism of action is that fetal steroids stimulate the release of precursors to prostaglandins, which in turn produce uterine labor contractions.[8] Shortly before labor, the sensitivity of the fetal adrenal to adrenocorticotropic hormone (ACTH), produced by the pituitary, increases. As a result, the production of cortisol increases. The release of corticosteroids during periods of stress has been suggested as one cause of premature labor. This may occur in situations where the fetus is compromised, such as preeclampsia or uterine overdistention due to multiple pregnancies or hydramnios.

Prostaglandin Theory

This theory hypothesizes that human labor is initiated by a sequence of events including the release of lipid precursors, possibly triggered by steroid action; release of arachidonic acid from these precursors, perhaps at the site of the fetal membranes; increased prostaglandin synthesis from the arachidonic acid; and increased uterine contractions as a consequence of prostaglandin action on the uterine muscle.[9,10] Study of the mechanisms of prostaglandin synthesis has shown that arachidonic acid, the obligatory precursor to prostaglandin, increases markedly in comparison to the other fatty acids in the amniotic fluid of women in labor.[11]

Research has shown prostaglandins to be effective in inducing uterine contractions at any stage of gestation.[3,12,13] Prostaglandins are formed by the uterine decidua, umbilical cord and the amnion, and their concentration in the amniotic fluid and blood of women increases just before and during labor and delivery.[14]

■ THE POWERS OF LABOR

In Chapter 20, the three necessary elements in labor and birth are described: the passageway, the passenger, and the force or powers. The first two are discussed in that chapter. As part of the phenomena of labor, the powers are discussed here.

Uterine Contractions

To expel the contents of conception, the uterus goes through a series of contractions (the intermittent shortening of a muscle). Each contraction presents three phases: a period during which the intensity of the contraction increases (increment), a period during which the contraction is at its height (acme), and a period of diminishing intensity (decrement). The increment, or crescendo phase, is longer than the other two combined.

The contractions of the uterus during labor are intermittent, with periods of relaxation between, resembling, in this respect, the systole and the diastole of the heart. The interval between contractions diminishes gradually from about 10 minutes early in labor to about 2 or 3 minutes in the second stage. These periods of relaxation not only provide rest for the uterine muscles and for the mother, but are also essential to the welfare of the fetus. Unremitting contractions may interfere with placental functions, and the resulting lack of oxygen may produce fetal distress.

Labor contractions are involuntary; their action is independent of the mother's will and of extrauterine nervous control. The efficiency of uterine contractions is facilitated by the existence of cell-to-cell contacts known as *gap junctions* in myometrial tissue. These communications promote synchronous contractions of smooth muscle cells. Prostaglandins assume a key regulatory role; PGE_2 and PGF_2 are powerful stimuli of myometrial contractions. These hormones act to cause the rapid appearance of myometrial gap junctions and induce the maturational changes of cervical ripening.[3]

During labor, the uterus is differentiated into two identifiable portions, the upper and lower uterine segments. The upper segment known as the *fundus* is the active, contractile portion of the uterus, which contains the greatest concentration of myometrial cells. Its function is to expel the uterine contents. The uterus displays a decreasing gradient of intensity of contractions from the fundus downward. As labor progresses, a passive lower segment is developed. With each contraction, the muscle fibers of the upper segment retract, becoming shorter as the fetus descends. The upper segment, therefore, becomes thicker. Fibers of the lower segment stretch, and consequently it becomes thinner. The distinct boundary between the upper and lower uterine segments is called a physiological *retraction ring*.

The degree of discomfort during labor varies considerably among clients. The woman who anticipates a painful experience generally has more pain than the woman who is properly prepared for what can be a good experience. To allay preexisting fear, one should refer to uterine contractions as *contractions*, not *pains*. The duration of these contractions ranges from 45 to 90 seconds, averaging about 1 minute.

Duration of Labor

Although there is usually some degree of variation in all labors, an estimate of the average length of labor can be based on studies of records of some several thousand primigravidas and multiparas.

The average duration of first labors is about 14 hours, approximately 13 hours in the first stage, 1 hour in the second stage, and 10 minutes in the third stage.

The average duration of multiparous labors is approximately 6 hours shorter than for first labors (e.g., 7 hours and 20 minutes in the first stage, ½ hour in the second stage, and 10 minutes in the third stage.)

During the first stage of labor, full dilatation of the cervix (10 cm) is accomplished, but for the greater part of this time the progress of cervical dilatation is slow (Fig. 21-1). This has been clearly demonstrated in Friedman's study of the labors of 500 primigravidas.[15] From his study, the first stage of labor is divided into the latent phase (*prodromal labor*) and the active phase. The *latent phase*, from the onset of uterine contractions, takes many hours and accomplishes cervical softening, effacement, and slight dilatation. With the beginning of the *active phase*, cervical dilatation proceeds at an accelerated rate and then reaches a deceleration phase shortly before the second stage of labor.

The first 4 cm of cervical dilatation occur during the slow, latent phase. The remainder of cervical dilatation is accomplished much more rapidly in the active phase. Hence, 5 cm of dilatation take the client well past the halfway point in labor, even though 10 cm represents full dilatation. In fact, at that point, the average labor is more than two thirds over.

The active period begins with the *acceleration phase*, proceeds to the *phase of maximum slope*, and ends with the *deceleration phase* (see Fig. 21-1). In the active phase of labor, the nulliparous woman's cervix should dilate at least 1.2 cm/h, and the multiparous woman's cervix should dilate at least 1.5 cm/h.

■ PREMONITORY SIGNS OF LABOR

During the last few weeks of pregnancy, a number of changes indicate that the time of labor is approaching.

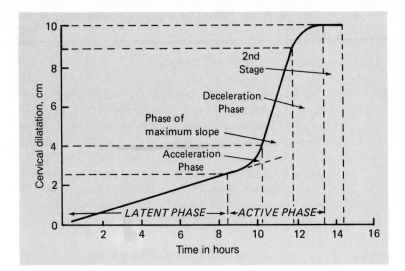

■ *Figure 21–1*

Composite of the average dilatation curve for nulliparous labor. The first stage is divided into a relatively flat latent phase and a rapidly progressive active phase. The active phase has three identifiable component parts: an acceleration phase, a linear phase of maximum slope, and a deceleration phase. (Friedman EA: Labor and Clinical Evaluation and Management, 2nd ed. New York, Appleton-Century-Crofts, 1978)

Lightening occurs about 10 to 14 days before delivery, particularly in primigravidas. This alteration is brought about by a settling of the fetal head into the pelvis. This may occur at any time during the last 4 weeks, but occasionally does not occur until labor actually begins. Lightening may take place suddenly, so that the expectant mother arises one morning entirely relieved of the abdominal tightness and diaphragmatic pressure that she had experienced previously.

But the relief in one direction often is followed by signs of greater pressure below, such as shooting pains down the legs from pressure on the sciatic nerves, an increase in the amount of vaginal discharge, and greater frequency of urination due to pressure on the bladder. In mothers who have had previous children, lightening is more likely to occur after labor begins.

True Labor vs False Labor

False contractions may begin as early as 3 or 4 weeks before the termination of pregnancy. They are merely an exaggeration of the intermittent uterine contractions that have occurred throughout the entire period of gestation, but now they may be accompanied by discomfort. The differences between false and true labor are described in the box.

Show

Another sign of impending labor is pink "show." After the discharge of the mucous plug that has filled the cervical canal during pregnancy, the pressure of the descending presenting part of the fetus causes the minute capillaries in the cervix to rupture. This blood is mixed with mucus and, therefore, has a pink tinge. It must be differentiated from substantial discharge of blood, which may indicate an obstetric complication.

Rupture of the Membranes

Occasionally, rupture of the membranes is the first indication of approaching labor. It was once thought that this was a grave sign, heralding a long and difficult dry labor, but present-day statistics show that this is not true. Nevertheless, the physician must be notified at once; under these circumstances, the client may be advised to enter the hospital immediately.

Premonitory Signs of Labor

"Lightening" or descent of fetal head into pelvis

Sciatic nerve pressure

Increased vaginal discharge

Greater frequency of urination

False Labor	*True Labor*
No change in cervix	Progressive cervical dilatation
Discomfort, usually in low abdomen and groin	Discomfort in back and abdomen
Contractions occur at irregular intervals	Contractions occur at regular intervals
No increase in frequency and intensity of contractions	Progressive increase in frequency, intensity, and duration of contractions

After the membranes rupture, there is always the possibility of a prolapsed cord if the presenting part does not adequately fill the pelvic inlet. This is more likely if the infant presents as a footling breech, or by the shoulder, or in the vertex presentation when the fetal head has not descended far enough into the true pelvis before the rupture of the membranes.

■ FOUR STAGES OF LABOR

The process of labor is divided into four stages (Table 21-1).

The *first stage of labor*, or the dilating stage, begins with the first true labor contraction and ends with the complete dilatation of the cervix. This stage may be further subdivided into the latent phase and active phase.

The *second stage of labor*, or the pelvic stage, begins with the complete dilatation of the cervix and ends with the delivery of the baby.

The *third stage of labor*, or the placental stage, begins with the delivery of the baby and terminates with the birth of the placenta.

The *fourth stage of labor*, the first hour postpartum, begins with the birth of the placenta. It is a critical period for mother and neonate.

First Stage of Labor

At the beginning of the first stage, the contractions are short, slight, 5 or 10 minutes or more apart, and lasting 20 to 30 seconds. The woman may not experience any particular discomfort and may be walking about comfortably between contractions. Early in the first stage, the sensation is usually located in the small of the back, but, as time goes on, it sweeps around, girdlelike, to the anterior part of the abdomen. The contractions recur at shortening intervals, every 3 to 5 minutes, and become stronger and last longer.

When labor has progressed to the active phase, the woman often prefers to remain in bed; ambulation may no longer be comfortable. She becomes intensely involved in the sensations within her body and tends to withdraw from the surrounding environment. The duration of each contraction ranges from 30 to 90 seconds, averaging about 1 minute.

As cervical dilatation progresses to 8 to 9 cm, the contractions reach peak intensity. This phase, between 8 and 10 cm dilatation, is called *transition* and is frequently the most difficult and painful time for the woman. There is usually a marked increase in the amount of show due to rupture of capillary vessels in the cervix and the lower uterine segment.

As the result of uterine contractions, two important changes occur in the cervix during the first stage of labor: *effacement* and *dilatation*.

CERVICAL EFFACEMENT

Cervical effacement is the shortening of the cervical canal from a structure 1 or 2 cm in length to one in which no canal at all exists, except a circular orifice with almost paper-thin edges. The edges of the internal os are drawn several centimeters upward, so that the former endocervical canal becomes part of the lower uterine segment (Fig. 21-2). In primigravidas, effacement is usually complete before dilatation begins, but in multiparas it is rarely complete; dilatation proceeds with rather thick cervical edges.

The terms *obliteration* and *taking up* of the cervix are synonymous with effacement. Effacement is measured during pelvic examination by estimating the percentage by which the cervical canal has shortened. For example, in a cervix 2 cm long before labor, 50% effacement has occurred when the cervix measures 1 cm in length.

DILATATION OF THE CERVIX

This means the enlargement of the cervical os from an orifice a few millimeters in size to an aperture large enough to permit the passage of the fetus (i.e., a diameter of about 10 cm). When the cervix can no longer be felt, dilatation is said to be complete.

Although the forces concerned in dilatation are not well understood, several factors appear to be involved. The muscle fibers about the cervix are so arranged that they pull on its edges and tend to draw it open. Mechanical stretching of the cervix intensifies uterine activity (*Ferguson reflex*). Release of endogenous oxytocin may mediate this process. The uterine contractions cause pressure on the amniotic sac, and this, in turn, burrows into the cervix in pouchlike fashion, exerting a dilating action (see Fig. 21-2). In the absence of the membranes, the pressure of the presenting part against the cervix and the lower uterine segment has a similar effect.

Measurement of cervical dilatation in terms of centimeters is done during pelvic examination through digital estimation of the diameter of the cervical opening.

Because dilatation of the cervix in the first stage of labor is solely the result of involuntary uterine contractions, the process cannot be expedited through maternal efforts such as bearing down. The mother should be discouraged from bearing-down efforts because the process may exhaust her and cause the cervix to become edematous.

INFLUENCE OF CATECHOLAMINES

During the process of labor, the human body produces stress hormones known as cathecholamines; examples

TABLE 21-1. SUMMARY OF STAGES OF LABOR

Stage	Definition	Duration	Uterine Activity	Maternal Behavior and Manifestations
First stage (dilating stage)	Period from first true labor contractions to complete cervical dilatation	Varies with phase and parity		
Latent phase	Begins at true labor onset and ends with onset of active labor	Approximately 8.6 h for the nullipara and 5.3 h for the multipara	Mild, often irregular contractions 5–30 min apart, 10–30 s duration; cervix becomes softer and thinner, 0 to 3–4 cm dilatation	Laboring woman is generally excited, alert, talkative or quiet, calm or anxious; may experience abdominal cramps, backache, rupture of membranes, pain controlled fairly well, may ambulate
Active phase	Begins with onset of active labor and ends with full dilatation	Approximately 4.6 h for the nullipara and 2.4 h for the multipara	Moderate to strong uterine contractions every 2–5 min; 30–90 s duration, cervical dilation for nulliparas of 1.2 cm/h and for the multipara 1.5 cm/h	Laboring woman generally feels increasing discomfort, perspiring, nausea and vomiting, flushed; experiences trembling of thighs and legs, pressure on bladder and rectum, backache, circumoral pallor, amnesia between contractions; may be more apprehensive, fear losing control, self-focused; may become irritable
Second stage (pelvic stage)	Period from complete cervical dilatation to delivery of infant	Approximately 1 h for the nullipara and ½ h for the multipara	Strong uterine contractions every 2–3 min, 45–90 s duration; intra-abdominal pressure is exerted	May experience decreased pain, feels pressure on rectum, bulging perineum, urge to bear down, often excited and eager, grunting sounds or expiratory vocalization
Third stage (placental stage)	Period from delivery of infant to delivery of placenta and membranes	5–30 min	Strong uterine contractions; uterus changing to globular shape; intra-abdominal pressure is exerted	Focus on newborn, excited about birth, feeling of relief
Fourth stage	Period from delivery of placenta and membranes to first hour postpartum	1 h	Uterus firm at level of two fingerbreadths above umbilicus	Exploration of newborn; family integration begins; infant alert and responsive

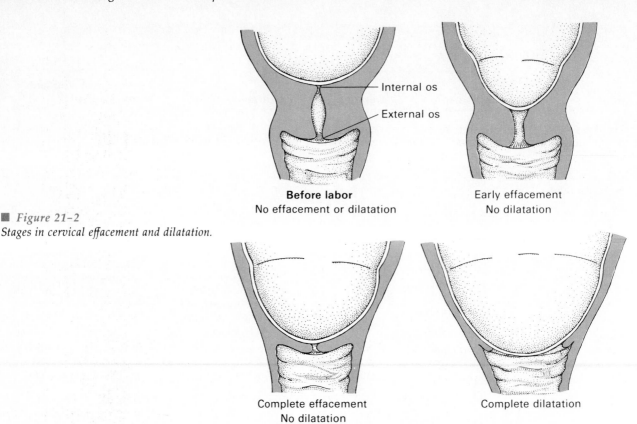

Internal os

External os

Before labor
No effacement or dilatation

Early effacement
No dilatation

Complete effacement
No dilatation

Complete dilatation

■ *Figure 21-2*
Stages in cervical effacement and dilatation.

of these hormones include epinephrine (adrenaline) and norepinephrine (noradrenaline), which are produced in the brain, nerve endings, adrenal medulla, and other body organs. The woman in early labor produces catecholamines at her usual prelabor level if she is relatively free of anxiety.[16–18] As labor advances, catecholamine levels are likely to rise in response to increasing stress, pain, or intrapartum complications.[18] Normal catecholamine production in the laboring woman is beneficial because it prepares the body for action and expenditure of energy; however, excessive amounts may have deleterious effects on labor and the fetus. These include decreased efficiency of uterine contractions, longer labor, and shunting of blood away from the uterus and placenta.[18,19]

The fetus also produces increasing amounts of catecholamines (predominantly norepinephrine) in response to the stress of normal labor and the temporary hypoxia caused by normal contractions. Production of fetal catecholamines causes more blood to shunt to vital organs, increases oxygen uptake, and helps to prevent fetal hypoglycemia.[20–22] A drop in fetal heart rate assists in oxygen conservation. The end result of these processes is that the fetus is able to obtain as much oxygen as before labor even though there is less oxygenated blood available during contractions.[18]

Maternal disorders of the antepartal or intrapartal period (see Chaps. 33, 34, and 38) may cause catecholamine production by the fetus to exceed physiological bounds. This can lead to postnatal problems such as respiratory distress, cold stress, metabolic acidosis, and hyperbilirubinemia.[18,22]

Second Stage of Labor

The contractions are strong and long, last 50 to 70 seconds, and occur at intervals of 2 or 3 minutes. Rupture of the membranes often occurs during the early part of this stage of labor, with a gush of amniotic fluid from the vagina. Sometimes, however, membranes rupture during the first stage and occasionally before labor begins. In rare cases, the baby is born in a *caul*, which is a piece of the amnion that sometimes envelops the baby's head.

During this stage, as if by reflex action, the muscles of the abdomen are brought into play, and when the contractions are in progress the woman strains, or "bears down," with all her strength so that her face becomes flushed and the large vessels in her neck become distended. As a result of this exertion, she may perspire profusely. During this stage, the mother directs all her energy toward expelling the contents of the uterus. There is a marked pressure in the area of the perineum and rectum, and the urge to bear down is usually beyond her control.

Toward the end of the second stage, when the head is well down in the vagina, its pressure causes the anus to become patulous and everted (Fig. 21-3), and often small particles of fecal material may be expelled from the rectum with each contraction. As the head descends still further, the perineal region begins to bulge, and the skin over it becomes tense and glistening. At this time, the scalp of the fetus may be detected through a slitlike vulvar opening. With each subsequent contraction, the perineum bulges more and more and the vulva becomes more dilated and distended by the head, so that the opening is gradually converted into an ovoid and at last into a circle. With the cessation of each contraction, the opening becomes smaller and the head recedes from it until it advances again with the next contraction.

The contractions occur rapidly, with scarcely any interval between. As the head becomes increasingly visible, the vulva is stretched further and finally encircles the largest diameter of the baby's head. This encirclement of the largest diameter of the baby's head by the vulvar ring is known as *crowning*. An episiotomy may be done at this time, while the tissues surrounding the perineum are supported and the head is delivered. One or two more contractions are normally enough to effect the birth of the baby.

Whereas in the first stage of labor the forces are limited to uterine action, during the second stage two forces are essential, namely, uterine contractions and intra-abdominal pressure, the latter being brought about by the bearing-down efforts of the mother. (The force exerted by the mother's bearing down can be likened to that used in forcing an evacuation of the bowels.) Both forces are essential to the successful spontaneous

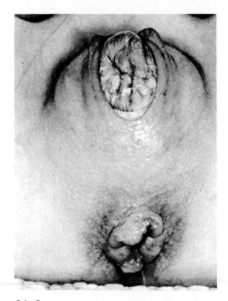

■ *Figure 21–3*
Extreme bulging of the perineum showing a patulous and everted anus.

outcome of the second stage of labor: uterine contractions without bearing-down efforts are of little avail in expelling the infant, whereas, conversely, bearing-down efforts in the absence of uterine contractions are futile. As explained in Chapter 22, these facts have important practical implications.

MECHANISM OF LABOR

In its passage through the birth canal, the presenting part of the fetus undergoes certain positional changes that constitute the mechanism of labor. These movements are designed to present the smallest possible diameters of the presenting part to the irregular shape of the pelvic canal, so that it encounters as little resistance as possible.

The mechanism of labor consists of a combination of movements, several of which may be going on at the same time. As they occur, the uterine contractions bring about important modifications in the attitude of the fetus, especially after the head has descended into the pelvis. This adaptation of the baby to the birth canal involves four processes: flexion, internal rotation, extension, and external rotation (Fig. 21-4).

For purposes of instruction, the various movements are described as if they occurred independently.

Descent. The first requisite for the birth of the infant is descent. When the fetal head has descended such that its greatest biparietal diameter is at, or has passed, the pelvic inlet, the head is said to be *engaged*. This provides a clear indication that the pelvic inlet is large enough to accommodate the widest portion of the fetal head and is, therefore, of adequate size. For the average fetal head, the linear distance between the occiput and the plane of the biparietal diameter is less than the distance between the pelvic inlet and the ischial spines. Thus, when the occiput is at the level of the spines, its biparietal diameter has usually passed the pelvic inlet, and the vertex is therefore engaged. However, one cannot assume that engagement has occurred simply because the vertex is at the spines. When the fetal head has been molded markedly, with consequent increase in the distance between the occiput and the biparietal diameter, the vertex may be felt at the spines but its greatest diameter may still be above the pelvic inlet.

The ischial spines are used as a landmark to describe the relative position of the fetal head in the pelvis (Fig. 21-5). This relationship is evaluated during the course of each pelvic examination and recorded, along with the assessment of cervical dilatation and effacement.

With primigravidas, engagement often precedes the onset of labor. This is the process of lightening, described earlier. Because the vertex is frequently deep in the pelvis at the onset of labor, further descent does not necessarily begin until the second stage of labor. In

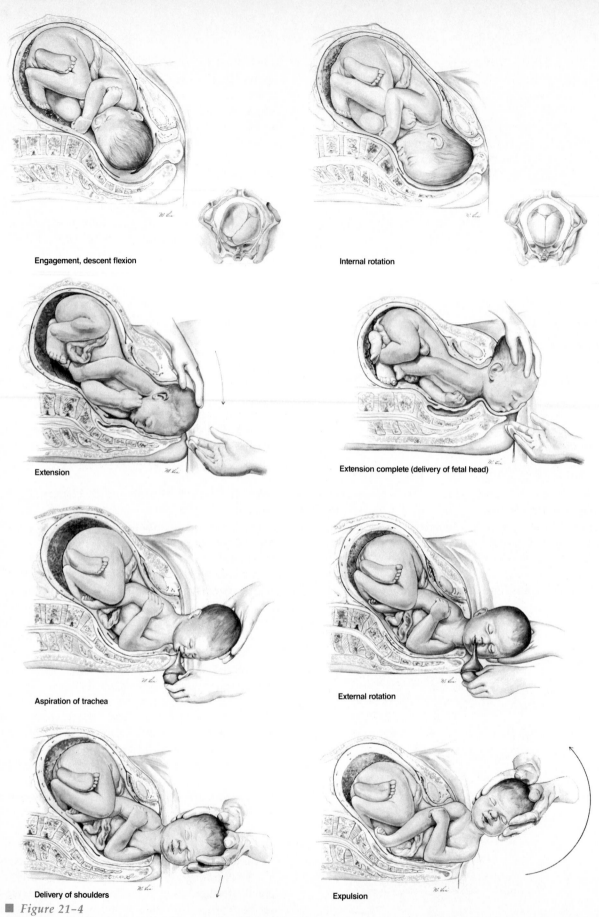

Engagement, descent flexion

Internal rotation

Extension

Extension complete (delivery of fetal head)

Aspiration of trachea

External rotation

Delivery of shoulders

Expulsion

■ *Figure 21–4*
Mechanism of delivery for a vertex presentation (Whitley N: A Manual of Clinical Obstetrics. Philadelphia, JB Lippincott, 1985)

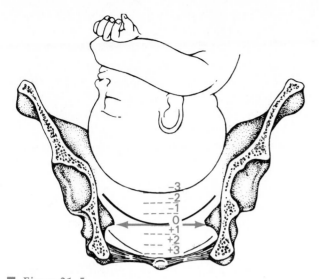

■ *Figure 21–5*
Stations of the fetal head:
−3 station—vertex is 3 cm above the spines.
−2 station—vertex is 2 cm above the spines.
−1 station—vertex is 1 cm above the spines.
0 station—vertex is at the level of the spines.
+1 station—vertex is 1 cm below the spines.
+2 station—vertex is 2 cm below the spines.
+3 station—vertex is 3 cm below the spines.

multiparas, on the other hand, descent often begins with engagement. Once having been inaugurated, descent is inevitably associated with the various movements of the mechanism of labor.

Flexion. Early in the process of descent, the head becomes so flexed that the chin is in contact with the sternum; as a consequence, the smallest anteroposterior diameter (the suboccipitobregmatic plane) is presented to the pelvis.

Internal Rotation. The head enters the pelvis in the transverse or diagonal position. When it reaches the pelvic floor, the occiput is rotated and comes to lie beneath the symphysis pubis. In other words, the sagittal suture is in the anteroposterior diameter of the outlet. Although the occiput usually rotates to the front, on occasion it may turn toward the hollow of the sacrum. If anterior rotation does not take place at all, the occiput usually rotates to the direct occiput posterior position, a condition known as persistent occiput posterior. Because this represents a deviation from the normal mechanism of labor, it is considered in Chapter 38, in the section on abnormal fetal positions.

Extension. After the occiput emerges from the pelvis, the nape of the neck becomes arrested beneath the pubic arch and acts as a pivotal point for the rest of the head.

Extension of the head ensues, and the frontal portion of the head, the face, and the chin are born.

External Rotation. After the birth of the head, it remains in the anteroposterior position only a short time, then turns to one or another side of its own accord, *restitution.* When the occiput originally has been directed toward the left of the mother's pelvis, it rotates toward the left. If it originally has been to the right, then it rotates toward the right. This is known as external rotation and is due to the fact that the shoulders, having entered the pelvis in the transverse position, undergo internal rotation to the anteroposterior position, as did the head. This brings about a corresponding rotation of the head, which is on the outside.

The shoulders are born in a manner somewhat similar to that of the head. Almost immediately after the occurrence of external rotation, the anterior shoulder appears under the symphysis pubis and becomes arrested temporarily beneath the pubic arch to act as a pivotal point for the other shoulder. As the anterior margin of the perineum becomes distended, the posterior shoulder is born, assisted by an upward lateral flexion of the infant's body. Once the shoulders are delivered, the infant's body is quickly extruded (*expulsion*).

Third Stage of Labor

The third stage of labor is made up of two phases, *the phase of placental separation* and *the phase of placental expulsion.*

Immediately after the birth of the infant, the remainder of the amniotic fluid escapes, after which there is usually a slight flow of blood. The uterus can be felt as a firm globular mass just below the level of the umbilicus. Shortly thereafter, the uterus relaxes and assumes a discoid shape. With each subsequent contraction or relaxation the uterine shape changes from globular to discoid until the placenta has separated, after which the globular shape persists.

PLACENTAL SEPARATION

As the uterus contracts down at regular intervals on its diminishing content, the area of placental attachment is greatly reduced. The great disproportion between the reduced size of the placental site and the size of the placenta brings about a folding or festooning of the maternal surface of the placenta, and separation takes place. Meanwhile, bleeding takes place within these placental folds, which expedites separation of the organ. The placenta sinks into the lower uterine segment or upper vagina as an unattached body. The signs that indicate placental separation usually occur within 5 minutes after the delivery of the infant.

Signs of Placental Separation

Globular and firmer uterus

Rise of uterus in abdomen

Descent of umbilical cord 3 in or more out of vagina

Sudden gush of blood

PLACENTAL EXPULSION

Actual expulsion of the placenta may be brought about by the mother bearing down if she is not anesthetized. If this cannot be accomplished, it is usually effected through gentle pressure on the uterine fundus. Excessive pressure should be avoided to obviate the rare possibility of inversion of the uterus (see Chap. 38).

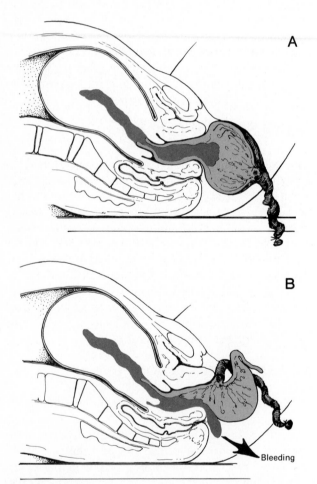

A

B

■ *Figure 21–6*
Expulsion of the placenta by (A) Schultze's mechanism, whereby the placenta is turned inside out within the vagina and is delivered with the glistening fetal surfaces to the outside, and by (B) the Duncan mechanism, whereby the placenta is rolled up in the vagina and is delivered with the maternal surface to the outside.

The extrusion of the placenta may take place by one of two mechanisms (Fig. 21-6). Schultze's mechanism, evident in approximately 80% of deliveries, signifies that the placenta has become detached first at its center, and usually a collection of blood and clots is found in the sac of membranes. The Duncan mechanism is seen in about 20% of deliveries and suggests that the placenta has separated first at its edges. Bleeding usually occurs at the time of separation with the Duncan mechanism. No clinical significance has been ascribed to either mechanism.

The contraction of the uterus after delivery serves not only to produce placental separation but also to control uterine hemorrhage. As the result of this contraction of the uterine muscle fibers, the countless blood vessels within their interstices are clamped shut. Even then, a certain amount of blood loss in the third stage is unavoidable, commonly amounting to about 500 ml or less. It is one of the aims of labor management to keep this bleeding to a minimum.

Fourth Stage of Labor

The first hour postpartum, sometimes referred to as the fourth stage of labor, is the time that *restoration of physiological stability* is established. During this period, myometrial contractions and retraction, accompanied by vessel thrombosis, operate effectively to control bleeding from the placenta site. However, potential risks exist for hemorrhage, urinary retention, hypotension, and side-effects of anesthesia.

The first hour after birth is also considered important for initial formation of the mother–child relationship and consolidation of the family unit. Early parental interactions with the new baby and each other are believed to affect subsequently the quality of their relationships (see Chap. 22).

■ REFERENCES

1. MacDonald PC, Porter JC (eds): Fourth Ross Conference on Obstetric Research. Columbus, OH, Ross Laboratories, 1983
2. Casey ML, Winkel CA, Porter JC et al: Endocrine regulation of parturition. Clin Perinatol 10:709–721, 1983
3. Cunningham FG, MacDonald PC, Gant NF: Williams Obstetrics, 18th ed. Norwalk CT, Appleton & Lange, 1989
4. Fuchs AR, Fuchs F, Husslein P et al: Oxytocin receptors and human parturition: A dual role of oxytocin in the initiation of labor. Science 215:1396–1398, March 12, 1982
5. Soloff MS: The role of oxytocin in the initiation of labor, and oxytocin–prostaglandin interactions. In Mc-

Nellis D, Challis JRG, MacDonald PC et al (eds): Cellular and Integrative Mechanisms in the Onset of labor. An NICHD workshop. Ithaca, NY, Perinatology Press, 1988

6. Chard T: The role of the posterior pituitaries of mother and fetus in spontaneous parturition. In Camline KS, Cross KW, Dawes GS (eds): Fetal and Neonatal Physiology. New York, Cambridge University Press, 1973

7. Padayachi T, Norman RJ, Ohavaraj K et al: Serial oxytocin levels in amniotic fluid and maternal plasma during normal and induced labour. Br J Obstet Gynaecol 96(9):888–893, 1988

8. Casey ML, MacDonald PC: Initiation of labor in women. In Hugzar G (ed): The Biochemistry and Physiology of the Uterus and Labor. Cleveland, CRC Press, 1985

9. Bennett PR, Chamberlain GV, Patel L et al: Mechanisms of parturition: The transfer of prostaglandin E_2 and 5-hydroxyeicosatetraenoic acid across fetal membranes. Am J Obstet Gynecol 162(3):683–687, 1990

10. Sahmay S, Coke A, Hekim N et al: Maternal, umbilical, uterine and amniotic prostaglandin E and F_2 alpha levels in labour. J Int Med Res 16(4):280–205, 1988

11. Reddi K, Norman RJ, Dappe WM et al: Amniotic membrane production of prostaglandin F_2 alpha is reduced in dysfunctional human labor: Results of in vivo and in vitro studies. J Clin Endocrinol Metab 65(5):1000–1005, November 1987

12. Granstrom L, Akman G, Ulmsten U: Myometrial activity after local application of prostaglandin E_2 for cervical ripening and term labor induction. Am J Obstet Gynecol 162(3):691, 1990

13. Shaala S, Darwish E, Anwar M et al: Cervical prostaglandin injection: A novel method of administration for ripening the cervix and induction of labor. Int J Gynaecol Obstet 30(3):221–223, 1989

14. Ilancheran A, Ratnam SS: Effect of oxytocics on prostaglandin levels in the third stage of labour. Gynecol Obstet Invest 29(3):177–180, 1990

15. Friedman EA: Labor and Clinical Evaluation and Management, 2nd ed. New York, Appleton-Century-Crofts, 1978

16. Lederman RP, Lederman E, Work BA et al: The relationship of maternal anxiety, plasma catecholamines, and plasma cortisol to progress in labor. Am J Obstet Gynecol 132:495–500, 1978

17. Sosa R, Kennell J, Klaus M et al: The effect of a supportive companion on perinatal problems, length of labor, and mother–infant interaction. N Engl J Med 303(11):597–600, 1980

18. Simkin P: Stress, pain, and catecholamines in labor: Part 1. A review. Birth 13:227–240, 1986

19. Lederman RP, Lederman E, Work BA et al: Relationship of physiological factors in pregnancy to progress in labor. Nurs Res 28(2):94–97, 1979

20. Lagercrantz H, Slotkin TA: The "stress" of being born. Sci Am 12:100–107, 1985

21. Phillippe M: Fetal catecholamines. Am J Obstet Gynecol 146(7):840–855, 1983

22. Fox HA: The effects of catecholamines and drug treatment on the fetus and newborn. Birth Fam J 6:157–165, 1979

■ SUGGESTED READINGS

Hariharan S, Takahashi K, Burd L: Initiation of labor. In Sciarri JJ (ed): Gynecology and Obstetrics. Philadelphia, WB Saunders, 1986

Liggins GC: Initiation of labour. Biol Neonate 55:366–375, 1989

Lopez BA, Hansell DJ, Alexander S et al: Steroid conversion and prostaglandin production by chorionic and decidual cells in relation to term and preterm labour. Br J Obstet Gynaecol 94(11):1052–1058, November 1987

Moore JJ, Dubyak GR, Moore RM et al: Oxytocin activates the inositol-phospholipid-protein-kinase-C system and stimulates prostaglandin production in human amnion cells. Endocrinology 123(4):1771–1777, October 1988

Nagata I, Furuya K, Imaizumi E et al: Changes in plasma cyclic AMP and cyclic GMP during spontaneous labor and labor induced by oxytocin, prostaglandin F_2 alpha and prostaglandin E_2. Gynecol Obstet Invest 26(1):21–28, 1988

Scott JR, DeSaia PJ, Hammond CB et al: Danforth's Obstetrics and Gynecology, 6th ed. Philadelphia, JB Lippincott, 1990

Willson JR, Carrington ER, Ledger WJ: Obstetrics and Gynecology, 8th ed. St Louis, CV Mosby, 1988

22

Management of Normal Labor

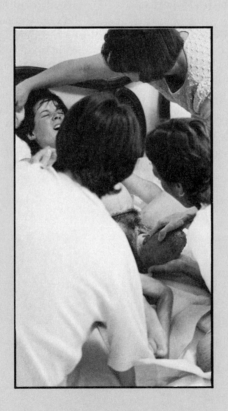

Parturition is a unique and humbling experience not only for the mother and the father, the main participants, but also for the health-care staff who shares this experience. From the couple's point of view, labor looms as a critical period in the process of child-bearing; often it is considered by them, and especially by the mother, as the end of a long drawn-out process rather than the beginning of a new role. Hence, they attribute enormous significance to events and people who are necessary and helpful to them at this time.

■ DIMENSIONS OF EFFECTIVE NURSING CARE

The goal of nursing during the birth process is to instill maximum physical and emotional well-being in both the woman and the fetus. This goal extends to include the transitions of woman to mother and fetus to newborn. At the same time, the nurse should facilitate the participation of the father or support persons in the birth. The nursing interventions used to achieve this goal are purposeful but flexible, based on thorough assessments and nursing diagnoses to meet the individual needs of the mother, newborn, and family. To implement such care, the nurse must be familiar with the normal physiology of labor and deviations from the norm (both discussed in Chapters 20, 21, and 38), and must have the judgment, self-confidence, and skills required to cope with stressful and emergency conditions. Additional attributes include a mastery of certain technical and communicative skills, which can be applied appropriately to meet the exigencies of the situation. These skills are used both with the client and in participating as a member of the health team in the labor and delivery unit. However, knowledge and technical ability are not sufficient; the nurse must also address the psychosocial aspects of care by conveying warmth and empathy. The empathic nurse is able to enter into the feelings of the client and at the same time retain a sense of separateness. Thus, objectivity is maintained, which contributes to more effective care. Yet the worth and the individuality of each mother are always recognized.

The labor nurse is concerned with two clients, mother and fetus, and this concern is reflected in the assessments, nursing diagnoses, interventions, and evaluation of care done on each individual client. The ability of the nurse to assume these responsibilities is contingent on competent guidance and instructions. To help the student or new graduate prepare for these responsibilities, we focus on both the woman and the nurse as they move through the successive stages of labor. Although it is the woman who truly delivers her infant, the other important people in this event—the father, the nurse, the physician or nurse–midwife, and ancillary personnel—are not to be forgotten; they also play important roles.

In this chapter we describe the environment and care that accompany a labor and delivery carried out in a conventional labor and delivery unit within a hospital setting. The care given in a conventional setting varies depending on each facility's policies and procedures but tends to be accompanied by more technological interventions and more restriction on the client's activity. The concept of labor–delivery–recovery–postpartum (LDRP) has become popular in the United States. In this type of delivery system, the client is admitted into her room and stays there for her entire maternity admission. The client does not have to change rooms as she goes through each phase of care. Hospitals have had to remodel to accommodate these changes and cross train their staff to be proficient in all areas of care.

Many hospitals have variations in this concept with the most common being labor–delivery–recovery (LDR) rooms in what was previously the labor and delivery unit. After recovery is complete, the client is transferred to a postpartum unit.

Professional organizations are publishing documents supporting changes in perinatal care to incorporate family-centered care concepts in every aspect of perinatal service.[1,2] Medical center personnel must look at the traditional procedures and determine whether they are based on sound scientific research and are in the best interest of the client and her family. Above all, the family should not lose their rights when they enter the hospital. They have choices and options in care, and the professional is there to support those choices that are not life threatening.

The nursing-service personnel within the medical centers who are responsible for perinatal care need to work with the medical staff in the revision of protocols. The combined efforts of the professionals who deliver perinatal care should provide quality health care while recognizing both physical and psychosocial needs of the mother, the family, and the newborn.

■ LABOR

Prelude to Labor

The prodromal signs that herald the onset of labor begin several weeks before true labor commences. As indicated in Chapter 21, lightening may occur any time during the last 4 weeks of pregnancy; in primigravidas, it usually occurs about 10 to 14 days before labor. This phenomenon causes a sensation of decreased abdominal

Research Highlight

Stolte's study explored women's birth experiences to see what aspects were described as different from or the same as their expectations before labor. A convenience sample of 70 women were interviewed within 24 to 72 hours postpartum using a semistructured questionnaire. Patients were asked to rate and then describe how similar their expectations were to actual experiences in the following areas: pain medication, ability to cope with labor, support from hospital staff and others, and length and quality of labor. One limitation of this study was that subjects were asked to recall events after they occurred and accuracy of recall could be challenged.

Seventy-three percent of the patients had experiences in labor and delivery that differed, either worse or better, from what they expected. In only three areas, expectations about procedures, the support person, and help from doctors and nurses, did 50% of the subjects rate their experiences "about what they expected." Overall, multiparas' birth experiences were more similar to the actual event than primiparas'. Thirty-percent of the women felt their ability to cope with labor was "worse than expected."

Primiparas described the effects of analgesia "not like" what they expected more often than multiparas. Data from content analysis of the open-ended questions showed that pain in labor was discussed both in terms of the presence and absence of it and the pain relief effects of analgesia and anesthesia. The most common response was "less effective than expected." When asked if anything occurred during the birth that was unexpected, women who had taken prepared childbirth classes were more likely to report unexpected events than unprepared women. The three most frequent areas reported were length of labor, anesthesia and analgesia, and the infant.

Primiparas were more likely to have questions after delivery than multiparas regardless of the type of hospital, private or public, and overall, women delivering in the public hospital had more questions than women who delivered in the private hospital. Women did not enter labor with the expectation of a one-to-one relationship with the nurse and expected to be left alone during their labor. Most said the doctor did as expected, but many rated the nurses' help as "much higher than expected." Sixty-one percent of the women rated the help they received from their support person or coach as expected and a common response was that the support person was just there and that presence was important.

Looking at this study, nurses can be aware that 73% of the women had different labor experiences than what they expected. Surprisingly, women who had childbirth classes were more likely to report unexpected events. One intervention would be to assess during pregnancy the client's expectations and confirm or clarify with her those expectations and to again assess and explain what will be happening when she is admitted during labor.

Another two areas that may go hand in hand were responses to pain and the ability to cope. Women need to be prepared that contractions are painful and what to expect in pain relief from analgesia and anesthesia. Also giving positive feedback and praise to the laboring mother may assist her in coping during her labor.

Stolte K: A comparison of women's expectations of labor with the actual event. Birth 14:2,99–103 June 1987.

distention produced by the descent of the presenting part of the baby into the pelvis. In multigravidas, this may not occur until the labor has begun. The usually painless Braxton Hicks contractions that have occurred intermittently throughout the latter part of pregnancy may increase so much that they become annoying. They may cause the mother many restless or sleepless nights that contribute to her gradually increasing tension and fatigue. Because the rise in the anxiety level contributes to heightened awareness, the mother becomes more sensitive to various stimuli—if the fetus is generally less active, she may worry; if the baby moves more than usual, she may worry. She wonders about the 2- to 3-lb weight loss that may occur 3 to 4 days before the onset of labor. Ordinarily, this might be an occasion of

great rejoicing, but it may give her some concern. Even the increased vaginal mucous discharge may have an ominous significance for her. The spurt of energy that may occur 1 to 2 days before labor begins often leads her into activities that are overfatiguing. She needs anticipatory guidance from the nurse and the physician to help her to set limits on activity.

This is the time for the mother to finish packing her suitcase and to simplify her housekeeping duties. She may want to complete meal preparations for the family's use when she is in the hospital; if this is done daily, little by little, it should not become bothersome. Last-minute details for the care of the other children or the functioning of the household can be taken care of at this time. Walks in the fresh air are a good way to release extra tension without overfatigue. The mother should be encouraged to achieve a happy balance between activity and rest. As term approaches, it is wise for the nurse to explore with the mother her preparations for coming to the hospital. The parents should know approximately how long it takes them to reach the hospital and what alternate means of transportation are available if the father is not able to take her. What entrance to the hospital they should use and what admission procedures they must go through also are important. A tour of the ward for the parents can be arranged during the antenatal period so that they can become more familiar with the surroundings.

Onset of Labor

Early in the third trimester, the client should be apprised of what to do when labor starts and of certain situations that would necessitate a visit to the hospital for evaluation. The client should be encouraged to report early in labor and not wait at home to see if it is true or false labor. Most physicians instruct their clients to notify them if the labor contractions become regular. A primigravida, for instance, may be given instructions to wait at home until contractions are every 5 minutes for 2 hours, whereas the multigravida would be instructed to come to the hospital much sooner. Other situations of which the mother needs to be advised include breaking of the bag of waters and any vaginal bleeding. Further instruction needs to be given to clarify the breaking of the amniotic sac, in which the woman may experience anything from only a small intermittent leak to a gush of fluid from her vagina. However, in either situation the physician should be notified and the mother should come to the hospital.

When the mother first becomes aware of the contractions, they may be 15 to 20 minutes apart and may last perhaps 20 to 30 seconds. Because these are of mild intensity, she usually can continue with whatever she is doing, except that she must be alert to time the subsequent contractions to have specific information when she calls the physician. It is important for the client to

know when it is appropriate to go to the hospital in relation to her uterine contraction pattern.

■ ADMISSION TO THE HOSPITAL

As previously stated, the mother who has been given adequate antepartal care has also received instruction on what to anticipate when she comes to the hospital to have her baby. If this is the mother's first hospital experience, it will be much easier for her if she has been told about the necessary preliminary procedures, such as any vulvar and perineal preparation, the methods of examination employed to ascertain the progress of labor, and the usual routines exercised for her care in the course of labor.

If the mother has not had adequate antepartal care to prepare her, her labor may be rather advanced on admission and she may not know what to expect. It falls to the nurse to reassure this mother and orient her as quickly as possible to the process of labor and the physical environment. In these instances, the ability to make decisive clinical judgments, especially with regard to establishing priorities of care, is extremely helpful and necessary.

The preparation for delivery varies in different hospitals, because every hospital has its own admission procedure. Many of the details of management may be accomplished in a number of ways. Few institutions employ precisely the same technique in preparing a mother for delivery. Actually, the differences are in details only, because the principles are the same everywhere, namely, asepsis and antisepsis, together with careful observation of the mother for any deviations from the normal, and meticulous supportive care.

Admission Information

After making the mother comfortable in the labor room, the nurse needs to proceed with the admission as quickly as possible, It may be remembered that the mother's labor usually becomes progressively stronger; therefore, when admitting procedures are done early in labor, when she can be more responsive with relative ease, the client's comfort and well-being are enhanced. Also, there are generally several other people concerned with the care of the mother (physician, nurse–midwife, and laboratory technician). Often they cannot carry out their duties until the client has been fully admitted.

The nurse initiates the admitting process with information that needs to be determined quickly to evaluate the following:

Labor Evaluation Guidelines

Client needs to go to hospital for evaluation when the following occur:

- There is a regular uterine contraction pattern, increasing in intensity
- The bag of water breaks
- There is bright-red vaginal bleeding
- There is a decrease in fetal movement (less than three movements per hour)

1. Is the client in true labor and, if so, how far has she progressed?
2. What is the general condition of mother and fetus?
3. What preparation has she done for childbirth and what are support systems to assist her through labor?

Each one encompasses those nursing skills specific to labor and delivery that take time for the new nurse to master.

As part of the admission procedure determined by hospital policies and physician orders, the nurse may be doing perineal shaves, enemas, and electronic fetal monitoring, starting intravenous therapy, and ordering laboratory tests (e.g., hematocrit, hemoglobin, type and screens, and urinalysis, or a minimum of dipstick test for protein, glucose, and acetone). A detailed look at admitting the laboring woman follows.

Assessment

NURSING HISTORY

Nursing practice is governed by standards, and in the course of admitting the laboring woman, the nurse must document the name of the client, the reason for admission, the date and time of arrival, the time the physician was notified, and the time the client was seen by the physician.[1,2] The prenatal record is sent from the doctor's office or clinic to the labor and delivery unit at approximately 36 weeks and should be checked by the admitting nurse. The following pertinent information is usually transcribed from the prenatal record to the admission form: blood group and Rh factor, irregular antibody detection, serology, hepatitis screen, and any diagnostic or therapeutic measures.

By taking a good nursing history and physical the admitting nurse evaluates the client in relation to high-risk factors. If any factors are found that place the mother or fetus at risk, the physician is notified, because they may alter the type of labor and delivery experience the client desires. (Refer to other chapters for further discussion of high-risk factors and how they influence perinatal outcome.) Clients who are not at high risk should have a more directed history, obtaining the following information: onset of contractions, status of membranes, bleeding, fetal activity, history of allergies, time and content of last ingestion, and current medications. The fetus is also evaluated by noting the gestational age, fetal position, and heart rate. Trained nursing personnel may perform the initial pelvic examination (first noting that there is no abnormal bleeding, status of membranes, and fetal position) to determine cervical dilatation, effacement, and fetal position

and station. These were discussed in Chapters 20 and 21. See the sample admitting form for general information required.

The nurse, as the person who spends a great deal of time with the client after admission, is expected to report on the general character of the labor contractions as well as the other manifestations of labor. First, it must be determined whether the client is actually in labor. Friedman has pointed out that there are no fixed or uniformly applicable rules that can be used at the bedside. We can assume that the client is in true labor if her contractions continue uninterruptedly and result in dilatation of the cervix.[3] In practice, however, a variety of types of contractions may be apparent; thus, the differential points between true and false labor contained in Table 25-1 are to be used only as *guidelines* for assessing the state of the mother's labor.

TABLE 22–1. DIFFERENTIAL FACTORS IN TRUE AND FALSE LABOR

True Labor	False Labor
Contractions	
Occur at regular intervals	Occur at irregular intervals
Start in the back and sweep around to the abdomen	Located chiefly in abdomen
Increase in intensity and duration	Intensity remains the same, or is variable
Intervals gradually shorten	Intervals remain long
Intensify by walking	Walking has no intensifying effect; often gives relief
Show	
Usually present; pink-tinged mucus released from the cervical canal as labor starts	Usually not present or if present is usally brownish. May be due to recent pelvic examination by her doctor or to intercourse
Cervix	
Becomes effaced and dilated	No change
Ambulation	
Increases the intensity of contractions	No change
Sedation	
Does not stop contractions	Tends to decrease number of contractions

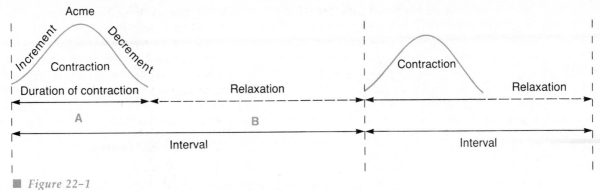

■ *Figure 22–1*

The interval and the duration of uterine contractions. The frequency of contractions is the interval timed from the beginning of one contraction to the beginning of the next contraction. The interval consists of two parts: (A) the duration of the contraction and (B) the period of relaxation. The broken line indicates an indeterminate period, because the time (B) is usually of longer duration than the actual contraction (A).

CHARACTERISTICS OF CONTRACTIONS

The frequency, duration, and intensity of the contractions should be watched closely and recorded whether a monitor is used or not.

The *frequency* of contractions is timed from the beginning of one contraction to the beginning of the next.

The *duration* of a contraction is timed from the moment the uterus first begins to tighten until it relaxes again (Fig. 22-1).

The *intensity* of a contraction may be mild, moderate, or strong at its acme. Because this is a relative factor if measured without the aid of the internal uterine pressure catheter, intensity is difficult to interpret unless one is at the mother's bedside palpating the uterus during contractions. The nurse uses the palmar surface of the fingertips, palpating different parts of the uterus during the contraction, to judge intensity.

During a *mild* contraction, the uterine muscle becomes somewhat tense, but can be indented with gentle pressure. During a *moderate* contraction, the uterus becomes moderately firm and a firmer pressure is needed to indent. During a *strong* contraction, the uterus becomes so firm that it has the feel of woodlike hardness, and at the height of the contraction, the uterus cannot be indented when pressure is applied by the examiner's finger.

GENERAL PHYSICAL CONDITION

Chief Complaint. The client should be asked why she came to the hospital. The nurse should not assume that it was the onset of regular contractions that made her come in, because it could be a complaint of leaking amniotic fluid or decrease in fetal activity that prompted her to come to the unit. The mother should be given time to express in her own words to the nurse her reason for admission. The use of open-ended questions to elicit this information is beneficial, although more direct questions may be necessary later to clarify information.

VITAL SIGNS

Temperature, Pulse, and Respiration. Temperature and respiration should be normal. If there is an elevation in temperature over 99.6°F (37.2°C) orally or if the pulse and respiration become rapid, the physician is to be notified. The temperature and respiration rates are taken every 4 hours, or more frequently if indicated.[2] Conditions that warrant closer observation are rupture of the membranes and the presence of a fetal tachycardia.

The pulse in normal labor is usually in the 70s or 80s and rarely exceeds 100. Sometimes the pulse rate on admission is slightly increased because of the excitement of coming to the hospital, but this returns to normal shortly thereafter. A persistent pulse over 100 suggests exhaustion or dehydration. Pulse rates are recorded every 4 hours.[2]

Blood Pressure. There are significant hemodynamic occurrences observed during labor and delivery that affect the blood pressure value. With the contraction of the uterus, approximately 300 to 500 ml of blood are shifted to the central blood volume, causing increases in cardiac output.[4] Other conditions leading to significant increase in cardiac output are anxiety and pain, especially in the primigravida. Hendricks and Quilligan have shown that pain and anxiety alone can increase cardiac output by 50% to 60%.[5]

For the most part, the minimal requirement for taking blood pressures during labor is every hour for the client without recognized high-risk factors and just before the delivery. To obtain accurate blood pressure, the nurse needs to be aware of the hemodynamic alterations involved with contractions and must work with the client to relieve her pain and anxiety as much as she is able. Blood pressures start to rise approximately 5 to 8 seconds preceding a contraction, returning to resting level when the contraction subsides.[6] Hence, the nurse should be taking the client's blood pressure and pulse after a contraction, well before the next one starts.

There are no recommendations based on research to help the nurse with the position of choice when obtaining a blood pressure. Most experts agree that the blood pressure taken with the client on her left side is the one to use for clinical diagnosis and management. If the nurse gets a blood pressure reading initially that needs to be reevaluated, either higher or lower than expected, the cuff should be deflated and a waiting period of 2 minutes observed. At this time, the nurse should assess factors that may be contributing to the reading. Is the reading elevated because of pain or anxiety or is it low as the result of regional anesthesia, supine position, or hemorrhage? The second reading can be taken in the same arm, and if the deviation from the expected norm still exists, this information is reported. The student needs to begin to realize that the person told the information, physician or staff nurse, will want other information to best evaluate the client. For instance, for an elevation in blood pressure, the experienced nurse evaluates the client for signs and symptoms of pregnancy-induced hypertension, knowing that a certain number of women are asymptomatic during their pregnancy but develop the disease when in labor.

When epidural anesthesia is given in labor, blood pressures are evaluated every 5 minutes for the first 15 to 20 minutes, or until stable. The client may be on an every-30-minutes blood pressure schedule or as directed by the Department of Anesthesia at that particular hospital. The minimal requirements for evaluating a client after epidural anesthesia are usually present in the labor and delivery policy book, which guides the nurse in giving care.

FETAL EVALUATION

It cannot be stressed enough that when caring for the pregnant woman, the nurse is treating two clients, mother and fetus. This is especially important to remember when admitting the laboring woman. The nurse must assess fetal health as well as maternal health. The assessments to establish fetal well-being are as follows:

1. Determine the estimated date of confinement (EDC).
2. Measure the fundal height of the uterus and correlate the height with the gestational age.
3. Determine fetal position by abdominal palpation.
4. Auscultate fetal heart tones to determine the baseline and any periodic changes.

Estimated Date of Confinement. The EDC can be obtained from the prenatal record. A term pregnancy is one that has achieved 37 weeks of gestation and has not exceeded 42 weeks. As explained in Chapter 19, the date of the client's last normal menstrual period allows the nurse to calculate the EDC by using Nägele's rule. The EDC is truly an estimate, influenced by factors such as nutrition, cultural differences, and climate; fewer than 5% of the pregnancies deliver on the due date.[7]

Fundal Height. Even though determination of fundal height using a tape measure is not a common practice on admission, the labor and delivery nurse should be able to perform this measurement and know its significance (see Chap. 19). Another method used by experienced nurses is to palpate the fundal height and to be cognizant of the relationship of fundal height to gestational age. Finding an abnormally low or excessively high fundal height does not necessarily indicate an unhealthy fetus, but cues the nurse to look for the reason of the deviation from the norm.

Abdominal Palpation: Leopold Maneuvers. Confirmation of fetal position before the initial vaginal examination is a recommended practice.[1,2,8] Performing Leopold maneuvers in a systematic manner enables the nurse to assess fetal position and makes locating the fetal heart tone easier. In the cephalic and breech presentations, the fetal heart is best heard through the back because it is the fetal part in closest contact with the uterine wall (see Chap. 19 for procedure and illustrations).

Fetal Heart Rate. Determination of fetal heart rate (FHR) should be done early in the admission process. Under normal circumstances, the heart rate of a term fetus, determined by the atrial pacemaker, usually ranges between 120 and 160 beats per minute.[9] The evaluation of the fetal heart rate in labor is of great importance. If the nurse works in a facility where electronic fetal monitoring is available, obtaining a 15- to 20-minute fetal monitoring strip before administering an enema or ambulation of the client gives her time to evaluate fetal health status.

The heart rate can be monitored in a number of ways. The simplest, and still an effective method, is by frequent auscultation using a fetoscope (Fig. 22-3). The widely used DeLee-Hillis fetoscope and the Leff fetal heart stethoscope are satisfactory for this purpose.

When checking the fetal heart sounds with fetoscope, the nurse listens and counts the rate for 1 full minute. Checking the rate before, during, and after a contraction is important so that any slowing or irregularities may be detected.

It may be difficult to hear the sounds during a contraction because the uterine wall is tense, and, in ad-

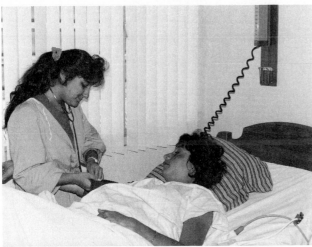

■ *Figure 22–2*
The nurse takes the initial blood pressure during admission.
(Courtesy of San Pedro Peninsula Hospital, San Pedro, CA)

dition, it is more difficult for the mother to lie still during this period. But it is particularly important to listen at this time because these observations inform the listener on how the fetus reacts to the contraction.

The student in the clinical area should be working with a staff nurse and not be totally responsible for evaluation of the fetal heart rate. To learn interpretation of fetal monitor strips, the registered nurse usually attends a separate class on fetal monitoring, with periodic updates to maintain clinical skill. If the student nurse notices a slowing of the fetal heart rate, the student should notify the staff nurse for further evaluation of the fetus, and the staff nurse determines if the pattern warrants notification of the physician. The passage of meconium can also indicate fetal distress; its presence, color, and consistency are documented in the nursing notes, and the physician is notified. Interpretation of fetal heart rate patterns and appropriate nursing interventions for decelerations are covered in Chapter 43.

AMNIOTIC FLUID STATUS

It is important to establish whether the mother's membranes are intact or not. Ruptured membranes are significant for the following three reasons:

- If the presenting part is not fixed in the pelvis, the possibility of prolapse of the cord and consequent cord compression is maximized.
- Labor is likely to occur soon after rupture if the pregnancy is at or near term.
- If the fetus remains in the uterus 24 hours or more after the membranes rupture, there is an increased probability of intrauterine infection that is especially harmful to the fetus even though the mother is given antibiotics.

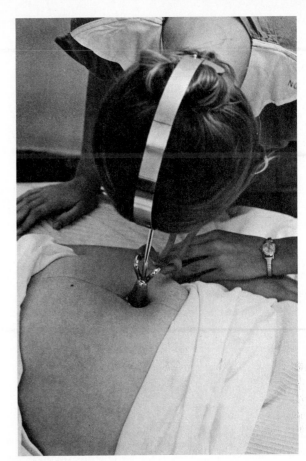

■ *Figure 22–3*
Auscultation of the fetal heartbeat using the fetoscope.

Ruptured membranes are often difficult to diagnose unless the fluid is seen escaping from the vagina. Moreover, there are no tests that are completely reliable. Those most widely employed involve testing the acidity or alkalinity of the vaginal fluid. The amniotic fluid pH is generally 7 to 7.5, whereas vaginal secretions are in the range of 4.5 to 5.5. The nitrazine tests use test papers similar to the Clinitest. These papers are impregnated with a dye that reacts with the vaginal material and can be compared to a standard color chart. Bloody show can confound the reading, giving a false reading or ruptured membranes when in fact the membranes are intact, because blood, like amniotic fluid, is not acidic.[8]

Some clients come in wearing a peripad or wet underclothing that may be tested with the nitrazine. If the client presents to the unit with a term gestation and a history of leaking fluid from the vagina and is not in obvious labor, the choice procedure is a sterile speculum examination for the determination of ruptured membranes.

The nurse may be assisting the physician with this procedure, or if instructed properly on the technique the nurse may be incorporating it into his or her practice. The procedure uses a sterile speculum inserted into the vagina and visualization of the cervix. At this time, ster-

Nitrazine Test Color Interpretations

Membranes Probably Intact

Yellow	pH 5.0
Olive yellow	pH 5.5
Olive green	pH 6.0

Ruptured Membranes

Blue green	pH 6.5
Blue gray	pH 7.0
Deep blue	pH 7.5

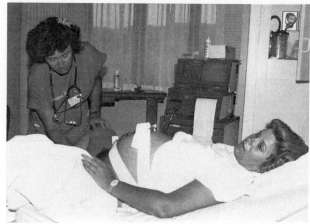

■ *Figure 22–4*

Initial examination. Performing Leopold maneuvers and assessment of abnormal vaginal bleeding and amniotic fluid status are important before performing the initial vaginal examination. The nurse performs a gentle but thorough examination while talking to the mother and encouraging relaxation. (Courtesy of Good Samaritan Hospital, San Jose, CA)

ile cotton swabs are used to take samples of vaginal secretions from the cervical os to test with nitrazine and make a slide to check for ferning. The practitioner also looks for fluid leaking from the cervix, vaginal pooling, color of the fluid, and any cervical dilatation. When the procedure is over, the woman is made comfortable. The slide prepared for the fern test needs to dry for 5 to 7 minutes before it is examined under the microscope. Because of the sodium chloride content in amniotic fluid, the dried specimen, if truly amniotic fluid, looks like clusters of fern leaves. The client and support person should be informed of the test results; if the membranes are ruptured, the report will be a positive fern test, and if they are not ruptured, the report will be a negative fern test.

Some physicians may wait, up to a certain time, for labor to start on its own; others may desire the starting of an oxytocin infusion. In either management, delaying or minimizing the number of vaginal examinations can lower the chance of introducing bacteria into the uterine cavity.[10]

INITIAL VAGINAL EXAMINATION

Abdominally assessing fetal position, assessing for abnormal vaginal bleeding, and assessing amniotic fluid status are all recommended nursing practices before the initial vaginal examination. Historically, rectal examinations were the primary method used to assess the pregnant woman, but almost universally the vaginal examination is the preferred method. In many teaching institutions, the physician or resident primarily assumes this responsibility of examination, but in any other facility it is common for the nurse to perform the vaginal examination (Fig. 22-4).

For this procedure, the client lies on her back with her knees flexed and heels together; her knees fall outward laterally. The nurse drapes the client so that she is well protected, leaving the perineal region exposed. Sterile gloves are donned by the examiner. Before the

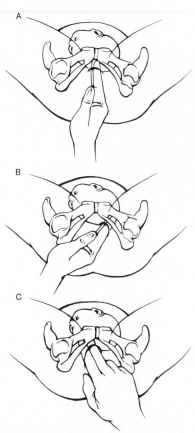

■ *Figure 22–5*

Vaginal examination. (A) Determining the station and palpating the sagittal suture. (B) Identifying the posterior fontanel. (C) Identifying the anterior fontanel. Note the first and second fingers are the examining fingers. The examiner must be careful not to touch the rectal area with the fourth and fifth fingers. The examiner must also be careful with placement of the thumb by not applying too much pressure to the mons pubis.

fingers are introduced into the vagina, the labia are opened widely to minimize possible contamination of the examining fingers if they should come in contact with the inner surfaces of the labia and the margins of the hymen. The index and middle fingers are lubricated with K-Y Jelly; it is important not to touch the lubricant tube with the fingers. An assistant can squeeze the lubricant onto the examiner's fingers. The index and second fingers of the examining hand are gently introduced into the vagina (Fig. 22-5).

Nursing Diagnosis

Admission process is the time the nurse starts assessing the client and initiates the care plan. The following is a list of potential nursing diagnoses that may be used:

1. Alteration in comfort: acute pain related to uterine contractions
2. Fear related to hospital surroundings
3. Fear related to impending labor and birth
4. Alteration in tissue perfusion: placental perfusion to fetus decreased due to supine position
5. Sleep pattern disturbance
6. Knowledge deficit related to expectations in labor
7. Knowledge deficit related to hospital procedures
8. Knowledge deficit related to the process of labor and appropriate relaxation techniques
9. Ineffective individual coping related to lack of support systems

The birth of a baby is viewed as a major event in life so that the labor and delivery nurse may be addressing the care plan not only for the mother and fetus but for other family members such as father, grandparents, aunts, uncles, and friends. From the above list of diagnoses, numbers 2, 3, 5, 6, and 7 might apply to the other family members.

Planning and Intervention

PSYCHOSOCIAL CONSIDERATIONS

Because contact with the client during the labor and delivery process is short term, the nurse is faced with the problem of providing high-quality care in a short space of time. The key appears to be the ability to use whatever time is available, whether it be 5 minutes or an hour, to provide an atmosphere of receptivity to the client's needs. The ability to determine needs lies in the perceptions that underlie the assessment and diagnosis portions of the nursing process. When effective care is implemented, the nurse's facility with therapeutic communication plus technical understanding and skill are key issues.

A good deal of time and effort has been spent in nursing research to determine the needs of clients, especially the needs above and beyond those related directly to physiological and pathological conditions. These needs have generally been classified as "emotional" or "psychosocial." Whatever their label, they are especially important for consideration with the maternity client and support system.

Establishment of the Nurse–Client Relationship. For many young women in labor, admission to the maternity unit may mark her first acquaintance with hospitals as a patient. Her immediate reaction may be one of strangeness, loneliness, and homesickness, particularly if the father is not permitted to stay with her in the labor room. Regardless of the amount of preparation for this event, whether she is happy or unhappy, whether she wants the baby or not, every mother enters labor with a certain amount of normal tension and anxiety. Moreover, some mothers are thoroughly afraid of the whole process. This may be attributed in part to the fact that the mother's preparation for childbearing has been limited, or, she may have been reared in an environment fraught with mysteries and old wives' tales about childbirth. If she has had children previously, she may have had unfortunate and fear-producing experiences. All these factors make her fear understandable.

First Impressions. The kind of greeting the client receives as she enters the labor and delivery unit is extremely important and sets the tone for future interaction with the health team. When the father is present, the nurse should be mindful that he is to be considered and welcomed in an appropriate way, as is the mother.

The mother needs to be made to feel welcomed, expected, and necessary. More hospitals are allowing not only the father to accompany the mother, but also other support persons whom the mother may want to have with her during labor and delivery.

Support Person. Rarely do we see women having their babies without some sort of support person present. This person can be the father of the baby, a family member (e.g., mother or sister), or a close friend. This person may have attended prepared childbirth classes with the client and may be ready to assume the role of coach during the labor and delivery. The converse is also true; the support person may not have attended classes and needs, as does the client, teaching on ways to relax and cope with labor.

Culture may dictate the amount of involvement the father is to have in the birth experience. Nursing needs to assess the family and be respectful of their choice and not judgmental if it differs from what the staff feels is the appropriate way for the father and family to act.

Orientation. The mother and the father need to know what is expected of them and what they, in turn, can expect. The mother can be helped, if necessary, to change to the hospital gown and can be made comfortable in a chair or, if she wishes, in bed.

The nurse can begin an orientation to the process of labor as well as to the general environment. There is no set form or content for this orientation and no set time for the introduction and the continuation of this process; rather, the nurse must first explore what the parents do know about the environment and the labor process, to judge what needs to be introduced, reinforced, and so on, and when the most appropriate time to do this would be. An easy conversational manner may be employed rather than a rapid-fire explanation of dos and don'ts.

The rationale for any procedures or restrictions is always given. The client must not be overloaded with too many stimuli at one time and should be allowed to absorb any new information and explanation before additional material is presented. The nurse can structure the situation to allow the client to "feed back" information, so as to reveal how much the mother really understands.

Generally, the couple should know the limits of the mother's activity and what restrictions of food and fluids there will be. What the client and the father can expect regarding the progress of labor should be included also (e.g., what will be happening physically, how the mother will be feeling, and how she and her partner can participate in the labor experience). Keeping the patient informed as to her progress in labor is foremost in nursing intervention.

As implied, this orientation continues throughout the entire course of labor and delivery. The nurse determines when and how each phase is to be instituted, according to the cues given by the mother and father.

PHYSICAL PREPARATION

Vulvar and Perineal Preparation. The aim in shaving or clipping and washing the vulva is to cleanse and disinfect the immediate area around the vagina, to visualize the perineal area better, and to prevent any contamination from entering the birth canal. During labor, pathogenic bacteria can ascend the birth canal; thus, every effort is made to protect the client from intrapartum infection. Research over the years has demonstrated that shaving the perineum actually enhances the possibility of infection, probably owing to the myriad of nicks that can occur in the shaving process. When clipping the hair is compared with not clipping, data indicate no difference in infection rates.[11-16] Nevertheless, in many institutions, shaving or clipping the perineal hair continues. Some physicians do not require that the mons pubis be shaved because of the discomfort that the regrowth of the hair causes; they feel that clipping the hair suffices. Other physicians do not order the perineum shaved and simply have the area washed well with a bacteriostatic soap.

When the perineum is to be shaved, a pad is placed under the buttocks and the client assumes the same position she was in for the vaginal examination. Lighting must be optimal, and the nurse asks the woman if she has any warts or moles that she should be made aware of before shaving. The nurse should put on gloves for this procedure.

The vulvar hair is lathered before shaving to facilitate the procedure and to make it more comfortable for the client. An ordinary safety razor is used. The shave is started at the top of the labia majora. The direction of the stroke goes from above downward as the area of the vulva is shaved. The skin can be stretched above each downward stroke and the razor permitted to move smoothly over the skin without undue pressure.

When the entire area anterior to an imaginary line drawn through the base of the perineal body has been shaved, the client can turn to her side to allow the anal area to be completely shaved. With the upper leg well flexed, the anal area is lathered and shaved, again with a front to back stroke. It must always be remembered that anything that has passed over the anal region must not be returned near the vulvar orifice. If an enema is to be given, it is at this time, with the client positioned on her left side (see next section).

In washing the genitals, the nurse first thoroughly cleanses the surrounding areas, using sterile sponges or disposable washcloths for each area, and gradually works in toward the vestibule. The strokes must be from above downward and away from the introitus. Special attention should be paid to separating the vulvar folds to remove the smegma that may have accumulated in the folds of the labia minora or at the base of the clitoris. Finally, the region around the anus is cleansed. The client is instructed not to touch the genital area after being cleansed.

Enema. Until recently, an enema was a routine admission procedure. It was deemed a necessity to prevent the presence of stool in the rectum, which might impede the descent of the presenting part, and also to ensure that no stool would be expelled during delivery, which might contaminate the sterile field. It was also thought to enhance the strength of the contractions.

However, experience and research indicate that the enema is not as necessary as once believed and enemas given solely to stimulate labor are not warranted in modern maternity care.

In some institutions, the decision to give an enema is left to the nurses on the basis of their clinical judgment. In other hospitals, an enema is still required as prescribed. In any case, it is wise for the nurse to ascertain, during the history taking, if the client has had a recent bowel movement. If she had a normal evacuation that day, an enema is probably not necessary. If the client is constipated, an enema can be helpful. However, if she is having diarrhea, the procedure is certainly not necessary and the possibility of an infection must be considered.

In addition to the above assessments, the nurse also must be aware that there are clinical conditions that warrant a contraindication to administering an enema. The following are examples of clinical conditions in which administrating an enema would be contraindicated: unengaged vertex, nonvertex lie, abnormal amount of vaginal bleeding or the history of placenta previa or abruptio, advanced labor, nonreassuring fetal heart rate. At any time the nurse feels the benefits of an enema do not outweigh the risk of administration the physician should be notified and the enema should not given.

The type of enema may vary from warm tap water using an enema can or bag to a disposable type that comes with the solution prepared and with a prelubricated tip. The nurse uses the same principles in administering the enema as for any other client. However, it may be more difficult to insert the tube because of the pressure of the presenting part of the fetus or because of hemorrhoids that may accompany pregnancy.

Hemorrhoids or the strength of the contractions may make the enema uncomfortable for the client, and it is essential that she be informed that the nurse is aware of the possible discomfort. To aid in comfort, the nurse can stop the enema infusion during the contractions by pinching the tubing or ceasing to squeeze the disposable enema container. The client is encouraged to hold the enema as long as possible before expelling. The nurse needs to chart that the procedure has been done and the results of the enema.

Soapsuds enemas should not be used and have been associated with acute colitis, bowel perforation, gangrene, and even anaphylaxis.[17]

UNIVERSAL PRECAUTIONS

The Centers for Disease Control (CDC) recommended in 1987 that blood and body precautions be used for all patients regardless of their bloodborne infection status.[18] This policy is referred to as "Universal Precautions." The intention of universal precautions is to prevent exposure of the health-care worker to bloodborne pathogens. Protection is achieved by the health-care worker using protective barriers to decrease the risk of exposure of the worker's skin or mucous membranes to potentially infective material. Protective barriers include the use of gloves, gowns, masks, and protective eyewear (Fig. 22-6).

Blood is the single most important source of human immunodeficiency virus (HIV), hepatitis B virus (HBV), and other bloodborne pathogens in the occupational setting.[18] Other body fluids to which universal precau-

tions apply that specifically relate to care in maternity are vaginal secretions, semen, and amniotic fluid.

Nurses working with women in labor and newborn infants must follow "Universal Precautions" policies to prevent exposure to HIV, HBV, and other bloodborne pathogens. Receiving HBV immunization is another way health-care workers can protect themselves.

■ FIRST STAGE OF LABOR

The first stage of labor (dilating stage) begins with the first symptoms of true labor and ends with the complete dilatation of the cervix. The physician examines the client early in labor and sees her from time to time throughout the first stage but may not be in constant attendance at this time.

During labor, assessments of the fetal heart rate and vaginal examinations determine whether the fetus is in good condition and that the mother is making steady progress. Furthermore, the rate of progress often gives some indication as to when delivery is to be expected. During this stage, the nurse is in constant attendance, safeguarding the welfare of the mother and fetus and notifying the physician of the progress of labor.

Assessment

VAGINAL EXAMINATIONS

The frequency with which vaginal examinations are required during labor depends on the individual case; often one or two such examinations are sufficient, whereas in some instances more are required. The nurse who stays with the mother constantly becomes increasingly skillful in the ability to follow the progress of labor by careful evaluation of the character of the uterine contractions, the amount of show, the progressive descent of the area on the abdomen where fetal heart sounds are heard, and the mother's overall response to her physical labor.

UTERINE CONTRACTIONS

Many young women approach childbirth with fear of pain. It is no easy task to dispel this age-old fear, but throughout the childbirth experience a conscious effort must be made to instill a wholesome point of view in the mother. The nurse should avoid the use of the word *pain* whenever possible because of the connotation of the word.

Sociocultural factors play an important part in the meaning and interpretation and expression of pain for

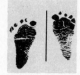

Nursing Care Plan

Admission of the Woman Into Labor Unit

Client Goals

1. Client and fetus are assessed for a state of well-being and maintain an uncompromised physical and emotional state as demonstrated by normal and appropriate maternal physical and emotional findings and reassuring FHR.
2. Client and father indicate a sense of being welcomed to the hospital during the admission.
3. Client and family demonstrate adequate knowledge of physical surroundings, procedures, expectations of them, and so forth.

Assessment	Potential Nursing Diagnosis	Planning and Intervention	Evaluation
Assess knowledge of: Preparation for labor process Hospital procedures Hospital surroundings	Knowledge deficit related to: Expectations during labor Hospital procedures and surroundings Preparation for labor relaxation methods Fear	Establish relationship with client and father Find out how client wants to be referred to (e.g., first name) Provide an orientation to unit and labor process Convey that the couple is expected and welcomed Individualize teaching plan to cover expectations and restrictions of the environment, review or teach relaxation methods, answer questions	Client and father are familiar with the new environment and settle in Client understands equipment, procedures, expectations Client uses appropriate relaxation methods for stage of labor Client and family feel rapport with staff
Maternal			
Frequency, duration, intensity of contractions Status of bag of waters Character and amount of show Vital signs Bowel and bladder patterns Allergies to medication Time of last ingestion	Alteration in comfort: acute pain related to uterine contractions	Take nursing history Record and report findings as appropriate Begin to provide comfort measures as needed Discuss choice of anesthesia for delivery and use of analgesia in labor	Client understands use of analgesia and anesthesia Client chooses type to be used Appropriate comfort measures are provided
Fetal			
EDC fundal height Fetal position, FHR		Document EDC and appropriateness of fundal height to gestational age, record FHR/fetoscope/Doppler/fetal monitor	Fetus at term, vertex position, appropriate fundal height, FHR within normal limits

(continued)

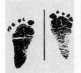

Nursing Care Plan *(continued)*

Assessment	Potential Nursing Diagnosis	Planning and Intervention	Evaluation
Admission Procedures			
General physical assessment	Alteration in tissue perfusion: placental perfusion to fetus decreased secondary to maternal supine position	Discourage supine position	Client avoids supine position and FHR is maintained
Vaginal exam, perineal clip or enema, if ordered		Perform physical assessment	Client rests, if needed
	Sleep pattern disturbance	Complete admitting procedures, as indicated	Support person is at bedside
	Ineffective individual coping related to lack of support systems	Provide quiet environment for resting, if indicated	
		Encourage presence of support person(s); if none available, provide support	

clients. Although pain is basically a physiological phenomenon, the meaning pain has and the kinds of responses to pain that are deemed appropriate are partly matters of cultural prescription. Cultural orientations, social conditioning, and sociocultural sanctioning play a large part in molding patterns of response to painful experiences that are modal (i.e., occur most frequently) in a group, and these modal patterns are meaningful in terms of the values and beliefs of a particular group.

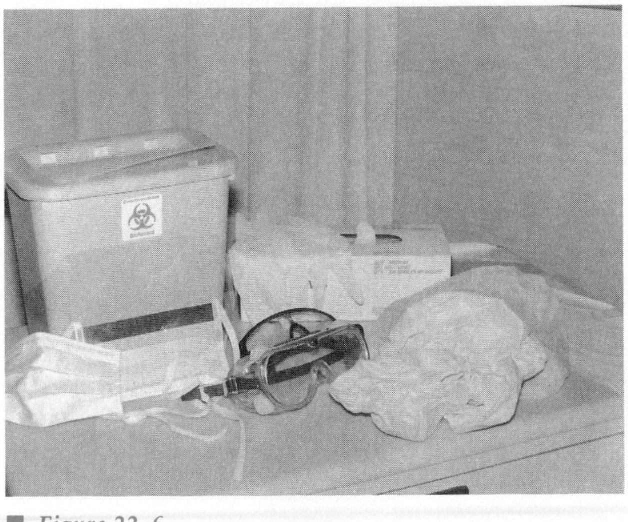

Therefore, the culture or subculture from which a person comes conditions the formation of her particular reaction patterns to pain, and a knowledge of a group's attitudes toward pain is extremely important to the understanding of the reaction of a particular member of that group.

It is important to remember, however, that as labor progresses, the contractions become increasingly painful. Therefore, it is the nurse's responsibility to help the mother distinguish between the *fear and anticipation* of pain and the *discomfort or actual pain* that she may be experiencing, and to help her cope effectively.

Timing the Contractions. Frequency, duration, and intensity of the contractions should be watched closely and recorded whether or not an electronic fetal monitor is used. As labor progresses, the character of the contractions changes. They become stronger in intensity, last longer (30–60 seconds), and come closer together (every 2–3 minutes). If the monitor is not being used, one effective method the nurse can employ to time contractions is to keep her fingers lightly on the fundus. The fingers are recommended because they are more sensitive than the palm. However, for some people the whole hand is helpful. It should be emphasized that enough of the fingers should be used to ensure adequate contact with the abdomen; too slight a contact does not enable the nurse to ascertain the contractions accurately.

Assessing contractions in this manner enables the nurse to detect the contraction, as it begins, by the gradual tensing and rising forward of the fundus and to feel the contraction through its three phases until the uterus relaxes again. The inexperienced nurse can get some

■ *Figure 22–6*

Examples of items available for universal precautions—gloves, masks with and without splash protection, apron, and disposal container for sharps. (Courtesy of Long Beach Memorial Medical Center, Long Beach, CA)

idea of how a contraction feels under her fingertips by contracting her own biceps. First, the forearm should be extended and the fingertips of the hand on the opposite side placed on the biceps. The arm is gradually flexed until the muscle becomes hard, held a few seconds, and gradually extended. This should take about 30 seconds to simulate a uterine contraction.

The nurse should not rely on the mother to indicate when a contraction begins, because often she is unaware of it for perhaps 5 or 10 seconds, sometimes even until the contraction reaches its acme. It is important to observe the frequency and duration of the contractions and to be assured that the uterine muscle relaxes completely after each contraction.

As the labor approaches the transition, the contractions become strong, last about 60 seconds, and occur at 2- to 3-minute intervals.

If any contraction lasts longer than 90 seconds and is not followed by a rest interval with complete relaxation of the uterine muscle, this should be reported to the physician immediately. The implications for both the mother and her infant can be severe (see Chap. 38).

SHOW

Show is a mucoid discharge from the cervix that is present after the mucous plug has been dislodged. As progressive effacement and dilatation of the cervix occur, the show becomes blood tinged owing to the rupture of the superficial capillaries. The presence of an increased amount of bloody show, blood-stained mucus and not actual bleeding, suggests that rapid progress may be taking place and the client should be assessed. Often in conjunction with the increase in bloody show are strong uterine contractions and the urge to push. If by vaginal examination the woman is found to be close to delivery, the physician is notified.

VITAL SIGNS

It is recommended that blood pressure be evaluated every hour and temperature, pulse, and respiration rate every 4 hours, or more frequently as necessary, depending on the clinical situation.

FETAL HEART RATE

Assessment of fetal heart rate (FHR) constitutes one of the most important responsibilities during the intrapartum period. The selection of method and frequency of assessment should reflect the patient's condition, department policy, and recommendations of professional organizations. Whether using electronic fetal heart rate monitoring or intermittent auscultation with uterine palpation it is recommended for low-risk patients to assess, evaluate and record FHR every 30 minutes after a contraction in the active phase of the first stage of labor and every 15 minutes in the second stage of labor.[2] With high-risk patients the recommendations are different, but the practitioner still has the choice to use electronic fetal monitoring or intermittent auscultation. During the active phase of the first stage of labor, the FHR is evaluated and recorded at least every 15 minutes. During the second stage of labor, the FHR is evaluated and recorded every 5 minutes.[2]

As discussed earlier, it is important to assess the fetus before ambulation, enema administration, artificial rupture of membranes, and the administration of analgesia or anesthesia. Equally important is the reassessment after all the events just listed. It is an important nursing function to assess FHR immediately after the rupture of membranes regardless of whether they rupture spontaneously or are artificially ruptured by the physician. With the gush of water that ensues, there is a possibility that the cord may be prolapsed, and any indication of fetal distress from the pressure on the umbilical cord can be detected by a decrease in the FHR. The electronic fetal monitor is widely used in the hospital setting for the assessment of fetal well-being and evaluation of uterine contractions during labor. A thorough discussion of this device can be found in Chapter 43.

Nursing Diagnosis

Updating the nursing care plan is an ongoing process that is done in correlation with the client's progress in labor. Attending to the immediate needs of the client, assuring comfort, and maintaining maternal and fetal well-being may be the primary areas the nurse is addressing, whereas other identified diagnoses may not be readdressed until the fourth stage of labor or during the postpartum period. Below is a list of potential nursing diagnoses; nursing interventions and evaluation criteria are found in the nursing care plan on pages 484 and 485.

1. Alteration in comfort: pain related to uterine contractions
2. Fear related to impending labor and birth
3. Alteration in tissue perfusion: placental, decreased, secondary to maternal position
4. Sleep pattern disturbance
5. Fluid volume deficit related to decreased fluid intake
6. Alteration in oral mucous membrane related to mouth breathing
7. Alteration in nutrition: less than body requirements related to onset of labor and need to decrease oral intake

8. Self-care deficit related to immobility during labor (toileting, hygiene)
9. Ineffective individual and family coping related to hospitalization
10. Ineffective individual coping related to inappropriate relaxation and breathing patterns
11. Ineffective individual coping related to lack of support systems
12. Ineffective family coping related to client being in pain
13. Knowledge deficit related to the process of labor and appropriate relaxation techniques

Planning and Intervention

PSYCHOSOCIAL CONSIDERATIONS

As already emphasized, it is important for the nurse to have an empathic supportive attitude toward the mother to interpret the progress of labor and perform certain technical procedures skillfully. It should be pointed out that "supportive care" includes not only emotional support but also aspects of physical care that, in the total context of care, contribute to the well-being and the comfort of the mother and hence to her emotional equilibrium. Thus, a sponge bath, oral hygiene, a back rub, an explanation before a procedure, and so on all enhance the mother's comfort and help her to feel that she is a special, worthwhile person. The nursing staff must not just walk into the labor room, review the fetal monitor, and walk out.

The Effective Use of Touch. Many of the physical care activities that nurses perform consist, in part at least, in "laying on of hands," which is known to be necessary and helpful to clients in maintaining or receiving good health. This type of communication can be a way of demonstrating the nurse's concern and empathy; especially when verbal communication is difficult or impossible. This contact can take the form of a back rub, stroking the client's brow, and so on. Many of the relaxation techniques practiced in the prepared childbirth classes rely on the use of this sense. Even the intrusive procedures that are so often painful or distasteful, if done with gentleness and skill, show the client that her dignity and integrity are respected.

However, touch should not be used indiscriminately; excessive or inappropriate touching is offensive to many people. The need varies from person to person and the woman indicates which type of touch is helpful and who is the most appropriate person to give it. The nurse must use professional judgment regarding its use, and rapport with the client helps to indicate a correct decision. It is also an effective means of incorporating the partner into the care and the support of his mate.

Providing Assurance. The mother who has attended antepartal classes that have included exercise and relaxation techniques is usually better prepared for labor, but nevertheless she needs to be coached in using the techniques that enable her to cooperate with the natural forces of labor. During early labor, the client usually prefers to move about the room and frequently is more at ease sitting in a comfortable chair. She can be permitted and encouraged to do this and whatever else seems to be most relaxing and pleasant to her.

Once labor is well established, the mother should not be left alone. The morale of women in labor is sometimes hopelessly shattered, regardless of whether or not they have been prepared for labor during pregnancy, when they are left by themselves over long periods. During labor, the mother is more sensitive to the behavior of those about her, particularly in relation to her perception of how much concern the personnel about her show for her safety and well-being. As labor progresses, there is a normal narrowing of the phenomenal field, an "inward turning," which results in easy distortion of stimuli and perception. For instance, careless remarks dropped in conversation often are misinterpreted as indicative of negligence or lack of feeling. It is important to remember that comments and laughter overheard in the corridor outside the client's room may contribute to her uneasiness. Therefore, the nurse must be on guard against unfortunate happenings of this kind.

The nurse should be aware that her own anxieties in the situation may be communicated to the client. The process of labor and the forthcoming delivery produce normal anxieties that are no more than a healthy anticipation of the events to come (in both client and nurse). *Thus, most clients tolerate their labor better if they are told the kind of progress that is being made and are assured that they are doing a good job working with their contractions.* This is part and parcel of the continuing orientation to the labor process that was mentioned earlier.

Another point that is apropos here is the usefulness and the effectiveness of suggestion for the mother in labor. The nurse can use this suggestibility to great advantage in her supportive care, because the mother responds readily to suggestions, especially in early labor. The groundwork can be laid at this time for the more complicated instructions that may be necessary later in labor concerning relaxation, breathing techniques, and the management of pain.

Psychosocial Support During Contractions. Particularly during the late active phase there is a need for human contact—someone to hold onto—during the severe contractions. The mother responds less well to other physical contact, stroking, sponging, and so on; she may even say, "Leave me alone," meaning, of

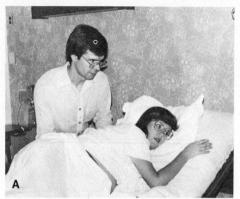
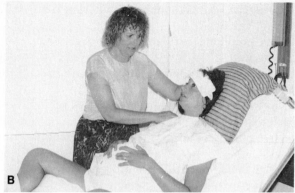

■ *Figure 22–7*
Nursing diagnosis—Alteration in comfort related to uterine contractions and descent of the fetus. Examples of nursing interventions include assisting the mother in position changes that provide the most comfort. (Courtesy of Long Beach Memorial Medical Center, Long Beach, CA, and San Pedro Peninsula Hospital, San Pedro, CA)

course, "Don't disturb me." However, if it is helpful for her to have someone's hand to hold, she should be allowed to do this if she indicates the need.

PHYSICAL COMFORT

Positioning. Since the introduction of the electronic fetal monitor, many hospitals attach the monitor to the client routinely for fetal assessment during labor. The mother must be in bed for this equipment to function appropriately. This, of course, limits the mother's mobility. The reason for the use of the monitor needs to be explained to the client so that she can understand why her activity is restricted and will not become unduly alarmed. If the client is requesting to ambulate, it is important to get an order from the physician. Most facilities allow ambulation if the presenting part is engaged or the bag of waters is intact. The mother should come back to the labor room for periodic auscultation of the FHR (i.e., every 30 minutes). It should be noted that the newer fetal monitors with improved electronics allow for better tracings on the external mode and allow more maternal movement to positions of comfort. Changes in position and transducer adjustments are noted on the strip chart.

If monitors are not employed, the client can be encouraged to assume any position that is comfortable for her, such as side, squatting, all fours, sitting (Fig. 22-7). A woman should not labor on her back. These other positions have been found to enhance the efficacy of the labor contractions, whereas in the supine position there is less uteroplacental perfusion, causing contractions to be more frequent but less intense (Fig. 22-8).[9,19,20,21]

Dealing with Contractions. The contribution that the nurse can make in the management of pain during labor

and delivery is discussed in Chapter 23. However, a few of the major points are reiterated here to reinforce them. Studies of pain have demonstrated that the anticipation of pain can raise the anxiety level significantly so as to lower pain tolerance. Thus, the client reacts sooner to even minimal pain stimuli. The pain is subjectively intensified and even a slight amount of pain seems to be much greater. Furthermore, other sensations may be misinterpreted as pain (e.g., pressure, stretching), which explains why the digital examinations and even the pressure of the nurse's fingers on the abdomen as she manually times contractions "hurt." Therefore, "everything" is painful, and the heightening of the anticipation of pain in turn increases the response to pain, and soon a vicious cycle is established.

The nurse can help to break this cycle or prevent it from becoming established by intervening at the anticipation–anxiety junction. This is done by reminding the client that a contraction is over (and the pain is gone) and that because another contraction is not expected for several minutes this is the time for her to rest and to relax. The anxiety related to the anticipation of pain is lowered or eliminated (the mother knows that she will be free from pain for several minutes and can rest), and the subjective intensification is diminished. It is obvious that the nurse or some other reliable person must be in continuous attendance to do this.

Breathing Techniques. Because during the first stage of labor the uterine contractions are involuntary and uncontrolled by the client, it is futile for her to "bear down" with her abdominal muscles, because this only leads to exhaustion. The mother who has been prepared for childbirth has been schooled in breathing techniques, such as diaphragmatic breathing or rapid, shallow costal breathing, and with coaching from her partner or her nurse is usually able to accomplish conscious relaxation.

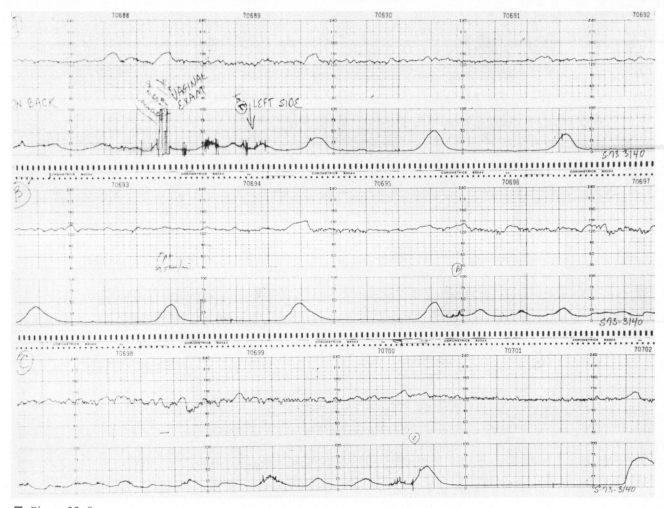

■ *Figure 22–8*

Uterine contractions. (A) Frequent uterine contractions are occurring. When the client is turned to her left side, the contractions become less frequent and increase in strength. (B) The woman has turned and is lying on her back; the contractions have become frequent and smaller. (C) Again on her left side, the contractions are spaced out as before, in A. (Freeman R, Garite T: Fetal Heart Rate Monitoring. Baltimore, Williams & Wilkins, © 1981)

The Unprepared Mother. A different situation exists with the unprepared mother. These mothers are often best helped to relax by encouraging and coaching them to keep breathing slowly and evenly during the early contractions and to assume a pattern of more rapid and shallow breathing that is most comfortable to them during the late active phase. They often need to be reminded not to hold their breath during the contractions.

One cannot expect perfection in breathing techniques with these clients; however, this activity gives the inexperienced mother a point of concentration, and her feeling that she is actually participating and "controlling" her labor to some degree is helpful to her. Most mothers in labor, whether they are "prepared" or not, want to cooperate, and the calm, kind, firm guidance of an interested nurse can do much to help the mother use her contractions effectively.

The practice regarding the intake of fluid and food varies greatly both in the literature and clinical practice. Therefore, the medical orders of the physician in charge and in some cases anesthesiologist need to be ascertained before proceeding. In the hospital setting, it is customary to limit oral intake to ice chips. If the client is admitted in the latent phase of labor, the physician may order a clear liquid diet. The client in active labor is usually not given solid or liquid foods because many women experience nausea and vomiting in labor. The other concern is the potential risk of aspiration of gastric contents. Gastric emptying is slower in pregnancy than the nonpregnant state, and labor may contribute to a slowing in gastric contents.[22] Proponents of allowing women in labor to eat might consider limiting this practice to healthy women with no risk factors and those labors that are unmedicated.[23] It seems to be common

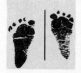

Nursing Care Plan

The Woman/Family During First Stage of Labor

Client Goals

1. Client is able to verbalize her progress in labor.
2. Client acknowledges increase in comfort by verbal and nonverbal communication when comfort measures are done by the nurse and support person(s).
3. Client, support person, and family continue to demonstrate adequate knowledge of physical surroundings, procedures, and expectations.
4. Support person and family indicate knowledge of client's progress in labor.

Assessment	Potential Nursing Diagnosis	Planning and Intervention	Evaluation
Monitor labor, contractions, FHR, vital signs	Alteration in tissue perfusion: placental, secondary to maternal position	Check vital signs regularly per hospital policy and clinical needs Attach fetal monitor or time contractions Check FHR for rate, accelerations, variability, decelerations Avoid supine position	Woman has vital signs within normal limits FHR maintains normal rate Woman's labor progresses
Monitor intake and output	Fluid volume deficit related to decreased fluid intake Alteration in oral mucous membrane related to mouth breathing Alteration in nutrition less than body requirement related to restriction of intake during labor	Give ice chips prn Maintain adequate parenteral intake (125 ml/h) Encourage voiding q2–3 h; catheterize if needed Record intake and output Encourage use of lip balm Provide mouth care Instruct and reinforce proper breathing techniques	Woman's mouth and lips are moist Woman's bladder remains normal
Determine which comfort measures are most helpful	Alteration in comfort; acute pain related to labor contractions Self-care deficit related to immobility during labor (toileting, hygiene)	Rub back and change client's position and linen as necessary Apply cool washcloth to face Encourage rest Encourage frequent voiding, giving assistance to bathroom or with bedpan Give analgesia if client requests and as ordered by physician	Client breathes appropriately with contractions Client relaxes between contractions Client states what comfort measures are most helpful
Determine client's need for explanations and emotional support as indicated	Sleep pattern disturbance related to labor Ineffective individual cop-	Keep explanations and instructions short and simple	Couple changes breathing patterns to coincide with stage of labor

(continued)

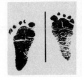

Nursing Care Plan   (continued)

Assessment	Potential Nursing Diagnosis	Planning and Intervention	Evaluation
	ing related to inappropriate relaxation and breathing patterns	Encourage mother to sleep and rest between contractions	Couple follows instruction with minimum of difficulty
		Decrease environmental stimulus	Client rests when able
Determine support person's ability to coach and support the client	Knowledge deficit related to coaching role	Allow couple time together	Support person assists mother in coping with labor
Determine support person's needs	Ineffective individual and family coping related to hospitalization for the onset of labor	Encourage support person's participation in care	Support person feels a part of the labor process
	Ineffective family coping related to client being in pain	Explain labor process as things progress to client and support person	Client benefits from support person's presence and support
		Keep support person(s) in waiting room up to date	
		Assist client in changing breathing techniques as labor progresses	
		Identify and reinforce adaptive coping behavior	
		Provide support to the coach (refreshments, breaks) and reinforce appropriate behavior	

practice in U.S. hospitals to limit the oral intake to women in labor to ice chips, clear fluids, and even NPO.

Nursing interventions to combat the dry mouth and potential for dehydration are to provide mouth care and offer the clear fluids or ice chips. The nurse may increase client comfort by using a washcloth to moisten the mouth and lips; using lip balm is also encouraged (Fig. 22-9).

Intravenous fluid administration for all labors is common practice in hospitals. Administration of an IV in early labor is probably not necessary, and delayed start of an IV may be an intervention that allows women more freedom for ambulation. The reasons intravenous solutions are started include: (1) prevention of dehydration, electrolyte imbalance, and acidosis; (2) having a "life line" for emergencies; (3) usually required before the administration of analgesia, anesthesia; (4) administration of oxytocin prophylactically after the delivery to prevent uterine atony.

Bladder. The client can be asked to void at least every 2 to 3 hours. The mother laboring often attributes all of her discomfort to the intensity of uterine contractions and therefore is unaware that it is the pressure of a full bladder that has increased her discomfort. In addition to causing unnecessary discomfort, a full bladder may be a serious impediment to labor or the cause of urinary retention in the puerperium. If the distended bladder can be palpated above the symphysis pubis and the client is unable to void, the physician is to be so informed. Straight catheterization may be prescribed in such cases.

Progression of Active Phase of Labor. As labor progresses into the active phase, the woman's mood changes and she "gets down to business." She begins to concentrate on her breathing techniques and needs assistance from the father. She needs help to get in a position of comfort. Regardless of how diligently the

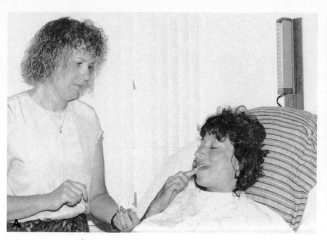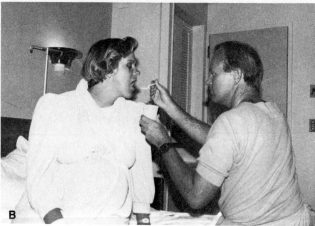

■ *Figure 22–9*
Nursing diagnosis—High risk for fluid volume deficit related to decreased fluid intake and for alteration in oral mucous membrane related to mouth breathing. Examples of high risk nursing interventions include reminding the woman to use lip balm and taking ice chips prn. (Courtesy of San Pedro Peninsula Hospital, San Pedro, CA, and Good Samaritan Hospital, San Jose, CA)

mother has practiced the various breathing and relaxing techniques during pregnancy, or the level of her understanding about the physiology of labor, the situation is changed somewhat during active labor. Encouragement should be given to both the mother and the father. The nurse remains with the client, providing care in an organized, calm manner; instructions need to be short and direct. Nursing care measures include mouth care, keeping ice chips available, placing a cool washcloth on the mother's forehead, keeping the perineum clean and dry, lowering the lights and keeping the environment quiet, providing counterpressure on the sacral area during contractions, and updating the physician and family members on the progress. Also, the nurse may

---

Signs and Symptoms of Second Stage

1. The client begins to bear down of her own accord; this is caused by a reflex when the head begins to press on the perineal floor.
2. Her mood of increasing apprehension, which has been building since the contractions began, deepens; she becomes more serious and may appear bewildered by the force of the contractions.
3. There is usually a sudden increase in show, which is more blood tinged.
4. The client may become increasingly irritable and unwilling to be touched; she may cry if disturbed.
5. The mother thinks that she needs to defecate. This symptom is due to pressure of the head on the perineal floor and consequently against the rectum.
6. Although she has been "working" successfully with her contractions during most of her labor, the uncertainty that she has been experiencing (since 6–8 cm cervical dilatation) as to her ability to cope with the contractions may become overwhelming; she is frustrated and feels unable to manage if left alone.
7. The membranes may rupture, with discharge of amniotic fluid. This, of course, may take place any time but occurs most frequently at the beginning of the second stage.
8. The mother may be saying at this time that she wants to be "put to sleep" or have a cesarean section owing to the increased pain and the desire for labor to be done. It is important to remember that the mother's consciousness is somewhat altered because of the pain, her enforced concentration, and possibly medication; therefore, any coaching needs to be short and explicit and may need to be repeated with each contraction. The nurse also must be firm but gentle in setting limits with the mother, so that she can conserve her energy for the second stage. Thrashing about and continued crying only lead to exhaustion, and the mother needs the firm guidance of a skillful person to help her to maintain control.
9. The perineum begins to bulge and the anal orifice begins to dilate. This is a late sign, but if signs numbered 1, 3, 5, and 7 occur, it should be watched for with every contraction. Only a vaginal examination or the appearance of the head can definitely confirm the suspicion.

want to suggest that the father take some nourishment for himself before the actual birth. As labor progresses (i.e., 8–10 cm), the nurse should continue to encourage correct breathing techniques and assist the client not to bear down prematurely. The client should be reassured that she will shortly be completely dilated and will be ready to start to push.

■ SECOND STAGE OF LABOR

The second stage of labor begins with complete dilatation of the cervix and ends with delivery of the baby. The complete dilatation of the cervix can be definitely confirmed only by a vaginal examination. However, the experienced nurse is often able to suspect complete dilatation by observing changes in her client's behavior, particularly if these findings are correlated with knowledge of the client's parity, the speed of any previous labors and the present labor, and the anticipated size of the baby. The median duration of the second stage of labor has been shown to be 50 minutes for the primigravida and 20 minutes for the multipara.[8] The length of the second stage can vary considerably.

Assessment

There are certain signs and symptoms, both behavioral and physical, that herald the onset of the second stage of labor. These are to be watched for carefully (see Signs and Symptoms of Second Stage). Reporting any or all of these manifestations promptly allows enough time to prepare the mother for the delivery without rushing and provides an opportunity to cleanse and drape the mother properly. If these signs are overlooked, a precipitous delivery may occur without benefit of medical attention. In the traditional setting, in which different rooms are used for labor and the delivery, the primigravida is usually not taken to the delivery room when the cervix is fully dilated and in fact may push in the labor room for some time before transfer. In contrast, the multipara should be taken to the delivery room much sooner, often at 7 to 8 cm of dilatation. The use of epidural anesthesia during labor usually delays transfer of the multipara also and she may even push in the labor room for a while, much like the primigravida.

Nursing Diagnosis

As the client begins the second stage of labor, she begins to realize that the dilatation phase of labor is done. The final part of labor, the pushing stage, is about to begin. Below is a list of potential nursing diagnoses.

1. Ineffective individual coping related to physical exhaustion in response to labor
2. Alteration in comfort: increased pain related to lower fetal position and uterine contractions
3. Fear related to new surroundings.

Nursing interventions and evaluation criteria are found in the nursing care plan, The Woman During Second Stage of Labor.

Planning and Intervention

METHODS FOR BEARING DOWN

During this period, the client is requested to exert her abdominal forces and bear down. In most cases, bearing-down efforts are reflexive and spontaneous in the second stage of labor, but occasionally the mother does not employ her expulsive forces to good advantage, particularly if she has had epidural anesthesia.

Positions and Pushing Efforts. The positions used during the second stage of labor must be such that the presenting part is in alignment with the axis of the pelvis. The student may find that in the hospital setting the semi-Fowler and lateral positions are frequently used. Other positions, such as squatting, kneeling, standing, and semisitting, are becoming more popular but require the staff to be flexible in their delivery of care (Fig. 22-10).

Previously, the bearing-down efforts were thought to be best when the client used long and sustained pushes with no audible sounds made. This methodology is being changed in conjunction with research showing the disadvantage on mother and fetus with repetitive Valsalva maneuvers. Caldeyro-Barcia's recommendations include the following:[21]

- Short pushes of no longer than 6 to 7 seconds
- Physiological pushing: pushing only with the urge to push or approximately three to five times during each contraction
- Pushing with an open glottis and slight exhale

The woman should be encouraged to listen to her body. Caregivers may treat all clients the same in this stage, but it is incorrect to assume that all labors are the same. It is the uterus that decides the amount of effort and the timing of that effort during the second stage.[24] The nurse should review with the couple the type of pushing method they learned in prepared childbirth classes and adapt as necessary. The nurse should facilitate a quiet environment and encourage total relaxation between contractions. Muscular cramps in the legs are

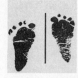

Nursing Care Plan

The Woman During Second Stage of Labor

Client Goals

1. Client continues to progress in labor as evidenced by descent of presenting part and dilatation.
2. Client maintains control by pushing effectively and resting between contractions.
3. Preparation for aseptic delivery is done by following correct infection control procedures.

Assessment	Potential Nursing Diagnosis	Planning and Intervention	Evaluation
Continue to monitor client's labor	Ineffective individual coping related to physical exhaustion in response to labor	Record and report as before; evaluate and record FHR every 15 min in low-risk mothers, every 5 min in high-risk mothers	Client continues with stable blood pressure and FHR
Determine appropriateness of bearing down		Monitor maternal blood pressure	Support person(s) participate actively
Assess client and support person's present coping status		Position client for pushing	Client relaxes her body between contractions
		Encourage active participation of support system	Client stays in control through the support given to her by the nurse and support person
		Praise client's pushing efforts	Client pushes effectively
		Promote complete rest between contractions	
		Assist in promoting constructive coping behaviors	
		Provide quiet environment	
Transfer to delivery room and prepare LDR	Fear related to new surroundings	Explain procedures and equipment	Client understands and verbalizes her role and upcoming procedures
		Instruct support person in delivery room procedures and policies	Support person understands delivery room procedures and policies and coaches mother correctly
		Check resuscitation equipment	
Assist with anesthesia	Alteration in comfort: increased pain related to lower fetal position and uterine contractions	Help with positioning for anesthesia, if necessary	Client experiences a decrease in pain
		Assist with supplies	Client expresses comfort
		Monitor vital signs and intravenous infusions	
Assist with delivery		Continue coaching of client in pushing and panting, when appropriate	Client positions herself appropriately for birth
		Prepare delivery room and LDR	Client delivers a healthy infant
		Position client for delivery	

(continued)

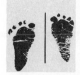

Nursing Care Plan *(continued)*

Assessment	Potential Nursing Diagnosis	Planning and Intervention	Evaluation
		Do perineal prep	
		Monitor FHR (see above)	
		Take blood pressure immediately before delivery	
		Prepare warm environment for newborn	

common in the second stage because of pressure exerted by the baby's head on certain nerves in the pelvis. To relieve these cramps, the leg can be straightened and the ankle dorsiflexed by exerting pressure upward against the ball of the foot until the cramp subsides. Meanwhile, the knee is stabilized with the other hand. These cramps cause excruciating pain and must never be ignored.

The following is a description of how the nurse can assist the client during second stage in the semi-Fowler position:

1. The mother's head and shoulders can be raised to a 45-degree angle and supported firmly during the contraction. The father is of great help in this regard and can provide the strength needed for this physical support.
2. The mother's thighs are flexed on the abdomen, with hands grasped just below the knees when a contraction begins.
3. The client can be encouraged to work with the urge to push, using short, 5-second pushes, with glottis open. She should be instructed that the action is similar to straining during a bowel movement. The long breath-holding pushes may be used if needed to hasten delivery, but should be avoided if possible.
4. Pulling on the knees at this time, as well as flexing the chin on the chest, is a helpful adjunct to maintain downward pressure of the diaphragm and to stabilize the chest and the abdominal musculature.
5. In addition, maintaining the legs flexed as for the "push" position deters the mother from pushing her feet against the table or bed. Avoiding such pressure on the feet is important because it discourages tensing of the gluteal muscles and contributes to further relaxation of the pelvic floor.

PSYCHOSOCIAL SUPPORT

The nurse notices that the mother has become increasingly involved in the whole birth process. The seemingly panicky frustration of the late active phase subsides a bit (with appropriate coaching and reassurance), and the client may experience a sense of relief that the expulsive stage has begun. The desire to push and to bear down is very strong—uncontrollable, in fact—and the client generally gets enormous satisfaction with each push. Some clients, however, experience acute pain and need all available help and encouragement to continue bearing down. In most instances there is complete exhaustion after each expulsive effort, and the mother often drops off to sleep, only to be roused by the next contraction. Because consciousness is still altered, it may

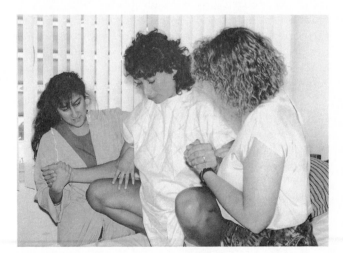

■ *Figure 22–10*
Squatting during second stage. (Courtesy of San Pedro Peninsula Hospital, San Pedro, CA)

be difficult for the mother to follow directions readily even though she may want to. Again, repeated, short, explicit directions are required to encourage her to rest or to work, but especially to prepare the mother for the expulsive effort if she is sleeping between contractions and awakens abruptly. Continue to praise her for her hard work.

Preparation for Delivery

As the second stage progresses, the nurse notices changes in the perineum such as bulging and anal orifice dilatation; if a fetal scalp electrode is in place, the wire comes out as the presenting part descends.

Regardless of the type of delivery system, the nurse at this time has certain responsibilities:

- Notifying the delivery attendant
- Setting up for the delivery
- Providing a warm environment for the newborn
- Checking to see that infant resuscitation equipment is present and functioning
- Checking that the adult emergency equipment is available
- Preparing for the type of anesthesia the client is requesting
- Assisting the father and other support persons to get ready for the delivery; this includes changing into scrub clothes, washing hands, getting camera or video equipment prepared, and setting out eyeglasses for the client if she needs them for the delivery.

All of this is done in addition to being supportive of the efforts of the client and father, pointing up the multifaceted role of the labor and delivery nurse. Preparation for delivery demands the closest teamwork among the physician, nurse, and anesthetist, if required, to best meet the needs of the client, newborn, and support person. By previous understanding, or more often by established hospital routine, each has his or her own responsibilities in the delivery room.

The primary focus for the nurse has been on direct client care. Now she must enlarge her focus to include the physician and other allied professionals (i.e., there are more activities that require the actual assistance of these people than was necessary during the first stage of labor). Thus, the nurse must be sensitive not only to the cues sent by the mother but also to those relayed by the other personnel.

PREPARATION OF THE DELIVERY ROOM

There are no two hospitals in which the delivery room setup or the procedure for delivery is precisely the same.

Therefore, observation and experience in a particular institution serves as the basis for becoming acquainted with the physical layout and the method of care offered. The following, however, gives a general idea of the equipment and materials used in the typical setting.

The delivery table is designed so that its surface is actually composed of two adjoining sections, each covered with its own mattress. This permits the client to lie on her back in the supine position or with her head and back elevated by using the table's hand crank, if the bed model has that feature; if that is not possible, a large wedge-type pillow or regular bed pillows can be used until she must put her legs up into stirrups or the lithotomy position. A word of caution: the mother is still at risk for hypotension due to compression of the gravid uterus on the inferior vena cava. To avoid this, the nurse may want to wedge or tilt the woman using folded towels or a sandbag under her right hip to shift the uterus off the vein and maintain venous return. The table is "broken" by a mechanical device. The retractable or lower end of the table drops and is rolled under the main section of the table. Thus, ready access is given to the perineal region. Or, if it is desired to deliver the client in the dorsal recumbent position, the lower portion of the table can remain in place.

The table opposite the foot of the delivery table, referred to as the back table, contains the principal sterile supplies and instruments needed for normal delivery, including sterile gowns, drapes, towels, sponges, basins, and cord set. The cord set is a group of instruments used for clamping and cutting the umbilical cord: two Kelly clamps, a pair of bandage scissors, and a cord clamp. Other instruments often are included because it may be necessary for the birth attendant to perform an episiotomy or to repair lacerations. Other instruments frequently included are two Kelly clamps, two Allis clamps, one mouse-tooth tissue forceps, two sponge sticks, two tenacula, one needle holder, and straight scissors. The nurse adds to this setup sterile gloves of the correct size, bulb syringe, syringe with large-bore needle for cord blood sample, and, if needed, local anesthesia tray with anesthetic solution, catheter, and suture (Fig. 22-11).

A single- or double-bowl solution stand or basin rack is used to hold warm sterile water or normal saline. Depending on the birth attendant's preference, the nurse may be asked to put into the basin an antimicrobial solution. If the double-bowl stand is used, the other basin may be used to place the placenta; again, this depends on the facility's preference. A prep set used to prepare the perineal area needs to be set up. Prep sets range from a small basin with sponges, to which the nurse must add antimicrobial solution and warm sterile water, to a prep set that the manufacturer prepares, requiring only that the nurse open it, put on the sterile gloves, and do the prep. To prepare for the newborn,

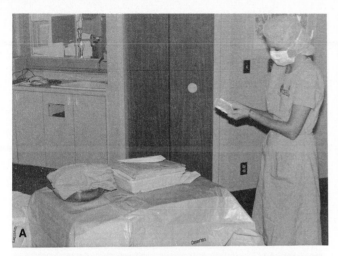

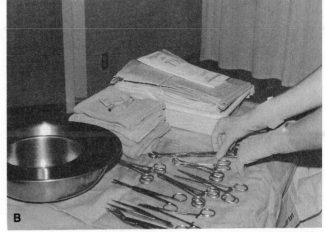

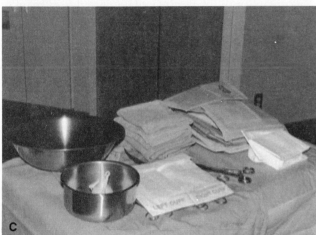

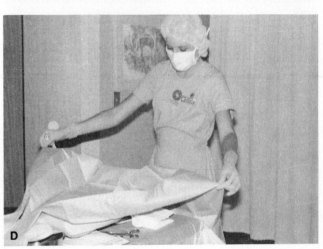

■ *Figure 22-11*
(A) The nurse prepares the LDR for delivery by opening the table and (B) arranging the
instruments. (C) The table is ready to be covered with items specific for the physician or nurse
midwife and bulb syringe and cord clamp for the infant. (D) The table is covered until needed
for the birth. (Courtesy of Long Beach Memorial Medical Center, Long Beach, CA)

a radiant warmer and a resuscitator are present with the necessary emergency equipment (Fig. 22-12).

ASEPSIS AND ANTISEPSIS

People who have a communicable disease or people who have been in contact with a communicable disease should be excluded from maternity service until examined by a physician. Only after a physician has certified that the employee is free from infections should he or she be allowed to return to duty. Personnel with evidence of upper respiratory tract infections or open skin lesions, diarrhea, or any other infectious disease also should be excluded. Furthermore, it is recommended that all people working in the maternity area should have a preemployment physical examination and rubella titers and such interim examinations as may be required by the hospital.

Of prime importance in the conduct of the second stage of labor are strict asepsis and antisepsis throughout the entire delivery. To this end, everyone in the delivery room wears clean scrubs, cap, and mask and those actually participating in the delivery are in sterile attire. Masking includes both nose and mouth, but some facilities are reevaluating the need for a mask for a normal delivery. Caps are to be adjusted to keep *all* hair covered. If the nurse scrubs to assist the doctor, the strict aseptic technique is observed. The hands are scrubbed as carefully as for a surgical operation. Scrubbing the hands should be started sufficiently early to allot full time for the scrub, as well as to don gown and gloves.

TRANSFER OF THE MOTHER TO THE DELIVERY ROOM

When birth appears imminent, the mother is transferred to the delivery room and prepared for delivery. Transfer

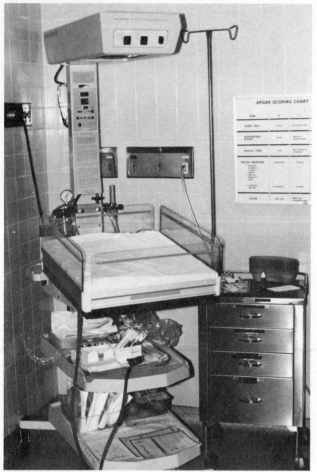

■ *Figure 22–12*
An infant resuscitation cart with an overhead radiant warmer for use in the delivery room. The overhead radiant heater provides a thermal environment for the infant and allows access to and full visualization of the infant. The lower shelves and metal cabinet to the side of the resuscitation cart are used to store infant supplies including equipment and drugs needed in an infant resuscitation. (Courtesy of Long Beach Memorial Medical Center, Long Beach, CA. Photograph by M. Sheridan)

to the delivery room can be a stressful time for the mother; contributing factors include temperature, environment, bed, and potential staff changes. Maternity centers who have changed to the LDR method of care alleviate this transfer to the delivery room.

If the father has chosen not to accompany the mother to the delivery room, time is allowed for them to bid each other a temporary goodbye. This kind of planning not only is supportive but also enables both to cooperate more fully. If the father is going to the delivery room, he should be changed in appropriate scrubs, cap, and mask, if needed, and ready with camera equipment, if appropriate.

Care should be taken to have only one person instruct or coach the mother at any one time. When de-

livery is imminent, her attention is limited, as already illustrated, and the sound of several voices at one time is confusing.

Before the actual transfer to the delivery room, the nurse finds out what type of anesthesia will be used. Because the immediate positioning of the client in the delivery room depends on the type of anesthesia used, this preplanning expedites activities during delivery and promotes smoother functioning of the team.

POSITIONING

For Anesthesia. If regional anesthesia is to be administered, the client is usually turned on her side. If she is given a saddle block, she may be placed on her side or assisted to a sitting position on the side of the delivery table, with her feet supported on a stool and her body leaning forward against the nurse. Her back should be toward the operator and bowed (the position requires flexion of the neck and the lumbar spine). This principle of cervical and lumbar flexion is used also in the side-lying position (see Chap. 24). A caudal or epidural anesthesia may be started in the labor room.

Although the positioning and the administration of the anesthesia take only a few minutes, the mother may be extremely uncomfortable owing to the severity of the contractions at this time; she can be assured that this discomfort is only temporary. The FHR and the maternal blood pressure are checked frequently, every 5 minutes or so. In addition, the mother's head should be elevated with at least two pillows to help prevent the anesthetic level from rising beyond the desired height. To allow the anesthetic level to stabilize, the nurse waits for instructions from the anesthetist before putting the mother's legs in stirrups or performing any other manipulations.

Local or pudendal anesthesia is administered with the mother in the lithotomy position.

As previously stated, anesthesia should be administered by a qualified physician or a nurse–anesthetist. This subject is discussed in detail in Chapter 24.

For Delivery. Some hospitals and physicians do not require that the mother be placed in the lithotomy position for delivery. She simply grasps her legs at the knees as she did during the pushing phase of the second stage. This position allows visualization of the perineum and adequate prepping and draping of the area. Before the mother's legs are placed in stirrups or leg holders of some type, cotton flannel boots that cover the entire leg are put on. When the legs are placed in the stirrups or holders, care is taken not to separate the legs too widely or to have one leg higher than the other. Both legs are raised or lowered at the same time, with a nurse supporting each leg if the mother is unable to help in the positioning. Failure to observe these principles may

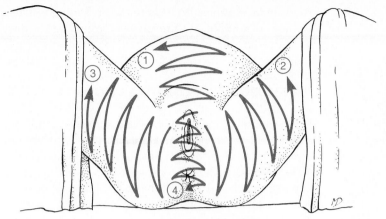

■ *Figure 22-13*
Perineal preparation. A recommended method when cleansing the perineum. Use a new sponge or gauze square for each numbered area; clean the rectal area last. To finish the procedure, blot the perineum dry with a sterile towel or rinse with warm sterile water.

strain the ligaments of the pelvis, with consequent discomfort in the puerperium. Care should be taken to avoid pressure on the popliteal space and to angle the stirrups so that the feet are not dependent.

If stirrups are used during the delivery, the mother can be given handles to grip and pull on, which aid her in her bearing-down efforts.

PREPARING THE PERINEUM

After the client is placed in the lithotomy position, the nurse carries out the procedure for cleansing the vulva and the surrounding area (Fig. 22-13). If the delivery is to be conducted with the mother in the recumbent position, this may be carried out with the knees drawn up slightly and the legs separated. Once the physician has scrubbed and donned sterile gown and gloves, the client is draped with towels and sheets appropriate for the purpose.

After the client has been prepared for delivery, catheterization, if needed, is carried out by the physician. Sometimes it is difficult to catheterize a client in the second stage of labor because the fetus's head may compress the urethra. If the catheter does not pass easily, it should not be forced. The mirror may be positioned for viewing of the delivery by the couple.

Delivery

As the infant descends the birth canal, pressure against the rectum may cause fecal material to be expelled. Sponges (as a rule with saline solution) may be used to remove any fecal material that may escape from the rectum.

Fundal pressure should not be used to accomplish spontaneous delivery or to bring the head deeper into the birth canal. Severe fundal pressure may cause uterine damage or rupture.

As soon as the head distends the perineum to a diameter of 6 or 8 cm (crowning; Fig. 22-14), a towel

may be placed over the rectum while forward pressure is exerted on the baby's chin with one hand, at the same time that downward pressure is applied to the occiput by the other hand. This technique, called the Ritgen maneuver (Fig. 22-15), provides control of the head as it is emerging and directs the extension phase of delivery so that the head is born with the smallest diameter presenting. The head is usually delivered between contractions and as slowly as possible. At this time, the mother may complain about a "splitting" sensation caused by the extreme vaginal stretching as the head is born. Birth is illustrated in Figure 22-16.

Control of the head by the Ritgen maneuver, extension, and slow delivery between contractions help to prevent lacerations. If a tear seems to be inevitable, an incision called an episiotomy may be made in the perineum. This not only prevents lacerations but also facilitates the delivery.

Immediately after the birth of the infant's head, the mouth and nose are suctioned with the bulb syringe,

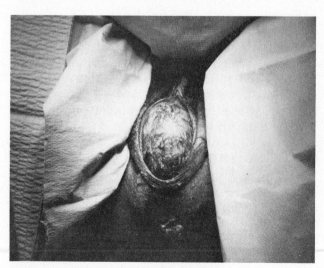

■ *Figure 22-14*
Note crowning, encirclement of the largest diameter of the baby's head by the vulvar ring.

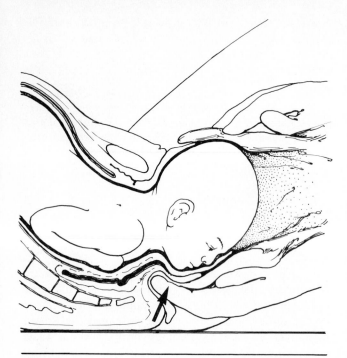

■ *Figure 22–15*
Ritgen's maneuver as it appears in median section. Arrow shows direction of pressure.

then a finger is passed along the occiput to the infant's neck to feel whether a loop or more of umbilical cord encircles it. If such a coil is felt, it should be gently drawn down and, if loose enough, slipped over the infant's head. This is done to prevent interference with the infant's oxygen supply, which could result from pressure of its shoulder on the umbilical cord. If the cord is too tightly coiled to permit this procedure, it must be clamped and cut before the shoulders are delivered; the infant must be extracted immediately before asphyxiation results. The anterior shoulder is usually brought under the symphysis pubis first and then the posterior shoulder is delivered, after which the remainder of the body follows without particular mechanism. The exact time of the baby's birth should be noted. The infant usually cries immediately, and the lungs gradually become expanded. The pulsations in the umbilical cord begin to diminish about this time.

CLAMPING THE CORD

The cord usually is clamped before pulsations cease to prevent transfusion from the placenta and, consequently, hyperviscosity in the infant. The cord is cut between the two Kelly clamps, which have been placed a few inches from the umbilicus; then the umbilical clamp is applied (Figs. 22-17 and 22-18). There are several types of umbilical clamps, such as the Kane, the Hollister, and the Hesseltine, which are used extensively

in many institutions. With these the possibility of hemorrhage is minimized. The delivery room nurse must assess and document the numbers of vessels present in the cord.

PSYCHOSOCIAL CONSIDERATIONS

If the mother is awake, she is usually eager to have a closer look at her baby and hold it. The nurse should remember that, although she is tired, she is usually elated, proud of her accomplishment of giving birth, and eager to share this with the baby's father. Whenever possible, all efforts should be made to allow the mother, father, and infant to share this momentous time together if they so desire. More hospitals are allowing the mother to hold her infant immediately after delivery and put it to breast if she is breast-feeding. Other institutions have the mother wait to hold the infant or nurse it until she has been transferred to the recovery room. These kinds of arrangements provide more opportunities for the parents to have a close, thorough look at their baby and to let the triad begin the necessary process of bonding and integrating the new member into the family constellation.

■ THIRD STAGE OF LABOR

The third stage of labor, the placental stage, begins after the delivery of the baby and terminates with the birth of the placenta. Immediately after delivery of the infant, the height of the uterine fundus and its consistency are ascertained by palpating the uterus through a sterile towel placed on the lower abdomen. The physician places his or her hand on top of the sterile drape and holds the uterus gently, with the fingers behind the fundus and the thumb in front. So long as the uterus remains hard and there is no bleeding, the policy is ordinarily one of watchful waiting until the placenta is separated. No massage is practiced; the hand simply rests on the fundus to make certain that the organ does not balloon out with blood.

Placental Separation and Delivery

Because attempts to deliver the placenta before its separation from the uterine wall are not only futile but may be dangerous, it is most important that the signs of placental separation be well understood. The signs that suggest that the placenta has separated are as follows:

1. The uterus rises upward in the abdomen because the placenta, having been separated, passes

downward into the lower uterine segment and the vagina, where its bulk pushes the uterus upward.

2. The umbilical cord protrudes 3 in or more farther out of the vagina, indicating that the placenta also has descended.
3. The uterus changes from a discoid to a globular shape and becomes, as a rule, more firm.
4. A sudden trickle or spurt of blood often occurs.

These signs are apparent sometimes within a minute or so after delivery of the infant and usually within 5 minutes. When the placenta has separated and the uterus is firmly contracted, the client is asked to bear down so that the intra-abdominal pressure so produced may expel the placenta. If this fails, or if it is not practicable because of anesthesia, gentle pressure is exerted downward with the hand on the fundus and the placenta is gently guided out of the vagina. This procedure, known as placental *expression,* must be done gently and without squeezing (Figs. 22-19 and 22-20). It never should be attempted unless the uterus is hard; otherwise, the organ may be turned inside out. This is one of the gravest complications of obstetrics and is known as inversion of the uterus. Once the placenta is expelled, it is carefully inspected to make sure that it is intact (see Fig. 25-20); if a piece is left in the uterus, it may cause subsequent hemorrhage (Fig. 22-21).

Use of Oxytocics

With the separation and delivery of the placenta in the third stage of labor, hemostasis is achieved at the placenta site by vasoconstriction of the myometrium. Oxytocin (Pitocin, Syntocinon), ergonovine maleate (Ergotrate), and methylergonovine maleate (Methergine) may be administered, at the physician's request, to stimulate uterine contractions and control bleeding. These agents are employed widely in the conduct of the normal third stage of labor, but the timing of their administration differs greatly in various hospitals. These oxytocics are not necessary in most cases, but their use is considered ideal from the viewpoint of minimizing blood loss and the general safety of the mother.

The oxytocic fraction separated from posterior pituitary extract is called oxytocin; it is widely used because it does not possess the strong vasopressor effects of Pituitrin, which was used more extensively in former years.

Oxytocin causes marked uterine contractions for the first 5 to 10 minutes, after which normal rhythmic contractions of amplified degree return with intermittent periods of relaxation.

It is the most frequently used drug, administered only with an order of the physician usually after the delivery of the placenta.

Oxytocin's most important side-effect is its antidiuretic effect, which can cause water intoxication if administered intravenously in a large volume of electrolyte-free aqueous dextrose solution. Fortunately, the antidiuretic effect disappears within a few minutes after the infusion is discontinued.

On the physician's order the nurse administers oxytocin intramuscularly or adds the medication to the intravenous fluid. The average dose is as follows: 10 units (1 ml) IM or 20 units added to 1000 ml intravenous solution.

Ergonovine is an alkaloid of ergot and is a powerful oxytocic; it stimulates uterine contractions and exerts an effect that may persist for several hours. When it is administered intravenously, the uterine response is almost immediate, within a few minutes of intramuscular or oral administration. This response is sustained with no tendency toward relaxation. *However, this drug does cause an elevation in blood pressure.* Intravenous route should be considered only with emergencies.

More recently, a semisynthetic derivative of ergonovine, *methylergonovine maleate,* has been employed. It is thought to cause less elevation in blood pressure when given parenterally.

Both drugs when given intravenously may cause transient headache and, to a lesser extent, temporary chest pain, palpation, and dyspnea. These side-effects are less likely to occur with intramuscular administration of the drug, which is the usual route of administration. The usual doses are ergonovine, 0.2 mg IM or IV, and methylergonovine, 0.2 mg IM or IV.

The choice of the oxytocic usually depends on the anesthetic agent administered. Oxytocin is contraindicated for use with drugs that have a sympathomimetic action.

Lacerations of the Birth Canal

During the process of a normal delivery, lacerations of the perineum and the vagina may be caused by rapid and sudden expulsion of the head, excessive size of the infant, and friable maternal tissues. In other circumstances, they may be caused by difficult forceps deliveries, breech extractions, or contraction of the pelvic outlet in which the head is forced posteriorly. Some tears are unavoidable, even in the most skilled hands, but control of the head is extremely important to deter perineal lacerations.

Perineal lacerations usually are classified in three degrees, according to the extent of the tear.

- First-degree lacerations are those that involve the fourchette, the perineal skin, and the vaginal mucous membrane without involving any of the muscles.

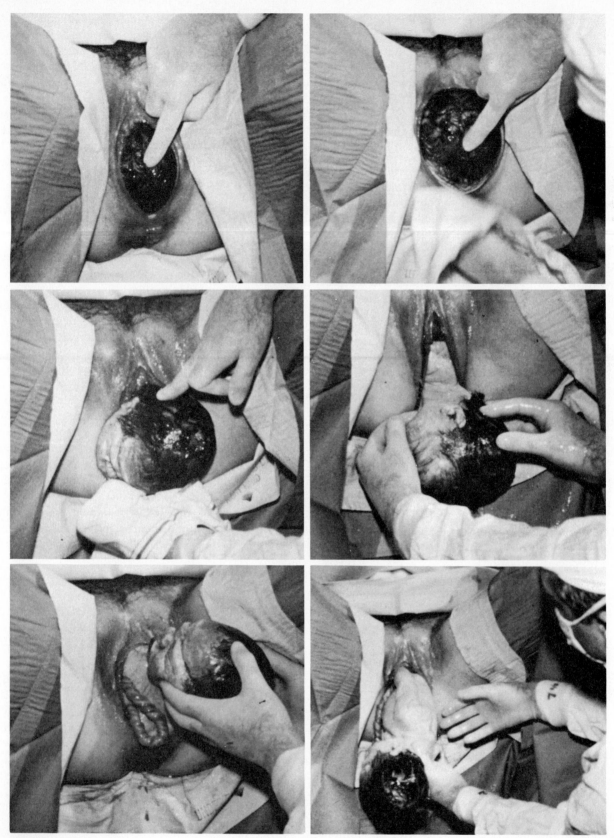

■ *Figure 22–16*
The normal birth process. (From the film Human Birth, published by JB Lippincott, Philadelphia, PA)

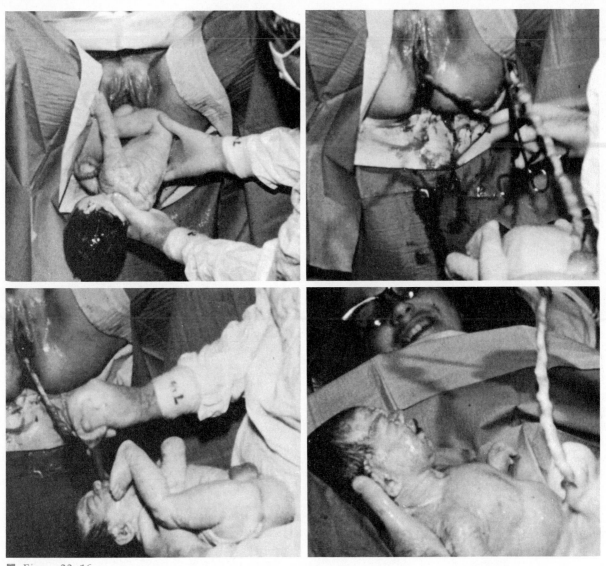

■ *Figure 22–16*
(Continued)

- Second-degree lacerations are those that involve (in addition to skin and mucous membrane) the muscles of the perineal body but not the rectal sphincter. These tears usually extend upward on one or both sides of the vagina, making a triangular injury.
- Third-degree lacerations are those that extend completely through the skin, the mucous membrane, the perineal body, and the rectal sphincter. This type is often referred to as a complete tear. Frequently these third-degree lacerations extend a certain distance up the anterior wall of the rectum.

Some classifications refer to a laceration that extends into the rectum as a fourth-degree tear.

First- and second-degree lacerations are extremely common in primigravidas; their high incidence is one

of the reasons that episiotomy is widely employed. Fortunately, third-degree lacerations are far less common. All three types of lacerations are repaired by the physician immediately after the delivery to ensure that the perineal structures are returned approximately to their former condition. The technique employed for the repair of a laceration is virtually the same as that used for episiotomy incisions, although the former is more difficult to do because of the irregular lines of tissue that must be approximated.

Episiotomy and Repair

An episiotomy is an incision of the perineum made to facilitate delivery (Fig. 22-22). The incision is made with blunt-pointed straight scissors about the time that the

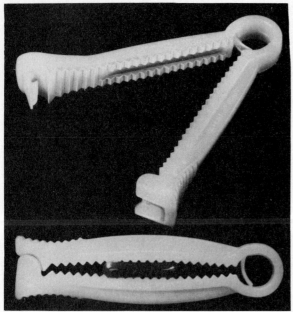

■ *Figure 22–17*
A double-grip umbilical cord clamp in the opened and closed positions. (Courtesy of Hollister, Inc., Chicago, IL)

head distends the vulva and is visible to a diameter of several centimeters. The incision may be made in the midline of the perineum, a median episiotomy, or it may be begun in the midline and directed downward and laterally away from the rectum, a mediolateral episiotomy. In the latter instance, the incision may be directed to either the right or the left side of the mother's pelvis.

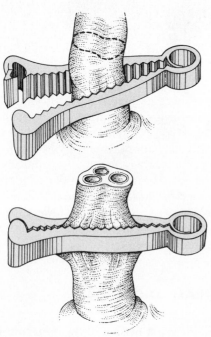

■ *Figure 22–18*
Umbilical clamp applied to cord.

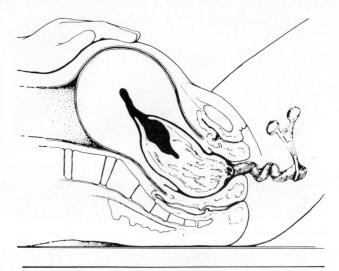

■ *Figure 22–19*
Placental expression.

If a laceration seems to be inevitable as the infant's head distends the vulva, the physician undoubtedly chooses to incise the perineum rather than allow that structure to sustain a traumatic tear. This operation serves the following purposes:

- It substitutes a straight, clean-cut surgical incision for the ragged, contused laceration that otherwise may ensue; such an incision is easier to repair and heals better than a tear.
- The direction of the episiotomy can be controlled, whereas a tear may extend in any direction, sometimes involving the anal sphincter and the rectum.
- Inordinate stretching and tearing of the perineal musculature is avoided, and the incidence of subsequent perineal relaxation with cystocele–rectocele may be reduced.
- The operation shortens the duration of the second stage of labor.

In view of these advantages, many physicians employ episiotomy routinely in the delivery of the primigravida, although routine use is being evaluated.

There are many equally satisfactory methods used for episiotomy repair (Fig. 22-23). The suture material ordinarily used is a fine chromic catgut, either 2–0 or 3–0.

A round needle and continuous suture are used to close the vaginal mucosa and fourchette; the continuous suture is set aside while several interrupted sutures are placed in the levator ani muscle and the fascia. The continuous suture is again picked up and used to unite the subcutaneous fascia. Finally, the round needle is replaced by a large, straight cutting needle, and the running suture is continued upward as a subcuticular stitch.

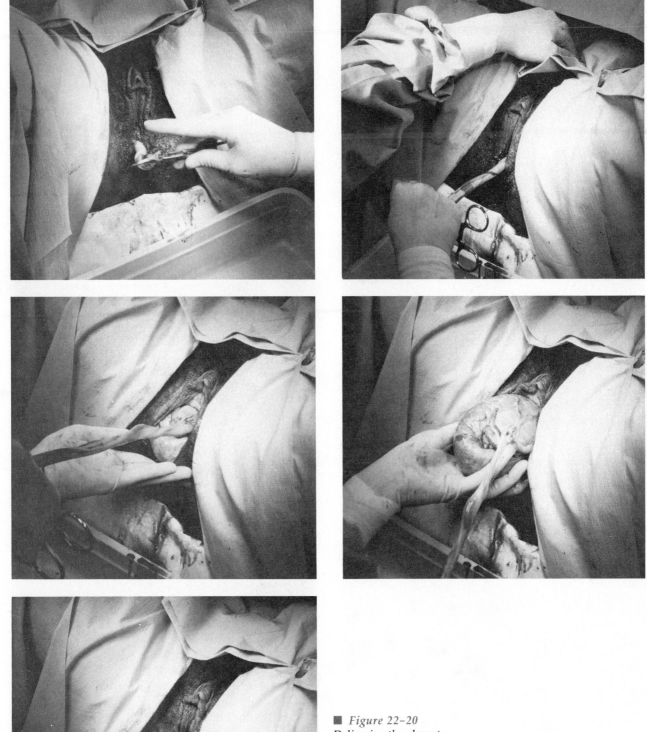

■ Figure 22–20
Delivering the placenta.

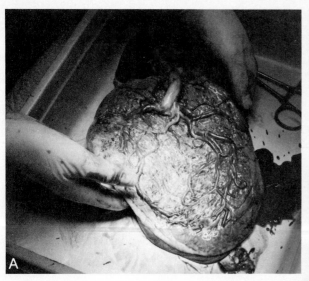

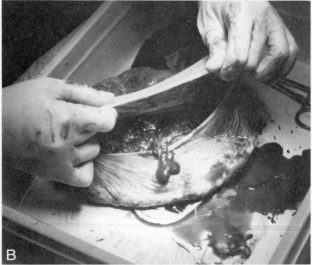

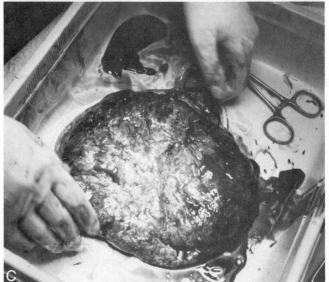

■ *Figure 22–21*
Inspecting the placenta. (A) Fetal surface. (B) The placenta is carefully turned inside out. (C) Maternal surface.

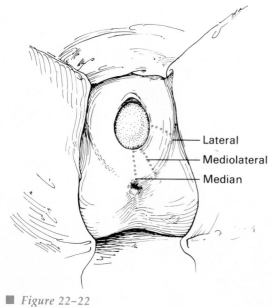

Lateral
Mediolateral
Median

■ *Figure 22–22*
Types of episiotomies.

■ FOURTH STAGE OF LABOR

The fourth stage can be defined as starting after the delivery of the placenta and ending when the mother's physical status has stabilized. This usually occurs within 1 to 2 hours. The weary work of labor is completed, and the mother and father should be commended by the nurse on the good job they did. Questions can be answered, and any labor occurrences can be clarified. This may not be adequate, and at a later time the couple may still need their delivery nurse to clarify the labor and birth process. This stage is a transitional period for the new parents, and many important physical and psychological tasks begin at this time. A couple making the transition to a three-member family is shown in Figure 22-24.

After the delivery has been completed and the episiotomy, if needed, has been repaired, the drapes

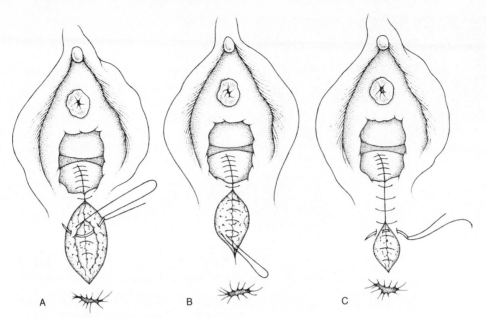

■ *Figure 22–23*

Repair of median episiotomy. (A) Chromic catgut 2-0, or preferably 3-0, is used as a continuous suture to close the vaginal mucosa and submucosa. (B) After closing the vaginal incision and reapproximating the cut margins of the hymenal ring, the suture is tied and cut. Next, three or four interrupted sutures of 2-0 or 3-0 catgut are placed in the fascia and muscle of the incised perineum. (C) Repair of complete perineal tear. The rectal mucosa has been repaired with interrupted, fine chromic catgut sutures. The torn ends of the sphincter ani are next approximated with two or three interrupted chromic catgut sutures. The wound is then repaired, as in a second-degree laceration or an episiotomy.

and the soiled linen are removed and the lower end of the delivery table is replaced. If stirrups have been used, the mother's legs are lowered simultaneously to prevent cramping or twisting of the extremities. A sterile perineal pad is applied, and the mother is given a clean gown and covered with a warm blanket to avoid chilling. Usually mother, infant, and father go to the postpartum recovery area (Fig. 22-25). Some institutions still require that all infants be taken to the nursery at this time, and mother and infant are recovered separately.

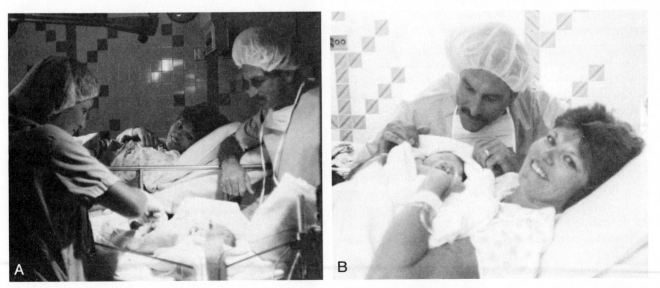

■ *Figure 22–24*

Psychosocial tasks begin after birth. (A) Both parents watch intently as the nurse cares for the newborn. (B) The father gazes fondly at the newborn while the mother shows pride in her accomplishment. (Courtesy of Long Beach Memorial Medical Center, Long Beach, CA

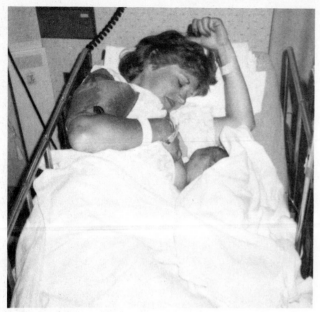

■ *Figure 22–25*
In the recovery area, the mother and newborn have quiet time together during breast-feeding, while the father announces the birth to family and friends. (Courtesy of Long Beach Memorial Medical Center, Long Beach, CA)

Assessment

Postpartum care begins immediately after the delivery; both mother and newborn are making adjustments that need to be assessed. If problems arise, actions need to be taken promptly to ensure well-being. Care of the newborn is addressed in Chapter 25. The first maternal assessment is to be done in the delivery room before transfer. If the delivery has taken place in the LDR, as soon as the mother's legs are down and the warm blanket has been placed the assessment is done. The immediate postpartum checks, done every 15 minutes, include blood pressure, pulse, respirations, massaging the fundus and observing the vaginal flow, inspecting the perineum, and assessing for bladder distention. A temperature reading is usually taken within the first hour.

To be assured of well-being, scrupulous assessment needs to be done, because the mother is at great risk at this time for postpartum hemorrhage and development of a hematoma. If a change in nursing staff occurs, in that the labor and delivery nurse is not the recovery room nurse, a complete report is given. The report includes name of the physician who delivered, method of delivery, presence of an episiotomy, presence of lacerations, type of anesthesia, IV bottle solution and number, amount of oxytocin in the bottle (or if not used, any medications she received to decrease bleeding), method of infant feeding, time of last voiding, sex of the infant, summary of the labor, any pertinent items

that need to be observed for and any pertinent medical history, and any medical orders that need to be carried out immediately.

During the first hour, with every assessment the fundus is massaged and its condition and position are documented (e.g., one fingerbreadth above the umbilicus and firm or boggy and massaged to firm). Refer to Figure 22-26 for the correct procedure when massaging the fundus. Vaginal bleeding is assessed in relation to amount, color, and presence of clots or foul odor. Documentation of the amount of bleeding is done: scant, light, moderate, or heavy. Problems arise when amounts are not standardized and when measurement differs among nurses. The following is a suggested standardized method to record vaginal flow. It can be implemented to ensure accurate documentation of the flow and reflection of the client's condition.[25]

- Scant: blood on tissue only when wiped, or less than 1-in stain on peripad
- Light: less than 4-in stain on peripad
- Moderate: less than 6-in stain on peripad
- Heavy: saturated peripad within 1 hour

The subject is discussed further in Chapter 28, with an illustration of peripads.

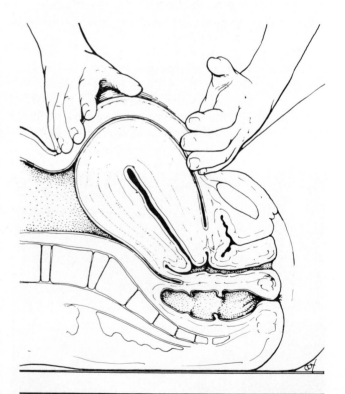

■ *Figure 22–26*
Proper method of palpating fundus of uterus during first hour after delivery to guard against relaxation and hemorrhage. The right hand is placed just above the symphysis pubis to act as a guard; meanwhile, the other hand is cupped around the fundus of the uterus.

Fourth-Stage Assessments

- Vital signs
- Fundus
- Amount of lochia, presence of clots
- Perineum
- Bladder distention
- Family interaction

Nursing Diagnosis

During the third and fourth stages of labor, the nursing goal of maintaining maternal and newborn well-being is ongoing. At this time, the nurse may be able to address and plan for some of the diagnoses identified in the admitting process that she was unable to attend to during the actual labor and birth of the newborn. Assuring her that physical systems are stabilized and providing comfort prepare the client for the new role of mothering.

1. Alteration in comfort or discomfort related to involution of uterus, episiotomy
2. Sleep pattern disturbance
3. Alteration in nutrition: less than body requirements
4. Alteration in parenting related to inexperience, lack of role models
5. Grieving related to labor and delivery not occurring the way client wanted it to be, baby not desired sex, pregnancy over
6. Infection: vaginal, perineal, related to bacterial invasion secondary to trauma during labor and delivery and episiotomy
7. Alteration in parenting related to inexperience, lack of role models
8. Knowledge deficit related to infant care, infant behavior, self-care, normal postpartum physiological occurrences

Planning and Intervention

MANAGEMENT OF POTENTIAL COMPLICATIONS

Hypothermic Reactions. Chilling accompanied by uncontrollable shaking often occurs in this early period after delivery. It is uncomfortable and sometimes embarrassing or frightening for the client, but it is self-limiting (usually not over 15 min) and is not considered an ominous sign. The exact etiology of this chilling has not been determined, although several explanations have been offered, which include sudden release of intra-abdominal pressure after delivery, nervous and exhaustion responses related to the stress of childbirth, disequilibrium in the internal and external body temperature resulting from the waste products of muscular exertion, break in aseptic technique (which predisposes to infection), minute circulatory amniotic fluid emboli, and previous maternal sensitization to elements of fetal blood.

Clean, dry, warm gowns and blankets and a warm, nondrafty environment help in the prevention and control of this phenomenon. Warm fluids by mouth can be given and are much appreciated for their hydrating and energy-giving effects.

Postpartum Hemorrhage. Constant massage of the uterus during this period immediately after delivery is unnecessary and undesirable. However, if the organ shows any tendency to relax, it is to be massaged immediately with firm but gentle circular strokes until it contracts effectively. *Relaxation of the uterus is a prime cause of postpartum hemorrhage, and surveillance of the uterus and the amount of bleeding is of extreme importance at this time.*

Because the prevention of postpartum hemorrhage is such a crucial factor in the health and well-being of the mother, clients at risk to develop this condition should be identified quickly. The most predictive factors associated with postpartum bleeding are:

Advanced maternal age and high parity
Rapid labor
Prolonged first and second stages of labor
Operative delivery (i.e., forceps extraction)
Overdistention of the uterus (hydramnios, multiple pregnancy, overly large infant)
Previous uterine atony or associated previous postpartum hemorrhage
Other hemorrhagic complications such as abruptio placentae or placenta previa
Induced labor
Heavy medication during labor or general anesthesia
Preeclampsia and eclampsia

The nurse has an intravenous infusion with an oxytocic for immediate administration ready in the event that the attendants suspect hemorrhage is imminent.

PSYCHOSOCIAL CONSIDERATIONS

Emotional Reactions. Immediately after delivery, or perhaps later, the parents, particularly the mother, may relieve tension by giving way to some emotional displays such as laughing, crying, talking incessantly, or expressing anger (if all has not gone well or as expected). These emotions often are unexpected and a calm, accepting, nonjudgmental attitude on the part of the nurse is effective in allaying any embarrassment.

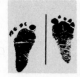

Nursing Care Plan

The Woman and Family During Third and Fourth Stages of Labor

Client Goals   1. Client achieves stabilization of physical systems by the second hour postpartum as evidenced by stable vital signs, firm fundus, appropriate lochia flow.

Assessments	Potential Nursing Diagnosis	Planning and Intervention	Evaluation

Observe post delivery
  Fundus
  Flow
  Bladder
  Vital signs
  Perineum
Complications
  Hemorrhage
  Hematoma
  Infection
	Alteration in comfort: pain related to:
	  Involution of uterus
	  Episiotomy
	Potential for infection: vaginal, perineal, related to bacterial invasion secondary to trauma during labor and delivery and episiotomy
		Administer oxytocin after delivery of placenta as ordered
		Gently massage fundus; if boggy express clots as necessary
		Wash hands when doing pericare
		Take pad off front to back
		Record and report amount and character of flow, vital signs, hematoma and bleeding from episiotomy
		Record temperature
			Client maintains normal temperature and vital signs

Determine need for comfort, rest, and nourishment	Sleep pattern disturbance Alteration in nutrition: less than body requirements	Reposition mother as needed: give warm, dry gown and blanket Provide adequate explanations, answers to questions; provide quiet environment for rest; provide light nourishment as indicated	Client is warm and comfortable Client takes nourishment Client rests

Assess family interaction	Alteration in parenting related to:
	  Inexperience
	  Lack of role models
	Grieving related to:
	  Labor and delivery not the way client wanted it to be
	  Infant not the desired sex
	  Pregnancy over
		Facilitate family interaction in the delivery and recovery rooms
		Answer any questions parents have about newborn
		Refer to Chapters 28 and 30 for more interventions
		Allow woman to ventilate feelings over loss
		Clarify when necessary
			Client verbalizes feelings to nurse
			Client satisfied with outcome

The nurse must remember that the client is beginning a period that is enormously important; she is, in fact, a "mother" with all its concomitant responsibilities. This is not the end but only the beginning of a whole new role. In addition, she is physically and emotionally exhausted from the labor and birth and is at risk for potential sleep and rest disturbance.

Several comfort measures can be employed to restore calm and to help the mother relax enough to get some much needed rest and sleep. A soothing back rub, change of gown and linen, a quiet conversation with the nurse or the father in which the client is allowed to ventilate her feelings, an environment conducive to rest—all are helpful. In addition, if she is stable after the first hour, a warm beverage can be offered to help relaxation. Because the mother is apt to be extremely hungry and thirsty; this is welcome nourishment as well as a therapeutic soporific.

Many mothers do not have an emotional outburst *per se*, although the majority do experience some degree of excitement and elation when the delivery is accomplished. Any of the above nursing activities are also suitable for them. Some clients experience a great need for sleep and drop off as soon as they know that the baby is normal and healthy. If the client is sleeping continuously or intermittently, she should be allowed to do so, being disturbed only for those nursing observations that are necessary. When she indicates readiness, her baby can be presented and she can be allowed to examine and to explore it to her heart's content.

Mothers who have not been conscious during the delivery may have rather different reactions from those who have participated in the birth process. Often they do not seem to believe that delivery has taken place or that the baby shown to them is really theirs. They question again and again, "Is it really all over?" "Tell me again, is it a boy or a girl?" "Did I have the baby?" The apparent alteration in awareness seems to be related to the anesthesia and the unconsciousness. These mothers may need more firm reassurance and contact with their infants to help them realize that they have had a baby. Even though the repeated questioning may become annoying, the nurse must recognize that this is necessary for the mother to begin the important process of disengagement from the symbiotic relationship that she had with her infant during pregnancy. She must establish the baby as a real entity outside her body rather than inside. All mothers have this task to perform, but it may be harder for the mother who has been delivered under heavy anesthesia, because as far as she is concerned, she was not "there" when it all happened.

Family Interactions. As we know, the couple's attachment for the new infant does not spring unbound at the time of delivery. At the birth, there may be excitement over the sex, the color and amount of hair, and other physical characteristics, but attachment develops over time, as in any other relationship. Attachment is defined as a "unique relationship between two people which is specific and endures through time."[26] Parental attachment may have started before conception and continued through the pregnancy; it is enhanced with the actual birth and intensifies during the next weeks.[26]

The nurse attending the delivery and giving care in recovery can assist the couple with the first interactions. The nurse may help the mother with her first breast-feeding or the father as he holds the infant the first time. These interactions are important as the beginning foundation for their family relationship continues to develop.

Assessment of Family Integration. Rising has pointed out that there is a certain openness about the fourth stage of labor that may not occur again during the postpartum period. This openness allows the nurse to make assessments regarding the couple's ability to proceed with integrating the infant smoothly into the family.[27] If family units are identified for potential alteration in parenting, the nurse should set aside more time to be with the couple to reinforce any positive responses that they might demonstrate and to give encouragement. Listening attentively as the couple relive their recent experience and encouraging verbalization of these feelings can be helpful. Most importantly, the nurse should pass on the client's care plan to ensure continuity in care. The postpartum nursing staff can work closely with community-health nurses or arrange for other followup care to encourage appropriate adjustment for the family. This is a time when the nurse needs to use all the observational skills, time, and laying on of the hands to foster initial integration and to begin prescribing future care aimed at consolidating the family unit. The topic of parent–infant attachment is discussed more thoroughly in Chapter 27.

■ REFERENCES

1. Nurses Association of the American College of Obstetricians and Gynecologists: Standards for Obstetric, Gynecologic, and Neonatal Nursing, 2nd ed, 1981
2. American Academy of Pediatrics, The American College of Obstetricians and Gynecologists: Guidelines for Perinatal Care, 2nd ed, 1988
3. Friedman EA: Labor, Clinical Evaluation and Management, 2nd ed. New York, Appleton-Century-Crofts, 1978
4. Adams JQ, Alexander AM: Alterations in cardiovascular physiology during labor. Am J Obstet Gynecol 12: 542–549, 1958
5. Hendricks CH, Quilligan EJ: Cardiac output during labor. Am J Obstet Gynecol 71:953–972, May 1956
6. Elkayam V, Gleicher N (eds): Cardiac Problems in Pregnancy. New York, Alan R Liss, 1982
7. Martin J, Miller J, Heins H et al (eds): Intrapartum Assessment and Management Module, Perinatal Education Program for Community Hospital. Charleston, Medical University of South Carolina, 1982
8. Pritchard JA, MacDonald PC, Gant NF: Williams' Obstetrics. Norwalk, CT, Appleton-Century-Crofts, 1985

9. Freeman RF, Garite TJ: Fetal Heart Rate Monitoring. Baltimore, Williams & Wilkins, 1981

10. Garite TJ: Achieving good outcomes when membranes rupture prematurely. Contemp OB/GYN 25:96–105, February 1985

11. Kantor HI, Rember R, Tabio P et al: Value of shaving the pudendal-perineal area in delivery preparation. Obstet Gynecol 25:509–512, April 1965

12. Johnston RA, Sidall RS: Is the usual method of preparing patients for delivery beneficial or necessary? Am J Obstet Gynecol 4:645–650, December 1922

13. Sweeney WJ III: Perineal shaves and bladder catheterization: Necessary and benign or unnecessary and potentially injurious? Obstet Gynecol 21:291–294, March 1963

14. Long AE: Unshaved perineum at parturition. Am J Obstet Gynecol 99:333–336, October 1, 1967

15. Seropian R, Reynolds BM: Wound infections after preoperative depilatory versus razor preparation. Am J Surg 121:251–254, March 1971

16. Landry KE, Kilpatrick DM: Why shave a mother before she gives birth? MCN 2(3):189–190, May/June 1977

17. Mahan CS, McKay S: Preps and enemas: Keep or discard? Contemp OB/GYN 22(5):241, November 1983

18. Centers for Disease Control: Morbidity and mortality weekly report. MMWR 37(24): 377–382, June 24, 1988

19. Liu YC: Effects of the upright position during labor. Am J Nurs 74:2202–2205, December 1974

20. Roberts JE: Maternal positions for childbirth: A historical review of nursing care practices. JOGN Nurs 8:24–32, January/February 1979

21. Caldeyro-Barcia R: The influence of maternal bearing-down efforts during second stage on fetal well-being. Birth Fam J 6(1):17–21, Spring 1979

22. Wilson J: Gastric emptying in labor: Some recent findings and their clinical significance. J Int Med Res 6:54–62, 1978

23. Douglas MJ: Commentary: The case against a more liberal food and fluid policy in labor. Birth 15(2):93–94, June 1988

24. Carr KC: Management of the second stage of labor. NAACOG Update Series, Lesson 9(1), 1983

25. Jacobson H: A standard for assessing lochia volume. MCN 10:174–175, May/June 1985

26. Klaus M, Kennell J: Parent–Infant Bonding. St Louis, CV Mosby, 1982

27. Rising S: The fourth stage of labor: Family integration. Am J Nurs 74:870–874, May 1974

■ SUGGESTED READINGS

Carpenito LJ: Nursing Diagnosis Application to Clinical Practice. Philadelphia, JB Lippincott, 1983

Carr KC: Management of the second stage of labor. NAACOG Update Series, Lesson 9(1), 1983

Cronenwett LR, Newmark LL: Father's responses to childbirth. Nurs Res 23:210–217, May/June 1974

Highley BL, Mercer RT: Safeguarding the laboring woman's sense of control. MCN 3(1):39–41, January/February 1978

Huprich PA: Assisting the couple through a Lamaze labor and delivery. MCN 2(4):245–253, July/August 1977

Jacobson H: A standard for assessing lochia volume. MCN 10:174–175, May/June 1985

Malinowski J: Nursing Care of the Labor Patient, 2nd ed. Philadelphia, FA Davis, 1983

Martin J, Miller J, Heins H et al (eds): Intrapartum Assessment and Management Module, Perinatal Education Program for Community Hospital. Charleston, Medical University of South Carolina, 1990

McDonough M, Sheriff D, Zimmel P: Parents' responses to fetal monitoring. MCN 6(1):32–34, January/February 1981

McKay S, Roberts J: Second stage labor: What is normal? JOGNN 14(2):101–106, March/June 1985.

Moore ML: Potential alterations in attachment: Maternal and/or neonatal illness. NAACOG Update Series, Lesson 7(1), 1983

Newel NJ: Grandparents: The overlooked support system for new parents during the fourth trimester. NAACOG Update Series, Lesson 21(1), 1984

Roberts JE, Goldstein SA, Gruener JS et al: A descriptive analysis of involuntary bearing-down efforts during the expulsive phase of labor. JOGNN 16(1):48–55, January/February 1987.

Walker MM: Siblings in the childbearing experience. NAACOG Update Series, Lesson 17(1), 1984

Wheeler L: Intrapartal measurement of blood pressure. NAACOG Update Series, Lesson 20(1), 1984

23

The Nurse's Contribution to Pain Relief During Labor

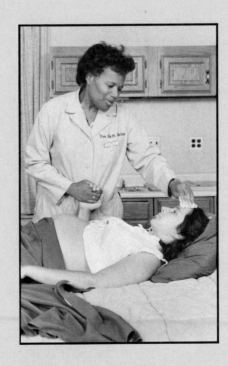

Unique among physiological muscle contractions, those of labor are usually painful. The generally accepted hypotheses of the physiological causes of labor pain include hypoxia of the uterine muscle; stretching and traction of the uterine ligaments; traction on the ovaries, fallopian tubes, and peritoneum; pressure on the urethra, bladder, and rectum; and distension of the pelvic floor muscles and perineum.[1] Other causes will be discussed in this chapter.

Nurses who provide care for the family in labor have a special and unique role. Unlike nurses who work in other hospital settings, they are privileged to watch a normal physiological process culminating in the miracle of birth, an event that transforms both the lives of the parents and of those who assist in the process. Nurses, in return, have the responsibility of helping to decrease the pain that usually accompanies this process. The varied ways nurses can help decrease labor pain is the focus of this chapter.

■ PAIN MECHANISMS

Gate Control Theory

The mystery and complexity of pain are especially well demonstrated by the fact that no one really knows what neurophysiological mechanism underlies the sensation of pain. Among the more recent theories is the *gate control theory*. It was first proposed in 1965 by Melzack and Wall[2] and has since been debated and expanded.[2-5] Like all theories, it is not absolute truth. Rather, it uses available information to explain the phenomenon of pain, suggesting reasons for known facts and offering possibilities when facts are absent.

There are numerous facets to the theory and many ways to categorize them. The following discussion focuses only on those aspects that are most pertinent to a basic understanding of the mechanisms of pain and its relief in childbirth.

As its name implies, the gate control theory proposes that there is a gating mechanism involved in the transmission of pain impulses. A closed gate results in no pain; an open gate results in pain; and a partially open gate results in less pain. This gating mechanism is probably located in various places throughout the central nervous system. When the gate is closed, the transmission of pain impulses is stopped and pain does not reach the level of awareness.

The transmission of pain impulses to the level of cortical awareness can be affected in the following ways:

- *The activity in large and small sensory nerve fibers.* The gate is opened by excitation of small-diameter fibers that carry pain impulses. However, these pain signals can be blocked (i.e., the gate can be closed to prevent or decrease their transmission to the cortex) by stimulation of large-diameter fibers. Because many cutaneous fibers are large-diameter fibers, stimulation of the skin by rubbing or other means may result in pain relief (Fig. 23-1).

- *Projections from the brain stem reticular formation.* The reticular activating system regulates or adjusts incoming and outgoing signals, including the amount of sensory input. Somatic inputs from all parts of the body, as well as visual and auditory inputs, are monitored by the reticular system. Although the process is not well understood, it appears that a sufficient amount of sensory input may cause the reticular system to project inhibitory signals to the gate (i.e., the reticular formation may cause the gate to be closed to the transmission of pain impulses). Hence, pain signals would not reach the level of cortical awareness (no pain), or fewer pain signals would reach the brain (less intense pain). Thus, distraction, for example, may inhibit pain impulses, whereas monotony (unvarying sensory input) would increase pain.

- *Projections from the cerebral cortex and thalamus.* Signals from the cortex or thalamus can open or close the gate to transmission of pain impulses, either indirectly by projecting through the reticular formation or directly by projecting to the gate. Cognitive and affective processes are subserved at least in part by neural activity in the cortex and thalamus. Therefore, the person's unique thoughts and feelings can influence the transmission of pain impulses from the gate to the level of cortical awareness. Such thoughts and feelings may include the meaning of the pain; the person's beliefs, anxieties, memories of past painful experiences; and any number of other factors. Thus, input to the gating mechanism is evaluated by the person *before* it is felt as a sensation as well as after.

Perhaps the most important contribution of the gate control theory is the possible explanation it offers for the individuality of the pain experience (Fig. 23-1). One conclusion has been clear for many years: comparable stimuli (or lesions) in different people do not produce comparable sensations of pain. In other words, when comparable stimuli are applied to several people, one person may perceive intense pain, another moderate pain, and still another no pain at all. The gate control theory suggests mechanisms by which a myriad of factors may determine the existence of pain and influence the nature of a painful experience. In summary, these factors may include not only stimulation of pain fibers but also cutaneous stimulation, other sensory input, thoughts, and feelings.

Research Highlight

The study of childbirth pain began more then 35 years ago, yet a review of the literature in this area reveals few studies. Although many variables have been found to influence the pain of childbirth, only two have been found to be significant in more than one study. The significant variables are anxiety about the pain of childbirth and anxiety in general. All other variables have been examined in one study only or have had conflicting results across studies.

After examining the literature, Wallach selected 21 variables for her study. One hundred sixteen primiparous women giving birth in Metropolitan Toronto hospitals participated in the study. The women in the study were divided into two groups: (1) women who received an epidural before transition and (2) women who did not receive an epidural before transition. In Wallach's study, the mean pain ratings for these two groups were not substantially different.

The individual variables that correlated significantly with pain were complications, length of labor, and medication. Women who had longer labors with more complications and received more medication experienced more pain. Extroverted women with an external locus of control experienced more pain. Other variables were more fear for themselves, presence of father, less accurate information, and expecting less pain.

The nurse may be able to assist women with the last four variables prenatally. Fears for self correlated with increased pain. The author found this interesting because most of the women in the study had participated in childbirth classes. The author suggests that health-care providers use a questionnare, discussion, or interview to determine each woman's specific fears and then work on dispelling them.

The presence of the father increased the pain experience. The author suggests further research on this issue, but meanwhile fathers should not be pressured into participating if they don't want to. Also, the couple should be allowed to decide on their own if the father will be present. The nurse can help the couple with suggestions to deal with any hospital staff who may not support the father's presence, which would undermine any positive effects he might have on helping relieve his partner's pain in labor.

Lack of accurate information about what to expect during labor also is an interesting variable. Although most of these women attended childbirth classes, most felt labor was either harder, longer, or more painful than they expected. This caused an increase in the pain felt during labor. Conversely, the more pain the women expected the less their pain seemed to be. It is very important for nurses who have contact with pregnant women prenatally to give an accurate picture of labor and the pain experience. This may be difficult without increasing her fears, which in turn increases pain. The author suggests that one way to deal with this is to give an accurate picture of the labor experience along with a choice of labor-coping strategies. This also may increase the woman's feeling of control over her pain and decrease the pain experienced.

Wallach H: Prenatal preparation: Suggestion for modification. Pre- and Peri-Natal Psychology 1(3), 1987

The gate control theory also provides a basis for understanding and devising pain relief measures (Table 23-1).

There are three other pain theories that are probably part of the overall theoretical model of the gate control theory. Melzak has defined these three interacting components of pain as the sensory-discriminative system, the motivational-affective component, and the cognitive-evaluative component.[6] A person's response to pain is affected by each of these components, as follows:[6]

1. Sensory-discriminative system—This component communicates information to the brain regarding physical sensations, for example, pain caused by physical changes in labor. This system can be used in pain management when pain information from the body is changed so that the brain receives a decreased pain message.
2. Motivational-affective system—Once the brain receives the message of pain, a central interpretation of the message occurs. The person's feelings, memories, past experiences, and culture affect how this message is interpreted.
3. Cognitive-evaluative system—Also affecting the central interpretation of the pain messages are the person's knowledge, attention, use of cognitive strategies, and cognitive evaluation of the situation.

Figure 23-2 shows these systems' interacting relationships. How the nurse can devise pain reduction strategies using these interacting systems will be discussed later in the chapter.

■ *Figure 23-1*
One influence on the gating mechanism is the ratio of large/small fibers activated. (A) Impulses traveling on small-diameter nerve fibers cause the gate to be held open. (B) Impulses traveling on large-diameter fibers generate feedback to the gate, almost closing it. (Hassid P: Textbook for Childbirth Educators, 2nd ed. New York, Harper & Row, 1987

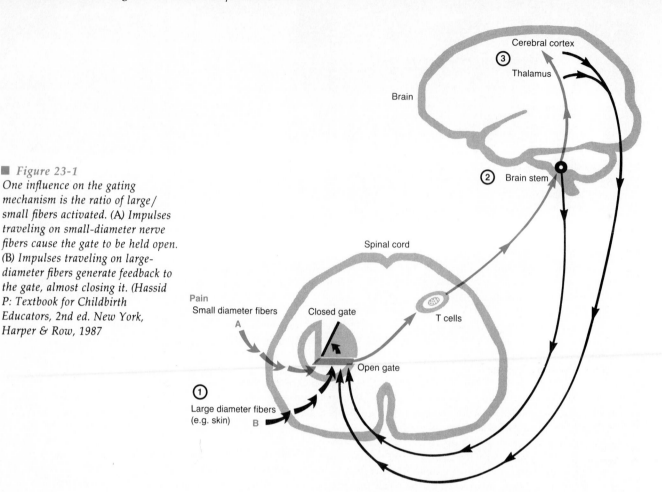

Endorphins

In 1975 it was discovered that opiatelike substances occur naturally within the body.[7] These substances have been called *endorphins*, a combination of the words *endogenous* and *morphine*. To date, several endorphins have been isolated, but it is clear that many more exist. Their role in the cause and alleviation of pain has not yet been clarified. An overview of the possible ways

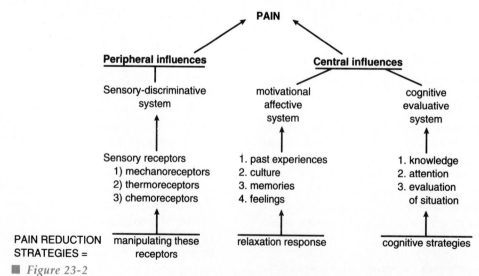

■ *Figure 23-2*
Cognitive-evaluative system. (Adapted from Hilbers S, Gennaro S: Nonpharmacologic pain relief. NAACOG Update Series, vol. 5, lesson 15. Princeton, NJ, Continuing Professional Center, 1986)

TABLE 23-1. NURSING PRACTICE ASPECTS OF THE GATE CONTROL THEORY OF PAIN

Major Contributions

1. An integrated conceptual model for appreciating the many factors that contribute to individual differences in the experience of pain
2. Conceptualization of categories of activity that may form a theoretical base for developing various pain relief measures

Nature of the Gate

The transmission of potentially painful impulses to the level of conscious awareness may be affected by a gating mechanism, possibly located at the spinal cord level of the central nervous system.

Structures Involved	No Pain or Decreased Intensity of Pain	Pain
Spinal cord (?)	Results from closing the gate in one of the following ways:	Results from opening the gate in one of the following ways:
Nerve fibers	1. Activity in the *large-diameter nerve fibers* (e.g., caused by skin stimulation)	1. Activity in the *small-diameter nerve fibers* (e.g., caused by tissue damage)
Brain stem	2. Inhibitory impulses from the *brain stem* (e.g., caused by sufficient or maximum sensory input arriving through distraction or guided imagery)	2. Facilitory impulses from the *brain stem* (e.g., caused by insufficient input from a monotonous environment)
Cerebral cortex and thalamus	3. Inhibitory impulses from the *cerebral cortex* and *thalamus* (e.g., caused by anxiety reduction based on learning when the pain will end and how to relieve it)	3. Facilitory impulses from the *cerebral cortex* and *thalamus* (e.g., caused by fear that the intensity of pain will escalate and will be associated with death)

(McCaffery M: Nursing Management of the Patient With Pain, 2nd ed. Philadelphia, JB Lippincott, 1979)

endorphins affect pain such as that felt in labor and birth follows.

Endorphins influence the transmission of impulses interpreted as painful. Endorphins possibly may act as either neurotransmitters or neuromodulators that inhibit the transmission of pain messages. Thus, the presence of endorphin at the synapse of nerve cells results in a decrease in the sensation of pain. Failure to release endorphin allows pain to occur. Opiates, such as morphine or endorphin (sometimes referred to as *enkephalin*), probably inhibit transmission of pain messages by attaching to opiate receptor sites of nerves in the brain and spinal cord (Fig. 23-3).[8]

Endorphin levels differ from one person to another, explaining in part why some people feel more pain than others. People with a high endorphin level obviously feel less pain. Also, it has been found, for example, that people with a low endorphin level prior to surgery require more analgesia postoperatively than people with a higher level of endorphin. Differences in endorphin levels may be inherited, which may explain cultural differences in pain sensitivity.[9]

Certain situations, such as stress and pregnancy, cause an increase in endorphin levels. Therefore, the endorphin level varies within the individual from one situation to another. During pregnancy and birth, both mother and infant may have a decreased sensitivity to pain because of increased endorphin levels.[9]

At 36 weeks of pregnancy, women with positive attitudes toward their pregnancies had higher blood endorphin levels. Women at delivery were found to have an endorphin blood level 30 times that of nonpregnant women,[10] and those levels have been found to be 20 times higher in women with prolonged, difficult labor than those with uncomplicated labor.[11]

Various pain relief measures may be dependent on the endorphin systems. For example, it is possible that certain kinds of patient teaching or stimulation of the skin, such as massage, can cause an increase in endorphin, which in turn relieves pain.[12]

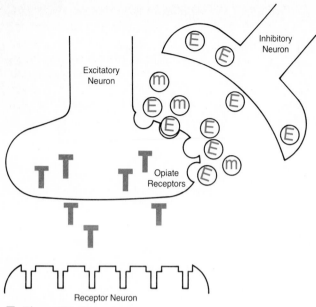

■ *Figure 23-3*

The opiate receptor is thought to be located on the endings of excitatory neurons. Binding of endorphin, or enkephalin (E), or opiates such as morphine (m) may inhibit release of transmitter (T) and thereby lead to alteration in pain perception. (Adapted from Pittman AW, Rudd GD: Analgesic Therapy, Part 2: Analgesia for Severe Pain, p 8. Chapel Hill, NC, Health Sciences Consortium, 1980)

Some people speculate that acupressure decreases pain by releasing endorphins, but there has been no research to support this hypothesis.

■ UNIQUENESS OF PAIN DURING CHILDBIRTH

The discomfort and pain of childbirth are unique. Hence, the childbirth experience has a high potential for the achievement of satisfactory pain relief. Studies suggest that anxiety is reduced if the person knows when a painful event will occur and how long the discomfort will last. Ordinarily, the woman knows the approximate date of confinement, and she has some idea of the approximate length of labor. In other words, she knows labor will occur, she knows the expected date within a few weeks, and she knows labor usually lasts a matter of hours, not days.

Even more helpful is the information the woman has once labor actually has begun. With the assistance of a watch, she can determine the usual length of her contractions and predict when the next one will occur. In addition, she knows that contractions generally become more intense and more frequent as labor pro-

gresses. Further, although her discomfort may increase in intensity, she is not usually in constant discomfort. Between contractions there are periods of relative comfort, even during the final phase of labor contractions.

The woman also knows the cause of her discomfort. At least she knows it is a normal process that has something to do with the birth of her baby and that parts of her body are contracting and stretching to accomplish this event. Most women recognize the onset of labor and do not fear that something harmful or life threatening is happening.

The discomfort of labor is also unique in that there is a tangible end product—the baby. The birth of the baby is something in which there has been deep personal involvement, both emotional and physiological. The involvement may have been positive and desirable or unpleasant and unwanted. Nevertheless, when the baby is born, the discomfort of labor subsides markedly and the event is characterized by physical and psychological closure. Few episodes of pain end so dramatically.

The commonly held belief that pain management is the key to satisfaction in childbirth is challenged by Hummenick and Bugen.[13] Several research studies that compared the amount of pain reported by women found no correlation between reported pain and satisfaction with their childbirth experience.[14–16] Another study found that the amount of medication was inversely related to positive ratings of the birth experience as well as positive initial descriptions of the baby.[17] Hummenick and Bugen believe that pain management is not the only variable in childbirth satisfaction. Several studies have shown that the major factor associated with birth satisfaction was the women's ability to influence decisions made and not giving all decisions and responsibilities to care providers.[13]

■ DEFINITIONS OF PAIN

Pain

Pain defies definition. It is a personal and subjective experience, differing from one person to another and varying within the same person from one time to the next. Quite simply, pain is a localized sensation of hurt. For the sake of both the nurse and the patient who work together to relieve pain, however, it seems more productive for the nurse to adopt the patient's definition of pain.

In this context, the definition of pain may be stated as whatever the experiencing person says it is, existing whenever she says it does.[18] A crucial aspect of this definition is that the nurse believes what the patient tells her. Of course, the patient may communicate the

---

pain experience in any number of ways besides verbalization. For example, in some patients, a marked increase in rate and depth of respirations may alert the nurse to the intensification of discomfort.

Pain Experience

The phrase *pain experience* encompasses all the patient's sensations, feelings, and behavioral responses, including physiological activities such as blood pressure changes. The pain experience may also refer to any or all of the three phases of pain: anticipation, presence, and aftermath. It may include not only the patient's actions but the impact that others have on the patient during the pain experience.

Pain Expressions

The manner in which a person responds to pain depends on numerous and varied factors, such as the culture in which the person lives, the personal meaning of the pain, and the intensity of the pain. Hence, pain expressions may be absent, minimal, or not easily observed. For example, a slight and momentary frown may be the only sign that the client is experiencing pain. Or the client may be more expressive and engage in prolonged moaning.

Expressions of pain are usually observed in one or more of the following categories of behavioral response: physiological, verbal, vocal, facial, body movement, physical contact with others, and general response to the environment.[18]

Reports of how childbirth is handled in some other cultures, especially the more primitive ones, often emphasize the lack of any expression of pain. Some women are noted to have their babies in the fields and resume work immediately after delivery. Other women are observed to remain quiet with relaxed facial expressions during childbirth. However, *lack of expression of pain does not necessarily mean that pain is absent.*

Pain Intensity

The *intensity* of pain refers to the severity of the sensation itself. To determine the degree of pain, the patient may be asked to rate the intensity on a numerical scale such as zero to ten, with zero being no pain at all and ten being the worst possible pain. An alternative is a series of words for rating pain intensity, such as none, mild, moderate, severe, and very severe.

When a patient does not exhibit many expressions of pain, it is helpful to ask her to use a rating scale to convey the intensity of pain, because it cannot be easily observed. If the use of a scale is explained early in labor, the woman may be able to use that method throughout labor and delivery whenever she is requested to.

Pain Tolerance

It is important to differentiate between the presence and intensity of a pain sensation, as indicated by expressions of pain, and the patient's tolerance for that pain. Pain *tolerance* may be defined as the duration or intensity of pain that the patient is willing to endure without pain relief.

Pain tolerance differs markedly from one person to another. Some patients state that the pain sensation is severe, yet they are willing to tolerate the pain and do not request pain relief. Other patients request pain relief measures when they rate the pain as mild. The latter group may be said to have a low tolerance for pain. Although a high pain tolerance is valued by many people, the nurse should realize that a patient's tolerance for pain is not a matter of good or bad, or right or wrong. Indeed, none of the patient's responses to pain are to be judged in this way.

During childbirth, the woman is expected to endure or tolerate a certain amount of pain to ensure her own and her baby's good health. Some women have a low pain tolerance, however, so it is especially important for the nurse to help these women find a way to cope with their discomfort. Admonishing the woman to cope with the discomfort or leaving the room when she complains certainly is not helpful. Other techniques can be called on in such instances. The nonpharmacologic measures discussed in this chapter are especially appropriate for the woman with a low pain tolerance.

Suffering

Suffering is an affective state that may accompany pain. Copp, a nurse–researcher in the field of pain, pointedly uses the term *suffering* in reference to pain and defines it as "the state of anguish of one who bears pain, injury, or loss."[19] When pain cannot be eliminated, it is imperative that the patient receive whatever assistance is necessary to prevent or diminish feelings of suffering. Although a painful experience is only unpleasant at best, in most instances it need not be unrelenting agony.

It is the suffering aspect of pain that women fear most and the aspect that nurses can most affect.

■ THE NURSING PROCESS

The nursing process is crucial in assisting women to decrease pain in labor by nonpharmacologic methods. In fact, the nursing process will likely be repeated many times during a specific labor as the nurse assesses the pain experience; forms a potential nursing diagnosis; plans, implements, and evaluates strategies; and continues in the feedback loop of the process.

Nursing Assessment

Before the nurse assesses the individual woman's expectations about pain or her actual experience with pain during childbirth, it is helpful to know the wide range of beliefs and experience that may be encountered. Precautions must be taken to avoid certain prejudices that may hamper the nurse's assessment of the pain experience.

SIGNS OF ACUTE PAIN

There is a tendency to recognize the existence of pain only in those patients who show signs of acute pain, such as perspiration, muscle tension, or moaning. The absence of these expressions of pain, as noted previously, does not necessarily mean the patient is not in pain. In fact, the patient may suffer greatly but exhibit only minimal pain expression.[18]

In childbirth the two major reasons for minimal pain expressions are (1) the woman may have learned that minimal pain expressions are the expectations of the culture; or (2) activities learned from a method of prepared childbirth may preclude expressions of pain. For example, practicing relaxation techniques may preclude muscle tension as a sign of acute pain; use of a breathing pattern or mouthing the words of a song may preclude the behavior of moaning.

It is often quite difficult, if not impossible, to rely on signs of acute pain in assessing the laboring woman who is using one of the methods of prepared childbirth. Usually she simply is too busy to show signs of acute pain, and a small percentage of women in fact do not have pain.

PHYSICAL CAUSE OF PAIN

We also tend to be prejudiced in favor of believing patients only when we know the physical cause of pain.[18] This hampers our understanding of the subjective pain experience. Hence, when the woman states, for instance, that she feels severe pain, her statement must be believed even if there seems to be no physical cause for such a painful labor. The temptation to judge the woman's discomfort by the results of electronic monitoring of intrauterine pressure also must be avoided.

VALUES OF MOTHER OR FATHER

The mother or father also may harbor prejudices or values that make it difficult for the nurse to assess the pain experience. Either or both of the parents may think that responses to pain should be minimized. The only appropriate response may be a verbal description of the pain. Some women may not even volunteer this much, so they have to be questioned directly and at regular intervals. Other women may want to avoid using the word *pain* or resist any tendency to say they feel pain. They may prefer to use other terms, which may be deceptive if taken at face value. For example, the woman may verbalize feeling "enormous pressure" but refuse to call it painful. Yet the woman may need assistance in coping with this sensation so that measures designed to relieve severe pain may be appropriate.

Another type of problem may arise with a father who forcefully tries to impose his own goals on the mother, who does not share his values. In the situation in which the father does not want the mother to admit pain or to seek assistance with pain relief measures, the nurse may find that she obtains more accurate information when the father is absent from the room. Of course, the opposite type of situation may exist. The mother may feel perfectly capable of handling the pain and discomforts of labor, but the father may become insistent that she be "put out of this misery."

It is difficult for some men to watch someone they love in pain. Sometimes it is the father who is put out of misery when the woman is given pain medications. The nurse can be a great reassurance if this is the problem.

DESCRIPTION OF PAINFUL SENSATIONS

Factually, probably only 9% to 14% of untreated labors are painless or minimally uncomfortable.[20] In a study of both multiparas and primiparas using the McGill Pain Questionnaire, the intensity of labor pain showed a wide variation but was found to rank among the most intense of pains. Further, pain intensity was significantly higher for primiparas than for multiparas.[21] In a study of primiparas, only 35% rated their pain as intolerable; 37% rated it as severe; and 28% rated it as moderate. Various studies of both primiparas and multiparas reveal that from about 35% to 61% of the women report pain that is intolerable or severe.[20]

Variability is probably the most striking feature of pain during labor. There is variability not only in overall intensity, as noted above, but also in the progression of pain intensity and the location of pain during labor. In one study, some women showed the expected rising curve of pain intensity, but others experienced increases and decreases in pain intensity throughout labor; some had high levels early in labor, and others had a low level pain up to the time of delivery. Location of pain also varied; some women had widespread pain over a large part of the abdomen, back, and perineum, whereas others had localized areas of pain (Fig. 23-4).[20]

During the first stage of normal labor, pain or discomfort may result from the involuntary contraction of the uterine muscle. The contraction tends to be felt in the lower back at the beginning of labor. As labor progresses, the sensation encircles the lower torso, covering both back and abdomen.

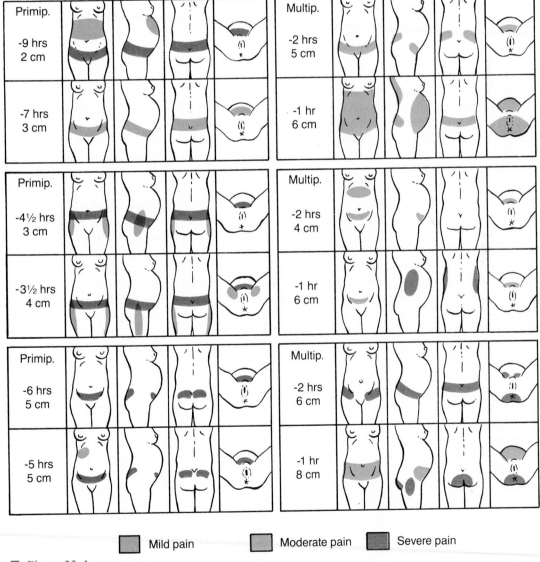

■ *Figure 23-4*

Distribution and intensity of pain during labor. Shaded areas show the distribution of pain at six points during labor prior to delivery. Pain intensity is indicated in the key. (Adapted from Melzack R, et al: Severity of labour pain: Influence of physical as well as psychological variables. Can Med Assoc J 130: 579–584, 1984)

Contractions are frequently described as wavelike: they come and go rhythmically, each one increasing to a certain height or intensity and then decreasing and, finally, disappearing. Contractions last from about 45 to 90 seconds. In early labor, the contractions are not necessarily uncomfortable. As labor progresses, the intensity of each contraction increases, resulting in a greater possibility of intensity of discomfort.

The quality of the discomfort is difficult to describe and certainly is varied. The possible qualities to any painful sensation include burning, pricking, and aching. Also, pain can be either deep or superficial. Consequently, one may say that a labor contraction is felt as deep aching. Words commonly chosen by women in labor to describe their pain are *sharp, cramping, aching, throbbing, stabbing, hot, shooting, heavy, tiring, exhausting, intense,* and *tight.*[20]

The intervals between contractions shorten as labor proceeds. Early labor contractions are about 5 to 20 minutes apart. Then, for several hours, they occur 3 to 5 minutes apart. During about the last hour prior to delivery, the intervals between contractions may be only a few seconds long. This period, when the cervix is dilating from about 7 to 10 cm, is referred to as *transition.*

Uterine contractions are at their highest intensity and greatest frequency during transition. This is usually when the woman experiences the most discomfort and has the most difficulty handling her discomfort.

Of course, the woman certainly may experience discomfort during birth, but it is generally much less intense than what she felt during transition.

The predominant sensations during birth occur in the vaginal and perineal area and can be described as pressure, stretching or splitting, and sometimes burning. Most of the time the woman has an overwhelming desire to push. Pushing may relieve whatever discomfort is felt. Also, the pressure of the baby's head causes a degree of numbness in the perineum.

In addition to uterine contractions, approximately 25% of women in labor also have to cope with the discomfort of back labor. This occurs when the fetus is in a posterior occipital position (see Chap. 38). With each contraction the occiput presses on the woman's sacrum, causing extreme discomfort as the intensity of contractions increases. Back labor is considerably more painful for the woman than is labor in which there is an anterior occipital position.

ASSESSMENT OF THE INDIVIDUAL WOMAN'S CONTRACTIONS

When labor is discussed with the woman, the sensations should be referred to as *contractions,* not pains. The initial contractions are not necessarily uncomfortable, and pain is usually a misnomer. Later in labor, the contractions may be painful, but it is preferable to call them what they are, contractions. Most women probably are not so suggestible that they would actually feel unbearable pain during contractions simply because the nurse used the term *pains* rather than *contractions.* But the use of the term *pains* may generate needless anxiety.

When the characteristics of uterine contractions (onset, frequency, duration, intensity, description of sensation, and attitude toward contractions) are assessed, it is important to note the time when labor began (*onset*), because prolonged labor intensifies the painful experience. Not only is a longer time spent in discomfort, but a lengthy labor often fatigues and discourages the parents, making it more difficult to cope with labor (see Part I of the Assessment Tool).

Regularity and *increase* in frequency of contractions that also increase in intensity indicate a normal labor. Such information can be used to assure the parents that progress is being made.

To obtain more detailed and useful information about *intensity of contraction,* the nurse may ask the woman to rate the contraction on a scale of mild, moderate, intense (strong), or very intense (very strong).

It is also helpful to encourage the woman to describe other characteristics of the contraction, such as where the sensation begins and where it is felt most intensely. This information often suggests the need for specific pain relief measures. For example, if the contraction begins in the lower back and is felt most intensely there, rubbing that area and applying pressure may provide considerable comfort.

As the woman is discussing her contractions, she may reveal her *attitude* toward labor in general. The degree of fear or anxiety experienced is of special importance, because these feelings have a profound effect on pain. They decrease pain tolerance and increase the perceived intensity of pain. Anxiety or fear also increases muscle tension and may increase painful stimuli during labor by interfering with contractions.

Anxiety or fear during labor may be related to worry about how pain will be managed and how labor is progressing. To alleviate such anxiety, the nurse may inform the mother of the various pain relief measures that may be employed. Concern about the progression of labor or the effectiveness of the contractions may be partially diminished if the nurse keeps the woman informed of signs of progress, such as increasing cervical dilatation or regularity of contractions. It is sometimes helpful to assure the woman that it is possible to stop or correct ineffective or dysfunctional uterine contractions.

Assessment of Pain Relief Methods Employed by Parents

Because a thorough assessment of the woman in labor is inextricably related to intervention, some pain relief measures are mentioned in this discussion of assessment. Actually, the manner in which the nurse assesses

Assessment Tool

Factors in Assessing the Pain Experience During Labor

I. Contractions:
Onset
Frequency
Duration
Intensity
Description of sensation, location
Attitude toward contractions

II. Pain Relief Methods Employed by Parents for Labor:
Relaxation techniques
Breathing patterns
Positioning
Other strategies
Persons to assist or be present during labor
Medication
Physical activities
Distraction (or concentration) methods

III. Current Discomforts of Woman Other Than Labor
Pregnancy
Chronic illness
Recent illness or injury
Methods of handling above; effectiveness of methods

IV. Parents' Current Concerns Other Than Labor:
Activities or plans interrupted by labor
Care of children at home
Financial arrangements
Condition of woman or unborn child
Plans for care of infant
Unexpected change in childbirth plans
Plans and needs for assistance regarding above

V. Parents' Goals and Expectations Regarding Labor:
Presence and intensity of pain
Provisions for pain relief (if any)
Father's (coach's) presence
Episiotomy
Differences between mother and father regarding above
Which of the above not possible or not discussed with physician

the client is often a pain relief measure. When the nurse conveys to the woman that she believes the woman and that she desires to understand the woman's experience as completely as possible, anxiety may be reduced and the pain thereby relieved.

RELAXATION

Numerous techniques are used to achieve and maintain total skeletal muscle relaxation. A pillow may be placed between the woman's legs to support the limbs when she is on her side. For general relaxation, the woman may smile, yawn, or take deep breaths at regular intervals. The father may aid by giving tactile or verbal cues to induce relaxation.

Again, the nurse finds out what techniques are used for relaxation so she can accurately interpret the woman's behavior. (See Chap. 17 for a review of relaxation as it is taught by the nurse–educator and Appendix C for the technique.)

BREATHING PATTERNS

The nurse may find many regional differences in breathing techniques. *What* is done is not as important as long as it meets the objectives of oxygenation, relaxation, open airways, and attention focusing and reduces response patterns to pain and stress.

The nurse may be able to obtain information about the breathing patterns from some women simply by asking. Other women may not be aware of the breathing pattern they are using. In such instances, the woman should be observed closely to ascertain the breathing patterns being used. (A thorough assessment of breathing pattern helps the nurse anticipate the needs of the woman.) If a breathing pattern is not helpful, the nurse can suggest another pattern. If the mother uses rapid breathing, the nurse can remind her to report any tingling in the hands and other initial signs of hyperventilation, or carbon dioxide insufficiency.

POSITIONING

When the woman is admitted to the labor room, the nurse asks her which positions have been comfortable and which have not and which positions she may wish to consider later in labor. Some positions require additional pillows, which the nurse can then obtain in advance. Positioning is discussed in Chapter 22.

The nurse should encourage frequent position changes to find those that are associated with less pain and more efficient labor.

OTHER PAIN-REDUCING STRATEGIES

Distraction and concentration are frequently used for coping with pain. Distraction techniques are also the most individualized and, therefore, the most varied of all the techniques a woman may employ during childbirth. For example, some women bring with them a personal "concentration point," an object to be stared at during a contraction (see also Distraction, later in this chapter).

Physical activities other than those that fit in the above categories may be used during labor. During a contraction, the mother or father may rhythmically massage the abdomen, using some preparation such as cornstarch or talcum powder to keep the skin smooth. The father may rub the mother's lower back between and during contractions. The mother may rock her pelvis while standing or lying on her side. The latter appears to be particularly helpful during back labor. Counterpressure is also useful. To achieve this, the father may place tennis balls, a rolling pin, paint roller, his knee, or his fist against the lower back.

LABOR SUPPORT PERSONS

The father almost always is the support person during labor if the couple has attended classes in one of the methods of prepared childbirth. When the father is absent, the person in attendance may be a childbirth educator or the woman's friend or relative. After identifying the support person, the nurse finds out if that person has been with the woman prior to hospital admission and if the woman wants the person to remain with her in the labor and delivery rooms. The nurse also assesses the attending person's attitude and desires. It is possible, for instance, that the mother might want the father to remain with her, but the father may be quite reluctant and fearful. (For convenience, the person the mother brings to the hospital to be with her during labor henceforth will be referred to as the father).

In addition, the nurse determines what the father has done for the mother prior to admission, what is planned for the remainder of labor, what (if any) preparation the mother and father have had, and whether they have practiced what they plan to do. Sometimes the father simply stays near the mother, touching her gently and offering verbal encouragement. In other instances the father is expected to take an active role in pain relief measures, such as massaging the back or abdomen or applying counterpressure (see Part II of the Assessment Tool).

MEDICATIONS

When the woman is admitted, the nurse also asks whether she has taken medication or any other substance for pain relief, such as aspirin, codeine, or an alcoholic beverage. If medication was taken, the nurse notes the time, type, and amount.

It is always possible that the woman has taken some illegal drug, such as marijuana, heroin, or a black-market drug of unknown composition. The woman who uses illegal drugs may fear legal action against her or disdain from the health team. Therefore, to increase the likelihood of obtaining an honest answer from a woman who has used an illegal drug, the nurse should always stress that the questions about medication are asked for important reasons, such as determining what other medication can be used safely.

It is also important to inquire about what analgesics and anesthetics are being considered for use during labor. The woman may have no knowledge about the medication process, or she and the father may have discussed several possibilities with the physician.

Assessment of Problems Other Than Labor

CURRENT DISCOMFORTS

The process of labor may not be the only source of discomfort for the woman. Indeed, there are other diseases or symptoms that may be much more irritating and painful than the concurrent labor. Such discomforts may be associated with the pregnancy itself or may represent a chronic illness or a recent illness or injury (see Part III of the Assessment Tool). For example, pregnancy may cause or increase heartburn, hemorrhoids, or varicose veins in the legs or vagina, all of which can be extremely uncomfortable.

As for chronic illness, any one of a number of disorders (e.g., arthritis, allergy) may result in pain and discomfort. The same is true of a recent illness or injury, such as influenza or an accident resulting in a broken bone, lacerations, or a sprained ankle.

The nurse assesses sources of discomfort extraneous to labor so that appropriate actions can be taken to provide relief. At the same time, any treatment instituted prior to the onset of labor should be identified. If the woman has found effective means of handling discomforts, it obviously is expedient for her to use the same methods during labor whenever possible.

CURRENT CONCERNS

Because the precise time for the onset of labor is rarely predictable, significant activities or plans may be interrupted by labor (see Part IV of the Assessment Tool). For example, the onset of labor may interfere with the requirements of the father's occupation and cause him to worry over the possibility of losing his job if he does not report to work. If the parents have other children, they may be anxious about what will happen to the children during their absence. The parents may also be concerned about financial arrangements related to hospitalization and the physician's fee, particularly if complications arise.

For some reason, realistic or not, the parents may be fearful about the condition of the woman or the unborn infant. The mother or father may be considering giving up the baby for adoption. Onset of labor may precipitate many feelings about this.

There may have been an unexpected change in some aspect of the parents' plans for childbirth. Their physician may be out of town, or labor may have progressed so rapidly that they were unable to reach the hospital of their choice.

It is important for the nurse to realize that such concerns can stir anxiety and interfere with the parents' ability to concentrate on handling discomforts, respond to directions, cooperate with examinations, and deal with all the other aspects of labor. Any of these difficulties should be noted on the assessment.

Assessment of Goals and Expectations Regarding Labor

Parents generally have certain expectations regarding labor. The nurse may encounter extremes in parents' expectations related to pain and pain relief. One woman may expect severe pain and desire that the physician render her practically unconscious throughout labor. Another woman may expect no pain at all and, therefore, no pain relief measures. When discomfort and pain are expected, the parents may believe that the techniques they have been taught to use during labor, such as breathing patterns, are sufficient assistance for the woman. Their goal may be a completely unmedicated labor, or the parents may expect to use the methods they were taught in combination with medication if they desire it.

In some instances, the father remains with the mother from the beginning of labor, during birth, and through the recovery period after delivery. In other instances, the mother does not want the father present. Parents' expectations of the nurse and physician also need to be determined.

Some parents, particularly mothers, want to observe the effects of their pushing and the birth of the baby. Many delivery rooms have mirrors for this purpose. The parents may have brought a camera to take pictures in the labor and delivery rooms. They may also want someone to take a picture of them with their baby immediately after birth. Some parents want to tape record or videotape the birth.

A fully conscious mother almost always wants to touch the newborn as soon as possible. The mother may plan on holding the baby before the cord is cut. She may also expect to be allowed to breast-feed the baby immediately after birth.

In helping the parents express their goals and expectations, the nurse is alert to differences between the desires of the mother and father. For example, the father may not want to witness the delivery although the mother wants him in the delivery room. Or the father may think the mother is unrealistic in her plans for little or no medication. When the nurse observes such differences, she helps the parents become aware of them and formulate compatible goals.

In the assessment of the parents' goals, the nurse also notes whether these goals have been discussed with the physician. Some goals may be contraindicated for medical reasons. Other goals may require the awareness and cooperation of the physician. In addition, hospital policy sometimes places limitations on the parents. For instance, some labor rooms are so small that the hospital must have a policy of including only the father.

As labor progresses, the nurse continues to monitor the client for any changes in the items listed in Part V of the Assessment Tool. Some aspects of the labor situation may change dramatically, such as the nature of the contractions. There may be a sudden need for modification of pain relief methods. Also, the discomforts and concerns extraneous to labor may be resolved or suddenly may appear when none had existed before.

Potential Nursing Diagnoses

Because we are concerned with pain in this chapter, nursing diagnoses are related to pain and its relief. Possible diagnoses, then, are alteration in comfort (pain) related to contractions, knowledge deficit of methods to relieve pain related to nonparticipation in childbirth classes, and disturbance in self-concept related to guilt about inability to handle pain during labor.

Nursing Planning and Intervention

Good pain relief does not necessarily mean the total elimination of painful sensations. In fact, complete abolition of pain is rarely a realistic goal. It is significantly helpful to the woman and often more reasonable to aim at a decrease in the intensity of pain or a decrease in the degree to which pain bothers the woman. The latter is closely related to another possible goal of increasing the woman's tolerance for pain.

Two important principles that underlie the accomplishment of these goals are decreasing the pain impulses that reach the cortex of the brain and managing anxiety. The transmission of pain signals may be interrupted in a number of ways, such as decreasing the source of noxious stimuli or closing the gate (see Gate Control Theory, discussed earlier in the chapter).

The interaction between anxiety and pain may become a spiraling process. Pain may cause anxiety, which may increase the intensity of pain by causing muscle tension or by opening the gate to pain impulses. In this way, mild pain and anxiety can eventually become severe pain and panic.

The nurse may use the sensory-discriminative, the motivational-affective, or the cognitive-evaluative systems, discussed earlier as well as in the following sections, to help the laboring woman decrease pain.

USING THE MOTIVATIONAL-AFFECTIVE SYSTEM

The motivational-affective system causes a fight-or-flight response to pain. Thus, none of the pain reduction techniques of the other systems will be as effective if this fight-or-flight response is not managed. The opposite is the physiological relaxation response, which is a primary goal of pain management in labor.[6]

Relaxation. Virtually every method of prepared childbirth heavily emphasizes total skeletal muscle relaxation during labor. Relaxation relieves pain by interrupting the spiraling process of pain and anxiety. Muscle tension is a response to pain and anxiety. Because relaxation is the opposite of muscle tension, it prevents or diminishes tension. The behavioral response of relaxation, therefore, is incompatible with pain-anxiety responses. Some

---

> ### *Nursing Guidelines for Pain Relief Measures*
>
> - Use a variety of pain relief measures.
> - Use pain relief measures *before* pain becomes severe. (It is easier to prevent severe pain and panic than to alleviate them once they occur.)
> - Include those pain relief measures that the patient believes will be effective.
> - Take into account the patient's ability to be active or passive in the application of the pain relief measure.
> - Regarding the potency of the pain relief measure needed, rely on the patient's experience of the severity of pain rather than the known physical stimuli.
> - If a pain relief measure is ineffective the first time it is used during a contraction, encourage the woman to try it at least one or two more times before abandoning it.

research suggests that people's evaluation of the intensity of pain is in part a function of their evaluation of their own overt behavioral response to pain.[22] Possibly, when patients observe themselves relaxed instead of tense, they evaluate their pain as less intense, or relaxation may cause the cortex to send signals to close the gate to the transmission of pain impulses.

Relaxation undoubtedly provides pain relief for other reasons, depending on the individual person. For some women in labor, efforts to relax can serve as a distraction from pain. The teaching of relaxation is discussed in Chapter 17, and techniques for relaxation are presented in Appendix C.

When the nurse encounters a woman who has been trained in relaxation techniques, she simply finds out how best to assist her. It is particularly helpful to identify cues that will encourage relaxation if the woman becomes tense. These cues may be verbal, such as "relax," or tactile-kinesthetic, such as touching or moving the tense body part.

If the woman has not been trained in relaxation, the nurse may use some simple techniques that can make a significant difference in the woman's level of relaxation. The nurse first explains to the woman that relaxing during a contraction is important because it can decrease abdominal pressure on the uterus and also help her feel more calm and generally comfortable. The quickest and easiest way to promote relaxation is to instruct the woman to take a deep breath or to yawn and to "go limp" or relax as she exhales. The nurse suggests that the woman try one or both of these at the beginning and end of contractions and any time during contractions that she feels the need to relax. (The patient who chooses to yawn may find it becomes spontaneous

Nursing Care Plan

The Woman With Increased Pain During Labor

Patient Goals

1. Woman says coping strategies with periodic changes make pain bearable.
2. Woman states back pain much better.

Assessment	Potential Nursing Diagnosis	Planning/Assessment	Evaluation
Identify or describe the presence or absence of: Consistent person for support during labor	Alteration in comfort/pain related to contractions	Identify one person who will remain with woman for support throughout remainder of labor	Patient's contraction pain is more bearable when active listening and breathing are used and support person is present
Woman's statement about intensity, tolerability, or other characteristics of discomfort from contraction and other sources	Knowledge deficit of methods of relieving back pain related to nonattendance of childbirth classes	Keep woman and support person informed of progress of labor	Patient's back pain decreases with use of cold
Concerns other than labor		Teach an appropriate breathing pattern	
Ability to fulfill goals and expectations regarding labor		Try position other than current one (e.g., up on all fours, standing and leaning on bed or partner, sitting on chair)	
		Give deep back massage; apply cold, heat, or firm pressure to lower back	
		Suggest abdominal massage by woman or support person	
		Encourage active listening with music and headset	
		Teach simple relaxation technique	
		Change coping strategies periodically to maintain effectiveness (e.g., change positions, change music, alternate heat and cold, vary breathing techniques)	

and more frequent.) These techniques are effective because they take advantage of conditioned responses. Both a big sigh (deep breath) and a yawn are associated with relaxation.

Relaxation may be furthered by providing support to extremities that are comfortably positioned and slightly flexed.

Jaw relaxation is an abbreviated form of progressive relaxation that is easy for the nurse to teach the untrained (or even trained) patient to use. Its effectiveness may be attributed to relaxation of one area of the body leading to relaxation of other areas of the body. It is useful for brief, moderate to severe pain, such as in contractions, especially if taught in the absence of severe pain and tension, that is, between contractions or during early labor.[23] The following statements made be used to teach jaw relaxation:

1. Let your lower jaw drop slightly, as though you were starting a small yawn.

2. Keep your tongue quiet in the bottom of your mouth.
3. Let your lips get soft.
4. Breathe slowly, evenly, and rhythmically: inhale, exhale, rest.
5. Allow yourself to stop forming words with your lips and stop thinking words.

USING THE COGNITIVE-EVALUATIVE SYSTEM

To use the cognitive-evaluative system to decrease pain, the nurse must first understand the differences between the functioning of the left and right hemispheres of the brain (see Chap. 17, Table 17-8). Both hemispheres receive and process pain and sensory information, but in different ways. The nurse may assist the laboring woman to use cognitive strategies that involve either one or both of the brain hemispheres.[6] The strategies are presented in the Table 23-2.

Breathing Techniques. Women who have taken childbirth education classes are easily identified by the labor nurse from their use of specific breathing techniques.

Although techniques may vary, the nurse needs to observe the various techniques so she can assist the woman later, if necessary, by breathing with her or help the labor support person to do so. (For a more complete description of Lamaze breathing techniques, see Chap. 17 and Appendix C.)

The untrained woman and her partner can usually be taught some simple breathing techniques but often need the nurse to breathe with them more than a pair who have been trained together prior to labor. (For more information on teaching untrained women breathing techniques, see Chap. 17.)

Attention Focusing. The power of imagery is considered by some theorists to be the image's physiological affect on the body and may decrease pain by altering the physical cause of pain. Although the scientific basis of imagery in unknown, the professional literature refers to imagery as a technique that is useful and that fits within the scope of nursing practice.[23]

Imagery is a well-known function of the mind and an activity that people actually do on and off during the day on a regular basis. It is a temporary shift away from the here and now and may be referred to by some people as *daydreaming* or *zoning out*. Unlike daydreaming, the conscious experience of imagery involves a cer-

TABLE 23–2. USING THE COGNITIVE-EVALUATIVE SYSTEM TO DECREASE PAIN PERCEPTION IN LABOR

Pain Management Technique	Left Hemisphere	Right Hemisphere
Breathing techniques	Listening to the sound of breathing and counting	Rhythm of breathing
	Patterns learned in class	Changing breathing in response to body symptoms
	Cleansing breaths	Changing and adapting patterns learned in class
		Intuitive sighs, yawns, or deep breaths not at beginning or end of contractions
Attention focusing	Focal points of word(s)	Picture focal point(s)
		Imagery
Patterned physical movements		Walking
		Rocking
Music	Words	Melody
		Rhythm
Verbal coaching	Relax your left arm	Positive affirmations
		Rhythm of words

(Data from Hilbers S, Gennaro S: Nonpharmaceutical pain relief. NAACOG Update Series, Vol. 5. Princeton, NJ, Continuing Professional Education Center, 1986)

tain level of discipline.[24] Guided imagery is commonly taught in childbirth education classes so the nurse may "see" this used as a coping strategy for labor. The nurse may want to find out if the couple have already chosen an imagery and, if not, may teach them one to use.

The nurse can also assist untrained women to use this by verbally guiding them through the process using any of the three "Guided Imagery Exercises" in Appendix C. The nurse may want to perform the exercise between contractions initially and then move gradually to doing it during the woman's contractions. Coupled with relaxation and paced breathing, imagery can be a powerful adjunct to helping women cope with labor pain.

Patterned Physical Movements. It is not unusual to see people in pain using patterned movement, such as rocking the body from side to side or rhythmic head motions. Women in labor also seem to benefit from patterned physical movement such as walking; even more popular is the rocking chair. Many hospitals have moved rocking chairs into labor rooms and are encouraging women to try them in labor.

Music. Another strategy that is becoming more popular in many clinical areas, including labor, is active listening, or auditory stimulation, through a headset or earphone. The equipment required is a battery-operated cassette player; headset or earphone; and one or more cassettes of music chosen by the woman. The music may be relaxing, soft, and familiar, or it may be fast and lively. Some women may use a combination of both. Usually during the contraction, and between contractions if she wants, the woman listens to the preselected music through the earphone or headset. This provides a demanding auditory stimulus very difficult to ignore. For visual input, she may focus on an object or close her eyes and imagine something suggested by the music. Often the woman taps out the beat to the music to help increase her concentration on the distraction. She may also move her body or parts of her body in rhythm to the music. To avoid what may possibly be habituation, a variety of music tapes can be used or the music may be used intermittently.

The equipment for active listening is usually brought by the woman. This is such a simple and effective distraction, however, that hospitals might well consider making the equipment available, especially if many women come to the hospital in labor and without previous childbirth education.

Verbal Coaching. From the beginning of labor, the woman needs to have someone with her at increasingly frequent intervals and to know that someone is available at all times. Toward the end of labor, she needs to have someone with her constantly. The presence, actions, and words of this person can be supportive to the woman. This person may be the nurse, the father, or someone else. At times the nurse's greatest contribution is to support the father so that he can support the mother in turn.

As mentioned previously, part of the uniqueness of labor pain is that the woman may possess anxiety-reducing knowledge. If the woman does not obtain this information for herself, the nurse can supply it. For example, the nurse may tell the woman approximately how long it will be before the next contraction and how long that contraction will last. During intense contractions, the nurse may count down at 15-second intervals until the end of the contraction, telling the woman how long it will be until the contraction is over. Or the nurse may time the contraction so she can reassure the woman by telling her when the contraction has reached its peak and will begin to subside. Information about the progress of labor, such as cervical dilatation and descent of the baby, is also important. It serves as a reminder that there is a purpose to labor, that labor does end, and that the end is getting closer and closer.

Such information not only reduces anxiety but may motivate the woman to tolerate pain. Especially toward the end of labor, when discomfort increases, the knowledge that the ordeal is almost over may enable the woman to tolerate an intensity of pain that she would otherwise find unbearable.

Knowing that she and her baby are not in danger also reduces anxiety. Sometimes the woman finds the forces of labor so unexpectedly powerful that she is fearful of harm. The nurse should periodically reassure the woman that she and her baby are doing well (provided, of course, that this is true). The nurse may say, for example, that the baby's heart beat is strong and regular. Remembering that discomfort is associated with a normal process and not a life-threatening illness may be helpful to the woman. Briefly and simply, the nurse can remind the woman of what is happening (e.g., that each contraction enlarges the opening for the baby).

Understanding what is happening during labor seems to increase the woman's sense of control over the event. Feelings of powerlessness can provoke anxiety, so it is important to further feelings of control. This may be done through instructions and explanations that help the woman cooperate with examinations and with the process of labor, such as effective pushing. In particular, the woman's feelings of control can be strengthened by teaching her about pain relief measures as early as possible. When this teaching has not been done prior to the onset of labor, the nurse can begin in early labor to explain certain of the pain relief measures. The woman then knows that pain relief is available, that there are several possibilities, and that to some extent she may choose from among them.

USING THE SENSORY-DISCRIMINATIVE SYSTEM

To decrease pain using the sensory-discriminative system, three peripheral receptors can be used—mechanoreceptors, thermoreceptors, and chemoreceptors. All three receptors are supplied by nerve fibers that differ in their speed of conduction to the cortex. Pain perception is decreased because the sensory information reaches the brain before the pain information[6] (see Gate Control Theory, discussed earlier in the chapter). Table 23-3 lists possible pain-reducing strategies the nurse can use to assist the laboring woman.

Positioning. In the past decade, professionals as well as parents have begun to understand the benefits of various positions a women uses during labor. The findings of researchers concerning the benefits of being upright and mobile during labor have contributed to this understanding. Roberts et al[25] studied position changes, and the overall results indicated that changing positions is important for efficient uterine contractions. Diaz et al[26] found that 95% of the women chose to be sitting, standing, or walking when given the choice.

Standing or walking during labor has been shown to contribute to shorter duration of labor with decreased pain and increased comfort levels.[26–28] Flynn et al[27] found ambulation during the first stage shortens labor by 30% and reduces the need for analgesia by the same amount. The nurse can encourage women to try getting out of bed and see if that helps. Another position that may provide comfort during labor is the lateral Sims' position.

Roberts et al[25] found that women preferred sitting in the first half of labor and sidelying in late labor.

Positioning is an especially important and effective pain relief measure when the woman experiences back labor (i.e., when the occiput of the fetus presses on the woman's sacrum).

An unusual but increasingly popular position for women with back labor is the up-on-all-fours position. This position may even succeed in rotating the baby's head to an anterior position. If the baby's head is not in the posterior position, this crawl position may still relieve pain, especially during transition, when labor is so often felt in the back.

Unless there are complications, the woman should be allowed to choose the position she finds most comfortable. If she wants to lie on her back, however, the head of the bed should be elevated and her thighs slightly flexed with pillows. The nurse should encourage frequent position changes to find those that are associated with less pain and more efficient labor.

Cutaneous Stimulation. The underlying mechanisms of pain relief from cutaneous stimulation are usually

unknown. Gate control theory suggests that stimulation of the skin may activate the large diameter fibers, which may cause an inhibition of the pain messages carried by the smaller fibers. Another possibility is that certain types of skin stimulation may increase the endorphin level. The effectiveness of some methods of cutaneous stimulation may be related to therapeutic touch.[23]

HEAT AND COLD. For centuries heat and cold have been used for pain relief, but the mechanisms that explain the effects are still largely a matter of speculation.[23] The application of heat or cold (with the physician's permission) may be especially comforting to the laboring woman.

Heat is good for decreasing tension and promoting overall relaxation. It dilates blood vessels and is usually recommended for low to moderate pain. An increasing number of hospitals have remodeled and have added larger showers and "warm" tubs to their labor areas. Many women present glowing reports about the pain-relieving benefits of a warm tub bath during labor (if membranes have not ruptured) or long warm showers if membranes have ruptured. For women in labor who do not have access to a tub or shower, the nurse can also try a hot water bottle, heating pad, or hot washcloths on the womens' lower abdomen, groin, back, perineum, or thighs. Heat should be used at least 5 to 10 minutes but may be used for 20 to 30 minutes or longer.[23] Cold penetrates two to three times more deeply than heat. Cold receptors in the skin far outnumber heat receptors. Cold numbs painful areas and constricts blood vessels. Cold also slows the pain impulse transmission along nerve pathways and is usually recommended for acute pain. For severe back pain, cold may feel better than heat. The nurse can put ice in a glove to try on the patients' back or back of her neck. A cold washcloth may also feel good.[29]

Cold is usually applied for 20 to 30 minutes or longer. The minimal effective time is 5 to 10 minutes. If cold relieves the pain, cold will likely work better than heat because cold relieves pain faster and relieves more pain and relief lasts longer after removal of the cold.[23]

The nurse may also encourage the woman to try alternating heat and cold or using either intermittently. Alternating heat and cold may be more effective with severe pain.[23]

MASSAGE. Several types of cutaneous stimulation may be used during labor and may prove to be effective pain relief measures. One of the more common of these is effleurage, or abdominal massage (Fig. 23-5). Rubbing the lower back is also common (Fig. 23-6). Rubbing a painful body part is a universal means of relieving pain.

The above methods are examples of relatively moderate stimulation of cutaneous fibers. Mild to moderate stimulation is ordinarily more effective than intense stimulation. One notable exception, however, is

TABLE 23–3. USING THE SENSORY DISCRIMINATIVE SYSTEM TO DECREASE PAIN PERCEPTION IN LABOR

Receptors	Nerve Endings	Location in Body	Transmission	Activities to Try With Laboring Woman
Mechanoreceptors	Merkel's disks (take physical stimuli and transform them into electrical energy that is transmitted to the brain)	Epidermis—most numerous in skin of the palms, soles of feet, and external genitalia	Well-mylelinated, fast-transmitting, large-diameter fibers. Do not habituate rapidly so techniques can be effective for long periods of time. Lips and index finger have large interpretive area in the brain	Pressure on lips by using Chapstick, kissing Pressure maintained over upper lip with index finger Partner hold her hands, she can sit on her hands Hold bed rails or squeeze hands or objects Standing or placing soles of feet on other hard surface, e.g., a stool Sitting on firm surface Warm baths
	Meissner's corpuscles	Fingertips and hairless skin	Also transmits faster than pain	Move her fingertips in circles on the sheets Feel soft textures like velvet, fur Feel her partner's face Effleurage with firm pressure Play with her hair Slow, firm pressure along a tense area in the same direction as hair grows Warm shower
	Pacinian corpuscles	Deeper layer of skin	Detect deep, rapid pressure sensations and vibrations. The largest and most widely distributed receptors in the body. Are slow to habituate so can be used over long periods of time	Lean against warm, vibrating clothes dryer Feet in devices that vibrate warm water Vibrating pillows or cordless vibrators Vibrating shower massage

	Tactile hair end organs	Base of each individual hair; fired by hair movement	Detect light touch. Stimulation can increase pain as they travel on some of same fibers as pain	Avoid:
				  Tickling
				  Light moving touch *against* hair follicles (i.e., rubbing someone the wrong way) Eq. light effleurage
				  Some movements of sheets, clothing, and air may irritate

(continued)

TABLE 23–3. USING THE SENSORY DISCRIMINATIVE SYSTEM TO DECREASE PAIN PERCEPTION
(continued)

Receptors	Nerve Endings	Location in Body	Transmission	Activities to Try With Laboring Woman
	Joint receptors	Found in joint capsules, ligaments, synovial membrane	Slow to habituate. Joint movement and pressure into joints will fire these receptors and decrease pain	Frequent changes of position Standing, walking, hugging, rocking Gently shaking joints Pelvic rock on all fours Breathing techniques may cause rib-cage movement Avoid: Lying quietly in bed with little joint movement
Chemoreceptors (take chemical stimuli and transform them into energy transmitted to brain)	Olefactory	Upper part of each nostril	Unmyeliniated small-diameter fibers	Familiar *positive* smells, e.g., her own pillow case, herbs, special foods, body odor of significant other
	Taste	Mouth		Familiar *positive tastes*, e.g., own mouthwash, special teas
Thermoreceptors (transmit information about temperature to the brain)		Skin	Not as well understood as other receptors. Rapidly habituate and respond greatly to temperature changes	Alternating hot and cold packs* Ice in plastic bag* Socks if feet are cool Neutral body warmth may be calming* Warm showers, bath* Warm hair dryer*

* Do not apply heat or cold to anesthestized or ischemic areas as tissues may be damaged.
(Data from Hilbers S, Gennaro S: Nonpharmaceutical pain relief. NAACOG Update Series, Vol. 5. Princeton, NJ; Continuing Professional Center, 1986)

the use of intense pressure over the sacrum during a contraction. The pressure may be applied with the knee or fist (Fig. 23-7), or the mother may lean back (in a semisitting position) on a tennis ball or rolling pin. It has been estimated that applying pressure during a contraction is equivalent to the pain relief potential of 50 to 100 mg of meperidine.[30]

Rubbing of any part of the body, even between contractions, possibly may contribute to pain relief. This not only encourages relaxation, but experimentation with cutaneous stimulation shows that it may help close the gate to painful impulses long after its use and that the painful area need not always be the area of stimulation.[18] For example, if an external monitor prevents abdominal massage, the thighs may be massaged instead. Some mothers find that foot massage by the father or nurse brings considerable comfort.

TRANSCUTANEOUS ELECTRIC NERVE STIMULATION. Transcutaneous electric nerve stimulation (TENS) is a newer form of cutaneous stimulation that has been used successfully for pain relief during the first stage of labor. The mechanisms behind the effectiveness of TENS in relieving pain are unclear. Some types of TENS appear to relieve pain by increasing endorphins. Other types may act as a counterirritant, masking the pain or activating a complex neural inhibiting system.[23]

In TENS, a mild electric current is applied to the skin by way of electrodes connected to a battery-operated device with controls to regulate the sensation. The patient is usually taught before labor how to control the unit herself, and she uses it in conjunction with prepared childbirth techniques. The patient usually feels a buzzing, tingling, or vibrating sensation. In one study of labor pain, two pairs of electrodes were placed on

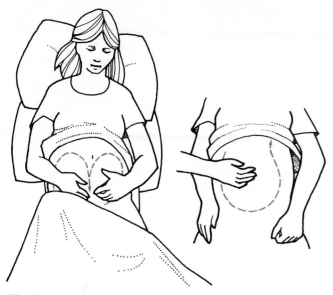

■ *Figure 23-5*
Two types of effleurage, or abdominal massage.

either side of the spinal column over the sacral and thoracic regions. Low-intensity stimulation was provided continuously, and the woman increased the stimulation during a contraction. No complications occurred except that in a few cases sacral stimulation interfered with fetal heart rate monitoring. The researchers recommended TENS as a primary method of pain relief during labor, noting that it is a low-risk, nonpharmacologic method that can be interrupted at any moment.[31] Comparable results have been obtained in studies of Egyptian and Italian mothers during childbirth.[32,33]

Other studies show good pain relief in 30% to 44% of women, moderate pain relief in another 30% to 44%, and no relief in 10% to 12%.[34–36]

TENS is also useful for postoperative (cesarean) incisional pain, with effectiveness rate of 70% to 90%.[23]

Nursing responsibilities when TENS is used might

include placing and securing the electrodes, explaining the use of the controls to the woman, and evaluating the effectiveness of TENS in relieving pain.

ACUPRESSURE. Acupressure is another possible way the nurse or labor partner can help decrease a womens' labor pain. It is believed by some that acupressure may release endorphins and other neurotransmitters associated with pain relief, but not all experts agree on this. There are several pressure points that may be helpful in labor. (Because pressure on some points may strengthen contractions, they should not be used before labor begins). Several of the pressure points are shown in Figure 23-8. It is best for the nurse or labor partner to apply moderate pressure at the acupressure points on both sides simultaneously for up to a minute at a time. The points can also be massaged with small, circular movements of 2 to 3 cycles per second also for up to a minute at a time.[29] Pressure may be applied with the tips of the index fingers or thumbs or the finger or thumb nails.

THERAPEUTIC TOUCH. Therapeutic touch is based on the folk-healing practice known as *laying on of hands.* Healers place themselves in a meditative state, hold their hands just above the patient, and transfer their energy to the patient to relieve pain or other problems. Therapeutic touch is the special province of nurses, and Delores Krieger, Professor of Nursing at New York University, has taught the technique to thousands of health professionals. Therapeutic touch is one more method nurses trained in its use have to help their patients in labor.[29]

DISTRACTION. We have not yet begun to uncover and understand fully the various strategies people use to cope with pain.

Some of the techniques discussed earlier in other frameworks are also useful as distracters. "Research and clinical observations show that distraction strategies are powerful techniques for making even severe pain bear-

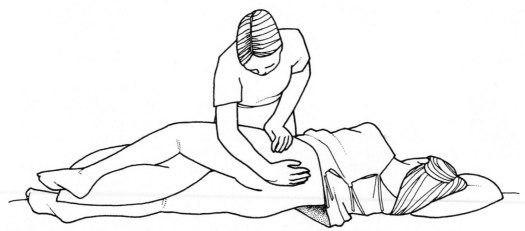

■ *Figure 23-6*
Deep back massage, while the mother lies on her side, relieves back pain during labor.

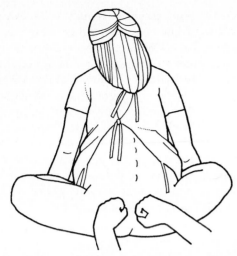

■ *Figure 23-7*
Firm counterpressure of the fists on the lower back, while the mother is in the tailor sitting position, effectively relieves back pain during labor.

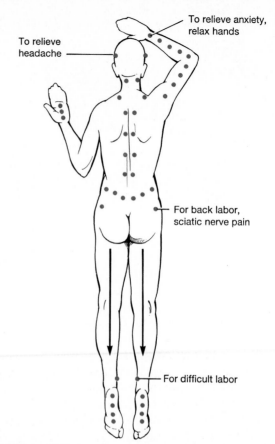

■ *Figure 23-8*
Acupressure points for back massage. From Jungman R: Education for Childbirth: A New Lamaze Handbook. Published privately by Education for Childbirth, 6102 Broadway, San Antonio, Texas 78209)

able for the patient."[23] Within the area of distraction, there are numerous approaches.

The nurse needs to be familiar with a variety of distracters that she may suggest to the woman. What is sufficiently distracting for one woman may not be for another. A woman may need assistance with distracters even if she has attended prepared childbirth classes. Instructors of methods of prepared childbirth have devised and taught many means of distraction for use during contractions. It is interesting to note that a large number of these are rhythmic, such as "riding the wave," tapping out the rhythm of a song, rhythmic head movements, and rhythmic breathing.

Emphasis is placed on distracters that are of some proven effectiveness and are also relatively easy to teach the woman. Most of the techniques taught in the Lamaze method meet these criteria. The Lamaze method reveals some of the ideas common to most methods of prepared childbirth: concentration on relaxation and a rhythmic breathing pattern during contractions. (A review of the information in Chapter 17 and in Table 23-4 will assist the reader in the following discussion of these distracters.) Some distracters used in the various methods of prepared childbirth are extremely distracting but difficult to teach quickly once labor is in progress.

Many of these activities serve double purposes. The breathing rhythms and purposeful thoughts undoubtedly serve as distracters, but maintenance of rhythmic breathing is also thought to relieve pain by providing adequate oxygenation of the uterus.

Although relaxation serves such purposes as decreasing the fight-or-flight response, the woman may find that her concentrated efforts to relax provide a significant distraction. Changing positions and massaging

the abdomen require both motor and cognitive effort and therefore may be distracting. Keeping the eyes open and focused on a particular point is perhaps the purest and simplest distracter. Altogether, the Lamaze-trained woman consciously performs several varied activities, with the end result of distraction from pain.

Whatever type of distracters the woman may choose during a contraction, the nurse and others must take care not to prevent her from using them. Early in labor, it may be a helpful distraction to the woman to have someone to talk with during a contraction, but, later, she may find this irritating because it interferes with other strategies for coping with pain. In any event, the nurse needs to find out from the woman what, if anything, she wants the nurse to do for her during a contraction.

When the nurse wishes to assist the laboring woman with pain relief measures in the form of distracters, it is only reasonable to approach the woman between, not during, contractions. The nurse can describe briefly one or two possibilities. The woman should be asked to decide which one she would like to try first. It usually is most helpful if the nurse first demonstrates and then has the woman do it. If a song or counting is to be used, it is often much easier for the woman if the nurse counts or sings for her during the first contractions in which the pattern is used. If the woman does not like any of the distracters, the nurse may creatively invent some others or simply ask the woman for suggestions.

When discomfort intensifies or possible habituation develops and a more powerful form of distraction is needed, the nurse may teach the woman the "modified or patterned paced breathing" of the Lamaze method. Either of these if done incorrectly may result in hyperventilation. Hyperventilation may be treated by having the woman breathe into a paper bag and suggesting that henceforth she breathe more slowly. Again, more distraction may be added to these breathing patterns by incorporating one or more of the distracters of the Lamaze method: the concentration point, abdominal massage, silent counting, or singing in rhythm with breathing. Another effective and relatively easy distracter to employ is finger tapping the rhythm to a 4/4 song, coordinating the rhythm with breathing.

During transition, the woman's focus tends to become extremely narrow because of the great increase in the intensity of contractions. Whereas earlier in labor the distracters could be suggested and taught between contractions, there is little time now and it is difficult for the woman to focus on anything but labor. Therefore, distracters used during transition should be more simple and must be taught prior to the onset of transition.

Toward the end of the accelerated phase of labor or in transition, most couples need increasing support from the labor nurse. When a woman requests medication, she often is asking not necessarily for medication alone but for help. It is important to know that a woman who panics during a contraction often feels like she is drowning. The waves keep coming, there is no letup, and it is hard for her to catch her breath. Holding her hand and saying, "Relax, it's okay," won't be much help. It is necessary for the nurse to know exactly what to do to make an effective "rescue." There are a few simple steps to the "panic routine":[37]

1. Stand up (especially important for a labor support person, who is usually seated). This action says, "I'm here and I'm in charge."
2. Hold her wrist. This action says, "I'm not going to let you be swept away. I'm here for you."
3. Bombard her senses with input. Your goal is to engage her total attention.
   a. Bring your face close to hers and make her look at you (if she turns her head from side to side, give up wristholding and grasp her face, one hand on each side).
   b. Do your breathing with a throaty, loud sound

so you will attract her attention. It is important to start where she is, no matter how fast, noisy or irregular, and then "bring her down."
   c. Move your free hand up and down to reinforce the breathing rhythm and rate.

This routine is confirmed by McCaffery.[23] As pain increases in intensity, increase the complexity of the stimuli. Try to provide stimuli through all the major sensory modalities, as follows:

1. Auditory (throaty breathing)
2. Visual (face of partner)
3. Tactile (hold her wrist or face)
4. Kinesthetic (not mentioned by Langendoen but could be having woman nod or tap out breathing rhythm)

McCaffery and Beebe mention, however, that with very high pain intensities, consider simpler distractions if the patient has limited energy to concentrate.[23]

HABITUATION. When the gate control theory is used as a conceptual framework to devise pain relief strategies, it is important to note that insufficient input or monotonous stimuli may also open the gate. If pain returns or increases, it may be due to advancing labor or it may be due to habituation. Therefore it is important for the nurse to know how to avoid habituation. Changing to different strategies may help; for example, changing positions, changing from imagery to eyes on external focal point, changing music, changing to a different breathing technique, or adding effleurage can be tried. The combinations of strategies are practically limitless. If and when the new strategies become less effective, the woman probably can go back to some of those methods used previously.

ASSISTANCE WITH CHANGE IN EXPECTATIONS AND GOALS

During the relatively brief and rapidly moving events of labor, any unexpected change in the parents' goals or expectations must be handled quickly; otherwise, anxiety may persist or increase, resulting in an increased intensity of pain. Some items listed in Part V of the Assessment Tool (earlier in the chapter) are examples of areas in which a disturbing change may occur. Several examples of changes are the following: because of unforeseen circumstances there is a physician unknown to the parents in attendance at labor and delivery or the father is unable to attend the birth; crowding of the labor section at this time limits use of planned facilities; internal or external monitors may be used, which may signify complications or limit movement; and pain relief medications may be necessary.

When a situation occurs that disturbs the parents, the nurse encourages them to express their feelings and

(Text continues on page 532)

TABLE 23–4. SUMMARY OF PAIN RELIEF MEASURES USED BY LAMAZE-TRAINED PARENTS DURING LABOR

Approximate Progress of Labor	Position	Eye Focus
Onset to 3 cm, or contractions 5–20 min apart	Supported with pillows sitting or lying on side; may walk between contractions; may stand and lean on object during contractions; may prefer rocking chair; should change positions at least hourly to facilitate labor and decrease pain	Eyes open and focused on one particular object or person's face ("concentration point," focal point"), or eyes may be closed while doing imagery during contractions
Dilates from 4 to 7 cm, or contractions 2–4 min apart	Same as above	Same as above
Dilates from 8 to 10 cm, or contractions 1 min apart	Same as above, but most women prefer to be in bed now	Same as above, but focusing eyes on another person may be more helpful to some at this stage
Birth (fully dilated)	For pushing in labor room, ABC room, or LDR may be sitting and holding legs to 90-deg angle with body, squatting holding bed rails, squat bar or support from people or on all fours (to rotate posterior baby); or be lying on side with back curved and top knee pulled up; if no progress in 20 min, change position For birth in delivery room, ABC room, or LDR, semipropped sitting position; if legs not in stirrups, she may put feet on bed or may give birth on her side	For pushing may focus on mirror or perineum, if visible, to see results of pushing

ABC = alternative birthing center; LDR = labor, delivery, recovery.

Breathing Patterns	Woman's Possible Thoughts	Labor Partner's Activities Through All Phases of Labor
Inhales deeply at beginning of contraction and relaxes totally on exhalation; takes a deep breath at end of each contraction Slow-paced breathing (inhale through nose or mouth, exhale through nose or mouth) *Minimum* rate is half individual woman's resting respiration rate	On inhalation, "In, 1, 2," on exhalation, "Out, 1, 2" or Concentrate on imagery or Concentrate on music	Times frequency of contractions Help woman get in comfortable positions, changing positions at least hourly As need arises, may do abdominal massage for her or rub her lower back Reminds her to urinate—a full bladder can slow labor progress Gives love, support, encouragement, hugs, holding
May continue slow-paced breathing or use modified paced breathing (may accelerate as contraction intensifies, decelerate as contraction subsides); breathing is maximum rate of twice woman's resting respiration rate Breathing may be inhale nose, exhale nose; inhale nose, exhale mouth; or inhale mouth, exhale mouth Breathing may be in 4/4 or other rhythm Modified paced breathing used only to break habituation, then may be able to return to slow paced	Counts each breath in 4/4 rhythm, emphasizing count of 1 (e.g., "1, 2, 3, 4, 1, 2, 3, 4," etc., or silently sings "Yankee Doodle," a 4/4 song) or Concentration on imagery or Concentrate on music	Same as above plus the following: During contractions at 15-sec intervals he calls off time that elapses (i.e., "15 seconds, 30 seconds, 45 seconds, 60 seconds") until contraction is over As need arises, may breathe in rhythm with her, count aloud in rhythm to her breathing, or sing song in rhythm; remind her of eye focus; remind her to breathe deeply at end of contraction If back labor or backache, may try deep counterpressure with heat/ice to lower back and position changes
Patterned paced breathing through mouth or nose (rhythm of 1–6 breaths and then 1 blow), (may accelerate and decelerate with intensity of contraction) breathing is maximum rate of twice woman's resting respiration rate If not allowed to push but feels urge to push, blows repeatedly If uncomfortable between contractions, uses slow-paced breathing	Counts each breath according to rhythm selected (e.g., "1, 2, 3, 4, 5, 6, blow") or Concentrates on imagery or Concentrates on music	Between contractions offers encouragement; wipes face with cool, wet cloth; moistens lips and mouth with water, ice chips, mouthwash, or Chapstick May use "panic routine;" keep environment safe and calm; other activities in previous phases Pressure on area of buttocks or squeeze buttocks together to make urge to push more tolerable
For pushing; 2 deep breaths, inhale, hold breath, hold 5–7 sec, release breath; repeat inhalation and continue as before until contraction is over or until instructed to stop pushing Alternate method: 2 deep breaths, on 3rd breath blow out slowly and bear down; repeat as necessary Making grunting noises is OK	Same as above, except when pushing For pushing may visualize baby slowly coming out of uterus and through birth canal	For pushing may stand at woman's back to support her in pushing position if no back rest, help hold legs or support in squat Counts aloud 5–7 sec during each breath holding, tells her "exhale, take a deep breath, and hold it," then counts to 5–7 again Reminds her to relax pelvic floor or "bulge" pelvic floor or "open up" Helps her to change to other positions as necessary; if no progress in 20 min, change position Offers cold cloth, love, encouragement

indicates an appreciation of their disappointment. The nurse then explains the reasons for any rules, policies, or circumstances that prevent the parents from achieving their goals or expectations.

One of the more difficult problems is assisting couples who are not able to achieve their ideal of labor and birth. This ideal may vary considerably from one couple to another. Inability to achieve this ideal labor may cause profound feelings of failure in the mother or father. Also, the couple may refuse or be reluctant to accept measures incompatible with their ideal.

Patients who have specific expectations or goals associated with an ideal labor may have arrived at these ideas in a number of ways. A recent study found that women who expected labor to be very painful were likely to find that it was, whereas women who preferred to cope without drugs were more likely to do so and had higher satisfaction scores. Women who expected relaxation and breathing techniques to be helpful were more likely to find that this was true and to be more satisfied than other women. The study also found that womens' expectations of being in control (both self-control and control of what was done to them) were positively associated with achieving that goal and "emotional well-being" scores[38] (see Chap. 17 for content about birth planning).

How does the nurse help the couple minimize feelings of failure and accept a change in their goals? Throughout childbirth, and particularly when goals must change, the nurse praises the mother and father for their efforts and abilities to handle labor. This promotes feelings of success. For example, the woman may have the goal of an unmedicated labor, but she may find the discomfort intolerable and request medication. If medication is given, the nurse can say that she knows medication was not planned. She can allow the woman to express her feelings and then praise the woman for the success of her efforts up to now and for the length of time medication was not necessary. She may add that the woman's continuing effort may reduce the amount of medication required. She may also stress to the man that his approval and support are extremely valuable.

AFTERMATH ASSIMILATION

After anticipation of pain and the presence of pain, a third and final phase of the pain experience occurs: the aftermath. The pain experience does not end with the cessation of the painful sensations. The patient does not necessarily immediately forget about the pain, especially if it was severe, frightening, or in any way disconcerting.

On the maternity unit, it is a common observation that women talk a great deal about their childbirth experiences. It is a frequent topic of conversation, regardless of whether the woman had an easy or difficult labor. Not only may the woman want to talk about the pain, but a variety of feelings resulting from the pain may be present, such as nausea, vomiting, chills, anger, or embarrassment. The woman may even have nightmares about the pain.

Clearly, at least some women need assistance during the aftermath phase of the pain experience. The most appropriate nursing action may be to assist the woman with the intellectual and emotional assimilation of her childbirth experience. In a sense, the nurse helps the woman relive her labor. The nurse can ask the woman questions that help her discuss her discomforts, emotions, thoughts, and overt responses and the reactions of others during her labor. The nurse needs to be particularly alert and responsive to the woman's needs for support, such as praise, confirmation that her perceptions of discomfort are believed by others, or reassurance that her behavior was acceptable. Some women need information to help them fill in memory gaps or to correct understandings that are inaccurate and anxiety provoking.[18]

It is particularly important to encourage assimilation in women who may harbor feelings of failure about childbirth. But assimilation may help maintain or restore a positive self-concept for any woman and enhance her ability to deal with mothering and other impending tasks.

Most prepared childbirth instructors encourage the parents to write a "birth report" about their experiences during labor and birth. This writing is not only treasured for years to come but is an excellent way for the couple to fill in the missing pieces and provide closure so they can move on to the new challenges of parenting.

Evaluation

SPECIFIC PAIN STRATEGIES

On-the-spot evaluation of pain-reducing strategies will be necessary if the nurse is to be effective in helping the woman in labor. The woman should be encouraged to try any new strategies for several contractions before deciding whether it is helpful. After the same strategies are used for a time, the nurse will know that habituation may be likely, with a resultant increase in pain, and the nursing process begins anew.

PHYSIOLOGICAL BENEFITS

The adequate relief of pain also results in physiological benefits (Table 23-5). The woman who experiences tol-

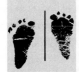

Nursing Care Plan

The Woman in the Process of Aftermath Assimilation of Labor

Patient Goals

1. Woman shares with nurse and others about how she felt when labor became too difficult to handle.
2. Woman understands reasons for increased pain beyond limits to realistically cope.
3. Woman expresses pride at ability to cope as well as she did.

Assessment	Potential Nursing Diagnosis	Nursing Planning/ Assessment	Evaluation
Encourage the woman to talk about all aspects of any discomfort experienced during labor Identify the presence of any feelings of guilt, lack of information, anxiety, or failure	Disturbance in self-concept related to guilt about her perception that she was unable to use breathing methods to handle discomfort during the latter portion of labor	Assist the woman to relive those moments when she felt unable to be effective in using breathing methods Praise her ability to resume use of breathing method after she occasionally failed to use the method Give information about reasons for increased pain at that time Point out positive attitude of others toward her efforts Remind her that she successfully delivered a healthy baby	Woman shares with nurse and others about how hard she worked at breathing methods when pain increased Woman talks less about negative feelings related to handling pain during labor Woman expresses pride in how she handled labor

erable discomforts in labor is able to cooperate with examinations and to work with her contractions. Consequently, she facilitates labor. After childbirth, she is less fatigued.

If she is able to use pain relief measures other than medication, she may eliminate the need for medication or reduce the amount necessary. This is of enormous physiological benefit to the infant because many analgesics and anesthetics, including regional anesthesia, have untoward effects on the fetus, such as respiratory depression and bradycardia, or indirect effects on the fetus, such as increased use of pitocin, forceps, or vacuum. There simply is no drug that has been proven entirely safe for the unborn child.

Pain and stress may cause exaggerated effects on respiration, circulation, endocrine function, and other body functions. A further reason to minimize pain during labor and delivery is to avoid the following specific problems that Bonica believes could occur as a result of severe pain during labor:[39]

- Severe respiratory alkalosis, because the pain of uterine contraction may cause a 5- to 20-fold increase in respirations.
- A 50% to 150% increase in cardiac output and a 20% to 40% increase in blood pressure, because of a significant increase in sympathetic activity and norepinephrine release.
- Significant increase in metabolism and oxygen consumption.
- Decrease in gastrointestinal and urinary bladder motility and, at times, uterine contractility.
- Progressive metabolic acidosis that may be deleterious to mother and fetus, because of increased

TABLE 23-5. BENEFITS OF PAIN CONTROL IN LABOR AND DELIVERY

Physiological Advantages	Emotional Advantages
Woman can cooperate with examinations	Positive experience with a significant step toward parenthood
Woman can work with contractions	Feeling of actual participation in birth of own child with possible increase in self-esteem
Woman is less fatigued after labor and birth	
Successful use of nonpharmacologic pain relief reduces risk to infant	Fostering growth of relationship between parent and child
Complications, such as pain-related decrease in oxygen, can be avoided in the fetus already at risk	Fostering growth of relationship between parents

oxygen consumption, loss of bicarbonate from the kidney as compensation for respiratory alkalosis, and possible reduction in carbohydrate intake.

- Increased risk of aspiration of gastric contents, because of decreased gastrointestinal motility and retention of fluid and food in the stomach.
- An increase in catecholamines.

EMOTIONAL BENEFITS

Identifying whether certain emotional benefits have occurred is another way of evaluating the success of the nurse, woman, and others involved in efforts to provide as much comfort as possible during labor.

Control or relief of pain potentially allows the significant step toward becoming parents to be a positive experience for the mother and father (Table 23-5). Ultimately, one or both parents may be able to witness that moment that remains miraculous and awesome

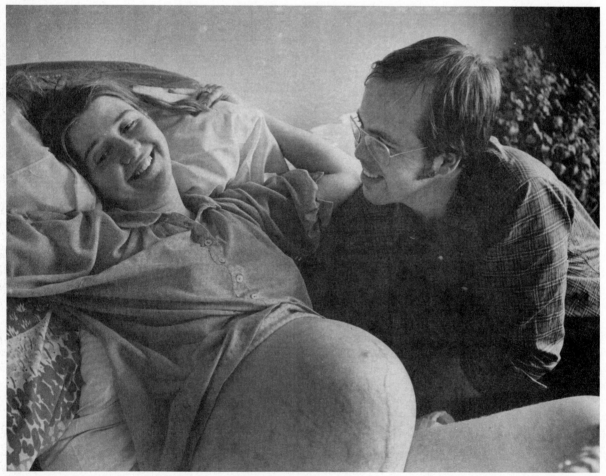

■ *Figure 23-9*
This mother and father work together throughout labor and birth in an alternative birthing center. Such experiences can foster a closer relationship between the parents and contribute significantly to successful parent–infant attachment.

even to many obstetricians: the emergence of a new human being into the world. Even when the parents do not observe the birth, there are other desirable outcomes. If the mother and father can handle the discomforts during childbirth, they can feel they are active participants in the actual birth of their own child. When people jointly plan for an event such as childbirth and are then able to carry through with these plans, the event will probably foster growth in the relationship between them. In the case of childbirth, a satisfying labor experience for both parents probably also fosters their relationship with their baby (Fig. 23-9).

Assisting women in labor to decrease pain by non-pharmacologic means is a real challenge to nurses, one that is all but lost in some clinical areas. It is one that brings special rewards not only for the woman but also to the nurse. There is a special closeness and bond that develop between patient and nurse, and both know the nurse has made a difference. The woman's labor and birth experience is one that can empower her and increase her self-esteem, and it is an event that she will always remember. The significance of the nurse's contribution to these outcomes can hardly be underestimated.

■ REFERENCES

1. Oxorn H: Foote Human Labor and Birth, 5th ed. Norwalk, CT, Appleton-Century-Crofts, 1986
2. Melzack R, Wall PD: Pain mechanisms: A new theory. Science 150:971–979, 1965
3. Melzack R: The Puzzle of Pain, pp 153–190. New York, Basic Books, 1973
4. Nathan PW: The gate-control theory of pain: A critical review. Brain 99:213–258, 1976
5. Wall PD: Modulation of pain by nonpainful events. In Bonica JJ, Albe-Fessard D (eds): Advances in Pain Research and Therapy, Vol 1, pp 1–16. New York, Raven Press, 1976
6. Hilbers S, Gennaro S: Nonpharmacological Pain relief. NAACOG Update Series, Vol 5, Lesson 15. Princeton NJ, Continuing Professional Education Center, 1986
7. Snyder SH: Opiate receptors and internal opiates. Sci Am 236:44–56, March 1977
8. Pittman AW, Rudd GD: Analgesic Therapy, Part 2: Analgesia for Severe Pain. Chapel Hill, NC, Health Sciences Consortium, 1980
9. Terenius L: Endorphins and pain. Front Horm Res 8: 162–177, 1981
10. Newnham J: A study of the relationship between beta-endorphin-like immunoreactivity postpartum blues. Clin Endocrinol 20:169, 1984
11. Kimball C: Do endorphin residues of beta-lipotrophin in hormone reinforce reproductive functions? Am J Obstet Gynecol 134:127, 1979
12. West A: Understanding endorphins: Our natural pain relief system. Nursing 81(11):50–53, February 1981
13. Hummenick S, Bugen L: Mastery: The key to childbirth Satisfaction? A Study. Birth Fam J 8:2, 1981
14. Davenport-Slack B, Boylan C: Psychological correlates of childbirth and Pain. Psychosom Med 36:215, 1974
15. Frank S: The effect of husbands' presence at delivery and childbirth preparation classes on the experience of childbirth (dissertation). Dissert Abstr Int, 1974 34, 6208-B (Univ microfilm No 74-13895). East Lansing, Michigan State University, 1973
16. Wilmuth L: Prepared childbirth and the concept of control. JOGN Nurs 4:38, 1975
17. Doering S, Entwistle D: Preparation during pregnancy and ability to cope with labor and delivery. Am J Orthopsychiatry 45:825, 1975
18. McCaffery M: Nursing Management of the Patient with Pain, 2nd ed. Philadelphia, JB Lippincott, 1979
19. Copp LA: The spectrum of suffering. Am J Nurs 74: 491, March 1974
20. Melzack R: The myth of painless childbirth. Pain 19: 321–337, 1984
21. Melzack R, Taenzer P, Kinch RA: Labor pain: Nature of the experience and the role of prepared childbirth training. Pain (Suppl) 1:S271, 1981
22. Bandler RJ Jr, Madaras GR, Bem DJ: Self-observation as a source of pain perception. J Pers Soc Psychol 9:205–209, July 1968
23. McCaffery M, Beebe A: Pain: Clinical Manual For Nursing Practice. St Louis, CV Mosby, 1989
24. Nichols F, Hummenick S: Childbirth Education: Practice, Research, and Theory. Philadelphia, WB Saunders, 1988
25. Roberts J Mendez-Bauer C Wodell D: The effects of maternal position on uterine contractility and efficiency: Birth 10:243, 1983
26. Diaz AG, Schwarez R, Fescina R, et al: Vertical position during first stage of the course of labor, and neonatal outcome. Eur J Obstet Gynaecol 11:1, 1988
27. Flynn AM, Kelly J, Hollins G, et al: The effect of ambulation in labor uterine action, analgesia and fetal well-being. Gynecol Obstet 512:981, 1980
28. Mendez-Bauer C, Arroyo J, Ramos C, et al: Effects of standing position, spontaneous uterine contractility and other aspects of labor. J Perinat Med 3:89, 1975
29. Lieberman A: Easing Labor Pain. Garden City, NY, Doubleday, 1987
30. Pace JB: Psychophysiology of pain: Diagnostic and therapeutic implications. J Fam Pract 1:4, May 1974
31. Augustinsson L-E, Bohlin P, Bundsen P, et al: Pain relief during delivery by transcutaneous electrical nerve stimulation. Pain 4:59–65, October 1977
32. Tawfik MO, Badraoui MHH: The value of transcutaneous nerve stimulation (TNS) during labour in Egyptian mothers. Pain (Suppl) 1:S146, 1981
33. Piva L: Transcutaneous electrical stimulation as a safe and useful method for pain relief in labour. Pain (Suppl) 1:S142, 1981
34. Augustinsson L: Pain relief during delivery by transcutaneous electrical nerve stimulation. Pain 4:1, 1977
35. Bundsen P, Ericsson K: Pain relief in labor by transcu-

taneous electrical nerve stimulation: Safety aspects. Acta Obstet Gynecol Scand 61:1, 1982

36. Bundsen P: Pain relief in labor by transcutaneous electrical nerve stimulation: A prospective matched study. Acta Obstet Gynecol Scand 60:459, 1981

37. Langendoen S: To expectant fathers: What to do if she panics in labor. Am Baby Mag November, 26, 1978

38. Green J, Coupland V, Kitzinger J, et al: Expectations, experiences, and psychological outcomes of childbirth: A prospective study of 825 women. Birth 17:1, 1990

39. Bonica JJ: Obstetric Analgesia and Anesthesia. Amsterdam, World Federation of Societies of Anaesthesiologists, 1980

■ SUGGESTED READING

Hilbers S, Gennaro S: Nonpharmacological pain relief. NAACOG Update Series, Vol 5, Lesson 15. Princeton, NJ, Continuing Professional Education Center, 1986

Lieberman A: Easing Labor Pain. Garden City, NY, Doubleday, 1987 (This book is also excellent for expectant parents to read)

McCaffery M: Nursing Management of the Patient with Pain, 2nd ed. Philadelphia, JB Lippincott, 1979

McCaffery M: Relieving pain with noninvasive techniques. Nurs 80 10:55–57, December 1980

McCaffery M: When your patient's still in pain don't just do something: Sit there. Nursing 81(11):58–61, June 1981

McCaffery M, Beebe A: Pain: Clinical Manual for Nursing Practice, St Louis, CV Mosby, 1989

Meinhart NT, McCaffery M: Pain: A Nursing Approach to Assessment and Analysis. New York, Appleton-Century-Crofts, 1983

Melzack R: The myth of painless childbirth. Pain 19:321–337, 1984

Nichols FH, Hummenick S: Childbirth Education: Practice, Research, and Theory, Philadelphia, WB Saunders, 1988

Reading AE, Cox DN: Psychosocial predictors of labor pain. Pain 22:309–315, July 1985

The Pregnant Patient's Bill of Rights. Distributed by Committee on Patient's Rights, Box 1900, New York, NY 10001

Wilson RW, Elmassian BJ: Endorphins. Am J Nurs 81:722–725, April 1981

24

Analgesia and Anesthesia During Childbirth

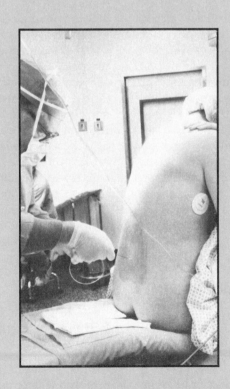

■ THE UNIQUE NATURE OF ANESTHESIA CARE IN OBSTETRICS

The anesthetic care of the obstetric patient potentially involves the most complex and multidimensional challenges afforded the nurse. The challenges are largely predicated on an appreciation of factors that differentiate the parturient from the normal surgical population.

Few other surgical populations require such extensively coordinated, labor-intensive efforts by a broad range of practitioners. That is, the labor and delivery nurse, nurse anesthetist, anesthesiologist, nursery personnel, perinatologist, nurse–midwife, and obstetrician may all be directly involved in patient care activities requiring critical and differentiated skills. Effective communication between practitioners is requisite as are team approaches to planning, decision making, and patient monitoring to ensure optimal care. One must also consider that, unlike the general surgical population, all decision making must take into account the effects nursing interventions will have on both the mother and the fetus. This compels all practitioners to have a detailed understanding of the extensive changes in maternal physiology at term as well as the chronology of fetal development and physiologic modes of adaptation to extrauterine life.

Two other factors remain paramount in our appreciation of the unique requirements of the parturient. First, maternal care usually involves extensive participation of family members throughout the course of labor and delivery. Therefore, each health care team member must be an astute teacher and must be able to direct and support the family member in ways that are productive to the patient and promote a successful course of labor and delivery. In addition, labor and delivery nurses should never fail to appreciate their role as a patient advocate, as many mothers who have not had comprehensive prenatal care and teaching feel inadequate or too uninformed to make competent decisions relative to their personal care or that of their unborn child. Consequently, the nurse acts as a primary source of information and support in the decision-making process about analgesic modalities and communicates those needs and concerns to other providers who will be involved in the woman's care.

Finally, the area of obstetrics continues to be one in which litigation over untoward maternal and fetal outcomes remains high, requiring all providers be highly skilled in areas of decision making, family communication, chart documentation, and risk management techniques.

Considering these several issues that clearly demonstrate that the anesthetic care of obstetric patients in the United States should be equal to none, it is ironic to learn that too often this is not the case. Standards of anesthetic care, although strictly adhered to in many institutions, are often less stringently applied in others. In 1988, the American Society of Anesthesiologists and the American College of Obstetricians and Gynecologists issued a joint set of standards governing the care of the gravid patient.[1] Unfortunately, these standards are, according to most practitioners involved in obstetric care, woefully inadequate in relation to other published standards of anesthesia care for the routine surgical patient. Future refinements in these and other standards of obstetric care should address the potentially critical and comprehensive nature of care required by the mother and infant, including a concerted effort to recruit sufficient numbers of professional personnel to this critical area of health care.

Within the last two decades, there have been significant advances in the field of obstetric anesthesia. These changes are in stark contrast to the practices found in seventeenth and eighteenth century Europe and America where women were strictly prohibited from using any method of pain relief during childbirth. Not until 1853 did John Snow, noted by some as the Father of Anesthesia, afford Queen Victoria chloroform analgesia for the birth of Prince Leopold. Even with this introduction, anesthesia administration was too often provided by the least well-trained participant (with attendant maternal mortality) in the birthing process. In later years, these duties were relegated to medical students or interns to administer while they were learning delivery or surgical techniques from the obstetrician.

Today, many health care facilities offer the full range of analgesic–anesthetic services provided by highly qualified certified registered nurse anesthetists (CRNAs) and physician anesthesiologists. These services range from administration of light sedation and systemic narcotics, usually by the labor and delivery nurse, to regional anesthesia. In particular, continuous lumbar epidural anesthesia has achieved great popularity because it offers the mother a nearly pain-free labor and delivery and minimal transplacental drug effects on the fetus. If general anesthesia is required, particularly in emergency situations, it can be induced rapidly and the patient maintained in light planes of anesthesia until delivery to minimize the deleterious impact of systemic drugs on the fetus.

The Role of the Labor and Delivery Nurse in Anesthesia Care

For many reasons, labor and delivery nurses assume a professional role quite different from their counterpart in any other intensive care setting. Chief among these

Research Highlight

Soluble oral antacids are commonly used before anesthesia for cesarean section. The purpose of this prospective, single-institution, randomized, experimental study was to examine the relationship of oral administration of Bicitra to the incidence of nausea and vomiting in patients undergoing elective cesarean section using regional anesthesia and to evaluate Bicitra's effectiveness in neutralizing gastric acid. Eighty-six patients were studied (39 in a control group and 47 in a Bicitra treatment group) to ascertain if there was any difference in regard to height, weight, parity, gravity, age, race, incidence of heartburn with pregnancy, incidence of nausea with pregnancy, length of NPO status, preoperative systolic blood pressure (SBP), perioperative low level of SBP, and cumulative drop in SBP. Pearson chi square analysis showed no significant difference between the two groups for all variables or the incidence of nausea and vomiting. No significant difference was noted in the mean pH and volume of emesis of seven subjects analyzed using pooled *t* tests. After initial hypothesis testing was concluded, the sample was divided into two groups: those who experienced nausea and those free from nausea. The nausea group demonstrated a significantly greater cumulative decrease in SBP than the non-nausea group. Larger patients (mean cube root weight index of 2.78) tended to become nauseated more frequently.

(Palmer AW, Waugaman WR, Conklin KA, Kotelko DM: Does the administration of oral Bicitra® prior to elective cesarean section affect the incidence of nausea and vomiting in the parturient? Nurse Anesthesia, 2: September 1991)

reasons is that much of the nursing care provided during the course of labor and delivery will be coincident to the administration of analgesic or anesthetic therapies. Consequently, the labor and delivery nurse must plan and implement most of the patient care activities that incorporate a clear understanding of pain management techniques, including anatomical and physiological mechanisms of pain, techniques of pain relief, drug administration, management of complications, patient monitoring, and standards of anesthetic care.

Because nurses may be the single provider who is in constant attendance with the patient, they will necessarily become the one clinician who is most familiar with assessing the patient's need for pain relief, assessing levels of pain tolerance, observing the patient's methods of adaptation or accommodation of painful stimuli, and monitoring the general course of labor as

it relates to anesthetic interventions. These are all factors of paramount importance to the anesthesia provider when selecting, administering, managing, and assessing the effectiveness of anesthetic interventions.

There have been some reports that some types of obstetric anesthesia can actually benefit the fetus.[2] Numerous animal studies as well as studies of women in labor indicate that lumbar epidural analgesia actually decreases plasma catecholamines and, therefore, improves uterine blood flow.[2,3] Skillful obstetric anesthesia, including psychological and emotional support of the mother, may make birth less stressful not only for her but for her baby as well.[4] There are a variety of anesthetic techniques and services available to the patient. Clearly, when the mother can make an informed decision regarding choice of anesthesia and feels comfortable with that decision, her overall birth experience can be enhanced.

■ ANALGESIA FOR LABOR AND VAGINAL DELIVERY

Techniques of Analgesia–Anesthesia

The mother has a variety of options available when selecting the particular type of analgesic support best suited for her labor and delivery. Some of these techniques do not involve pharmacologic intervention; however, the nurse should make clear to the patient that no particular preference is irrevocable. Many mothers may choose to use methods of natural childbirth, Lamaze, Bradley, or other psychophysiological support techniques for the duration of their labor and delivery (see Chaps. 17 and 23). Patients, however, should also clearly understand that their decision to change from these techniques to more direct means of pharmacologic intervention will be respected and supported. Many mothers, for instance, will accept minimal doses of intramuscular (IM) or intravenous (IV) narcotics during labor; however, as cervical dilation proceeds, they often request placement of a lumbar epidural catheter for more complete pain relief. It should also be stressed that, barring a strict contraindication to a particular drug or technique, the choice should remain ultimately an independent one made by the mother in consultation with the anesthesia provider. Although the wishes of the husband may be considered, it is not appropriate for him or other family members to dictate to the mother the type or extent of analgesia–anesthesia required or sought.

There are four general categories under which most techniques of analgesia–anesthesia fall: (1) systemic medications using narcotics, sedatives, and tranquilizers, either by IV or IM routes; (2) inhalation anesthetics using subanesthetic concentrations of drugs; (3) regional anesthesia using continuous lumbar epidural analgesia–anesthesia, spinal anesthesia, sacral epidural anesthesia (caudal), or obstetrician-administered paracervical or pudendal block; and (4) general anesthesia.

Characteristics of Analgesic–Anesthetic Techniques

Before proceeding further, some attempt at definitions should be made relative to the terms *analgesia* and *anesthesia*. This is an admittedly difficult distinction, as analgesia and anesthesia are considered to represent two distinct poles of a continuum. Consequently, establishing a distinct demarcation between the two is difficult at best. Most anesthesia practitioners generally accept the notion that analgesia (usually administered IV or IM) represents a mild to moderate attenuation or obtundation of central nervous system function, thereby rendering the patient conscious but sedated and experiencing a decreased level of pain. Lack of sensory perception of pain may also be achieved with epidural analgesia. Vital organ functions, such as ventilation, are not usually compromised, and protective airway reflexes remain intact. Patients should otherwise be able to respond to verbal command and have full, purposeful motor function.

Anesthesia describes a total loss of sensory capability, whether imposed regionally to the pelvic area via epidural anesthesia or centrally to the brain as in a general anesthesia, where consciousness is lost. Anesthesia usually implies that one or more vital organ functions are under partial or total control of the anesthesia provider, thus temporarily lost to the patient. It becomes obvious then, that analgesic techniques can rapidly and unexpectedly progress to an anesthetic state, such as in the case of inadvertent overdose or miscalculation of the mother's level of drug tolerance. In addition, it is well documented that the gravid patient will require less medication than the nongravid patient to achieve a similar therapeutic effect.[5] Consequently, it is required that the nurse be prepared to sustain vital functions of the mother or fetus should patients progress through planes of analgesia to anesthesia. All regional block or conduction techniques will be discussed under the category of anesthesia, although some would consider regional block an analgesic technique.

Selection of an Anesthetic

Several factors should be considered in planning and selecting the anesthetic for labor and delivery. Ideally, this process should begin early in the prenatal period, with information usually introduced by the obstetrician or office nurse or through prenatal classes conducted by qualified personnel. Obviously, these professionals must be well versed on all possible techniques and be able to provide answers to patient questions capably. They should also be able to provide other resources, such as prepared reading material outlining the variety of anesthetic options or early referrals to professional anesthesia providers. Too often, patients receive incomplete or inaccurate information that promotes certain unfounded biases or predispositions toward certain anesthetic techniques, which may not be in the best interest of the mother or fetus. For instance, patients may often say "I'm afraid of a needle in my back. It may paralyze me." Unfortunately, in this instance, the patient may not have received sufficient information to make an informed decision concerning regional anesthesia, including the relative risks of the technique, the benefits of allowing more maternal participation in the delivery by avoiding systemic medications, and the level of profound pain relief to the mother and avoidance of depressant medication on the fetus.

Once the patient is admitted to the labor and delivery suite, the CRNA or physician anesthesiologist should perform a history and physical and interview the patient personally to assist her in determining which type of anesthetic is best suited to her needs as well as those of the infant. Even in the event a mother should choose not to use any type of analgesic or anesthetic for delivery, she should nevertheless be interviewed by a qualified anesthesia provider early in the labor process in case circumstances arise that require immediate anesthetic intervention on behalf of the patient or fetus. Consent forms for anesthesia should be signed by the patient at the time of interview that delineate the type of anesthesia selected and alternative plans in case of emergency. An ideal analgesic or anesthetic experience should be tailored to the individual patient, one based on her personal physical and surgical history, prenatal course, and personal preferences. Although there is no single modality of pain relief that encompasses all desired outcomes, the following objectives should be kept in mind when helping a patient select an anesthetic:

- The mother should never be coerced into accepting an anesthetic technique promoted only by the preferences or biases of the nurse, obstetrician, or anesthesia provider.
- The anesthetic should provide satisfactory pain relief for the mother that will maximize her active participation and satisfaction with the process of labor and delivery.
- The anesthetic technique should be one that promotes patient safety, does not unduly interfere with the normal progression of labor and deliv-

ery, and provides optimal surgical or delivery conditions.

- The anesthetic should not be associated with undue risks to the mother or excessively depressant effects on the infant.
- The anesthetic should allow sufficient flexibility so that if emergent measures are required to deliver the infant, induction can proceed smoothly with minimal time delays. The mother should always be informed of any alternative plans for anesthesia should they become necessary as a result of unexpected complications.

Nursing Considerations

The nurse plays an important role in the selection of anesthesia and preparation of the patient for delivery. The nurse should be conversant with the range of anesthesia services available and provide informed counsel to the patient. The nurse should also appreciate the fact that pregnancy alters the normal physiological state of patients and often exacerbates many preexisting diseases such that the patient's normal homeostatic mechanisms or organ systems may be significantly compromised. Although parturients are usually healthy young adults, and birth usually is a normal physiological function, these patients can be at risk for complications during labor and delivery. If such complications arise, swift and deliberate nursing and medical interventions are required. The nurse must be knowledgeable of and prepared for such complications should the need arise.

■ SYSTEMIC MEDICATIONS FOR ANALGESIA

Systemic medications are most often used to attenuate pain and allay anxiety in the first stage of labor. In many instances, these drugs are the only pharmacologic intervention required by mothers to afford adequate pain relief during the course of labor, especially when supplemented with paracervical or pudendal blocks administered close to or immediately prior to delivery. Systemic drugs are most often administered either by IV or IM routes. Brief mention will be made, however, regarding analgesic techniques involving the use of nitrous oxide via inhalation, usually reserved for administration in the delivery suite.

The goal of systemic pain medication is to provide maximum pain relief to the parturient while minimizing depressive effects on the fetus and uterine function. At the least, systemic medications have been found par-

ticularly useful in helping the mother relax sufficiently to regain control of breathing techniques and allow labor to proceed expeditiously. Titrated doses of systemic narcotics, for instance, are usually well tolerated by the mother and have little deleterious effect on the fetus.

Systemic medications are also of benefit in maintaining greater maternal physiological homeostasis during labor. Endogenous catecholamines, such as epinephrine and norepinephrine, are elevated during labor and delivery, largely from the body's response to pain. These high levels of circulating catecholamines can cause uterine artery vasoconstriction and resultant decreases in uterine blood flow. Catecholamines are also known to contribute to maternal metabolic acidosis. This acid–base derangement may cause a shift of the oxygen dissociation curve, which inhibits the release of oxygen from hemoglobin, thus generally decreasing oxygen availability to the fetus. Narcotic use can effectively decrease these stress responses and return the patient to a state of normoventilation, thus obviating conditions that may compromise perfusion and oxygenation of the fetus.

Narcotics: Agents and Indications

Opioids remain the most commonly used and effective analgesic agents for the parturient. Although these drugs will effect the mother and fetus equally in terms of respiratory depression and sedation, none has been shown to have significant fetal effects as demonstrated by neurobehavioral studies or long-term effects on intelligence or subsequent infant development. Opioids, however, cross the placenta rapidly and may be accountable for temporary postnatal ventilatory depression. It becomes important, therefore, when administering these drugs, to take into account the last drug injection-to-delivery interval to avoid excessive neonatal depression from delivery that coincides with the drug's peak effect.

Meperidine remains the most popular of this drug class as it has dependable effects and less ventilatory depression than morphine. Meperidine is usually titrated IV in doses not to exceed 25 mg, which can be repeated in smaller increments to achieve the desired level of analgesia. The drug can also be administered IM in somewhat higher doses; however, the rate of uptake is much less dependable and onset is slower. Meperidine can precipitate maternal nausea and vomiting and cause decreases in fetal beat-to-beat variability as well as tachycardia. Morphine may cause significant ventilatory depression attributable to the drug's long half-life and, consequently, is not often used in the laboring mother. Morphine, when given IV, is usually administered in doses of 1 to 2 mg titrated over several minutes. IM doses of morphine are usually 5 to 10 mg. Onset of action of morphine IV occurs within 2 to 3 minutes and will last for several hours, depending on the total dose administered and intensity of the contractions.

Other shorter acting synthetic narcotics are now being used to a greater extent in those circumstances requiring short but intensive pain relief. Fentanyl and sufentanil can be used successfully when uterine manipulation by the surgeon is required to correct fetal presentation or when a forceps delivery is anticipated. Fentanyl is equianalgesic to morphine in the ratio of 100 μg:10 mg, respectively.[6] The duration of effect of IV doses of fentanyl is 30 to 60 minutes. Both of these drugs should be used with extreme caution and by qualified providers when in the delivery suite, as their potency is quite high. Fentanyl, in small doses, can also be used by the nurse for the laboring mother when relief is required for severe pain. The dose is 25 to 50 μg IV and can be repeated once. Again, extreme caution should be used to assess maternal ventilation and fetal well-being when this drug is used. In exchange for the benefits of high potency, the nurse must be ever vigilant for respiratory depression. Fentanyl usually does not result in significant cardiovascular depression. Butorphanol (Stadol) and nalbuphine (Nubain), both agonist–antagonist non-narcotic analgesics, have also been used for labor because in theory they maintain their analgesic effect yet demonstrate less ventilatory depression than the more traditional narcotics. The IV dose of butorphanol is 0.5 to 1 mg given in titrated doses, and IM is 2 mg every 4 hours. Nalbuphine doses are 3 to 5 mg IV or 10 to 20 mg IM.

NURSING IMPLICATIONS

Generally speaking, the judicious use of narcotics both in the first and early second stage of labor can be safe with minimal side effects to the mother or fetus. When administering these drugs by IV routes, the nurse should be in constant attendance with the mother to assess ventilatory and cardiovascular effects. The patient's blood pressure, pulse, and ventilatory rate should be taken every 5 minutes during titration and for 15 to 20 minutes (up to 1 hour) after administration to determine general patient stability. When maternal pain has subsided after drug administration, hypotension and hypercarbia can readily occur as endogenous catecholamines subside and the drug induces some element of direct myocardial depression as well as decreases in peripheral vascular resistance and dilation of capacitance vasculature. In addition, electronic fetal monitoring should always be used during drug administration to observe any changes in fetal heart rate, pattern, or variability.

If required, reversal of the effects of all narcotic analgesics it can be accomplished with maternal administration of naloxone in incremental doses of 0.1 to 0.4 mg IV or 0.2 to 0.4 mg IM. Infant doses should be initiated at 0.01 mg/kg.[4] One should not attempt to reverse narcotic effects in the mother immediately prior to delivery, unless absolutely necessary, as antagonism is quick and complete. Reversal will increase maternal pain and the risk for nausea and vomiting if other forms of pain relief, such as local anesthetics via infiltration or epidural, are not instituted prior to narcotic reversal. Extreme caution should be exercised in the use of reversal agents in mothers who have a documented history of drug abuse and/or methadone therapy as symptoms of withdrawal are likely to ensue in both the mother and fetus. These same precautions should be applied to the use of the agonist–antagonist drugs.

Sedatives and Tranquilizers: Agents and Indications

Medications within the sedative and tranquilizer classifications are most often used for their anxiolytic properties, potentiation of narcotics, and promotion of sleep, especially when parturients experience protracted initial stages of labor. They are also quite effective in attenuating nausea and vomiting common during this period. Drugs in common use are the benzodiazepines, phenothiazine derivatives, hydroxyzine, buterophenones and, to a lesser extent, barbiturates.

BENZODIAZEPINES

The benzodiazepines such as diazepam and midazolam can reduce maternal anxiety and narcotic requirements without prolonging labor. In doses exceeding 30 mg over the course of labor, however, fetal hypotonia, lethargy, hypothermia, and feeding problems may result.[6] Benzodiazepines can exacerbate respiratory depression when given in combination with narcotics; consequently, drugs within this classification are used minimally, as narcotics remain the agents of choice, even for properties of mild sedation. Administration of diazepam by IV bolus is largely reserved to treat convulsive disorders associated with eclampsia. However, doses of diazepam not to exceed 5 to 10 mg IV or midazolam 2 to 3 mg IV may be helpful in decreasing maternal anxiety and aiding progression of labor.[6] Midazolam, however, may be the preferred drug because it causes less venous irritation after IV administration than diazepam. Fetal drug effects generally manifest with decreases in beat-to-beat variability; however, neonatal acid–base balance is not affected.

PHENOTHIAZINES AND HYDROXYZINE

All drugs in this category act similarly to allay anxiety, promote relaxation, control emesis, and prolong narcotic effect. Promethazine (Phenergan) and prochlorperazine (Compazine) are the most commonly used of these drugs, especially for their antiemetic properties. Prochlorperazine has been reported to produce hypotension by blockade of alpha receptors.[6] These drugs are normally given in conjunction with small doses of narcotics, because in the presence of pain not otherwise controlled with analgesics, some patients exhibit confusion and delirium, making control of labor much more problematic. Hydroxyzine (Vistaril), a minor tranquilizer, is frequently used in conjunction with IM narcotics to reduce the narcotic requirement. It also exhibits potent antihistaminic and antiemetic effects.

BUTEROPHENONES

The prototype of the buterophenone group is droperidol, a long-acting major tranquilizer. In normal sedative doses of 2.5 to 5 mg IV, its use is often reserved for the operating room suite as an adjunct to anesthesia to provide profound amnesia and postoperative sedation. During labor it can be used in small, single doses of 0.625 mg IV to ablate nausea and vomiting. Higher doses should be avoided as they will lead to a significant alpha-receptor blockade producing hypotension.

KETAMINE

Ketamine is a dissociative anesthetic agent that should be used only in the operating room or where there is capability of mechanical support of ventilation. Ketamine, although used primarily as an induction agent for general anesthesia, can be used in low doses as an analgesic adjunct in special circumstances, such as retained placenta or protracted repairs of cervical or vaginal tears subsequent to delivery of a large infant or trauma due to malpresentation. Other indications include use during a difficult low or midforceps delivery when substantial pain relief is required. In a forceps delivery, ketamine may have to be supplemented by a pudendal block as this drug does not block visceral pain. Ketamine can be used on these occasions in doses of 10 mg to a total dose of 20 to 30 mg, which permits the patient to remain conscious and in control of her breathing and other reflexes.[7]

Ketamine will cause some patients to become dysphoric and hallucinatory, requiring postoperative recovery in a quiet surrounding devoid of extraneous auditory and visual stimulation. Consequent with induction, the administration of 1 to 2 mg of diazepam or midazolam usually limits these unpleasant episodes or eliminates their occurrence entirely.[5] In addition, ketamine is a powerful amnestic agent that may have the undesirable side effect of memory loss for the mother for part or all of the labor and delivery process.

NURSING IMPLICATIONS

The primary untoward effect of sedative medication is lack of diligent titration of the drug and subsequent overdose. Some mothers may also exhibit dysphoria as an idiosyncratic reaction to the drug and become confused or agitated. Many of these drugs can cause temporary amnesia if doses are too high, and the mother will be unable to cooperate or manage her breathing techniques or pushing, when required. The normal progress of labor may also be slowed if doses are too high.

Equal caution should be given to the administration of sedative hypnotics or tranquilizers as are given for narcotics. The nurse should be in constant attendance during drug administration and record vital signs every 5 minutes during IV drug titration. It should also be recognized that many of these drugs have a synergistic effect with narcotics, and respiratory depression can be compounded if the mother has recently received narcotics. In this instance, it is also likely that the patient may experience significant decreases in blood pressure. Every attempt should be made to keep maternal systolic blood pressure above 100 mmHg, as below that point fetal perfusion may be compromised. This critical perfusion pressure assumes that the mother is healthy and does not suffer from chronic hypertension or eclampsia, in which case the critical systolic pressures for perfusion would naturally be higher. As a general rule, blood pressure should not decrease for any significant time 20% below the mother's normal, resting blood pressure. In the case when sustained hypotension occurs, the nurse may consider increasing IV infusion rates, placing the patient in a head-down, left-lateral position and administering oxygen. If hypotension does not resolve, pharmacologic intervention may be required, such as ephedrine in an initial IV dose of 5 to 10 mg.

Maternal overdose with systemic medications is possible as parturients have been found to require less drug on a per weight basis than the nonpregnant patient. IV drugs should always be titrated slowly to effect, that is, administer only what is required by the mother for ablation of her discomfort or to afford sedation. As most drugs can be identified in colostrum (albeit in very small quantities) for up to 14 days after administration, this may have some relevance for nursing mothers; however, such effects appear to have minimal clinical relevance.

A list of potential maternal and fetal effects secondary to the administration of systemic medications is provided below that may require vigilant nursing assessment and possible interventions. Major complications however, depend largely on the degree to which fetal perfusion and maternal ventilation are compromised. The following actions screen for the potential effects:

- Monitor for loss of fetal variability and arrhythmias, most commonly atrial in origin.

- Monitor for respiratory depression of neonate at birth if peak or cumulative effect of drug is coincidence with delivery.
- Monitor maternal nausea and vomiting.
- Monitor fetal hypotonus at delivery.
- Monitor maternal hypoventilation and hypotension.
- Monitor for urinary retention from narcotics.

Inhalation Analgesia: Agents and Indications

The inhalation method of analgesia for the parturient is becoming less frequently used primarily because it has been supplanted by the increased acceptance and popularity of regional techniques. For those patients who are fearful of needles or complications attendant to blocks or who arrive at the hospital with delivery eminent, inhalation anesthesia may still find some use. It is often used as a supplement to other analgesic techniques, particularly regional anesthesia when the block is incomplete or waning. Most inhalation anesthetics can be administered at an analgesic concentration (subanesthetic concentration) sufficient to allow adequate pain relief, yet the mother remains conscious during birth and can take directions from her coach or delivery room personnel.

Nitrous oxide (N_2O) is perhaps the most widely used inhalation agent for analgesia in obstetrics. It is administered during delivery from the anesthetic machine breathing circuit usually on an intermittent basis coincident to the peak of contractions. It can also be used effectively during manual extraction of a placenta or minor repairs of the vagina or cervix or as an adjunct to pudendal block for episiotomy repair. Concentrations of the drug, usually between 30% and 50%, are adjusted according to the patient's need, state of consciousness, and ability to push. N_2O has little deleterious effect on the fetus as the drug is cleared from maternal circulation via the pulmonary system rapidly. Other techniques of inhalation analgesia for childbirth include the combination of N_2O and subanesthetic concentrations of potent inhalation agents, such as enflurane and isoflurane. Analgesic concentrations of inhalation agents are usually relatively benign to the fetus and only cause transient depression after protracted maternal administration.

NURSING IMPLICATIONS

For decades patients have chosen to use inhalation analgesia for childbirth as testament to its ease of application, low cost, reasonable effectiveness, and minimal complications. The primary problems of this technique of anesthetic delivery are those associated with depressant effects exerted on maternal airway reflexes, predisposing the patient to vomiting and aspiration of gastric contents, loss of ability to swallow and ventilatory depression. Loss of airway reflexes mandates endotracheal intubation of the patient and possible decompression of the stomach via nasogastric tube. Caution should always be employed in the use of these agents, as loss of airway reflexes prior to establishment of airway patency could portend disaster. All inhalation agents should be administered by clinicians certified or licensed to practice anesthesia.

■ ANESTHESIA FOR LABOR AND VAGINAL DELIVERY

Regional Blockade: Characteristics and Indications

Regional blocks for laboring mothers now enjoy increasing popularity as the preferred form of pain relief for both labor and vaginal delivery. Use of this technique allows the patient to be fully awake and to participate in all facets of the birthing process. Additionally, this technique is not usually associated with the depressive effects of systemic agents, consequently allowing the mother and infant to proceed immediately with the bonding process and initial trials at breast feeding. When properly administered, regional epidural techniques provide a favorable physiological environment for the fetus as drug uptake is minimal or of short duration and effect.

Epidural analgesia does not impede the normal progression of labor or the mother's ability to push the infant down the birth canal. Pelvic muscle tone is sustained so that rotation of the fetal head is possible. Because the patient is awake, there is no concern for potential airway reflex obtundation, which predisposes the mother to gastric aspiration. It may also be a preferred technique for those patients with severe preexisting cardiac or pulmonary disease such as asthma, when a general anesthetic would more likely compromise the preexisting condition. Perhaps the most compelling argument for the selection of regional anesthesia is that the quality of the block can afford near-complete pain relief in selected areas of the body yet not normally interfere with motor function unless an intrathecal (spinal) anesthetic is used (Fig. 24-1). This is in sharp contrast to systemic analgesic methods that, although effective, provide pain relief by altering the perception patients have of pain to a more accommodating level of tolerance.

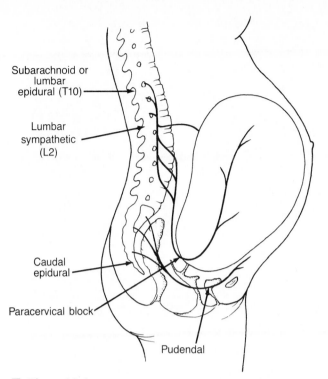

Subarachnoid or
lumbar
epidural (T10)

Lumbar
sympathetic
(L2)

Caudal
epidural

Paracervical block

Pudendal

■ *Figure 24-1*
Pain pathways during labor and techniques of nerve block.

The most prevalent techniques of regional anesthesia include lumbar epidural blocks, spinal, caudal, pudendal, paracervical, and local infiltration of the perineum. Regardless of the type of regional technique selected, the nurse should have available all requisite equipment required to treat respiratory or cardiovascular complications, including airways, endotracheal tubes, laryngoscope, an oxygen source, capability of positive-pressure ventilation, and medications to treat arrhythmias and hypotension. In spite of the benefits of regional blockade, there are some contraindications to the technique, including refusal by the mother, coagulation defects, previous spinal injuries resulting in chronic back pain, skin lesions at the site of needle entry, possibly previous surgery for back injuries that has altered normal spinal anatomy, or morbid obesity, which may present formidable logistic obstacles in block placement.

LUMBAR EPIDURAL ANESTHESIA

After appropriate patient teaching, signing procedure consent forms, and insertion of an IV infusion line, administration of the epidural can proceed when effective labor is established and the cervix is 5 to 6 cm dilated in the primigravida.[6] The catheter can be placed earlier and a dose of local anesthetic administered if the mother is multiparous, not tolerating labor well, or an oxytocin drip has been instituted. The patient should have received 500 to 1000 ml of a crystalloid solution prior to

the injection of the drug into the epidural space to attenuate hypotensive episodes secondary to sympathetic blockade.

The primary objective of this technique is to place a volume of local anesthetic into the epidural space that, through diffusion to surrounding nerve fibers, temporarily interrupts normal transmission of pain impulses from the pelvic area and provides an anesthetized state for those dermatome areas preselected to block (Fig. 24-2). In carefully titrated doses, the patient's motor function is usually uninterrupted, but sensory block is complete.

The epidural space is termed a *potential space*. It is normally filled with segments of nerve roots from the spinal cord, fatty tissue, and an intricate networking of blood vessels. It is surrounded by a series of protective and supportive ligaments as well as the bony vertebral column. The space also serves as an outer covering to the several layers of dura, spinal fluid, and cord (Fig. 24-3).

Under sterile technique, the patient is placed in a sitting or lateral decubitus position with knees tucked to best expose the vertebrae to the anesthetist. After infiltration of local anesthetic between the L3–4, or L4–5 vertebral interspaces, the needle is placed in the epidural space by using a loss of resistance or a hanging-drop technique (Fig. 24-4). A small amount of air or sterile water is injected to widen the epidural space, and the needle is aspirated to ensure that its placement is not in an epidural vein. One or more test doses of local anesthetic containing minute doses of epinephrine is injected into the space, again to confirm that the needle is not in a vein or that the dura has not been inadvertently punctured.

After confirmation of correct placement has been achieved, the epidural catheter is guided through the needle to be left in the space and the needle pulled out over the catheter. The catheter is then protectively padded with sponge at the site of entry and is taped to the mother's back and brought over her shoulder for easy accessibility of the injection port. The patient reassumes a supine position with her head up slightly. Subsequent doses of local anesthetics can be administered as boluses through the catheter or connected to continuous infusion pumps to maintain a steady state of drug in the plasma, allowing lower concentrations of drug to be used.

The objective of incremental dosing is to achieve a sensory block to a level of approximately T10 for the first stages of labor, eliminating pain of uterine contractions and dilation of the cervix. This would involve blockade of the T10, T11, T12, and L1 segments. During the second stage, the level of block can be elevated to alleviate pain from perineal stretching by blocking pudendal nerves at the S2, S3, and S4 segments. Dosing can also be augmented to accommodate cesarean section

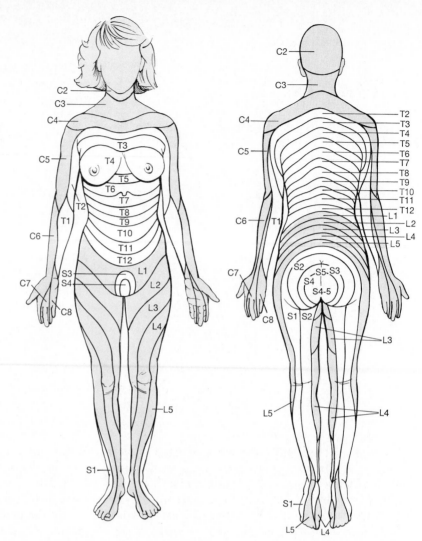

■ Figure 24-2
Dermatome levels. (Cousins MJ, Bromage PR: Epidural neural blockade. In Cousins MJ, Bridenbaugh PO (eds): Neural Blockade in Clinical Anesthesia and Management of Pain, 2nd ed, p 344. Philadelphia, JB Lippincott, 1988)

when the level of block reaches T4. Thus, in an emergency situation, the epidural can still be used when "top off" doses of short-acting local anesthetics, such as 2-chloroprocaine or lidocaine, are administered in a timely manner. The most commonly used local anesthetics for

epidural anesthesia are lidocaine 1% to 1.5%, bupivacaine 0.25% to 0.5%, and chloroprocaine 2% to 3% (Table 24-1).

More recently, the addition of small amounts of synthetic narcotics, such as fentanyl and butorphanol,

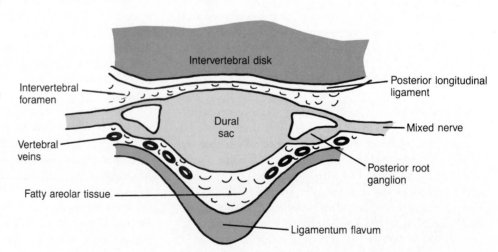

■ Figure 24-3
Diagrammatic cross section of the vertebral canal showing the contents of the epidural space. Note the prominent epidural veins. Local anesthetic injected into the epidural space primarily blocks conduction of nerve roots as they traverse the epidural space.

LUMBAR EPIDURAL

(a) Midline   (b) Paraspinous

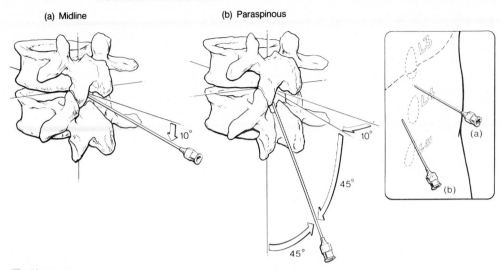

■ *Figure 24-4*
Epidural needle placement. (Cousins MJ, Bromage PR: Epidural neural blockade. In Cousins MJ, Bridenbaugh PO (eds): Neural Blockade in Clinical Anesthesia and Management of Pain, 2nd ed, p 323. Philadelphia, JB Lippincott, 1988

which significantly decrease required doses of local anesthetics, has been incorporated into practice.[4,6] Analgesia produced by narcotics, such as fentanyl and morphine, epidurally and intrathecally, are segmental and effective for visceral pain but not usually effective for severe surgical or somatic pain, especially when used as the sole agent, without accompaniment of local anesthetics. Administration of epidural and intrathecal narcotics is becoming more widely employed in spite of the relatively high incidence of pruritus and incidental nausea and vomiting, both of which can be attenuated with a partial or total reversal of the narcotic with bolus or drip reversal agents, such as naloxone. These symptoms can also be treated with diphenhydramine and appropriate antiemetics such as droperidol if reversal of analgesia is not desired.

SPINAL BLOCKADE

Subarachnoid blockade (spinal anesthesia) is used predominately for cesarean section when an epidural technique is not otherwise employed. Because onset of the block takes only a few minutes and affects sensory as well as motor function, spinal anesthesia is not a viable option for labor. It is technically easier and in some hands quicker to administer than an epidural. Dosing requires 20% of the local anesthetic one would expect to administer for an epidural, and anesthetic toxicity is normally not a problem. Selective spinal blockade, such as a saddle block, can be used for a forceps delivery or repair of an extensive episiotomy when spinal segments S1 through S5 are blocked. A spinal block, appropriate for a cesarean section, can be achieved when a level of

T4 is achieved, although it has the disadvantage of allowing only a single dose as there is no catheter (as with the epidural) that would allow redosing should initial levels be inadequate for surgical anesthesia.

The technique for administration of a spinal block is virtually the same as for epidural, except that the dura is purposefully entered and local anesthetic injected directly into the spinal fluid. Injection of drugs for both spinal and epidural should not take place during uterine contractions as the level of the block may be pushed to unacceptably high levels. Lidocaine and tetracaine are the predominate local anesthetic agents used for spinals, with effective anesthetic durations of 1 and 3 hours, respectively. In spinal anesthesia, 2-chloroprocaine is contraindicated because of its reported incidence of neurotoxic effects.

PUDENDAL AND PARACERVICAL BLOCK

The paracervical block is most often administered by the obstetrician during the first stage of labor (Fig. 24-5). It is accomplished transvaginally and requires only 1 to 2 minutes to execute. Administration of the block involves a submucosal injection of local anesthetic near uterine nerve fibers, at the vaginal fornix lateral to the cervix. It most often obliterates visceral pain from the uterus, cervix, and upper vagina. Neither hypotension nor loss of urge to push results. The block is somewhat less popular today than in the past as it has been associated with fetal distress in about 10% to 40% of cases and poor neonatal outcome.[7] Most assume that fetal effects result from the high concentration of local anesthetics in fetal blood or decreased uterine blood flow

TABLE 24–1. LOCAL ANESTHETICS COMMONLY USED IN OBSTETRICS

Local Anesthetic and Trade Name	Characteristics	Maximum Safe Initial Dose (mg)		Epidural	
		Without Epinephrine	*With Epinephrine*	*Dose* Vaginal Delivery*	*Dose* Cesarean Section*
2 chloroprocaine (Nesacaine)	Very low toxicity, most rapidly metabolized with little accumulation, rapid onset but poor spread	600	1000	1–2% 8–12 ml	3% 15–25 ml
Tetracine (Pontocaine)	5 times toxicity but 10 times potency of procaine. Today used only for spinal and topical. Poor spread, very slow onset	100	200	Not available	
Lidocaine (Xylocaine)	Most versatile local anesthetic, moderate toxicity, rapid onset, moderate duration, excellent spread	300	500	1–1½% 8–12 ml	1½–2% 15–25 ml
Bupivacaine (Marcaine, Sensorcaine)	Slow onset, long duration, marked cardiac toxicity, low concentrations give excellent sensory and little motor block; ideal for obstetrics	175	225	⅛–½% 8–12 ml	½% 20–25 ml

* Doses are given as suggested concentration and milliliters required.
† Lower dose represents minimum duration without epinephrine; upper dose represents maximum duration using epinephrine.
‡ All solutions described have a higher specific gravity than cerebrospinal fluid, because they are weighted with local anesthetic and dextrose.
§ Given as concentration of solution and milligrams of local anesthetic used. Note the low dose of local anesthetic required for subarachnoid block as compared with epidural block.
∥ Addition of epinephrine to subarachnoid bupivacaine does not significantly prolong the duration of block.

secondary to local-anesthetic–mediated uterine vasoconstriction. All anesthetics except bupivacaine are appropriate.

The pudendal nerve block involves interruption of sacral nerve transmission that supplies the vaginal vault, perineum, and rectum (Fig. 24-6). Local anesthetic, usually 10 ml of 1% lidocaine, is administered transvaginally behind each sacrospinous ligament.[6] The block is administered immediately prior to delivery and is ideal for episiotomy repair or to facilitate a forceps delivery.

Complications of Regional Blockade

MATERNAL HYPOTENSION

Hypotension is still the most frequently encountered complication of regional blockade consequent to a sympathetic block that may transiently diminish vasomotor tone. Many factors influence the extent to which systemic blood pressure is compromised, including the current state of maternal hydration, level of the block achieved, and whether epinephrine is used in the anesthetic solution. Prophylactic measures should always be instituted prior to administration of the block to attenuate severe hypotensive episodes. These maneuvers include administration of 1000 to 1500 ml of a balanced salt solution 30 minutes prior to block to supplement vascular volume and left uterine displacement, and some suggest preemptory treatment with IM ephedrine for its predominate beta-agonist effects (Fig. 24-7). Transient maternal hypotension is usually without severe fetal effects if corrected within several minutes. If hypotension is protracted, incremental doses of 5 to 10 mg of ephedrine should be administered IV and further uterine displacement attempted. Drugs such as meth-

| Block | Bilateral Pudendal Block | | Hyperbaric Subarachnoid (Spinal)‡ | | | Comments |
| | | | Dose§ | | | |
Duration† (min)	Dose*	Duration† (min)	Vaginal Delivery	Cesarean Section	Duration‡ (min)	
30–60	1–2% 10–20 ml	30–60	Not available			Large inadvertent subarachnoid injection associated with neurologic residual. Its rapid onset and metabolism make it an ideal drug for epidural in the obstetric client. Extremely low maternal and fetal toxicity
	Not available		0.2–0.5% 3–6 mg	0.3–0.5% 6–10 mg	120–200	In past was used for epidural and local infiltration, but has been replaced by others owing to poor spread and slow onset. Now manufactured only for subarachnoid block
60–90	1% 10–20 ml	60–90	1.5% or 5% 15–50 mg	5% 60–90 mg	60–120	Epidural use in past was thought to be associated with depressed neonatal muscle tone. Recent studies question this.
90–180	¼% 10–20 ml	180–720	0.75% 4–6 mg	0.75% 7–12 mg	100–150‖	Inadvertent intravascular injection associated with cardiovascular collapse

oxamine and phenylephrine should be avoided as their vasoconstrictive (predominate alpha) effects on the uterine artery will likely compromise placental and fetal circulation. In severe cases of hypotension, the mother should be placed in Trendelenburg position and an additional peripheral IV placed if necessary to infuse crystalloid or colloid solutions rapidly.

SPINAL HEADACHE

The malady of postspinal headache is not uncommon in the obstetric population, especially in those patients who have sustained an inadvertent puncture of the dura mater while an epidural catheter was being placed. Leakage of cerebral spinal fluid out of the spinal canal allows the brain stem to impinge on the cranial foramen, resulting in mild to incapacitating headaches. The incidence of headache occurs within 24 to 72 hours after delivery. It is dependent on the gauge of the needle used and the subsequent size of the dural tear. It has

been reported that the incidence is 2% when a 25-gauge needle is used to well over 70% when a larger bore (16-gauge) needle is employed.[6] Treatment for mild symptoms usually consists of having the patient lie flat or in a slight head-down position, infusing ample crystalloid solutions, and requiring the patient to use a tight abdominal binder when upright to increase pressure on the epidural space and slow cerebral spinal fluid leakage.

In more severe cases, the anesthesia provider may administer an epidural blood patch to alleviate symptoms. This involves careful replacement of the epidural at the site of previous skin puncture and injecting 10 to 20 ml of the patient's own, unclotted blood into the epidural space to "patch" the original defect. This modality has been found to be quite effective, eliminating symptoms usually within a few minutes or at least within several hours. Clinical case reports demonstrate that there are few complications, such as infection or recurrence of the headache after this procedure. Blood patching can be done immediately after delivery, even

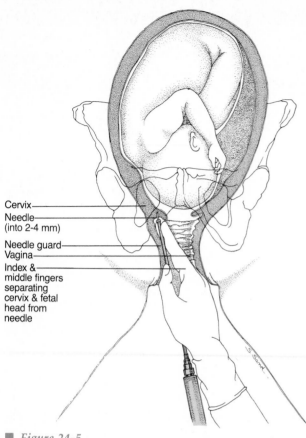

Cervix
Needle
(into 2-4 mm)
Needle guard
Vagina
Index &
middle fingers
separating
cervix & fetal
head from
needle

■ *Figure 24-5*
Technique of paracervical block.

in the absence of headache, if the dura was punctured on initial attempts at placement.

TOTAL SPINAL

On the rare occasion that too large a volume of local anesthetic was administered or excessive spread of the local results from administration of the drug during a contraction, immediate attention should be given to maintaining maternal blood pressure and ventilatory integrity. The patient's trachea should be intubated and the cuff of the endotracheal tube inflated immediately to prevent aspiration of gastric contents. Oxygen should be administered and ventilation controlled with positive pressure. The patient should then be placed in Trendelenburg and left-lateral position to facilitate venous return to the right heart. The rate of IV fluids should be increased and appropriate vasopressors employed to maintain maternal systolic pressure above 100 mmHg. The anesthesia care provider and labor and delivery nurse should always maintain reassuring verbal contact with the patient, explaining the sudden changes required for her proper care. In many instances, low doses of ketamine or midazolam may be advantageous to sedate the patient and afford amnesia of the event. With proper care, the block will recede and delivery can be accomplished by cesarean section or forceps with little deleterious effect on the infant.

LOCAL-ANESTHESIA–INDUCED CONVULSIONS

In the parturient, convulsions most often occur when systemic concentrations of local anesthetic reach toxic levels in the brain. This situation occurs rarely; however, immediate action must be taken to stop convulsive episodes that could potentially result in fetal and maternal hypoxia, acidosis, and death. High plasma concentrations of local anesthetics can result when repeated, high concentrations of anesthetics are administered in a short period of time, when an inadvertent arterial injection is given (during pudendal, epidural, paracervical blockade), or when rapid absorption of the local results from injection into highly vascular areas.

Most often, high concentrations of agent result when aspiration during block placement fails to reveal blood, otherwise indicating intravascular placement or the epidural catheter migrates into a vein, which may occur during protracted courses of labor. Within the epidural space, the epidural veins are plentiful, dilated, and easily ruptured by the trauma of an adjacent catheter during excessive patient movement or catheter migration. Consequently, it is possible that a previously patent epidural catheter may, during the course of labor, find IV access. Because of this probability, each therapeutic redose of the catheter is always preceded by careful aspiration for blood followed by titration of drug.

For the astute nurse, certain prodromal signs may appear that indicate toxic levels of local anesthetics are about to be reached. First, verbal contact with the patient is required. Should slurred speech, ringing in the ears, visual disturbances, or anything of substance that is not normal to their sensorium occur, the injection should be stopped (if germane to the situation), oxygen applied, and vital signs taken. If convulsions ensue, the airway should be maintained either with the aid of a bite block, oral airway, or potentially an endotracheal tube if the episode is protracted and there is difficulty in maintaining the airway. The nurse may be required to administer diazepam 5 to 10 mg or sodium thiopental 50 to 75 mg IV to abort the seizure. Positive-pressure ventilation and oral suction should be immediately available. Again, patients should be placed in a supine and lateral position, with rapid administration of fluids. Cardiotoxicity has been reported with inadvertent intravascular injection of bupivacaine (usually with concentrations of 0.75%), a common and widely used local anesthetic.[5] Bupivacaine has been found to be 16 times more cardiotoxic than lidocaine as well as of longer duration. In addition, several case reports in the early 1980s de-

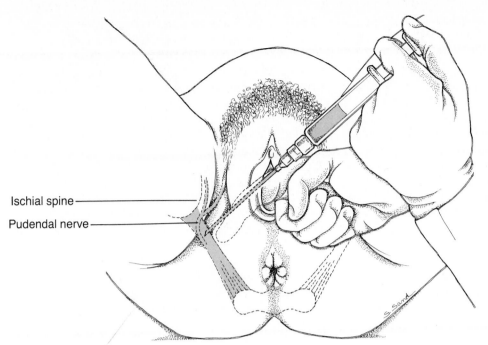

■ *Figure 24-6*
Pudendal block technique by the transvaginal approach. The examiner's fingers guide the needle to the ischial spine; the pudendal nerve is lateral to the spine at its tip.

Ischial spine
Pudendal nerve

scribed cardiovascular collapse resulting from these injections that were protracted and not amenable to traditional methods of resuscitation or drug therapy. This concentration is no longer recommended for obstetrics, as 0.5% provides adequate epidural anesthesia with minimal motor block. With careful administration and technique, however, bupivacaine remains one of the mainstays of epidural anesthesia in the United States.

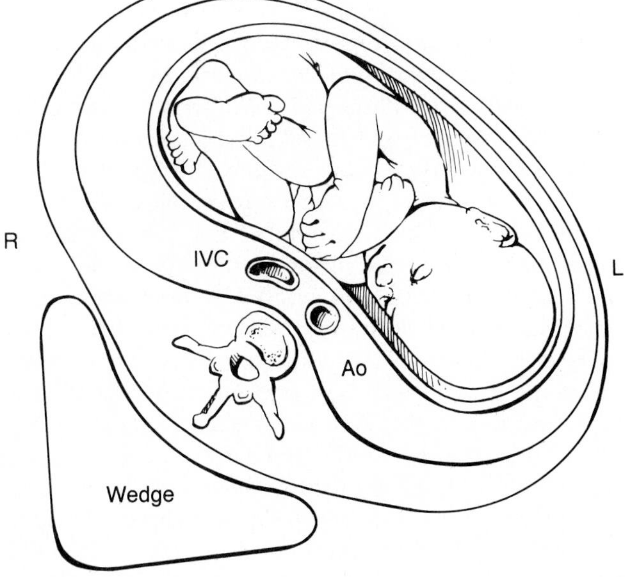

■ *Figure 24-7*
Lateral decubitus position with lateral pelvic tilt. (Stoelting RK, Miller RD: Basics of Anesthesia, 2nd ed, p 372. New York, Churchill Livingstone, 1989)

R

IVC

Ao

L

Wedge

NERVE DAMAGE

Nerve damage accountable directly to the placement of a spinal or epidural catheter is exceptionally rare, in fact highly unlikely as a direct cause, because needle trauma on a spinal nerve root is so exquisitely painful that the needle would be immediately withdrawn. Injury is more likely caused by leg supports and subsequent pressure to the peroneal or femoral nerves while the patient is in the lithotomy position. This injury would likely take 12 to 16 weeks to heal and the patient to regain function.[6] The inadvertent administration of 2-chloroprocaine into the subarachnoid space has resulted in permanent neurologic damage, including incontinence and foot drop.

Nursing Implications for Regional Blockade

The labor and delivery nurse fulfills a series of important functions relative to the administration and monitoring of either an epidural or spinal block. These can be considered more easily when divided into three distinct time intervals: preblock preparation, block administration, and block maintenance. These implications for patient care should be viewed primarily as effects or consequences that may occur secondary to the technique, not the technique itself.

During preblock preparation of the patient, the nurse will provide some or most of the primary teaching about the block and must be able to clarify expectations or concerns the patient may have about undergoing the procedure. This would most likely include a description of the procedure and associated risks as well as benefits to the mother and fetus. The nurse may secure IV lines to administer crystalloid solution prior to the block, have requisite resuscitation equipment available, obtain preliminary vital signs prior to the procedure, and generally make the patient as comfortable as possible during administration.

During administration of the block, the nurse will most likely be present in the room to help initially position and maintain the patient so that the block can be administered most efficaciously. The nurse may help communicate special instructions to the patient from the anesthetist during the procedure and monitor fetal and maternal responses from intermittent epidural drug injections. The nurse should continue to monitor the patient for signs of inadvertent intravascular injection and prodromal seizure behavior. The nurse will also be responsible for assessing the extent of hypotension and subsequent hypoxia that may result from the sympathetic block. Interventions include monitoring oxygen saturation by pulse oximetry, increasing IV fluids as indicated, or administering oxygen. The nurse must also begin to evaluate the quality of the block and the extent to which it is providing adequate pain relief.

During the postblock phase, the nurse will have primary responsibility for determining the patient's cardiovascular and ventilatory integrity by assessing vital signs intermittently. It may be necessary for the nurse to reposition the patient side to side to assure bilateral distribution of the local anesthetic and to prevent or treat signs of supine hypotensive syndrome. The nurse will monitor the integrity of the epidural catheter to make certain that positional changes of the patient after the block is in place do not dislodge the catheter. It is possible that the nurse will have to discontinue continuous infusions of local anesthetics if the block level becomes too high or if the patient's motor function is significantly impaired or signs of toxicity appear. Finally, most nurses will remove the epidural catheter after delivery and check for patency of the entire length of the catheter and document findings on the patient's medical record. If epidural narcotics are used, an apnea monitor may be indicated during postoperative recovery.

General Anesthesia

General anesthetics are rarely used for routine vaginal delivery as risks of complications, availability of regional and systemic techniques of pain relief, and the mother's desire to be awake for delivery do not justify its use. A general anesthetic is indicated however, in emergent situations, including the need for uterine relaxation to relieve tetanic contractions, fetal manipulation for mal-

presentation, some footling and complete breech extractions, emergency hysterectomy for placenta accreta, reinversion of a prolapsed uterus, excessive hemorrhage from a placental abruptio or previa, precipitous fetal distress and of course, elective cesarean section, which will be discussed in the following section. A general anesthetic is most often elected when regional anesthesia is contraindicated, rapid maternal physiologic control is required (in the case of hemorrhage), or time limitations to delivery (as in eminent fetal demise) require immediate delivery or surgical intervention.

Complications of general anesthesia are considered minimal as recent advances in monitoring modalities, including mass spectrometry, capnometry, and pulse oximetry, have greatly reduced anesthetic morbidity and mortality in all surgical populations. Gastric acid aspiration and failed intubation still account for the highest number of maternal complications associated with the administration of general anesthesia.[8]

■ ANESTHESIA FOR CESAREAN SECTION

Cesarean delivery can be accomplished using spinal, epidural, or general anesthesia. Depending on the mother's desires and the circumstances for which the cesarean section is being performed, any technique has desirable attributes and will yield satisfactory outcomes.

Elective Cesarean Section

In this scenario, the obstetrician, mother, and the mother's family have preplanned the birth of their child by cesarean section. Ideally, the mother will have learned of the procedure from her physician prior to admission or by the anesthesia provider during the preoperative interview in the hospital. Cesarean section accounts for nearly 20% to 25% of all deliveries in the United States.[4] This high number may be due in part to the malpractice crisis plaguing the obstetric field and the consequent defensive practice of medicine. Many obstetricians have been more inclined to deliver by this route at the first sign of failure to progress or of complications, rather than "wait out" the labor process, potentially exposing the mother and fetus to complications that could otherwise be avoided by an earlier, more controlled cesarean birth. More recent statistics show that this number may be decreasing in response to public and governmental inquiries regarding this unusually high incidence and the suspicion of a number of unnecessary procedures.

Usual indications for elective cesarean section are cephalopelvic disproportion, failure to progress, malpresentation, previous uterine surgery, history of vaginal herpes, anticipation of hemorrhage (placental previa), fetal distress, or any other related fetal condition that calls into question the ability of the fetus to tolerate a vaginal delivery. It is common practice in some institutions, when multiple births are anticipated, to allow the patient a trial spontaneous vaginal delivery with the operating room supplies, equipment, and sterile procedures established and ready for an immediate cesarean section if complications arise with the birth of subsequent children. This same scenario is followed for women who have had previous cesarean section, who heretofore underwent a cesarean section automatically. It has been suggested that as many as 60% of the women who have had previous cesarean sections can deliver vaginally and uneventfully with this double setup in readiness.

Epidural and Spinal Anesthesia

Spinal anesthesia remains the most popular anesthesia technique for cesarean section throughout the country, although those medical facilities that maintain an active obstetric epidural service are using that technique virtually exclusively. Spinal anesthesia has achieved widespread use because of its ease and rapidity of administration, usually within 5 minutes. Analgesia and motor block are profound. It has an induction to delivery time of 10 to 15 minutes if required, and many suggest that a spinal can be a likely alternative to general anesthesia for emergency cesarean section if there is a contraindication to the latter. Lidocaine 50 to 75 mg is the most widely used agent for the block, although tetracaine 8 mg can be used if a longer duration is required. A full complement of monitoring should be employed, including electrocardiogram, precordial stethoscope, a blood pressure cuff, and a pulse oximeter to measure oxygen saturation.

The primary disadvantage to this technique is the sudden hypotension that can occur consequent to the sympathetic block resulting from the introduction of local anesthetic into the spinal fluid. In view of concerns that the maternal blood pressure stay above 100 mmHg systolic to ensure uteroplacental perfusion, patients should receive at least 1, if not 2 L of crystalloid solution prior to the procedure to minimize hypotension. Prophylactic use of ephedrine 25 to 50 mg IM or 10 mg IV after placement of the block, as well as extracellular fluid enhancement, can be effective therapy.[4] In addition to these measures, lateral displacement of the uterus may also be required after the block is set to alleviate hypotension. Although the block (spinal or epidural) is usually brought to the T4 level (nipple line), the patient may still experience some discomforting "pulling sensations" when the surgeon exteriorizes the uterus for

surgical repair and closure. If the patient does not tolerate this procedure, the anesthetic can be supplemented with 5 to 10 mg IV of morphine or 50 to 100 μg IV of fentanyl to obtund these temporary sensations of discomfort.

Epidural anesthesia has the advantage of allowing a more controlled rise of the anesthetic and consequently less chance of encountering hypotensive problems from the sympathetic blockade. Drug administration can be titrated to the exact level required by the patient. There is also a lessened chance of postspinal headache from dural tears. In addition, a labor epidural can be used for a cesarean section by "topping off" the block with larger volumes of local anesthetics that have a faster onset, thus greatly reducing the time to cesarean section. The normal time of initial administration of the block to delivery is 20 to 30 minutes. Chloroprocaine 2% is the local anesthetic of choice in emergency situations where fetal acidosis is suspected and rapid onset is required. Monitoring of the patient and supplemental narcotic therapy are the same for epidural as with spinal anesthesia.

General Anesthesia

Prior to the induction of general anesthesia, the mother should receive nonparticulate antacids, such as 30 ml of sodium citrate, to increase the pH of gastric fluid. Particulate antacids should be avoided as aspiration of these products into the lung have been shown to cause more severe inflammatory changes in lung parenchyma. Patients should be monitored as described before, with the inclusion of capnometry or preferentially the availability of mass spectrometry to monitor the concentrations of all exhaled gases. Induction proceeds with rapid sequence procedures employed including cricoid pressure applied by the circulating nurse or anesthesia assistant (Fig. 24-8). An endotracheal tube is then inserted into the trachea, the tube balloon inflated and auscultation of breath sounds conducted to confirm proper placement of the endotracheal tube. Until the infant is delivered, the mother should receive 100% oxygen and a low concentration of a potent inhalation agent such as isoflurane 0.5%. After delivery, anesthesia can be deepened by supplementing the anesthetic with higher concentrations of potent volatile inhalation agents or narcotics such as fentanyl, alfentanyl, sufentanil, or morphine.

Emergency Cesarean Section

When fetal or maternal complications requiring immediate delivery arise during the period of labor, general anesthesia is usually the technique of choice. General

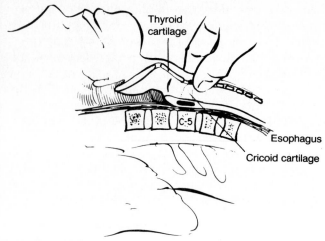

■ *Figure 24-8*
Technique of cricothyroid pressure (Sellick's maneuver).

anesthesia can be induced within 1 to 2 minutes after IV access is established. Emphasis is placed on maintaining basic anesthetic safety requirements, effective speed, affording the mother and infant high concentrations of oxygen, and maintaining acceptable perfusion pressures in the brain and other vital organs. Regional techniques can be used if the anesthetist is adept at placement and time limitations are such that the level and intensity of the block are acceptable.

Postoperative Pain Relief

In addition to traditional routes of IM and IV injection of narcotics for postoperative pain relief, the use of epidural injections of narcotics has become increasingly popular for control of pain after cesarean section. Clinicians report the use of a dilute solution of epidural morphine (Duramorph) 5 mg to be the most effective, with therapeutic effects lasting 24 to 36 hours.[6] Fentanyl 50 to 100 μg has also proven to be effective.[6] These drugs are generally administered through the epidural catheter after delivery of the infant and then the epidural catheter is removed. Patient-controlled analgesia has also been used successfully in the postoperative period to ameliorate surgical pain. This mechanism allows the mother to self-administer, within pre-set limitations, small doses of narcotics through an IV access according to her own needs.

Nursing Implications

All patients who have undergone a cesarean section, whether by general or regional techniques, should be recovered in a similar fashion to other surgical patients. The labor and delivery nurse, therefore, must apply the same principles of patient care as would the recovery room nurse. On the patient's arrival to the recovery area after a general anesthetic, the nurse should obtain initial vital signs and continue to take them every 15 minutes for 2 hours or until the patient is stable. The nurse should check the surgical incision for drainage and bleeding and make certain that the IV is patent. In most instances, the patient should have oxygen administered through a face mask at a concentration of 40% and have recorded oxygen saturation levels by pulse oximetry every 15 minutes. The nurse should also evaluate the patient's need for further postoperative medication.

If a regional anesthetic has been employed, vital signs should be taken in a similar fashion and notations placed on the medical record relative to the extent both sensory and motor function have returned. If epidural narcotics have been used for postoperative pain relief, the nurse should be especially vigilant in monitoring potential respiratory depression. This can be accomplished via an apnea monitor or by systematic, observational monitoring by the nurse.

A frequent side effect of epidural narcotic use is pruritus, which occurs in over 60% of patients. IV administration of naloxone effectively attenuates this problem by reversing the narcotic effects. However, if continued analgesia is required, symptoms can be treated with diphenhydramine. The nurse should also be ever mindful that respiratory or cardiac depression may be further exacerbated by the concomitant use of other central nervous system depressant medications when combined with intraspinal narcotics. In addition, the site of epidural placement should be checked periodically for the first 24 hours for any type of drainage or bleeding subsequent to removal of the catheter.

■ LEGAL IMPLICATIONS OF PRACTICE IN ANESTHESIA CARE

There is no doubt that the labor and delivery nurse is assuming increased responsibilities as a team member in the provision of anesthesia care of the obstetric patient. The nurse should also appreciate that there is great diversity among institutions as to the policies that exist governing the scope of practice labor and delivery nurses can assume in the provision of anesthesia care. Consequently, it is incumbent on nurses to be aware of the those locally determined limitations as well as the rights and privileges granted by their license to practice as a registered nurse. It is increasingly the practice of state boards of nursing to broaden the scope of practice of nurses such that there are fewer rather than more restrictions on clinical practice prerogatives. Statutory stipulations for the practice of advanced nursing, however, often require formal training and credentialing that verifies to the public competence in the field.[9] Thus, nurses often find themselves in the dilemma of being encouraged on the one hand to assume greater responsibilities, yet on the other hand having to deal with state statute or precedent that fails to clearly define the limits of practice. As the boundaries of care are expanded further for nursing, the legal authority for assumption of those rights will be less clear, at least until they become standards of practice.

This calls into question the issue of liability for the nurse should some negative patient outcome result directly from an action of a nurse not normally considered a traditional prerogative of a labor and delivery nurse. Even though the state board of nursing may tend to rule that such action is within the general scope of nursing practice, that does not necessarily mean that an insurance carrier or a court of law will agree with them. Quite the contrary, a nurse may be found negligent or practicing beyond the scope of authority as determined by common community practice and adequacy of educational preparation to assume new responsibilities. For instance, a nurse may be found liable in certain circumstances for a negative patient outcome resulting from an independent decision to manipulate local anesthetic concentrations or rates of infusion in a continuous epidural infusion pump. The question is not whether the nurse is culpable for patient harm or capable in the technical or judgmental skills to make the changes, rather that the nurse lacks the publicly accepted or mandated authority to make such changes if they are not in concert with community practice standards and based on clear evidence that through credentialing or other educational preparation the nurse is qualified to manipulate the drug.

Circumstances such as these will no doubt proliferate in the years ahead as nursing expands it practice and inevitably impinges on the traditional practice rights of medical and other specialized nursing personnel. These issues, are in fact, not new to nursing and will continue to be discussed as long the public expectation of nursing requires that they care for patients of increasing acuity as well as demonstrating increased facility with technologically advanced equipment and new therapeutic modalities. Above all, resolution of these issues is a responsibility nursing must assume as a consequence of our continued growth and sophistication as a profession; one that requires effective communication within nursing and our best efforts to protect the public interest and safety.

The labor and delivery nurse should understand not only the scope of professional responsibilities as they have been traditionally practiced but also those grayer areas in which practice is expanding and less well defined. These trends have a way of eventually finding their way into a more permanent practice pattern; however, until then, the nurse should be aware of hospital or departmental policy, state nurse practice acts, as well as professional and legal trends that will all assist in providing a clearer definition of nursing practice in the challenging and dynamic field of obstetrics.

■ APPLYING THE NURSING PROCESS TO THE USE OF ANALGESIA–ANESTHESIA

Anesthesia, unfortunately, still accounts for one of the parturient's major sources of anxiety on admission to the delivery unit. This fear can be do to many sources: from other family members who have had particularly unpleasant anesthetic experiences in the past, insufficient educational material or expert advice on which to make decisions, concern over drug effects on the fetus, loss of physical or emotional control under anesthesia, inability to understand the technical nature of anesthesia, or the fear that someone else will decide for them what is best. Mothers express these frustrations differently, ranging from total silence and unwillingness to make decisions to denial that they will need any anesthesia support at all. The approach to all mothers by the labor and delivery nurse or the anesthesia provider should be one of competent teaching and calm reassurance that emphasizes the range of anesthetic techniques available, the fact that the mother can select different analgesic methods as labor proceeds, and that the discomforts of labor can be reduced significantly, if not completely obviated, without significant impact on fetal well-being. The many decisions required of the expectant mother relative to her analgesic or anesthetic experience should be explored prior to her admission to the hospital. Many hospitals provide access by families to the labor and delivery suite during the final stages of pregnancy and an opportunity to talk with the anesthesia care provider so that preliminary plans can be made, questions asked, and issues discussed to the satisfaction of the expectant mother and father.

Nursing Assessment

Although labor and delivery nurses are not directly responsible for the administration of many modalities of analgesic or anesthetic drugs, they are required to provide expert observation skills for those mothers who

NAME: JANE DOE
HOSP # 256-01-8974

AGE 26	HT (cm) 157	WT (kg) 60	BP 115/80	P 84	T 99°	DATE

		GRAVIDA: 1
LABS HCT	10.9 Hbg 32.7 Hct	PARA: 0
		WKS GEST:

MEDS/PREMED		E ①2 3 4 5
Fe# supp. qd Bronchoinhaler prn	/ Demerol 50 IV }800pm / Phenergan 25 IV	TIME: START FINISH
		ANES 8³⁰P 2⁰⁰A
ALLERGIES NKA		SURG 1⁰⁰H 1⁴⁵A

CHEST X-RAY	Clear	☒ PT ID ☒ CONSENT	Pt seen preop at 8:30 pm. H+P
ECG	NSR	DATE: 4/9/90	Obtained. Procedures explained
TEETH	Good denten.	ATTENDING: LSB	

OXYGEN	L/MIN.	TOTALS								
8L NRB MASK										
TEST DONE: 3cc	Xylo	Epi 15ng								
1/4% Bupivacaine										
(cc)		8+2			6			6+3		

FLUIDS: LR
F₁ −1000CC
PITOCIN:
EST. BLOOD LOSS

MONITOR		EtCO₂								
ECG L-II		O₂ SAT	96	98	94	96	96	96	96
BP R ✓ L		TEMP							
PRECORD ✓ ESOPH									
TEMP A X E S PA		TIME	9⁰⁰ 15 30 45 10⁰⁰ 15 30 45 11⁰⁰ 15 30 45 12⁰⁰ 15 30 45 1¹⁵ 30 45 2⁰⁰ 15						
NERVE STIM NO									
O₂ ANALYZER SB		FHR							
PULSE OXIMETER YES		X							
AIRWAY CO₂ NO									
IA NO		150							
CVP NO									
PA CATH NO		INCIS							
INTRP ABG ∅ 1 2 3		⊙							

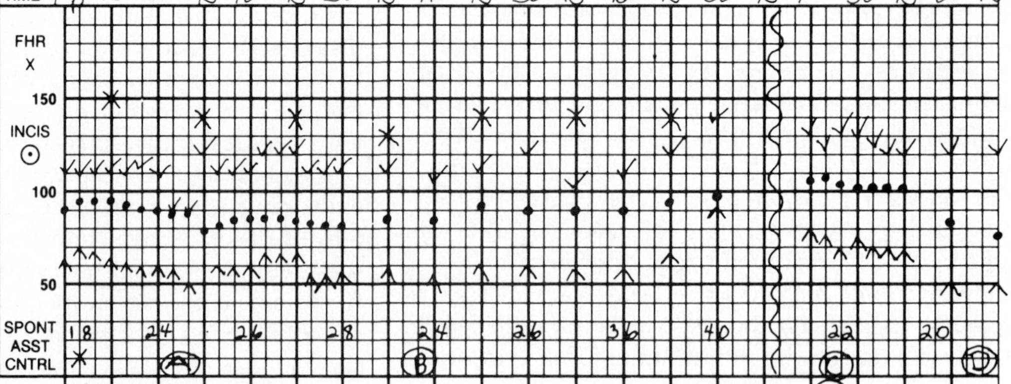

TECHNIQUE		100							
IV #20 L wrist								
AIRWAY ∅ O N								
ENDOTUBE ∅ O N T		50						
CUFF ∅								
MAC ∅								
SPINAL								
EPIDURAL ✓ Lumbar		SPONT	18	24	26	28	24	26	36	40	22	20
GENERAL ∅		ASST							
DURAMORPH EPID SA		CNTRL	✻	Ⓐ		Ⓑ			Ⓒ	Ⓓ

POSITION	LAT→ L LITH →
CERVICAL DILATATION/STATION	5/0 6/ 8/ 9/ 10/
SENSORY LEVEL	AWAKE + ALERT →

TIME BORN: 1³⁰A	NOTES: ☒ EQUIP CHECK
SEX M Ⓕ	X = placement of epidural catheter; I₂ prep; Loc Infiltration 1°
WEIGHT (gm) 4 Kg	needle placement at L3-4, LOR technique (Tuohy Needle) #18; cath
PLACENTA TIME: 1³⁵A	inserted easily – needle removed; no BLD or ESF aspir. Test doses

	1 MIN	5 MIN
HEART RATE	2	2
RESPIR EFFORT	2	2
REFLEX IRRIT.	2	2
MUSCLE TONE	1	2
COLOR	1	2
APGAR SCORE	8	10

x2 s̄ effect. Catheter secured + patent. Ⓐ Ephed. 10 mg
hypotension Ⓑ F₂ 1000 LR Ⓒ Delivery viable infant
Ⓓ catheter removed intact

POST ANES RECOVERY	RECOVERY ROOM DISCHARGE NOTE	PROCEDURES	ATTENDING
BP 134/80 P90 R20	Stable Condit.	1. Lumbar	
COLOR GOOD (AWAKE) REACTIVE ASLEEP	Full Motor + Sen.	2. epidural	RESIDENT ∅
SENSORY LEVEL Lucid	ATTENDING LSB	0.25% 3. Bupivacaine	OBSTETRICIAN SDS

■ *Figure 24-9*
Sample obstetric anesthesia record.

556

have received medications. These skills range from assessment of the effects of traditional IV and IM narcotics and tranquilizers to assessing the effects such agents have on the fetus via recorded electronic mechanisms now in popular use. In addition, they provide valuable insights into the patients history and physical condition both prior to and during pregnancy, including drug and allergy histories. When regional anesthesia is used, required nursing assessment skills necessarily become more sophisticated and incorporate management and interpretation of pulse oximetry data; observation and recording of vital signs (Fig. 24-9), physical signs and symptoms of allergic or untoward reactions of local anesthetic drugs for seizure activity; and, of course, frequent observation of cardiovascular and respiratory parameters. Most important are the skills required to anticipate and recognize early the range of complications that can occur with drug therapy and to intervene with supportive measures that assure maternal and fetal well-being until anesthesia or other support staff arrive. In the care of the high-risk obstetric patient, these responsibilities are compounded by the additional requirements of managing complex medical problems, such as those associated with toxemia, previa, abruptio, diabetes, or fetal distress.

Nursing Diagnosis

Nursing personnel perform a key role in diagnosis and early intervention of a range of problems that the parturient will present. These problems include the following:

- Maternal coping and adaptation mechanisms to pain of labor and delivery
- Patient understanding of anesthetic procedures and compliance with same
- Extent of pain relief
- Fetal distress secondary to any endogenous or exogenous source
- Maternal complications secondary to progression of labor
- Maternal complications secondary to anesthetic agents
- Changing parameters related to maternal physical homeostasis
- Normal patient progression from recovery after anesthetic procedures

Planning and Intervention

It is important that the expectant mother and father perceive that they are active participants in the process of labor and delivery, that they are not just bystanders to the birth while events are happening to them that are beyond their control. This requires that the labor and delivery nurse, physician, and anesthetist involve parents in all facets of the birth process. These efforts would normally include establishing a free flow of information that incorporates their ability to ask questions, clarify expectations, and make decisions when appropriate. It is also important that they understanding the normal progression of labor (and its variations) so that they can see the correlation between their efforts and continued progress toward delivery. It is most important that nurses explain what expectations the parents can have of their care, essentially establishing what both the nurse's role is as well as that of the parents. This will help the parents maintain a sense of control and determination and will promote full parental participation.

When labor has progressed sufficiently that the administration of systemic medication is indicated, the nurse can suggest that medication may now be helpful in allowing the mother to relax and regain better control of breathing techniques, thus promoting cervical dilation. The mother should be asked to first empty her bladder prior to receiving medication as narcotics may precipitate urinary retention in some patients. Fetal heart rates are recorded as well as baseline maternal vital signs, which can be used for comparison after the medication is administered. After the medication is given, the mother should be given reassurances that the nurse will be immediately available, side rails of the bed raised, and the room made quieter and more restful. Once the medication is administered, the patient should either be NPO or receive only small amounts of ice chips to prevent any episodes of nausea. The nurse should check the patient intermittently to evaluate vital signs as well as the patency of the IV line and the efficacy of the medication. All obstetric patients, regardless of the type of analgesia or anesthesia received during labor and delivery, should always have a patent IV line established prior to the receipt of any medication. It is the nature of obstetric care that fetal and maternal conditions can change abruptly, which may require IV access for medication or fluid.

Nurses often find themselves in the position of counseling the patient in regard to the initial acceptance of systemic (IV or IM) agents. This may occur when the mother is concerned about the effect medications will have on her baby. Reassurances need to be given that the fetus will not be unduly affected and that in the rare event that the baby is pharmacologically depressed, these effects are easily reversed. Many mothers will attempt to manage the entire course of delivery without medication of any sort and then find they are unable to tolerate more intense contractions. On these occa-

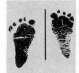

Nursing Care Plan

Lumbar Epidural Anesthesia

A 24-year-old woman, gravida 3, para 2, is admitted to the labor and delivery suite in active labor. She is somewhat relaxed except during contractions and is actively attempting to establish appropriate breathing techniques. On physical examination, the cervix is found to be dilated to 3 cm. Vital signs of the mother and infant fetal monitoring strips indicate both are stable. The mother states a friend suggested she should have an epidural anesthetic and wants it administered as soon as possible.

Nursing Goals

1. To facilitate patient understanding of analgesia options for labor and delivery
2. To prepare for implementation of the epidural procedure that will facilitate patient compliance, understanding and safety
3. To provide conditions during the anesthetic procedure to affect minimal disruption to the laboring process and maximize pain relief
4. To competently assess extent of pain relief from epidural anesthetic

Assessment	Nursing diagnosis	Implementation	Evaluation
Patient and fetus stable/early labor/requests epidural/exhibits moderate pain	Patient demonstrates knowledge deficit relative to epidural procedure/unaware of other pain relief modalities	Explain other anesthesia alternatives/explain epidural procedure/demonstration of epidural technique/nurse seeks anesthesia consult/allays patient concerns about the procedure	Patient understands alternatives/understands epidural benefits and risks/signs procedural consent forms.
Establish extent of cervical dilation (5–6 cm)/assess state of patient extracellular hydration/assess fetal condition and maternal stability via vital signs and electronic monitoring/assess degree of patient discomfort efficacy of coping mechanisms	Potential for alterations in maternal ability to cope with stress of labor and potential unfulfilled expectations of anesthesia	Acquire resuscitation equipment/have patient empty bladder/establish IV line of non-dextrose solution for preload/take and record vital signs and fetal monitoring for baseline data	Patient communicates satisfaction and confidence with decision to have epidural anesthesia
Patient exhibits acute pain/active labor established	Potential for alterations in physical regulation, circulation and oxygenation	Position patient in left lateral/knee/chest position/continue fetal monitoring/ongoing communication with patient to answer questions/observe for signs of local anesthetic toxicity (tinnitus, hypotension, metallic taste in mouth, altered sensorium/continue to coach patient relative to breathing techniques/record vital signs every 5 minutes	Patient exhibits stable vital signs/block is bilateral and provides pain relief/fetus and mother are stable.

(continued)

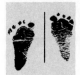

Nursing Care Plan *(continued)*

Assessment	Nursing diagnosis	Implementation	Evaluation
		after block secure and pad epidural catheter	
Patient complains of continued pain in fundal area of uterus and predominance of right sided pain relief in hip and thigh	Potential alteration in patient comfort	Take patient vital signs/ test motor function by having patient move legs and feet/test sensory function by sequential pin prick from knees to upper abdomen to identify level of dermatome blocked/ turn patient to non-anesthetized side/lower head to facilitate cephalad movement of local anesthetic/check integrity of epidural catheter/seek anesthesia consult after preliminary interventions	Block becomes bilateral/ patient blood pressure returns to normal limits/patient states pain is becoming relieved

sions, the nurse should support the notion that new choices can and should be made due to changing circumstances, that the mother has not failed in her attempt to avoid medications. These feelings of failure may also become prominent in the postpartum period, especially if the patient had desired a natural childbirth but fetal crisis required a cesarean section. Efforts should be made on the part of all personnel to dispel the patient's feelings of guilt and any potential anger directed at the infant.

Evaluation and Reassessment

The efficacy of drug therapy can be determined by a variety of criteria, all of which should be considered in the evaluation of the intervention. Failure of a drug to achieve a desired effect may be caused by an inadequate dose, administration during peak periods of pain rather than in earlier stages of labor, inappropriate routes of administration, excessive anxiety of the mother, or too much activity in the room by the family or nursing staff. Factors that indicate successful intervention with analgesics include patient satisfaction with the drug effect,

moderate decreases in maternal heart rate and blood pressure, decreased maternal ventilatory rate, progressive cervical dilation, and maintenance of fetal heart rate and beat-to-beat variability.

■ REFERENCES

1. American Society of Anesthesiologists, American College of Obstetricians and Gynecologists: Joint statement on the optimal goals for anesthesia care in obstetrics. ACOG Newsletter 9–10, September 1988.
2. Jouppila R, Jouppila P, Hollmen A: Effect of segmental extradural analgesia on placental blood flow during normal labour. Br J Anesth 50:563, 1978
3. Shnider SM, Abboud TK, Artal R, et al: Maternal catecholamines decrease during labor after lumbar epidural anesthesia. Am J Obstet Gynecol 147:13, 1983
4. Pedersen H, Santos AC, Finster M: Obstetric anesthesia. In Barash PG, Cullen BF, Stoelting RK (eds): Clinical Anesthesia, pp 1215–1251. Philadelphia, JB Lippincott, 1989
5. Stoelting RK: Pharmacology and Physiology in Anes-

thetic Practice, pp 134–144, 148–161. Philadelphia, JB Lippincott, 1987

6. Shnider SM, Levinson G: Anesthesia for obstetrics. In Miller RD (ed): Anesthesia, 3rd ed, pp 1829–1873. New York, Churchill Livingstone, 1990

7. Blass NH, Skerman JH: Obstetric anesthesia and analgesia. In Waugaman WR, Rigor BM, Katz LE, Bradshaw HW, Garde JF (eds): Principles and Practice of Nurse Anesthesia, pp 410–423. Norwalk, CT, Appleton and Lange, 1988

8. Stoelting RK, Miller RD: Basics of Anesthesia, 2nd ed, pp 369–392. New York, Churchill Livingstone, 1989

9. Mannino MJ: The Nurse Anesthetist and the Law, pp 13–31. New York, Grune and Stratton, 1982

■ SUGGESTED READING

Shnider SM, Levinson G: Anesthesia for Obstetrics, 2nd ed. Baltimore, Williams & Wilkins, 1987

25

Immediate Care of the Newborn

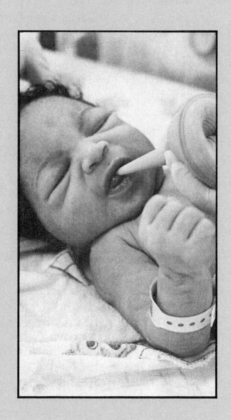

During the first and second stages of labor, the mother has been the primary center of attention, whereas the fetus has been assessed and cared for only indirectly. As the newborn emerges into the outside world, the term *fetus* no longer applies. The newborn *infant* receives direct attention as physicians and nurses care for its immediate needs, and the mother and father ask, "Is it a boy or a girl? Is it OK?" and other questions to identify its characteristics and to verify its well-being.

A typical hospital birth of a normal full-term newborn might proceed as follows: the physician uses a bulb syringe to suction the infant's mouth and nose as the head is born. When expulsion of the infant is complete, the nurse notes and records the time and the sex and sets the 1-minute timer. The physician holds the infant at about the level of the uterus, with the head slightly dependent, to facilitate drainage of fluid and mucus from the nose and mouth while continuing to use the bulb syringe. The physician then places two clamps on the cord and cuts between them. By this time, the infant is crying vigorously and the physician holds him or her up for the parents to see. When the timer goes off at 1 minute, the nurse assesses and records the infant's 1-minute Apgar score and resets the timer for the 5-minute score.

The nurse picks up a sterile blanket and places it across his or her chest and arms, making sure the side away from him or her remains sterile. The physician places the infant in his or her outstretched arms and the nurse then brings the infant in close to the body to hold him securely, grasping one leg through the blanket. The nurse shows the infant to the parents, and the mother may hold him for a few minutes; he is then placed under the preheated radiant warmer. When he has been dried off well, the nurse places a clean, dry, warm blanket under him and leaves him uncovered, with the temperature probe on his abdomen to regulate the radiant heat. The nurse places a cord clamp on the cord, 0.5 to 1 inch from the umbilicus and cuts off the excess cord with sterile scissors. Identification bands are made up. Two are placed on the infant's extremities, and one is placed on the mother's wrist. Erythromycin ointment might be placed in the infant's eyes and an injection of vitamin K given at this time, or these procedures might be deferred until the infant is in the nursery.

While caring for the infant, the nurse does a brief physical examination to detect any problems or defects and continues to keep the airway clear by suctioning as necessary. The 5-minute Apgar score is done at the appropriate time and recorded. When initial care of the

This chapter covers briefly the immediate care of the newborn. Various aspects of this care are discussed in more detail in Chapter 29 and 30, Assessment of the Newborn and Nursing Care of the Newborn.

infant is completed, the nurse places a stockinette cap on his head and wraps him in a warm blanket before giving him to one of the parents to hold. By the time the infant leaves the delivery room, the nurse should have the newborn record completed, with all pertinent information recorded. The nurse who takes the infant to the nursery gives the record and a verbal report to the nursery nurse and checks the infant's identification bands with him or her.

Most newborns adapt readily to extrauterine life, as in the above example, and the infant can soon be shown to or placed in the arms of the new parents. Because this transitional period can be hazardous for the newborn, however, nurses must be aware of the potential problems and alert to the infant's changing condition to intervene appropriately when necessary.

■ GOALS FOR IMMEDIATE CARE

To assist the infant in this transition, goals for the initial care of the newborn include the following (see also Nursing Care Plan at the end of the chapter):

- Establish and maintain an airway and respiratory effort.
- Provide warmth and prevent hypothermia.
- Provide safety from injury or infection.
- Identify actual or potential problems that might require immediate attention.

How these goals are accomplished may vary according to the setting, agency policy, parents' wishes, and condition of mother and infant. Delivery room nurses use the nursing process and their knowledge of the newborn's transitional changes to play an important role in meeting these goals.

■ ASSESSMENT OF THE NEWBORN

The importance of accurate assessment of the newborn immediately after birth and continued observation during the first critical hours cannot be stressed enough. The information about the infant's condition and responses that nurses gather at this time provides valuable baseline data for subsequent care in the nursery. All assessment and care should be well documented and should be reported to those caring for the infant after he or she leaves the birth area.

Research Highlight

In attempting to meet the goal of preventing cold stress in the newborn, many facilities place a stockinette cap on the infant's head soon after birth. Because of the proportionately large surface area of the infant's head, it is expected that the uncovered head is a significant source of heat loss. To help evaluate the effectiveness of the use of head coverings, Greer conducted a study comparing three groups of full-term, healthy newborns randomly assigned to three head-covering methods: no head covering, a stockinette cap, or a fabric-insulated bonnet. A radiant warmer was used for all infants.

Temperatures were taken at 5, 15, and 30 minutes after birth. The study showed that the temperatures of all infants declined during this 30-minute period but did remain within normal range. The temperatures of infants with stockinette caps dropped the fastest. There was no significant difference between the no-hat group and the group with the insulated bonnet. Although there were limitations to the study, the author recommends the stockinette caps not be used when an infant is under a radiant warmer. Further research is suggested to determine the effect of head coverings on preterm newborns. Nurses need to be aware that covering the head of a newborn under a radiant warmer is not necessarily beneficial in reducing heat loss and maintaining body temperature.

Greer PS: Head coverings for newborns under radiant warmers. JOGNN 17(4):265–271, July/August 1988

Risk Assessment

Ongoing risk assessment plays an important part in the newborn's care by alerting the health care professionals to potential problems and allowing them time to prepare for these problems. Although nurses often identify risk factors for individual patients and are aware of their significance, without a planned method of reporting and recording, this information is not always transmitted from one health care giver to the next. Standardized risk assessment systems used in many hospitals use forms that follow the obstetric patient throughout her antepartal, intrapartal, and postpartal course and include copies for the newborn's chart to improve continuity of care.

Most factors that cause the mother to be identified as high risk also place the fetus–newborn at increased risk. The mother's age, marital status, family history, and previous obstetric history are some of the general factors to be considered. Factors that should be noted from the present pregnancy and the intrapartal period are shown in Table 25-1. Examples are given of specific conditions or situations that would alert the nurse to the need to call a special resuscitation team or additional staff to assist with resuscitation.

After the baby's birth, information about analgesia or anesthesia given to the mother during the first and second stage of labor is of particular importance as a risk factor. The timing and amount of medication used influence the infant's responses immediately and for some time after birth. Ahls and Brazelton[1] have made the point that infants whose mothers have been heavily premedicated may respond at delivery with excellent function and optimal Apgar scores. About 30 minutes later, however, these same infants may be in a dangerously depressed state and require special nursing care to help them keep their airways clear of mucus.[1]

Apgar Scoring System

The *Apgar score*, developed by the late Dr. Virginia Apgar, provides a valuable index for assessing the newborn's condition at birth. The score is usually determined for each infant at 1 and 5 minutes after birth. For a 5-minute Apgar score less than 7, the American Academy of Pediatrics suggests that additional scores be obtained every 5 minutes for up to 20 minutes, unless there are two successive scores of 8 or greater.[2] It is helpful for all nurses who are responsible for the care of newborns, not merely those in the delivery room, to be familiar with the principles set forth by Apgar for infant assessment. These provide a simple, accurate, and safe means of quickly appraising the infant's condition.

The Apgar scoring system focuses attention on the following five signs ranked in order of importance. Each sign is evaluated according to the degree to which it is present and is given a score of 0, 1, or 2 (Table 25-2). The scores of each of the signs are then added to give a total score, with 10 being the maximum.

COMPONENTS

Heart Rate. The heart rate is the most important sign and the last to be absent when the infant's condition is

TABLE 25–1. PERINATAL RISK ASSESSMENT

Areas to be Assessed	Conditions Associated With Increased Risk
Antepartal Course	
General prenatal information	Lack of prenatal care
	Weight gain ≤15 lb or ≥35 lb
Maternal health	Medical conditions:
	Diabetes
	*Insulin-dependent
	Heart disease
	Habits:
	Smoking
	Substance abuse
	Infections during pregnancy:
	Rubella
	Venereal disease
	Complications of pregnancy:
	Pregnancy-induced hypertension
	*3rd-trimester bleeding
	Rh sensitization
	*Severe
	*Multiple fetuses
Results of antepartal tests	Estriol levels: ↓ or no ↑ after 36 wk
	Ultrasound: growth retardation ≥2 wk
	Amniocentesis:
	Bilirubin or meconium present
	L/S ratio < 2:1
	Nonstress test: nonreactive
	Stress test: positive
Intrapartum Course	
Length of pregnancy	≥37 wk; ≥42 wk; *<34 wk
Duration and character of labor	*Prolonged 1st or 2nd stage
	Precipitous labor or delivery
	PROM > 24 hr
	*Difficult labor
	Cephalopelvic disproportion
Maternal conditions	Preexisting problems (see antepartal course)
	Progressive hypotension
	Progressive hypertension
	*Excessive bleeding
	Signs of infection
	*Severe
Fetal presentation and position	*Breech
	*Transverse lie
Events indicating possible fetal distress	Fetal monitoring
	*Persistent late decelerations
	*Severe variable decelerations
	Heart rate <120 or >160 for >30 min
	*Poor beat-to-beat variability
	*Scalp *p*H ≤ 7.25
	*Meconium-stained fluid

(continued)

TABLE 25-1. PERINATAL RISK ASSESSMENT *(continued)*

Areas to be Assessed	Conditions Associated With Increased Risk
	*Prolapsed cord
Analgesia	Large or repeated doses of analgesia
	IM analgesia within 1 hr of delivery
	IV analgesia within ½ hr of delivery
Anesthesia	General anesthesia
	Conduction anesthesia with maternal hypotension
Method of delivery	*Cesarean delivery
	*Mid forceps or high forceps delivery
	*Failed vacuum extraction

* Conditions usually requiring presence at delivery of someone skilled in resuscitation.
L/S ratio = lecithin–sphingomyelin ratio; PROM = prolonged rupture of membranes; IM = intramuscular; IV = intravenous.

grave. It may be evaluated by palpating the pulsation of the cord or by observing the pulsation where the cord joins the abdomen. Listening to the heartbeat with a stethoscope is the most accurate method of ascertaining the beat. The beat may range from 150 to 180 beats per minute during the first few minutes of life; later, within the hour, it usually slows to between 130 and 140 beats per minute. Crying or increased activity will increase the number of beats. If the rate is 100 beats per minute or less, asphyxia is present and resuscitation is indicated.

Respiratory Effort. An infant who is responding well cries vigorously and has no difficulty in breathing. "Regular" respiration usually is established in a minute or so. Slow, irregular respiration or apnea indicates that respiratory difficulty or depression is present, and these signs should be reported immediately so that prompt treatment may be instituted.

Muscle Tone. An infant who has excellent tonus will keep the extremities flexed and resist efforts to extend them. An infant who does not keep the extremities flexed consistently usually has only moderate tonus; one who is flaccid is in extremely poor condition.

Reflex Irritability. Although there are several ways to test reflex irritability, the one most frequently used is a gentle slap on the sole of the infant's foot. This sign can also be observed when a vigorous infant is suctioned for mucus by the way in which it resists the catheter. A newborn who is in excellent condition will respond with a vigorous cry. An infant is judged to have a poor response if it cries weakly or merely makes a grimace.

TABLE 25-2. APGAR SCORING CHART

Sign	Score		
	0	1	2
Heart rate	Absent	Slow (less than 100)	Over 100
Respiratory effort	Absent	Slow, irregular	Good, crying
Muscle tone	Flaccid	Some flexion of extremities	Active motion
Reflex irritability	No response	Weak cry or grimace	Vigorous cry
Color	Blue, pale	Body pink, extremities blue	Completely pink

If there is a good deal of central nervous system depression, the infant does not respond at all.

Color. Cyanosis is seen in almost all infants at the moment of birth. As the infant's circulation makes the change from fetal to extrauterine existence and breathing begins, the body of a healthy infant usually becomes pink within 3 minutes. Because acrocyanosis usually is present for a short while, even in infants who are in excellent condition, those who have scored 2 for each of the other signs may receive only a score of 1 for this part of the evaluation.

INTERPRETATION

An Apgar score of 7 to 10 indicates that the infant's condition is good. If the infant breathes and cries (or coughs) seconds after delivery, there are usually no special procedures necessary other than those of routine close observation, maintaining a clear airway, and supplying warmth as necessary.

A score of 4 to 6 means that the infant is in fair condition. There may be moderate central nervous system depression, some muscle flaccidity, and cyanosis; respiration is not readily established. *These infants must have the air passage cleared and must be given oxygen promptly.* Sometimes directing a stream of oxygen toward the infant's face while suctioning is being done will be sufficient, but administration of oxygen can best be done by mask, and the flow should not exceed 4 L/min. Gentle patting and rubbing with the receiving blanket to dry the infant's body usually acts as an additional stimulus.

A score of 0 to 3 denotes an extremely poor condition. Resuscitation is needed immediately (see Chap. 44). If an infant is obviously depressed at birth, resuscitative measures should begin even before the 1-minute evaluation. For the depressed neonate, scores repeated at intervals provide an index of recovery.[3]

General Assessment

Initial assessment of the newborn should include a brief, general physical assessment. Hospitals may have different policies as to what is to be checked in this brief initial physical examination, but the following basic areas should be covered:

1. Inspection
   a. Head and face, anterior of body, posterior of body, or extremities for any obvious defects or evidence of trauma
   b. Skin: for color, staining, peeling
   c. General appearance: for anything unusual
   d. Nostrils: for patency
   e. Cord: for three vessels
2. Auscultation
   a. Heart: for rate and quality of sounds
   b. Lungs on each side: for comparison and to evaluate efficiency of respiratory exchange
3. Palpation
   a. Liver: for enlargement
   b. Chest: for position of maximum impulse of heart

Although not of critical importance for immediate intervention, checking the cord for three vessels should be done as soon as possible after the cord is cut, because the edges of the vessels are more difficult to see as the cord begins to dry. When first cut, the edges of the arteries are seen as two white papular structures, which usually stand out slightly from the surface. The vein is larger, often gaping, so that the lumen and thin wall are easily seen. The presence of only one artery is suggestive of congenital abnormalities.

Prompt detection of congenital anomalies or other problems is important to facilitate early treatment, and knowledge that there are no problems allows more leisurely time for parents and infant to get acquainted. Some congenital anomalies would be obvious, but others require some knowledge of what to look for. The practice of dimming the delivery room lights for a Le Boyer-type birth would increase the need to look more closely at the infant at birth. Newborn physical assessment is covered in more detail in Chapter 29, and congenital anomalies are covered in Chapter 45.

Gestational Age Assessment

Estimation of gestational age during the prenatal period is usually based on the mother's expected date of delivery as calculated from her last menstrual period. After birth, a more accurate estimation can be made by physical examination of the infant. The complete gestational age assessment is usually done in the nursery (see Chap. 29), but it is often helpful to use a shorter version during the immediate newborn period, especially if the infant appears smaller or larger than expected from the mother's dates. A rapid estimation of gestational age includes examination of sole creases, breast nodules, scalp hair, earlobes, and, in the male infant, testes and scrotum (Table 25-3).[4]

■ NURSING DIAGNOSIS

By using the previously noted assessment methods, nurses are able to assist in identifying problems and

TABLE 25–3. RAPID ESTIMATION OF GESTATIONAL AGE OF THE NEWBORN

| Sites | Gestational Age | | |
	36 Wk or Less	37–38 Wk	39 Wk or More
Sole creases	Anterior transverse crease only	Occasional creases anterior two thirds	Sole covered with creases
Breast nodule diameter	2 mm	4 mm	7 mm
Scalp hair	Fine and fuzzy	Fine and fuzzy	Coarse and silky
Earlobe	Pliable, no cartilage	Some cartilage	Stiffened by thick cartilage
Testes and scrotum	Testes in lower canal, scrotum small, few rugae	Intermediate	Testes pendulous, scrotum full, extensive rugae

(Cunningham FG, MacDonald PC, Gant NF: William's Obstetrics, 18th ed. Norwalk, CT, Appleton & Lange, 1989)

potential problems that require early intervention. In the immediate care of the newborn, certain potential nursing diagnoses are kept in mind during assessment to assist with early identification and intervention if problems are present or developing. Problems that are possible during this early neonatal period include ineffective breathing patterns related to alteration in response to extrauterine life; ineffective airway clearance related to excess mucus; impaired gas exchange; alteration in temperature (hypothermia) related to newborn status; high risk for infection related to immature immune system; and high risk for alteration in parenting (maternal–infant attachment process).

■ PLANNING AND INTERVENTION

While caring for the infant immediately after birth, nurses use their assessment of the preceding areas and the appropriate nursing diagnoses to plan and implement care to meet the stated goals.

Establishing and Maintaining an Airway

At birth neonates undergo profound and rapid physiological changes as the fetoplacental circulation ceases to function. The infant's survival depends on the rapidity and efficiency of these changes. The fluid-filled alveoli of the infant's lungs must fill with air, and respiratory motion must occur to exchange that air.

As soon as the infant is born, measures are taken to promote a clear air passage. As the head is delivered, the mucus and fluid are wiped or suctioned from the infant's nose and mouth to avoid aspiration of more fluid and mucus into the lungs with the first breath. A bulb syringe is usually used for this purpose. The infant is then observed to make sure respiratory efforts begin and are maintained. The first cry is eagerly awaited, because crying is one way the infant demonstrates its respiratory effort. The infant may not cry at once, but the removal of the mucus and the stimulation provided by the suctioning usually elicit a gasp or cry.

Some infants cry very little but are alert, active, and breathing well. Others seem to need to cry to force mucus from the nose and throat. If it is necessary to stimulate the infant to cry, this should be done with care. Vigorous external irritants, including spanking, forcible rubbing of the skin along the spine, alternate hot and cold tubbing, and dilatation of the anal sphincter are no longer considered necessary or effective and can be dangerous and shocking to the infant. Drying the infant with the blanket or gently rubbing the back or soles of the feet is usually sufficient stimulus to initiate crying (Fig. 25-1).

At first the infant should be kept in a modified Trendelenburg position to facilitate drainage of mucus. An exaggerated Trendelenburg position should be avoided, because the relatively large amount of abdominal contents will press against the diaphragm and the partially expanded lungs and may impede the infant's respiratory efforts. The bulb syringe should be used as needed. Collapsing the bulb before inserting it into the baby's mouth will prevent the material in the oropharynx from being forced into the bronchi and lungs when the bulb is squeezed (Fig. 25-2). If the bulb syringe is not adequate to remove the mucus, a suction catheter

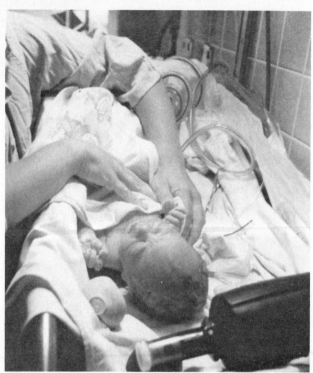

■ *Figure 25-1*
The baby may be stimulated to cry by rubbing it gently with a blanket. (Courtesy of Booth Maternity Center, Philadelphia)

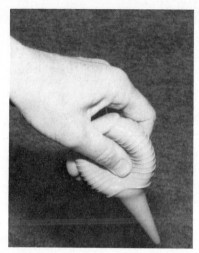

■ *Figure 25-2*
To prevent mucus from being forced into the bronchi and lungs, the bulb syringe is collapsed before it is inserted into the newborn's nostrils and mouth.

attached to mechanical suction or to a DeLee mucus trap, which uses the nurse's mouth to provide suction for aspirating the mucus (Fig. 25-3) may be used. It is important not to oversuction, because this may deprive the infant of oxygen by interfering with breathing. Deep, prolonged suctioning can also cause vagal stimulation, which can result in bradycardia.[2] Care should be taken not to traumatize the tissues of the oropharynx with the tip of the catheter or bulb syringe or with forceful suction. The mouth should be suctioned before the nose. If it is necessary to remove mucus through the nostrils, force should be avoided and the catheter should not be inserted far back. If the catheter is directed horizontally, as if passing over the roof of the mouth, instead of directed upward as for the adult patient, it usually slips into the tiny infant nostril with more ease.

RESUSCITATION

For most normal newborns, there is little need for resuscitative measures beyond clearing the airway and applying warmth and gentle tactile stimulation. A small percentage of newborns do require assistance, and for them the immediate availability of this assistance may be lifesaving. Successful active resuscitation requires skilled personnel who have been trained in the procedures, an adequate work area that is warm and well lighted, and appropriate equipment (Fig. 25-4), includ-

ing the means to deliver oxygen by positive pressure. It is important for any facility where births occur to have a plan that can be implemented immediately when emergency resuscitation of a newborn is anticipated or needed.[2] Part of this plan should be a list of maternal and fetal conditions that, when identified, would require someone specifically trained in newborn resuscitation to be present at the birth. The items starred in Table 25-1 are samples of conditions that might be included on the list. An additional item might be "request by the pediatrician or obstetrician."

Respiratory depression, the inability to initiate respirations, is the most common cause of perinatal asphyxia. Maternal analgesia and anesthesia are among the most frequent contributors to respiratory depression, because they can reduce the responsiveness of the respiratory center in the brain of the neonate. Inadequate respirations that persist beyond a minute severely compromise the infant by leading to a falling heart rate, decreased muscle tone, and greater possibility of acidosis.[3] A schematic approach for resuscitation is presented in Figure 25-5. Before beginning resuscitative efforts with positive-pressure oxygen, the airway must be cleared well by suctioning, because oxygen delivered under pressure may force any foreign material present in the airway deep into the infant's lungs. A well-fitting mask is placed over the infant's mouth and nose, and oxygen is administered by bag and mask ventilation at a rate of 40 to 60 breaths per minute to deliver the oxygen into the bronchi. If this procedure (called *bagging*) does not promptly stimulate breathing and correct the evidence of hypoxia, endotracheal intubation will be necessary under direct visualization with a laryngoscope.[5] Further details of resuscitative measures can be found in Chapter 44.

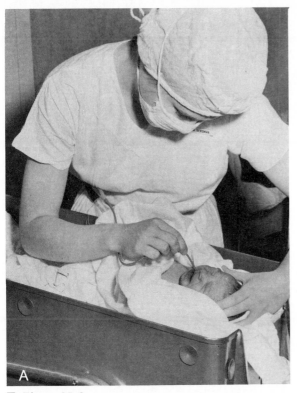

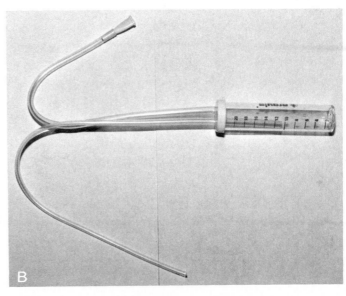

■ *Figure 25-3*
Suctioning the newborn in the delivery room. (A) The suctioning may be done mechanically. (B)
A DeLee mucus trap in which the nurse's mouth provides suction for aspiration.

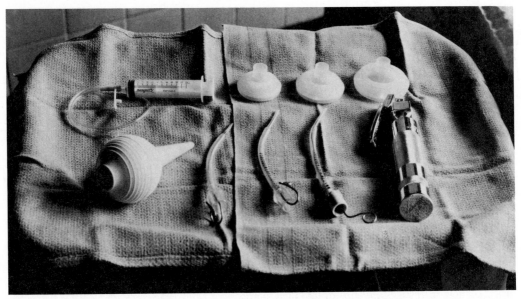

■ *Figure 25-4*
Close-up view of a sterile tray for management of the airway. Counterclockwise from top left
are a sterile, disposable syringe and tube for suctioning the stomach; a bulb syringe for
suctioning the mouth; Cole endotracheal tubes (three sizes); an infant laryngoscope; and Bennett
masks (three sizes).

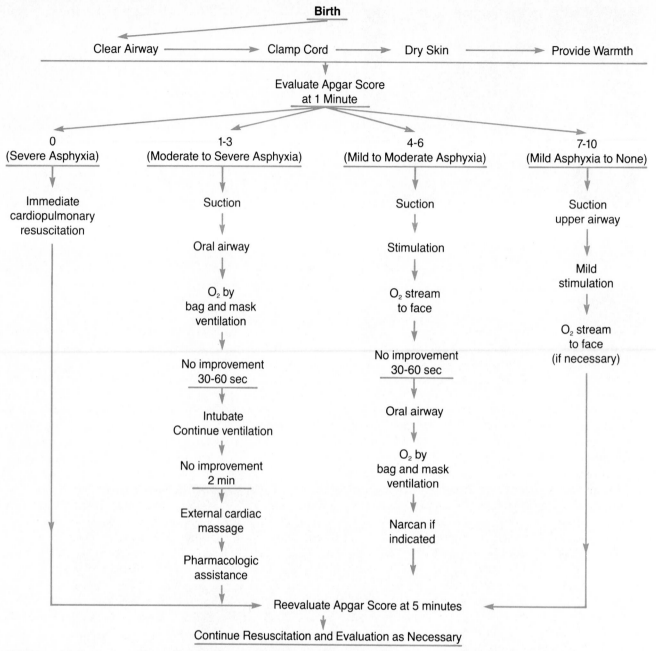

■ *Figure 25-5*
Schematic approach for resuscitation based on 1-minute Apgar score.

When resuscitative measures are needed and used in the delivery room, it can be a frightening time for the parents. In the rush to resuscitate the infant, it is important not to ignore the parents and their concern. The nurse should explain what is happening, as much as possible, and assure the parents that, although the baby has a problem, measures are being taken to correct it.

Maintaining a Neutral Thermal Environment

An important aspect of the newborn's immediate care is the prevention of hypothermia. The environmental temperature in the delivery room is much cooler than the intrauterine temperature and the infant is wet, which

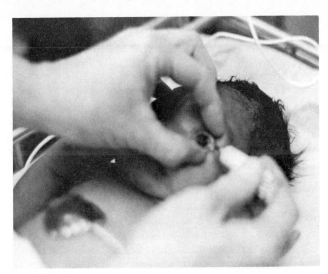
■ *Figure 25-6*
Ointment is applied to the eyes to prevent infection.

further increases the chilling effects of the transition to the outside world. Wiping the amniotic fluid from the newborn's head and body as soon as possible will help to minimize heat loss by evaporation. A stockinette cap is often placed on the infant's head to help prevent heat loss from this area. Use of a radiant warmer and a pre-warmed mattress for the infant's initial care provides a heat-gaining rather than a heat-losing environment. Prevention of hypothermia and cold stress in the neonate is related to the amount of oxygen needed by the infant and to the control of apnea and the acid–base balance (see Chap. 29).

Providing a Safe Environment

Safety for the newborn is not always considered as a separate entity and is sometimes taken for granted. The newborn is vulnerable to environmental hazards, including infection or physical harm. When handling the infant immediately after birth, nurses should be aware that newborns are slippery and that a firm grip is essential. The infant should be placed in a safe area for care. Following initial care, nurses will need to observe the infant frequently for any change in condition.

Infection control in the delivery room is important for both mother and infant. The newborn has an immature immune system and is susceptible to acquiring an infection when exposed to a variety of organisms. Nurses should consider handwashing an integral part of the procedure before handling the baby. Personnel who are ill should stay out of the delivery room. The umbilical cord stump is a potential portal of entry for infection, especially while still moist. Although it should be left uncovered, care should be taken that it is not contaminated. Further measures to prevent infection of the cord are usually implemented in the newborn nursery (see Chap. 30).

CARE OF THE EYES

Another aspect of preventing infection is eye care. The eyes of the newborn are at risk for becoming infected by a variety of infectious agents that might be present in the mother's vagina. For about 100 years, instillation of silver nitrate solution into the eyes of newborns has been used as a preventive measure against gonococcal ophthalmia neonatorum, or infectious conjunctivitis of the newborn (Fig. 25-6). In the United States, the use of some form of prophylaxis against eye infections is required by law. Although silver nitrate was used almost exclusively for years, other antiinfective agents are now acceptable. Two of the reasons for replacing silver nitrate as the agent of choice are that it often causes a chemical conjunctivitis and that it is not effective against *Chlamydia*, another infectious agent sometimes responsible for ophthalmia neonatorum.[2]

The Committee on Ophthalmia Neonatorum of the National Society to Prevent Blindness states that the prevention of both gonococcal and chlamydial infections must be considered (see Recommendations for Prevention and Treatment of Ophthalmia Neonatorum).

Although both tetracycline and erythromycin are acceptable for use, erythromycin ointment is usually the drug of choice, because it is less expensive than tetracycline and is more effective against *Chlamydia*.[7] It is recommended that infants born by cesarean delivery also receive eye prophylaxis. Even though they did not pass through the vagina, it is possible that these infants have been infected by ascending organisms.[2]

Eye prophylaxis may be done in the delivery room or may be delayed until the infant is taken to the nursery. This allows the parents to see the infant with the eyes open, because the infant is less likely to open the eyes for awhile after having drops or ointment instilled.

Other Aspects of Care

PROPHYLAXIS AGAINST HYPOPROTHROMBINEMIA

A single 0.5 to 1.0-mg dose of phytonadione solution (AquaMEPHYTON) is administered intramuscularly to the newborn in the delivery room or on admission to the nursery (see Fig. 30-5). This water-soluble form of vitamin K_1 acts as a preventive measure against neonatal hemorrhagic disease. Amounts of the medication in excess of

Recommendations for Prevention and Treatment of Ophthalmia Neonatorum

1. A prophylactic agent should be instilled in the eyes of all newborns.
2. Acceptable prophylactic agents that prevent gonococcal ophthalmia neonatorum include the following:
   a. Silver nitrate solution (1%) in single-dose ampules
   b. Erythromycin (0.5%) ophthalmic ointment or drops in single-use tubes or ampules
   c. Tetracycline (1%) ophthalmic ointment or drops in single-use tubes or ampules
3. Acceptable prophylactic agents that prevent chlamydial ophthalmia neonatorum include the following:
   a. Erythromycin (0.5%) ophthalmic ointment or drops in single-use tubes or ampules
   b. Tetracycline (1%) ophthalmic ointment or drops in single-use tubes or ampules
   Silver nitrate does not prevent chlamydial infections.
4. Prophylactic agents should be given shortly after birth. A delay of up to 1 hour is probably acceptable and may facilitate initial maternal–infant bonding.
5. The importance of performing the instillation so the agent reaches all parts of the conjunctival surface is stressed. This can be accomplished by careful manipulation of the lids with fingers to ensure spreading of the agent. If medication strikes only the eyelids and lid margins but fails to reach the cornea, the instillation should be repeated. Prophylaxis should be applied as follows:
   a. Silver nitrate
      (1) Carefully clean eyelids and surrounding skin with sterile cotton, which may be moistened with sterile water.
      (2) Gently open infant's eyelids and instill 2 drops of silver nitrate on the conjunctival sac. Allow the silver nitrate to run across the whole conjunctival sac. Carefully manipulate lids to ensure spread of the drops. Repeat in the other eye. Use 2 ampules, one for each eye.

      (3) After 1 minute, genly wipe excess silver nitrate from eyelids and surrounding skin with sterile water. Do not irrigate eyes.
   b. Ophthalmic ointment (erythromycin or tetracycline)
      (1) Carefully clean eyelids and surrounding skin with sterile cotton, which may be moistened with sterile water.
      (2) Gently open infant's eyelids and place a thin line of ointment, at least ½ in (1–2 cm), along the junction of the bulbar and palpebral conjunctiva of the lower lid. Try to cover the whole lower conjunctival area. Carefully manipulate lids to ensure spread of the ointment. Be careful not to touch the eyelid or eyeball with the tip of the tube. Repeat in other eye. Use one tube per baby (Fig. 28–6).
      (3) After 1 minute, gently wipe excess ointment from eyelids and surrounding skin with sterile water. Do not irrigate eyes.
   c. Ophthalmic drops (erythromycin or tetracycline). Apply as silver nitrate.
6. The eye *should not* be irrigated after instillation of a prophylactic agent. Irrigation may reduce the efficacy of prophylaxis and probably does not decrease the incidence of chemical conjunctivitis.
7. Infants born to mothers infected with agents that cause ophthalmia neonatorum may require special attention and systemic therapy, as well as prophylaxis. A single dose of aqueous crystalline penicillin G, 50,000 units/kg body weight for term and 20,000 units for low-birth-weight infants, should be administered intravenously to infants born to mothers with gonorrhea.
8. The detection and appropriate treatment of infections in pregnant women, which may result in ophthalmia neonatorum, are encouraged.
9. All physicians and hospitals should be required to report cases of ophthalmia neonatorum and etiologic agent to state and local health departments so that incidence data may be obtained to determine the effectiveness of the control measures.[6]

(After Committee on Prevention and Treatment of Ophthalmia Neonatorum: Prevention and treatment of ophthalmia neonatorum. New York, National Society to Prevent Blindness, 1981)

1 mg may predispose to the development of hyperbilirubinemia and are to be avoided (see Chap. 29).

IDENTIFICATION METHODS

While the newborn is still in the delivery room, it is the nurse's responsibility to prepare and apply some means of identification. Most hospitals use flexible plastic bands that come in sets of three with identical numbers on them. The mother's name and admission number, the physician's name, the date, the time of birth, and the sex of the baby are written on a special insert, which is put into each band. Two bands are placed on the infant, usually one on a wrist and one on an ankle, and the

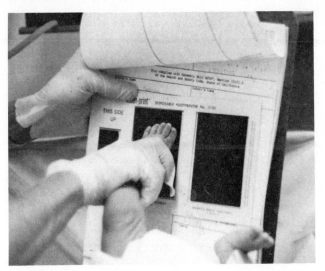

■ *Figure 25-7*
One method of footprinting includes a disposable plastic frame with the ink side away from the infant's foot. The foot is "walked" across the form just as it is when using the ink pad style. By using this method, the infant's foot does not get ink on it.

other band is placed on the mother's wrist. The number on the bands should be entered on the infant's record, and the information on the bands should be verified with the mother as soon as possible. The bands are checked with the nursery nurse when the infant is admitted to the nursery and are rechecked with the mother's band each time the infant is brought to her, to make sure they match.

Footprints and fingerprints are sometimes used and have at times been required as methods of newborn identification. Although they are no longer recommended as a universal practice, many hospitals still use them. If the infant's footprints are to be made, care should be taken to get a good print.

The infant's foot should be clean and dry and must be pressed firmly against the ink pad and then gently on the footprint form, "walking it on," beginning with the heel. The excess ink should be wiped from the infant's feet.

A newer alternative to the ink pad for footprinting is a disposable cardboard frame with squares of ink-coated plastic to press the infant's feet and mother's thumb against. The frame, with ink side down, is placed over the identification form on a clipboard (Fig. 25-7). As with the ink pad method, the feet must be clean and dry and each foot walked onto the form with gentle pressure, beginning at the heel. Nurses must be careful not to move the infant's foot while pressing it down on the frame. Because the ink does not come in contact with the infant's feet, no clean-up is required.

PROMOTION OF EARLY MATERNAL–INFANT ATTACHMENT

It is important for the new mother to see and hold her infant as soon as possible after birth. Many women will be eager to do this and will ask. Others may want to hold the infant but will not know that it is permitted and may hesitate to ask. Still others may be too tired or too uncomfortable or for some other reason may not be as eager for contact with the baby. Although the reluctant mother should not be forced to hold her baby, by bringing the newborn to the mother's side and showing it to her, nurses may help to initiate the attachment process. When desired and the condition of mother and infant are favorable, allowing the mother to breast-feed or have skin-to-skin contact with the infant in the delivery room is an excellent way to promote attachment.[8] Provision for warmth should be made by using a radiant warmer or warm blanket. Allowing time for parents and infant to be alone together, with the nurse near enough to provide assistance if needed, is another way of getting the new family off to a good start.

When there are problems with mother or infant and early contact is not possible, it is particularly important that the infant be shown to the mother before being taken from the delivery room and that she be given information about the infant's condition.

BAPTISM OF THE INFANT

If there is any probability that the infant is in imminent danger and may not live, consideration should be given to the question of baptism. This is particularly important if the family is Roman Catholic, and it also applies to some other denominations of the Christian church. Baptism often means a great deal to the family of a critically ill newborn, and the nurse's assistance is usually greatly appreciated. If time allows, a member of the clergy should be called, but if this is not possible, anyone, preferably of the same faith or who has been baptized, may baptize the infant. The following form may be used:

> Pour the water on the child (preferably the head) saying at the same time, "I baptize you in the name of the Father and of the Son and of the Holy Ghost." The water should be pure and may be warmed, if necessary. Care should be taken to make the water flow. If there is any doubt whether the child is alive or dead, it should be baptized conditionally (i.e., "If you are alive, I baptize you . . .").

The baptism should be reported to the parents, and recorded on the chart.

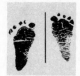

Nursing Care Plan

Immediate Care of the Newborn

Patient Goals and Patient Behavioral Outcomes

1. Apgar score between 7 and 10 at 1 and 5 minutes
2. Vital signs remain within normal limits:
    (a) Apical pulse between 120 and 160 beats per minute
    (b) Respiratory rate between 40 and 60 breaths per minute
3. Infant's airway remains clear
4. Infant does not develop cold stress
5. Infant has appropriate identification (i.e., band) before leaving birthing area
6. Infant does not develop ophthalmia neonatorum
7. Infant and parent demonstrate appropriate beginning attachment behaviors

Assessment	Potential Nursing Diagnosis	Planning/Intervention	Evaluation

Apgar score
  Heart rate
  Respiratory effort
  Muscle tone
  Reflex irritability
  Color
	Ineffective breathing patterns related to alteration in response to extrauterine life	Have resuscitation equipment available and in good working order
		
		Alert resuscitation team when problems anticipated, and summon when necessary
		
		Place infant in a modified Trendelenberg position
			Newborn scores 7 to 10 at 1 and 5 minutes

Ongoing general assessment of airway and responsiveness	Ineffective airway clearance related to excess mucus	Gently bulb suction mouth and nose Use other suctioning methods as needed Proceed with resuscitation measures if necessary	Infant breathes without difficulty
	Impaired gas exchange	Gently stimulate by rubbing body with towel. Use O₂ or resuscitative measures as needed	Infant is reactive, is pink, and cries lustily when stimulated
Continuous temperature monitoring	Alteration in temperature: (hypothermia) related to newborn status	Dry head and body well Place stockinette cap on head Place in radiant warmer on top of warm blanket Tape temperature probe on abdomen for monitoring heat regulation	Newborn maintains stable temperature

Determine general status
  Size
  Maturation
		Weigh; measure length and head circumference	Infant adapts to extrauterine life with minimal trauma

(continued)

Nursing Care Plan (continued)

Assessment	Potential Nursing Diagnosis	Planning/Intervention	Evaluation
Normality of body systems Vital signs		Perform gestational age assessment Examine body systems by thorough observation, inspection, auscultation, and palpation Record, report as appropriate	Infant has good color and good muscle tone Infant remains free of trauma
Recognize needs of newborn	High risk for infection related to immature immune system	Use good handwashing and aseptic technique when caring for newborn	Infant remains free of infection
Protection from infection Protection from hypoprothrombinemia		Provide prophylaxis against ophthalmia neonatorum Administer vitamin K	Infant's clotting time is normal
Proper identification		Apply matching identification bands to infant and mother Check numbers and information with mother	Mother has correct infant
Family interaction	High risk for alteration in parenting (maternal–infant attachment process)	Encourage father or support person to be with mother Allow couple to hold and explore infant as soon as possible Point out infant's features; explain normal variations, Observe for inappropriate behaviors (e.g., reluctance to touch baby, lack of eye contact, inappropriate remarks)	Family interacts favorably

■ EVALUATION

Nurses evaluate the effectiveness of their care of the newborn by monitoring the infant and family for attainment of the evaluative criteria. Apgar scores of 7 to 10, vital signs within normal limits, absence of trauma or infection, and evidence of good parent-infant attachment are all indications that the early newborn period has been negotiated successfully. Identification of deviations from these criteria would lead to revisions in the nursing care plan to meet the needs of the individual infant and family.

■ REFERENCES

1. Ahls H, Brazelton TB: Comprehensive neonatal assessment. Birth Fam J 2:3–9, Winter 1974–1975

2. Frigoletto FD, Little GA (eds): Guidelines for Perinatal Care, 2nd ed. Elk Grove Village, IL, American Academy of Pediatrics and American College of Obstetrics and Gynecology, 1988

3. James LS: Emergencies in the delivery room. In Fanaroff AA, Martin RJ (eds): Neonatal–Perinatal Medicine, 4th ed, pp 360–378. St. Louis, CV Mosby, 1987

4. Cunningham FG, MacDonald PC, Gant NF (eds): Williams' Obstetrics, 18th ed, pp 235–244. Norwalk, CT, Appleton & Lange, 1989

5. Ehrenkranz RA: Delivery room emergencies and resuscitation. In Warshaw JB, Hobbins JC: Principles and Practice of Perinatal Medicine, pp 209–225. Menlo Park, CA.Addison Wesley, 1983

6. Committee on Ophthalmia Neonatorum: Prevention and Treatment of Ophthalmia Neonatorum. New York, National Society to Prevent Blindness, 1981

7. Bryant BG: Unit dose erythromycin ophthalmic ointment for neonatal ocular prophylaxis. JOGN Nurs 13(2):83–87, March/April 1984

8. Klaus MH, Kennell JH: Care of the mother, father and Infant. In Fanaroff AA, Martin RJ (eds): Neonatal–Perinatal Medicine, 4th ed, pp 379–392. St. Louis, CV Mosby, 1987

Study Aids

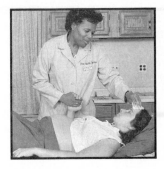

Unit V
Assessment and Management in the Intrapartum Period

CONFERENCE MATERIAL

1. Your client is a gravida 1, para 0, who is now dilated to 9 cm and 100% effaced, and the presenting part is at 0 station. Her husband is present and assisting well with her relaxation in labor. In the waiting room are both grandparents and the client's sister, who have visited the couple during labor but now decided it best to wait and not disturb the couple's concentration. Describe what the nurse's responsibilities are as delivery approaches.

2. An 18-year-old woman who is having her first baby is admitted to the hospital in early labor. It is obvious from her behavior that she has no preparation for this experience and is frightened and apprehensive. What are your nursing diagnoses and what interventions would you include in your nursing plan for her care?

3. The nurse has two clients to assess and to determine the well-being of both mothers and fetuses on admission to the labor and delivery unit. Discuss the nursing actions done to assess for fetal well-being on admission.

4. A couple who have attended Lamaze childbirth education classes find that all patients must be monitored externally during labor at the hospital they have chosen for delivery. What explanation would you give the couple for this practice? What specific measures would you include in your care plan to help the couple practice their relaxation and concentration and still maintain monitoring?

5. Why is prophylaxis for the eyes of the newborn required by law in all states? How would you go about securing the desired information concerning such legislation in the various states of the United States?

6. A 21-year-old mother at term who attended prepared childbirth classes for a previous pregnancy comes to the hospital on her birth attendant's instructions because her membranes have ruptured. She is apologetic because no contractions have started and states that she "should not really be here yet." Discuss your nursing care plan if this were your client, outlining how you would document the rupture of membranes, rule out infection, and establish both maternal and fetal well-being, and describe the explanation you would give in response to her statement about coming to the hospital when contractions have not started.

7. Your hospital does not permit the infant to stay with the mother during recovery. What specific steps might you take to help get this policy changed? Who would you have to talk to in order to implement the change?

8. What arguments would you put forth to institute a policy of putting the newborn to breast immediately after birth?

9. You are attending a mother in the recovery room who was heavily medicated immediately before delivery. She has her infant in the bed with her. What precautions should you take to ensure the safety of *both* the mother and infant? What signs should you be especially alert for in the couple?

10. A mother is dilated 6 cm and states that she is experiencing severe discomfort in the lower back during contractions and some discomfort in that area between contractions. What comfort measures can you consider using to relieve the discomfort?

11. Describe and contrast the behavioral changes the nurse may observe in a pregnant woman as she progresses through stage 1 and stage 2 of labor. Explain the underlying physiological adaptations occurring as they relate to the identified behaviors.

12. A primigravida is admitted to the labor and delivery suite in early labor. She expresses to the nurse her fear of anesthesia and the desire on the part of her family that she undergo childbirth naturally. What options can the nurse offer this patient regarding analgesia for labor and delivery? How can the nurse effectively facilitate communications between the patient and family regarding techniques of analgesia and anesthesia?

MULTIPLE CHOICE

Read through the entire question and place your answer on the line to the right.

1. After a protracted labor and a difficult delivery, the mother, upon seeing her baby, was shocked at the elongated appearance of the infant's head. The nurse could correctly reassure the client by saying
   A. "The newborn's head is molded during delivery and will return to normal in a few days."

B. "All newborn babies' heads are shaped this way."

C. "The newborn's head was traumatized during delivery, and it will take about 3 months for it to return to normal."

D. "After the 'soft spot' closes, the head will return to normal." ____

2. The character and the frequency of uterine contractions and the location of the discomfort experienced by the mother during labor often provide pertinent information regarding the labor.

Situation No. 1:
In the case of a multipara who is having discomfort but is not in true labor, which of these symptoms would most probably serve to identify false labor contractions?

A. Discomfort begins as early as 3 to 4 weeks before the onset of true labor.

B. Discomfort occurs 3 to 4 days before the onset of true labor.

C. Contractions occur at regular intervals.

D. Contractions occur at irregular intervals.

E. Discomfort is confined to the lower abdomen and the groin.

F. Discomfort is felt in the upper abdomen and the back.

Select the number corresponding to the correct letter or letters.

1. A only
2. A and C
3. A, D, and E
4. B, D, and F ____

Situation No. 2:
In the case of a primigravida in the beginning of the first stage of labor, which of the following symptoms would most probably describe her labor contractions?

A. Contractions occur at regular intervals.

B. Contractions occur at irregular intervals.

C. Discomfort is confined to the lower abdomen and the groin.

D. Discomfort is located in the lower back and the abdomen.

E. Contractions occur at intervals of from 2 minutes to 3 minutes.

F. Contractions occur at intervals of from 10 minutes to 15 minutes.

Select the number corresponding to the correct letters

1. A and C
2. A, D, and F
3. B, C, and E
4. All of the above ____

Situation No. 3:
In the case of a primigravida approaching the end of the first stage of labor, which of the following symptoms would most probably give an accurate description of her labor?

A. Contractions occur at regular intervals.

B. Contractions occur at irregular intervals.

C. Contractions occur at 1- to 1½-minute intervals.

D. Contractions occur at 2- to 3-minute intervals.

E. Duration of contraction is from 35 to 50 seconds.

F. Duration of contraction is from 50 to 60 seconds.

Select the number corresponding to the correct letters.

1. A, C, and E
2. A, D, and F
3. B, D, and E
4. All of the above ____

3. Labor is divided into the first, the second, the third, and the fourth stage.

A. When is the first stage of labor considered to be terminated?
   1. When contractions occur at 5 minute intervals
   2. When the cervix is completely dilated
   3. When the baby is delivered ____

B. When is the second stage of labor considered to be terminated?
   1. When the cervix is completely dilated
   2. When contractions occur at 2- to 3-minute intervals
   3. When the baby is delivered
   4. When the placenta is delivered ____

C. When is the third stage of labor considered to be terminated?
   1. When the baby is delivered
   2. When the placenta is delivered
   3. After the uterus has remained firm for 1 hour
   4. When the baby is 1 hour of postdelivery ____

D. When is the fourth stage of labor considered to be terminated?
   1. When the placenta is delivered
   2. One hour following delivery
   3. Twenty-four hours following delivery
   4. When the mother is transferred to the postpartum unit ____

4. In the typical vertex presentation, the sequence of events by which the fetal head adapts to the birth canal during descent is

A. Flexion, external rotation, internal rotation, and extension

B. External rotation, internal rotation, extension, and flexion

C. Flexion, internal rotation, extension, and external rotation

D. External rotation, extension, flexion, and internal rotation ____

5. The signs that suggest that the placenta has separated include

A. The uterus becomes firmer and globular in shape.

B. The umbilical cord descends further out of the vagina.

C. There is often a sudden gush of blood.

D. The mother exhibits deep respirations.

Select the number corresponding to the correct letter or letters.

1. A only
2. B and D
3. A, B, and C
4. All of the above   _____

6. The nurse is caring for a mother in the active phase of labor who is being internally monitored both for fetal heart rate and uterine pressure. She is 42 weeks' gestation with suspected fetal distress, and meconium staining is present in the amniotic fluid. Which of the following observations would you report promptly to the birth attendant?

A. Minimal variability with periodic late decelerations

B. Reactive fetal heart rate baseline that is fluctuating more than 5 beats per minute with periodic accelerations

C. Minimal amount of bloody show

D. Increasing thickness in the meconium-stained amniotic fluid

E. Uterine contraction frequency of every 70 seconds, with rising resting tone

Select the number corresponding to the correct letters.

1. A and C
2. A, C, and E
3. B, D, and E
4. A, D, and E   _____

7. Why is an enema sometimes ordered for a mother during the early part of the first stage of labor?

A. To obtain a stool specimen

B. To avoid straining as the mother bears down with contractions

C. To cleanse the lower bowel   _____

8. Often it is the nurse's responsibility to decide when the mother is ready to be moved from the labor room to the delivery room. Which of the following signs would signify to the nurse that the time of delivery is near?

A. The mother has a desire to defecate.

B. Increase in frequency, duration, and intensity of uterine contractions.

C. The mother begins to bear down spontaneously with uterine contractions.

D. The perineum bulges.

E. Amount of blood-stained mucus from the vagina increases.

Select the number corresponding to the correct letter or letters.

1. D only
2. A, C, and E
3. B, D, and E
4. All of the above   _____

9. Which of the following are indications that the placenta is beginning to separate?

A. Gradual descent of the uterus into the pelvis

B. Protrusion of several more inches of umbilical cord

C. Uterus becomes more firm and rounded

D. A sudden gush of blood from the vagina

E. Large clots of blood coming out of the vagina

Select the number corresponding to the correct letters.

1. A and C
2. B, C, and D
3. B, C, and E
4. A and D   _____

10. The nurse who is caring for the mother during the fourth stage of labor would include which of the following in her nursing care plan?

A. Keep the mother warm and out of drafts.

B. Massage the uterus every 15 minutes or more often if needed.

C. Massage the uterus continuously.

D. Administer oxytocin medication, as ordered.

E. Check maternal vital signs every 15 minutes during the first hour after delivery.

Select the number corresponding to the correct letter or letters.

1. B
2. A and C
3. A, B, D, and E
4. All of the above   _____

11. The most common cause of postpartal hemorrhage is atony of the uterus. What is the first thing to do as a preventive measure if the uterus appears to be atonic?

A. Take a firm grasp on the uterus.

B. Massage the uterus firmly.

C. Administer an oxytocic drug.   _____

12. Soon after delivery, a new mother complains of feeling cold. Which of the following are common practices that should occur after every delivery and will assist this mother from feeling cold?

A. Changing the client's gown

B. Giving oxygen per mask

C. Placing a warm blanket on the client

D. Removing the linen wet from the delivery

E. Placing the mother in Trendelenburg position

Select the number corresponding to the correct letter or letters.

1. A
2. A and C
3. A, B, and C
4. A, C, and D   _____

13. Which of the following are reasons to place the infant in the mother's arms right after delivery?

A. Prevent chilling in the infant

B. Allow the bonding process to begin in the sensitive period

C. Prevent infection in the mother and infant

D. Allow the mother to begin identifying her infant

Select the number corresponding to the correct letter or letters.

1. A, C, and D
2. A and B
3. B and D
4. B, C, and D
5. All of the above _____

14. After the physician clamps and cuts the umbilical cord and hands the infant to the nurse, which of the following acts would the nurse perform in the immediate care of the infant?
   A. Suction mucus from the infant's mouth with a bulb syringe.
   B. Hold the infant up by the heels to allow gravity to assist in removal of mucus.
   C. Slap the infant's back and soles of the feet sharply to stimulate crying.
   D. Dry the infant's body and head with the receiving blanket.
   Select the number corresponding to the correct letter or letters.
   1. A only
   2. A and B
   3. A and D
   4. B, C, and D
   5. All of the above _____

15. Which of the following may relieve pain during labor contractions by distracting the mother from pain?
   A. Walking and talking
   B. Slow rhythmic breathing
   C. Focusing eyes on an object
   D. Firm pressure to the lower back
   Select the number corresponding to the correct letter or letters.
   1. A only
   2. B only
   3. A, B, and C
   4. D only _____

16. One method of helping a mother who is untrained in relaxation to relax quickly at the beginning or end of a contraction is to suggest that she
   A. Stare at an object
   B. Count backwards from 100
   C. Take a slow, deep breath
   D. Massage her abdomen _____

17. What is the main objective in prophylactic eye care in the newborn?
   A. To enhance and protect the infant's vision in the immediate period after birth
   B. To prevent candidiasis neonatorum
   C. To prevent ophthalmia neonatorum
   D. To prevent staphylococcus colonization
   Select the number corresponding to the correct letter or letters.
   1. A only
   2. B only
   3. C only
   4. A, B, and C

5. B, C, and D
6. All of the above _____

18. Which of the following are needed for successful resuscitation of the newborn immediately after birth?
   A. Skilled personnel trained in resuscitation
   B. Well lighted area
   C. Equipment to deliver O_2 by positive pressure
   D. Drug therapy
   E. Intubation as necessary
   Select the number corresponding to the correct letter or letters.
   1. A, C, and E
   2. A, B, C, and D
   3. A, C, and D
   4. C only
   5. All of the above _____

19. The factors that should be considered in selection of an anesthetic for labor and delivery include
   A. The amount of discomfort experienced
   B. Experience of the personnel available and the facilities available
   C. The desires of the mother
   D. The dictum that no anesthesia is the safer course of action in all circumstances
   Select the number corresponding to the correct letters.
   1. A and B
   2. A, B, and C
   3. A and D
   4. All of the above _____

20. The discomfort caused by uterine contractions and cervical dilatation is conveyed to the spinal cord
   A. At levels T10 to T12
   B. At L3 to L5
   C. At S1 to S4
   D. At T8 to T10 _____

21. Identify and match the most important risks of the various methods of obstetrical anesthesia listed below.
   A. General anesthesia _____
   B. Conduction anesthesia _____
   C. Paracervical block _____
   1. Aspiration of stomach contents
   2. Fetal bradycardia
   3. Maternal hypotension

22. Under anesthesia, maternal systolic blood pressure below what level may be detrimental to fetal perfusion?
   A. 120 mm Hg
   B. 100 mm Hg
   C. 80 mm Hg
   D. 60 mm Hg _____

23. The most critical factor in planning a parturient's general anesthetic is
   A. Risk of postoperative bleeding
   B. Potential neonatal depression

C. Decreased uterine contractility

D. Prevention of aspiration ____

24. In the treatment of maternal hypotension following a spinal or epidural anesthetic, the following measures are correct *except*

A. A rapid infusion of Ringer's lactate solution

B. Oxygen by face mask

C. Left uterine displacement

D. Place the patient in the head-up position ____

25. Which change does *not* occur in the gastrointestinal system of the woman in labor?

A. Faster emptying time of stomach contents

B. Decreased lower esophageal sphincter tone

C. Increased intragastric pressure

D. Increased incidence of "heartburn" ____

COMPLETION

26. On admission of the mother to the labor suite, which of the following procedures are usually carried out on every client and which procedures are done in relation to the client's birth attendant's specific orders? Fill in the appropriate answer.

A. Check mother's vital signs. ____

B. Take the mother to the bathroom to void. ____

C. Do a perineal shave. ____

D. Listen to the fetal heart rate. ____

E. Prepare the mother for vaginal examination. ____

F. Give an enema. ____

27. Indicate the abbreviations that might be used on a client's chart to represent each of the positions and the presentations described.

A. Back of head directed straight to the left ____

B. Back of head directed toward the left side and the front quadrant of the pelvis ____

C. Back of head directed toward the left side and the back quadrant of the pelvis ____

D. Breech presentation, buttocks at the left back quadrant ____

E. Face presentation, chin at the right front quadrant ____

28. Give the term or the phrase that best fits each of the following statements.

A. Enlargement of the external os to 10 cm in diameter ____

B. Maximum shortening of the cervical canal ____

C. A condition caused by failure of the uterine muscle to stay contracted after delivery ____

D. A surgical incision of the perineum during second stage of labor ____

E. Settling of the baby's head into the brim of the true pelvis ____

29. In each of the following, write the term or the phrase by which the pelvic measurement described is commonly called.

A. From the lower margin of the symphysis pubis to the sacral promontory ____

B. The posterior portion of the symphysis pubis to the promontory of the sacrum ____

C. From the inner aspects of the ischial tuberosities ____

30. By using the letter of the measurements described in question 25, indicate the following.

A. The one that must be estimated rather than measured directly ____

B. The one that represents the most important measurement ____

C. The one that represents a transverse diameter ____

31. A client's chart shows pelvic measurements of 10.5 cm for the diagonal conjugate and 9 cm for the true conjugate; therefore, the nursing care for the patient in the labor room should anticipate that the patient might have which of the following?

A. An easy, rapid delivery

B. A labor and delivery of reasonable duration

C. A protracted labor with difficult delivery

D. An emergency cesarean section ____

UNIT VI

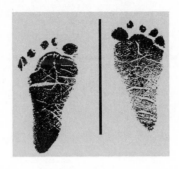

*Assessment
and
Management
in the
Postpartum
Period*

26

Biophysical Aspects of the Postpartum Period

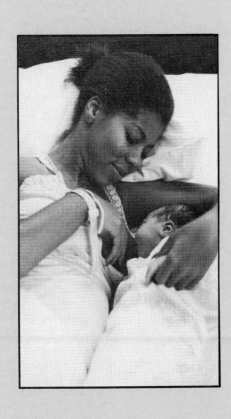

he postpartum period encompasses the time between delivery until the reproductive organs have returned to their prepregnant state. Marked anatomical and physiological changes occur during this period, as the processes undergone during pregnancy are reversed (Table 26-1). Knowledge of the reproductive process in pregnancy and labor serves as a basis for understanding how the generative organs and the various systems of the human body adapt after the delivery.

The term *puerperium* (*puer*, a child, plus *parere*, to bring forth) refers to the 6-week period elapsing between the termination of labor and the return of the reproductive organs to their normal condition. This includes both the *progressive changes* in the breasts for lactation and *involution* of the internal reproductive organs. The changes brought about by involution are normal physiological processes; however, such marked and rapid involution of tissues does not occur in other circumstances without a departure from a state of health. For this reason, the quality of the mother's care at this time is important to ensure her immediate as well as her future health. This chapter provides a basis for understanding these changes. Chapter 28 covers postpartum nursing care.

■ ANATOMICAL AND PHYSIOLOGICAL CHANGES

Uterus

Immediately following the delivery of the placenta, the uterus becomes an almost solid mass of tissue. Its thick

TABLE 26-1. POSTPARTUM PHYSIOLOGIC CHANGES

Organ or System	Changes and Time Frame
Uterus	Undergoes involution at rate of 1 fingerbreadth per day; becomes pelvic organ in 9–10 days (nonpalpable); placental site heals by 6 weeks
Cervix	Os closes to 1 cm by 1 week; endocervical glands regress by day 4; edema remains 3–4 months
Vagina	Rugae reappear by 3 weeks; normal estrogen levels and lubrication return by 6–10 weeks
Ovulation	Wide variation; affected by lactation; average first ovulation 10–12 weeks for nonlactating women, 12–36 weeks for nursing mothers
Breasts	Secrete colostrum after delivery; milk produced by 3–4 days; may have transient engorgement
Cardiovascular system	Transient increase in blood volume after delivery, declines by day 3 and attains nonpregnant levels by week 4; increased cardiac output and stroke volume at delivery, decreases after 48 hr with normal levels by week 3
Blood constituents	Early hemodilution followed by increased hematocrit days 3–7 and normal values by 4–5 weeks, leukocytosis first 10–12 days that returns to normal by 2 weeks; increased fibrinogen and clotting factors at delivery are normal by 3 weeks; increased protein, lipids, and electrolytes return to normal by 2 weeks
Respiratory system	Increased residual volume, resting capacity, and oxygen consumption; decreased inspiratory capacity, vital capacity, and maximum capacity; returns to nonpregnant pulmonary function by 6 months
Urinary system	Diuresis in 12 hr of delivery, output 3000 ml for 4–5 days, return to nonpregnant renal function by 6 weeks; bladder tone restored by end of 1 week
Gastrointestinal system	Constipation and difficulty eliminating for 2–3 days, restored intestinal tone by end of 1 week
Neuromuscular system	Numbness of thighs, fingers, or hands disappears in several days; backache improves in 6–8 weeks

Research Highlight

Changes in Functional Status After Childbirth

According to role theory, the woman s functional status in various aspects of life will change as the maternal role is taken on. This study explored changes in and variables associated with role performance, in the form of functional status, during the first 6 months following childbirth. Functional status was defined as the woman's readiness to assume infant care responsibilities and to resume usual household, social and community, self-care, and occupational activities.

A sample of 110 women was recruited from prepared childbirth classes and postpartum units (final N = 97). Subjects were married, English-speaking, over 18 years old, had delivered healthy, full-term infants, had no major prenatal or postpartal complications, and had no medical problems. They were followed longitudinally, with data collected at 3 weeks, 6 weeks, 3 months, and 6 months postpartum. Research instruments included (1) Inventory of Functional Status After Childbirth, which tested various dimensions of function; (2) Postpartum Self-Evaluation Questionnaire, which tested psychosocial variables; (3) Infant Characteristics Questionnaire, which measured infant temperament; and (4) background data sheets for health and demographic variables. Reliability and validity of the instruments were demonstrated.

The subjects were homogenous; most were white, well-educated, and middle class. About half had professional or managerial positions. Slightly under half were primiparas, and women with cesarean births were oversampled (40 of 97) for comparison purposes. Results revealed significant changes in total functional status over the 6 months following childbirth. By the traditional 6-week postpartum recovery period, less than 30% of women had fully resumed their usual levels of household or social and community activities. At this time, 25% still had not fully assumed their desired level of infant care responsibilities. In general, infant care responsibilities were fully assumed more rapidly than household, social and community, self-care, or occupational activities.

By 6 months' postpartum, almost 20% of women had not fully resumed their usual level of household activities, and 30% had not fully resumed their usual level of social and community activities. None had fully assumed self-care activities by 3 weeks, and less than 20% had done so by 6 months. More than 60% of women who had returned to work by 6 months were not yet assuming full occupational activities. Variables most related to fuller functional status included energy level, vaginal delivery, increased parity, confidence in coping ability, father's support, and having an infant with predictable temperament. Recovery of functional status after childbirth takes at least 3 to 6 months.

(Tulman L, Fawcett J, Groblewski L, et al: Changes in functional status after childbirth. Nurs Res 39(2):70–75, 1990.)

anterior and posterior walls lie in close opposition, leaving the center cavity flattened. The uterus remains about the same size for the first 2 days after delivery but then rapidly decreases in size by a process called *involution*. This is effected partly by the contraction of the uterus, with decrease in size of individual myometrial cells, and partly by autolytic processes, in which some of the protein material of the uterine wall is broken down into simpler components that are then absorbed.

Constriction and occlusion of underlying blood vessels occur at the placental site. This accomplishes hemostasis (to control postpartal bleeding) and causes some endometrial necrosis. Involution occurs by the extension and downward growth of marginal endometrium and by endometrial regeneration from the glands and stroma in the decidua basalis. Except for the placental site, where involution is not complete until 6

weeks after delivery, the process is completed in the remainder of the uterine cavity by the end of the third postpartum week.

AFTERPAINS

Afterpains are intermittent uterine contractions after delivery that are of varying intensity. These are most common in multiparas, whose uterine musculature does not sustain steady retraction because of decreased tone from prior childbearing. In primiparas, uterine tone is increased and the musculature remains in a state of tonic contraction and retraction; thus, primiparas usually do not experience afterpains. However, if the uterus has been markedly distended, as with multiple pregnancy or polyhydramnios, intermittent contractions will occur, producing afterpains.

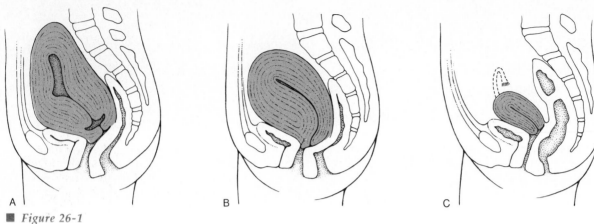

■ *Figure 26-1*
Changes in uterus size and shape following delivery. (A) Uterus after delivery. (B) Uterus at sixth day. (C) Nongravid uterus.

Afterpains frequently occur also with breastfeeding, when the posterior pituitary releases oxytocin as a result of infant suckling. Oxytocin causes contractions of the lacteal ducts in the breasts, expressing colostrum or milk and also causes the uterine muscles to contract. The sensation of afterpains can occur during active uterine contractions to expel blood clots from the uterine cavity.

PROCESS OF INVOLUTION

The separation of the placenta and the membranes from the uterine wall takes place in the outer portion of the spongy layer of the decidua. Remnants of this layer remain in the uterus to be partly cast off in a vaginal discharge called the *lochia*. Within 2 or 3 days after labor, this remaining portion of decidua becomes differentiated into two layers, leaving the deeper or unaltered layer attached to the muscular wall, from which the new endometrial lining is generated. The layer adjoining the uterine cavity becomes necrotic and is cast off in the lochia. The process is like the healing of any surface: blood oozes from the small vessels on this surface. The bleeding from the larger vessels is controlled by compression of the retracted uterine muscle fibers.

The process of regeneration is rapid, except at the site of former placental attachment, which requires 6 or 7 weeks to heal completely. Elsewhere, the free surface of the endometrium is restored in half that time.

PROGRESS OF INVOLUTION

The normal process of involution requires 5 or 6 weeks, and at the end of that time, the uterus regains its normal size, although it never returns exactly to its nulliparous state.

One can realize more fully the rapidity of this process by comparing the changes that occur in the weight of this organ. Immediately following the delivery, the uterus weighs approximately 1 kg (2 lb); at the end of the first week, about 500 g (1 lb); at the end of the second week, about 350 g (12 oz); and by the time involution is complete, only approximately 40 to 60 g (1.5–2 oz).

By observing the height of the fundus, which may be felt through the abdominal wall, the nurse is able to appreciate more fully these remarkable changes. Immediately after the delivery of the placenta, the uterus sinks into the pelvis and the fundus is felt midway between the umbilicus and the symphysis,[1] but it soon rises to the level of the umbilicus (12–14 cm, 5–5.5 in, above the pubes); 12 hours later, it is probably found a little higher (Figs. 26-1 and 26-2).

LOCHIA

A knowledge of the healing process by which the lining of the uterus becomes regenerated is valuable in understanding and interpreting the lochial discharge. At first the discharge consists almost entirely of blood, with a small amount of mucus, particles of decidua, and cellular debris that escape from the placental site. It should not contain large clots or membrane or be excessive in amount. The discharge lasts about 3 days and is called *lochia rubra*.

As the oozing of blood from the healing surface diminishes, the discharge becomes more serous or watery and gradually changes to a pinkish color; this discharge is called *lochia serosa*. Toward the tenth day, the lochia is thinner, greatly decreased, and almost colorless; this is called *lochia alba*. By the end of the third week, the discharge usually disappears, although a brownish mucoid discharge may persist a little longer.[2] Lochia possesses a peculiar animal scent that is quite characteristic and should never, at any time, have an offensive odor. Standards for assessing lochia character and volume are described in Chapter 28.

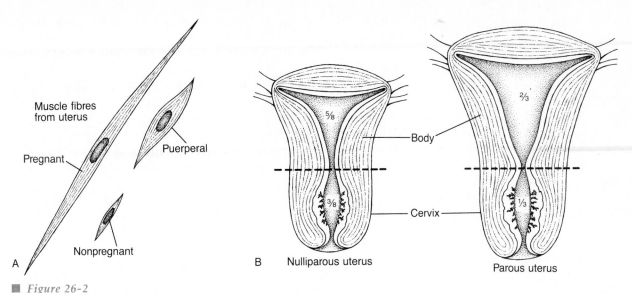

■ *Figure 26-2*

(A) *Changes in the size and shape of myometrial cells during the nonpregnant, pregnant, and puerperal states. (B) Size and relationship of the cervix and fundus in the nulliparous and parous uterus.*

Other Organs and Structures of Reproduction

CERVIX

Immediately following delivery, the cervix collapses and has little tone; it appears soft and edematous and has multiple small lacerations. It can admit two fingers and is about 1 cm thick. Within 24 hours, it rapidly shortens and becomes firmer and thicker. The cervical os closes gradually to 2 to 3 cm after a few days and by 1 week is only about 1 cm dilated. Histologic examination immediately after birth reveals almost universal edema and hemorrhage. The endocervical epithelium remains generally intact, with occasional areas of partial denudation. As early as the fourth day, there is regression of glandular hypertrophy and hyperplasia seen during pregnancy and reabsorption of interstitial hemorrhage. Cervical involution is still proceeding beyond 6 weeks, however, with edema and round cell infiltration persisting as long as 3 to 4 months.

Examination of the cervix with a colposcope (a viewing instrument similar to a microscope, with low magnification and binocular viewing, designed to fit a speculum for close viewing of the cervix) shows ulceration, laceration, bruising, and yellow areas within several days of delivery. These lesions, which are usually smaller than 4 mm, are seen more often in primiparas. Repeat examination 6 to 12 weeks later usually shows complete healing; this indicates rapid reepithelialization of the injured tissue.[3] Cervical lacerations heal by proliferation of fibroblasts.[4] There is variable retraction of everted columnar epithelium (ectropion) beginning early in the postpartum period. Not every cervix regains its prepregnant appearance; some have more ectropion, and the os is generally wider, shaped in a transverse slit, and may gape if there have been lacerations of clinical significance (Fig. 26-3).

VAGINA AND INTROITUS

The vagina is smooth and swollen and has poor tone following delivery. After 3 weeks the vascularity, edema, and hypertrophy resulting from pregnancy and birth are markedly decreased. When vaginal cells are examined microscopically on a smear, the epithelium appears atrophic by the third to fourth week but regains its proper estrogen index by 6 to 10 weeks' postpartum. This relative estrogen deficiency contributes to poor vaginal lubrication and decreased vasocongestion, which leads to a diminished sexual response in the weeks following delivery. The lower vagina usually has multiple superficial lacera-

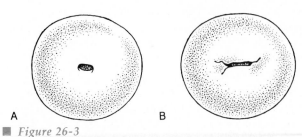

■ *Figure 26-3*

The perfectly round os of the nulliparous cervix becomes elongated after childbirth. The cervical os may gape if there have been significant lacerations during delivery. (A) Round os of nulliparous cervix. (B) Transverse slit of os in parous cervix.

tions after birth; primiparas may have small tears of underlying fascia and musculature.[4] Most of these are resolved by 6 weeks postpartum.

Vaginal rugae reappear by the fourth week postpartum, but many remain permanently flattened. After birth, rugae are not as thick as in nulliparas. The vaginal mucosa thickens when ovarian function returns and often remains atrophic in lactating women until they begin to menstruate.

Immediately following delivery, the introitus is edematous and erythematous. If lacerations or an episiotomy is present, this condition may be exaggerated in the area of repair. In the absence of infections or hematomas, the introitus heals rapidly.

Most women are free of perineal pain by 1 month postpartum, although for some discomfort may persist up to 6 months. Over half of postpartum women have resumed sexual intercourse by 2 months, with the median time for comfortable intercourse about 3 months' postpartum. A delay in restoration of perineal and introital integrity, with persistence of discomfort beyond median time periods, is associated with vaginal lacerations, forceps delivery, perineal edema more than 4 days after birth, and vaginal infection.[5]

FALLOPIAN TUBES AND LIGAMENTS

Histologic changes in the *fallopian tubes* reveal reduction in the size of secretory cells, decrease in size and number of ciliated cells, and atrophy of the tubal epithelium. After 6 to 8 weeks, the epithelium reaches the condition of the early follicular phase of the menstrual cycle. There is transient nonbacterial inflammation of the tubal lumina appearing about the fourth day.

The *ligaments* that support the uterus, the ovaries, and the fallopian tubes, which have also undergone great tension and stretching, are relaxed following delivery. It takes a considerable time for them to return to their normal size and position.

PELVIC MUSCULAR AND FASCIAL SUPPORT

The muscular and fascial support structures of the uterus and vagina may be injured during childbirth. This injury can lead to pelvic relaxation and the weakening and lengthening of support structures for the uterus, vaginal wall, rectum, urethra, and bladder. Although relaxation of pelvic structures can occur in women who have not experienced childbirth or sexual activity, it is most often a delayed result of injuries during the birth process. Symptoms and signs of pelvic relaxation usually appear around menopause, when atrophic changes in fascia occur and the tonic effects of estrogens on pelvic tissues decrease.

The most common types of pelvic relaxation include rectocele, enterocele, uterine prolapse, urethrocele, and cystocele. These defects are due to distention and separation of muscle bundles, fascial lacerations, and stretching and tearing of support structures. They tend to be progressive over time.

The pelvic muscles are critical to maintenance of urinary continence when there is a sudden increase in intraabdominal pressure, such as with coughing and sneezing. The various pelvic muscles, which are under voluntary control, combine with the smooth muscle of the urethra to maintain continence in women with intact muscle tone.[6]

Repeated childbearing places women at increased risk of pelvic muscle relaxation. Women who have greater antepartal pelvic muscle strength tend to demonstrate greater strength following vaginal delivery. Postpartal women who practice pelvic muscle exercises show greater improvement in pelvic muscle strength than those who do not exercise.[6,7] Exercises to aid restoration of pelvic and vaginal muscle tone were first recommended by Kegel;[8] the effectiveness of these exercises has been supported by subsequent studies.[9,10]

Chapter 19 describes Kegel's exercises; approaches to teaching these exercises to postpartal patients are discussed in Chapter 28.

ABDOMINAL WALL

The abdominal wall recovers partially from the overstretching but remains soft and flabby for some time. The skin regains its elasticity in time, but the striae persist, because of the rupture of the elastic fibers of the cutis. The striae become less conspicuous because of their silvery appearance. The process of involution in the abdominal structures requires at least 6 weeks. The abdominal walls regain their muscle tone and gradually return to their original condition, depending on prepregnancy tone, exercise, and amount of adipose tissue. However, if these muscles are overdistended or if they have lost their tone, there may be a marked separation or *diastasis of the recti muscles*, so that the abdominal organs are not properly supported. Rest, diet, prescribed exercises, good body mechanics, and good posture may do much to restore the tone of the abdominal wall muscles.

HORMONAL CHANGES: OVULATION AND MENSTRUATION

Circulating levels of *estrogen* and *progesterone* decline rapidly after delivery as the placenta is no longer present to produce these hormones. The woman's usual hypothalamic-pituitary-ovarian cycle is reactivated. Follicle-stimulating hormone (FSH) levels are low in postpartum women for 10 to 12 days then increase to follicular phase concentrations by the third week. Estrogen reaches follicular phase levels in about 3 weeks in nonlactating women, but it takes longer in those who are lactating. Ovulation and menstruation following childbirth are influenced by whether the woman is breastfeeding. Menses that occur within the first 6 weeks are rarely ovulatory; the longer after delivery the first menses occur, the greater the likelihood that they will be ovulatory. Once menstruation begins, the percentage of subsequent menses that are ovulatory rises rapidly.

The first ovulation after delivery in nonlactating women occurs, on an average, at 10.2 weeks. Among women lactating for at least 3 months, the first ovulation occurs at 17 weeks, on an average. With increased duration of lactation, the average time of ovulation rises, and among women lactating for 6 months, ovulation occurs at 28 weeks. Nonlactating women may ovulate as early as 27 days after delivery.

The return of menstruation after delivery follows a linear pattern. By 12 weeks postpartum, 70% of nonlactating women will have their first menses; over the next 24 weeks this rises to 80%. In lactating women, menses return more gradually, with only 45% menstruating by 12 weeks. Between 55% and 75% of women menstruate by 36 weeks. The average time until the first menses in nonlactating women is 7 to 9 weeks, with longer times in women who breast-feed. (Table 26-2).

Women who breast-feed for less than 1 month have a similar time for return of ovulation and menses as nonlactating women.[11] The time of initial postdelivery ovulation varies greatly, however, among both nonlactating and breastfeeding mothers. This underscores the importance of prompt initiation of contraception following delivery.

The basis for postdelivery amenorrhea is not completely understood. The hormone *prolactin* (associated with lactation) reaches peak concentration around delivery, then declines erratically over the next 2 weeks in nonlactating women. In nursing mothers, prolactin increases in the early puerperium, then diminishes.

TABLE 26-2. RETURN OF MENSTRUATION

	Average Time of First Ovulation (weeks)	Average Time of First Menstruation (weeks)
Nonlactating Women	10.2	7–9‡
Lactating Women	17.0*	30–36§
	28.0†	

* Lactating for 3 months.
† Lactating for 6 months.
‡ First menses usually anovulatory.
§ Depends on duration of lactation.

Levels of luteinizing hormone (LH) and human chorionic gonadotropin decline rapidly after delivery to low follicular phase by 2 weeks and do not change again until ovulation occurs. FSH levels are low until they reach normal levels by 3 weeks. This return of gonadotropins occurs whether or not the woman is lactating, although return to normal estrogen levels is delayed by lactation. This is interpreted to mean that lactation causes a temporary refractory state of the ovaries to pituitary gonadotropins.

Breasts

During pregnancy, progressive changes occur in the breasts in preparation for lactation. The breast lobules develop under the stimulation of the estrogen and progesterone produced by the placenta, and the lactiferous ducts undergo further branching and elongation. Prolactin, released from the anterior pituitary; cortisol from the maternal adrenal gland; human placental lactogen (hPL); and insulin, all of which appear in increasing amounts during gestation, also contribute to breast changes. Prolactin has a central role in the initiation of lactation, but its actions are inhibited during pregnancy as a result of high levels of estrogen and progesterone.[11]

In the last month of pregnancy, the parenchymal cells in the alveoli of the breasts hypertrophy and produce colostrum, a thin, yellow fluid. With delivery and loss of the placenta, the resulting abrupt drop in estrogen and progesterone levels appears to initiate lactation. The breasts produce increasing amounts of colostrum after delivery, containing more protein and inorganic salts but less fat and carbohydrate than breast milk. Colostrum also provides immunoglobulin A, an important gastrointestinal antibody that the newborn infant lacks.

PHYSIOLOGY OF LACTATION

At least six pituitary hormones play a role in mammary development and lactation. These include prolactin, adrenocorticotropic hormone, human growth hormone, thyroid-stimulating hormone, FSH, and LH. In addition, human chorionic somatotropin, hPL, and steroid hormones secreted by the adrenal glands, the ovaries, and the placenta play a part, as does pancreatic insulin. Prolactin prepares the breasts for lactation through an increase in breast size and in the number and complexity of the ducts and alveoli during pregnancy. As pregnancy progresses, prolactin stimulates secretion by mammary alveolar cells, and estrogen and progesterone stimulate ductal and alveolar growth, but these latter two paradoxically inhibit milk secretion.

With the delivery of the placenta, the source of most estrogen and progesterone during pregnancy, as well as of all hPL, is suddenly removed. The blood levels of these hormones fall rapidly, but the secretion of prolactin by the anterior pituitary gland continues. The appearance of milk postpartally has been demonstrated to coincide with falling estrogen and progesterone levels in the presence of elevated prolactin. The synthesis and secretion of milk is thus initiated when the inhibitory effects of estrogen and progesterone are removed and under the continuing effects of prolactin.

The secretion of milk begins at the base of the alveolar cells, where small droplets are formed and then migrate to the cell membrane; these are extruded into the alveolar ducts for storage. Milk ejection is the process by which contraction of myoepithelial cells in the breasts propels milk along the ducts into the lactiferous sinuses. These sinuses are located beneath the areola, and milk is removed from them by infant suckling. A neurohormonal reflex controls milk ejection and works through afferent nerve pathways to the hypothalamus. Suckling is the primary afferent stimulus, but the ejection reflex can be activated by auditory (infant crying) and visual (seeing the infant) stimuli. The efferent limb of this pathway is clearly hormonal, because oxytocin that is released from the posterior pituitary causes contraction of the myoepithelial cells of the breasts.[11]

The importance of higher cortical centers in the brain is demonstrated by the sensitivity of the ejection reflex to various noxious stimuli. Anxiety and tension, severe cold, and pain inhibit the ejection reflex and decrease milk ejection. This points to the need for the mother to have a comfortable, relaxed setting in which to breastfeed her infant. Chronic stress in life situations contributes to an ineffective lactation response. The nurse needs to assess the mother's psychosocial situation carefully and to plan approaches to alleviate factors that increase stress if successful breastfeeding is to be accomplished.

Prolactin appears to be more critical for initiation of lactation than for its maintenance once it is established. With continued nursing, levels of prolactin released in response to suckling increase less dramatically than in the beginning. Eventually, prolactin levels may not rise at all with suckling. The pathways by which lactation and milk ejection are brought about are illustrated in Figure 26-4.

COLOSTRUM

After delivery, the breast produces increased amounts of colostrum for the first 3 to 4 days. Women who carry out breast-care preparation during the last weeks of

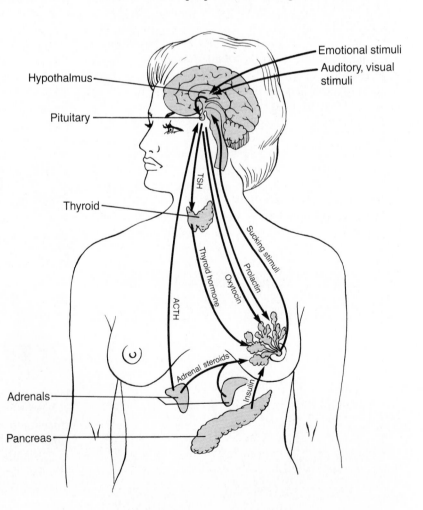

■ *Figure 26-4*
Neurohormonal pathways influencing lactation and milk ejection. (Redrawn from Hytten FE, Leitch I: The Physiology of Human Pregnancy, 2nd ed. Oxford, Blackwell Scientific Publications, 1971)

pregnancy often are able to express manually small amounts before birth.

Although the nutritive value of colostrum is lower than that of breast milk, it is particularly suited to the newborn infant's digestive system and provides important immunological protection.

LACTATION

On the third or fourth postpartum day the breast milk usually "comes in." There is an obvious change in the color of the secretion from the nipples: it becomes bluish white, the usual color of normal breast milk. At this time the breasts suddenly become larger, firmer, and more tender as lacteal secretion is established, causing the mother to experience throbbing pains in the breasts that extend into the axillae. This congestion, which usually subsides in 1 or 2 days, is caused in part by pressure from the increased amounts of milk in the lobules and the ducts but, even more, by the increased circulation of blood and lymph in the mammary gland, producing tension on the extremely sensitive surrounding tissues. This is sometimes referred to as *primary engorgement* (see Chap. 32).

The efficiency and maintenance of milk production is, in large measure, controlled by the stimulus of repetitive nursing. The neurohormonal mechanism involving prolactin and oxytocin release, which triggers the milk ejection reflex, has been discussed previously. The oxytocin released by suckling also stimulates uterine contractions, which explains the mild abdominal cramps often associated with the initiation of breastfeeding.

SUPPLY OF BREAST MILK

Breast milk varies markedly in its quality and quantity, not only in different people, but also in the same person at various times. In general, the amount of breast milk increases as the infant's need for it increases. Nature seems to have carefully coordinated the mother's need for rest and the infant's need for food during the first few days, when only colostrum is secreted. But during this time, lactation is definitely stimulated by the infant's suckling, and, although the secretion of breast milk would occur naturally, without this stimulation and the complete emptying of the breasts the secretion of breast milk would not continue for more than a few days.

If the infant is put to breast consistently, by the end of the first week a healthy mother usually has about 200 to 300 ml (6–10 oz) of breast milk a day. By the end of 4 weeks, this amount almost doubles, so that she produces about 600 ml (20 oz) a day. Breast milk is produced on the basis of supply and demand (i.e., the amount secreted gradually adjusts in relation to what the baby takes at an average feeding). In time, as the baby grows, the mother may have about 900 ml (30 oz) of breast milk a day.

The supply of breast milk is dependent on several factors, such as the mother's diet, the amount of exercise and rest she gets, and her level of contentment. An adequate diet for lactation requires increased amounts of protein, calcium, iron, and vitamins, as well as an ample fluid intake. The mother who is breastfeeding needs a good night's sleep, a rest period in the middle of the day, and normal exercise. Worry, emotional tension, and too much activity (overexertion and fatigue) have an adverse effect on lactation (see Chap. 32).

In relation to lactation, the actual size of the breast is not as important as the amount of glandular tissue, because the secreting tissues of the mammary gland and not the fatty tissues produce the breast milk.

LACTATION SUPPRESSION

The production and ejection of milk may be suppressed at the level of the breast, the pituitary, or the hypothalamus. The most simple, natural method is to avoid stimulation of the breast, which reduces the milk ejection reflex and decreases the stimulation of prolactin required for continuation of milk production. When the milk ejection reflex is inhibited in this way, over the course of several days the distended alveoli suppress lactation. However, some women experience engorged breasts during this time and have considerable discomfort. Lactation can be suppressed with natural methods in about 60% to 70% of postpartum women by wearing a tight brassiere and avoiding stimulation of the nipples and breasts.

Prolactin secretion can be inhibited with synthetic ergot alkaloids, such as bromocriptine mesylate (Parlodel). Administered orally twice a day for 14 to 21 days, this drug is quite effective in inhibiting lactation. Rebound congestion, breast secretion, or engorgement occur in some women using bromocriptine, but the breast symptoms are usually mild to moderate. Continuing mechanical and natural methods usually provides relief of symptoms.

The administration of estrogens or androgens to suppress lactation is infrequently used because of the risk of thromboembolic or neoplastic disorders.

Other Systemic Changes

CARDIOVASCULAR SYSTEM

Most of the significant cardiovascular changes produced by pregnancy disappear by the end of the second postpartal week. Within a few days of delivery, blood pressure, heart rate, oxygen consumption, and total body fluids generally return to prepregnant levels. Other changes require several weeks to resolve.

Blood Volume. During pregnancy, blood volume has increased 40%, or by about 1000 ml, with a total volume of 5 to 6 L. Changes in blood volume after delivery are related to blood loss and extent of postdelivery diuresis. The average blood loss for normal vaginal delivery is 400 to 500 ml; for cesearean delivery it often exceeds 1000 ml. Postpartum physiological changes mediate the response to blood loss and exercise a protective effect. Loss of the endocrine functions of the placenta reduces vasodilation; the maternal vascular bed is reduced by 10% to 15% when uteroplacental circulation is eliminated; and extravascular fluid is mobilized for excretion by the kidneys.

Postpartum changes in blood volume occur rapidly. There is a transient 15% to 30% increase in circulating blood volume between 12 to 48 hours after delivery because of mobilization of extravascular fluid and diuresis. This produces a hemodilutional effect, with a decrease in hematocrit and increase in cardiac output. By the third postpartum day, blood volume has declined 16% from pregnancy-related increases.[11] Total blood volume decreases to nonpregnant levels of 4 L by the fourth postpartum week.

Cardiac Output. Cardiac output, which increases during labor, peaks immediately after placental separation as uterine contractions force a large volume of blood into the circulation.[12] The increased stroke volume produced by pregnancy continues about 48 hours after delivery as a result of increased venous return that results from loss of placental circulation and reduced uterine blood flow. With postpartum diuresis causing a transient increase in blood volume, these combined effects increase cardiac output by about 35% in the early postdelivery period.

Within 2 weeks after delivery, cardiac output decreases by about 30%.[13] Gradual reduction in blood volume occurs during the second to the fourth postpartal weeks, permitting cardiac output to return to nonpregnant levels by about the third week postpartum.[14]

Blood Pressure and Pulse Rate. Blood pressure undergoes little change under normal conditions. Orthostatic hypotension may occur in the first 48 hours after delivery because of splanchnic engorgement. After delivery, there often is transient physiological bradycardia, lasting 24 to 48 hours, with pulse rates of 40 to 50 beats per minute. This results from hemodynamic changes, including increased stroke volume and cardiac output, and a vagal response to increased sympathetic nervous system activity during labor.[11] Milder bradycardia of 50 to 70 beats per minute may continue for about 1 week.

The pulse rate returns to nonpregnant levels by about 3 months' postpartum.

Blood Constituents. Following early hemodilution caused by interstitial fluid mobilization, the hematocrit rises in 3 to 7 days because of the hemoconcentration that accompanies diuresis with a greater loss of plasma volume than blood cells. The increase in red blood cell mass during pregnancy also contributes to an increased hematocrit. There is no red blood cell (RBC) destruction during the postpartum period, but the RBC count gradually returns to normal levels as the increased RBCs of pregnancy reach the end of their lifespan. Hematocrit values return to prepregnant levels by the fourth or fifth postpartum week.

The white blood cell (WBC) count normally increases to 12,000/mm^3 during pregnancy. A pronounced leukocytosis occurs during the first 10 to 12 days after delivery with values of 20,000 to 30,000/mm^3. This leukocytosis is characterized by increased neutrophils and eosinophils and decreased lymphocytes. This shift to the left in the WBC count is also typical of infections, and combined with the increased erythrocyte sedimentation rate typical after delivery, it may make postpartum infection hard to distinguish.

Coagulation Factors. The increase in coagulation factors that occurs with pregnancy continues into the postpartum period. Clotting factors I, II, VIII, IX, and X are activated extensively after delivery; these decrease within a few days to prepregnant levels, but fibrinogen and thromboplastin remain elevated until the end of the third week postpartum. These increased clotting factors can interact with immobility, sepsis, or trauma to predispose women to postpartum thromboembolism.

Other Constituents. Effects of high estrogen levels during pregnancy on protein and fat synthesis result in increased production of fatty acids, cholesterol, triglycerides, lipoproteins, and clotting factors. These constituents return to prepregnant levels by 2 to 3 weeks' postpartum. Serum electrolytes are altered after delivery, with a negative chloride balance resulting from rapid excretion of extracellular fluid during diuresis. Serum sodium rises in part because of falling steroid hormones as well as relatively greater loss of water than sodium. Increased serum potassium levels are probably caused by catabolism of tissues during involution. These changes are reversed by about 2 weeks' postpartum.

RESPIRATORY SYSTEM

Changes in abdominal pressure and thoracic cage capacity after delivery result in rapid alterations of pulmonary function. Increases are found in residual volume, resting ventilation, and oxygen consumption. There are decreases in inspiratory capacity, vital capacity, and maximum breathing capacity. By 6 months' postpartum, pulmonary functions return to nonpregnant levels. During this time, however, women have less efficient responses to exercise.

Acid–base balance changes during labor and in the early postpartum period. Progesterone during pregnancy creates a type of hyperventilation at the alveolar level increasing oxygen saturation without changing respiratory rate. Pregnancy is characterized by respiratory alkalosis (caused by decreased carbon dioxide concentration in alveoli) and a compensated metabolic acidosis. During labor, these begin to change with rising blood lactate, falling pH, and hypocapnia (<30 mm Hg) toward the end of the first stage. These conditions continue into the early puerperium, but more normal nonpregnant values (P_{CO_2} 35–40 mm Hg) appear within a few days. Falling progesterone levels affect this postpartum hypercapnia, which is accompanied by elevated base excess and plasma bicarbonate. Gradually, the pH and base excess increase until normal values are reached, about 3 weeks after delivery. The basic metabolic rate remains increased for 1 to 2 weeks following delivery.

Oxygen saturation and P_{O_2} are higher during pregnancy than in nonpregnant women. In labor, women may experience decreases in oxygen saturation, especially when supine. This may be a result of decreased cardiac output in this position. Oxygen saturation rises rapidly after delivery, to 95% during the first postpartal day. An oxygen debt in the postdelivery period may occur, apparently related to the length and difficulty of the second stage of labor. There is increased resting oxygen consumption during this time, which may also be affected by lactation, anemia, and emotional and psychological factors.

URINARY SYSTEM

The bladder mucosa following delivery shows varying degrees of edema and hyperemia, with diminished bladder tone. This results in decreased sensation to increased pressure, increased capacity, overdistention with overflow incontinence, and incomplete emptying of the bladder. It is important that postpartum nursing care include careful monitoring of the condition of the bladder, as distention and urinary retention are common occurrences and can cause discomfort as well as predispose to infection. With adequate emptying of the bladder, tone is usually restored within 5 to 7 days.

Reversal of the water metabolism of pregnancy results from decreased steroid hormones and the involutional processes of the puerperium. Catabolic processes contribute to increased values for blood urea nitrogen, proteinuria, and, occasionally, acetonuria. Changes in blood volume and hormone levels affect postpartum diuresis, the glomerular filtration rate (GFR), and serum electrolytes.

The GFR remains elevated during the first postpartum week, and combined with increased blood volume, it causes marked diuresis of up to 3000 ml/day for the first 4 to 5 days. Fluid is lost from the body tissues; combined with involutional changes, this contributes to a loss of about 9 lb of weight during the puerperium. Glycosuria occurs about 20% of the time, and proteinuria for 1 to 2 days occurs up to 50% of the time. The ureters and renal pelvis of the kidneys remain dilated after delivery and return to normal in 3 to 6 weeks, although this may occasionally take as long as 8 to 12 weeks. This must be kept in mind in interpreting intravenous pyelography during this time. By 6 weeks' postpartum, the renal plasma flow, GFR, plasma creatinine, and nitrogen usually return to nonpregnant levels.

GASTROINTESTINAL SYSTEM

The motility and tone of the gastrointestinal system usually returns to normal within 2 weeks after delivery. Most women are quite thirsty the first 2 to 3 days, probably because fluids are restricted during labor and because of fluid shifts between interstitial spaces and circulation associated with diuresis. Most women are hungry a short time after delivery and can enjoy a light meal and fluids. After recovery from the fatigue of labor and effects of analgesia and anesthesia, most mothers are have a markedly increased appetite and will eat large portions of food.

Bowel Elimination. Constipation is common during the early postpartum period. This results from the relaxation of the intestines caused by pregnancy (adynamic ileus) and the distended abdominal muscles, which provide less assistance with elimination. These physiological processes are exacerbated by the effects of food and fluid restriction during labor, predelivery enema (if given), and medications used during labor and delivery.

Bowel evacuation may be delayed for 2 to 3 days following delivery. Pain from hemorrhoids, episiotomy, or perineal lacerations, which commonly are present, further deters defecation. Most postpartum women are given stool softeners or laxatives such as docusate sodium (DSS), bisacodyl (Dulcolax), or milk of magnesia to aid elimination. The mother must reestablish regular bowel habits after bowel tone is restored.

Weight Loss. Following delivery, weight loss is about 12 lb and includes the weight of the fetus, placenta, amniotic fluid, and blood loss. Another 9 to 10 lb is lost due to uterine involution, lochia, perspiration, and diuresis during the first postpartum week. The mother's total weight loss related to delivery and postpartum processes is about 22 lb (Table 26-3). Many women gain 30 lb or more during pregnancy, and this additional weight may be retained, especially during lactation.

NEUROMUSCULAR SYSTEMS

After delivery, there is a reversal of neurologic adaptations caused by pregnancy. Discomforts resulting from nerve compression disappear as mechanical pressure from the enlarged uterus and pressure from fluid retention are relieved. Numbness of the thighs due to compression of nerves against the pelvic sidewall or beneath the inguinal ligament during pregnancy improves. Periodic numbness and tingling of the fingers, which affect 5% of pregnant women as a result of brachial plexus traction, are relieved. Elimination of edema and reversal of physiological changes in fascia, tendons, and connective tissue during pregnancy relieve pressure on the median nerve and improve carpal tunnel syndrome (pain, numbness, and tingling in sides of hands and fingers). Depending on their cause, leg cramps may improve after delivery.

Endocrine effects on fibrocartilage during pregnancy are gradually reversed during the postpartum period. The relative relaxation and increased mobility of pelvic articulations are restored to nonpregnant stability by about 6 to 8 weeks after delivery. This often relieves backache characteristic of pregnancy, although a new source of strain from lifting the infant may confound symptomatic improvement. Postural changes caused by the enlarged uterus are reversed, improving lumbar lordosis and compensatory dorsal kyphosis. However, enlarged lactating breasts and weakened abdominal wall muscles may contribute to poor posture after delivery.

INTEGUMENTARY SYSTEM

The increased melanin activity of pregnancy causing hyperpigmentation of nipples, areola, and linea nigra gradually decreases after delivery. Although darker coloration of these areas regresses, color may not return to prepregnant character, and some women have persistent darker pigment. Chloasma (mask of pregnancy) usually improves, although it may not disappear completely.

Vascular effects during pregnancy causing spider angiomas, darker nevi, palmar erythema, and epulis regress as estrogen levels decline rapidly following delivery. Spider angiomas, which occur in 10% to 15% of women, may become permanent although smaller. Increased fine hair distribution seen in pregnancy usually disappears; coarse, bristly hair usually remains. Pruritus associated with hyperestrogen states improves postpartum.

Perspiration. Elimination of waste products through the skin is accelerated in the early puerperium, often to such a degree that the mother is drenched with perspiration. These episodes of profuse sweating, which frequently occur in the night, gradually subside and do not require any specific treatment aside from protecting the mother from chilling when they occur and ensuring adequate skin cleansing.

TEMPERATURE

Slight rises in temperature may occur without apparent cause following the delivery, but, in general, the mother's temperature should remain within normal limits during the puerperium, that is, below 38°C (100.4°F) when taken orally. Any mother whose temperature exceeds this limit in any two consecutive 24-hour periods of the puerperium (excluding the first 24 hours' postpartum) is considered to be febrile.

Occasionally, peak of fever for several hours may be caused by extreme vascular and lymphatic engorgement of the breasts, but this does not last longer than 12 hours.

In judging the significance of a rise in temperature, the pulse rate is a helpful guide because a slow pulse and a slightly elevated temperature are not likely to signify a complication. Any sustained rise in temperature postpartally may indicate endometritis (see Chap. 40).

TABLE 26-3. SOURCES AND AMOUNT OF WEIGHT LOSS DURING THE POSTPARTUM PERIOD

Source of Weight Loss	Amount of Weight Loss	
	Pounds	*Kilograms*
Fetus and placenta; amniotic fluid and blood loss at delivery	12–13	5.5–6
Perspiration and diuresis during the first postpartum week	5–8	2.5–4
Uterine involution and lochia	2–3	1
Total weight loss	19–24	9–10

∎ REFERENCES

1. Cunninghan F, MacDonald PC, Gant NF, et al: Williams' Obstetrics, 18th ed. Norwalk, CT, Appleton & Lange, 1989

2. Oppenheimer L, et al: The duration of lochia. Br J Obstet Gynaecol 93(7):754–757, July 1986
3. Monheit AG, Cousins L, Resnik R: The puerperium: Anatomic and physiologic readjustments. Clin Obstet Gynecol 23(4):973–984, December 1980
4. Willson R: The puerperium. In Willson JR, Carrington ER, (eds): Obstetrics and Gynecology, 8th ed. St. Louis, CV Mosby, 1987
5. Abraham S, Child A, Ferry J, et al: Recovery after childbirth: A preliminary prospective study. Med J Aust 152:9–12, 1990
6. Sampselle CM, Brink CA: Pelvic muscle relaxation: Assessment and management. J Nurs Midwif 35:127–132, 1990
7. Dougherty MC, Bishop K, Abrams R, et al: The effect of exercise on the circumvaginal muscles in postpartum women. J Nurs Midwif 34:8–14, 1989
8. Kegel A: Progressive resistance exercise in the functional restoration of the perineal muscles. Am J Obstet Gynecol 56:238–258, 1956
9. Burgio K, Robinson J, Engel B: The role of biofeedback in Kegel exercise training for stress urinary incontinence. Am J Obstet Gynecol 154:58–64, 1986
10. Burns P, Marecki M, Dittmar S, et al: Kegel's exercises with biofeedback therapy in treatment of stress incontinence. Nurse Pract 10:28–34, 1985
11. Resnick R: The puerperium. In Creasey R, Resnick R: Maternal-Fetal Medicine: Principles and Practice, 2nd ed. Philadelphia, WB Saunders, 1989
12. Laros RK: Physiology of normal pregnancy. In Willson JR, Carrington ER (eds): Obstetrics and Gynecology, 8th ed. St. Louis, CV Mosby, 1987
13. Robson S, et al: Haemodynamic changes during the early puerperium. Br Med J 294:106, 1987
14. Easterling W, Herbert W: The puerperium. In Danforth D, Scott J: Obstetrics and Gynecology, 5th ed. Philadelphia, JB Lippincott, 1986

■ SUGGESTED READING

Gordon H, Logue M: Perineal muscle function after childbirth. Lancet 11:123–125, 1985
Jacobson H: A standard for assessing lochia volume. MCN 10(3):174, 1985
Longo LD, Hardesty JS: Maternal blood volume: Measurement, hypothesis of control, and clinical considerations. Rev Perinat Med 5:35–59, 1984
McKey PL, Dougherty MC: The circumvaginal musculature: The correlation between pressure and physical assessment. Nurs Res 35:307–309, 1986
Metheny NM: Fluid Balance. Philadelphia, JB Lippincott, 1984
Moise KJ, Cotton DB: Colloid osmotic pressure and pregnancy. In Clark SL, Phelan JP, Cotton DB (eds): Critical Care Obstetrics. Oradell, NJ, Medical Economics Books, 1987
Tilkian SM: Clinical Implications of Laboratory Tests, 3rd ed. St. Louis, CV Mosby, 1983
Tulman L, Fawcett J, et al: Changes in of functional status after childbirth. Nurs Res 39(2):70–75, 1990

27

Psychosocial Aspects of the Postpartum Period

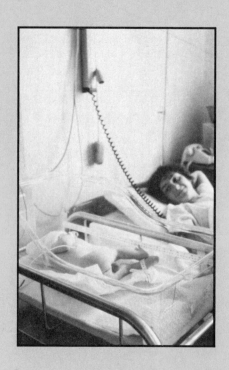

In discussing the psychosocial aspects of pregnancy in Chapter 16, we made the point that pregnancy and parenthood can be thought of as a role transition. We noted the tremendous change that comes with childbirth and the assumption of the new role together with the concomitant instability that can occur until new roles are allocated and the new member is integrated. In this chapter, we continue our exploration of the psychosocial needs of the new, expanding responsibilities of the parents.

■ PARENTHOOD: A CONTINUING PROCESS OF TRANSITION

Assumptions About Parenthood

The present discussion is based on the underlying assumption that the degree of ease and satisfaction with which people make the transition to parenthood depends mostly on how successfully they have defined and accepted their relationship with each other. If they have developed an ability to see each other as they are (not as they ought to be) and if they can allow for divergence of values and behaviors, work collaboratively toward a flexible power base for each, and develop norms that allow for mutual growth, then they are more likely to move smoothly into the new role.[1] The student will remember that we view the transition to parenthood as a process, rather than a state, that begins in pregnancy and flowers with the assumption of parental responsibilities.

This assumption is identified specifically here because much of the literature on parenting, particularly the early writings that relied heavily on a psychoanalytical orientation, singles out either the content of the parent-child relationship, per se, or the parents' own childhood relationships as the primary determinants of the family s progression through this phase. This neglects three other vital areas: (1) the needs of each person within the system as an individual; (2) the needs of the

parents as a couple; and (3) the influence of the couple's (and the infant's) interaction over time. Use of these assumptions does not negate the importance of the parent-child relationship or the parents' own background, but it does provide some focus on the marital couple as an entity. In reality, it is the balancing of the three areas of needs within the family that is the ultimate task of the new family. Moreover, it is these areas that the nurse must be aware of and respect when working with families undergoing the transition to parenthood.[2,3]

Role Supplementation and Role Mastery

One integrative conceptual framework for the care and support of couples experiencing role transition to parenthood is role supplementation.[4,5] By using this framework, health providers can help the parents and their significant others gain the necessary information or experience to bring them to a full awareness of the anticipated behavior patterns, sensations, and goals involved in the complementary roles of mother and father. In essence, this approach assists the parents-to-be in moving to role mastery of parenthood. The student will recall that we said previously that pregnancy is the anticipatory phase of the transition to parenthood. The impending role must be at least partly rehearsed, modeled, and clarified through a process of communication with significant others. In so doing, the role expectations become clearer and the couple begin to put themselves into the role of parents (role take). As this is done, there is a better "fit" to the impending role, with increased confidence leading to role mastery. A schematic drawing of the role mastery process is shown in Figure 27-1. Ideally, this process should be begun during pregnancy. A similar modified process, however, can be instituted or reinforced in the important early postpartum period by the nurse.

■ OTHER CONCEPTUALIZATIONS OF PARENTHOOD

Parenthood as a Negative Change in the Quality of Life

La Rossa and La Rossa[2] and others[6] have pointed out that the majority of the studies on the assumption of the parenting role focus on how the quality of personal or marital life changes after the birth of a child. More-

---

Vital Areas in the Transition to Parenthood

- The needs of each person in the system as an individual
- The needs of the parents as a couple
- The influence of parent-child interaction over time

Research Highlight

Research has suggested that stress is associated with family dysfunction, appearing to have an impact on parenting behaviors. Concern about the potential long-term effects of antepartal stress on family functioning led Mercer and Ferketich to test a theoretical, causal model explaining family functioning. High- and low-risk mothers and fathers during pregnancy; early postpartum; and 1-, 4-, and 8-months following birth were examined.

The 593 subjects consisted of 153 high-risk women (HRW), 75 male partners of HRW (HRM), 218 low-risk women (LRW), and 147 male partners of the LRW (LRM). All HRW were hospitalized during the 24th to 34th weeks of pregnancy. There were no perceived differences in family functioning at 8 months after birth between risk groups, however LRW viewed family functioning less optimally than LRM. Conclusions while testing the theoretical model were not predictive as hypothesized, resulting in respecification of the model. Final results in HRW suggested that less depression, greater perceived support, less stress from negative life events during early parenthood, being married, younger age, and more close friends were associated with optimal family functioning. LRW differed from the HRW by implying that poorer health perception and lower parent–infant attachment were associated with more optimal family functioning. Analyses for men showed the HRW's pregnancy risk had long-term direct effects on family functioning; while the LRM perceived support after birth, medical treatment during pregnancy, and relationship with their fathers had direct effects on family functioning.

Nurses must be aware that high- and low-risk pregnancies may have less than optimal family functioning. Incorporation of the infant into the family may be more difficult than expected, leading to an increased risk of child abuse. Assessment for depression, health perception, parent–infant attachment, negative life events, and social support can assist the nurse in identifying the families at greater risk for family dysfunction. Counseling concerning incorporation of the infant into the family should include all expectant families. Referrals for follow-up visits should be incorporated to include high- and low-risk families to ensure optimal family functioning.

Mercer RT, Ferketich SL: Predictors of family functioning eight months following birth. Nurs Research 39(2):76–82, March/April 1990

over, these studies tend to perceive and define quality of life in individualistic terms. An individualistic measure of the quality of life focuses on the degree to which a person succeeds in accomplishing his or her desires and goals despite the constraints of a variety of forces, including an indifferent or hostile nature and the social order.[2,7] An individualistic measure of health care, for instance, would focus on how personally inconvenienced a mother might feel who has to be hospitalized periodically for diabetes during her pregnancy. The less the inconvenience, the better the health care. This formulation suffers from three major flaws. First, the individualistic approach stresses attitudes at the expense of behavior; thus, interaction patterns are often ignored altogether. Second, the approach looks at the variable under study (e.g., health, parenthood) as a "status" rather than a process and therefore fails to consider the reciprocal relationship between it and other aspects of the persons' lives. Third, the individualistic approach is laden with administrative bias that dictates that researchers be more concerned with bureaucratic efficiency: if complaints can be reduced, then the best goal has been achieved.[2,8]

Parenthood as Crises Versus Transition

Probably the best-known series of studies on the assumption of the parenting role is the "parenthood as crises" series. This line of research began with the Le Masters article in 1957 and continued with Dyer, Russell, and the various reports of Hobbs and his colleagues.[9-15] The principal question that these studies pursued has been: To what extent does becoming a parent constitute a "crisis?" It was assumed that this life change constituted a crisis, i.e., extreme negative change. With the exception of the Le Masters and Dyer articles, the only criterion for answering this question has been a 23-item checklist originally developed by Hobbs.[2,12-15] Moreover, the checklist did not focus on the patterns (or changed patterns) of interaction between the couple; rather it stressed the coping ability of the parents. For instance, the parents were not asked if there was an interruption of routine, a change in their sex life and sleeping patterns, and the like. Instead, they were asked to indicate whether each item in the checklist bothered

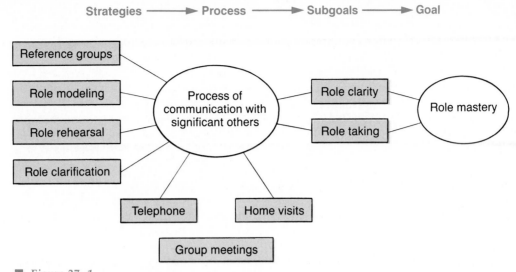

■ *Figure 27–1*
Conceptual framework of preventive role supplementation leading to role mastery. (After Swendsen LA, Meleis A, Jones D: Role supplementation for new parents: A role mastery plan. MCN 3(2):84–91, March/April 1978)

them by choosing from three choices: "not at all," "somewhat," and "very much." Thus, it was difficult to determine from these types of answers whether or not there were changes in the couple's interactions. For example, in response to the item, "decreased sexual responsiveness of spouse," if marked "not at all," one would not know whether there had been change in the couple's sexual pattern or whether they simply were not bothered by such a change. From an individualistic standpoint, those using the checklist have been interested in how well their subjects were doing in spite of the *assumed* crisis brought on by the constraints of parenthood.[2] As early as 1969, Jacoby called attention to the conceptual limitations of this formulation by pointing out that this body of research allowed little opportunity or stimulus for the reporting of affectively positive (or neutral) attitudes toward the adjustments required by parenthood.[16] In addition, there was no attempt to delineate any behavioral changes as distinct from attitudes that might accompany the behavioral changes. Interestingly, his critique appeared not to be taken seriously, and this criticism obtains today when researchers continue this line of investigation.

We have already pointed out the many methodological problems inherent in this research, namely, small, skewed samples and the lack of sophisticated analyses. Although this body of research has grave limitations and is essentially nonvalid, it is important to remember that it was "pioneering" in a sense. Current difficulties arise when health providers accept these studies uncritically and proceed on the faulty assumption that parenthood for everyone is a time of crisis or extreme stress.

In future research, there needs to be greater attention to determining the social processes and patterns involved in the transition and a teasing out of attitudes toward the phenomena as opposed to behavior associated with the transition. The importance of social networks and supports, the input of the infant, including temperament, how couples define their stressors and resources, and how they communicate and modify their existing social roles are all important aspects to be considered.

■ TRANSITION TO PARENTHOOD

We used Rossi's formulation of phases in the process of role transition. Specifically, these were the anticipatory phase, the honeymoon phase, the plateau phase, and the disengagement phase (see Chap. 16).[17] In the puerperium, it is the honeymoon phase of the transition that has the most bearing on the nursing care that the maternity nurse must render. We shall also review briefly the anticipatory phase, however, because we previously focused primarily on its relevance to pregnancy rather than to parenthood (see Nursing Care Plan: Couples in Transition to Parenthood).

Anticipatory Phase

Pregnancy is an anticipatory stage to becoming a parent, and parents need to accomplish certain tasks during this time. We already discussed decision making and expectations that influence later parenting. Another important aspect is the division of labor in the family. This becomes extremely crucial when the baby arrives. Observing how the mundane activities of family maintenance are carried out often indicates how well the parents accept their changing roles. This also gives a clue as to what role assignments the child may later assume in the family. The nurse should note whether there is any negotiation or flexibility between the couple in allocating and sharing of tasks. If one partner unilaterally appoints the other to manage a responsibility or if there is a rigid conceptions of "his work" and "her work," there may be subtle sabotage or task overload as responsibilities mount with the addition of the infant.[2,3,7] Thus, how the family uses the time of pregnancy to work out or rework their division of labor in the family has a large impact on their transition.

Couples in the anticipatory phase experience many intense feelings, challenges, and responsibilities. If used correctly, this can be an opportune time to test skills in preparing to accept and integrate the new family member into the system. The nurse can be helpful in aiding the couple to examine and understand what they are experiencing by providing accurate information and feedback of perceptions and offering validation of the dynamics that are emerging.[3,7]

Honeymoon Phase

The *honeymoon phase* refers to the postchildbirth period during which an attachment between the parents and child is achieved through prolonged contact and intimacy.[17] This is a "psychic honeymoon" and not necessarily a time of romanticized peace and joy. Rather, it is an intense period when both the mother and the father explore their new family member and their relationships to the infant, who, in turn, is working out a complicated communication system with the parents so that his or her survival is assured. The couple's personal relationship is no less important, but most of their energies at this time are focused on developing the new relationship with the infant.

RECIPROCAL INTERACTION

With newer technology and more sophisticated research on brain physiology as well as infant behavior, we have come to recognize the amazing talents the newborn possesses for capturing the attention of the parents and holding them in real communicative interaction.[18]

We now know that the child learns to organize in response to positive stimuli and experiences. Overstimulation and noncontingent care (care that is not synchronized with the infant's responses) hinders both the organization of the infant's central nervous system and development of a positive parent-infant interaction.[7,18,19] Parents should be cautioned to avoid trying to do things strictly "by the book" or by schedules organized to expedite routines and procedures. Care for the newborn needs to be timed to the infant's activity and responses, not to preordained schedules.[7,19,20-22]

Neonates have a repertoire of adaptive responses that enable them to survive and to capture the attention of the important adults around them. Research shows that newborns demonstrate a marked ability to habituate to different visual, auditory, and seminoxious stimuli. Research also shows there are definite auditory and visual orienting responses. For example, if one talks and begins to play with the baby, the infant responds by becoming alert and searching for a face (Fig. 27-2). When he finds it, he softens, and as long as the face moves, the infant follows it. If it becomes still, however, the infant frowns and turns away.

Responses to auditory stimuli also demonstrate the ability of the neonate to make choices. It has been shown that when a man and woman stand on opposite sides of the baby and begin to talk, the infant will stop moving, his face knits, and he turns toward the female's voice again and again. When presented with a nonhuman sound, babies who are sucking will stop, then quickly resume; on hearing a human sound, infants will stop sucking and then resume with a complex sucking pattern that researchers believe indicates a preference for the human sound. Infants' ability to control and console themselves by such behaviors are powerful reinforcers for parents who are ready to move beyond the initial bonding and continue their attachment.[18,19-22] See Chapter 31 for a more detailed discussion of the newborn's abilities.

BONDING AND ATTACHMENT

Three major theoretical perspectives have contributed to attachment theory: psychoanalytical, ethological, and learning theory. Psychoanalytical theory postulates that attachment arises from instinctual drives and object relations. From the ethological standpoint, attachment consists of specific behaviors such as imprinting, clinging when afraid, crying, and the like, which promote proximity in humans. Learning theorists claim that attachment is formed through secondary drives when the mother meets the needs of the infant and the infant, in turn, associates need satisfaction with her.

In the 1970s, the concept of the "fourth stage of labor" developed. This time immediately after delivery was thought to be optimal for close contact between parents and child to initiate the process of bonding the trio together. Currently, the terms *bonding* and *attachment* are often used interchangeably to describe this process of parent-child affiliation.[23] Some believe there

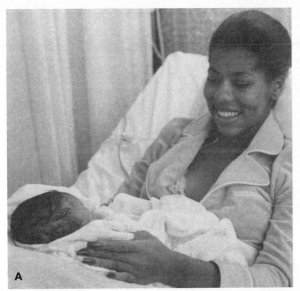

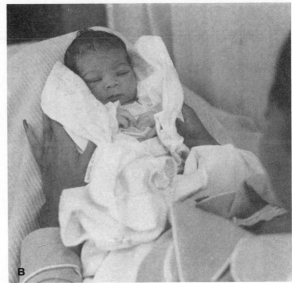

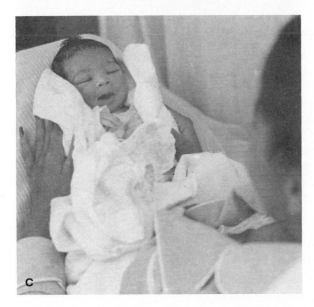

■ *Figure 27-2*
(A) An infant responds to an animated smiling face. (B) The infant establishes eye contact with the mother. (C) The infant begins to move his mouth as the mother smiles and talks.

is a distinction between the terms and define *bonding* as the initial attraction and desire to get to know another person and *attachment* as the long, hard work of *staying in love.*[18] Thus, bonding can be thought of as the initial step in a process in which the mutual attractiveness and response between parents and child develops and paves the way for the later development of love and affiliation.

Factors Associated With Attachment. Research has shed much light on the fascinating subject of how infants and parents first develop their acquaintance.[23,24] Although much of the early findings were hampered by small, self-selected samples and many of the studies have undergone considerable revision over time,[23–26] the initial research efforts did result in a much more flexible management of parental interaction during and after labor.

Although we still do not have definitive answers and some of the information must still be considered tentative, we do know there are several important factors associated with the process of attachment.[29] They are explained in the box below.

Health care providers should be cautious in advising patients so as not to instill feelings of guilt in parents if they cannot or do not participate in the birth process and if they do not immediately bond with the infant. This attachment process varies from situation to situation and from culture to culture. The nurse must remember that attachment is a process—just as is the development of the parental role. It does not occur instantaneously at birth.[29] This process takes time and can be impeded or facilitated by a variety of variables, some of which are discussed in the box, Factors Associated With Attachment. As the research continues in this area, perhaps we will learn more about factors influencing this bonding process.

■ ASSUMPTION OF THE PARENTAL ROLE

The honeymoon phase continues as the parents continue in their transition. Certain behaviors become apparent. It is important to note that there is much more information on maternal behavior than on paternal be-

havior. Again, as with attachment principles, these observations and findings are not to be considered definitive.

Paternal Behavior

Although most researchers agree that more studies need to be done regarding paternal behavior, we are still in the early stages of this type of research. Early research in the 1970s concluded that there was no significant behavioral difference between fathers alone with their infants and mothers alone with their infant, but if the trio were together, the father tended to hold, touch, and vocalize more than the mother but smile significantly less. These and more recent findings established that the father plays a far more active role than the passive cultural stereotype suggests.[30–33]

CATALYSTS IN THE ATTACHMENT PROCESS

Jordan[34] has delineated several experiences both during pregnancy and after the birth ("reality boosters") that serve as catalysts to aid the father in his attachment to his infant and his transition to fatherhood (see box: Experiences That Aid the Father in Attachment).

Fathers must work at the business of attachment. Grappling with the reality of the pregnancy and the child is central. The child becomes more real as the pregnancy progresses and through the first months' postpartum. Like the mother, the father needs hands-on contact and interaction with the infant during the first days and months to feel that the child is "real" and theirs. Fathers must make strong efforts to become involved in both the childbearing experience and in "fathering" to overcome society's obstacles that have previously excluded fathers from this process.

Recent research shows that, in most instances, fathers bond to their offspring and are highly sensitive to their infants' signals.[33,34] Fathers' responses after birth include perceiving the newborn as attractive, having a desire to hold and touch the newborn, and a tendency to focus attention on the newborn. Observations of the father's behaviors with their newborns have documented a high degree of verbal and nonverbal interaction in the first several postnatal days.[32-35]

The term *engrossment* has been used by Greenberg and Morris to describe the behavior pattern noted in

---

Maternal Tasks According to Rubin

- Identifying the new child
- Determining one's relationship to the child
- Guiding and reconstructing the family constellation to include a new member

---

fathers when they are involved and interacting with their newborn. This refers to the absorption of the father in the interaction[35] (Fig. 27-3). Jones and Thomas, in a study monitoring cardiovascular changes in the father during engrossed infant interaction, found that fathers appeared highly sensitive to the stimuli of interacting

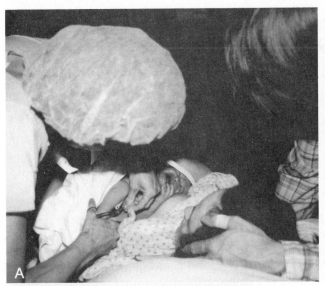

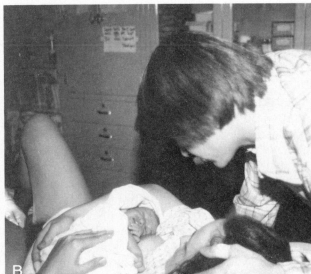

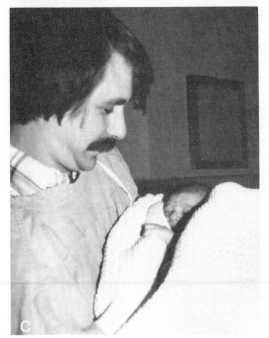

■ *Figure 27–3*
Parents should be given the opportunity to hold the infant soon after birth. (A) The naked newborn is placed on the mother's abdomen while the midwife cuts the cord. (B) Wrapped with a blanket for warmth, the newborn remains on the mother's abdomen while the placenta is delivered, and the parents can begin their bonding. (C) After the baby has had its initial assessment, the father holds the baby. (Courtesy of Booth Maternity Center, Philadelphia)

with their newborns and responded in a complex manner to infant signals. They conclude that there may be an autonomic balance that is situationally specific and may be predictive of parental response just as other psychosocial measures are.[33]

CONTROVERSIES ABOUT PATERNAL BONDING

Some controversy exists as to whether maternal and paternal attachment behaviors should be considered separately or as "parental" behaviors. Similarities have been found between paternal and maternal interaction behaviors.[32,33,35] As research accrues, however, it appears that differences as well as similarities continue to be noted.[32,34] Rather than being compelled to define categories or list behaviors, it is appropriate to acknowledge these similarities and differences and design research to determine under what conditions they might pertain, particularly as society moves toward a more flexible masculine-feminine role definition.

Maternal Behavior

A pioneer in delineating maternal behavior was Reva Rubin, who focused on the mother and identified various phases of maternal behavior, particularly relating to maternal touch and the infant. She contended that mothering is composed of a set of interpersonal and production skills designed to foster the emotional, intellectual, and physical development of the child.[36] Rubin's tasks of mothering are described below. Although subsequent research has called into question the rigor of her methodology and her sample size as well as her findings regarding touch and the time of its progression, her basic thesis regarding the mothering tasks is still relevant.[36-38]

Subsequent researchers have attributed the changes in observed maternal behavior to a changed philosophy surrounding maternity care and to changed hospital practices that involve the mother and parents in the infant's care immediately, as well as to much shorter hospital stays. For instance, the slower progression of touch and the extreme dependency of the "taking in phase" as described by Rubin are seen to be telescoped in modern hospitals.[37-39] The student is referred to the classic maternal behavior articles by Rubin noted in the Suggested Reading list.

MATERNAL ROLE ATTAINMENT

There still remains a progression in the mother-infant interactions that facilitates bonding and attachment and leads ultimately to what Mercer had called "maternal role attainment." In Mercer's formulation, maternal role attainment is a process that occurs over a 3- to 10-month period and that includes attachment to the infant through identifying, claiming, and interacting with him or her, thereby gaining gratification and competence in mothering behaviors and mother-infant interactions. Mercer also suggests that maternal attachment and adaptation may be delayed or hampered if the woman's health status is less than optimal because of chronic illness and complications from childbirth.[28]

Mother-infant interactions tend to be of a progressive nature but are less structured than previously described. Also, the surroundings can facilitate (or impede) interactions. In an environment where free interaction, holding, and nursing can proceed without restraint, the fingertip to enfolding progression of touch proceeds quickly as do the eye-to-eye contact and other interactive activities.

PHASES OF MATERNAL ROLE ATTAINMENT

In what is called an *introductory and acquaintance phase*, touching activities begin. Fingertip exploration, palmar contact, and gradual enfolding of the infant are all noted. This may take minutes to hours (or even days if delay is experienced) depending on ease of interaction, physical proximity, clothing constraints, and physical condition of the mother and infant. Culture and ethnic variations can also be noted. When the mother holds her infant, she will move him around until she has eye contact and can see him face to face (en face position; Fig. 27-4).

She also uses her other senses, sight, smell, and hearing, to become acquainted and identify her infant.[40] Studies have found that the mother can distinguish her infant's odor, and this aids in the claiming process. The mother's emotions play a part as well as she begins to identify and incorporate similarities and dissimilarities of the infant to her husband, herself, and family.[41]

As she becomes more acquainted with her infant, she first identifies him as her own and is interested in clarifying her emerging feelings for the infant. She then relates the infant's appearance and behavior to people and things that have meaning for her and are familiar. Finally, she interprets what the behavior and characteristics mean and will mean. She may anticipate that the curly hair will be wonderful for her girlchild or that the infant's immediate rooting for food portends a hearty, robust nature.

As attachment progresses, a *mutual regulation and reciprocity phase* can be seen. The infant and the mother develop a cuing system, which hopefully results in both the infant's and mother's needs being met. The mother must become sensitive to the infant's states, and the infant must learn to send out signals and cues that can

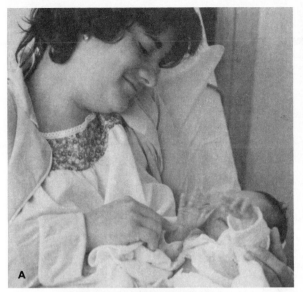

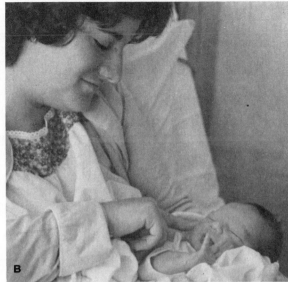

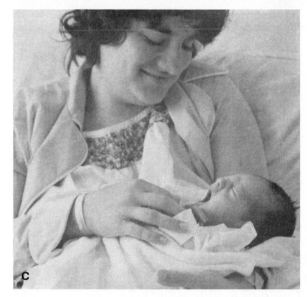

■ *Figure 27–4*
Identification process through maternal touch. (A) Exploring the infant with fingertip touch. (B) The mother continues her exploration, progressing to the infant's face. (C) The baby is finally enfolded by the mother.

be interpreted by the mother. It is during this time of mutual adjustment that negative feelings may surface in the mother. She may feel that the infant is too demanding and his or her cues not readable. Mutual regulation is never instantaneous and continues through infancy and, to some degree, childhood. If the mother's feelings are denied by health providers and family, the mother will feel inadequate and guilty, which will only intensify the negative feelings. The nurses's support during this time in acknowledging that these feelings are natural can be a great encouragement to the mother-infant interaction.[42]

Researchers have described the concept of *reciprocity* as interactional cycles that occur simultaneously between the mother and infant that are rhythmic and form the basis for communication. Several phases in the reciprocal–interactional cycles have been delineated.[18,42] They are summarized in Figure 27-5.

POSTPARTUM BLUES AND DEPRESSION

As can be seen from the changes and stressors that accompany the birth process, the transition to parenthood can be a stressful time for the parents, particularly the mother. She is dealing not only with a role change but also with her body's return to a prepregnant state, with all of the attendant physiological and hormonal changes. Thus, in the early postpartum period, for no apparent reason (the mother thinks) she may experience a let-down feeling accompanied by irritability, tears, and

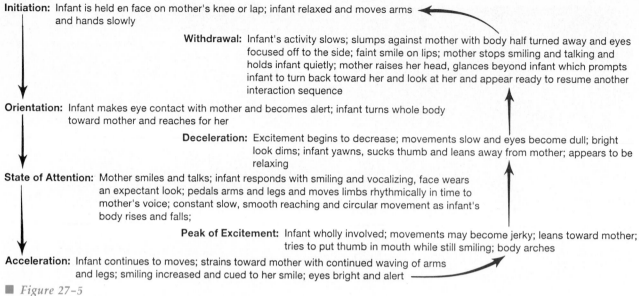

Initiation: Infant is held en face on mother's knee or lap; infant relaxed and moves arms and hands slowly

Withdrawal: Infant's activity slows; slumps against mother with body half turned away and eyes focused off to the side; faint smile on lips; mother stops smiling and talking and holds infant quietly; mother raises her head, glances beyond infant which prompts infant to turn back toward her and look at her and appear ready to resume another interaction sequence

Orientation: Infant makes eye contact with mother and becomes alert; infant turns whole body toward mother and reaches for her

Deceleration: Excitement begins to decrease; movements slow and eyes become dull; bright look dims; infant yawns, sucks thumb and leans away from mother; appears to be relaxing

State of Attention: Mother smiles and talks; infant responds with smiling and vocalizing, face wears an expectant look; pedals arms and legs and moves limbs rhythmically in time to mother's voice; constant slow, smooth reaching and circular movement as infant's body rises and falls;

Peak of Excitement: Infant wholly involved; movements may become jerky; leans toward mother; tries to put thumb in mouth while still smiling; body arches

Acceleration: Infant continues to moves; strains toward mother with continued waving of arms and legs; smiling increased and cued to her smile; eyes bright and alert

■ *Figure 27–5*
Phases in establishing maternal–infant reciprocity.

feelings of inadequacy. Occasionally, her appetite and sleep are disturbed. These symptoms are manifestations of the "baby or maternity blues" and are generally temporary. They are thought to be related in part to the physiological and hormonal changes as well as the other ego and social adjustments that accompany this crucial role transition. Discomfort, fatigue, and exhaustion certainly contribute largely to this condition. Crying often relieves the tension, and rest and support are extremely important. Anticipatory guidance and support by the nurse are important in helping the parents understand this condition as transitory.[43]

Occasionally, the woman experiences a true postpartum depression, which may begin in the first weeks after delivery and persist for months. The mother feels extremely fatigued (even with rest) inadequate, unable to cope, and gradually withdraws. This state may progress to a frank psychosis. The symptoms mentioned above are exacerbated and prolonged. Diagnosis and treatment are important, and the nurse should be watchful and refer the mother if symptoms persist.[43] This condition and its care are discussed more fully in Chapter 28.

Plateau and Disengagement Phases

We would note that the perinatal nurse does not often have the opportunity to observe the couple in the plateau phase of the transition to parenthood. The student will recall this is the protracted middle period of a role cycle in which the role is fully exercised and the parents validate themselves as competent or not, depending on how well they and others perceive their parenting efforts.[17] Similarly, unless there is a perinatal or infant death, the disengagement–termination phase of the role cycle is not seen by the hospital-based maternity provider.

■ INFLUENCES ON PARENTAL BEHAVIOR

Once again, it is important to note that new parents face a major decision regarding the enactment of their sex roles in addition to the myriad of other large and small decisions they must make. For instance, will the woman assume the more traditional role of total homemaker-mother or will she attempt to combine a career with parenthood? Similarly, will the father extend his role to active involvement in homemaking and childrearing or choose the traditional "breadwinner" role (Fig. 27-6)? The choice of either nontraditional parental role is accompanied by a certain amount of stress. There is little support for either mother or father from employers, and there may be little support from significant others. On the other hand, assuming the traditional parental roles can also be stressful because this course of action may be thwarting the potential and actualization of the parents. Researchers have found that, in the case of fathers' adjustment to parenthood, it does not matter so much whether they choose a traditional fathering role or nontraditional fathering role but rather whether they assume the role in a consistent and coherent manner.[44,45] As more research is done on this fascinating topic, we should gain more insight into how we can better help the family make the parental role transition more smoothly.

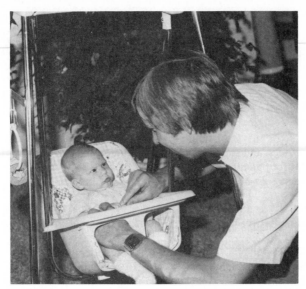

■ *Figure 27–6*
Fathering. Paternal involvement is engrossing and can be satisfying to everyone.

■ APPLYING THE NURSING PROCESS TO THE DEVELOPING FAMILY

Assessment and Nursing Diagnosis

Assessment and nursing diagnosis are based on careful observation and interviewing. Nurses will want to keep in mind that they are assisting with role supplementation that will lead to role mastery in the parents (see Fig. 27-1). Nurses can enhance the communication process with themselves and the parents' significant others by assessing and clarifying questions, concerns, and issues with them and encouraging them to use knowledgeable persons in their networks. Apprising them of the availability of parenting support groups and the telephone for information purposes (hot lines and so forth) as well as arranging home visits will also contribute to role supplementation.

The nurse may find that knowledge deficit may be a primary diagnosis for the parents. Learning needs can be determined by assessing the following areas: expectations of children's performance ability, lags in developmental task fulfillment, social isolation, immobilization due to role overload, and ability to set limits and carry them out. When these learning needs are diagnosed, the nurse can develop a teaching plan aimed at preventing and alleviating problems in these areas. Strengths of the couple should always be delineated and worked with. When deficits are found, verbal and behavioral skills can be developed to cope with the problem. If the deficit is related to outside institutions,

the nurse will want to be aware of community institutions and agencies to which she can refer the parents.[40] The student is referred to the inserts for additional areas of assessment, diagnoses, and intervention.

Planning and Intervention

Intervention with the parents begins immediately in the early postpartum hours. The nurse, during both the immediate and the later postpartum period, can be helpful to parents and facilitate bonding by pointing out and reinforcing parents' perceptions of their infant's ability to interact with them. One reinforcer to attachment that can be shown to the mother and father is the manner of consoling the baby. When a baby is crying, even at the top of his voice, he can be quieted by insistently saying "baby, baby, baby." Simply by using the voice, one can get the infant to turn his head, put his fist in his mouth, and start looking for the speaker.

Another key element of nursing intervention with the expanding family is the teaching of parenting skills that promote the child's maturity, autonomy, and competence. If the parents have a realistic conception of the infant's needs and their resources, they need not expend all their energy on their parenting responsibilities at the expense of their own personal needs and growth.

Nursing's involvement in the recent trend toward health maintenance and promotion has set the stage for classes that include information and skill development needed after the infant is born. Teaching styles and format for parenting classes resemble those in prenatal instruction. Nurses will want to be aware of what is available in their institution and/or the community so that they may make referrals when appropriate.

It is impossible to teach all of the skills necessary to parenting. If nurses can help parents sort out problems, examine options and resources, and negotiate outcomes, however, they have accomplished a great deal and have been instrumental in this momentous role transition.

Evaluation

Nurses will know whether their nursing interventions have been successful if the mother and father verbalize their questions and concerns and indicate appropriate methods for solution. If they indicate realistic expectations for themselves and their infants, manage their time successfully, and enlarge, maintain, and use their social supports, nurses will know that the role transition is proceeding in a healthy manner. A care plan for dealing with learning needs during this transition is presented earlier in the chapter.

Assessment and Management in the Postpartum Period

POSTI

PE:

Initial a
process
of bleed
neum (s
Physiol
that it r
serves t
is
pad and
taken to
function
matom;
observa
hour af
the first
Her
immedi
the uter
Pulse ra
by low

Ob
ian
per
of
mc
an
is
ble
de
an

be
pe:
tur
are
W
ou

of
the
na
of
an
to
siz

Nu

Are

Vita
T
P
B
R

Invc
U
L

Abc

Peri

Brea
C
N
L

Legs

Elim
V
D

Disc

Ene

App

Emc

TABLE 28-4. POSTPARTUM RISK FACTORS

Risk factor	Complication	Assessment Data
Uterine overdistention	Hemorrhage	Fundus boggy, atonic; excessive bleeding; low blood pressure; high pulse
Prolonged labor	Infection, dehydration	Fever, high pulse
Lacerations or episiotomy	Hemorrhage	Excessive bleeding, low blood pressure, high pulse
	Infection	Fever, high pulse, redness, edema
	Hematoma	Swelling, ecchymosis pain, dark mass
Premature rupture of membranes	Infection (endometritis)	Fever, high pulse, subinvolution
Prolonged second stage of labor	Thrombophlebitis	Unilateral calf pain, swelling, redness, Homan's positive
	Impaired urination (trigone edema)	Unable to void, small voiding, distended bladder
Retained placental fragments	Delayed hemorrhage	Fresh red lochia, low blood pressure, high pulse
Breastfeeding	Infection (mastitis)	Nipples red, sore; breasts hot, red, tender

Reaction to Childbirth Process. Most women have a need to review the birth experience.[9] This allows them to integrate the experience and serves as a method of critical self-evaluation that is part of an important psychological task of the postpartum period. The woman's perceptions of the fit between her actual and expected or desired intrapartal behaviors provide indications of positive self-regard or potential problems in self-esteem. Embarrassment, apologies for behaviors, and feelings of failure may be expressed and serve as cues to decreased self-esteem.

Adaptations to Parenting and Caretaking. A number of maternal behaviors can be observed that indicate adaptive responses to the infant and caretaking responsibilities (see Chap. 27 for approaches to assessment). New mothers who are relatively inexperienced may encounter some difficulties in caretaking due to knowledge and experience deficits. With practice, their abilities improve and their self-esteem increases, supporting a positive emotional response to the baby.

Parents with significant life stresses, socioeconomic difficulties, health problems, and pregnancy-related complications may not adapt as effectively to parenting. Maladaptive behavior occurs when parents respond in-effectively or inappropriately to their infant's needs. Those who have not developed a sense of self-competence and feel little personal control in their lives often experience parenting difficulties.[10]

Fathers also will exhibit adaptive or maladaptive responses to parenthood. Many of the same behaviors can be assessed to determine the level of paternal adaptation. The effects of different cultural practices on the paternal and maternal roles must be considered (see Cultural Beliefs and Practices in the Postpartum Period).

Cultural Variations. Ethnic and cultural beliefs and practices influence parenting behaviors during the postpartum period (see Chap. 6). The model of illness as resulting from body imbalances is common in non-Western cultures. Balance may be perceived in terms of energy flows, hot and cold, or yin and yang (feminine-receptive–masculine-active principles). The postpartum woman is perceived to be in a state of imbalance and is vulnerable to illness unless she follows specific practices usually related to rest and seclusion, avoidance of cold, and diet[11-15] (see Cultural Beliefs and Practices in the Postpartum Period).

Cultural practices may restrict the father's role in childbirth and postpartal experiences and may establish

Nursing Guidelines: Postpartum Catheteriza[...]

Nursing Intervention

Explain procedure and rationale, reassure about gentleness.

Have equipment positioned, put sterile gloves on.

Inform of each step in procedure, encourage deep breathing.

Provide perineal care.

Gently separate vulva, cleanse vestibule.

Place sterile cotton ball in introitus.

Exposing urinary meatus, gently insert small-gauge flexible catheter until urine flows.

If bladder markedly distended, pinch catheter after each 300 ml, wait 10–15 sec, then allow flow to continue.

Withdraw catheter or inflate baloon if indwelling.

Replace perineal pad, help client reposition.

Measure amount of urine, note color and character, record, send specimen to laboratory if ordered.

Remove gloves, discard bloody items in containers according to agency protocol.

Medication. Anesthetic sprays, ointments, or witch hazel pads (Tucks) may be applied directly to sutured areas on the perineum. These relieve pain and promote comfort. Analgesic medications are sometimes needed when pain is severe. Women with extensive perineal repair may need medication every 4 hours for the first 1 or 2 postpartum days. If medications are needed, they should be given about 30 to 40 minutes before the infant's feeding period. This relieves the mother's pain and allows her to concentrate her energies and attention on the infant.

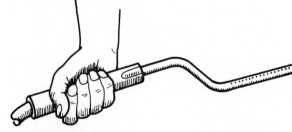

■ *Figure 28–6*
Surgitator for perineal care. With client seated on toilet, hold nozzle several inches from perineum, start flow, and direct against perineum. Do not touch nozzle to perineum; use a new nozzle for each client. Dry perineum with gentle front-to-back blotting motion.

Cultural Beliefs and Practices in the Postpartum Period

Beliefs

Imbalance related to energy flows, hot/cold, yin/yang. Postpartum women are in state of imbalance (decreased energy flows, cold state, excessive yin)

Practices

Rest and seclusion: Postpartally women need a long period of rest, avoiding physical activity and sex, and limiting contact with others. Household responsibilities and infant care often provided by female relatives
  40 days—Mexican Americans, Southeast Asians
      (Laotian, Vietnamese, Cambodians)
  1 month—Chinese, Japanese
  2 weeks—Filipino

Avoid cold, maintain warmth: To restore balance, postpartum women must avoid chilling activities or foods, or increase external heat
  Avoid bathing—Chinese, Mexican Americans,
      Southeast Asians, Japanese, Shinto
      (may shower, ritual bath at end of
      seclusion period)
  Cannot wash hair—Chinese, Raza/Latina
  Avoid exposure to breeze or wind—Chinese, Southern blacks, Mexican Americans,
      Filipino, Southeast Asian
  Add external heat—Hispanics, Filipinos, Asians (remain covered at all times, use
      extra blankets, slippers)

Dietary prescriptions/restrictions: Usually based on which foods are "hot" and "cold" by cultural definition
  Chinese—Eat 5–6 meals daily, hot herbal teas, hot
      foods encouraged (rice, eggs, organ meats,
      chicken); cold foods avoided (water, raw
      and cold foods)
  Hispanics—Avoid cold foods (fresh fruit and vegetables, sour, acidic, cold foods)

specific types of parenting activities. Applying Western expectations and methods of assessment to paternal behaviors is inappropriate in these cultures.

Nursing Diagnosis

Nursing assessment may lead to a variety of nursing diagnoses related to the mother's and family's postpartum experiences. Physiological adaptations frequently lead to diagnosis of altered bowel elimination (constipation) related to decreased bowel motility and abdominal muscle tone, dehydration, and painful defecation. Women often have altered patterns of urinary elimi-

nation related to postpartum diuresis and urinary retention from postdelivery edema. Pain related to uterine contractions (afterpains), episiotomy or lacerations, hemorrhoids, or breast engorgement is common. When there has been a surgical incision (episiotomy, cesarean birth) or laceration, the diagnosis of impaired skin integrity can be made.

Many postpartum women have a high risk for infection, related to impaired skin integrity and tissue trauma from childbirth or lactation. There may be fluid-volume deficits related to decreased oral intake or blood loss. Altered nutrition may occur that is less than body requirements for lactation.

Mothers may experience sleep-pattern disturbances related to postpartum discomforts or the infant's feeding needs. There often is knowledge deficit regarding infant care, self-care, health maintenance, and prevention of infections and complications. Bathing and hygiene self-care deficit may exist related to knowledge deficits or altered functional ability in the early postpartum period.

Situational low self-esteem may be diagnosed related to knowledge deficits of physiological processes, self and infant care, altered body image, emotional moodiness ("baby blues"), and changes in personal and role identities. The new mother may have a disturbance in self-concept related to body changes or parenting abilities. There are changes in family coping with potential for growth, as the infant is integrated into the family. Altered parenting may occur due to fatigue, difficult labor, feelings of incompetence, or disappointment or conflict over the baby. Parents may have anxiety related to undertaking parenting, the mother or baby's condition, and family adaptations. Family processes often are altered, related to role and life-style changes, stresses of new parenthood, and family reorganization. Ineffective coping may occur when parents use maladaptive behaviors related to infant or personal needs.

Nursing Planning and Intervention

Based on the assessment and diagnosis, plans are made to alter or alleviate the problem and nursing interventions are carried out. Interventions can include providing direct care, teaching, supporting the mother in carrying out self-care and infant care, providing a supportive and health-promoting environment, coordinating care, working with family adaptations, and making referrals for other medical or social services.

The goals of nursing care are to promote effective recovery and postpartum physiological adaptations and to facilitate the family's transition as a new member is added. With a shorter time in which to provide postpartum care due to the trend toward early discharge, nurses must carefully prioritize their interventions. Greater emphasis is placed on client teaching in support

of self an
physical c
Durin
care enco
is assisted
ambulatic
be maxir
concept a
mation ai
partum S
about th
motherhc

Client

Physic;

Involt
Bathii
Perini
Breas'
  sure
Nutri
Rest ;
Exerc
  cises
Bowe
Dang

Psychc

Emot
  blue
Famil
Role
Sexu;
Expec
Deali
Comr
  hou
  brea
  ing

Infant

Feedi
Posit
Bathi
Cord
Diap;
Infar
Infar
  tion
Temj
Sucti
Safet
  ing,
Signs

fundal height, boggy or tender fundus, persistent or new bright-red bleeding, and foul-smelling lochia. The importance of seeking medical attention for these deviations is explained and emphasized.

AFTERPAINS

Uterine contractions similar to menstrual cramps often occur for about 2 days after delivery in multiparas and in women with an overdistended uterus. Nursing mothers experience more severe afterpains during nursing, which releases oxytocin and stimulates the uterus to contract. Client teaching includes an explanation of the cause and purpose of afterpains, with reassurance that they serve a helpful function and will disappear in a short time. Self-care measures are taught, such as emptying the bladder, fundal massage, using a heating pad, lying on the stomach, or doing leg-lift exercises. These actions increase circulation and uterine tone, which reduces discomfort. Analgesics may be ordered if afterpains are severe; the nurse can advise taking these about 30 minutes before nursing and periodically as needed for comfort.

BLADDER DISTENTION

Some mothers have difficulty in voiding after delivery and may develop a distended bladder if not assisted to void. Incomplete emptying of the bladder (voiding < 300 ml) can also lead to distention and predispose to infection. To encourage spontaneous voiding, the nurse assesses the bladder frequently for fullness and explains the importance of voiding. The client is assisted to the bathroom or provided a bedpan with privacy. Running water in the sink, having the woman dip her fingers in warm water, or pouring warm water over the perineum often stimulates voiding. If voiding does occur, it is measured (subtracting the amount poured over the perineum) whenever possible; the bladder is assessed for any remaining fullness.

If there is significant perineal or afterpain discomfort, the nurse may administer analgesics 15 to 30 minutes before voiding is attempted. This may help the women relax and encourage voiding. Warm fluids shortly before may also be helpful.

If voiding is unsuccessful after using these approaches, catheterization will be necessary. It is important that the woman empty her bladder within 8 hours of delivery or sooner if significant distention develops. An intermittent or indwelling catheter may be ordered (see Nursing Guidelines: Postpartum Catheterization). There is risk of infection from either approach; this is less with intermittent catheterization. If an indwelling catheter is used, it is kept in place a minimum of time (usually 48 hours), and a urine specimen is taken for

cult
with

PEF

Som
to p
The
wate
vulv
Equi
peri
won
care
are j
onst
deliv
dispc
perir
cauti

Cold
imme
icant
apy i
and j
edem
An ic
partal
with
lowec
to col
ondar
in wh
in the
ature
for 24
wounc
H
comfc
have i
perine
comm
flow si
are av;
mainta
times j
of the
moist-l
Dr
lamp p
while t
and wa
times p
with a
fortabh

Client Teaching: Perineal Self-Care

Procedure or Action	*Rationale*
Wash hands.	Reduce risk of infection by removing microorganisms
Remove used pad from front to back.	Reduce risk of transferring microorganisms from rectum to vagina
Without separating labia, pour or squeeze solution over vulva and perineum.	Rinse away lochia, cleanse vulva, reduce risk of transferring organisms from vulva to vagina
Pat dry with tissue from front to back.	Reduce friction, reduce risk of transferring organisms from rectum to vagina
Apply Tucks, spray, or ointment as directed	Promote comfort
Apply fresh perineal pad from front to back, do not touch inner surface of pad, secure with sanitary belt or pantie	Promote comfort, reduce risk of infection and organism transfer, prevent pad from sliding
Wash hands.	As above

breasts in the breastfeeding mother is covered in Chapter 32.

The mother who is bottle-feeding her infant can bathe her breasts daily with mild soap and water; this is done most conveniently at the time of the daily shower or bath. No other special care is needed except that of breast support with a well-fitted brassiere. Usually these mothers are given lactation-suppressing medication, and engorgement usually is not a problem.

Engorgement. Engorgement occasionally occurs in both breastfeeding and nonlactating mothers. They may experience throbbing pains in the breasts that extend into the axillae. During this time, analgesic medication may be required for pain relief until the condition subsides in 1 or 2 days. Ice bags to the breasts and axillae and firm pressure to the breasts also are often helpful for nonlactating mothers (see Chap. 32).

HEALTH MAINTENANCE

Nutrition. Shortly after the delivery, the woman may express a desire for something to eat. Unless she has received a general anesthetic or is nauseated, there is usually no contraindication to giving her some nourishment. The diet postpartally should provide for balanced nutrition and enough nourishing foods to supply the additional calories and nutrients required during lactation. If these nutritional requirements are provided for, the mother's convalescence is more rapid, her strength is recovered more quickly, and the quality and quantity of her milk is better. She is also more able to resist infections. Mothers usually have good appetites and become hungry between meals, especially if breastfeeding. They should be provided between-meal

snacks, including milk or milk products, which help to incorporate the additional milk requirements nursing mothers need (see Chap. 32).

Rest and Sleep. During the puerperium, the mother needs adequate rest and can be encouraged to relax and sleep whenever possible. Rest is facilitated by reducing worry and anxiety-producing situations and promoting comfort. Rest is especially significant for the mother who is breastfeeding, because worry and fatigue inhibit her milk supply. Fatigue enlarges worries over minor concerns, and emotional problems are often precipitated by sleeplessness and fatigue.

The nurse adjusts the hospital routine whenever possible to provide the mother with uninterrupted periods of rest. Routine procedures can be delayed or rearranged to meet the mother's needs. A bottle-fed infant may be fed occasionally by the nurse if the mother is sleeping and does not want to be awakened. If the mother is unable to nap during the day, she can be encouraged to rest as quietly as possible at various times. The need for rest and sleep may need reinforcement, especially during the "taking-hold" phase, when the mother is eager to assume care responsibilities.

Early Ambulation. The mother is encouraged to be out of bed within 4 to 8 hours of delivery, unless there are contraindications. Early ambulation promotes circulation and reduces the risk of thrombophlebitis. Bladder and bowel functions are improved by ambulation, reducing the need for catheterization and improving abdominal distention and constipation.

Women who had local, epidural, or caudal anesthesia during delivery can ambulate as soon as they feel able. If the mother had intrathecal subarachnoid spinal anesthesia, she should remain flat in bed for at least 8 hours before ambulating. This helps to prevent leakage of spinal fluid through the needle puncture site in the dural membrane, reducing the incidence of postspinal headache. This recumbent position must be maintained while taking fluids and interacting with the infant. The nurse reminds the mother to remain flat and not lift her head and positions the infant so the mother can look and touch without lifting her head.

The first time the mother gets up she should dangle her legs over the side of the bed for a few minutes. The nurse assesses her status, checking for dizziness or weakness. She is then assisted to stand, then walk a few steps to determine balance. The nurse accompanies her to the bathroom or chair and remains close at hand to give immediate assistance if the mother becomes weak or faint.

The nurse explains the purpose and value of early ambulation to the mother or other decision makers. Activity should be gradually increased according to the mother's strength.

Bathing. Postpartum women often have marked diaphoresis as interstitial fluids retained during pregnancy are excreted. Taking a shower is refreshing and promotes hygiene. Mothers with no complications are allowed to shower within a few hours of delivery. The first time the mother takes a shower, the nurse should remain nearby for safety. Tub baths usually are allowed in 2 weeks. In association with showers, the nurse provides self-care instructions for bathing and breast care. As the mother is able to absorb the information, the nurse can explain about other aspects of self-care, such as perineal care and elimination.

Constipation. Measures are generally instituted to prevent constipation, such as a stool softener or laxative the first few days after delivery. The nurse explains the purpose of these medications and encourages intake of fluids and dietary roughage. The presence of bowel sounds indicates increasing bowel activity. Bowel sounds and the first stool are recorded by the nurse.

If a bowel evacuation has not occurred by the second or third day, a cleansing enema or a rectal suppository may be prescribed. Should these measures not result in stool passage, an oil retention enema, followed some hours later by a cleansing enema, may be ordered. The mother who is breastfeeding is advised to follow her physician's directions regarding use of laxatives, as some laxatives are excreted in breast milk and therefore affect the infant (see Chap. 32). Client teaching for self-care emphasizes dietary approaches to encourage regular bowel elimination, such as good bowel habits, adequate fluid intake, and foods providing roughage. Prevention of constipation is discussed in Chapter 19.

Hemorrhoids. Hemorrhoids are a common problem for women during the postpartum period. They are most painful during the first 2 to 3 days after delivery, then gradually reduce in size and regress. Painful hemorrhoids are treated with sitz baths, anesthetic sprays or ointments, and cool astringent compresses (such as witch hazel [Tucks]). Comfort is promoted by wearing perineal pads loosely and lying on the side in Sims's position while in bed. Prevention of constipation is the main measure to relieve ongoing difficulties with hemorrhoids.

PREVENTION OF INFECTION

Thrombophlebitis. Postpartum women are instructed in measures to reduce the risk of thrombophlebitis. The importance of early and regular ambulation is emphasized, and the mother is advised to avoid constricting garters or clothing that interferes with circulation. Signs of thrombosis and infection are described (severe unilateral calf or thigh pain, redness, swelling, heat), and the mother is instructed to report these immediately to the physician.

Perineal or Breast Infections. Proper techniques for applying and removing perineal pads and for wiping after voiding and defecation (front-to-back, single wipe, then discard tissue), are taught to reduce the risk of infection when an episiotomy or lacerations are present. Breast cleansing and support measures are discussed to minimize potential for mastitis (see Breast Care, Chap. 32). Signs of infection (redness, heat, swelling, pain) are taught, and the mother is instructed to report the presence of any signs to the physician immediately.

POSTPARTUM DEPRESSION ("BLUES")

Many mothers experience a transitory depression beginning the second or third day after birth. Postpartum depression reduces the level of family functioning and is related to the woman's lower self-esteem. Symptoms of transitory depression include crying easily, feelings of despondency, loss of appetite, poor concentration, difficulty sleeping, feeling let down, and anxiety. These usually disappear within 1 to 2 weeks, although some women remain mildly depressed much longer. About one fourth of women report high levels of depression at 8 months' postpartum.[1] Severe depressive psychosis occurs in only 1% to 2% of all normal childbirths.[20] Causes of postpartum blues are discussed in Chapter 27.

Mild postpartum blues usually respond to empathy, support, and acceptance by the nurse. The nurse can provide opportunities for the mother to express her anxiety, despondent feelings, and other concerns. Sharing these with an empathetic listener is often therapeutic in itself. Helping the mother put her responses in perspective and understand that this is a common experience can help alleviate her concerns about having an inappropriate or abnormal reaction to childbirth. It is also helpful to encourage adequate rest and nutrition and to assist the mother to be successful in early mothering tasks. Seldom are psychotropic drugs necessary in transitory depression. Persistent and severe depression, however, requires psychotherapy.

POSTPARTUM EXERCISES

Exercises may be initiated postpartally to hasten recovery, prevent complications, and strengthen the muscles of the back, pelvic floor, and abdomen. By toning the muscles, these exercises assist the mother to restore her figure and can be psychologically beneficial. Exercises can be started on the first postpartum day and increased gradually. The mother is counseled not to overexercise and to allow slow progression in adding to the routine. A new exercise can be added daily, with each done five to ten times per day for at least 6 weeks after delivery (see Chap. 17 and Appendix *A* for postpartum exercises).

Kegel's exercises can be taught to increase vaginal tone, which may be flaccid and distended after delivery. This exercise consists of contracting the muscles of the perineum with enough force to stop a stream of urine. The contraction is held for a few seconds and then released. The exercise is repeated 50 to 100 times and can be done several times per day (see Chap. 19).

Kegel's exercises facilitate perineal healing and help restore muscle tone by increasing circulation and through isometric muscle activity. The pubococcygeal muscle is strengthened, which helps prevent urinary stress incontinence and pelvic relaxation and enhances orgasmic capacity. Recovery of pelvic muscle tone after delivery is enhanced by regular practice of Kegel's exercises. Postpartum women who do regular Kegel's exercises show greater improvement in pelvic muscle strength than those who do not exercise.[21,22]

SEXUALITY AND CONTRACEPTION

Postpartum sexuality is affected by the degree of perineal trauma during birth and the decrease in the mother's steroid hormones, which is characteristic of the early postpartum period. Postpartum sexuality is discussed more fully in Chapter 11. Nurses must approach discussion of postpartum sexuality and contraception with sensitivity to cultural values and determine the appropriateness of counseling on an individual basis. Sexual adjustment after birth of a baby often is a major concern of new parents and can be a source of conflict and confusion. The mother's interest in intercourse is usually less than her partner's in the first few months after delivery, and her physiological responses are diminished because of low hormonal levels, the adjustment to the maternal role, and fatigue due to lack of sleep and rest. The nurse provides information about the normality of these responses, supports expression of concerns, and clarifies misunderstandings.

Lochia has generally ceased or progressed to the alba stage by 2 to 4 weeks postpartum, and the perineal area and episiotomy are well healed and not painful. Client teaching includes when to resume intercourse; the couple is advised that sex is appropriate after lochia has ceased and the perineum has healed to the point that intercourse is not painful, as long as there are no contraindicating factors, such as hematoma or infection. If intercourse causes discomfort, the couple should wait somewhat longer or use noncoital sexual practices if they find this acceptable. Positions for intercourse that avoid the penile shaft pressing posteriorly on the perineum can also alleviate discomfort.

For most couples, intercourse is resumed by the third postpartum week, so it is important to provide contraceptive information before the mother leaves the hospital. Although it is unlikely that she will ovulate and become fertile before 6 weeks, it is possible. Menses usually resume by about 9 weeks in the nonlactating woman and by 30 weeks to 36 weeks in the lactating woman. The time of return of fertility, however, is unpredictable, and all postpartum women are counseled to use contraception if they desire to avoid pregnancy (see Chaps. 11 and 26). Many hospitals provide a supply of contraceptive vaginal cream and condoms; the nurse instructs the parents on using these before discharge. Clients are encouraged to make an appointment for follow-up care with their provider, during which additional methods of contraception can be discussed.

IMMUNIZATIONS

During the postpartum period, immunizations may be administered to the mother, including rubella vaccine and Rho (D) immune globulin as indicated. The nurse discusses the infant's immunization schedule with the mother; infants born to mothers with hepatitis B receive an injection of hepatitis B immune globulin shortly after birth, followed later by vaccine.

Rubella Vaccine. Postpartum women who are serologically negative for rubella (titer 1:8 or less) or who have a negative history for rubella infection are advised to have rubella vaccination before discharge. Nursing mothers can be vaccinated, because the vaccine uses attenuated live virus and is not communicable. Women with hypersensitivity to egg protein may have allergic reactions. Pregnancy should be avoided for 2 to 3 months after vaccination, because the rubella vaccine may be teratogenic to the fetus.

Rho (D) Immune Globulin. Rh-negative women who have not been previously sensitized receive Rho (D) immune globulin within 72 hours of delivery to prevent Rh sensitization. Criteria for this immunization include an Rh-negative mother with a negative indirect Coombs test (no Rh antibodies), an Rh-positive infant, and a negative direct Coombs test (no Rh antibodies) on cord blood. Women who meet these criteria receive 300 μg of cross-matched Rho (D) immune globulin. This dosage causes lysis of any fetal red blood cells that might have entered maternal circulation (fetomaternal transfusion) before the mother has time to build up antibodies against this foreign protein.

LACTATION SUPPRESSION

Mothers who are not nursing usually need measures to suppress lactation, even in the absence of suckling. Mechanical measures frequently used include tight compression of the breasts with a breast binder or a well-fitted support brassiere and application of ice packs. Fluids should not be restricted, as these are important to postpartum recovery. The mother is instructed to avoid any stimulus to the breasts, such as suckling the infant, expressing or pumping the breasts, or putting warm water on the breasts. Some women experience breast firmness, tenderness, and temporary engorgement. The postdelivery stimulus to lactation and discomfort from temporary engorgement usually decrease after 3 days.

To prevent the secretion of prolactin, the physician may order bromocriptine mesylate (Parlodel) 2.5 mg, one tablet twice per day with meals, beginning at least 4 hours after delivery. One side effect of this drug is hypotension, and the nurse monitors blood pressure every 4 hours for 72 hours. Bromocriptine is continued for 14 to 21 days. Occasionally, there may be rebound breast secretion, congestion, and tenderness when the medication is discontinued; these usually are mild and resolve shortly. Other antilactogenic medications include estrogens and androgens, but these are infrequently used because of the risk of thromboembolism and potential relationship to endometrial cancer.

EVALUATION FOR DISCHARGE

Many mothers are discharged home on the second or third day, although increasingly early discharge is chosen by parents. Regardless of when discharge occurs, the nurse evaluates readiness and prepares mothers and families for self and infant care at home. The condition of the mother is confirmed before she is discharged from the hospital or birth center to determine satisfactory progress physiologically and psychosocially. Nursing assessments in all areas should be normal, including vital signs, involution, perineal healing, elimination (bowel, bladder), lactation or lactation suppression, ambulation, laboratory tests, and immunization status.

The nurse identifies knowledge and skill levels, reviewing points as needed, for self-care and infant care activities, return of ovulation and menstruation, contraception, resumption of sexual intercourse, medications that have been prescribed, and danger signs to be immediately reported. The parents are assisted to identify support systems for household help with child care, cooking and cleaning, shopping, and other activities. The need for referrals to community resources is assessed, and recommendations are made. Printed instruction sheets and brochures are helpful and should include danger signs and phone numbers for assistance with questions or problems (see Client Teaching: Postpartum Danger Signs). Follow-up care for both mother and infant is emphasized, and the first postpartum visit is scheduled if possible.

EARLY DISCHARGE

Low-risk mothers and infants may be discharged from the hospital or birth unit within the first day, as early as 2 to 6 hours after delivery.[23] Both mother and infant are evaluated carefully, usually beginning during the prenatal period, and again following labor and delivery. All assessment findings must be normal, remaining within established limits throughout the postpartum recovery period until the time of discharge (see Nursing Guidelines: Evaluation for Early Discharge).

Data indicate that families with adequate economic resources, immediate access to health care, stable home environments, good support systems at home, who meet early discharge criteria, and who are well prepared for parenthood have few unfavorable outcomes when discharged early.[23–25] After early discharge, the mother and infant are seen within 48 to 72 hours in the physician's

---

Client Teaching: Postpartum Danger Signs

The following physical signs could indicate infection or hemorrhage and should be reported to the physician or primary care provider at once.

Heavy vaginal bleeding or bright-red lochia (after lochia has become dark red-brown or pale)

Fever (with or without chills)

Increased vaginal discharge, especially foul smelling

Swollen, tender, red, or hot area on one leg

Area of swelling or tender, red, hot area on breast

Burning or pain with urination, inability to void

Persistent perineal or pelvic pain

Nursing Guidelines: Evaluation for Early Discharge

Normal, uncomplicated term pregnancy (38–42 wk)

Normal, uncomplicated labor and vaginal delivery

Blood loss not excessive; normal hemoglobin and hematocrit

All assessment findings within normal limits:
  Mother:
    Vital signs stable
    Fundus firm
    Moderate lochia rubra
    Perineum intact, no hematoma
    Voiding in adequate amounts
    Taking fluids without difficulty
    Homan's sign negative
    Ambulating without assistance
    No weakness or dizziness
  Infant:
    Appropriate weight for gestational age (>2500 g)
    Normal cry and reflexes
    Vital signs stable
    Mucus not excessive
    Sucking well at initial feedings
    Initial voiding and stool normal
    Normal cord blood bilirubin
    Negative Coombs' test (if Rh incompatibility)
  Caretaking:
    Signs of parental attachment
    Handles infant competently
    Able to initiate feeding without difficulty
Client teaching for self and infant care completed
  Accurate return demonstration of fundal check, perineal care, infant care (feeding, diapering, cord care, suctioning)
  Verbal and written instructions provided for self and infant care, limiting activities, family adjustments
  Accurate repeating of danger signs to report immediately
  Telephone numbers provided for obstetrician, pediatrician, or primary provider, hospital maternity unit, emergency services
Appointment made for office visit within 48–72 h, or home visit scheduled by nurse within this time

---

Further testing is reinforced, such as the second phenylketonuria test and thyroid screening. Additional home visits are made as needed.[24] Problems must be identified early and action taken to prevent further complications. Skilled nurses can handle many common problems, particularly related to inadequate knowledge, comfort, and self or infant care needs. Only a small number of mothers and infants will need physician attention within the first several days of delivery, if careful prenatal screening for early postpartum discharge is carried out.

Evaluation

Evaluation of the effectiveness of postpartum nursing care is a continuous process that feeds back into reassessment. The nurse uses specific outcomes to determine the success of interventions. Outcomes for physiological care include attainment of the purpose of the intervention, such as control of bleeding, relief of discomfort, initiation of voiding and defecation, successful ambulation, prevention of infection, normal progression of involution, and adequate nutrition and hydration.

Psychosocial care is evaluated also in terms of outcomes that accomplish goals. Teaching is evaluated according to how well the mother carries out self and infant care activities, whether she feels her questions have been adequately answered, and her ability to state knowledge (i.e., danger signs, when to contact physician, resources available, infant behavior, family adjustments to anticipate). Supportive care is evaluated by the mother's stated or apparent positive adaptations during the postpartum period, her ability to express feelings and share perceptions, and her sense of being in a caring environment.

When evaluation of nursing care indicates that anticipated outcomes have not been met, the nurse reassesses the situation by gathering additional data, arrives at a new or modified nursing diagnosis, and develops additional plans to accomplish the goals of care. These plans are implemented through appropriate nursing interventions, which are again evaluated for accomplishment of their purposes in terms of outcomes for the client (see Nursing Care Plan).

office, or a home visit is made by the nurse. Skilled nursing assessment and teaching in the home is an important factor in successful family adaptations and includes evaluation of the mother's physiological and psychological responses to childbirth and parenting, self-care and infant care skills, family coping, sexuality and contraception, and use of resources.

The nurse identifies high-risk problems and takes appropriate preventive action or institutes referrals.

■ FIRST WEEKS AT HOME

The process of integration of a new baby into the family is challenging and often stressful. Many parents have limited contact with health providers during the time between discharge and the first postpartum office visit, although they are contending with major changes and

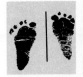

Nursing Care Plan

Postpartum Care

Nursing Goals   The woman and family will experience a normal postpartum course that includes:
1. Normal progress of involution.
2. Effective healing and restoration of usual body functions.
3. Prevention or minimization of complications.
4. Optimal comfort, balanced rest and activity.
5. Appropriate nourishment for lactation and restoration.
6. Development of knowledge and skills for self and infant care.
7. Understanding of physiological and emotional changes.
8. Family adaptation and integration of the infant.

Assessment	Potential Nursing Diagnosis	Planning and Intervention	Evaluation
Physiological Adaptations Conditions of fundus, lochia, vital signs, perineum Bladder and intestinal elimination Breasts and lactation Lower extremities Afterpains, perineal pain Ambulation and rest	High risk for injury: uterine atony, hemorrhage, hematoma Fluid volume deficit: related to excessive blood loss Altered patterns of urinary elimination: urinary retention Altered patterns of bowel elimination: constipation Altered comfort: pain related to perineal trauma, engorgement Impaired skin integrity: episiotomy, lacerations, nipple fissures Altered nutrition: less than body requirements for lactation High risk for infection: mastitis, endometritis, cystitis High risk for injury: thrombophlebitis Sleep pattern disturbances: related to discomfort, infant feeding schedule	Monitor vital signs, condition of fundus and perineum, bleeding at scheduled frequencies Begin fundal message for atony, heavy bleeding Initiate emergency measures for hemorrhage Assess bladder regularly, encourage first void in 6–8 h, measure for adequacy, perform catheterization if indicated Encourage fluids and roughage, assess for bowel sounds, administer stool softeners or laxatives Apply comfort measures for pain (sitz baths, perineal care, ice packs, heat lamp, breast expression); administer pain medications Monitor skin integrity, use preventive measures (nipple shield, cleansing, proper hygiene); teach infection prevention Encourage frequent, nutritious meals and snacks,	Fundus contracted, lochia moderate, vital signs stable, perineum intact Voids within 6–8 h, adequate amount; continues urinary elimination without problems Bowel movement in 2–3 days, without significant discomfort No signs of thrombophlebitis in legs Adequate relief or absence of afterpains, perineal pain Ambulates within a few hours without dizziness or weakness, balances activity with adequate rest, feels enough energy.

(continued)

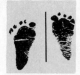

Nursing Care Plan (continued)

Assessment	Potential Nursing Diagnosis	Planning and Intervention	Evaluation
Physiological Adaptations			
	Health-seeking behaviors: related to postpartum recovery	beverages; teach need for adequate nutrition	
		Identify and report early signs of infection, institute medical regimen for treatment	
		Monitor condition of extremities, encourage ambulation, report early signs of thrombophlebitis	
		Apply comfort measures to decrease pain, administer pain medications before nursing or activity, at bedtime, advise nursery feeding if appropriate	
		Explain physiological changes; teach comfort measure techniques, infection prevention, need for nutrition, activity and rest	
Self and Infant Care			
Mother-infant interactions	Alterations in parenting: related to fatigue, disappointment with infant, feelings of incompetence	Encourage expression of feelings about infant, promote rest, assist to acquire parenting skills	Mother interacts frequently and affectionately with infant; begins to identify behavior patterns, characteristics
Infant caretaking knowledge and skills			
Self-care knowledge and skills	Anxiety: related to mother–baby condition, parenting responsibilities, family adaptations	Explain mother–baby condition, reassure as appropriate, listen empathetically, teach and explore coping with caretaking and family adaptations	Mother performs infant caretaking appropriately (bathing, feeding, diapering, handling, comforting)
Nutrition and hydration			
Understanding of physiological and psychological changes	Disturbance in self-concept: related to body changes, parenting abilities	Explain expected recovery of body shape and tone, self-care to aid recovery; teach parenting skills	Mother performs self-care appropriately (perineal care, sitz bath, heat lamp, perineal pad placement and removal, breast care, bathing)
Knowledge of signs of postpartum complications	Situational low self-esteem: knowledge deficits, altered body image, emotional changes, role changes	Provide information to increase knowledge, listen and discuss feelings, help normalize experiences,	Mother had adequate intake of nutrients and fluids, hunger is satisfied,
	Knowledge deficits: post-		

(continued)

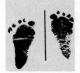

Nursing Care Plan *(continued)*

Assessment	Potential Nursing Diagnosis	Planning and Intervention	Evaluation
Self and Infant Care	partal processes, self and infant care, health maintenance, prevention of complications	provide anticipatory guidance	reports feeling replenished
		Provide information to reduce specific deficits	Mother expresses understanding and acceptance of postpartal changes
	Bathing and hygiene self-care deficit: related to knowledge deficits, altered functional status	Assist with bathing and hygiene initially, encourage self-care when able, provide information	Mother describes danger signs for postpartum complications, what to do if these occur
	Health-seeking behaviors: related to competence in self and infant care, early identification of complications	Support and acknowledge development of competence in self and infant care, teach and review danger signs to report immediately	Mother states plans for postpartum follow-up visit after discharge
Family Adaptation			
Planning for infant care at home	Family coping: potential for growth by integrating infant	Support family incorporation of infant through frequent parental caretaking and interaction	Parents describe realistic plans for infant care at home, have made appropriate preparations
Integrating infant into family	Altered parenting: related to home and infant care stresses	Assist parents to identify stresses when infant is home; develop plans for coping, using available resources	Parents interact positively with infant, discuss changes in family structure and functioning with acceptance, no major problems anticipated
Resources for assistance with home, infant, child care	Altered family processes: related to stress of childbirth, infant care, role and life-style changes		
Parents' reactions to infant, caretaking	Ineffective family coping: related to difficult family adjustments, parental conflicts, siblings rivalry	Identify ineffective family processes, provide teaching and support for conflicts and problems, refer if maladaptive	Parents report knowledge or plans for use of resources according to their needs
Knowledge and concerns about sexuality			
Contraceptive needs and preferences	Ineffective individual coping: related to responses to family stresses, adjustment difficulties	Identify ineffective individual coping, provide teaching and support for more effective responses, refer if severe	Parents reactions to infant caretaking reflect effective coping, realistic understanding of stresses, concrete plans for dealing with difficulties
Relationship between parents	Altered sexuality patterns: related to postpartum discomforts, decreased sexuality of mother, ineffective coping, fatigue	Teach parents expected alterations in sexuality, factors that affect sexual expression postpartally, when to resume sex	Relationship between parents appears mutually caring and supportive (within cultural contexts), no significant conflicts/problems
	Knowledge deficit: family adjustments, household	Provide information to reduce specific deficits	

(continued)

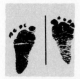

Nursing Care Plan   *(continued)*

Assessment	Potential Nursing Diagnosis	Planning and Intervention	Evaluation
Family Adaptation			
	management, use of resources, parenthood stresses, changes in sexuality		Parents express understanding and are accepting of altered sexuality during postpartum
			Parents state intention to use contraceptives, know method and how to use in first few weeks (if desire to avoid pregnancy)

adjustments in what is often a new experience in their lives. Parents may find the first few weeks at home characterized by a disorganized household and greatly increased work related to diapers, feeding, and care of the new baby. The mother usually is coping with fatigue and may feel frustrated in trying to learn the baby's patterns and ways of communicating.

Nursing Assessment

The concerns of new mothers in the first weeks after delivery cover a wide range. The nurse assesses the mother's and family's concerns and responses during this time. The most common concerns expressed by new mothers are in the following areas: changes in their figures, fatigue and lack of sleep, infant care, changing roles and life-styles, and infant feeding.

Whether pregnancy was high risk or low risk, families experience changes in functioning during the transition to parenthood (see Research Highlight: Family Functioning in the Months After Birth). More optimal family functioning appears related to less depression, greater social support, and less stress from negative life events during the year preceding pregnancy. At 8 months after birth, family functioning remains relatively disorganized and incorporation of the new infant is not yet completely resolved. Among high-risk families, family functioning tends to get worse by 8 months after birth.[1]

CHANGES IN BODY IMAGE AND MARITAL RELATIONSHIP

One of the mother's most frequently expressed concerns of the postpartum period involves return of the figure to normal. This appears to be more than just a minor anxiety. Although new mothers are initially delighted when their abdomens decrease in size after delivery, this positive feeling turns to dismay when the abdominal wall remains soft and flabby and part of the weight gained during pregnancy is retained, making it impossible to wear clothes that fit before pregnancy. Frequently, the mother feels as though she is still several months pregnant.

Although mothers may want to lose weight and tighten up muscles, they often find that the baby's demands and their own fatigue interfere with these attempts. A flabby postpartum figure and the feeling of lack of ability to improve it can be depressing. Fathers, too, are often disappointed because of the time it takes for the mother's figure to become slim again, and both partners may fear that the figure changes are permanent.

Persistent discomforts from episiotomy pain, which may last 2 to 3 weeks, breast engorgement, and nipple soreness, continued lochial discharge, and the annoyance of leaking milk can decrease energy and affect the couple's relationship. Another source of concern is the lack of vaginal tone, which may affect the couple's sexual relationship (see Assessment Tool: Sexual History During Postpartum). The quality of the couple's rela-

Assessment Tool

Sexual History During Postpartum

As part of postpartum nursing assessment, these questions about sexual experiences and concerns can be included. Several can be asked of both partners, and joint history taking is recommended.

1. How do you feel about the changes in appearance and emotions following birth?
2. How do you feel about each other's experience of the birth process?
3. How are you managing with the baby's care at home?
4. Have you resumed sexual intercourse or other sexual activity?
5. Are you comfortable during intercourse and has the episiotomy (if present) healed?
6. Do you have adequate vaginal lubrication during intercourse?
7. If breastfeeding, has this altered your sexual experiences or your relationship with your partner?
8. Are you using contraception? If not, are you concerned about getting pregnant again?
9. How has the new baby affected your sexual relationship and experiences?

tionship often declines through the ninth month postpartum.[26] Strain on the marital relationship varies, but by 1 year most couples report their relationship as unchanged from prepregnant quality.[27]

FATIGUE AND LACK OF SLEEP

Fatigue appears to be a consistent problem for new mothers. Labor and delivery are hard, exhausting work, followed immediately by the demands of caring for a totally dependent infant. The short stay in the hospital is insufficient to restore energy levels, because excitement, the strange environment, and physical discomforts often interfere with rest and sleep. Most women have also not slept well during the last weeks of pregnancy. This leaves them with a deficit of energy and sleep, which increases sharply during the first weeks at home with the baby.

Sleep deprivation is to some degree a part of living for all new mothers, and it can be severe. The mother's sleep needs are curtailed by the baby's needs for food and attention. It may be difficult for new mothers to obtain more than 30 to 45 minutes of uninterrupted sleep per night, particularly if there are other small children who frequently need attention. Increased bodily tension as a result can lead to insomnia when there is the opportunity to sleep. Sleep deprivation can produce changes in mood and mental functioning, with the parents experiencing increased anxiety, irritability, illogical thought patterns, and mental confusion.

INFANT CARE

Infants are quite different in their patterns, and the new mother must learn her baby's particular behaviors and ways of communicating. Mothers are often concerned about how normal their infant's behaviors are, especially regarding weight gain, crying, bowel movements, feeding, and sleep patterns. Parents may be surprised at the wide range of behaviors among infants. Conflicting advice regarding how frequently the baby should be fed, when to add solid food, when to pick up a crying baby, what clothes to put on the baby, who should be allowed to visit and when, and so forth, leads to further confusion.

The way a mother perceives and relates to her infant has an impact on the child's subsequent growth and development and reflects the mother's satisfaction with her interaction with the infant. If she feels satisfied, she has a more positive perception of the infant and reinforcement of her own identity as a mother. This, in turn, fosters a nurturing relationship.

About 25% to 30% of women who are breastfeeding when discharged have weaned their babies by 1 month postpartum. The use of bottle supplementation in the hospital and lower satisfaction with breastfeeding are associated with problems in the early postpartum period.[28] Breastfeeding for more than 13 weeks has a protective effect against gastrointestinal and respiratory infections in the infant.[29] The mother's enjoyment of breastfeeding in a relaxed atmosphere is important in continuation and supports the need for flexibility and responsiveness to the infant's needs that are related to successful breastfeeding.[30]

CHANGING ROLES AND LIFE-STYLES

Parents may not be completely prepared for the amount of change required in their roles, relationships, and lifestyles as the infant is integrated into the family. Many parents may actually "grieve" over the passing of former life patterns. The mother particularly may have to make major changes in career and other activities, although the gratifications of motherhood may be enough to compensate for these relinquishments. Alterations take place in the family constellation, and problems related to jealousy or rivalry among the other children may occur. Marital problems between spouses may arise from relative neglect of their relationship. With less time for each other and possible strain in their sexual relations, many couples report stress in their relationship following the birth of a new baby. Social isolation, lack of recreational activities, and financial concerns can compound family stresses.

Nursing Planning and Intervention

The nurse can provide anticipatory care during the prenatal and postpartal periods. During the third trimester, the expectant mother has increased interest in caretaking activities, and teaching related to infant behavior and care can be productive at this time. The nurse can include such topics as preparing other children for the new baby, exploring ways to meet the increased demands of a new baby for attention and continuous care, and considering sources of potential stress to the marital and family relations and ways of coping with these problems.

Reinforcing the importance of help with household tasks during the first few postpartum weeks at home may encourage the mother to make arrangements. This can help to alleviate fatigue and sleep deprivation. Knowing that she will need time to regain her energy level will help the mother to be more realistic in her expectations. Also knowing that her figure will take time to return to its prepregnant form and that physical discomforts will exist for a time after delivery will prepare the parents and reduce stress from unrealistic expectations.

Nursing intervention is aimed at increasing the mother's sense of mastery and satisfaction in infant care, thereby promoting healthier mother-infant relationships and infant development. Mothers can be assisted to recognize and respond appropriately to their baby's unique patterns, ways of communicating, and particular needs for stimulation, sleep, and feeding. When able to respond more smoothly to her infant, the mother's satisfactions are increased and the development of a healthy relationship is encouraged.

Community health nurses may be available to visit new mothers and provide teaching and support during the first few weeks at home. With early discharge, a home visit by the nurse is usually scheduled. Providing professional assistance by telephone is usually part of postdischarge care. Various methods and groups for postpartum teaching are discussed in Chapter 17.

Evaluation

Nursing care is successful when the mother is able to cope adequately with self and infant care during the first few weeks at home. Family adaptations that provide for the needs of other children, the parents, and the new baby are positive outcomes. The nurse may observe family functioning and maternal-infant interactions during a home visit or may rely on the mother's reports by telephone or at an office visit. When difficulties arise, families who can identify and use appropriate resources have benefitted from nursing care.

■ POSTPARTUM FOLLOW-UP VISIT

A follow-up visit is scheduled, depending on the mother's condition and needs for careful monitoring. Because most reproductive organs have returned to their nonpregnant condition within 6 to 8 weeks after delivery, a visit usually is planned for 4 to 6 weeks postpartum.

Visits are scheduled earlier when problems or complications of the mother or infant are present. The progress of involutional changes, the mother's physical condition and recovery, the family's adaptation to the new baby, the parent's sexual relations and need for contraception, and the infant's growth and development are assessed.

Nursing Assessment

During the visit, the weight and the blood pressure are taken and a urinalysis and a complete blood count may be done (see Nursing Guidelines: Postpartum Follow-Up Visit). The condition of the abdominal wall is observed, and the breasts are inspected. If the mother is breastfeeding, the condition of the nipples and the degree of lacteal secretion are observed. If the mother is

and whether involution is complete. The presence, amount, and character of lochia are assessed. Questions about physiological status are elicited and discussed.

The family's response to the new baby is discussed, and questions related to behavior, patterns of feeding, sleep and elimination, crying, weight gain, and so forth are explored (see Nursing Care Plan).

Nursing Planning and Intervention

Problems with healing or infection are treated, if present, and arrangements are made for further examinations and treatments as necessary. This return examination provides an opportunity to discuss any other problems or concerns relating to the birth experience. The mother's concerns about rest and exercise, weight, diet, her energy level, household tasks, relations with relatives and friends, sexual relations, and physical needs or discomforts are discussed. If weight continues to be a problem, a suitable weight reduction diet and exercise program can be started. If desired, the woman can resume full employment or activities at this time, if there are no complications and she feels psychologically ready. The need for further care or referrals is identified.

Contraception is discussed at this visit, and a suitable method is decided on if the parents wish to prevent another pregnancy. The method is instituted at this time, and the couple is instructed in its uses and risks (see Chap. 11).

Evaluation

The effectiveness of nursing care is determined by outcomes for the mother and family. Physiological outcomes, such as normal progression of lochia and healing of the episiotomy, can be observed. Satisfactory interaction between mother and infant and development of mothering abilities signify effective outcomes in mother-infant relationships. The mother, father, and family may describe effective adaptation to the new infant; new routines are developed and stabilized. Referrals and other sources of assistance are used and provide effective help. The mother and family believe their questions have been answered and feel capable of managing their new family processes.

Nursing Guidelines: Postpartum Follow-up Visit

Involution Status

Vital signs and weight
Perineal examination
Amount and character of lochia
Condition of episiotomy or lacerations
Condition of anus, hemorrhoids
Pelvic examination
Size and position of uterus and cervix
Condition of vagina (musculature, lacerations)
Pap smear
Breast examination
Condition of breasts and nipples
Lactating or lactation suppression

Infant Development and Care

Growth and development of baby
Infant behavior
Patterns of feeding, sleep, and elimination
Crying
Weight gain
Family response to new baby
Reactions of siblings
Relatives, and friends' visits or assistance
Mother's response to caretaking, feeding, and reactions of others

Physical Recovery

Mother's physical condition and recovery
Rest and exercise
Weight loss
Diet
Energy level
Recreation and activities
Returning to work
Physical discomforts and remedies

Sexuality and Contraception

Sexual relations
Resumption of intercourse
Concerns or difficulties
Responses of mother and father
Contraception
Current contraceptive practice (if any)
Desires for regulating fertility and family planning
Contraceptive method selection and teaching

---

not breastfeeding, the breast should be observed to see that lactation suppression has occurred.

A pelvic examination is done to determine the condition of the uterus, the healing of the episiotomy or perineal lacerations, the tone of the pelvic floor muscles,

■ REFERENCES

1. Mercer T, Ferketich SL: Predictors of family functioning eight months following birth. Nurs Res 39(2):76–82, March/April 1990

2. Tulman L, Fawcett J, Groblewski L, et al: Changes in functional status after childbirth. Nurs Res 39(2):70–75, March/April 1990

3. Kunst-Wilson W, Cronenwett LR: Nursing care for the emerging family: Promoting paternal behavior. Res Nurs Health 4:201, 1981

4. Miles JF, Martin JN, Blake PG, et al: Postpartum eclampsia: A recurring perinatal dilemma. Obstet Gynecol 76(3):328–331, Part I, September 1990

5. Jacobson H: A standard for assessing lochia volume. MCN 10:174–175, May/June 1985

6. Cunningham F, MacDonald P, Gant N: Williams Obstetrics, 18th ed. Norwalk, CT, Appleton & Lange, 1989

7. Resnick R: The puerperium. In Creasey R, Resnick R: Maternal-Fetal Medicine: Principles and Practice, 2nd ed. Philadelphia, WB Saunders, 1989

8. Willson JR: The puerperium. In Willson JR, Carrington ER (eds): Obstetrics and Gynecology, 8th ed. St. Louis, CV Mosby, 1987

9. Mercer RT: The nurse and maternal tasks of early postpartum. MCN 6:341, September/October 1981

10. Turner RJ, Avison WR: Assessing risk factors for problem parenting: The significance of social support. J Marr Fam 47:881, November 1985

11. Pillsbury B: Doing the month: Confinement and convalescence of Chinese women after childbirth. In Kay MA (ed): Anthropology of Human Birth. Philadelphia, FA Davis, 1982

12. Bernstein GL, Kidd YA: Childbearing in Japan. In Kay MA (ed): Anthropology of Human Birth. Philadelphia, FA Davis, 1982

13. Wadd L: Vietnamese postpartum practices: Implications for nursing in the hospital setting. JOGN Nurs 12:252, July/August 1983

14. Orque M: Nursing care of Filipino American patients. In Orque M, Bloch B, Monrroy L (eds)): Ethnic Nursing Care. St. Louis, CV Mosby, 1983

15. Monrroy L: Nursing care of Raza/Latina patients. In Orque M, Bloch B, Monrroy L (eds): Ethnic Nursing Care. St. Louis, CV Mosby, 1983

16. Horn B: Cultural concepts and postpartal care. Nurs Health Care 11:516–517; 526–527, 1981

17. Davis J, Brucker M, MacMullen N: A study of mother's postpartum teaching priorities. MCN 15:41–51, 1985

18. Rutledge DL, Pridham KFK: Postpartum mother's perceptions of competence for infant care. JOGNN 16(3):185, 1987

19. Rhode MA, Barger MK: Perineal care: Then and now. J Nurs Midwif 35(4):220–229, July/August 1990

20. Landy S, Montgomery J, Walsh S: Postpartum depression: A clinical view. Matern Child Nurs J 18(1):1–29, Spring 1989

21. Sampselle CM, Brink CA: Pelvic muscle relaxation: Assessment and management. J Nurs Midwif 35:127–132, 1990

22. Dougherty MC, Bishop K, Abrams R, et al: The effect of exercise on the circumvaginal muscles in postpartum women. J Nurs Midwif 34:8–14, 1989

23. Norr K, Nacion K: Outcomes of postpartum early discharge, 1960–1986: A comparative review. Birth 14(3):135–141, September 1987

24. Jansson P: Early discharge. Am J Nurs 85(5):547–550, May 1985

25. Regan K: Early obstetrical discharge: A program that works. Can Nurse 80:32–35, October 1984

26. Belsky J, Lang ME, Rovine M: Stability and change in marriage across the transition to parenthood: A second study. J Marr Fam 47:855–865, 1985

27. Lewis JM: The transition to parenthood: II. Stability and change in marital structure. Fam Process 27:273–283, 1985

28. Kearney MH, Cronenwett LR, Barrett JA: Breast-feeding problems in the first week postpartum. Nurs Res 39(2):90–95, March/April 1990

29. Howie PW, Forsyth JS, Ogston SA, et al: Protective effect of breast feeding against infection. Br Med J 300:11, 1990

30. Pridham K, Knight CB, Stephenson G: Decision rules for infant feeding: The influence of maternal expertise, regulating functions, and feeding method. Matern Child Nurs J 19(1):31–47, Spring 1989

■ SUGGESTED READING

Anderson GC: Risk in mother-infant separation postbirth. Image 21(4):196–199, Winter 1989

Baisch MJ, Fox RA, Whitten E, et al: Comparison of breast-feeding attitudes and practices: Low-income adolescents and adult women. Matern Child Nurs J 18(1):61–71, Spring 1989

Bee HL, Hammond MA, Eyres SJ, et al: The impact of parental life change on early development of children. Res Nurs Health 9:65–74, 1986

Cronenwett LR: Parental network structure and perceived support after birth of first child. Nurs Res 34:347–352, 1985

Fishman SH, et al: Changes in sexual relationships in postpartum couples. JOGNN 15:58, January/February 1986

Konrad CJ: Helping mothers integrate the birth experience. MCN 14(4):268, December 1987

Pridham K: The meaning for mothers of a new infant: Relationship to maternal experience. Matern Child Nurs J 16(2):103–122, Summer 1987

Tomlinson PS: Spousal differences in marital satisfaction during transition to parenthood. Nurs Res 36:239–243, 1987

Vezeau TM, Hallsten DA: Making the transition to mother-baby care. Am J Matern Child Nurs 12:193–198, 1987

Walker LO: Stress process among mothers of infants: Preliminary model testing. Nurs Res 38(1):10–15, 1989

Walker LO, Crain H, Thompson F: Maternal role attainment and identity in the postpartum period: Stability and change. Nurs Res 35:68–71, 1986

Wilkerson NN, Barrows TL: Synchronizing care with mother-baby rhythms. Am J Matern Child Nurs 13:264–269, 1988

29

Assessment of the Newborn

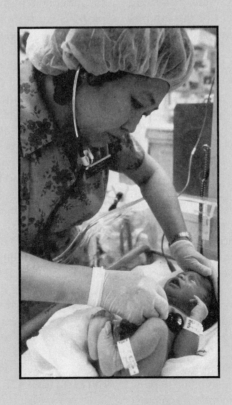

uring the first few days of life, the newborn undergoes more profound physiologic changes than at any other time in his life. Frequent assessments of the infant help to determine how well he or she is coping with the many changes that are occurring. The types of assessments that are done, and who does them, depend on the setting and the infant's condition. Registered nurses are usually the health-care professionals who have closest contact with the newborn during this period of transition to extrauterine life. Nurses need to possess the knowledge and skills to evaluate the newborn's status comprehensively during this period.

Assessments are ongoing throughout the time the infant remains in the hospital or birth center. Assessment of physical status, including vital signs, general activity, color changes, feeding status, elimination, and the condition of skin, eyes, and cord is usually done at least once every 8 hours, and the infant is usually weighed daily. With hospital stays sometimes as brief as 12 hours after birth, and birth center stays even shorter, accurate early assessment, and teaching the family what to watch for at home during the remainder of the transition period, become important aspects of nursing care.

In addition to assessing the newborn's physical condition and adaptation, nurses should also be familiar with other areas of assessment. For example, increasing attention is now placed on assessment of the infant's behavior and the interaction between the parents and the infant.

■ PHYSIOLOGIC BASIS OF ASSESSMENT

While undergoing the changes that lead to adaptation to extrauterine life, the infant passes through several phases. This transitional period must be negotiated successfully if the infant is to survive and to develop normally. The transition begins with labor when the fetus is stimulated by uterine contractions and pressure changes as a result of the rupture of the membranes. At birth, a variety of foreign stimuli are encountered, such as light, sound, heat, cold, and gravitation. Breathing then must start, and profound changes and reorganization in the functioning of the organ systems and metabolic processes begin. Respiration must be initiated, circulation must shift from fetal to neonatal, hepatic and renal function must be altered, and meconium must be passed. The final phase of the transition involves further reorganization of the metabolic processes to achieve a viable, steady state. This includes changes in blood oxygen saturation, reduction of enzymes, diminution in postnatal acidosis, and recovery of the neu-

rologic tissues from the trauma of labor and delivery. Because these changes take time, it is no wonder that the infant's natal day is so crucial to his or her life and future well-being.

Respiratory Changes

Prior to birth, the oxygen needs of the fetus are met by the placenta. Although the fetal lungs do not function as organs of respiration, it has been confirmed in recent years that respiratory-like movements do occur. The function of this "fetal breathing" is not known, but some of the hypotheses are that it may (1) represent "prenatal practice" for later breathing; (2) aid in the development of alveolar and bronchial structures; or (3) relate to the synthesis, release, and distribution of surfactant.[1,2]

For the newborn to survive extrauterine life, adequate maturation of the lungs is essential. The lungs are in a continuous state of development structurally throughout fetal life and early childhood. About the 17th week of gestation, canals begin to develop in the bronchial tree and, soon after, primitive air sacs begin to form. By 24 to 26 weeks' gestation, there is adequate vascularization and development of respiratory sacules for gas exchange to be possible so there is a potential for independent survival. Because surface-active lipoproteins (surfactant) are not available at this time and there is limited development of alveoli, however, the infant born this early is at high risk for respiratory problems and chances for long-term survival are not good.[3] (See Chap. 44 for discussion of respiratory problems of the preterm infant.)

At the time of birth, the normal, full-term fetus is ready for the initiation of effective breathing. For example, fetal respiratory movements have prepared the lungs for this activity and the complex interrelationships of swallowing and breathing have been developed. With everything in readiness, the question is often asked, "What keeps the fetus from taking real breaths before it is born?" Some important inhibitory mechanisms have been identified. One of these is facial immersion. Another is the inhibition of respiration by the presence of fluid in the laryngeal area. This emphasizes the importance of clearing fluid from this area after birth. Also, the fetal lungs are constantly filled with fluid that is thought to be secreted by the alveolar cells, and this fluid in the deep respiratory tracts stimulates inhibitory stretch receptors.[4]

INITIATION OF RESPIRATION

A multiplicity of factors is probably involved in stimulating the infant's initial respirations. This would seem to provide a margin of safety for the infant. Physical, sensory, and chemical factors are involved, but precisely how each of these influences the other and to what degree is not known exactly. Some evidence exists to indicate that the change in pressure from intrauterine to extrauterine life may produce enough physical stimulation to prompt respiration.

Of the sensory stimuli, such as cold, pain, touch, light, sound, and gravity, that have been thought to play a role in initiation of respiration, cold seems to play a most significant role. In animal studies, cold stimulation has induced breathing in fetal sheep.[2] This should not be taken to mean that the infant needs to be in a cold environment. Normal room air of about 22°C (72°F) is a decrease of more than 15°C (25°F) below the mother's normal body temperature that the neonate has been used to in utero, and should, therefore, be sufficient to stimulate respiration.

The chemical changes that occur in the blood as a result of transient asphyxia during delivery are also powerful stimuli for the first breath. These include a lowered oxygen level, increased carbon dioxide level, and a lowered *p*H, indicating respiratory acidosis. This presumably normal condition is characterized by the absence of metabolic acidosis. A vigorous infant usually breathes within seconds and certainly within 1 minute after birth. If the asphyxia is prolonged, metabolic acidosis does develop, depression of the respiratory center occurs rather than stimulation, and resuscitation is usually necessary (see Chap. 44).[2]

A great effort is required to expand the lungs and to fill the collapsed alveoli. Surface tension in the respiratory tract, as well as resistance in the lung tissue itself, the thorax, the diaphragm, and the respiratory muscles must be overcome. Moreover, any obstruction (i.e., mucus, and so on) in the air passages has to be cleared. The first active inspiration comes from a powerful contraction of the diaphragm, which creates a high negative intrathoracic pressure, causing a marked retraction of the ribs because of the pliability of the baby's thorax.

This first inspiration distends the alveolar spaces, and on expiration, a residual volume of nearly 20 ml of air remains as molecules of pulmonary surfactant diminish surface tension. Therefore, the second breath takes less effort than the first, and the third breath even less, because by this time most of the small airways are open. Fluid is rapidly removed from the lungs by drainage, swallowing, evaporation, and pulmonary, capillary, and lymphatic circulation. After several minutes of breathing, lung expansion is usually complete[5] (see Box: Initiation of Respiration).

RESPIRATION IN FIRST AND SECOND PERIODS OF REACTIVITY

A healthy infant begins life with intense activity. This phase has been designated by some authorities as the first period of reactivity. In this phase, the infant exhibits outbursts of diffuse, purposeless movements that alternate with periods of relative immobility. At this time respiration is rapid (reaching as high as 80 breaths per minute), and there may be *transient* flaring of the nostrils; retraction of the chest and grunting are not uncommon. Tachycardia also is present at times, and the heart rate may reach 180 beats per minute in the first minutes of life. Thereafter, it falls to an average of 120 to 140 beats per minute.

After this initial response, the baby becomes relatively quiet and does not respond intensely to either internal or external stimuli. He relaxes and may fall asleep. His first sleep occurs, on an average, at 2 hours after birth and may last anywhere from a few minutes to several hours.

When he awakes, he is again hyperresponsive to stimuli, and he begins his second period of reactivity. His color may change rapidly (from pink to moderately cyanotic), and his heart rate responds to stimulation and becomes rapid. Oral mucus may be a major problem in respiration during this period. Choking, gagging, and regurgitation alert the nurse to the presence of mucus, and appropriate intervention must be taken (see Chap. 44). Because the length of the second period of reactivity is variable, the nurse must be particularly alert for the occurrence of these problems during at least the first 12 to 18 hours of the infant's life[6] (Fig. 29-1).

Circulatory Changes

The anatomical changes that occur with birth have been discussed previously in Chapter 10. It will be recalled that a rapid change takes place, with closure of several fetal structures and with the redistribution of oxygenated blood to a circulation similar to that of an adult. Because all changes are not immediately complete, this time of conversion may be called a period of *transitional circulation*.

TOTAL BLOOD VOLUME

It is difficult to give accurate values for the total blood volume of the newborn because of the variables involved, such as time of clamping the umbilical cord, weight and gestational age of the infant, type of delivery (vaginal or cesarean), and time after delivery the determination is made.

For example, an additional 50 to 100 ml of blood may be added to the circulation if the infant is placed below the level of the placenta and the clamping of the cord is delayed several minutes until the cord stops pulsating. Many studies have been done to help decide the issue of early or late clamping, but it is still unclear whether this placental transfusion that occurs with late clamping is advantageous for the infant. The rapid increase in blood volume might stress the heart and pulmonary vasculature, but according to some reports, the

Initiation of Respiration

Factors in Stimulation of First Breath

Physical—Changes in pressure

Sensory—Cold, pain, touch, light, sound, gravity

Chemical—Changes in blood (decrease in O_2 level, increase in CO_2 level, decrease in pH)

Expansion of Alveoli

Must overcome the following:
  Surface tension in respiratory tract
  Resistance in lung tissue, thorax, diaphragm, and respiratory muscles

Must clear air passages of mucus

Fluid Removed From Lungs by the Following

Drainage

Swallowing

Evaporation

Pulmonary capillary circulation

Lymphatic circulation

Before 1st breath	1st breath	1st expiration	2nd breath
Fluid-filled alveolus	Fluid forced out Alveolus expanded	Residual air	Less effort required for expansion

incidence of neonatal respiratory distress is decreased with delayed clamping.[7] The infants who receive this extra blood gain an increased storage supply of iron, resulting from the breakdown of the additional hemoglobin. This may contribute to hyperbilirubinemia during the first week of life, but the iron stores may be used to good advantage later when iron is needed for rapid growth or when the dietary intake of iron is inadequate.[7]

PERIPHERAL CIRCULATION

Peripheral circulation in the newborn is somewhat sluggish. It is believed that this accounts for the residual cyanosis of the infant's hands, feet, and circumoral area. These areas often remain mildly cyanotic for 1 or 2 hours after delivery. The general circulatory lability probably accounts for the mottled appearance of the baby's skin when it is exposed to air and for the "chilliness" of the infant's hands and feet.

PULSE RATE

Like the rate of respiration, the pulse rate also is labile and generally follows a pattern similar to that of the respiration. When the respiration is rapid, the pulse tends to be rapid; similarly, when the respiration slows down, so does the pulse. Because the pulse is affected by both internal and external stimuli, taking the *apical* pulse rate while the baby is quiet provides a more accurate evaluation of the infant's heart rate. The normal rate is usually 120 to 150 beats per minute, but it may rise to 180 beats per minute for short periods with crying and other intense activity or drop to 100 beats per minute during deep sleep.

BLOOD PRESSURE

Accurate indirect assessment of arterial blood pressure is more difficult in the newborn; therefore, it has not always been checked routinely in the normal infant.

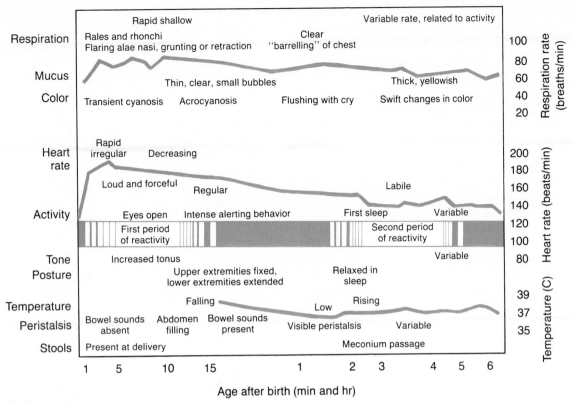

■ *Figure 29–1*
Periods of reactivity. (After Arnold HW, Putman NJ, Barnard BL, et al: Transition to extrauterine life. Am J Nurs 65(10):78, 1965)

Invasive methods using an arterial catheter for direct recording of the blood pressure are usually limited to the sick neonate who has an arterial line in place for other reasons (see Chap. 44). Indirect, noninvasive methods consisting of auscultation, palpation, and the color change (flush) method usually result in only the systolic pressure or the mean pressure and are not very precise. The advent of the Doppler reflected-ultrasound technique has made the estimation of systemic blood pressure more accurate, and taking the blood pressure has become part of the routine procedure in many normal newborn nurseries.

Blood pressure in the neonate is characteristically low, averaging 71/49 mm Hg at birth and rising slowly during the first week.[8] Pressure also varies according to the size and activity of the infant, with lower averages for the small, preterm infant and with the blood pressure rising when the infant is crying and active. Cause for concern and further investigation in the term neonate would include diastolic pressures lower than 25 mm Hg or higher than 60 mm Hg, and mean pressures of less than 30 mm Hg or greater than 70 mm Hg.[9]

The width of the cuff used in the procedure should be 25% greater than the diameter of the arm or leg where the blood pressure is being taken. Too small a cuff will give too high a reading. Either the arm or the leg can be used in obtaining the blood pressure. Leg pressure will be slightly higher but should be within 20 mm Hg of the arm pressure.[10]

ERYTHROCYTE COUNT AND HEMOGLOBIN CONCENTRATION

The newborn has much higher erythrocyte, hemoglobin, and hematocrit levels than the adult. The erythrocyte level ranges between 5 million and 7 million/μl, the hemoglobin level is usually 15 to 20 g/dl of blood, and the hematocrit values average about 55%.[7]

The following factors influence these values:

1. *Duration of gestation*—During the final weeks of intrauterine life, hemoglobin concentration rapidly increases. The infant born before term does not have the benefit of this increase and has a low concentration compared with the full-term infant.
2. *Time of cord clamping*—In infants who receive the additional blood that is added to the circulation with delayed cord clamping, increased hemoglobin and hematocrit levels can be demonstrated for at least 3 or 4 days.
3. *Site of blood sample*—In the first week of life, ow-

ing to peripheral venous stasis, capillary blood samples usually show markedly higher hemoglobin and hematocrit values than venous samples drawn at the same time. The venous samples are considered to be more accurate. If only heel sticks are used for assessing blood values, anemia could go undetected. Warming the infant's heel before the stick is suggested as a way of decreasing the difference between the two values.[7]

The higher blood values are needed by the fetus in utero for adequate oxygenation. After birth, the need no longer exists because the lungs are functioning and a gradual decrease takes place. Immediately after birth, there is an increase in erythrocyte count from cord blood levels because of a decrease in plasma volume. This reaches a maximum level 2 to 6 hours after birth, then it decreases to cord blood levels when the infant is about 1 week of age. Red blood cell production (erythropoiesis) is suppressed for several months after birth and this, added to the increased blood volume caused by the infant's rapid growth, results in a progressive decline in the hemoglobin concentration. A low point of 11 g/dl (±2.0) may be reached after 2 to 3 months, producing a physiologic anemia that does not represent any abnormality or nutritional deficiency in the infant and is not affected by giving iron or other hematinics. Active erythropoiesis resumes about this time and, if the iron supply is adequate, the hemoglobin concentration gradually increases to an average of 12.5 g/dl, where it stays during early childhood.[7]

PHYSIOLOGIC JAUNDICE

In the newborn period, there is a rise in the serum concentration of unconjugated bilirubin from approximately 2 mg/dl in cord blood to a mean peak of 6 mg/dl between 60 and 72 hours of age. Then there is usually a rapid decline to 2 mg/dl by the fifth day of life and a slower decline until normal adult levels of less than 1 mg/dl are reached by about the tenth day. Jaundice is the visible evidence of this rise in serum concentration of unconjugated bilirubin to levels of 5 to 7 mg/dl or

above.[11] Approximately 40% to 60% of full-term newborns (and a higher number of preterm infants) develop jaundice between the second and fourth days of life, and in the absence of disease or specific causes, this has been called *physiologic jaundice*. Bilirubin levels greater than 5 mg/dl, or the appearance of jaundice during the first 24 hours, or bilirubin levels greater than 12 mg/dl at any time are indications that the condition might be pathologic jaundice and that further investigation is needed to attempt to find the cause.[11] (See Chap. 46 for a discussion of pathologic jaundice and its treatment.)

The etiology of physiologic jaundice is not fully understood, nor are the hypotheses agreed on. The following are possible mechanisms in the development of this condition:

1. The newborn's high erythrocyte count and the shorter mean red blood cell life span lead to an increased breakdown of red blood cells, which contributes to the increased bilirubin load presented to the liver in the first days of life. Bilirubin from other sources such as myoglobin, a protein found in muscle, is also produced in increased amounts in the newborn.
2. The unconjugated, fat-soluble form of bilirubin that is produced when hemoglobin is broken down is usually changed in the liver to the conjugated, water-soluble form that can be excreted. In the newborn, there is interference with this conjugation, possibly owing to inhibition of the activity of the enzyme glucuronyl transferase.
3. Uptake of bilirubin from the plasma by the liver cells may be decreased because of immaturity of the liver.
4. Owing to the lack of intestinal bacterial flora in the newborn, bilirubin may be reabsorbed from the intestine and recirculated to the liver, rather than being excreted. Retention of meconium, which has a high bilirubin content, may add to the amount of bilirubin reabsorbed.[12]

Course of Hyperbilirubinemia in Normal Newborn

Unconjugated bilirubin in cord blood = approximately 2 mg/dl

Mean peak between 60 and 72 hours = 6 mg/dl

Rapid decline by 5th day to 2–3 mg/dl

Slower decline by about 10th day to <1 mg/dl

Possible Mechanisms Related to Development of Physiologic Jaundice

Increased production of bilirubin due to increased breakdown of red blood cells

Decreased clearance of bilirubin by the liver cells probably secondary to inhibition of glucuronyl transferase

Immaturity of the liver

Recirculation of increased amounts of bilirubin reabsorbed from the intestine

There seem to be some genetic and ethnic influences on the incidence of physiologic jaundice. Asian infants and some other isolated groups have mean maximal serum unconjugated bilirubin levels between 10 and 14 mg/dl, which is approximately double that of non-Asian populations. Kernicterus is also significantly increased in Asian neonates. The reasons for these increases are not known, but there may be a genetic predisposition to slower maturation of hepatic bilirubin metabolism or a possible relationship to ethnic food or herbal medicines.[11]

Nurses should not be lulled into a false sense of security by the term *physiologic*. Any baby who develops observable jaundice should be closely watched for symptoms of other possible problems. Parents of infants who are discharged early should be instructed on how to observe the infant for jaundice. If jaundice develops, the mother is usually instructed to bring the infant in for a blood test. A portable bilirubinometer used for noninvasive home testing has been found to be fairly accurate as a screening tool.[13]

BLOOD COAGULATION

At birth the vitamin K-dependent blood clotting factors (factors VII, IX, X, and prothrombin) are significantly decreased. The intestinal tract of the newborn does not harbor the bacteria necessary to help synthesize vitamin K; thus, the infant has a transitory deficiency in blood coagulation occurring between the second and the fifth postnatal days. This deficiency is sometimes severe enough to cause clinical bleeding. As a preventive measure, 0.5 to 1 mg of vitamin K is administered to the neonate during the first day of life.[7]

WHITE BLOOD CELLS

There is a wide range of normal for the leukocyte count at birth; the average is approximately 20,000 cells per microliter. Neutrophils comprise about 70% of this total. During the first few days after delivery there is a considerable decrease in the total count, as well as a shift in the type of predominant cell. The neutrophils decrease, and the lymphocytes increase, so that by the end of the first week the lymphocytes predominate and continue to do so until the child is 4 or 5 years old.[7]

Changes in the Immune System

The immune system begins to develop during fetal life but is still immature at birth. Nonspecific immunity is adversely affected by a number of differences from adult cell responses, including increased rigidity of leukocyte membranes and deficiency of complement and bacte-ricidal activity.[14] The ability of cells to ingest particles (phagocytosis), however, is close to normal adult levels.[7]

Specific immunity is also limited at birth. Development of immunity to specific organisms requires exposure to the antigen, by infection or immunization. In addition, ability to develop antibodies (immunocompetence) is necessary and develops sequentially, beginning in fetal life and continuing for months or years after birth. Antibody responses of newborns, therefore, are limited compared with those of older children or adults.[15] The fetus with an intrauterine infection does appear to develop IgM antibodies against the agents responsible, but IgA and IgE are seldom found at birth. Some maternal antibodies do cross the placenta, but not equally. IgG is most frequently found, but which IgG antibodies the infant receives depends on the mother's immune status. This passive immunity is transient. Because IgG has a half life of 20 to 30 days, the concentration falls rapidly and reaches its lowest level between the second and fourth months of life. Passive antibodies from placental transfer may interfere with active antibody formation, thus early immunization or infection may not result in long-lasting immunity.[14]

Temperature Regulation and Metabolic Changes

The infant is born into an environment that is considerably cooler than the one encountered in the uterus. Because of this rapid change in environmental conditions, the newborn's temperature may drop several degrees after birth. In recent years, attention has been focused on the effects of hypothermia on the newborn, and increasing efforts have been made to prevent this temperature drop in the delivery room and in the nursery. Neonates are predisposed to heat transfer between themselves and the environment because they have a limited supply of subcutaneous fat and a large surface area in relation to body weight.

Heat Loss. Evaporation, conduction, convection, and radiation are four ways in which the newborn can lose body heat to the environment. Excessive loss by *evaporation* occurs most often in the delivery room when the infant is wet (see Chap. 25), but it can also occur when the infant is being bathed. Heat evaporation may also occur from the lungs if the infant has tachypnea or if the humidity is low. Heat loss by *conduction* involves the transfer of heat from a warm object to a cooler one by direct contact and can occur when the infant is placed on a cold surface or when cool blankets or clothing are used. Through *convection*, the transference of heat is from a body to the surrounding air; the infant's temperature is affected by the air currents in the environment, such as those caused by air condi-

TABLE 29-1. THERMAL REGULATION IN THE NEWBORN

Mechanisms of Heat Loss	Prevention
Evaporation—loss of heat to air by way of moisture from skin or lungs	Dry well after delivery, especially head; protect from exposure while wet during bath; avoid very low humidity
Radiation—loss of heat to cool objects not in contact with infant	Avoid placing infant near cold outside walls or windows
Conduction—loss of heat from infant to cold surface	Do not place on cold surface; use warmed blankets in delivery room
Convection—loss of heat to air by way of drafts	Keep infant out of air flow currents
Mechanisms of Heat Production and Conservation	**Effects**
Nonshivering thermogenesis (metabolism of brown fat)	Increased metabolic consumption of calories
	Increased oxygen consumption
Increase in voluntary muscular activity (shivering is rare in the newborn)	Increased glucose consumption
Peripheral vasoconstriction	Conserve heat for body core
	Hands and feet may be blue, mottled, or cold to touch
Assumption of fetal position	Decreased surface area for loss of heat

tioners. The fourth mechanism, *radiation*, occurs when heat is transferred from a warm object to a cooler one when the objects are not in direct contact. This type of heat loss can occur in infants if the walls of an incubator are cool or if the crib is placed close to a cool outside wall or window. Each of these mechanisms, with the exception of evaporation, can be responsible for an increase in the infant's temperature as well as the losses described (Table 29-1).

Heat Production. To maintain a normal temperature when exposed to a cool environment, newborns increase their rate of heat production in an attempt to replace what is lost (see Table 29-1). Shivering is the most common mechanism of heat production in an adult, but the neonate rarely shivers, although there may be an increase in voluntary muscular activity. The primary mechanism of heat production in the newborn is nonshivering thermogenesis, whereby a chemical reaction occurs in brown fat, which breaks down triglycerides into glycerol and fatty acids and thereby produces heat. Brown fat cells contain many small fat vacuoles in contrast to the single, large vacuole of white fat. There is also a richer blood supply, which helps to account for its darker color and aids in the distribution of the heat produced. Brown fat is usually not found in adults, but in the newborn it accounts for approximately 1.5% of the total body weight. Significant deposits of brown fat are found at the nape of the neck, in the axillae, around the kidneys and adrenals, between the scapulae, and in the mediastinum[2] (Fig. 29-2).

Heat Conservation. Conservation of body heat in the infant occurs through peripheral vasoconstriction and through assumption of a flexed or fetal position, which decreases the surface area from which heat may be lost.

Effects of Cold Stress on the Newborn. The increased metabolic rate associated with nonshivering thermo-

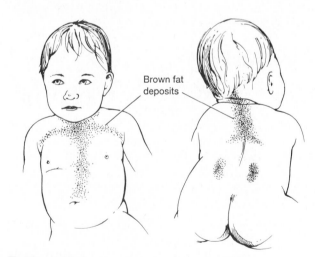

Brown fat deposits

■ *Figure 29–2*
Brown Fat. Deposits of brown fat are found between the scapulae, at the nape of the neck, in the axillae, in the mediastinum, and surrounding the kidneys and adrenals. The skin overlying brown fat deposits feels slightly warmer to the touch. Brown fat reserves usually persist for several weeks after birth unless depleted for heat production required by cold stress.

genesis necessitates an increase in both oxygen and calorie consumption. To replace the heat lost during a temperature drop of 3.5°C (6.3°F), it has been found that the infant requires a 100% increase in oxygen consumption for more than 1½ hours.[16] Even vigorous full-term infants may develop metabolic acidosis if allowed to become hypothermic. Prolonged cold stress may deplete brown fat stores and thus eliminate the infant's ability to produce heat by this mechanism.[2] It is obvious that cold stress can be detrimental or even fatal to an infant who is having difficulty with metabolism or oxygenation.

Efforts should be made to keep an infant in a neutral thermal environment, which means an environment where the infant's metabolic rate, and therefore oxygen consumption, is minimal but the body temperature remains within the normal range.

Neurologic Changes

The nervous system of the newborn is immature, that is, it is neither anatomically nor physiologically developed fully. Although all neurons are present, many remain immature for several months and some for years. Thus, infants are uncoordinated in their movements, are labile in their temperature regulation, and have poor control over their musculature—they "startle" easily, are subject to tremors of the extremities, and so on. However, during the neonatal period, development is rapid, and as the various nerve pathways controlling the muscles are used, the nerve fibers connect with one another. Gradually, more complex patterns of behavior emerge, and the higher cerebral levels begin to function.

Reflexes. The reflexes are important indices of the baby's normal development. Their presence or absence at certain times reflects the extent of normality in the functioning of the central nervous system (individual reflexes are discussed in Neurologic Assessment).

Gastrointestinal Changes

The gastrointestinal tract functions in a very limited capacity during fetal life. The fetus is known to swallow amniotic fluid, and a fecal material called *meconium* is formed, but the gastrointestinal tract is not responsible for the digestion or absorption of nutrients. By 36 to 38 weeks, though, it is mature enough to adapt readily to extrauterine life. The various enzymes necessary for digestion are active, and the muscular and reflex development provide the capability of transporting the food.[17]

For infants to swallow, food must be placed well back on the tongue, because they do not have the ability to transfer food from the lips to the pharynx. This means that the nipple should be placed well inside the infant's mouth. Sucking is facilitated by strong sucking muscles and ridges or corrugations in the anterior portion of the mouth. In addition, the *sucking pads* (deposits of fatty tissue in each cheek) prevent the collapse of the cheeks during nursing and further make sucking effective. This fatty tissue remains (even when fat is lost from the rest of the body) until sucking is no longer essential to the baby as a method of obtaining food. The salivary glands are immature at birth and manufacture little saliva until the infant is about 3 months old.

The newborn's intestinal tract is proportionately longer than that of an adult. Although it contains a large number of secretory glands and a large surface for absorption, its elastic tissue and supporting musculature are poor and not fully developed. This increases the likelihood of distention. Furthermore, nervous control is variable and inadequate. Nevertheless, the infant digests and absorbs a tremendous amount of food in proportion to body weight.

Most of the digestive enzymes seem to be present and adequate, with the exception of pancreatic amylase and lipase, which are somewhat deficient for several months but eventually reach a normal amount. Infants can digest simple foods easily but have a difficult time with the more complex starches. Protein and carbohydrates are easily absorbed, but fat absorption is poor.

Changes in Kidney Function and Urinary Excretion

The kidneys become functional during fetal life, as evidenced by the presence of urine in the bladder as early as the fourth month of gestation. Even at full term, however, the level of kidney function in the newborn is low. The full number of nephrons are present, but the surface area of the glomerular capillaries and the tubule length are about one tenth of adult size.[18]

Owing to the relatively low rate of glomerular filtration at birth, excess water and solute cannot be disposed of rapidly and efficiently. The limitations in tubular reabsorption that are also present may cause inappropriate substances from the glomerular filtrate, such as certain amino acids and bicarbonate, to appear in the urine.[18] In the healthy neonate these limitations do not have a detrimental effect, but they do restrict the ability of the newborn to respond to stress. As the kidneys grow and mature, function increases.

Ninety-two percent of healthy infants void within 24 hours, but the first voiding may occur shortly after delivery and not be noticed. Voidings during the first days after birth may be scanty and somewhat infrequent unless the infant was edematous at birth, but as the fluid intake increases, so does the output. Frequency usually increases from 2 to 6 times on the first and second day to 5 to 20 times per 24 hours after that until the infant begins to develop bladder control and the number of voidings per day decreases.

The urine of the newborn may appear cloudy owing to high mucus and urate content, but with increased fluid intake the urine becomes clear, straw colored, and nearly odorless. Uric acid crystals in the urine may cause a reddish "brick-dust" stain on the diaper that is sometimes confused with blood in the urine.

Changes in Hepatic Function

During fetal life, the liver performs an important role in blood formation, and it is thought that it continues this function to some degree after birth. Later in the neonatal period, the liver produces substances that are essential in the coagulation of the blood. If the mother's iron intake has been adequate during pregnancy, enough iron is stored in the infant's liver to carry over the first months of life when the diet (primarily milk) is iron deficient. About the fifth month, however, the baby's iron reserve is depleted, and unless foods containing iron are given, a deficiency will ensue.

■ PHYSICAL ASSESSMENT

The physical examination was traditionally done by the physician. In recent years, many nurses have learned physical assessment skills, and in some hospitals a pediatric nurse practitioner has the responsibility for part of the newborn physical examinations. Although all nurses do not possess practitioner skills, those who work with newborns should be able to do a basic assessment and recognize deviations from normal.

The Assessment Tool, Newborn Physical Assessment Guide, can be used in learning to assess the newborn. The discussion of newborn characteristics that follows and Table 29-2 are helpful in using the guide. Practice and experience also improve the nurse's ability to recognize the range of normal. Discussion of abnormalities is found in Chapters 44 to 46.

The format of the Newborn Physical Assessment Guide can be used for an admitting assessment or a later one. It is not intended to be a complete physical examination, but it should give the nurse a good idea of the status of the infant. The examiner can use any system of notation that is helpful to fill in the spaces on the form. A suggestion is to use a "check" to indicate "within normal limits" and a "plus" or "minus" to indicate whether something is present or absent. When appropriate, description can be written in the spaces or under "comments."

Methods used in physical examination are inspection, auscultation, palpation, and percussion, usually in that order. Percussion is not specifically used in this form. The examination is written for use in evaluating the infant in a cephalocaudal direction, but it may be best to begin with items, such as auscultation of the chest, that require the infant to be quiet, before performing procedures that might cause the infant to cry. Each examiner should establish a definite pattern and follow it each time so that nothing is missed. To avoid startling the infant, it is helpful for the nurse to have warm hands, talk to the infant quietly, and use slow, smooth movements. Having a pacifier available can also assist in quieting the infant for parts of the examination.

When any assessment of the newborn is carried out, the parents should be included as much as possible. If they cannot be present for the examination, it should at least be discussed with them. Being there, though, is a good way to help them get better acquainted with their infant. Also, it is important for the nurse to look at the baby from the parent's viewpoint. The healthy newborn has many characteristics that momentarily may look unusual to them. The nurse should be ready to talk with the parents about their baby and to answer their questions.

Physical assessment of the neonate begins at birth when the delivery room nurse observes the infant to assign the Apgar score and to detect any anomalies or problems (see Chap. 25). When the infant is brought to the nursery, pertinent information concerning the mother's antepartal history, the course of labor and delivery, the condition of the infant at and following birth, and any care given to the infant is reported to the nursery nurse.

After confirming the report by looking at the newborn's record, the next step is the nursery nurse's initial evaluation of the infant's general condition, including the following:

1. Observe the infant's appearance. Is the color ruddy, pale, cyanotic, or jaundiced? Is the color evenly distributed? The infant usually is in a flexed position with good muscle tone. A "floppy" baby or a very tense baby needs careful observation.
2. The infant's cry can also be an indicator of general condition. A lusty cry is usually a good sign, but a weak or shrill cry can be indicative of central nervous system problems, and grunting sounds mean that the infant is having to work harder to get oxygen.
3. Other signs of increased respiratory effort, such

Assessment Tool

<hr>

Newborn Physical Assessment Guide

Baby's Name _____ Date and Time of Birth _____
Mothers's Name _____ Date and Time of Exam _____

Initial Evaluation
1. General Appearance: Color _____ Muscle tone _____
2. Respiratory Effort: Retractions _____ Gasping _____
   Grunting _____ Quality of cry _____
3. Temperature: _____
Comments: _____
_____

Assessment of Head and Neck

1. Observe and palpate the infant's head for symmetry; note absence or presence of:
   Molding _____ Caput succedaneum _____ Cephalhematoma _____
2. Palpate the fontanels and sutures for: Fullness _____ Depression _____
   Overriding _____ Shape _____ Size _____
3. Measure circumference of head: _____
4. Evaluate ears: Position _____ Shape _____ Location _____
5. Evaluate symmetry of face: _____
6. Observe eyes for: Shape _____ Position _____ Size _____
   Appearance of pupils _____ Presence of hemorrhage _____ Red reflex _____
7. Evaluate mouth for: Clefts _____ Teeth _____ Frenulum linguae _____
8. Observe neck for: Length _____ Relationship to body _____
   Mobility _____ Presence of webbing or fat pad _____
9. Observe skin of scalp, face, and neck for: Abrasions or contusions _____
   Other breaks or marks _____
10. Observe nose for: Symmetry _____ Septum _____ Flaring _____
Comments: _____
_____
_____

Assessment of Body

General Appearance
1. Measurements: Weight _____ Length _____ Circumference of chest _____
2. Observe throughout evaluation for: General activity _____
   Posture _____ Responsiveness _____
3. Observe skin for: Lanugo _____ Vernix _____ Meconium staining _____
   Texture _____ Hydration _____ Color _____ Rashes _____
   Pigmentation _____
Comments: _____

Thorax

1. Palpate clavicles for masses and intactness: _____
2. Inspect thorax for: Size _____ Symmetry _____ Shape _____
3. Auscultate for: Breath sounds _____ Heart sounds _____ Rhythm _____
4. Count: respiratory rate _____ Apical pulse _____

(continued)

Assessment Tool   (continued)

Comments: _____

_____

Abdomen

1. Inspect shape of abdomen: _____
2. Palpate: Liver _____ Spleen _____ Kidneys _____
3. Observe cord for number of vessels: _____
4. Palpate: Femoral pulses _____
Comments: _____

Genitals

1. Observe visible genitals for: Appropriateness with stated sex _____
2. Observe female infant for: Maturation of labia _____ Vaginal discharge _____
3. Observe male infant for: Position of urethral opening _____
   Maturation of scrotum _____ Presence of testes _____
4. Note elimination: (should occur within 24 hours)
   Urine _____ Color _____ Amount/24 hours _____
   Stool _____ Color _____ Type _____ Number/24 hours _____
Comments: _____

Posterior of Body

1. Palpate and inspect spinal column for: Masses _____
   Symmetry of vertebrae _____ Intactness _____
2. Determine patency of anus: _____
3. Observe pilonidal dimple for intactness: _____
Comments: _____

Extremities

1. Note for all extremities: Symmetry _____ Abnormalities _____
   Ability to move _____
2. Count digits on: Hands _____ Feet _____
   Observe for polydactyly _____ Syndactyly _____
3. Evaluate rotation of hips: Abduct thighs to bed _____
   Rotate hips through full range of motion _____
   Observe leg length, front and back (Are they equal?) _____ Knee height _____
   Observe symmetry of leg creases _____
4. Note position of feet _____
   Can they passively be returned to normal? _____
Comments: _____

Assessment of Neurologic Function—Reflexes—Elicit and Evaluate:

1. Rooting and sucking: _____

(continued)

Assessment Tool (continued)

2. Grasp: Palmar _____ Plantar _____

3. Traction: (Pull to sitting position, note head and arm position) _____

4. Moro: _____

5. Stepping: _____

Comments: _____

Items that require manipulation, such as palpation of the abdomen and abduction of the hips, require care in performance to avoid injury to the infant and should not be attempted for the first time without supervision by a trained examiner.

(After NAACOG Technical Bulletin No. 2, ''Physical Assessment of the Neonate'')

as retractions, gasping, or flaring of the nostrils, should also be noted.

4. The vital signs should be taken.

From the foregoing observations the nurse can make a decision about whether the infant needs immediate treatment, if time is needed for the temperature to stabilize, or if the assessment can continue.

It is important to remember that certain symptoms that might be cause for concern in an older child (*e.g.,* rapid rate and irregular rhythm of respirations) may merely represent normal physiology in a newborn (see Newborn Physical Assessment Guide).

Assessment of Head and Neck

The infant's head is large, comprising about one quarter of his size and, with cephalic presentations, may initially appear to be asymmetrical because of the molding of the skull bones during labor (Fig. 29-3). If there has been extended pressure on the head, caput succedaneum (a swelling of the soft tissues) or cephalhematoma (an accumulation of blood between the bone and the periosteum) might be present (see Chap. 46).

The suture lines between the skull bones and the anterior and the posterior fontanels can usually be palpated easily (see Fig. 20-10). The fontanels should feel soft and be neither bulging nor depressed. The diamond-shaped anterior fontanel is normally about 2 to 3 cm wide and 3 to 4 cm long at birth. It may feel

smaller for the first day or two when there is marked overriding of the skull bones. Closure usually takes place by 12 to 18 months. The posterior fontanel is triangular and is located between the occipital and the parietal bones. It is smaller than the anterior fontanel and may be almost closed at birth and completely closed by the end of the second month.

(Text continues on page 656)

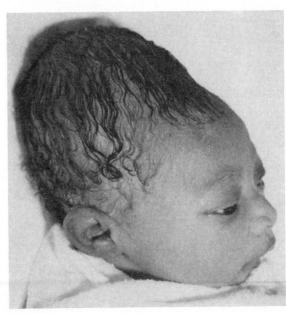

■ *Figure 29–3*
Molding of the head.

TABLE 29-2. SUMMARY OF NEWBORN PHYSICAL ASSESSMENT

Assessment Area	Usual Findings	Deviations
General Observations		
Muscle tone	Flexed position; good tone	"Floppy"; rigid or tense
Skin		
Color	Pink tone to ruddy when crying; appropriate to ethnic origin; acrocyanosis	Pallor; cyanosis; jaundice; ecchymosis; petechiae
Texture	Smooth; dryness with some peeling; lanugo on back; vernix	Excessive peeling or cracking; roughness
Rashes and pigmentation	Erythema toxicum; milia; mongolian spots	Impetigo; hemangiomas; nevus flammeus (port-wine stain)
Hydration	Skin pinch over abdomen immediately returns to original state	Skin maintains "tent" shape after pinch
Cry	Lusty	Shrill; weak; grunty
Measurements		
Weight	2700–4000 g (6–9 lb)	
Length	48–53 cm (19–21 in)	
Head circumference	33–37 cm (13–14.5 in)	
Chest circumference	31–35 cm (12.5–14 in)	
Vital Signs		
Temperature	Axillary (preferred method)—36.5–37°C (97.7–98.6°F)	Hypothermia; fever
	Rectal—36.5–37.2°C (97.7–99°F)	
Respirations	40–60 respirations/min; quiet and shallow; diaphragmatic; occasional periods of rapid breathing, alternating with short periods of apnea	Prolonged rapid breathing; apnea lasting longer than 10 sec; grunting; retractions; persistent slow rate
Heart rate (apical pulse)	120–160 beats/min; faster when crying (up to 180 beats/min); slower when sleeping (down to 100 beats/min)	Tachycardia—greater than 160 beats/min at rest Bradycardia—less than 120 beats/min when awake
Head	Vaginal delivery—elongated (molding) Breech or cesarean birth—round, symmetrical Size within normal range	Caput succedaneum; cephalhematoma; hydrocephaly; microcephaly
Fontanels	Flat; soft; firm	Bulging; sunken
Anterior	Diamond shaped; 2–3 cm wide; 3–4 cm long; smaller at birth with molding	Small; almost closed; closed (craniostenosis); widened
Posterior	Triangular shape; small; almost closed	Enlarged
Face	Small; round; symmetrical; fat pads in cheeks; receding chin	Asymmetrical; disorted
Eyes	Edematous lids; usually closed; blue or slate-gray color; no tears; red reflex present; pupils equal, round, react to light Common variations—subconjunctival hemorrhages; chemical conjunctivitis; occasional slight nystagmus or convergent strabismus	Elevation or ptosis of lids; epicanthal folds; absence of red reflex; unequal, dilated, or constricted pupils Purulent discharge; frequent nystagmus; constant, divergent, or unilateral strabismus
Mouth	Intact lips, gums, palate; epithelial pearls; "sucking blisters" on lips; tongue midline, mobile, appropriate size for mouth; can extend to alveolar ridge	Cleft lip or palate; white, cheesy patches on tongue, gums, or mucous membrane; large or protruding tongue

(continued)

TABLE 29–2. SUMMARY OF NEWBORN PHYSICAL ASSESSMENT *(continued)*

Assessment Area	Usual Findings	Deviations
Nose	In midline; even placement in relation to eyes and mouth; nares patent; septum intact, midline	Flattened or bruised; unusual placement or configuration; obstructed nares; deviated or perforated septum
Ears	Well-formed cartilage; appropriate size for head; upper attachment on line extended through inner and outer canthus of eye; external auditory canal patent	Floppy, large and protruding; malformed; low set; obstruction of canal
Neck	Short; thick; full range of motion; no masses	Webbing; abnormal shortening; limitation of motion; torticollis; masses
Clavicles	Straight; smooth; intact	Knot or lump; decreased movement of extremity on one side
Thorax	Round; symmetrical; protruding xiphoid process	Asymmetrical; funnel chest
Breath sounds	Loud; bronchial; bilaterally equal	Decreased breath sounds; increased breath sounds; absent breath sounds
Heart sounds	Regular rate and rhythm; first and second sounds clear and distinct	Murmurs; arrhythmias
Breasts	Symmetrical; flat with erect nipples; engorgement 2nd or 3rd day not unusual	Redness and firmness around nipple
Abdomen	Symmetrical; slightly protuberant; no masses	Scaphoid or concave shape; distention; palpable masses; asymmetrical
Liver	Palpable 2–3 cm below right costal margin	Enlargement
Spleen	Tip may be palpable in left upper quadrant	Enlargement
Kidneys	May be palpable at level of umbilicus	Enlargement
Femoral pulses	Bilaterally equal	Unequal or absent
Umbilicus	No extensive protrusion or herniation; no signs of infection	Umbilical hernia; omphalocele; redness; induration; foul-smelling discharge
	Cord—bluish white, moist → black, dry; 3 vessels; no oozing or bleeding	Two vessels; bleeding or oozing from stump
Genitalia	Appropriate for gender	Ambiguous genitalia
Female		
Labia	Edematous; labia majora cover labia minora; vernix in creases	Hematoma; lesions; fusion of labia
Vagina	Mucus discharge, possibly blood tinged	
Male		
Foreskin	Adherent to glans of penis	Opening below tip of penis (hypospadias)
Urethra	Opening at tip of penis	Opening above tip of penis (epispadias)
Testes	Palpable in each scrotal sac	Palpable in inguinal canal; not palpable

(continued)

TABLE 29–2. SUMMARY OF NEWBORN PHYSICAL ASSESSMENT *(continued)*

Assessment Area	Usual Findings	Deviations
Posterior of Body		
Spinal column	Straight, flexible; intact, no masses	Exaggerated curves; spina bifida; any masses; pilonidal cyst
Anus	Patent	Imperforate anus; anal fissures
Extremities	Symmetrical in size, shape, and movement	Unequal or abnormal size or shape; asymmetrical or limited movement of one or more extremities
Digits	Five on each hand and foot; appropriate size and shape	Missing digits; syndactyly (webbing); polydactyly (extra digits)
Hips	Even leg length, knee height, gluteal folds; no resistance or limitation to abduction	Uneven leg length, knee height, or gluteal folds; uneven or limited abduction; hip "click" or "clunk" on abduction
Feet	Straight, or postural deviation easily corrected with gentle pressure	Structural deformities—talipes equinovarus (clubfoot); metatarsus adductus
Reflexes		
Rooting and sucking	Turns toward object touching cheek, lips, or corner of mouth; opens mouth; begins sucking movements; strong suck, pulls object into mouth May be diminished or absent after eating	No rooting; weak, ineffective, or absent suck
Grasp Palmar	Fingers grasp object when palm stimulated and hang on briefly	Weak or absent
Plantar	Toes curl downward when soles of feet are stimulated	Weak or absent
Moro	Symmetrical response to sudden stimulus—lateral extension of arms with opening of hands, followed by flexion and adduction	Asymmetrical; absent; incomplete
Stepping	Stepping movements when infant held upright with sole of foot touching surface	Asymmetrical or absent

The circumference of the head is measured by placing a nonstretchable tape measure just above the eyebrows and over the most prominent part of the occiput (Fig. 29-4). Normally, the head circumference is 2 cm larger than the chest circumference, but an accurate measurement may not be obtained at first if molding is present. The normal range is 33 to 37 cm (13–14½ in), depending on the general size of the infant.

The face is small and round, and the lower jaw appears to recede. Facial asymmetry is sometimes seen, especially of the chin and mandible. This can be the result of posture *in utero* when the flexed head is tilted to one side and presses against the shoulder. The nose may also be asymmetrical or have a deviated septum from intrauterine pressure. It is important that the nose not be obstructed, because infants are nose breathers and have difficulty breathing through their mouths.

The scalp, face, and neck should be observed carefully for any abrasions, contusions, or breaks in the skin. These can result from application of internal fetal monitor electrodes, forceps, or other instruments used in delivery. Any opening in the skin is a potential site for bacterial invasion and should be watched for signs of infection.

Eyes. The eyes are closed much of the time but may open spontaneously if the infant's head is lifted or rocked gently (a valuable point to remember when one wants to inspect the eyes). From birth the infant can see and discriminate patterns as the basis for form perception. This capacity is rather limited by imperfect oculomotor coordination and inability to accommodate for varying distances. Moreover, the eye, the visual pathways, and the visual part of the brain are poorly

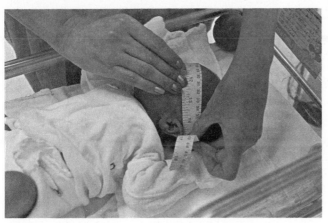

■ *Figure 29–4*
The circumference of the head is measured by placing a nonstretchable tape just above the eyebrows and over the most prominent part of the occiput.

developed at birth. Nevertheless, although the baby's vision is much less acute than an adult's, a good deal of visual experience is possible.

Many mothers do not realize the visual capabilities of their infants, and they appreciate being informed of this. In addition, some mothers become exceedingly anxious when they observe strabismus or nystagmus in their infants, but they should be reassured that this lack of coordination is normal during the first few months of life.

Most babies' eyes are blue or a slate-gray color at birth. By the time the infant is 3 months old, most have achieved their permanent color, although complete pigmentation of the iris does not occur until the infant is about 1 year old. Because the lacrimal glands may not be functioning at birth, babies do not usually shed tears when they cry. Tears may not appear for several weeks and sometimes for several months. There may be some edema of the lids or purulent discharge caused by the silver nitrate, if it was used. The changes in the vascular tension of the eyes during delivery sometimes cause small areas of subconjunctival hemorrhage. These areas disappear spontaneously in 1 or 2 weeks and are not significant.

If an ophthalmoscope is used in examining the eyes, the pupil should appear as a small, red-orange circular spot when the light is directed at it. This is the red reflex, which is caused by the light shining on the retina, and any opacities of the lens or other obstructions would be visible if present.

Ears and Hearing. The ears should be inspected for size, shape, position, malrotation, and anomaly. The point where the top of the ear is attached to the scalp should fall on or above an imaginary line drawn from the inner through the outer canthus of the eye (Fig. 29-5). Abnormal positioning of the ears is frequently associated with certain chromosomal abnormalities or kidney anomalies.

Otoscopic examination of the ear establishes the patency of the external auditory canal, but the tympanic membranes are usually difficult to visualize for the first 2 or 3 days of life owing to accumulated vernix caseosa. Phibbs suggests, however, that visualization should be attempted in the infant suspected of having an infection because otitis media can occur during these first days.[19] During the first few months, the light reflex is diffuse rather than cone shaped as it is later.

The ear and the nerve tracts for hearing are anatomically mature at birth, and newborns can hear after their first cry. Hearing apparently becomes acute within several days as the eustachian tubes become aerated and the mucus in the middle ear disappears.

Hearing can be tested by sounding a bell or rattle near the baby's head but out of eyesight. Hearing the sound causes blinking of the eyes, momentary cessation of activity, or a startle response. This is not an accurate

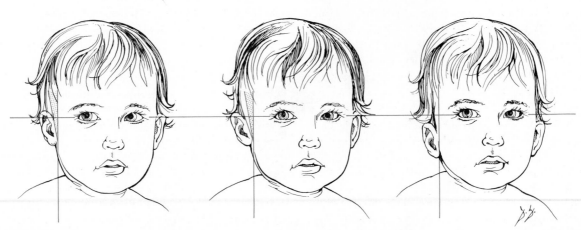

■ *Figure 29–5*
(A) Normal ear. (B) Abnormally angled ear. (C) Low-set ear.

test, but it may be helpful in alerting the examiner to a possible problem.

Neck. The newborn generally appears to have a short neck, which sometimes makes it difficult to tell if webbing or other problems are present. The head should be gently rotated to determine the range of motion of the neck, and the muscles should be palpated for any masses.

Lips, Mouth, and Cheeks. The rounded, thickened areas often present on the lips (particularly on the center of the upper lip) are known as labial tubercles or "sucking blisters," although they are not true blisters because there is no fluid in them. Sucking (fat) pads are usually present in the cheeks. The lips, gums, and palate should be examined to see that they are intact. Epstein's pearls, small white cysts that may be seen on the hard palate or gums, are not abnormal. Occasionally, a tooth is present, which may be pulled to avoid the possibility of its being aspirated.

At this early age, the tongue does not extend far beyond the margin of the gums because the frenulum is normally short. A mother's concern that her baby is tongue tied is usually unwarranted.

Assessment of Body

General Appearance. The average term infant weighs 3500 g (7½ lb), and 95% weigh between 2500 g (5½ lb) and 4250 g (9½ lb). There is usually some weight loss in the first 3 to 5 days, possibly as much as 10% of the infant's birth weight. This is usually regained by the eighth to twelfth day.

Length should also be measured soon after birth to serve as a baseline from which to judge future growth. The average length of a full-term infant at birth is 51 cm (20 in), with 95% between 46 and 56 cm (18 and 22 in). Because the newborn usually assumes a somewhat flexed position, it can be difficult to get an accurate measurement from the top of the head to the heels. Measurement is more accurate when done on a firm surface, and it is helpful to have an assistant hold the infant's head.

Color. The infant's color should be assessed early in the examination. The color may be pink, reddish, or pale, becoming more ruddy when the baby cries. The skin tends to be less pigmented in the neonatal period than later in life, so color changes may be noted even in darker-skinned babies. Initially, the hands and feet are usually blue (acrocyanosis) owing to the sluggish peripheral vascular circulation, but this cyanosis of the extremities is transient and often disappears in a few

hours. If more generalized cyanosis is present, the extent and circumstances of its appearance should be noted. The infant who is cyanotic at rest and pink only when crying may have choanal atresia. Cardiac or pulmonary problems may be suspected if crying increases the cyanosis. The infant who continues to be ruddy or plethoric even at rest should have a hematocrit done to rule out polycythemia. The very pale infant may be anemic or hypotensive and should be checked for these conditions.[20]

Frequent assessment of the newborn for jaundice is an important nursing responsibility, to help detect significant hyperbilirubinemia as early as possible. The red color of the blood or the pigment in the skin of dark-complected babies sometimes hides the yellow color. Blanching the skin over a bony area, such as the chest or forehead, by pressing with a finger and observing the area before the color comes back often allows the yellow to be seen. The sclera and the buccal mucosa are also good places to look.

Skin. The skin of the normal full-term newborn is soft, velvety, and wrinkled. At birth, it is covered to varying degrees with vernix caseosa, a white, cheesy material made up of sebum and desquamating cells. The vernix serves as a protection for the skin in utero and at term is found primarily in the body creases. After the vernix is removed or disappears, the skin is often dry and peeling. A fine, downy hair called *lanugo* may be found on the face, brow, and shoulders, especially in preterm infants.

A variety of rashes, discolorations, and other "birthmarks" appear on the skin in the newborn period. Many are considered normal variations, and most fade with time, but some can be indicative of genetic syndromes, and, depending on their location, some can be disfiguring (Table 29-3).

Small, flat hemangiomas may be apparent on the nape of the neck, on the eyelids, or over the bridge of the nose. These clusters of small capillaries are sometimes called *stork bites*. They usually disappear spontaneously during infancy, but some, especially those on the nape of the neck, may persist into adulthood.

Gray-blue pigmented areas are seen most often in dark-skinned infants, especially in the lumbosacral area, although other sites are not uncommon. These "mongolian spots" have no relationship to mongolism and usually disappear spontaneously during late infancy or early childhood.

ERYTHEMA TOXICUM. Erythema toxicum is a blotchy, erythematous rash that may appear in the first few days of life (Fig. 29-6). It is sometimes referred to as the *newborn rash* or as *"flea-bite" dermatitis* (although no fleas are involved). The erythematous areas, which develop most frequently on the back, shoulders, and buttocks, have a small, blanched wheal in the center. The cause

TABLE 29–3. BIRTHMARKS

Type	Characteristics
Vascular nevi	
Telangiectic nevi (stork bites)	Tiny pink to red spots found commonly on nape of the neck, eyelids, and bridge of the nose; do blanch on pressure; usually disappear spontaneously during infancy, but some persist into adulthood
Nevus flammeus (port-wine stain)	Flat, purple-red, sharply demarcated areas, often found on the face (on black infants, they are deep purple-black); do not blanch on pressure, increase in size, or fade over time; disfigurement varies with size and placement
	If the infant also displays epileptic-like seizures, may indicate Sturge-Weber syndrome, a serious genetic disorder
Nevus vasculosus (strawberry marks)	Dark red, rough-textured, sharply demarcated elevations usually found on head or face; continue to grow for several months, then shrink spontaneously and usually disappear by 7–10 yr of age
Pigmented nevi	
Mongolian spots	Gray-blue pigmented areas seen most often on lumbosacral region and buttocks of dark-skinned and Asian infants; usually spontaneously disappear during late infancy or early childhood; have no relationship to mongolism
Café au lait spots	Patchy, flat, brown areas that are lighter in color than the surrounding skin; commonly found on the face, chest, arms, hands; usually of no significance; however, if spots are >1.5 cm long or more than six are present, they may indicate certain genetic syndromes (e.g., Von Recklinghausen disease)

of this skin disturbance is obscure, and no treatment is necessary. The rash is transient, is likely to change appreciably within a few hours, and usually disappears entirely within a day or so.

MILIA. Milia are pinpoint-sized, pearly white spots that occur commonly on the nose, forehead, or chin of the newborn. When touched gently with the tip of the finger, these spots feel like tiny, firm seeds. They are due to retention of sebaceous material within the sebaceous glands and, if they are left alone, usually disappear spontaneously during the neonatal period.

Mothers often mistake milia for "whiteheads" and may attempt to squeeze them if the nurse or the physician has not warned them against such practice.

CAFÉ AU LAIT SPOTS. Café au lait spots or patches are flat, brown areas that are lighter in light-skinned people and darker in those with more pigmentation. Single, small lesions are not unusual in newborns and are of no significance, but if the spots are greater than 1.5 cm in length or more than six are present, they may be indicative of neurofibromatosis or certain genetic syndromes.[21]

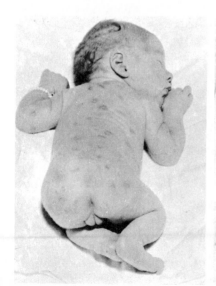 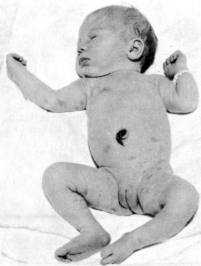

■ *Figure 29–6*
Erythema toxicum. This "newborn rash" develops more frequently on the back, the shoulders, and the buttocks. (Courtesy of MacDonald House, The University Hospitals of Cleveland, Cleveland, OH)

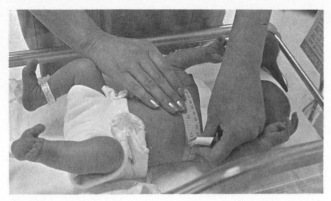

■ *Figure 29–7*
Measuring the infant's chest.

Thorax. The infant's chest is round with a transverse diameter that is approximately equal to the anteroposterior diameter. The circumference, measured just above the nipple line, is slightly smaller than the head (Fig. 29-7). The thorax is relatively short compared with the abdomen. The chest wall is thin with little musculature, and the rib cage is very soft and pliant. The tip of the xiphoid process often protrudes visibly.

Engorgement of the breasts is common during the neonatal period in both male and female infants (Fig. 29-8), owing to endocrine influence. The breasts have been acted on throughout pregnancy by the estrogenic hormone that passes to them through the placenta from the mother. This is the same hormone that prepares the mother's breasts for lactation. When it is withdrawn after birth, changes in the infant's breasts, similar to those in the mother, take place. Mammary engorgement in the newborn subsides without treatment, but many persist for 2 or 3 weeks.

Sometimes a small amount of fluid that has been called *"witches' milk"* is secreted. Mothers should be

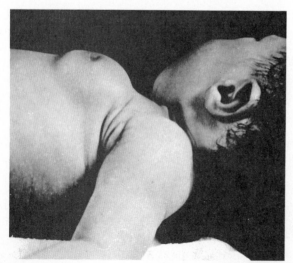

■ *Figure 29–8*
Hypertrophy of breast developing in the neonatal period.

cautioned against massaging the infant's breasts or trying to express the fluid because this could lead to an infection, such as breast abscess or mastitis.

ASSESSING RESPIRATION. As the infant adapts successfully to extrauterine life, the respiratory rate usually ranges from 40 to 60 breaths per minute and is easily altered by internal and external stimuli. Counting respirations in the newborn can be very frustrating, because the infant may have periods of rapid breathing alternating with short periods of apnea. Intermittent crying may also interfere with counting. Respirations should be counted for 1 full minute or longer if necessary. Because the infant primarily uses diaphragmatic breathing, it is easier to count abdominal rather than chest excursions. An alternate method is to count respirations by auscultation (Fig. 29-9).

The respiration is normally quiet and shallow, with the chest and abdomen moving together. Although retractions, mild expiratory grunting, and nasal flaring may be considered normal during the first few minutes after birth, presence after that time leads one to suspect obstruction or abnormality.

In auscultation of the infant's chest, it is best to use the bell or small diaphragm of the stethoscope, because the adult-sized diaphragm may not make complete contact with the small chest wall. Auscultation should be done in both upright and supine positions because breath sounds may be altered with changing positions. Bronchial breath sounds are normally heard over most of the chest and sound louder and harsher than in the adult because they are closer.

Periods of dyspnea and cyanosis may occur suddenly in an infant who is breathing normally, even after the transition period is over. This *may* indicate some anomaly or other pathologic condition and should be reported promptly. The nurse should notify the physician if the respiratory rate is persistently below 40 respirations per minute or if it increases beyond 60 respirations per minute when the infant is at rest, or if dyspnea or cyanosis occurs.

HEART. The heart rate is determined by counting the apical pulse (Fig. 29-10). It is normally between 120 and 160 beats per minute and, like the respiratory rate, changes with the infant's activity. It beats faster with crying, increased activity, or rapid breathing, and more slowly when the infant is quiet, especially during the short periods of no breathing.

The first and second heart sounds should be clear and well defined. Murmurs may be present in the newborn period. They may be heard more easily with the bell of the stethoscope held lightly against the chest wall. The areas of cardiac auscultation where murmurs are most likely to be heard are the right sternal border, the upper left sternal border, the lower left sternal border, and the apex. Any murmurs should be reported, recorded, and followed but may be less significant in

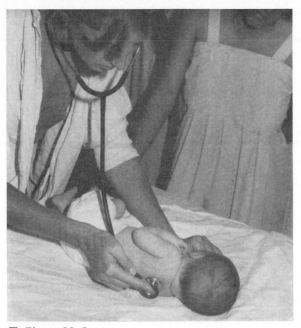
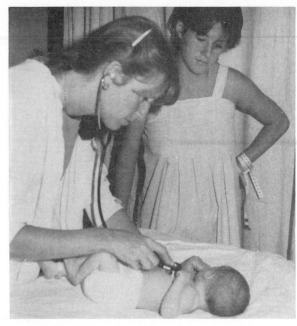

■ *Figure 29–9*
Auscultation of the newborn. The nurse practitioner performs a discharge physical examination while the mother observes.

the newborn period than at other times, because a closing ductus arteriosus may cause a loud murmur that soon disappears, whereas a serious heart anomaly may cause no murmur at all.

Early experiences in listening to the newborn's chest can be confusing because both the heart rate and respirations are so much faster than an adult's and the infant often wiggles and fusses. With practice the stu-

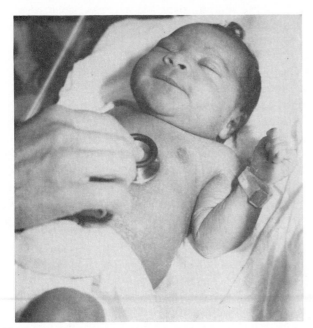

■ *Figure 29–10*
Taking an apical pulse.

dent will learn how to quiet the infant and to be able to distinguish between the different sounds.

Abdomen. The abdomen is round and slightly protuberant owing to the relative size of the abdominal organs and weak muscular structures. Superficial veins are often visible. Observation can be a valuable part of the examination of the abdomen, because outlines of the anterior organs may sometimes be seen. An abdomen that is asymmetrical, scaphoid (sunken), or grossly distended is suggestive of abnormalities and should be checked carefully.

Palpation should begin with gentle pressure or stroking of the abdomen upward, then deeper palpation may be done. The liver edge is usually palpable just below the right rib margin, but it is not sharp and may be missed if palpation is too high or too forceful. The tip of the spleen may sometimes be palpated in the left upper quadrant. The kidneys can usually be palpated during the first 4 to 6 hours after birth, but they are more difficult to locate after this. If palpable, the lower edges are usually located approximately at the level of the umbilicus, about half way between the infant's side and the midline.

The umbilical cord stump should be checked for bleeding or oozing (Fig. 29-11), and the number of vessels noted if not already recorded (see Chap. 25). The umbilicus and surrounding area should also be inspected carefully. Redness, induration, skin warmth, and foul-smelling discharge are signs of infection that should be reported. Infection in this area is potentially dangerous

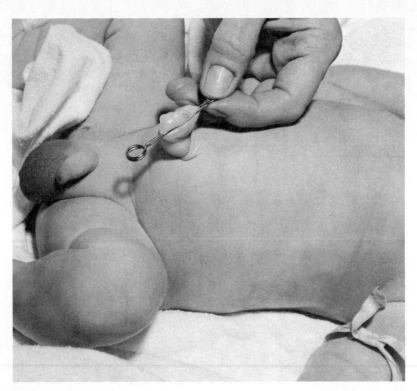

■ *Figure 29–11*
Inspection of the cord stump.

in the newborn because it can spread up the open arteries into the peritoneum. Serous or serosanguineous discharge continuing after separation of the cord stump may indicate a granuloma. This has the appearance of a small, red button deep in the umbilicus. It can be cauterized by the physician with a silver nitrate stick.[22]

Genitals. Female genitalia should be inspected for presence and size of the labia majora, labia minora, clitoris, and vaginal opening. Enlarged labia or vaginal discharge may be present due to *in utero* stimulation by maternal hormones. The discharge is sometimes blood tinged but need cause no special concern. The swelling and discharge disappear spontaneously.

In male babies, the scrotum usually appears relatively large and may have increased pigmentation at birth owing to maternal hormones. At term, the testes usually can be palpated in the scrotum or can be easily brought down. The prepuce (foreskin) covers the glans penis and is usually adherent at birth. When the opening in the foreskin is so small that it cannot be pulled back at all, the condition is called *phimosis.* If it is tight enough to interfere with urination, circumcision may be recommended. The penis should be inspected to determine the location of the urinary meatus. It is usually located at the tip of the penis. When it is located on the underside of the penis, the condition is known as *hypospadias;* location on the dorsum of the penis is called *epispadias.* If the meatus is covered by the foreskin, observation of the infant during voiding will help to determine its placement.

Posterior. With the infant in the prone position, the entire posterior surface of the body should be inspected and palpated. Any masses or abnormal curvatures of the spine should be noted. Tufts of hair or small indentations, especially in the sacral area, may be an indication of spina bifida occulta.

The perineal area should be inspected to determine the patency and location of the anus. A pilonidal "dimple" resulting from an irregular fold of skin is sometimes seen in the midline over the sacrococcygeal area. It should be examined for intactness to make sure no sinus is present.

Extremities. Throughout the examination, the infant's ability to move all four extremities is evaluated and the limbs are compared as to size, shape, and movement. Webbing (syndactyly) or extra digits (polydactyly) should be noted also.

To check for congenital problems of the hip, the infant is placed in the supine position and the legs are flexed on the abdomen and then abducted laterally toward the bed. With congenital dislocation, there may be uneven or limited abduction or uneven leg length or knee height, or a "hip click" might be felt (Fig. 29-12). Asymmetrical skin folds on the posterior aspect of the thigh are not diagnostic but may alert the examiner to this condition. Unusual positions of the feet can indicate congenital clubfoot or other foot and ankle deformities (see Chap. 45). If the foot can be moved to the normal position with ease, the condition may just be due to intrauterine malposition.

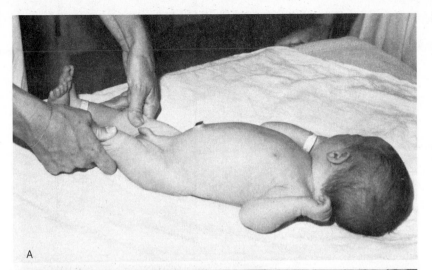

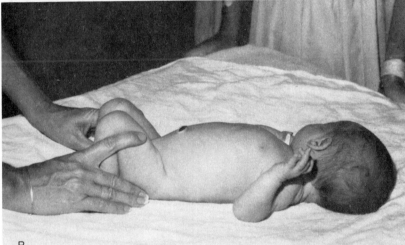

■ *Figure 29–12*
Assessment of the lower extremities. (A)
Comparing the length of the legs. (B)
Comparing the height of the knees. (C) Hip
abduction.

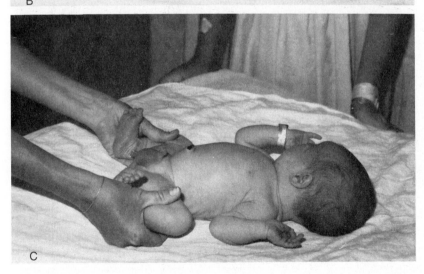

■ NEUROLOGIC ASSESSMENT

The neurologic assessment deals with the functioning of the infant's nervous system. Some of the items assessed in the physical, gestational age, and behavioral assessments are also indicators of nervous system functioning. For example, vital signs are part of the physical assessment but could also be included in the neurologic assessment because extreme lability of the temperature and blood pressure reflects immaturity of the autonomic neuromuscular mechanisms.[23] The focus in this section will be on the character of the infant's movements and on the reflexes that are usually present at birth.

Movements

At the beginning of the examination, the infant's movements should be observed before the infant is touched. The spontaneous movements of normal newborns usually involve all extremities and are random and symmetrical but not stereotyped. Sometimes jitteriness or tremors will be noted and might be interpreted as seizures. It is important to differentiate seizures from other movements, because neonatal seizures are usually treatable and brain damage might be avoided if they are identified early. The following clinical features are helpful in differentiating between tremors or jitteriness and seizures[24]:

- The rhythmic movements of jitteriness or tremors are equal in amplitude, but seizures have a fast and slow component to the movements.
- Jitteriness or tremors are provoked by external stimuli, such as noise or handling, but this is not true of seizures.
- The examiner can usually stop the movements that are caused by jitteriness or tremors by passively holding the affected limb still.

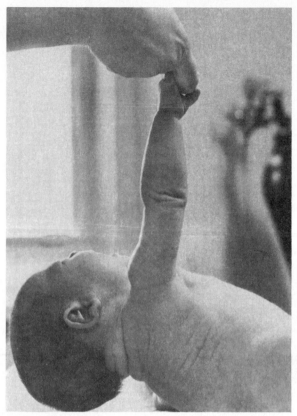

■ *Figure 29–14*
Grasp reflex. (A clinical review of concepts and characteristics in infant development. In Reflexes, Vol 2. Evansville, IN, Mead Johnson and Company. Copyright 1974.)

Reflexes

ROOTING AND SUCKING

Gently stroking the infant's cheek or corner of the mouth with a sterile nipple or clean finger causes the baby to open his mouth and turn toward the stimulus (Fig. 29-13). This is known as the *rooting reflex*. The *sucking reflex* can be evaluated by placing the nipple or finger in the baby's mouth and noting the strength of the sucking response. These reflexes may not be too active if the infant has eaten recently.

It is well known that during the first months of life newborns have a great need to suck and usually suck on anything that comes in contact with their lips. Newborns even suck while sleeping, and this nonnutritive sucking may have a quieting effect on excitable babies.

GRASP REFLEX

The *grasp reflex* is present at birth in both the hands and the feet (Fig. 29-14). Infants grasp any object placed in their hands, cling briefly, and then let go. Even at birth they may be able to hold onto an adult's forefinger

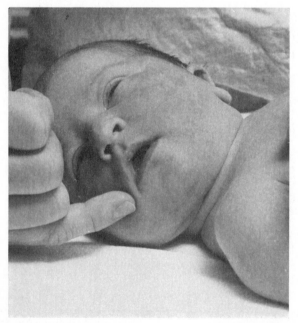

■ *Figure 29–13*
Rooting reflex. (Sullivan R, Foster J, Schreiner RL: Determining a newborn's gestational age. MCN, American Journal of Maternal/Child Nursing, January/February, 4:38–45, 1979)

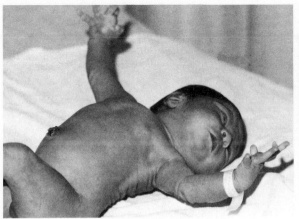

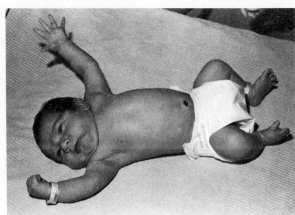

■ *Figure 29–15*
Moro reflex.

so securely that they can be lifted to a standing position. Although babies cannot actually grasp with their feet, stroking the soles causes the toes to turn downward as though trying to grasp. The grasping movements are a reflex action at birth, but with practice and experience, the hand grasp soon becomes voluntary and purposeful.

By grasping the infant's hands and arms, the examiner can gently pull the infant to a sitting position. The infant flexes the elbows to resist extension (traction response). The strength of the neck muscles can be assessed by noting the amount of head lag. Normal term newborns are able to support their heads momentarily.

MORO REFLEX

The *Moro* or *startle reflex* indicates an awareness of equilibrium in newborns (Fig. 29-15). The preferred method of eliciting this reflex is to hold the infant with head supported, then allow the head to drop backward a short distance. Alternately, the infant can be lying quietly and the mattress struck, or the head lifted a few inches and allowed to drop back. The reaction should consist of lateral extension of the upper extremities and opening of the hands, followed by anterior flexion and adduction of the arms in an embracing motion. The

movements should be symmetrical. If they are not, injury to the part that lags should be suspected.

The Moro reflex should be present at birth; normally it disappears by 3 months of age. If it cannot be elicited at birth, edema of or injury to the brain may be present. As the edema subsides, the reflex returns, and it should be demonstrable on the day following delivery. If frank brain damage has occurred, the reflex is absent for several days; if the damage is not too severe, the reflex returns in 3 or 4 days. Occasionally, the reflex is present at birth but disappears over the first days. Increasing cerebral edema or slow intracranial hemorrhage then is suspected.

TONIC NECK REFLEX

When the *tonic neck reflex* is elicited, infants assume a "fencing" position (*i.e.*, they lie on their back with their head rotated to one side). The arm and the leg on the side toward which they are facing are partially or completely extended, and the opposite arm and leg are flexed (Fig. 29-16). This reflex also disappears in a few months, because it is another manifestation of the immaturity of the newborn's nervous system.

STEPPING REFLEX

The *stepping* or *dancing reflex* is another action that is present at birth but soon disappears. This reflex causes infants to make little stepping or prancing movements when they are held upright with their feet touching a surface (Fig. 29-17). After this reflex diminishes, infants do not attempt stepping motions until they are ready to stand and walk. They do exercise their leg muscles a great deal, however, and seem to derive much enjoyment from waving and kicking their legs about.

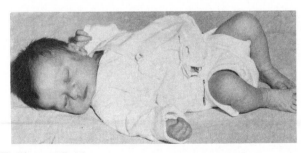

■ *Figure 29–16*
Tonic neck reflex.

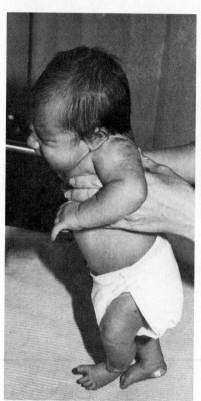
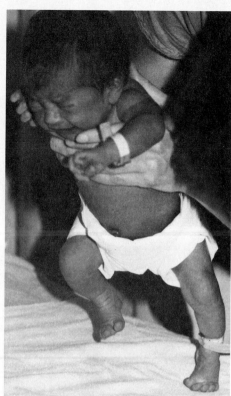

■ *Figure 29–17*
Stepping reflex.

OTHER REFLEXES

The next group of reflexes might be termed protective because they are necessary and at times essential to the preservation of the newborn's safety. The *blinking reflex* occurs when infants are subjected to a bright light. The *cough* and the *sneeze reflexes* clear their respiratory passages. The *yawn reflex* draws in additional oxygen. These, together with the infant's ability to cry when uncomfortable, to withdraw from painful stimuli, to resist restraint, and so on, are all defensive measures. As the baby grows and develops, these together with the other reflexes mentioned either diminish or become more highly developed according to the need. Thus, the infant's behavior patterns become more complex and highly developed.

■ GESTATIONAL AGE ASSESSMENT

Accurate assessment of an infant's gestational age is another important aspect of newborn assessment. *Gestational age* is the estimated age of the fetus or newborn, expressed in weeks, counting from the first day of the mother's last menstrual period. During the prenatal period, a variety of techniques can be used in the esti-

mation of the gestational age (see Chap 42). After the infant's birth, assessment of certain external physical characteristics and neurologic signs can result in a more accurate estimate. Knowing the approximate gestational age helps to determine whether the infant was born early (preterm), born on time (term), or born late (postterm), when compared with the expected gestation of 40 weeks. When gestational age is considered together with birth weight, infants can be designated as small, appropriate, or large for gestational age. Chapter 44 gives a more complete discussion of these categories, the potential problems they suggest, and the part they play in planning care for the newborn.

Assessment of gestational age by examination should be done in the first days of life, because the extrauterine environment leads to rapid changes in the characteristics of the newborn. The physical characteristics that are assessed are independent of the baby's health and ideally are evaluated within a few hours of the birth. The neurologic criteria can be altered by the infant's physical condition, and this part of the examination is deferred until later.[23]

The physical and neurologic criteria that have been identified as being useful in gestational age assessment are used in a variety of combinations in the different scoring systems that have been suggested. The Dubowitz scoring system uses a combination of physical, neurobehavioral, and reflex criteria to arrive at a gestational

(Text continues on page 670)

Dubowitz Scoring System

NAME		D.O.B./TIME		WEIGHT		E.D.D. L.N.M.P.		E.D.D. U/snd.
HOSP.	NO.	DATE OF EXAM		HEIGHT				
RACE	SEX	AGE		HEAD CIRC.				

GESTATIONAL SCORE WEEKS ASSESSMENT

STATES
1. Deep sleep, no movement, regular breathing.
2. Light sleep, eyes shut, some movement.
3. Dozing, eyes opening and closing.
4. Awake, eyes open, minimal movement.
5. Wide awake, vigorous movement.
6. Crying.

Columns at right: STATE | COMMENT | ASYMMETRY

HABITUATION (≤state 3)

LIGHT
Repetitive flashlight stimuli (10) with 5 sec. gap.
Shutdown = 2 consecutive negative responses

| No response | A. Blink response to first stimulus only. B. Tonic blink response. C. Variable response. | A. Shutdown of movement but blink persists 2-5 stimuli. B. Complete shutdown 2-5 stimuli. | A. Shutdown of movement but blink persists 6-10 stimuli. B. Complete shutdown 6-10 stimuli. | A. Equal response to 10 stimuli. B. Infant comes to fully alert state. C. Startles + major responses throughout. |

RATTLE
Repetitive stimuli (10) with 5 sec. gap.

| No response | A. Slight movement to first stimulus. B. Variable response. | Startle or movement 2-5 stimuli, then shutdown | Startle or movement 6-10 stimuli, then shutdown | A. B. C. Grading as above |

MOVEMENT & TONE
Undress infant

POSTURE * (At rest — predominant)

(hips abducted) / (hips adducted)

Abnormal postures:
A. Opisthotonus.
B. Unusual leg extension.
C. Asymm. tonic neck reflex

ARM RECOIL
Infant supine. Take both hands, extend parallel to the body; hold approx. 2 secs. and release.

| No flexion within 5 sec. | Partial flexion at elbow >100° within 4-5 sec. | Arms flex at elbow to <100° within 2-3 sec. | Sudden jerky flexion at elbow immediately after release to <60° | Difficult to extend; arm snaps back forcefully |

ARM TRACTION
Infant supine; head midline; grasp wrist, slowly pull arm to vertical. Angle of arm scored and resistance noted at moment infant is initially lifted off and watched until shoulder off mattress. Do other arm.

| Arm remains fully extended | Weak flexion maintained only momentarily | Arm flexed at elbow to 140° and maintained 5 sec. | Arm flexed at approx. 100° and maintained | Strong flexion of arm <100° and maintained |

LEG RECOIL
First flex hips for 5 secs, then extend both legs of infant by traction on ankles; hold down on the bed for 2 secs. and release.

| No flexion within 5 sec. | Incomplete flexion of hips within 5 sec. | Complete flexion within 5 sec. | Instantaneous complete flexion | Legs cannot be extended; snap back forcefully |

LEG TRACTION
Infant supine. Grasp leg near ankle and slowly pull toward vertical until buttocks 1-2" off. Note resistance at knee and score angle. Do other leg.

| No flexion | Partial flexion, rapidly lost | Knee flexion 140-160° and maintained | Knee flexion 100-140° and maintained | Strong resistance; flexion <100° |

POPLITEAL ANGLE
Infant supine. Approximate knee and thigh to abdomen; extend leg by gentle pressure with index finger behind ankle.

| 180-160° | 150-140° | 130-120° | 110-90° | <90° |

HEAD CONTROL (post. neck m.)
Grasp infant by shoulders and raise to sitting position; allow head to fall forward; wait 30 sec.

| No attempt to raise head | Unsuccessful attempt to raise head upright | Head raised smoothly to upright in 30 sec. but not maintained. | Head raised smoothly to upright in 30 sec. and maintained | Head cannot be flexed forward |

HEAD CONTROL (ant. neck m.)
Allow head to fall backward as you hold shoulders; wait 30 secs.

| Grading as above | Grading as above | Grading as above | Grading as above | |

HEAD LAG *
Pull infant toward sitting posture by traction on both wrists. Also note arm flexion.

VENTRAL SUSPENSION *
Hold infant in ventral suspension; observe curvature of back, flexion of limbs and relation of head to trunk.

HEAD RAISING IN PRONE POSITION
Infant in prone position with head in midline.

| No response | Rolls head to one side | Weak effort to raise head and turns raised head to one side | Infant lifts head, nose and chin off | Strong prolonged head lifting |

ARM RELEASE IN PRONE POSITION
Head in midline. Infant in prone position; arms extended alongside body with palms up.

| No effort | Some effort and wriggling | Flexion effort but neither wrist brought to nipple level | One or both wrists brought at least to nipple level without excessive body movement | Strong body movement with both wrists brought to face, or 'press-ups' |

SPONTANEOUS BODY MOVEMENT
during examination (supine). If no spont. movement try to induce by cutaneous stimulation.

| None or minimal / Induced | A. Sluggish. B. Random, incoordinated. C. Mainly stretching. | Smooth movements alternating with random, stretching, athetoid or jerky | Smooth alternating movements of arms and legs with medium speed and intensity | Mainly: A. Jerky movement. B. Athetoid movement. C. Other abnormal movement. |

(COMMENT column: 1 / 2)

TREMORS
Mark: Fast (>6/sec.) or Slow (<6/sec.)

| No tremor | Tremors only in state 5-6 | Tremors only in sleep or after Moro and startles | Some tremors in state 4 | Tremulousness in all states |

STARTLES

| No startles | Startles to sudden noise, Moro, bang on table only | Occasional spontaneous startle | 2-5 spontaneous startles | 6+ spontaneous startles |

ABNORMAL MOVEMENT OR POSTURE

| No abnormal movement | A. Hands clenched but open intermittently. B. Hands do not open with Moro. | A. Some mouthing movement. B. Intermittent adducted thumb. | A. Persistently adducted thumb. B. Hands clenched all the time. | A. Continuous mouthing movement. B. Convulsive movements. |

(continued)

						STATE	COMMENT	ASYMMETRY

REFLEXES

						STATE	COMMENT	ASYMMETRY
TENDON REFLEXES Biceps jerk Knee jerk Ankle jerk	Absent		Present	Exaggerated	Clonus			
PALMAR GRASP Head in midline. Put index finger from ulnar side into hand and gently press palmar surface. Never touch dorsal side of hand.	Absent	Short, weak flexion	Medium strength and sustained flexion for several secs.	Strong flexion; contraction spreads to forearm	Very strong grasp. Infant easily lifts off couch			
ROOTING Infant supine, head midline. Touch each corner of the mouth in turn (stroke laterally).	No response	A. Partial weak head turn but no mouth opening. B. Mouth opening, no head turn.	Mouth opening on stimulated side with partial head turning	Full head turning, with or without mouth opening	Mouth opening with very jerky head turning			
SUCKING Infant supine; place index finger (pad towards palate) in infant's mouth; judge power of sucking movement after 5 sec.	No attempt	Weak sucking movement: A. Regular. B. Irregular.	Strong sucking movement, poor stripping: A. Regular. B. Irregular.	Strong regular sucking movement with continuing sequence of 5 movements. Good stripping.	Clenching but no regular sucking.			
WALKING (state 4, 5) Hold infant upright, feet touching bed, neck held straight with fingers.	Absent		Some effort but not continuous with both legs	At least 2 steps with both legs	A. Stork posture; no movement. B. Automatic walking.			
MORO One hand supports infant's head in midline, the other the back. Raise infant to 45° and when infant is relaxed let his head fall through 10°. Note if jerky. Repeat 3 times.	No response, or opening of hands only	Full abduction at the shoulder and extension of the arm	Full abduction but only delayed or partial adduction	Partial abduction at shoulder and extension of arms followed by smooth adduction A. Abd>Add B. Abd=Add C. Abd<Add	A. No abduction or adduction; extension only. B. Marked adduction only.	J S		

NEUROBEHAVIOURAL ITEMS

						STATE	COMMENT	ASYMMETRY
EYE APPEARANCES	Sunset sign Nerve palsy	Transient nystagmus. Strabismus. Some roving eye movement.	Does not open eyes	Normal conjugate eye movement	A. Persistent nystagmus. B. Frequent roving movement C. Frequent rapid blinks.			
AUDITORY ORIENTATION (state 3, 4) To rattle. (Note presence of startle.)	A. No reaction. B. Auditory startle but no true orientation.	Brightens and stills; may turn toward stimuli with eyes closed	Alerting and shifting of eyes; head may or may not turn to source	Alerting; prolonged head turns to stimulus; search with eyes	Turning and alerting to stimulus each time on both sides		S	
VISUAL ORIENTATION (state 4) To red woollen ball	Does not focus or follow stimulus	Stills; focuses on stimulus; may follow 30° jerkily; does not find stimulus again spontaneously	Follows 30-60° horizontally; may lose stimulus but finds it again. Brief vertical glance	Follows with eyes and head horizontally and to some extent vertically, with frowning	Sustained fixation; follows vertically, horizontally, and in circle			
ALERTNESS (state 4)	Inattentive; rarely or never responds to direct stimulation	When alert, periods rather brief; rather variable response to orientation	When alert, alertness moderately sustained; may use stimulus to come to alert state	Sustained alertness; orientation frequent, reliable to visual but not auditory stimuli	Continuous alertness, which does not seem to tire, to both auditory and visual stimuli			
DEFENSIVE REACTION A cloth or hand is placed over the infant's face to partially occlude the nasal airway.	No response	A. General quietening. B. Non-specific activity with long latency.	Rooting; lateral neck turning; possibly neck stretching.	Swipes with arm	Swipes with arm with rather violent body movement			
PEAK OF EXCITEMENT	Low level arousal to all stimuli; never > state 3	Infant reaches state 4-5 briefly but predominantly in lower states	Infant predominantly state 4 or 5; may reach state 6 after stimulation but returns spontaneously to lower state	Infant reaches state 6 but can be consoled relatively easily	A. Mainly state 6. Difficult to console, if at all. B. Mainly state 4-5 but if reaches state 6 cannot be consoled.			
IRRITABILITY (states 3, 4, 5) Aversive stimuli: Uncover Ventral susp. Undress Moro Pull to sit Walking reflex Prone	No irritable crying to any of the stimuli	Cries to 1-2 stimuli	Cries to 3-4 stimuli	Cries to 5-6 stimuli	Cries to all stimuli			
CONSOLABILITY (state 6)	Never above state 5 during examination, therefore not needed	Consoling not needed. Consoles spontaneously	Consoled by talking, hand on belly or wrapping up	Consoled by picking up and holding; may need finger in mouth	Not consolable			
CRY	No cry at all	Only whimpering cry	Cries to stimuli but normal pitch	Lusty cry to offensive stimuli; normal pitch	High-pitched cry, often continuous			

NOTES ✱ If asymmetrical or atypical, draw in on nearest figure

Record any abnormal signs (e.g. facial palsy, contractures, etc.). Draw if possible.

Record time after feed:

EXAMINER:

Assessment Tool

Estimation of Gestational Age by Maturity Rating

Symbols: X - 1st Exam   O - 2nd Exam

NEUROMUSCULAR MATURITY

	0	1	2	3	4	5
Posture						
Square Window (Wrist)	90°	60°	45°	30°	0°	
Arm Recoil	180°		100°-180°	90°-100°	< 90°	
Popliteal Angle	180°	160°	130°	110°	90°	< 90°
Scarf Sign						
Heel to Ear						

Gestation by Dates _____ wks

Birth Date _____ Hour _____ am/pm

APGAR _____ 1 min _____ 5 min

MATURITY RATING

Score	Wks
5	26
10	28
15	30
20	32
25	34
30	36
35	38
40	40
45	42
50	44

PHYSICAL MATURITY

	0	1	2	3	4	5
SKIN	gelatinous red, transparent	smooth pink, visible veins	superficial peeling &/or rash, few veins	cracking pale area, rare veins	parchment, deep cracking, no vessels	leathery, cracked, wrinkled
LANUGO	none	abundant	thinning	bald areas	mostly bald	
PLANTAR CREASES	no crease	faint red marks	anterior transverse crease only	creases ant. 2/3	creases cover entire sole	
BREAST	barely percept.	flat areola, no bud	stippled areola, 1–2 mm bud	raised areola, 3–4 mm bud	full areola, 5–10 mm bud	
EAR	pinna flat, stays folded	sl. curved pinna, soft with slow recoil	well-curv. pinna, soft but ready recoil	formed & firm with instant recoil	thick cartilage, ear stiff	
GENITALS Male	scrotum empty, no rugae		testes descending, few rugae	testes down, good rugae	testes pendulous, deep rugae	
GENITALS Female	prominent clitoris & labia minora		majora & minora equally prominent	majora large, minora small	clitoris & minora completely covered	

SCORING SECTION

	1st Exam=X	2nd Exam=O
Estimating Gest Age by Maturity Rating	_____Weeks	_____Weeks
Time of Exam	Date _____ am Hour _____pm	Date _____ am Hour _____pm
Age at Exam	_____ Hours	_____ Hours
Signature of Examiner	_____ M.D.	_____ M.D.

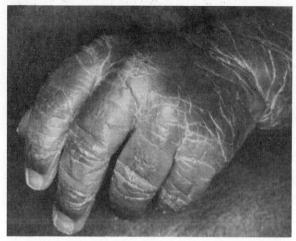

■ *Figure 29–18*
Postterm infant's hand. Note dry, peeling, cracked skin. (Sullivan R, Foster J, Schreiner RL: Determining a newborn's gestational age. MCN, American Journal of Maternal/Child Nursing, January/February, 4:38–45, 1979)

in an orderly manner. The presence, absence, or degree of development of these characteristics at birth is used to help determine gestational age.

Skin and Vernix. The skin of premature infants is thin, pink, smooth, almost transparent (with blood vessels visible), and thickly covered with vernix. Presence or absence of blood vessels is usually observed over the abdomen. The skin becomes thicker and more opaque with increasing age, until by 40 weeks it is pale with few vessels visible and sparse vernix often occurring only in skin creases. In the postmature infant, there may be extensive desquamation of skin and absence of vernix (Fig. 29-18).

Lanugo. Fine lanugo hair covers the infant's body at 20 weeks' gestation and begins to disappear first from the face, then the trunk, and then the extremities (Fig. 29-19). At term, lanugo, if present, tends to be located only over the shoulders.

age (see Assessment Tool: Dubowitz Scoring System).[25] This has the disadvantage of being rather long. An abbreviated system using seven physical and six neurologic signs, developed by Ballard and colleagues, is more widely used (see Assessment Tool: Estimation of Gestational Age by Maturity Rating).[26] Other combinations of criteria may be used in different settings. When learning to do the examination it may be helpful at first to check only five of the criteria, such as the breasts, ears, genitalia, sole creases, and posture, and then to expand to other areas as proficiency is achieved.[27]

Sole Creases. The soles of the feet become wrinkled first on the anterior portion and then in the area extending toward the heel as gestation progresses. At 32 weeks, one or two creases can be seen; they become more numerous, crisscrossed, and deeper, covering the anterior two thirds of the sole by 37 weeks. The entire sole, including the heel, is covered at 40 weeks (Fig. 29-20). In the postterm infant, creases are deeper and there may be desquamation of the soles.

Physical Characteristics

During the growth and development of the fetus, certain external physical characteristics develop and progress

Breast Tissue and Areola. The nipples are present early in gestation, but the areola is barely visible until 34 weeks. After this time, the areola becomes raised and hair follicles become evident. Infants of less than 36 weeks' gestation have no breast tissue. At 36 weeks, a 1- to 2-mm nodule of breast tissue becomes palpable. This increases with gestational age under hormonal

■ *Figure 29–19*
Cartilage is well developed in the term infant (A) and the ear is erect, away from the head, whereas the ears of the preterm infant (B) lie flat against the head. Also note the matted hair of the preterm infant. (Sullivan R, Foster J, Schreiner RL: Determining a newborn's gestational age. MCN, American Journal of Maternal/ Child Nursing, January/February, 4:38–45, 1979)

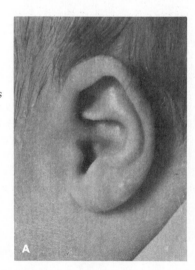

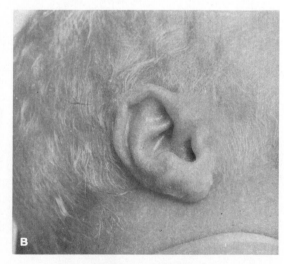

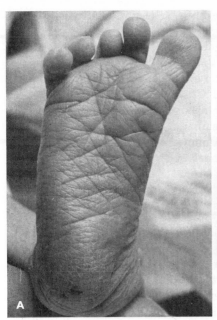
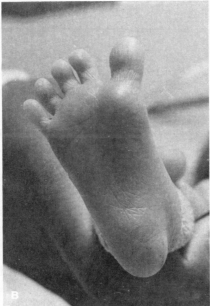

■ *Figure 29–20*
A comparison of the sole creases on the foot of a term infant (A) with those of a preterm infant (B). At 40 weeks' gestation, the entire foot, including the heel, is crisscrossed with creases. (Sullivan R, Foster J, Schreiner RL: Determining a newborn's gestational age. MCN, American Journal of Maternal/Child Nursing, January/February, 4:38–45, 1979)

stimulation until it reaches 7 to 10 mm at 40 weeks (Fig. 29-21).

Ear Form and Cartilage. Infants less than 33 weeks' gestation have relatively flat ears. After 34 weeks, the upper pinnae begin to curve inward. By 38 weeks, the upper two thirds of the pinnae are incurved; this extends to the earlobe by 39 to 40 weeks. Because ear form can vary widely from one individual to another, cartilage is more reliable than ear form in estimating gestational age. Owing to the absence of cartilage, the extremely premature infant's ear remains folded over if pressed. Cartilage begins to appear at 32 weeks, so the ear slowly returns to its original position when folded over. By 36 weeks, the pinnae spring back when folded, and at term they are firm, with the ear standing erect away from the head (see Fig. 29-19 *A* and *B*).

Genitalia. The characteristics of both male and female genitalia change with gestational age. In the female, the clitoris is prominent at 30 to 32 weeks, whereas the labia majora are small and widely separated. The labia majora increase in size and fullness with age, and at term they completely cover the labia minora and clitoris (Fig. 29-22).

In the male, the testes are high in the inguinal canal at about 30 weeks, gradually descend to be felt high in the scrotal sac at 37 weeks, and are well descended into the lower scrotal sac by 40 weeks. Rugae first appear on the scrotum anteriorly at 36 weeks and extend to cover the entire sac by 40 weeks. The postterm infant often has a pendulous scrotum covered with numerous rugae (Fig. 29-23).

Hair. Strands of hair are very fine in early gestation and tend to mat together like wool, with small bunches sticking out from the head. The full-term infant has silky hair that lies flat in single strands. In the postterm infant the hairline may recede. Important considerations to take into account when using hair as an assessment criterion are that hair varies in texture and characteristics with race and must be free of vernix before it is observed (see Fig. 29-19).

Nails. At about 20 weeks, the nails appear and gradually grow to cover the nail bed. At term, the nails extend beyond the fingertips slightly, but long nails well beyond the fingertips are characteristic of postmature infants.

Skull Firmness. The preterm infant has soft skull bones, particularly near the fontanels and sutures. The bones become firmer as gestation progresses, and at term the sutures are not easily displaced.

Neurologic Development

Gestational age may be assessed according to a number of neuromuscular responses of the newborn within the first few days of life. The infant's posture, the passive range of motion of certain parts, righting reactions, and various reflexes are evaluated. The development of muscle tone begins in the lower extremities and progresses in a cephalad direction.

The neurologic examination requires that the infant be in a quiet, rested state, although this may not be possible immediately after delivery. Most infants can

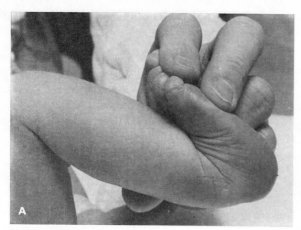
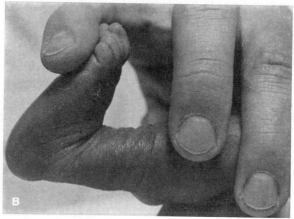

■ *Figure 29–25*

*Dorsiflexion of the ankle (A) In the term infant the foot can be flexed until it touches the leg.
(B) In the preterm infant the foot can be flexed only to an angle of 45 to 90 degrees. (Sullivan R,
Foster J, Schreiner RL: Determining a newborn's gestational age. MCN, American Journal of
Maternal/Child Nursing, January/February, 4:38–45, 1979)*

Ankle and Wrist Flexion. Pressure is applied to the foot to push it onto the anterior aspect of the leg, and the angle between the dorsum of the foot and the leg is measured. In premature infants this angle is 45 to 90 degrees, whereas in full-term infant the foot can be flexed until it touches the leg (Fig. 29-25). Similarly, the wrist is flexed with enough pressure to bring the hand as close to the forearm as possible (square window). The angle between the hypothenar eminence of the wrist and the ventral aspect of the forearm is measured, with care taken not to rotate the wrist. In the premature infant this angle is 90 degrees. In the full-term infant, the wrist can be flexed on the arm (Fig. 29-26).

Popliteal Angle. Passive movement of the leg reveals an inverse relationship between muscle tone and popliteal angle, with a smaller angle associated with greater tone. Premature infants have larger popliteal angles than full-term infants (Fig. 29-27).

Scarf Sign. The infant's arms are drawn across the neck as far across the opposite shoulder as possible (like a scarf). In the premature infant, there is less resistance and a greater draping (or scarf) effect. This maneuver is best carried out by lifting the elbow across the front of the body. Note how far across the chest the elbow will go. In the premature infant, the elbow reaches near or across the midline, whereas in the full-term infant it does not reach the midline (Fig. 29-28).

Heel to Ear. With the infant supine and hips flat, the foot is drawn as close to the ear as possible without forcing. In a premature infant, there is very little resis-

■ *Figure 29–26*

Wrist flexion. (A) In the term infant, the wrist can be flexed onto the arm. (B) In the preterm infant, the wrist only can be flexed to an angle of about 90 degrees. (Sullivan R, Foster J, Schreiner RL: Determining a newborn's gestational age. MCN, American Journal of Maternal/Child Nursing, January/February, 4:38–45, 1979)

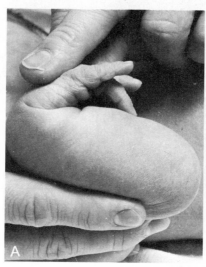
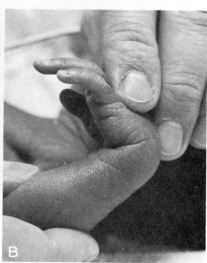

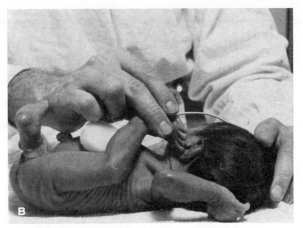
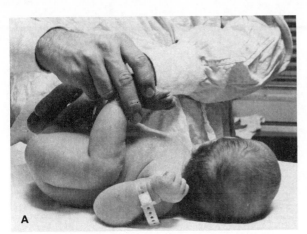

■ *Figure 29–27*

Heel to ear. (A) In the term infant, there is a marked resistance in the leg as the foot is gently drawn toward the ear. (B) In the preterm infant, very little resistance is noted. Note the difference in the popliteal angle. (Sullivan R, Foster J, Schreiner RL: Determining a newborn's gestational age. MCN, American Journal of Maternal/Child Nursing, January/February, 4:38–45, 1979)

tance and the foot may approximate the ear, with the leg well extended. There is marked resistance in the full-term infant, and it is impossible to draw the foot to the ear and extend the leg well (see Fig. 29-27).

Ventral Suspension. The infant is suspended in the prone position with the hand of the examiner supporting it under the chest (two hands may be used for a large infant). The degree of extension of the back and head, as well as the degree of flexion of the arms and legs, are noted. The premature infant hangs limply with arms and legs almost straight and back rounded. The full-term infant extends the head, straightens the back, and flexes the arms and legs (Fig. 29-29).

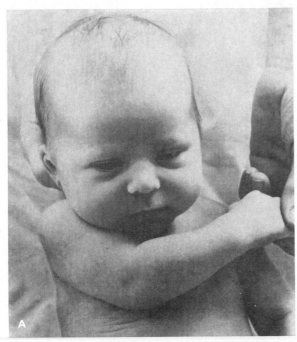
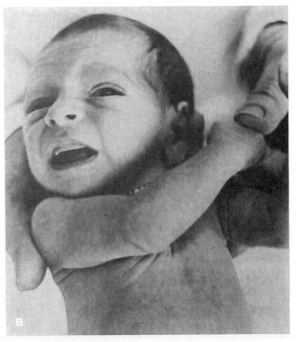

■ *Figure 29–28*

Scarf sign. (A) In the term infant, the elbow will not reach the midline. (B) In the preterm infant, the elbow will reach across the midline. (A clinical review of concepts and characteristics in infant development. In Reflexes, Vol 2. Evansville, IN, Mead Johnson and Company. Copyright 1974)

■ *Figure 29–29*
Ventral suspension. (A) When suspended in the prone position, the term infant's head extends, the back is straight, and the arms and legs flex. (B) However, the preterm infant hangs limply with the arms and legs almost straight. (Sullivan R, Foster J, Schreiner RL: Determining a newborn's gestational age. MCN, American Journal of Maternal/Child Nursing, January/February, 4:38–45, 1979)

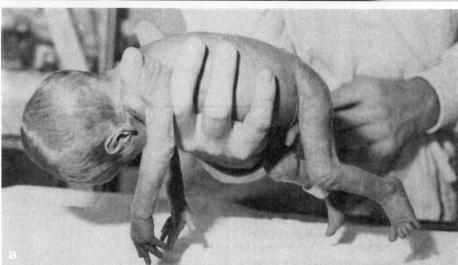

Head Lag. With the infant supine, the hands or arms are grasped and he is pulled slowly to a sitting position. The position of the head should be observed in relation to the trunk. The premature infant has no flexion of the neck. A gradual increase in flexion can be noted as gestation progresses. The full-term infant holds the head erect while being pulled to a sitting position (Fig. 29-30).

REFLEXES

Although there are differences in reflexes according to the infant's gestational age, these are not as age specific as the other signs described above and are less useful in determining gestational age. The reflexes of the normal newborn are discussed under Neurologic Assessment.

In the premature infant, the rooting reflex is less developed, as evidenced by the slower response in turning the head toward the stimulus. The sucking reflex is weak or absent, depending on prematurity and condition. The grasp reflex is weak, and the infant cannot be lifted off the bed while grasping the examiner's finger.

The Moro reflex is also weak, and the walking reflex is often absent. The sucking reflex, which is of particular importance because it is related to the ability to take adequate nourishment with nipple feedings, begins at about 34 weeks.

■ BEHAVIORAL ASSESSMENT

Newborns are often thought of as being essentially passive. It is generally recognized now, however, that infants interact actively with their environment from birth. Adding behavioral assessment to the overall newborn assessment contributes important information about an individual neonate's behavioral responses to his or her environment.

The Neonatal Behavioral Assessment Scale (NBAS), developed by Brazelton,[28] is useful in making a behavioral assessment. Although the scale is intended to be used by trained examiners in clinical practice, as a pre-

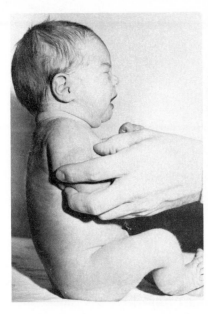

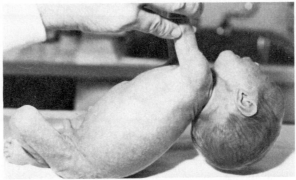

■ *Figure 29–30*
Head lag. (A) As the infant is slowly pulled from a supine to a sitting position, the term infant holds the head erect. (B) The preterm infant has no flexion in the neck. (Sullivan R, Foster J, Schreiner RL: Determining a newborn's gestational age. MCN, American Journal of Maternal/Child Nursing, January/February, 4:38–45, 1979)

dictive tool, or in research, knowledge of Brazelton's ideas can be useful to anyone working with newborns and their parents. It combines aspects of physical and neurologic assessment, with assessment of specific newborn behaviors. The scale measures a total of 27 items (see Box: Brazelton Scale Criteria). Each item is scored on a scale of one to nine, based on the infant's best rather than average performance. The items can be divided into the following six categories:[29]

1. Habituation—how soon the neonate diminishes responses to specific repeated stimuli
2. Orientation—how often and when the infant attends to auditory and visual stimuli
3. Motor maturity—how well the infant coordinates and controls motor activities
4. Variation—how often the infant exhibits alertness, state changes, color changes, activity, and peaks of excitement
5. Self-quieting abilities—how often, how soon, and how effectively the neonate can use his own resources to quiet and console himself when upset or distressed
6. Social behaviors—how often and how much the newborn smiles and cuddles

Essential to an understanding of an infant's behavior is the concept of sleeping and waking "states." The infant's state at the time any given item on the NBAS is tested is important. Some items require that the infant be in a certain state for valid testing. States of the newborn have been studied and classified in a number of ways during the past three decades. One such classification is the following described by Brazelton[28]:

Sleep States

1. Deep sleep—regular breathing, eyes closed, no spontaneous activity except startles or jerky movements at quite regular intervals; external stimuli produce startles with some delay; suppression of startles is rapid, and state changes are less likely than from other states; no eye movements
2. Light sleep—eyes closed, rapid eye movements can be observed under closed lids; low activity level, with random movements and startles or startle equivalents; movements are likely to be smoother and more monitored than in state 1; responds to internal and external stimuli with startle equivalents, often with a resulting change of state; irregular respirations; sucking movements occur off and on

Awake States

3. Drowsy or semidozing; eyes may be open or closed; eyelids fluttering; activity level variable with interspersed, mild startles from time to time; reactive to sensory stimuli, but response often delayed; state change after stimulation frequently noted; movements are usually smooth
4. Alert, with bright look; seems to focus attention on source of stimulation, such as an object to be sucked, or a visual or auditory stimulus; impinging stimuli may break through but with some delay in response; motor activity is minimal (Fig. 29-31).
5. Eyes open; considerable motor activity, with thrusting movements of the extremities and even a few spontaneous startles; reactive to external

Brazelton Scale Criteria

1. Response decrement to light
2. Response decrement to rattle
3. Response decrement to bell
4. Response decrement to pinprick
5. Orientation response—inanimate visual
6. Orientation response—inanimate auditory
7. Orientation—animate visual
8. Orientation—animate auditory
9. Orientation—animate visual and auditory
10. Alertness
11. General tonus
12. Motor maturity
13. Pull-to-sit
14. Cuddliness
15. Defensive movements
16. Consolability with intervention
17. Peak of excitement
18. Rapidity of buildup
19. Irritability (to aversive stimuli—uncover, undress, pull-to-sit, prone, pinprick, tonic neck response, Moro, defensive reaction)
20. Activity
21. Tremulousness
22. Amount of startle during examination
23. Lability of skin color
24. Lability of states
25. Self-quieting activity
26. Hand-to-mouth facility
27. Smiles

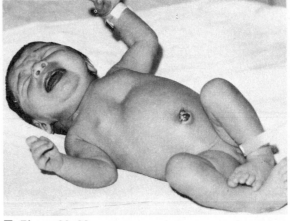
■ *Figure 29–32*
Active crying state.

Other classifications include similar components but add transition states between sleep and waking and within the sleep state.[30] Babies vary greatly in the amount of time they spend in the various states and in the ease or difficulty with which they make the transition from one state to another. Sleep cycles generally lengthen with maturation of the central nervous system, so that immature infants are more likely to have shorter, less well-defined cycles.[31]

Use of information from the NBAS for anticipatory guidance when teaching parents about their newborn can be helpful. Most parents are interested in what kinds of stimuli their infant will focus attention on. Some parents discover these things for themselves. Others need to be told that most infants will focus on a bright red ball and follow it briefly when they are in the quiet alert state (state 4) or that the infant particularly likes to follow a moving human face or a high-pitched voice.

Many people think that all infants are cuddly and that if an infant does not cuddle when held there is either something wrong with them or with the infant. In fact, infants respond in many different ways to being cuddled. Scores on "cuddliness" range from (1) "ac-

stimulation with increase in startles or motor activity, but discrete reactions difficult to distinguish because of general high activity level
6. Crying; characterized by intense crying that is difficult to break through with stimulation (Fig. 29-32)

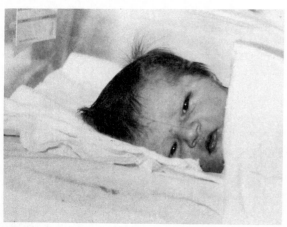
■ *Figure 29–31*
Quiet alert state.

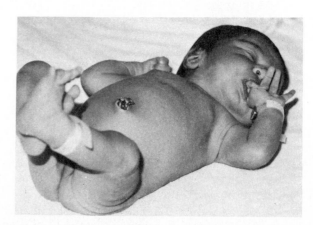
■ *Figure 29–33*
Self-consoling activity according to the Brazelton behavioral assessment scale: hand-to-mouth and sucking activity.

tually resists being held, continuously pushing away, thrashing or stiffening," to (9) "molds into arms and relaxes, turns toward examiner's body when held horizontally, or leans forward when held on the examiner's shoulder, all of the body participates and baby grasps examiner to cling to him."[28]

Infants also vary in their ability to be consoled or to console themselves. These items are scored when the infant is upset (state 6). Some babies only quiet down when they are dressed and left alone. Others need restraint to help them inhibit the startle reflex. These babies are the ones that usually do best when swaddled in a blanket.

Possible self-consoling activities that are counted in the assessment are hand-to-mouth efforts, sucking on fist or tongue (Fig. 29-33), or using visual or auditory stimuli from the environment to quiet self. Finding out ways in which their particular infant can console himself or be consoled can be helpful to the parents.

Babies often smile even in the first days, but the statement is usually made that it is just a reflex or "gas." Brazelton comments that he has "seen close replicas of 'social smiles' in the newborn period" and that, although they are hard to be sure of, "they surely are the precursors of such smiling behavior and a mother reinforces them as such."[28]

■ REFERENCES

1. Manning FA, Platt L, LeMay M: Fetal breathing. In McNall L, Galeener J (eds): Current Practice in Obstetrics and Gynecologic Nursing, Vol 2, pp 108–119. St. Louis, CV Mosby, 1977

2. Korones SB: High-risk newborn infants. The Basis for Intensive Nursing Care, 4th ed, pp 209–210. St. Louis, CV Mosby, 1986

3. Farrell PM, Perelman RH: The developmental biology of the lung. In Fanaroff AA, Martin RJ (eds): Neonatal-Perinatal Medicine, 4th ed, pp 557–571. St. Louis, CV Mosby, 1987

4. Harned H Jr: Respiration and the respiratory system. In Stave U (ed): Perinatal Physiology, pp 53–101. New York, Plenum Press, 1978

5. Nelson NM: Respiration and circulation after birth. In Smith CA, Nelson NM (eds): The Physiology of the Newborn Infant, 4th ed, pp 117–262. Springfield, IL, Charles C Thomas, 1976

6. Arnold HW, Putman NJ, Barnard BL, et al: Transition to extrauterine life. Am J Nurs 65(10):77–80, October 1965

7. Shurin SB: The blood and hematopoietic system. In Fanaroff AA, Martin RJ (eds): Neonatal-Perinatal Medicine, 4th ed, pp 825–869. St. Louis, CV Mosby, 1987

8. Hernandez A, Meyer DA, Goldring D: Blood pressure in neonates. Contemporary OB/GYN 5:34–37, March 1975

9. Cabal LA, Siassi B, Hodgman J: Neonatal clinical cardiopulmonary monitoring. In Fanaroff AA, Martin RJ (eds): Neonatal-Perinatal Medicine, 4th ed, pp 343–359. St Louis, CV Mosby, 1987

10. Lees MH, King DH: The cardiovascular system. In Fanaroff AA, Martin RJ (eds): Neonatal-Perinatal Medicine, 4th ed, pp 639–743. St. Louis, CV Mosby, 1987

11. Gartner LM, Lee KB: Jaundice and liver disease. In Fanaroff AA, Martin RJ (eds): Neonatal-Perinatal Medicine, 4th ed, pp 946–965. St. Louis, CV Mosby, 1987

12. Gartner LM: Hyperbilirubinemia. In Rudolph AM (ed): Pediatrics, 17th ed, pp 1007–1013. Norwalk, CT, Appleton-Century-Crofts, 1982

13. Brucker MC, MacMullen NJ: Neonatal jaundice in the home: Assessment with a noninvasive device. JOGNN 16(5):355–358, 1987

14. Bellanti JA, Boner AL, Valletta E: Immunology of the fetus and newborn. In Avery GB (ed): Neonatology: Pathophysiology and Management of the Newborn, 3rd ed. Philadelphia, JB Lippincott, 1987

15. Polmar SH, Manthel U: Immunology. In Fanaroff AA, Martin RJ (eds): Neonatal-Perinatal Medicine, 4th ed, pp 744–762. St. Louis, CV Mosby, 1987

16. Roberts FB: Perinatal Nursing. New York, McGraw-Hill, 1977

17. Bucuvalas JC, Balistreri WF: The neonatal gastrointestinal tract development. In Fanaroff AA, Martin RJ (eds): Neonatal-Perinatal Medicine, 4th ed, pp 894–899. St. Louis, CV Mosby, 1987

18. Spitzer A, Bernstein J, Edelman CM Jr, et al: The kidney and urinary tract. In Fanaroff AA, Martin RJ (eds): Neonatal-Perinatal Medicine, 4th ed, pp 981–1015. St Louis, CV Mosby, 1987

19. Phibbs RH: The newborn infant. In Rudolph AM (ed): Pediatrics, 17th ed, pp 119–166. Norwalk CT, Appleton-Century-Crofts, 1982

20. Gagliardi JV: Initial assessment of the newborn. In Warshaw JB, Hobbins JC: Principles and Practice of Perinatal Medicine, pp 197–208. Menlo Park, CA, Addison-Wesley, 1983

21. Easterly NB, Solomon LM: The skin. In Fanaroff AA, Martin RJ: Neonatal-Perinatal Medicine, 4th ed, pp 1172–1199. St. Louis, CV Mosby, 1987

22. Alexander MM, Brown MS: Pediatric Physical Diagnosis for Nurses, p 156. New York, McGraw-Hill, 1974

23. Farwell J: Maturational and neurobehavioral assessment of the newborn. In Warshaw JB, Hobbins JC: Principles and Practice of Perinatal Medicine, pp 226–247. Menlo Park, CA, Addison-Wesley, 1983

24. Brann AW Jr, Schwartz JF: Central nervous system disturbances. In Fanaroff AA, Martin RJ: Neonatal-Perinatal Medicine, pp 495–506. St. Louis, CV Mosby, 1987

25. Dubowitz L, et al: Clinical assessment of gestational age in the newborn infant. J Pediatr 77:1–10, 1970

26. Ballard J, et al: A simplified score for assessment of fetal maturation of newly born infants. J Pediatr 95:769–774, 1979

27. Sullivan R, Foster J, Schreiner RL: Determining a newborn's gestational age. MCN 4(1):38–45, January/February 1979

28. Brazelton TB: Neonatal behavioral assessment scale. Clin Dev Med 50: 1973

The care of the newborn presents an interesting challenge to those who work in maternity nursing. In a short period of time, usually a matter of seconds, the fetus, who has been completely dependent on the mother to supply all the physiological needs, suddenly becomes an "independent" being.

Although independent of the mother for vital functions, newborns are, of course, still very dependent in other ways. They could not survive long without a caretaker. In the immediate postnatal period, this caretaker is often the nurse.

Because these first days and weeks are so critical, the care given by the nurse is very important. The nurse must use the utmost care in handling the infants, keeping them warm and protecting them from exposure and injury, at the same time making accurate observations and recording and reporting them. Communication and teaching skills are used in contributing to the infant's future well-being by helping the parents to develop an understanding of their baby's needs and to acquire skill in his or her care. In this way their concept of themselves as adequate parents is reinforced. The nurse also must be aware that some parents need assistance in developing healthy attitudes regarding childbearing practices, so that the infant can make a satisfactory emotional and social adjustment. Opportunity must be provided in the hospital environment for the beginning development of a close parent–infant relationship. Also of importance is the maintenance of communication between the nurse and the parents.

Occurences That Should Be Reported to the Primary Health Care Provider

1. If the skin color changes:
   a. To blue (cyanosis), around the mouth or all over
   b. To yellow (jaundice)
2. Temperature above 38.4°C (101°F) or below 36.1°C (96°F)
3. Projectile vomiting two or more times
4. Refusal of two consecutive feedings
5. Periods of apnea (absence of breathing) longer than 15 seconds
6. Behavior changes, such as excessive crying, fussiness, lethargy, or difficulty in rousing the infant
7. Elimination pattern changes, such as two or more green, watery stools; hard stools; or decreased number of wet diapers (less than 5 per day)
8. Local signs of bleeding or infection:
   a. Swelling, redness or discharge from eyes
   b. Swelling, redness, discharge, or bleeding from umbilical cord stump
   c. Swelling, redness, discharge, or bleeding from circumcision

---

■ PROVIDING A SAFE ENVIRONMENT

As in the immediate newborn period (see Chap. 25), protection from injury and infection continues to be a major goal of nursing care throughout the infant's hospital stay.

Policies are formulated in each setting where newborns are cared for in an effort to provide safe, individualized care in a protective environment.

Preventing Infection

Prevention of infection is of paramount importance in caring for the newborn. Although the immune system begins to develop during fetal life, it is still very immature at birth (see Chap. 29). The neonate has come from a highly protected environment in utero to the outside world, where there is exposure to a wide variety of microorganisms. It is not surprising that organisms generally considered to be of low pathogenicity may cause infections in the neonate.[1]

It is important, therefore, to attempt to limit the number of organisms the infant comes in contact with in the early days of life.

MINIMIZING EXPOSURE TO ORGANISMS

The newborn's major source of exposure to organisms is the caretakers. Nurses and other staff members who care for newborn infants should be free from infectious diseases (i.e., respiratory, gastrointestinal, skin lesions) that could be transmitted to the neonates. Everyone who is in contact with the newborn, including parents and personnel, should assume responsibility for protecting the baby from infection. Parents may need help in reminding family and friends to postpone their visits if they are not well.

Handwashing. The basis for prevention of infection when handling the newborn is frequent, thorough handwashing with an antiseptic detergent or soap. The wash at the beginning of a shift, lasting approximately 2 minutes, should cover the forearms and elbows in addition to all areas of the hands, including between the fingers (see Guidelines for Handwashing). After the initial wash, staff members should be especially careful to wash their hands vigorously for 15 seconds before a feeding, after a diaper change, before going from one baby to another, and after touching anything that is not clean to that baby, such as a cabinet door or their own face or hair.[2] Studies of handwashing behavior in hospitals have indicated that the frequency of handwashing

tually resists being held, continuously pushing away, thrashing or stiffening," to (9) "molds into arms and relaxes, turns toward examiner's body when held horizontally, or leans forward when held on the examiner's shoulder, all of the body participates and baby grasps examiner to cling to him."[28]

Infants also vary in their ability to be consoled or to console themselves. These items are scored when the infant is upset (state 6). Some babies only quiet down when they are dressed and left alone. Others need restraint to help them inhibit the startle reflex. These babies are the ones that usually do best when swaddled in a blanket.

Possible self-consoling activities that are counted in the assessment are hand-to-mouth efforts, sucking on fist or tongue (Fig. 29-33), or using visual or auditory stimuli from the environment to quiet self. Finding out ways in which their particular infant can console himself or be consoled can be helpful to the parents.

Babies often smile even in the first days, but the statement is usually made that it is just a reflex or "gas." Brazelton comments that he has "seen close replicas of 'social smiles' in the newborn period" and that, although they are hard to be sure of, "they surely are the precursors of such smiling behavior and a mother reinforces them as such."[28]

■ REFERENCES

1. Manning FA, Platt L, LeMay M: Fetal breathing. In McNall L, Galeener J (eds): Current Practice in Obstetrics and Gynecologic Nursing, Vol 2, pp 108–119. St. Louis, CV Mosby, 1977
2. Korones SB: High-risk newborn infants. The Basis for Intensive Nursing Care, 4th ed, pp 209–210. St. Louis, CV Mosby, 1986
3. Farrell PM, Perelman RH: The developmental biology of the lung. In Fanaroff AA, Martin RJ (eds): Neonatal-Perinatal Medicine, 4th ed, pp 557–571. St. Louis, CV Mosby, 1987
4. Harned H Jr: Respiration and the respiratory system. In Stave U (ed): Perinatal Physiology, pp 53–101. New York, Plenum Press, 1978
5. Nelson NM: Respiration and circulation after birth. In Smith CA, Nelson NM (eds): The Physiology of the Newborn Infant, 4th ed, pp 117–262. Springfield, IL, Charles C Thomas, 1976
6. Arnold HW, Putman NJ, Barnard BL, et al: Transition to extrauterine life. Am J Nurs 65(10):77–80, October 1965
7. Shurin SB: The blood and hematopoietic system. In Fanaroff AA, Martin RJ (eds): Neonatal-Perinatal Medicine, 4th ed, pp 825–869. St. Louis, CV Mosby, 1987
8. Hernandez A, Meyer DA, Goldring D: Blood pressure in neonates. Contemporary OB/GYN 5:34–37, March 1975
9. Cabal LA, Siassi B, Hodgman J: Neonatal clinical cardiopulmonary monitoring. In Fanaroff AA, Martin RJ (eds): Neonatal-Perinatal Medicine, 4th ed, pp 343–359. St Louis, CV Mosby, 1987
10. Lees MH, King DH: The cardiovascular system. In Fanaroff AA, Martin RJ (eds): Neonatal-Perinatal Medicine, 4th ed, pp 639–743. St. Louis, CV Mosby, 1987
11. Gartner LM, Lee KB: Jaundice and liver disease. In Fanaroff AA, Martin RJ (eds): Neonatal-Perinatal Medicine, 4th ed, pp 946–965. St. Louis, CV Mosby, 1987
12. Gartner LM: Hyperbilirubinemia. In Rudolph AM (ed): Pediatrics, 17th ed, pp 1007–1013. Norwalk, CT, Appleton-Century-Crofts, 1982
13. Brucker MC, MacMullen NJ: Neonatal jaundice in the home: Assessment with a noninvasive device. JOGNN 16(5):355–358, 1987
14. Bellanti JA, Boner AL, Valletta E: Immunology of the fetus and newborn. In Avery GB (ed): Neonatology: Pathophysiology and Management of the Newborn, 3rd ed. Philadelphia, JB Lippincott, 1987
15. Polmar SH, Manthel U: Immunology. In Fanaroff AA, Martin RJ (eds): Neonatal-Perinatal Medicine, 4th ed, pp 744–762. St. Louis, CV Mosby, 1987
16. Roberts FB: Perinatal Nursing. New York, McGraw-Hill, 1977
17. Bucuvalas JC, Balistreri WF: The neonatal gastrointestinal tract development. In Fanaroff AA, Martin RJ (eds): Neonatal-Perinatal Medicine, 4th ed, pp 894–899. St. Louis, CV Mosby, 1987
18. Spitzer A, Bernstein J, Edelman CM Jr, et al: The kidney and urinary tract. In Fanaroff AA, Martin RJ (eds): Neonatal-Perinatal Medicine, 4th ed, pp 981–1015. St Louis, CV Mosby, 1987
19. Phibbs RH: The newborn infant. In Rudolph AM (ed): Pediatrics, 17th ed, pp 119–166. Norwalk CT, Appleton-Century-Crofts, 1982
20. Gagliardi JV: Initial assessment of the newborn. In Warshaw JB, Hobbins JC: Principles and Practice of Perinatal Medicine, pp 197–208. Menlo Park, CA, Addison-Wesley, 1983
21. Easterly NB, Solomon LM: The skin. In Fanaroff AA, Martin RJ: Neonatal-Perinatal Medicine, 4th ed, pp 1172–1199. St. Louis, CV Mosby, 1987
22. Alexander MM, Brown MS: Pediatric Physical Diagnosis for Nurses, p 156. New York, McGraw-Hill, 1974
23. Farwell J: Maturational and neurobehavioral assessment of the newborn. In Warshaw JB, Hobbins JC: Principles and Practice of Perinatal Medicine, pp 226–247. Menlo Park, CA, Addison-Wesley, 1983
24. Brann AW Jr, Schwartz JF: Central nervous system disturbances. In Fanaroff AA, Martin RJ: Neonatal-Perinatal Medicine, pp 495–506. St. Louis, CV Mosby, 1987
25. Dubowitz L, et al: Clinical assessment of gestational age in the newborn infant. J Pediatr 77:1–10, 1970
26. Ballard J, et al: A simplified score for assessment of fetal maturation of newly born infants. J Pediatr 95:769–774, 1979
27. Sullivan R, Foster J, Schreiner RL: Determining a newborn's gestational age. MCN 4(1):38–45, January/February 1979
28. Brazelton TB: Neonatal behavioral assessment scale. Clin Dev Med 50: 1973

29. Erickson MP: Trends in assessing the newborn and his parents. MCN 3(2):99–103, March/April 1978
30. Thoman EB: Sleeping and waking states in infants: A functional perspective. Neurosci Biobehav Rev 14(1): 93–107, 1990
31. Brazelton TB: Behavioral competence of the newborn infant. In Avery GB (ed): Neonatology: Pathophysiology and Management of the Newborn, 3rd ed. Philadelphia, JB Lippincott, 1987

■ SUGGESTED READING

Anderson C: Integration of the Brazelton neonatal behavioral assessment scale into routine neonatal nursing care. Iss Compr Pediatr Nurs 9:341–351, 1986

Brazelton TB: Neonatal behavioral assessment scale. Clin Dev Med 50: 1973

Brucker MC, MacMullen NJ: Neonatal jaundice in the home: Assessment with a noninvasive device. JOGNN 16(5): 355–358, September/October 1987

Coen RW, Fanaroff AA, Taylor PM: A fast, efficient newborn exam. Patient Care 22(10):192–207, June 15, 1988

Coen RW, Fanaroff AA, Taylor PM: The detailed newborn examination. Patient Care 22(12):90–112, July 15, 1988

Keefe MR, Kotzer AM, Reuss JL, et al: Development of a system for monitoring infant state behavior. Nurs Res 38(6):344–347, November/December 1989

NAACOG: Neonatal Thermoregulation. Washington, DC, OGN Nursing Practice Resource, 1990

NAACOG: Physical Assessment of the Neonate. Washington, DC, OGN Nursing Practice Resource, 1986

30

Nursing Care of the Normal Newborn

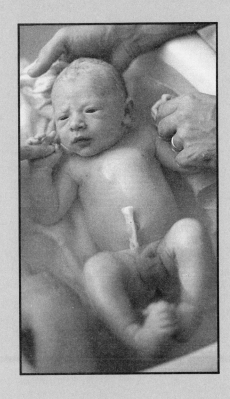

The care of the newborn presents an interesting challenge to those who work in maternity nursing. In a short period of time, usually a matter of seconds, the fetus, who has been completely dependent on the mother to supply all the physiological needs, suddenly becomes an "independent" being.

Although independent of the mother for vital functions, newborns are, of course, still very dependent in other ways. They could not survive long without a caretaker. In the immediate postnatal period, this caretaker is often the nurse.

Because these first days and weeks are so critical, the care given by the nurse is very important. The nurse must use the utmost care in handling the infants, keeping them warm and protecting them from exposure and injury, at the same time making accurate observations and recording and reporting them. Communication and teaching skills are used in contributing to the infant's future well-being by helping the parents to develop an understanding of their baby's needs and to acquire skill in his or her care. In this way their concept of themselves as adequate parents is reinforced. The nurse also must be aware that some parents need assistance in developing healthy attitudes regarding childbearing practices, so that the infant can make a satisfactory emotional and social adjustment. Opportunity must be provided in the hospital environment for the beginning development of a close parent–infant relationship. Also of importance is the maintenance of communication between the nurse and the parents.

Occurences That Should Be Reported to the Primary Health Care Provider

1. If the skin color changes:
   a. To blue (cyanosis), around the mouth or all over
   b. To yellow (jaundice)
2. Temperature above 38.4°C (101°F) or below 36.1°C (96°F)
3. Projectile vomiting two or more times
4. Refusal of two consecutive feedings
5. Periods of apnea (absence of breathing) longer than 15 seconds
6. Behavior changes, such as excessive crying, fussiness, lethargy, or difficulty in rousing the infant
7. Elimination pattern changes, such as two or more green, watery stools; hard stools; or decreased number of wet diapers (less than 5 per day)
8. Local signs of bleeding or infection:
   a. Swelling, redness or discharge from eyes
   b. Swelling, redness, discharge, or bleeding from umbilical cord stump
   c. Swelling, redness, discharge, or bleeding from circumcision

---

■ PROVIDING A SAFE ENVIRONMENT

As in the immediate newborn period (see Chap. 25), protection from injury and infection continues to be a major goal of nursing care throughout the infant's hospital stay.

Policies are formulated in each setting where newborns are cared for in an effort to provide safe, individualized care in a protective environment.

Preventing Infection

Prevention of infection is of paramount importance in caring for the newborn. Although the immune system begins to develop during fetal life, it is still very immature at birth (see Chap. 29). The neonate has come from a highly protected environment in utero to the outside world, where there is exposure to a wide variety of microorganisms. It is not surprising that organisms generally considered to be of low pathogenicity may cause infections in the neonate.[1]

It is important, therefore, to attempt to limit the number of organisms the infant comes in contact with in the early days of life.

MINIMIZING EXPOSURE TO ORGANISMS

The newborn's major source of exposure to organisms is the caretakers. Nurses and other staff members who care for newborn infants should be free from infectious diseases (i.e., respiratory, gastrointestinal, skin lesions) that could be transmitted to the neonates. Everyone who is in contact with the newborn, including parents and personnel, should assume responsibility for protecting the baby from infection. Parents may need help in reminding family and friends to postpone their visits if they are not well.

Handwashing. The basis for prevention of infection when handling the newborn is frequent, thorough handwashing with an antiseptic detergent or soap. The wash at the beginning of a shift, lasting approximately 2 minutes, should cover the forearms and elbows in addition to all areas of the hands, including between the fingers (see Guidelines for Handwashing). After the initial wash, staff members should be especially careful to wash their hands vigorously for 15 seconds before a feeding, after a diaper change, before going from one baby to another, and after touching anything that is not clean to that baby, such as a cabinet door or their own face or hair.[2] Studies of handwashing behavior in hospitals have indicated that the frequency of handwashing

Research Highlight

An important aspect of newborn care is the maintenance of the infant's temperature within a safe range. In choosing a site for temperature monitoring in the newborn, it is important to consider safety, accuracy, and the time needed to obtain an accurate reading. Although rectal temperature readings have been considered to be the standard, the safety of this method has been questioned because of the high risk for trauma to the rectal mucosa. Axillary temperatures have sometimes been questioned because of the possible effect of the proximity of the area to deposits of brown adipose tissue (BAT).

In a study by Bliss-Holtz, rectal, axillary, and inguinal temperatures were compared to determine the maximum temperature at each of the three sites, the correlation between readings at the various sites, and the time needed to reach a maximum temperature. A total of 120 full-term infants between 12 and 48 hours of age were used in the study. Rectal, axillary, and inguinal temperatures were taken, in randomized sequential order, for each infant. At each site, the temperature was recorded every 30 seconds until it remained constant for 90 seconds (stabilization).

The study found that temperature stabilization was reached by 95% of the subjects at all sites within 5½ minutes. Changes after 3 minutes for rectal and inguinal temperature readings, and after 4 minutes for axillary readings, were minimal. Axillary and inguinal readings showed a mean difference of 0.6°F; rectal and inguinal readings a mean difference of 0.8°F; and axillary and inguinal readings a mean difference of 0.2°F. Rectal and inguinal temperatures showed the highest correlation with each other.

The investigator concludes that 3 minutes is probably sufficient for the placement of rectal and inguinal thermometers and 4 minutes for axillary temperatures. In addition, the inguinal site may be preferable to the rectal site for safety reasons, and to the axillary site because of the absence of BAT in the area, and the shorter time of thermometer insertion.

Bliss-Holtz J: Comparison of rectal, axillary, and inguinal temperatures in full-term newborn infants. Nurs Res 38(2):85–87, 1989.

between patient contacts is very low.[3] Personnel may need frequent reminders of the importance of handwashing in preventing hospital-acquired infections in neonates. Parents also need instruction about the importance (and technique) of proper handwashing, and reinforcement should be given as necessary during the hospital stay.

Gloving. With increasing concern about potential transmission of infection from patients to health care providers, nonsterile gloves are advised for use in caring for all infants until amniotic fluid and blood are removed from the infant's skin, usually during the first bath. Gloves must be removed and the hands washed before going to a central area or giving care to another infant.[2]

Nursery Dress Code. Protecting the infant from infection has traditionally involved a dress code for those coming in contact with the newborn in the hospital. Most nursery nurses (and in many hospitals where rooming-in is practiced, the postpartum nurses as well) change to scrub suits or dresses when they come to work. These should be short sleeved so hands, forearms, and elbows can be washed more readily. An advantage of scrub clothes is the ease with which they can be changed when soiled, thus making the spread of infection from one infant to another less likely.

Other hospital personnel and visitors are usually expected to put cover gowns on over their street clothes before coming into the nursery or into the mother's room if the infant is there. If they are going to touch the baby, they should wash their hands and arms before putting on the gown. There are those who question whether cover gowns are necessary. Some studies have shown that bacterial colonization of the infant's nares or umbilicus has not increased when cover gowns were no

Guidelines for Handwashing at the Beginning of a Shift

1. Remove watch and rings.
2. Wash hands (including between the fingers), wrists, forearms, and elbows thoroughly with antiseptic handwashing agent.
3. Clean fingernails with a plastic or orangewood stick.
4. Wash hands again, using a soft brush, soap pad, or vigorous friction.
5. Rinse thoroughly.
6. Dry with paper towels.

longer used. In one study, colonization actually decreased significantly without the use of cover gowns for visitors.[4] The researchers speculated that the gowns may have provided a false sense of security for visitors and that, without them, better handwashing technique may have been used.

Caps, beard covers, and masks are no longer considered necessary for routine activities in the nursery.[2] Hair should be worn short, however, or long hair should be pulled back, to avoid allowing the hair to come in contact with the infant or equipment. If circumstances arise necessitating masks, they should cover the nose and mouth, should be changed frequently, and, when removed from the face, should be discarded, not pulled down around the neck. Masks can become a reservoir for bacteria when not applied properly or changed regularly.

Maternal Infection. Special problems are created when the mother has an infection. Which maternal infections would the infant be most likely to acquire if the two are not separated? Hospital policies vary in this matter. In many hospitals, the mother and infant are routinely separated if the mother is febrile. Some of the suggestions offered by the American Academy of Pediatrics and the American College of Obstetricians and Gynecologists are as follows:[2]

- Maternal genital infections are rarely spread to the infant postnatally. A mother who is febrile without a specific diagnosed site of infection may usually handle and feed her newborn if she feels well enough and uses good handwashing technique. Additionally, she should wear a clean cover gown and protect the infant from potentially contaminated items, such as her nightgown, bedclothes, and perineal pads.
- When a respiratory infection is present, the mother should be informed that these infections can be spread by hands or contaminated articles. She should also be instructed in careful handwashing techniques and appropriate handling of tissues and other items contaminated by secretions. Wearing a mask may be helpful in reducing the droplet spread of infection.
- A woman with a communicable disease that may be transmitted to her baby should be separated from the baby until the disease is no longer communicable.

The mother who must be separated from her infant needs special attention from the nurse. Making arrangements for the mother to see the baby through the nursery window, bringing her frequent reports about the infant, or providing a picture of the baby taken with an instant camera can help ease the frustration of the separation. The mother who is breast-feeding may need assistance in pumping her breasts to ensure stimulation and continued milk supply (see Chap. 32).

If the mother with an infection is allowed to care for her infant and is instructed to wear a mask, the nurse should make certain that the mother understands that she should do the following:

1. Avoid touching or adjusting the mask, to avoid contaminating her hands.
2. Wash her hands if the mask is touched.
3. Wear a clean mask on each occasion that a mask is needed.

Newborn Care Areas

Providing a safe environment also includes concern about the areas and equipment used for the newborn's care. Many hospitals today offer more than one setting for care of newborns alone or of mothers and newborns together. Whichever setting is used, attention is still required to the environmental aspects of safe care.

MOTHER–BABY CARE

Current interest in family-centered maternity care has led to having healthy newborns spend increasing amounts of time with their mothers and less time in central nurseries. In the free-standing birth centers, or in hospitals with labor–delivery–recovery–postpartum rooms, mother and infant are usually not separated at all. In these settings, initial newborn care is done in the birthing room and the family usually goes home within a few hours after the birth.

Some hospitals use newborn nurseries as admission nurseries, where the infant goes for initial care and observation for a set time and then goes to the mother's room until discharge. This is often referred to as "rooming-in" and may be either optional or mandatory. The family-centered approach to maternity care not only provides an environment that fosters a natural parent-child relationship from the beginning but it also affords opportunities for both parents to learn about and practice infant care (Fig. 30-1).

A variable in these situations is the staff responsibility for the infant's care. The nursery staff may still be responsible for meeting the rooming-in baby's needs and for educating the mother regarding the baby's care. An alternate plan is to have the infant and mother cared for by the same nurse. This may be called "mother–baby couple care" or "couplet care." Nurses are prepared to provide this type of care by cross training in nursery and postpartum. Advantages of having the same nurse care for both mother and newborn infant include facilitation of more flexible care routines and increased opportunities for parenting education.[5]

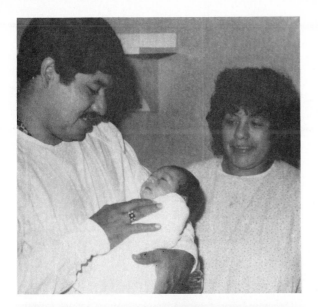

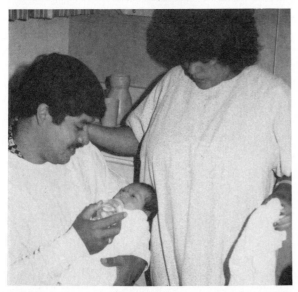

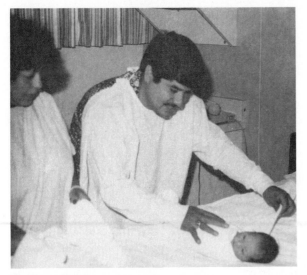

■ *Figure 30–1*

In the rooming-in unit the father has the opportunity to gain experience holding and caring for the new baby while the mother observes.

Infants must be protected from sources of infection regardless of where they are cared for. The same basic principles for asepsis employed in the nursery must be followed when infant care is provided in the mother's room. Plans for safe care of infants who are in the room with their mothers for extended periods need to include education of the mother about possible safety concerns. In addition to prevention of infection, these would include use of the bulb syringe, positioning the infant to avoid aspiration, keeping the infant in the bassinet when not being held, and not leaving the infant unattended in the room.

THE CENTRAL NURSERY

The central newborn nursery is designed for the care of a variable number of healthy newborns (Fig. 30-2). When this system is in use, infants are brought to their mothers at specified times during the day for feeding or visiting. The nursery staff assumes the responsibility for total care of the infants. Some type of central nursery is found in most hospitals, if only for those infants whose mothers cannot care for them.

To assure safe care for infants in the central nursery, certain recommendations are made. For instance, the area should be well lighted, have a large wall clock, and be equipped for emergency resuscitation. Handwashing facilities and materials should be readily available. There should be at least 3 ft between bassinets in all directions, and there should be one nursing staff member for each 6 to 8 infants.[2]

The precautions previously mentioned, such as handwashing, wearing scrub clothes, and following other aspects of nursery aseptic technique, afford additional protection.

It must be understood that there is a difference in nursery technique between what is considered to be nursery clean and what is considered to be baby clean (i.e., what is clean for an individual baby). There should be no common equipment, such as a common bath table, used in providing care for the babies. There should be provisions in the nursery for individual technique to be followed. Each infant should have his own crib and general supplies, so that he can be given such care as his daily inspection bath or be diapered or dressed in his own bed.

Most cribs are constructed with a built-in cabinet or drawers to hold clean diapers, shirts, linens, and small items such as the thermometer, lubricant, cotton balls, and applicators. When such cribs are not available, something should be improvised so that individualized care techniques can still be carried out.

The Cohort Nursery System. In hospitals in which the nursery area is comprised of more than one normal newborn nursery room, the cohort system is sometimes used to reduce cross-contamination between groups of newborns. All infants born during a designated time

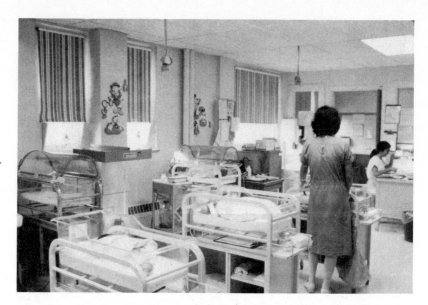

■ *Figure 30–2*
Term newborn nursery.

period are placed in one nursery room and, ideally, cared for by a group of personnel who do not care for infants from other nurseries during that shift. Mothers of the infants are placed with roommates who have infants in the same nursery. That particular nursery is closed to new admissions until all the cohort babies have been discharged. It is then cleaned and a new cohort is started.

THE NEWBORN REQUIRING ISOLATION

Maternity units have varying policies for infants who are suspected of or known to have infections. The infected neonate may be placed in a separate room in the nursery area, kept in the central nursery, allowed to room-in with the mother, or transferred to a pediatrics unit, depending on the type and manifestations of the infection, the staffing available, and hospital policy. Decisions are often made on an individualized basis.

Nurses must be alert for infants who show no signs of, or are at increased risk for developing, an infection, so that isolation procedures can be implemented if necessary. Infants who are born at home or on the way to the hospital should be bathed and observed for signs of infection, but separate isolation facilities are not required.[2]

Isolettes are sometimes used for isolating infants within the central nursery. This equipment may be helpful in keeping the infant separate and as a reminder of the isolation status, but it should not be assumed to provide adequate isolation for infected neonates. Although the air coming into the incubator is filtered, the air being discharged into the nursery is not. Also, the surface and portholes of the incubator are easily contaminated with organisms from the infected infant, so the hands and forearms of personnel are likely to be colonized.[2]

Infants segregated from the other neonates may require closer observation and additional care related to the infection, but they continue to need the usual care given to the healthy newborn. Also, their need for human contact, holding, and cuddling should not be forgotten.

■ NURSING CARE DURING THE TRANSITION PERIOD

In the delivery room, initial care has been given to the infant, and any early problems have been dealt with (see Chap. 25). From the delivery room, the infant may be taken to the recovery room and remain with the mother and father for a while, go to a transitional nursery, or be admitted directly to the regular nursery. Of course, if the infant has serious problems, a special-care nursery is indicated.

Because the day of birth is the most hazardous time for the infant, it is important that continuing observations be made during the first 24 hours. A receiving or transition nursery in the labor or nursery section provides an excellent physical environment for the extensive observations that are necessary, similar to that of recovery room care for adults. An infant whose mother has been heavily medicated during labor and delivery is particularly in need of this recovery care. If this kind of setup is not available, the new babies should be placed in an area of the regular nursery where they can be easily observed. Low-risk babies whose mothers had little or no medication can probably be safely left with their mothers for a time under close supervision of a

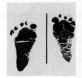

Nursing Care Plan

Care of the Newborn During the Transition Period

Patient Goals
1. Infant's airway remains clear.
2. Infant's temperature remains in the average range (97.7°–99.5°F).
3. Infant is not exposed to infection and receives appropriate prophylaxis.
4. Infant remains free of injury.
5. Infant's body systems adapt to extrauterine environment.

Assessment	Potential Nursing Diagnosis	Planning and Intervention	Evaluation
Respiratory status	Ineffective airway clearance related to excessive oropharyngeal mucus	Observe infant frequently during transition period Keep bulb syringe in basinet and use as necessary	Newborn remains free of respiratory difficulties
Temperature	Ineffective thermoregulation, related to newborn transition to extrauterine environment	Place in radiant warmer and monitor temperature continuously until stable Delay bath until temperature stable Dry well after bath and place back in warmer until temperature is again stable	Newborn's temperature stabilizes Infant does not develop hypothermia

Newborn's environment	High risk for infection related to maturational factors—immature immune system	Provide clean area with individual care items
		
		Maintain clean technique
		  Careful, frequent handwashing
		  Caretakers free from infection
		
		Provide eye prophylaxis
		
		Remove blood and meconium from skin
		
		Give cord care with tripple-dye
			Newborn remains free of infection
			
			Infant does not develop ophthalmia neonatorum
			
			Skin and umbilicus remain free of colonization

	High risk for injury related to maturational factors—unable to protect self	Maintain safe environment
		  Warm room without drafts
		  Handle gently, but firmly
		  Protect from falls
			Infant is not injured

General status
  Size
  Maturation
  Normality of body
	Potential complication: alteration in physiological responses related to problems with adaptation to extrauterine environment	Weigh; measure length and head circumference
		
		Perform gestational age assessment
			Newborn adapts to extrauterine life with minimal problems
			
			Newborn shows no evi-

(continued)

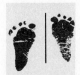

Nursing Care Plan (continued)

Assessment	Potential Nursing Diagnosis	Planning and Intervention	Evaluation
systems Vital signs		Examine body systems by thorough observation, inspection, auscultation, and palpation; monitor vital signs Record, report as appropriate	dence of trauma or abnormalities Newborn has good color and muscle tone Newborn retains stabilized vital signs
Blood sugar levels	Potential complication: hypoglycemia secondary to maternal diabetes, cold stress, or infant large or small for gestational age	Observe for signs of hypoglycemia: jitteriness, tremors, eye rolling, weakness, high-pitched cry, poor muscle tone Use Dextrostix: report to doctor if less than 40 mg/dl Feed infant: glucose water, formula, or breast, according to hospital policy	Newborn does not develop symptoms of hypoglycemia Newborn has blood glucose level above 40 mg/dl

nurse in case of presence of mucus or other sudden changes in the infant's condition. If the mother plans to have rooming-in, it is often delayed for several hours until the infant is considered stable, with no signs of excessive mucus.

Initial Assessment

When the infant is admitted to the nursery, the nursery nurse receives a report from the delivery room nurse, checks identification bands according to hospital policy, and checks the infant's record to note any additional important information. She then does an initial assessment of the infant (see Chap. 29). It is particularly important at this time to check the infant's respiratory status and temperature and to observe for any congenital anomalies that might have been missed at birth but need immediate care.

IMPORTANT OBSERVATIONS

The vital signs should be checked every half hour until they are stable or as indicated by hospital policy. Apical heart rate and respirations should each be counted for a full minute. The pulse may vary with the infant's activity, but a persistent rate below 120 beats per minute or above 150 beats per minute should be reported. The infant's temperature is checked on admission, then usually monitored frequently until the axillary reading reaches about 36.6°C (97.8°F). Axillary temperature (Fig. 30-3) is preferred because it eliminates the potential danger of perforation of the rectum with the rectal thermometer. In some settings, however, an initial rectal temperature is taken to determine rectal patency. The axillary reading is usually slightly lower than the rectal temperature, but occasionally, if the infant has been chilled and brown fat stimulated, it may be higher[6] (see Chap. 29).

The infant's color and respiratory pattern are good indices of whether or not the newborn is experiencing respiratory insufficiency. Dyspnea, rapid respiration exceeding 50 breaths per minute, and persistent cyanosis should be reported. Because mucus in the nasopharynx often causes respiratory distress, the nurse should be particularly watchful for its presence. Gagging, vomiting, breath holding, retraction of the head, choking, and cyanosis all may be signs of the presence of mucus,

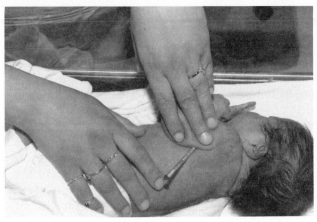

■ *Figure 30–3*
Taking an axillary temperature. The infant's arm is held gently but firmly against his side while the thermometer is in place to ensure a more accurate temperature reading.

which is particularly prone to develop in the second period of reactivity following the first sleep.

Breathing difficulties or excessive mucus may also be evidence of congenital anomalies, such as choanal atresia or tracheoesophageal fistula. Observing for the timing of the breathing difficulties will help determine the cause. In some nurseries, especially those with high-risk populations, gastric contents are routinely aspirated to screen for anomalies of the gastrointestinal tract. Other nurseries do this only when there is evidence of a problem.

In a vigorous, normal infant, the cry should be lusty and will occur especially when the baby is handled or moved. If the infant doesn't cry at all when disturbed or seems unusually sleepy or depressed, or if the pulse and respiratory rate are slow, the condition should be

reported. It may be necessary to stimulate the infant to cry periodically by rubbing the back, head, or feet or changing his position. Brief tremors and twitching are not unusual in the transition period, but if they are prolonged or occur frequently, they may indicate a problem and the physician should be notified (see Chap. 29).

TESTING FOR HYPOGLYCEMIA

Many infants are at risk for becoming hypoglycemic in the first few hours after birth. Assessment for this condition can now be done by the nursery nurse using the Dextrostix to estimate blood sugar levels. The test, using blood from a heel stick, is done routinely on all newborns in some nurseries. In other nurseries, it is done according to a protocol defining infants most likely to become hypoglycemic soon after birth, such as infants of diabetic mothers or those who are large or small for gestational age. If routine testing is not done, the nurse should be aware that such central nervous system symptoms as poor muscle tone, weakness, tremors, eye rolling, high-pitched cry, and, as a late symptom, even convulsions may indicate low blood sugar levels.

When a heel stick is to be done for a Dextrostix or to obtain blood for other tests, surface blood flow should first be improved by warming the infant's foot. This can sometimes be done by holding the infant's heel in the palm of the nurse's hand[7] or by wrapping the foot in a warm, moist compress for 3 to 5 minutes. After cleaning the heel with alcohol and allowing it to dry, a quick, clean stick is made in the outer surface of the heel with a disposable lancet (Fig. 30-4). The area is then wiped off with a sterile gauze square, and when the blood starts to flow again, it is dropped on the Dextrostix or collected in a capillary tube, depending on the intended purpose.

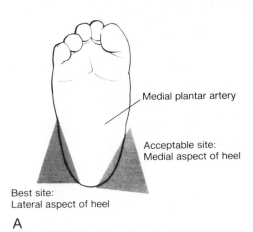

Medial plantar artery

Acceptable site:
Medial aspect of heel

Best site:
Lateral aspect of heel

A

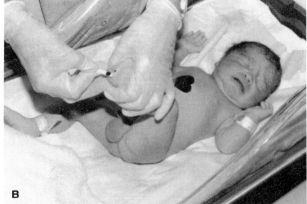

B

■ *Figure 30–4*
The heelstick procedure is used to test for blood glucose. (A) Appropriate sites for the heelstick procedure. (B) After the site is punctured with a pediatric microlancet and after elimination of the first drop of blood, the nurse holds the Dextrostix under the heel to collect the second drop of blood.

It is important to follow the Dextrostix package directions precisely, especially in regard to the 60-second lapsed time before wiping or washing off the blood. Care should be taken not to squeeze the foot too vigorously when obtaining the sample, because this may dilute the blood with tissue fluid or cause hemolysis. If the blood flow diminishes or stops before an adequate amount is obtained, wiping the area with a sterile gauze square will sometimes result in increased blood flow. Positioning the infant with the foot in a dependent position (lower than the body) may also increase blood flow. Following the procedure, a small sterile bandage may be applied to the area. Use of a Glucometer adds to the accuracy of timing the procedure and interpreting the results.

ASSESSING ELIMINATION

The time of the infant's first stool and voiding should be noted to indicate proper excretory function. It is sometimes necessary for the nursery nurse to review the delivery record or check with the delivery room nurse to see whether the infant voided or defecated before being brought to the nursery.

CONDITION OF THE CORD

The cord should be checked periodically. Any oozing or bleeding should be reported immediately, and the cord should be reclamped or retied as indicated. Oozing occurs most often between the second and sixth hour of life and is frequently associated with crying or the passage of meconium.

Nursing Diagnosis

Initial assessment of the newborn, coupled with the nurse's knowledge of the expected physiological status of the newborn, will lead to formulation of a number of potential or actual nursing diagnoses, such as the following:

Ineffective airway clearance related to excessive oropharyngeal mucus
Ineffective thermoregulation, related to newborn transition to extrauterine environment
High risk for infection related to maturational factors—immature immune system
High risk for injury related to maturational factors—
unable to protect self

The nurse will also monitor the infant for potential complications that would lead to identification of problems that would require collaboration between the nurse and physician.

Planning and Intervention

Nurseries vary as to what is included in routine admission care. Certain procedures such as eye prophylaxis (see Chap. 25) and vitamin K injection (see Chap. 29) are done in the nursery if they are not included in the delivery room care. The injection technique is shown in Figure 30-5. Results of the assessment procedures noted in the previous section guide the planning and intervention for each individual infant. Equipment for suctioning and resuscitation must be on hand, and someone who is trained in its use should be immediately available. A bulb syringe should be in each infant's bassinet.

PREVENTING HYPOTHERMIA

Hypothermia is a major concern in the transition period. When a radiant warmer is used, the servocontrol should be set to maintain the abdominal skin temperature at 36.5°C. The skin probe (thermistor) should be taped securely to the anterior abdominal wall and covered with an aluminum patch to shield it from the radiant heat source.[2] The patch used in many nurseries is heart shaped, with gold-colored aluminum on one side and adhesive to hold the probe in place on the other (see Fig. 30-5). The skin probe should be checked periodically to make sure it is in contact with the skin. A probe not touching the skin causes the warmer to misinterpret the infant's temperature and continue to radiate heat after the desired infant temperature is reached. The infant can become overheated or possibly even burned. Hyperthermia, like hypothermia, increases the infant's

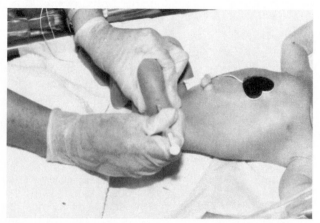

■ *Figure 30–5*
The infant's thigh is grasped firmly, bunching up the muscle (vastus lateralis). The needle is inserted quickly at a 90° angle into the middle third of the muscle. After aspirating (with no blood return), the medication is injected slowly to distribute it evenly and minimize discomfort. The rectus femoris muscle is an alternate site.

metabolic requirements and oxygen consumption.[8] The temperature of an isolette being used as a warmer should also be checked periodically, because it also can rise higher than expected and cause overheating.

INITIAL BATH

The first bath is usually delayed until after the temperature has stabilized. Bathing is often done under the radiant warmer, because wetting the skin causes heat loss by evaporation. Because some degree of temperature drop usually occurs, the temperature is rechecked after the bath, and the infant remains under the warmer until the temperature is stable again.

The type of initial bath given and the agents used depend on hospital policy. Warm water may be used with sterile cotton sponges to wash any blood, meconium, and amniotic fluid from the newborn's face, head, and body, or a mild soap can be used followed by careful rinsing. Soap containing hexachlorophene may still be used in some hospitals for the initial bath, because of its effectiveness against staphylococcal infections. It should be rinsed off completely and not be used on a daily basis because of its potential neurotoxicity in neonates.[2]

There is no recognized need to remove the vernix caseosa from the newborn's skin completely, unless it is stained with blood or meconium. There is some indication that the vernix serves a protective function and may be bactericidal.[9] It usually disappears spontaneously in about 24 hours. If it remains in the creases and folds of the skin longer than 2 days or appears to cause irritation, gentle wiping will usually remove it. (For more information on infant bathing, see later section.)

SPECIFIC PROPHYLAXIS AGAINST INFECTION

Several procedures routinely done for the newborn are directed toward prevention of specific types of infection. Within the first few hours after birth, a prophylactic agent is placed in the eyes to prevent ophthalmia neonatorum (see Chap. 25). Initial skin and cord care is done to help prevent colonization of the skin and umbilical area with potentially pathogenic bacteria. In choosing an agent to cleanse the skin, care must be taken that the agent does not have an adverse effect on the skin, is not toxic if absorbed, and does not give rise to new infection problems by altering the skin flora.[2] For cord care, triple dye or an antimicrobial agent such as bacitracin ointment are currently recommended to prevent colonization.[2] Alcohol, which has been used for years to care for the cord, hastens drying of the stump but is probably not very effective in preventing cord colonization or umbilical infection.[2]

The cord care may be done following the bath. Triple dye, usually a one-time treatment, is applied to the cord and over the junction between the cord stump and the skin (Fig. 30-6). It leaves a temporary purple stain on the abdomen that may last several days. This should be explained to the parents so they don't worry about the stain. If an ointment such as bacitracin is used, it should not be applied until the infant no longer needs to be under the radiant warmer. The oily substance tends to concentrate the heat and could possibly cause a burn.

Evaluation

The nurse will evaluate her care by determining whether the nursing goals for the transition period have been met. The infant who has a clear airway, stable vital signs, is free of injury, and has received all planned measures to prevent infection is progressing appropriately to a period when less intensive observation is needed. If any goals are not met, the nurse reassesses her care plan to determine possible revisions to meet the infant's needs.

■ CONTINUING CARE AND PARENT TEACHING

Assessment

Ongoing assessment during the newborn's hospital stay varies according to hospital policy. The nurse will be expected to assess not only the infant's physical condition but also his behavioral patterns, interaction with

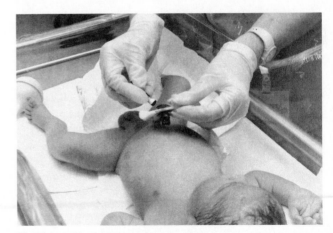

■ *Figure 30–6*
Initial cord care. Tripple-Dye is applied to the cord stump and approximately 1 in of skin around the umbilicus.

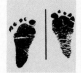

Nursing Care Plan

Continuing Care of the Newborn

Patient Goals

1. Infant is not exposed to and does not develop signs of infection.
2. Infant body systems continue to adapt to extrauterine environment.
3. Infant's skin and umbilical cord stump are clean and free of infection.
4. Parents demonstrate ability to handle and care for infant.
5. Parents demonstrate appropriate attachment behaviors and understanding of newborn characteristics during interactions with infant.

Assessment	Potential Nursing Diagnosis	Planning and Intervention	Evaluation

General status
  Vital signs
  Color
  Responsiveness
  Activity
	High risk for infection related to maturational factors—immature immune system
	
	Potential for injury related to maturational factors—unable to protect self
		Make observations according to hospital policy
		
		Note any changes in infant's condition and report and record as appropriate
		
		Use good handwashing and invdividual clean technique when caring for newborn
			Newborn has stabilized vital signs
			
			Newborn does not develop hypothermia or hyperthermia
			
			Newborn remains free of evidence of jaundice or cyanosis
			
			Newborn alternates sleep and activity
			
			Newborn's skin remains intact

Condition of skin, umbilical cord stump and umbilicus	Alteration in skin integrity, related to peeling, cracking skin, moist umbilical cord stump, or recent circumcision	Observe umbilical area for inflammation or odor and cord stump for moistness or oozing Observe skin for peeling or cracking For long, moist cord, obtain permission to cut shorter Apply antiinfective agent (tripple dye, antibiotic ointment, or alcohol) according to hospital policy	Newborn remains free of infection
Elimination: stools and urine	Alteration in bowel elimination: lack of stool related to possible imperforate anus Alteration in patterns of urinary elimination: decreased related to insufficient fluid intake	Record passage of first and subsequent stools: describe color, consistency, and amount Report if no stool in first 24 h Record number of wet diapers	Newborn passes meconium stool within first 24 h Newborn voids within first 24 h and has at least 6–10 wet diapers per day after first 24 h

(continued)

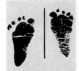

Nursing Care Plan (continued)

Assessment	Potential Nursing Diagnosis	Planning and Intervention	Evaluation
		Report if number decreases	
		Encourage more frequent feedings	
Parent's knowledge of infant care	Parental knowledge deficit related to inexperience in infant care	Develop teaching plan for individual couple, based on assessment of knowledge	Parents express and demonstrate ability to care for infant before discharge from hospital
		Provide information, demonstrations, practice opportunities, and other teaching modalities as appropriate	
		Provide assistance as needed without taking over	
Parent's coping behaviors when dealing with infant	High risk for ineffective parental coping related to new parent's inexperience and feelings of incompetence	Observe infant's behavior patterns, assist parents in recognizing and understanding their infant	Parents express their comfort in handling the infant
		Teach comfort measures for infant: holding, swaddling, gentle voice and touch	
Family interactions	High risk for alteration in parenting related to potential for impaired parent-infant attachment	Provide opportunities for parents to handle and get acquainted with infant	Parents demonstrate attachment behaviors: en face position, touching, enfolding
		Encourage and reinforce attachment behaviors	

the parents, and the parent's need for information about the newborn and his care (see Chap. 29). Early detection of problems in any of these areas is of primary concern. Most nurseries use some type of flow sheet to record specific nursing assessments. These usually include the infant's daily weight, vital signs, skin color and integrity, condition of cord, circumcision, activity level, intake, and elimination. Besides these observations, done at predetermined intervals, nurses should be alert for and report any changes in the infant that they might notice at any time while giving care. For example, subtle changes in color, activity, posture, or vital signs in the newborn can indicate beginning infection or possible abnormalities.

Nursing Diagnosis

Awareness of potential nursing diagnoses, based on areas of assessment, will assist the nurse in planning care for the newborn. Ineffective airway clearance, ineffective thermoregulation, high risk for infection, and high risk for injury, as in the transition period, would still be of concern. Examples of additional nursing diagnoses include the following:

Alteration in skin integrity, related to peeling and cracking of skin, moist umbilical cord stump, or circumcision

Parental knowledge deficit related to possible lack of
experience with infant care

High risk for ineffective parental coping related to
new parents' inexperience and feelings of
incompetence

High risk for alteration in parenting related to
impaired parent–infant attachment

Following her assessment, the nurse would be able
to identify actual nursing diagnoses for the individual
infant. Examples include the following:

Alteration in elimination or lack of stool in first 24
hours, related to possible rectal anomaly

Alteration in urinary elimination decreased, related to
insufficient fluid intake

Maternal knowledge deficit regarding infant care
(handling, bathing, feeding) related to mother
having first baby.

Planning and Intervention

During the infant's hospital stay, the nurse is responsible
for planning and providing daily care. The mother
should be involved with as much of this care as possible
to help her prepare for taking over the responsibility
when she gets home. This is easiest when mother and
baby are cared for together, but it can also be arranged
when a central nursery is used.

It is important that the nurse assess the mother's
understanding and her skill in caring for her infant.
Any basic principles or procedures related to infant care
that the mother finds necessary and useful should be
part of the nurse's teaching plan for the mother during
her hospital stay. A written plan or checklist of what
the mother wants to learn and what teaching has been
done is helpful in providing continuity between health-

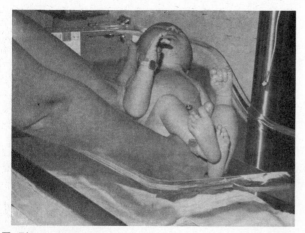

■ *Figure 30–7*
One method of lifting the baby is to place one hand under the
infant's neck and the other under the buttocks.

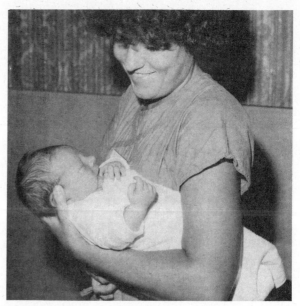

■ *Figure 30–8*
Football hold for carrying the infant.

care providers. Consistency in what is taught is necessary to avoid confusing the parents.

If the parents' primary language is not English, it
is important to assure that they are able to understand
what is being said, and, if not, that an interpreter is
present to assist them.

The following guidelines for infant care can be
helpful for the nurse and also can be used for teaching
the mother and the father, if he is present.

HANDLING AND POSITIONING THE INFANT

Although they are small, newborns are not as fragile
as they sometimes seem. They should be treated gently,
of course, but firm, smooth handling helps them feel
secure. There is no one right way of turning, lifting, or
holding a newborn, but the following points should be
kept in mind:

- The head and buttocks need to be supported.
- Babies are wiggly and can push themselves out of
  your grasp.
- It is easier to pick an infant up from the supine
  position than from the side-lying or prone
  position.

A suggested way to lift an infant is to place one
hand under the neck to support the head and shoulders
and the other hand under the buttocks to grasp the
opposite thigh (Fig. 30-7). The infant can then be lifted
up to a holding position or moved from one place to
another. A useful position for holding or carrying is the
"football hold" (Fig. 30-8). Mothers appreciate learning
about this position, because, like the nurse, they often

have times when they need to hold the baby and still have one hand free.

Positioning in the crib is usually on the side with a blanket roll at the infant's back for support. This should extend from shoulder to hip. If it is behind the infant's head, it pushes the head forward. An alternate position would be to place the infant on his abdomen. Both of these positions allow for drainage of secretions, such as mucus or regurgitation of milk from the infant's mouth. The back-lying position makes drainage of secretions difficult and should be avoided as a sleeping position, or when the infant is unattended, to reduce the danger of aspiration.

DRESSING, DIAPERING, AND WRAPPING

Feelings of confidence in dressing and undressing the baby come with practice. Putting on a shirt or gown should be done gently. Helpful hints include enlarging the neck opening to avoid dragging the garment over the infant's face and reaching through the sleeve with your fingers from the outside, when pulling the infant's hand through, to avoid snagging the fingers.

Diapering is fairly simple when disposable diapers that fasten with tapes are used. With increasing concern being expressed about the adverse effect of disposable diapers on the environment, however, many hospitals and new parents are now using cloth diapers. These can be held in place with pins or with diaper covers

that have Velcro closures. If pins are used, they should be inserted pointing toward the back of the infant so there is less danger that they will stick the infant if they come open.

Wrapping the infant snugly in a blanket (swaddling) makes the infant easier to handle and often quiets a fussy baby. Figure 30-9 illustrates a method that will keep the blanket around the baby securely and avoid loose ends. Some infants seem happier with their arms inside the blanket, and others like their arms free (see Fig. 30-8).

BATHING AND HYGIENE

The daily cleansing of the infant affords an excellent opportunity for making the observations that are necessary during the immediate postnatal period. How frequently a bath is given and what materials are used may vary from institution to institution.

In some hospitals, daily cleansing of the baby's skin is limited to washing the buttocks and perianal area with a mild soap and water during diaper changes and washing the face with warm water as needed. Many hospital nurseries, however, give the newborn a complete sponge bath with mild soap and water every day or every other day in addition to the periodic cleansing of face and buttocks (Fig. 30-10). The use of strong soap and scented baby oil or powder is discouraged because of the sensitivity of the newborn's skin.

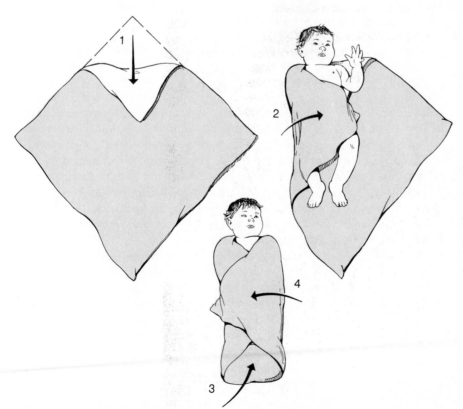

■ *Figure 30-9*

Swaddling an infant. 1. fold down top corner of blanket and place infant on blanket with neck near fold; 2. bring corner of blanket around from infant's right side and tuck under left side; 3. bring bottom corner up to chest 4. bring remaining corner around and tuck under right side. Wrap securely, but not too tightly—leave some room for infant to move.

Client Education

Basic Principles in Bathing an Infant

1. All equipment, clothing, and supplies should be assembled. Safety pins, if used, should be closed and placed out of the reach of the baby. Receptacles for soiled clothing, cotton balls, and so on should be available.
2. Care should be taken so that the environment is free from drafts and warm enough (i.e., 24°–27°C or 75°–80°F). The bath should not have to be interrupted to close a door or a window. The water for the bath should be about 37° to 38°C (98°–100°F). Water that feels warm to the elbow is approximately that temperature.
3. Proceed from the "cleanest" areas to those that are "most soiled." Thus, the eyes are bathed first, then the face, ears, scalp, neck, upper extremities, trunk, lower extremities, and finally the buttocks and the genitals (Fig. 30–10). Each of these in turn are washed, *rinsed well*, and dried. Particular attention should be paid to cleansing and drying the scalp and all creases at the neck, behind the ears, under the arms, the palms of the hands, and between the fingers and the toes, under the knees, and in the groin, the buttocks, and the genitals.
4. *The infant never should be left unattended*, even on a large work area; one hand should be kept on the infant at all times. If it is necessary to leave the area, even for a second, the infant should be taken along or placed in the crib.

Demonstration and Practice. Each mother should have an opportunity to observe a demonstration of a sponge bath and, if possible, to give a bath to her infant. If there is an opportunity for only one bath with the mother present, the nurse can combine the demonstration and return demonstration by discussing the bath with the mother first and then letting her give the bath, with the nurse there for moral support and assistance as necessary (Fig. 30-11). The father's participation is an added benefit.

The basic principles of bathing should be conveyed to the mother, for safety's sake, but she should not be made to feel that there is only one way to bathe the baby. Each mother develops her own manner of bathing the newborn according to her manual dexterity, the size and the activity of the infant, and the facilities available. By discussing with the mother what she already knows or has heard about bathing the baby, nurses can make their teaching more meaningful for the individual client.

Nurses should also explore with the mother what equipment and facilities are available in the home and instruct her in how the use of these might differ from what is available in the hospital. Usually the necessities can be met without undue expenses or difficulty. For instance, a large counter or table that can be washed and padded adequately (and is a comfortable height for handling the infant) can be used as the bath area. A large pan or basin serves well for the bathtub in the early weeks; it should be kept only for the baby's use. Thus, the extra expense of special equipment can be minimized. A soft towel and washcloth, for the baby's use only, and a mild soap are also needed.

Some mothers and babies enjoy the bath as a daily routine, but others do not or cannot always find the time. For these, as long as the face, neck creases, and diaper area are washed as needed, giving a bath every other day should be sufficient. A sponge bath should continue to be the type of bath given until the cord stump has fallen off and the area has healed. After this, a tub bath can be given.

Suggestions for Care of Specific Areas

EYES. The eyes should be wiped from the inner corner to the outer corner, using a clean cotton ball or clean area of the washcloth for each eye. No care, other than this cleansing with clean water, is necessary unless there is evidence of inflammation or infection. There may be some reaction from the medication used for prophylaxis against ophthalmia neonatorum beginning in the first few hours, and this condition does not usually require treatment. Any redness, swelling, or discharge, however, should be reported and recorded so that the eyes can be observed more closely and tests to rule out infection can be done if necessary.

NOSE AND EARS. Cotton-tipped applicators should not be used to clean inside the infant's nose or ears because the delicate tissues could be injured. The nose usually does not need cleaning because the infant sneezes to clear the nasal passages. If some dried mucus does need to be removed from the nose, a small twisted piece of cotton moistened with water may be used.

Twisted cotton, or a soft washcloth, can also be used to clean the *outer* ear. Nothing should be put *inside* the ear.

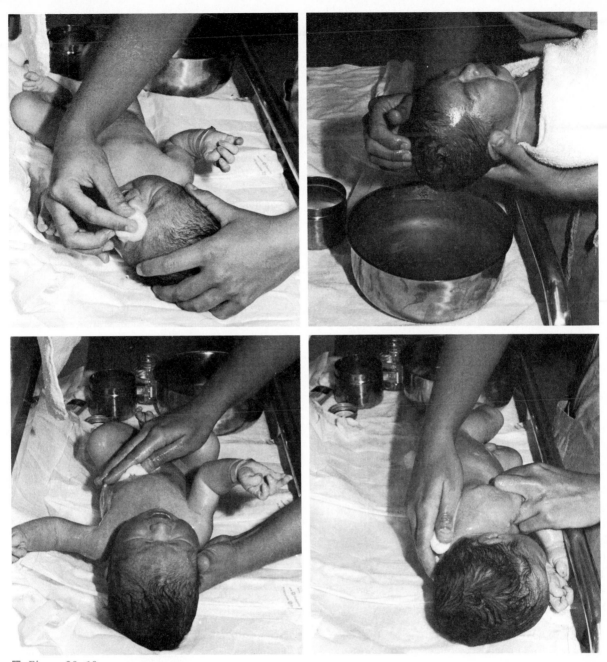

■ *Figure 30–10*
The cleanest areas of the infant are bathed first (eyes, head) before the chest and back.

HAIR. The head should be washed each time the baby is bathed. Swaddling the baby in a blanket or towel and using the football hold makes the job easier. The same soap the baby is washed with or any brand of baby shampoo can be used. Oil should not be put on the hair, as it may predispose to cradle cap.

SKIN. The newborn's skin is often dry and peeling within a few days after birth, and dry cracks may appear in the wrist and ankle areas. This is sometimes a cause of concern to mothers, and they want to put oil or some other preparation on the skin to get rid of the dryness.

They can be reassured that the flakiness and cracks will disappear in a few days and that oil and some lotions may make matters worse by causing a rash.

The skin is thin, delicate, extremely tender, and very easily irritated. Because the skin is a protective covering, breaks in its surface may lead to infection. Skin disturbances can constitute an actual threat to the infant's well-being.

The newborn does not usually perspire until after the first month. Warm weather or excessive clothing may cause the infant to develop prickly heat, a closely

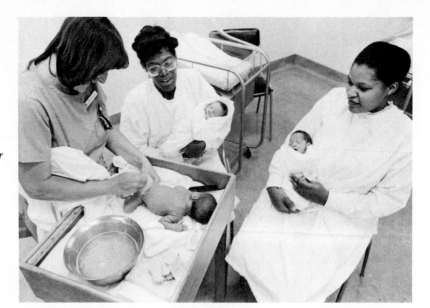

■ *Figure 30–11*

Basic care methods such as bathing the baby are taught by the nurse either individually or as a demonstration class for a small group. (Photo by Kathy Sloane)

grouped, pinhead-sized rash of papules and vesicles, on the face, the neck, and wherever skin surfaces touch. Fewer clothes and lower room temperature help to relieve the discomfort.

BUTTOCKS. Sometimes, despite good nursing care, the infant's buttocks become reddened and sore. A diaper rash that is caused by the reaction of bacteria with the urea in the urine may occur. This is turn causes an ammonia dermatitis. The most important prophylaxis is to keep the diaper area clean and dry. Sometimes petroleum jelly, baby oil, a bland protective ointment (such as vitamin A and D), or a commercial ointment is used to protect the area. Pastes may not be advised, because they are much more adhesive than ointments and thus create cleansing problems.

A simple treatment that is often effective is to expose the infant's reddened buttocks to air (Fig. 30-12) and light several times a day, using care to keep the infant covered otherwise. Air may be all that is necessary, although the use of a lamp treatment is more effective and at the same time provides a measure of warmth. An ordinary gooseneck lamp with a screened bulb (no stronger than 40 watts) can be placed on the table so that the bulb is a foot or more away from the infant's exposed buttocks. The light may be used for 30 minutes at a time. Because the already irritated skin is very sensitive, care should be exercised so that it is not burned by using too strong a bulb or by placing the light too close.

If the condition occurs at home, the treatment described above also is appropriate, and the mother can be so instructed. Boiling the diapers is another effective measure, because this destroys the bacteria. Many of the detergents and conditioners used today have antibacterial agents in them, however, and these may be effective in washing the diapers. Care should be taken to rinse the diapers thoroughly because the residue of the detergent can be irritating. In this respect, the modern diaper services are very effective in sterilizing diapers and preventing diaper rash. Disposable diapers are also less likely to cause diaper rash, but some brands may contain substances that are irritating to some babies.

CORD CARE. The cord clamp is removed when the umbilical stump has dried sufficiently, usually in about

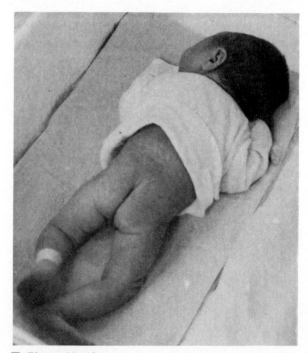

■ *Figure 30–12*

Exposing buttocks to air.

24 hours. More time may be needed for a cord that is cut long or that is thick and gelatinous. Depending on the initial care of the area, ongoing care of the umbilicus usually consists of cleaning around the junction between the cord stump and the skin with alcohol at each diaper change to encourage drying. In some hospitals, an antibiotic is used instead of alcohol, but alcohol is still recommended for home use. The mother should be taught how to care for the infant's cord (Fig. 30-13) while in the hospital so she will feel comfortable with the procedure when she gets home.

To further promote drying of the cord, infants do not receive a tub bath until the cord has separated and the umbilicus has healed. A cord dressing is considered to be unnecessary because exposure to the air enhances drying of the cord. A red, inflamed area around the stump or any discharge with an odor should be noted on the chart and reported to the physician.

The cord usually becomes detached from the body between the fifth and the eighth day after birth but may not detach until 14 days or later. Care should be taken not to dislodge the cord before it separates completely. When the cord drops off, the umbilicus should be free from any evidence of inflammation. Continued use of

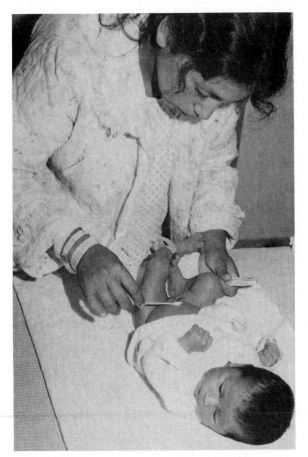

■ *Figure 30–13*

The mother can be encouraged to give cord care to her infant.

alcohol around the umbilical area, for a few days, can help keep the area clean and dry until healing is complete. The mother should be instructed to notify the physician if inflammation or discharge is present.

GENITALIA. For the uncircumcised male, it has often been recommended that the foreskin be retracted for cleansing purposes beginning a few days after birth. Because in most newborn males the still-developing prepuce is continuous with the epidermis of the glans, it is therefore nonretractable.[10] Forced retraction may cause adhesions to develop. If retraction is done, the foreskin should not be pushed any farther than it will go easily, and it must be replaced over the glans after cleaning or edema may occur.

Current recommendations are to wait until separation occurs naturally with further growth and development, sometime between the age of 3 years and puberty, before trying to retract the foreskin.[11,12] Most foreskins are retractable by 3 years of age and should be pushed back gently for cleaning about once a week. As the child learns to do more for himself, he should be taught to retract the foreskin and wash the penis, as he is taught to wash other areas of his body. As he gets older, cleaning should be done as part of his daily hygiene.[12]

In female infants, a curdy secretion, "smegma", may accumulate between the folds of the labia and should be carefully cleansed with moistened cotton balls, using the front-to-back direction and a clean cotton ball for each stroke. When demonstrating this technique to the mother, the nurse can underscore the importance of teaching a little girl to wipe herself from front to back to help prevent urinary tract infections.

CIRCUMCISION

Circumcision, the surgical excision of the end of the prepuce (foreskin) of the penis, is an elective procedure quite often performed in the neonatal period. For many years it was almost routine in US hospitals, but it is done less frequently in other parts of the world. Since the statement by the Committee on Fetus and Newborn of the American Academy of Pediatrics in the 1970s that there is "no absolute medical indication for routine circumcision,"[13] studies have shown that circumcision rates have dropped from 85% in 1978 to about 60% more recently.[14]

The value of circumcision is controversial. Some of the advantages that have been stated by advocates of the procedure are that circumcision decreases the risk of urinary tract infection in male infants, promotes better hygiene, and decreases the incidence of inflammation, infection, and cancer of the penis. Those who are opposed to routine circumcision contend that good personal hygiene practices by uncircumcised males can also prevent these problems. In addition, opponents of the procedure also list potential hazards such as pain, hemorrhage, infection, and mutilation as reasons for discouraging routine circumcision.[15]

This issue is still unresolved. A new task force on neonatal circumcision recently considered evidence in support of circumcision's role in the prevention of urinary tract infections in male infants and sexually transmitted diseases in young men.[16] In their report, evidence for and against circumcision was presented, but no final recommendations were made. More prospective studies are needed.[12,14]

Making a Decision and Giving Consent. The parents of the male infant are asked to make the decision about circumcision. Traditional, cultural, and religious factors may be involved in deciding whether the procedure should be done. Studies have shown that major influences on the decision are the physician's opinion and whether fathers and older brothers of the infant are circumcised.[15] Some mothers are concerned about having to clean the penis and retract the foreskin if circumcision is not done, and they choose circumcision for that reason. Receiving information during the prenatal period about the pros and cons of circumcision and about cleaning the circumcised and uncircumcised penis can be helpful to parents and can give them more time to make the decision. If not already given to them, however, the information should be made available soon after the baby's birth.

The decision concerning circumcision is becoming more of a dilemma for some parents. When it was a recommended procedure, parents found it easier to justify the possible risks and discomforts by saying, "It's the best thing to do." Now that the procedure is not encouraged by many physicians, the parents have to take more responsibility. The final decision is up to them, and a consent form must be signed by one parent before the circumcision is done. "Informed consent" often means listening to a long list of possible undesirable side effects of the procedure. Some mothers feel very guilty after deciding to have it done. It is important for the nurse to give the parents factual answers to their questions, then support them in their decision, whichever it may be.

Care During Circumcision. If the decision is made to circumcise the infant, the procedure is usually delayed for 12 to 24 hours until the infant has had time to stabilize. Because the infant will be restrained in a supine position for some time, it is best if he is not fed just prior to the circumcision, to avoid regurgitation. After checking to be sure the permit has been signed, the nurse prepares for the procedure by placing the infant on the restraint board (Fig. 30-14) and setting out the sterile gloves, instruments, and drapes that the physician will use.

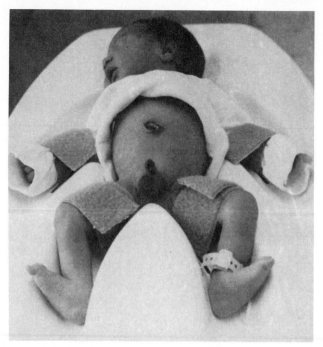

■ *Figure 30-14*
The infant is placed on a plastic restraining form to restrict movements during the circumcision procedure.

Several techniques have been devised for circumcising newborns. The most common methods currently in use are the Gomco (Yellen) clamp or the Plastibell. Further explanation of these techniques is given in Figures 30-15 and 30-16. The nurse should assess the infant's condition periodically during the procedure and be alert for any changes.

Although studies of behavioral and physiological responses of the infant during circumcision indicate that he does feel pain, the procedure is usually performed without anesthesia. Dorsal-penile nerve block has been shown to reduce these responses, but there have not been adequate studies of the long-term effects of this anesthetic on the infant.[14] Comfort measures, such as talking to him or stroking his head, may have a calming effect. In a study by Marchette et al, playing music or a tape of intrauterine sounds appeared to have a positive effect on infant heart rates during some phases of the circumcision procedure.[17] Although the infant undoubtedly feels pain during the procedure, it is difficult to tell how much of the crying results from pain and how much from being restrained.

Care Following Circumcision. When the newborn is circumcised, the main principles of postoperative care are to keep the wound clean and to observe it closely for bleeding (Fig. 30-17). For the first 24 hours, the area is covered with a sterile gauze dressing to which a liberal amount of sterile petroleum jelly has been added. If the

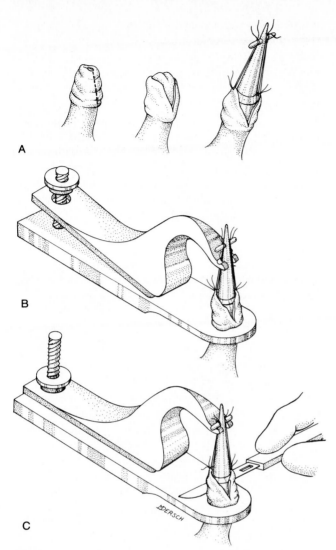

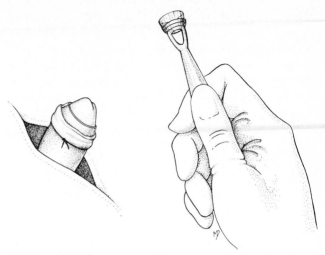

■ *Figure 30–16*
Circumcision using the Plastibell. The bell is fitted over the glands. Suture is tied around the rim of the bell. Excess prepuce is cut away. The plastic rim remains in place until it falls off, after healing has taken place.

In changing the infant's diaper, the nurse should hold his ankles with one hand so that he cannot kick against the operative area. Unless the physician orders otherwise, the circumcision dressing can be removed postoperatively when the infant voids for the first time.

■ *Figure 30–15*
Circumcision using Gomco clamp. (A) Prepuce is slit and drawn over cone. (B) Clamp is applied and pressure is maintained for 3 to 5 minutes. (C) Excess prepuce is cut away.

circumcision is done with the Plastibell, no dressing or petroleum jelly is used.

Mothers are naturally anxious about their babies at this time, so as soon as it is feasible after the circumcision has been done, the nurse should take the baby to his mother for a brief visit. It may be helpful to show her what the circumcision looks like and explain how it will look when healing, so that she can recognize any deviations from normal. With the Plastibell, there is a plastic ring and suture in place, which drops off with the foreskin in about 7 to 10 days.

The infant may be fed immediately after the circumcision, and both mother and baby seem to enjoy the comfort that the feeding and cuddling bring. If the infant is left in the mother's room for an extended length of time, the nurse should go in periodically to check the circumcision for bleeding.

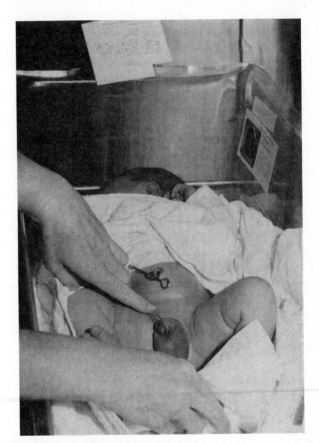

■ *Figure 30–17*
Postcircumcision inspection.

Cleansing must be done gently but can be accomplished as necessary with cotton balls moistened with warm tap water. A fresh sterile petroleum jelly dressing is usually applied to the penis each time the diaper is changed for the first day. The penis must be observed closely for bleeding and should be inspected every hour during the first 12 hours. It is advisable to place the infant's crib where he can be watched conveniently. Moreover, to keep all the nursing personnel alerted, some signal, such as a red tag, can be attached to the identification card on the crib. If bleeding occurs, it can usually be controlled with gentle pressure. If bleeding persists, the physician should be notified immediately.

Because the length of the maternity stay has been considerably shortened, circumcision may be done on the day of discharge; therefore, the nurse should ascertain the physician's wishes for aftercare and make certain that the mother knows how to care for her newly circumcised infant. Generally, the care is the same as that described.

OTHER AREAS OF CONCERN

Weight. The infant should be weighed on the day of birth and then daily or every other day while in the hospital. Infants who remain in the hospital longer than 5 days should be weighed at intervals prescribed by the medical staff, and the weight should be recorded accurately.

During the first few days after birth, the infant may lose 5% to 10% of the birth weight. This is due partly to the minimal intake of nutrients and fluid and partly to the loss of excess fluid and brown fat.[18] About the time the meconium begins to disappear from the stools, the weight begins to increase, and in normal infants does so regularly until about the tenth day of life, when it may equal the birth weight. Many infants regain their birth weight sooner. During the first 5 months, the weight gain should be from 4 to 6 oz per week. After this time, the gain is from 2 to 4 oz per week. At 6 months of age, the infant has usually doubled the birth weight, and by the first birthday it has tripled.

Keeping track of weight gain patterns is one way to note the infant's condition and progress. When the infant is not gaining weight, the physician should be notified. Besides gaining regularly in weight and strength, the infant should be happy and good natured when awake and inclined to sleep a good part of the time between feedings.

Sleeping. Infants who are well and comfortable usually sleep much of the time and wake and cry when they are hungry or uncomfortable. They may sleep as much as 20 out of 24 hours (although this varies considerably from infant to infant). It is not the sound sleep of the adult; rather, infants move a good deal, stretch, and at intervals awaken momentarily. Because they respond so readily to external stimuli (and this may make them restless), their clothing and coverings should be light in weight and warm, but not too warm. They should be placed in a different position each time they are returned to the crib. They can be placed on either side or on the abdomen, especially when it is time for sleep. When an infant is in the back-lying position, someone should be present, because aspiration is more likely if regurgitation occurs in this position. The importance of avoiding the back as a sleeping position should be emphasized to parents. As they get older and learn to roll over, infants will assume the position that they like most for sleep.

Crying. After infants are dressed and placed in a warm crib, they usually do not cry unless they are wet, hungry, ill, or uncomfortable for some reason, or are moved. One learns to distinguish an infant's condition and needs from the character of the cry, which may be described as follows:

- A fretful, hungry cry, with fingers in the mouth and flexed, tense extremities, is easily recognized as hunger.
- A fretful cry, accompanied by green stools and passing of gas, may indicate indigestion.
- A loud, insistent cry with drawing up and kicking of the legs usually denotes colicky pain.
- A whining cry is noticeable when the baby is ill, premature, or very frail.
- A peculiar, shrill, sharp-sounding cry suggests injury, especially to the central nervous system.

This information about the ways in which infants' cries give clues to their condition or needs can be helpful to the mother. Newborns have only their posture and their voice at this time to communicate their needs, so it is essential that the mother learn to interpret her infant's cues.

HYPERTONIC BABIES. Some infants seem to be fussy from birth. They appear very active, startle easily, cry readily and more frequently (and apparently for no reason), are alert and awake much of the time, and generally do not fit the usual newborn activity pattern of sleeping and eating.

These babies may be described as *hypertonic* (i.e., they do not seem to be able to relax as well as other infants).

The parents of hypertonic infants may find it difficult to adjust to their new baby and may experience a great deal of anxiety until they are informed (or learn by trial and error) that this is "normal behavior" for this child. Too often they assume they must be doing something "wrong," because despite their efforts, their baby remains fussy, tense, and crying. The nurse can be very helpful to the parents in giving them anticipatory guidance about their baby's behavior and helpful ways in which he or she can be soothed. The physician should also be informed of the nurse's observations so appropriate advice can be given to the parents.

These infants usually respond favorably to being held securely. Thus, wrapping them snugly with a receiving blanket, cuddling them securely, and changing their position slowly and surely rather than quickly all help to allay undue tenseness. Rocking babies and walking with them are particularly successful measures, but no parent can or should do this over protracted periods of time.

An automatic baby swing with a music box is often soothing, and even a young infant can be placed in one for a short time when supported by pillows. Additional ways of lulling a fretful infant to sleep include recorded heartbeat sounds, various types of music, or a ride in the car. The parents should be encouraged to experiment to find out which sounds have the best effect on their infant.

Any new activity or procedure should be introduced slowly to infants with this type of personality. For instance, when a tub bath is given for the first time, the infant should be placed very slowly in a small amount of water, and each lower extremity immersed gradually so as not to frighten or startle the infant too much. The parents should not consider an occasional evening out a luxury; it should be considered a necessary item in the care of their baby. These infants do place greater demands on their parents than do infants of a more placid nature, and a short time away from the baby does wonders in restoring the perspective and good humor of the parents.

Urinary Elimination. Urinary activity of the fetus is evidenced by the presence of urine in the amniotic fluid. The baby usually voids during delivery or immediately after birth, but the function may be suppressed for several hours. If the baby does not void within 24 hours, however, the condition should be reported to the physician; retention of the urine may be caused by an imperforate meatus. After the first 2 or 3 days, the infant voids from 10 to 15 times a day. When the urine is concentrated, red or rusty stains on the wet diaper may be due to uric acid crystals in the urine.

Intestinal Elimination. During fetal life, the content of the intestines is made up of greenish-black, tarlike material called *meconium*. It is composed of epithelial and epidermal cells and lanugo hair that probably were swallowed with the amniotic fluid. The color of the meconium is due to bile pigment. Before birth and for the first few hours after birth, the intestinal contents are sterile. Apparently, there is no peristalsis until after birth, because normally there is no discoloration of the amniotic fluid.

The newborn passes meconium stools for the first few days of life (Fig. 30-18). After this time, the stools gradually begin to change to greenish brown and then

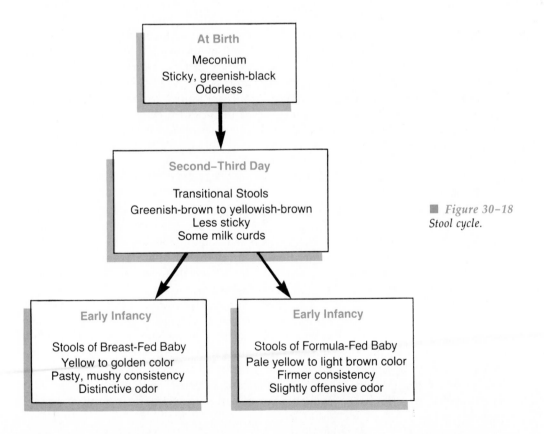

■ *Figure 30–18*
Stool cycle.

to yellowish brown. These "transitional stools" are less sticky than meconium and contain some milk curds. Following the transitional stools, the characteristics depend on whether the infant is fed breast milk or formula. The stools of the breast-fed infant tend to be a golden-yellow color with a distinctive odor, sometimes described as "sweet." Their consistency varies from loose to mushy, and they may be frequent or infrequent. If the infant is formula-fed, the stools may be pale yellow to light brown and of firmer consistency and may have a slightly offensive or foul odor.

Most newborns pass the first stool within 12 hours of birth; nearly all have a stool in 24 hours. If an infant has not passed a stool by this time, imperforate anus or intestinal obstruction must be considered as a possible reason for the delay, and the baby must be observed closely.

The daily number of stools on about the fifth day of life is usually four to six. As the infant grows, this number decreases to one or two each day. The type of stool of the breast-fed baby may be influenced by the mother's diet. Slight variations from the normal may have little significance if the baby appears to be comfortable and sleeps and nurses well. If the baby's stools have a watery consistency, are of a green color, contain much mucus, and have a foul odor and flatus is being passed, the condition may be evidence of some digestive or intestinal irritation or infection and should be reported to the physician.

The number, color, and consistency of stools should be recorded daily on the baby's record.

SCREENING FOR INBORN ERRORS OF METABOLISM

Certain disorders related to inborn errors of metabolism have been found to be detectable by blood tests soon after birth. Early detection and appropriate treatment can often prevent or decrease permanent defects resulting from these disorders. Although a number of tests have been developed, not all are used in mass screening. To be most useful, the test should be sensitive and specific, and effective intervention should be available for those who have positive tests.[19] Phenylketonuria (PKU), congenital hypothyroidism, and galactosemia meet these criteria and are the conditions most often tested for in government-funded neonatal screening programs. Additional tests that are included in some state programs are maple syrup urine disease and the hemoglobinopathies (sickle-cell anemia and thalassemia). Tests for other conditions may be done on the blood of infants at risk by family history.

Nurses often are responsible for obtaining the blood for the tests. This is usually done by heel stick, as described earlier in this chapter. The blood is dropped on absorbent paper to fill premarked circles, which must be completely saturated for best results. The blood sample for the tests should be taken before the infant leaves the hospital. Although the usual recommendation is to wait until 24 hours after birth, if the infant is discharged before this time it is better to obtain the blood early than to risk missing the tests altogether in case the mother doesn't bring the infant back. It is suggested that infants initially screened before 24 hours of age be rescreened for PKU by the third week of life for better reliability of this test. Because results are thought to be related to food intake by the infant, early testing may miss some affected newborns.[2] Recent information, however, indicates that most infants with PKU have an elevated blood phenylalanine concentration during the first day of life and probably will not be overlooked by early testing.[20]

Evaluation

Before the infant's discharge from the hospital, the nurse will evaluate both the effectiveness of the newborn's care and the effectiveness of parent teaching. The infant should be free of infection or any other complication, should be maintaining a stable temperature, and should be taking nourishment well, whether breast or bottle. Appropriate parent-infant attachment behaviors should be observed. The parent(s) should be able to demonstrate or return demonstrated skills in newborn care, including handwashing, use of bulb syringe, infant assessment, and bathing. They should also be able to repeat instructions or answer questions related to (1) response to emergency situations; (2) danger signs or changes in the infant requiring a call to the primary health care provider; (3) follow-up visits to the health care provider; and (4) infant safety measures, including use of a car seat. Any unmet goals would indicate the need for reassessment and further interventions, such as additional teaching or referrals.

Discharge From the Hospital

Discharge planning for the new mother and baby may begin in the prenatal class or clinic when discussions are held about planning for what happens after the baby comes home. During the hospital stay, nurses continue to assess the family's needs for assistance in planning for care of the baby at home. Early discharge (less than 24 hours after birth) for mothers and babies without complications is a reality in many places, owing either to the parents' desire or to hospital policy. Observations and care traditionally done by hospital personnel are now the responsibility of the new parents. This increases the need for adequate instruction but decreases the time available for teaching. Giving the parents a phone

---

Early Discharge Checklist

When a newborn is discharged to the care of the parents or a caretaker during the first 24 hours after birth, the nurse should assure that the caretaker understands the following instructions:

Recognizing signs of airway problems
  Excessive mucus
  Noisy respirations
  Cyanosis—circumoral or general
  Retractions

Suctioning and use of bulb syringe

Maintaining body temperature
  Prevention of cold stress
  Use of thermometer

Meeting needs for food and fluids
  Observation of necessary feeding reflexes
  Timing of feedings

Positioning and handling the infant

Bathing

Clothing and diapering

Cord and circumcision care

Infant behavior (e.g., crying, fussing, neuromuscular, eye movements)

Infant safety

---

number they can call at any hour if they need help or further information after they get home is often very helpful. For some new mothers, especially the inexperienced, a referral to a community-health agency for a home visit may be appropriate for follow-up. Some families with financial problems may need to be referred to a family-service agency.

As part of the plan for taking the infant home, the nurse should find out if the parents have and plan to use a car seat for the infant. Car seats, even in the states where they are mandatory, are not being used consistently by many parents. Nurses should be well informed about the use of car seats and should take the opportunity to advocate their use whenever possible. New parents are usually receptive to information that will help them provide good care for their baby, so discussing car seats is particularly appropriate at this time. A space on the discharge chart form to indicate the use of a car seat will encourage staff members to include this in their discharge planning and teaching.[21]

Plans for health-care follow-up of the infant should be discussed with the mother. A follow-up appointment should be made with a private physician or at a well-baby clinic. Most new mothers appreciate an opportunity to talk to the nurse regarding their concerns about taking the baby home. Taking time for such a talk is well worth the nurse's effort, because it can help make those first few days at home less frightening and more enjoyable for the new parents.

■ REFERENCES

1. Polmar SH, Manthel U: Immunology. In Fanaroff AA, Martin RJ (eds): Neonatal-Perinatal Medicine, 4th ed, pp 744–762. St. Louis, CV Mosby, 1987
2. Frigoletto FD, Little GA (eds): Guidelines for Perinatal Care, 2nd ed. Elk Grove Village, IL, American Academy of Pediatrics; and Washington, DC, American College of Obstetricians and Gynecologists, 1988
3. Larson E: Rituals in infection control: What works in the newborn nursery? JOGNN 16(6):411–416, November/December 1987
4. Renaud MT: Effects of discontinuing cover gowns on a postpartal ward upon cord colonization of the newborn. JOGN Nurs 12(6):399–401, November/December 1983
5. NAACOG Committee on Practice: OGN Nursing Practice Resource Mother-Baby Care (pamphlet). Washington, DC, NAACOG, March 1989
6. Phibbs RH: The newborn infant. In Rudolph AM (ed): Pediatrics, 17th ed, pp 119–166. New York, Appleton & Lange, 1982
7. Roberts FB: Perinatal Nursing. New York, McGraw-Hill, 1977
8. Hey E, Scopes JW: Thermoregulation in the newborn. In Avery GB (ed): Neonatology, 3rd ed, pp 201–211. Philadelphia, JB Lippincott, 1987
9. Coen RW, Koffler H: Primary Care of the Newborn. Boston, Little, Brown, 1987
10. NAACOG Committee on Practice: Nurse's Role in Neonatal Circumcision (pamphlet). Washington, DC, NAACOG, August 1985
11. Belman AB: Abnormalities of the genitourinary system. In Avery GB (ed): Neonatology, 3rd ed, pp 985–1011. Philadelphia, JB Lippincott, 1987
12. Poland RL: The question of routine circumcision. N Engl J Med 322(18):1311–1315, May 3, 1990
13. Committee on Fetus and Newborn, American Academy of Pediatrics: Report of the ad hoc task force on circumcision. Pediatrics 56:610–611, October 1975
14. Schoen EJ: The status of circumcision of newborns. N Engl J Med 322(18):1308–1311, May 3, 1990
15. Kaplan G: Circumcision: An overview. Curr Probl Pediatr 7:1–33, March 1977
16. Task Force on Circumcision: Report of the Task Force on Circumcision. Pediatrics 84:388–391, 1989
17. Marchette L, Main R, Redick E: Pain reduction during neonatal circumcision. Pediatr Nurs 15(2):207–210, March/April 1989
18. Brans YW: Neonatology in Obstetrical Practice. Philadelphia, JB Lippincott, 1987
19. Nicholson JF: Inborn errors of metabolism. In Fanaroff

AA, Martin RJ (eds): Neonatal-Perinatal Medicine, 4th ed, pp 1016–1048. St. Louis, CV Mosby, 1987
20. Hsia YE, Wolf B: Inherited metabolic disorders. In Avery GB (ed): Neonatology, 3rd ed, pp 724–752, 1987
21. Nachem B, Bass RA: Children still aren't being buckled up. MCN 9(5):320–323, September/October 1984

■ SUGGESTED READING

Becker L, Lagomarsino W: Isolation guidelines for perinatal patients: Creating a new protocol. MCN 12:400–404, November/December 1987

Care of the Uncircumcised Penis (pamphlet). Elk Grove, IL, American Academy of Pediatrics, 1984

Circumcision: A personal choice (pamphlet). Washington, DC, American College of Obstetricians and Gynecologists, 1984

NAACOG Committee on Practice: Mother-Baby Care (pamphlet). Washington, DC, NAACOG, March 1989

NAACOG Committee on Practice: Nurse's Role in Neonatal Circumcision (pamphlet). Washington, DC, NAACOG, 1985

Nachem B, Bass RA: Children still aren't being buckled up. MCN 9:320–323, September/October 1984

Newton LD: Helping parents cope with infant crying. JOGN Nurs 12:199–204, May/June 1983

Renaud MT: Effects of discontinuing cover gowns on a postpartal ward upon cord colonization of the newborn. JOGN Nurs 12:399–401, November/December 1983

31

Sensory Enrichment With the Newborn

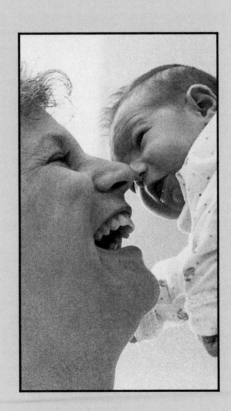

The senses are the primary source of information for the neonate brain until intentional thought develops 8 or 9 months later. Intentional thought is the deliberate creation of thoughts, which can in turn stimulate the mind.[1] All learning before this time is a result of sensory enrichment, using and challenging each sense. In this first year of life, the sensory and motor systems are used to navigate through the environment. Once thoughts are formed, infants no longer rely solely on their senses and motor abilities to learn and solve problems.

■ SENSORY ENRICHMENT

As soon as infants are born, they are capable of sensing and responding to all that they experience. At birth they can sense the brightness of the room, the drop in ambient temperature, and the presence of a warm embrace, and they listen to the familiar sound of their mother's heartbeat and their parents' voices. As they are cuddled, they relax their body and assume a posture of contentment. As they are spoken to, their face brightens and they gaze intently, conveying interest and pleasure in this contact.

A certain amount of sensory stimulation, such as feeding and swaddling for warmth, is necessary for proper maturation. Sensory experiences that transcend satisfaction of shelter, nutrition, warmth, and protection needs are enrichment experiences.

Enrichment experiences are designed to provide infants with pleasure and empower them to achieve mastery and self-esteem as they progress through infancy. Once an infant has seen a human face and established eye-to-eye contact, he learns to build up a repertoire of gestures that keep the caregiver entrained upon him, thereby being provided with additional sensory experiences. Empowered infants, then, are those who are able to precipitate and encourage caregiving and social interactions, not just passively receive enrichment.

Sensory enrichment is an important corollary to physical care of the newborn. Supervising and supporting the parents in their enrichment endeavors is an important maternal–newborn nursing intervention, especially if supervision can prevent an overzealous and inadvertent bombardment with multiple stimuli in hopes of accelerating the infant's development. Overstimulation and "pushing" an infant is always a potential risk when educating parents about sensory enrichment.

Support of the parent ultimately impacts on infants, enhancing their development. To support the parent, the nurse must first have an understanding of the rationale for sensory enrichment, the development of the central nervous system, the effects of sensory enrichment, maternal and infant assessments to prevent overstimulation, principles guiding active sensory enrichment interventions, and safe sensory enrichment interventions that can be incorporated into previously existing caregiving strategies with the newborn.

Rationale for Sensory Enrichment

The reasons for recommending incorporation of sensory enrichment in maternal–newborn nursing care are as follows:

- Sensory enrichment facilitates satisfaction with the maternal role.
- Sensory enrichment promotes positive interactions between parent and infant.
- Sensory enrichment is an integral force influencing infant development.

SATISFACTION WITH MATERNAL ROLE

Parents are driven by a desire to please their infant. This desire is fueled by the biologic drives known as maternal and paternal instincts, attachment and affection for the infant, and the extreme dependency of the infant on the caregivers. New parents often find their time is consumed by the feeding, changing, consoling, and cuddling needs of their infant. Overwhelmed by the demands, a perceived inequity in the giving and receiving of the parent–infant relationship may occur. When reciprocal giving and receiving is not present, either in reality or perception, mutual gratification is denied and maternal stress, anger, frustration, anxiety, and dissatisfaction with the maternal experience ensue.[2] Sensory enrichment offers the caregiver a repertoire of approaches that foster pleasure in the infant, an emotional response that the caregiver can then observe. When the mother is buttressed by knowledge and the ability to recognize her infant's cues, this positive feedback promotes satisfaction with the maternal experience.

POSITIVE INTERACTIONS BETWEEN PARENTS AND CHILD

Sensory enrichment fosters the positive interaction cycle demonstrated in Figure 31-1. In observing maternal reactions to her alert infant once she has called the infant's name, it may be noticed that the mother comes back with smiles, inflected vocalization, and caressing that brings the infant into a face-to-face orientation. The infant's behavior in response to her call has been detected, altering the mother's behavior into a pattern that is congruent with the infant's manifestations, changing the frequency, duration, intensity, and quality of the stimulation.

Research Highlight

Even though it is accepted that a mother needs close contact with her infant to facilitate bonding and provide reassurance to the infant, seldom is a mother allowed to hold her infant in skin-to-skin contact (SSC). Although the research reported here was conducted on healthy premature infants, the clinical concerns it answers and the benefits that exist with prematures also apply to full-term infants. The treatment is called Kangaroo Care (KC); this entails placement of the diaper-clad nude infant skin-to-skin, chest-to-chest upright between his or her mother's breasts. The study was designed to answer the following research questions: "Do infants lose body heat when held skin-to-skin?" and "Are there any benefits of skin-to-skin contact to the infant?"

Twelve infants were observed for 9 consecutive hours within 4 days of discharge from the hospital. The 9 hours were divided into pre-SSC, SSC, and post-SSC periods that began after one feeding and continued until the next, 2 to 3 hours later. In Pre- and Post-SSC, the infants lay clothed in head cap, t-shirt, diaper, and booties, swaddled in one blanket and tucked beneath another in an open-air crib lying on their left side. In SSC, the mothers sat at the bedside in a stationary chair and held their infant in the KC position for 2 to 3 hours, not rocking. Heart rate, respiratory rate, oxygen saturation, skin and rectal temperatures, and level of arousal (behavioral state) measures were taken every minute from monitors and observations.

The results showed that heart rate and temperatures increase when being held. Infants did not lose any body heat; instead they became much warmer when being held in SSC. Further, infants slept twice as long when in SSC, a finding that is very important because healing and brain maturation occur during sleep. Although SSC has not been tested with full-term infants, we hope that they will experience similar warmth and improvement in sleep.

Ludington SM, Hadeed AJ, Anderson GC: Physiological responses to skin-to-skin contact in hospitalized premature infants. J Perinatology 11 (March/April):19–24, 1991.

Infants actively participate in interactions. Babies initiate and regulate behavioral exchanges and communicate in accordance with rules.[3] They do so using gestures and prespeech movements and sound known as *protoconversations*.[4] Newborns effectively communicate in burst-pause patterns, expecting alternating interchanges with the caregiver. Communication begins with random movements at birth, and by 6 weeks of age, facial expressions and hand gesturing are employed to indicate "greeting" and withdrawal responses to both people and objects.

Many researchers support the precept that mutually enjoyable interactions between caregiver and infant constitute the foundation of optimum development.[5-7] Other researchers have found that stability and constancy of maternal stimulation of the infant are major factors in his or her cognitive development.[8] Even in mothers who have expressed concern about their mothering skills, maternal education and enrichment strategies have been instrumental in aiding normal infant development in potentially detrimental situations.[9] It is crucial to note that gratification and the beneficial effects of this interaction cycle can be thwarted if inappropriate or overstimulating activities occur. Cautious assessment to prevent their appearance is recommended and discussed as a nursing assessment.

FORCES INFLUENCING DEVELOPMENT

Barnard and coworkers propose an interactional model in which characteristics of the environment, mother, and child are forces that interact to influence the infant's development.[10] Brazelton[11] postulated that infants are equipped with reflexive responses that are organized into complex patterns of behavior, attention, and interaction with their world. The organization occurs once infants reach a state of homeostatic control (physiological balance and stability) and then devote their energies to a *quest for social stimuli*. This system, including the sensory enrichment provided, increases infants' availability to their world. Once available and interested in the environment, infants respond in such a way that they learn more about themselves and their world.[12]

Development of the Central Nervous System

In the first year of life, the brain grows faster than it will at any other time. The infant has obtained 25% of adult brain weight by birth, 50% by 6 months, and 70% by 1 year; this period is known as the *brain growth-spurt period*. (See Brain Growth Time Chart on page 711.)

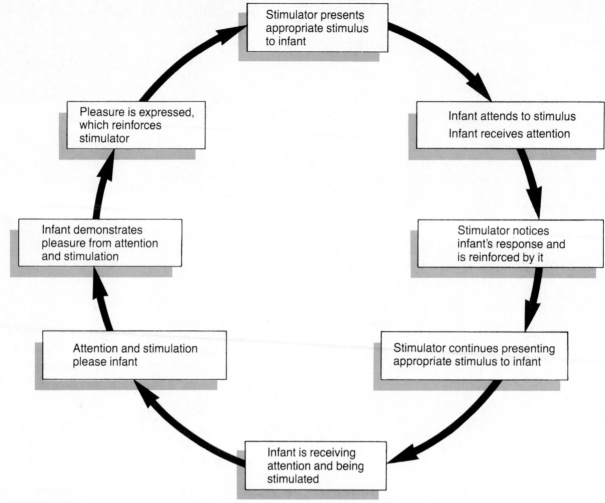

■ *Figure 31–1*
*Sensory enrichment interaction cycle. (Copyright 1982, 1986, Infant Development Education
Association, ISEA)*

This accelerated central nervous system development is influenced by three factors: *genetic endowment*, which may account for 25% to 70% of a child's optimal capabilities; *good nutrition*, especially a well-balanced diet with 20 to 40 g of extra protein per day during pregnancy if renal function is adequate;[13] and *environmental factors*, such as adversity or enrichment.[14]

The rapid growth period is thought to be one of increased vulnerability to nutrition restriction and environmental conditions, particularly adversity (e.g., drug and radiation exposure). Malnutrition is associated with a decreased number of brain cells, diminished size of the brain cells, and a reduction in the branching and synapses formed by each cell. Each of these conditions contributes negatively to mental function.

Environmental enrichment during the brain growth-spurt period also has dramatic effects. Enriched environments have conclusively been shown to alter the actual structure and function of brains of many mammals.[15] Animal studies strongly support the belief that there are critical and sensitive periods for brain development. Critical periods are those in which certain types of stimuli must be present for a particular structure or function to develop. Sensitive periods are those in which the brain's continuing function is particularly vulnerable to internal and external environmental conditions. It is postulated that the brain growth spurt is a critical and sensitive period in humans, but this can never be confirmed, because information about brain responses to environmental conditions can be derived only from animal studies.

DEVELOPMENT OF THE SENSES

Each of the six senses (visual, auditory, tactile, gustatory, olfactory, and vestibular proprioceptive) is receptive to sensory enrichment at birth. This capability is based on prenatal growth and development.

The senses are known to be functional by 25 weeks' gestation. It is not unreasonable to expect that the senses

---

Brain Growth Time Chart

10–18 Weeks' Gestation

Phase 1 (hyperplasia phase): number of brain cells is set 20 weeks' gestation to 2 years of age.

Phase 2 (brain growth spurt): neuron cells increase in size; nerve fibers insulated; dendrites develop 20 weeks' gestation to 4 years of age. Nerve fibers are insulated (myelinated) at rapid rate; process slows down after 4 years of age 8 months' gestation. Brain undergoes extra spurt of growth

8th and 9th Months of Pregnancy

Brain doubles in weight from 183 g to 365–392 g

Birth

Brain has attained 25% of its adult brain weight at 6 months of age. Brain has doubled its weight again, from 392 to 870 g; brain has attained 50% of its adult brain weight; brain growth after 6th month slows considerably

1 Year of Age

Brain weighs 1000 g; brain has attained 70% of its adult brain weight; majority of DNA deposited in brain cells has been set down by 1 year of age. Brain has attained more than 90% of its maximum size. The majority of brain growth occurs in the first year of life!

Adapted from Ludington-Hoe SM: Foundations of Infant Stimulation, p 12. Los Angeles, Infant Development Education Association, 1981.

---

turning devices and suck meters are used to analyze infant choices for various sensory stimuli and reactions to others. Babies selectively respond to the human voice and soft, rhythmical sounds.[18] The "mass of buzzing confusion," as infants were characterized prior to 1960, has become a competent infant who, in fact, thinks he is a human being.[19]

Effects of Sensory Enrichment

Common patterns of parenting are usually sufficient to guarantee normal development in healthy, full-term infants. Yet, the role of sensory enrichment in this development should not be negated.

According to Piaget, the first stage of infant development and cognitive growth is the sensorimotor period, spanning the age from birth to 2 years. This is a reflex stage in which infants learn to adapt to the sensory stimuli coming to them. This adaptation occurs through *assimilation*, acquisition of new knowledge from the environment, and *accommodation*, adjusting to the assimilated knowledge. Each sensory stimulus is a schema that will be joined with other schema to form schemata, units of thought that direct the infants' cognitive or physical reaction to their environment. In this way, programs for the anticipation, thinking, reasoning, logic, and problem-solving aspects of cognition are formed quite early. For example, following a few days of conditioning by being placed in a feeding position, newborns engaged in anticipatory sucking, having successfully been conditioned, which is a rudimentary form of learning.[20]

The role of early sensory enrichment in acceleration and broadening of cognitive ability in normal infants is not conclusively known. Sensory stimulation programs to date rarely report success in helping a normal infant achieve significantly higher intelligence quotient (IQ) scores; instead, infants in early intervention programs acquire distinct mental and motor development advantages compared with infants who were not in the early intervention program.[21,22] A "number" of intelligence is not as important as a "profile" of intelligence, infants' ability to master some tasks and feel powerful in influencing their immediate environment.

The positive cognitive effects of early sensory enrichment may be limited by a genetic ceiling. The genetic ceiling, or what is commonly called a child's potential, is not a definitive cutoff. It is instead a range of potential such as encountered when one has a gene for medium-to-tall height. A study investigating the long-term effects of daily skin-to-skin stroking and placement on a rocking hammock with simulated heartbeat sounds during the first 3 months of life found that the "enriched" infants performed similarly to the "unenriched" infants on mental and motor tests at birth and 1 month.[23] In

are capable of detecting changes in the intrauterine environment after 17 weeks' gestation. Mothers commonly report that the fetus kicks more when music is played or quiets down when she starts rocking. Some reports indicate that fetuses behave in a particular manner when classical music is played over the abdomen and bright lights and sounds induce specific fetal heart rate changes when the fetus becomes aware of their presence.

It is evident that the newborn is capable of perceiving environmental events at birth. The senses may be exquisitely sensitive at birth, as in the olfactory sense, or they may be relatively immature, as in the visual and auditory senses; however, even the immature senses perform well within their limitations.

Scientists now realize that infants can see at birth with good acuity within 10 to 20 in of their face, fixate longer on patterned than unpatterned stimuli, accommodate more easily to big items (3 in high by 3 in wide), and seek out high-contrast geometric shapes rather than pastel bunnies, butterflies, and balloons.[16,17] Head-

another study, full-term infants who were exposed to extra stimulation or handling have not shown evident acceleration, only an increased variability of performance within the accepted normal range, with perhaps more of them functioning at the upper limits of normal range than unstimulated full-term infants.[24] The genetic ceiling may have been exerting influence in these experiments, or development measurements may have been taken too early, because most cognitive gains from sensory enrichment do not appear until 24 months of age.[25] This means that manifestations of enhanced cognition may not appear until the child is at least 2 years old.

Many parents misinterpret enrichment to mean approaches to increase their offspring's IQ. This is not correct. Sensory enrichment is designed to foster development of a well-rounded, well-balanced baby, one who is equally comfortable, competent, and accomplished in mental, motor, social, and emotional skills. The "enhancing intelligence" motive has recently been associated with clinical observations that children who are "pushed" to improve their intelligence lose an inherent interest in learning[26] and suffer emotional setbacks.[27]

■ ASSESSMENT

Prior to the initiation of sensory enrichment with any infant, several assessments need to be made to determine the extent of knowledge, supervision, and support the parents need. These assessments prevent oversimplified, nonindividuated enrichment programs that may do more harm than good. Individuated programs have the potential of interacting with each infant in ways that address unique needs and will make the infant feel special.

Awareness of an infant's characteristic rhythm of interaction, maternal reciprocity, and signs of infant attention, habituation, fatigue, and engagement–disengagement cues ensures personalization of enrichment interventions and avoidance of overstimulation. Overstimulation is the threat or presence of physiological and alert-state compromise because of enrichment interventions that are too much, too intense, and poorly timed. Recognition of the signs of overstimulation can assist in the early reversal of this condition, should it occur.

In addition to assessments designed to personalize sensory enrichment interventions, there are some principles of enrichment that are applicable to all infants as a measure of safety. These principles are used to foster positive responses in the infant and apply interventions in nonirritating, physiologically supportive ways.

Infant Rhythms

In the first 2 days following delivery, there will be many opportunities to observe neonates display their rhythm of interaction. Infants move through the rhythm at their own individual rate, lingering at some stages while traversing others with such swiftness that its manifestations escape observation except in the most vigilant and astute nurse; however, the pattern is relatively similar. It is best to pick a peaceful interlude in which the infants are quietly lying in their crib with eyes open and an expression of interest on their face. This is the period of alert inactivity. At this time they are most receptive to the presentation of sensory stimuli and will demonstrate the stages of their rhythm.

- *Presentation.* The stimulus is presented by softly calling the infant's name. As the stimulus reaches his brain, there will be an alerting response and slight movements in the trunk, legs, and head as acknowledgment of the stimulus.
- *Orientation.* Once the stimulus has been received and recognized as something different from what existed a minute before its presentation, the infant makes attempts to orient toward the stimulus. Orientation is marked by trunk straightening, slight head righting or raising, head turning toward the stimulus, and fanning motions of the fingers and toes. Orientation is the infant's attempt to get the stimulus into the visual field and capture all of its sensory modalities.
- *Attentiveness.* The infant pays attention to the stimulus for the length of his attention span, which, in normal newborns, is about 4 to 10 seconds. Attention is different from arousal and alertness. Arousal is the change from a less alert state to a more alert state, such as going from drowsiness to alert inactivity. Alertness refers to eyes open rather than shut or half closed. Infants can have their eyes open and be inattentive, just as adults can go into a stare. Attentiveness, on the other hand, is an active process that makes demands on the infants' energy and concentration abilities. Pupil dilation; slowing of heart rate (by 6–8 beats per minute), respiratory rate (by 4–6 per minute), and sucking rate; cessation of gross arm and leg movements; and quiet gazing characterize this stage of rhythm, as does change in affect.[28]
- *Acceleration.* As infants reach the end of their attention span and exhaust their attentional energy supply and concentration ability, they accelerate their body movements, initially squirming and later flailing their arms and legs about, extending the fingers and toes, and twisting the torso. The acceleration of random, uncontrolled movements

adds sensory input, driving the infant toward sensory overload.

- *Peak of Excitement.* The input from attentiveness and aggressive movements surges toward the infant's threshold, the level at which no more input can be tolerated without jeopardizing the physiological status or behavioral balance. The only alternative left for this infant is withdrawal if sensory enrichment continues rather than subsides.

- *Withdrawal.* The infants attempt to shut out the sensory stimuli, to get away from it by turning their head away, averting their gaze, drowning out the sounds with their own wailing, or physically distancing themselves from the source. It is often best to allow infants to console themselves rather than adding to the sensory input with active consoling (cooing, rubbing, talking) by the mother.

- *Refractory.* This is a period of recovery that varies in duration for each infant but is generally 10 to 20 seconds long. Infants need some time to regroup their resources and organize themselves for another interaction. They will stop their crying, slow their movements, regain their posture and flaccid expression, and eventually become alert as they gain control over their autonomic functions, motor movements, state of alertness, and interactional faculties. Sustained human presence accompanied by silence will facilitate rapid recovery, making the infant available for another rhythmic interaction.

These stages should be highlighted for the parent and family members so that overstimulation can be avoided and interactions remain mutually gratifying.[29] Most mothers are relatively synchronous with their infant's rhythm within 3 months of delivery.

Reciprocity

Infants actively engage in interaction, but their ability to interact is marked by bursts and pauses. A neonate may undergo three or four cycles of attentiveness–recovery–attentiveness before fatiguing or reaching the point at which rest is advised. If the infant is still fascinated by the eye contact with mother, then mother can be reciprocal to the infant by maintaining her intent gaze. When the infant reaches acceleration, mother should gradually withdraw the intensity and number of stimuli involved in the interaction. Maternal responses that enable infants to regain attentiveness and control over their movements and physiological status are reciprocal behaviors. Reciprocity with the infant is to be reinforced whenever observed.[30]

Habituation

Habituation is the progressive decrease in response by an organism when repeatedly stimulated. Although this is a rudimentary form of learning and indicates intact central nervous system function,[31] it is also a potent indicator of the infant's waning interest or ability to attend. Each time an infant is shown the same picture, the intensity and extensiveness of his response decrease, undergoing diminution until the response is entirely extinguished. If one is timing the neonate's attention span for a stimulus, when the attention span starts to fall off, habituation or fatigue may be coming on. Habituation is very individual and may even vary within each infant, depending on his interest and state.[32]

Fatigue

Fatigue as a result of sensory enrichment can be successfully prevented when its signs are recognized early. Infants will signal that they are tiring and cannot engage in further interaction. Sagging cheeks, closing eyelids, drooping chin, limp extremities, and yawning are all signs of fatigue that can accompany sensory overload. Mother should modify the sensory components of the environment accordingly and permit the infant some quiet time.

Engagement and Disengagement Cues

Eye-to-eye contact is a potent nonverbal communication between infant and parent, one that acknowledges the existence of the other person and conveys a sense of worth to the person. As long as infants gaze, their mothers pay attention to them and a dialogue of eye movements, facial twitches, and sound emissions transpires. This cascade of interactions effectively keeps both parent and infant engaged, learning about each other's likes, dislikes, and needs. An infant who smiles receives attention in the form of a smiling face, a gentle rock, cooing noises, and engulfing arms. This infant eventually learns that smiles result in many pleasing sensory experiences. These behaviors are known as *cues*, little segments of nonverbal or verbal communication designed to influence the environment to which the infant is exposed, creating an interaction between infant, caregivers, and environment. Infants use engagement cues to initiate and sustain interactions and disengagement cues to detach from interactions. Examples of subtle disengagement cues are lip compression or grimace, pucker face, eyes clinched, gaze aversion, tongue show, and immobility. Examples of potent disengagement cues are crying, whining, fussing, spitting, vomiting, and pushing away.[33] The disengagement cues are activated when an infant is reaching the sensory threshold or desires to withdraw from sensory stimulation. Each of these behaviors, when considered singly, may not indicate a need for disengagement, but when followed or accompanied by others, the message should be clear. Sensory interactions need to be gradually withdrawn if overstimulation is to be avoided. Enraptured mothers who desire to engage the infant may not recognize the disengagement cues. Astute observation and gentle comment can improve a mother's sensitivity to her infant's communication. Two easily identified signs of disengagement are a furrowed brow and tightly fisted hands that may or may not be in the mouth (Tables 31-1 and 31-2).

Using these signals, the infant is a socially competent individual.[34] Interactions with people and objects refine this competency and enable infants to seek out pleasing experiences, shut out unpleasant ones, and keep people fascinated with them while they are de-pendent on them for their physical, cognitive, and emotional growth.

Overstimulation

Babies can be overstimulated. It is important that nurses use their keen observation skills to identify behaviors before this physiological, attentive, and behavioral compromise occurs. Distress; crying; skin color change; sudden, dramatic alteration in respiratory or cardiac rate; flaccid extremities; arching of the head, neck, and back; tongue thrusting; and a painful expression on the infant's face are all signs heralding the onset of overstimulation. If these signs fail to convey the message, the infant may be forced to close his eyes and drop off to sleep to shut out the relentless bombardment of the senses. This bombardment commonly occurs during medical procedures, nursing and medical rounds, and physical examinations.

TABLE 31-1. PHYSIOLOGICAL SIGNS OF FULL-TERM NEWBORNS

Parameter	Adaptive (Beneficial)	Maladaptive (Detrimental)
Heart	Rate 110–160 beats per minute Regular pattern Full, robust beat	Tachycardia, bradycardia Sudden change of 15 beats per minute up or down over baseline Irregular pattern Thready, weakening beat
Lungs	Rate 30–60 beats per minute Regular pattern Easy breathing	Tachypnea, bradypnea, apnea Sudden change of 10 beats per minute up or down over baseline Gasps, hiccups, sighs Labored breathing Irregular pattern Periodic breathing
Blood pressure	Systolic 42–66 mm Hg Diastolic 25–48 mm Hg Mean 36–58 mm Hg	Hypertension Hypotension Sudden change of 10 mm Hg in diastolic or systolic pressure
Skin color	Pink	Pale, mottled appearance Acrocyanosis Red, dusky, blue
Transcutaneous O_2 pressure	90%–100%	Hyperoxemia Hypoxemia
Oxygen saturation of arterial hemoglobin (SaO_2)	90% Normal R = 89%–100%	97% may be hyperoxemia 86% is hypoxemia

TABLE 31-2. BEHAVIORAL SIGNS OF FULL-TERM NEWBORNS

Parameter	Adaptive	Maladaptive
Brow	Relaxed, no creases	Furrowed
Ears	Relaxed, curving slightly forward	Retracted, tucked back
Eyes	Alert	Squinting, tightly closed
	Pupils dilated	Averting gaze
	Direct eye-to-eye gaze	Pupils shifting to avoid eye-to-eye contact (called *floating*)
Sounds	No crying	Crying
	Cooing	Grunting
		Sneezing
		Fussing noise
Mouth	Affectless face nonnutritive sucking on fingers, hands, fist, arm	Mouth hanging open
		Tongue protrusion, or mouth tightly closed
	Mouthing	Pursed appearance
	Smiling	Twitching
		Absence of mouthing
		Spitting out
		Gagging, grunting, grimacing
Head	En-face position	Turning away from stimulus
	Slight movements in direction of stimulus, flexed position, steady	Head rocking or shaking movement
		Extended position
Trunk	Relaxed, in alignment	Arched
	Slightly flexed	
Arms	Normotonic	Twitching
	Flexed and tucked	Startle posture
		Flaccid, hypotonic
		Extended, stretched out
Legs	Normotonic	Flaccid, hypotonic
	Flexed and tucked	Hypertonic
		Extended into air (called air sitting)
		Extended
Hand	Fisted posture	Clenched fist
	Slightly open	Hand closed within other hand (called *tactile reinforcement*)
		Praying position
Fingers	Relaxed	Extended
	Flexed	Pressing against each other (also called *tactile reinforcement*)
	Slightly open	

■ NURSING DIAGNOSIS

Based on the forgoing, several nursing diagnoses are possible. The most common one encountered in sensory enrichment nursing practice is that of the parents' and grandparents' knowledge deficit. The science of infancy has expanded so greatly in such a short time that the consumer is not always familiar with infants' sensory capabilities and the need to use these senses for learning in the first year of life. Parents require information about an infant's individual overtures and responses to interaction as well as sensory interventions. Other problems
(Text continues on page 719)

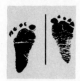

Nursing Care Plan

The Parents and Infant Participating in Sensory Interactions

Patient Goals

1. Visual
   1. Mutual gazing occurs for 10 to 15 seconds.
   2. Mother verbalizes infant's black and white preferences and shape preferences.
   3. Mother attends to alert infant, allows infant to withdraw when tired.

2. Auditory
   1. Mother uses melodic tone of voice and coos to baby.
   2. Mother acknowledges all vocalization by baby.
   3. Mother demonstrates "listening loop."

3. Tactile
   1. Gentle, soothing, caressing touch is given to receptive infant.
   2. Mother recognizes when infant is uncomfortable with touch.
   3. Embracing and rhythmic touch are provided.

4. Vestibular
   1. Mother recognizes the soothing qualities of vestibular stimulation.
   2. Mother provides variety of movements.

5. Gustatory
   1. Mother verbalizes that infants prefer sweet tastes and breast milk even though breast milk may seem bitter to adult.

6. Olfactory
   1. Mother recognizes that breast milk scents are pleasing to infant.
   2. Mother verbalizes two sweet smells she will allow her infant to experience when home.

Assessment	Potential Nursing Diagnosis	Intervention	Evaluation
Parental Assessment Factors			
Visual			
Eye-to-eye contact between mother and infant within 10 to 13 inches of infant's face	*High Risk for:* Knowledge deficit of infant stimulation strategies	Provide education on the potency of eye-to-eye contact and depth of newborn's visual field	Mother and infant maintain short-duration eye-to-eye contact
Face-to-face experiences with infant	Diversional activity deficit related to inappropriate stimuli or lack of individuation	Provide education on the appeal of human face to the infant	Parents aware of allure of the human face
	Alteration in parenting (bonding) related to separation of high-risk newborn and parents	Demonstrate attentiveness on infant's part to motionless, noiseless face and then to animated face	Parent repeats demonstration
	Noncompliance to sensory enrichment related to disinterest, misinformation		
Experiences with visual targets		Provide opportunities for infant to visually search high-contrast geometric shapes	Parent observes the appeal of such items
Auditory			
Inflected, modulating tone of parent used with atten-		Demonstrate pleasing, higher-pitched vocaliza-	Infant is attentive

(continued)

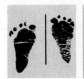

Nursing Care Plan (continued)

Assessment	Potential Nursing Diagnosis	Intervention	Evaluation
tive infant in face-to-face vocalizations		tions with alert, attentive infant	
		Provide education on the type of tone that appeals	Mother uses appealing tone of voice
Soothing cooing or humming with agitated infant		Provide education on individual infant's response to auditory enrichment when upset	Mother uses soothing approach
		Provide parent with a repertoire of auditory approaches to soothe agitated infant	
Little or no conversation with newborn during early breast-feeding experiences		Provide education about the fascination of human voice and its supremacy over breast-feeding for an infant who is still learning how to breast-feed	Mother allows infant to breast-feed
Speech and music (humming, singing) or other nonspeech sounds are provided		Provide education on benefits of speech and nonspeech sounds	Mother initiates mother–infant dialogue
Tactile			
Skin-to-skin contact between parent and infant is allowed		Provide education on human need for touch and special need for parental touch	Mother sees positive signs in infant in response to touch
		Provide skin-to-skin opportunities for both parents in a warm room	Mother expresses infant individuality that she sees
Quality of touch		Demonstrate firm, gentle touch for parents on their skin; allow return demonstration on infant's skin	Parent comments on infant's signs of pleasure or sensitivity to the type of touch experienced
		Encourage rhythmic, short stroking	Parent uses short, rhythmic strokes
Parent's holding patterns		Demonstrate swaddling of an infant who is flailing about	Parent holds infant securely, swaddling or embracing him as determined by infant's cues
Observe use of pacifiers and non-nutritive sucking		Provide education on importance of sucking and hand–mouth activity for self-consolation and self-control	Parent encourages or permits hand-to-mouth activity and sucking

(continued)

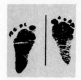

Nursing Care Plan (continued)

Assessment	Potential Nursing Diagnosis	Intervention	Evaluation
Vestibular			
Observe linear movement		Provide education on role of movement in motor development and proprioception	Parents provide linear movement of infant by lifting or lowering and walking with infant
Observe for violent, sudden, or accentuated movements of infant that cause exaggerated, independent head movement		Provide education on need to keep head from swinging about, which throws the brain against a hard, potentially bruising cranium	Parents hold infant securely and maintain head alignment
Gustatory			
Provision of breast milk or formula to satiety		Provide appropriate supervision and support of chosen feeding method	Mother expresses satisfaction with feeding experience
Olfactory			
Opportunities for close skin contact with parents are provided		Provide education on the influence of olfactory markers of the parent on helping an infant learn to whom he or she belongs	Parents are aware of reaction of infant to their olfactory markers
Infant Assessment Factors			
Signs of Attention 　Face brightens 　Pupils dilate 　Head orients toward 　stimulus 　Arm and leg movements 　cease 　Sucking rate decreases 　Heart rate decreases 　Respiratory rate 　decreases	*High Risk for:* Knowledge deficit of infant attention signs related to lack of experience in interaction Sensory perceptual alteration related to separation of newborn and parents	Provide education on differentiating alertness from attentiveness; on importance of frequent, short-duration enrichment episodes rather than infrequent, long-duration episodes; and that length and quality of attentiveness will increase as the infant matures	Parents determine length of infant's attentiveness
Signs of Fatigue 　Yawning 　Eyes closing, drooping 　Cheeks sagging 　Chin dropping 　Extremities limp 　Body collapses, doubles 　over	Activity intolerance related to overstimulation	Provide education for early recognition of fatigue	Parents can read the infant's cues
Interaction Pattern* Initiation–orientation– attention–acceleration–		Provide education on each infant's ability to create and alter his own pattern	Parents reciprocate to the infant's pattern

(continued)

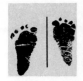

Nursing Care Plan   *(continued)*

Assessment	Potential Nursing Diagnosis	Intervention	Evaluation
peak of excitement–withdrawal–recovery–reorganization		Point out infant's behaviors and pattern during a social interaction; reinforce parent's ability to recognize infant's cues	
Engagement Behaviors Alerting, eyes opening Hands opening Head raising Babbling, cooing, clicking, giggling noises Smiling Mutual gazing Cyclic movements of the extremities	*High Risk for:* Knowledge deficit of engagement behaviors related to lack of experience in interaction	Provide education on infant's engagement behaviors; supervise an enrichment interaction, verbally acknowledging each behavior as it is observed	Parents verbally acknowledge these behaviors when they appear
Disengagement Behaviors Arching Fussing Crying Head turning away Gaze shifting Head shaking Arms and legs flailing Fingers extending Facial grimacing Facial swiping Hands clasping each other Hands in prayer position	*High Risk for:* Knowledge deficit of disengagement behaviors related to lack of experience in interaction	Provide education of these cues that convey the idea that it is time to slow-down and cease the interaction Verbally identify the behaviors when demonstrated by the infant Provide education on the importance of acknowledging these behaviors and acting accordingly	Parents able to read their infant's cues and respond appropriately

* This paradigm is explained by Ludington-Hoe (1977) and derived from Brazelton TB: Early Infant Reciprocity. In Vaughan VC, Brazelton TB (eds): The Family—Can It Be Saved?, pp 133–142. Chicago, Year Book Medical Publishers, 1975

involve lack of reciprocity and potential for overstimulation. Inappropriateness of stimuli may occur if individuation of sensory enrichment does not exist. Individuation can be learned best if it is modeled by nurses in their interactions with the infant as well as by the environment of the hospital nursery. Nursing diagnoses are stated in accepted terms in the nursing care plan at the end of the chapter.

■ INTERVENTION

Each sense can be appropriately stimulated to use and expand sensory capabilities. Sensory capabilities and appropriate enrichment strategies for each modality are enumerated in the following sections.

Principles Influencing Nursing Interventions

Sensory stimulation may be actively and passively provided by the environment. Active provision means that deliberate efforts to stimulate each sense are being made; passive infant stimulation occurs spontaneously without conscious intent. Fortunately, caregivers offer a plethora of passive stimulation, ensuring infant development within the normal range. Most of the unconscious sensory stimulation occurs during changing and feeding.[35]

These instinctual presentations of sensory stimuli are to be encouraged if they are in accordance with the principles of sensory enrichment.

Briefly, these principles are as follows:

1. All newborns have right-sided preferences during the first 3 months. The infant's right side is more sensitive to touch than the left, the right side conducts messages to the brain faster than the left, and infants turn their heads to the right more reliably than to the left. Stimulating experiences encourage more infant attention if they are begun on the infant's right side, regardless of the infant's eventual handedness.

2. If newborn attention or concentration is desired, it is best to present the stimulus during periods of alert inactivity, when infants are awake with their eyes open but their legs and arms still. During this restive phase, newborns can attend to and track with ease and sustained interest. The alert, inactive state characterizes the infant for an hour or two immediately after birth and for 5 to 10 minutes before and after feedings.

3. Newborns become alert for longer periods if they are in upright positions and are being held. Sitting in this manner increases infant gazing by 70%. When infants look around, they receive visual stimulation, which helps them learn how to relate to their environment.

4. Stimulating an infant to the point of agitation may not be wise, because agitation causes increased heart rate, increased respiratory rate, and prolonged inspiratory phases, which can induce aspiration. Some types of sensory stimulation will agitate some infants and please others. Each infant should be the guide, and his particular rhythm and readiness for stimulation, as manifested by engagement cues, should be respected.

5. Because of neuromuscular immaturity, the time for the brain to develop and send a message to the muscles for the muscle activity to be organized and expressed as a discernible behavior in response to a sensory event is called *latency to response* time. Generally, a response will be forthcoming 15 to 75 seconds after the stimulus in the newborn period. For example, auditory responsivity is eyes brightening when mother's voice is heard; visual attentiveness tends to emerge slowly over the course of a minute or two.

Once these principles are used to guide nursing interventions, administration of sensory enrichment will be beneficial to the infant. Because the nurse cannot provide continuity of enrichment once the infant goes home, it is vital that the mother be exposed to sensory enrichment techniques and given opportunities to practice them.

Visual Interventions

Visual Capabilities. The normal newborn has very good visual abilities. At 9 minutes of life, infants can turn their eyes and head significantly to follow schematic (black-and-white) faces[36] and they can remember high-contrast visual targets for 3 minutes.[37] An infant can see items with great clarity as long as they are within his visual field, which is 20 to 22 cm (9–12 in), the same distance from the breast-feeding infant's eyes to the mother's eyes.[16] Within this visual field, infants can see items distinctly (known as acuity), without blurriness, and can search the field to 30 degrees either side of midline before deciding the item of preference on which to gaze.[38] Gazing can be deliberately prolonged, depending on the amount of interest an item holds for the infant. Newborns have individual preferences and differences, so it is necessary to allow for variation.

Visual Strategies. The newborn prefers visual items that provide contrast between figure and background.[17] The greatest contrast occurs when black is placed against a white background. Newborns love faces,[39] especially eyes. Until they realize they are not the real thing, two big black dots on a white background (called *popsicle face*) will appeal to them. (See Client Education on page 721.)

Moving objects are more fascinating to an infant than are stationary ones,[40] and newborns prefer to maintain their gaze (fixate) on circular items because of their immature ocular movement ability.[41]

The newborn searches the visual field by moving across it with little jumps (saccades) rather than rolling both eyes simultaneously in the same direction. Eye-to-eye contact in the face-to-face position facilitates eye fixation for both parent and infant. If the mother's or the father's face is not available, black-and-white schematic faces or black-and-white glossy photos are the next best thing.

Infants also like to look at geometric figures, and they prefer cylinders and circles to rectangles and squares.[16] The geometric figures should be sharp rather than blurry and in a black-and-white configuration to enthrall the newborn. Newborns do not like to look at plain-colored walls or walls with little figures on them. Animals and cartoon characters are inappropriate visual stimuli for the full-term newborn. These patterns are not appreciated until the infant is more than 1 year of age. In the first 6 months of life, infants prefer to look at big geometric figures (2×2 in) rather than small ones ($\frac{1}{2} \times \frac{1}{2}$ in).[42] After the first 3 weeks of life, the size of the geometric figures can be decreased to accommodate the newborn's preference for increasing complexity and visual information processing. Stripes (especially good for the first 3–4 weeks of life), black-and-white checkerboards, bull's eyes, dots, and triangles are appealing

Client Education

What Your Infant Likes to Look At in the First Month of Life

Age	Stimulator (Held 10–13 in From Baby's Face)
Newborn to 2 weeks	• Your animated face, smiling and talking • Your eyes • The breast as nursing • Simple black-and-white drawing of your smiling face on a paper plate • Black stripes (8 in long by 2 in high) pasted or drawn on white 8 × 11 cardboard background • A 4-square black-and-white checkerboard, each square 3 × 3 in • One black dot, 3 in diameter, pasted on white 8 × 11 background
2 to 4 weeks	Add (held 10–13 in from baby's face): • Simple bold drawing of two round faces, each at least 6 in in diameter—one male and one female—done in heavy black ink on white 11 × 14 background • A 4- to 6-square checkerboard, each square 2½ × 2½ in • Black or red stripes (3 in long by 1½ in high) pasted or drawn on white 8 × 11 cardboard background or crocheted • Two black dots, 3 in in diameter, pasted or drawn on 8 × 11 white background • Simple black-and-white bull's eye: one 3-in black dot in the center, surrounded by a 2-in white band and a 1-in black outline at the edge drawn on a paper plate • Simple two-dimensional mobile made from 4 dessert-size paper plates with drawings of stripes, 4-square checkerboard, a black dot, and a simple bull's-eye, hung so that the plates face down 10 to 13 in from baby's eyes • Simple drawing of face on paper plate glued onto popsicle stick (popsicle face)

Ludington-Hoe SM, Golant S: How to Have a Smarter Baby. New York, Bantam Books, 1988.

geometric shapes. Cards containing these items can be used separately as stimuli or used in mobiles and crib hangings. Black-and-white geometric-shaped mobiles may be made from other materials also (Fig. 31-2).

Auditory Interventions

Auditory Capabilities. The newborn has the capacity to hear all sounds greater than 55 dB,[43] with slightly higher sensitivity to the lower frequencies.[44] This sensitivity may be a reflection of the smaller degree of attenuation of low-frequency sounds during transmission through the amniotic sac. Immediately after birth, infants may alert to their father's voice more readily than to their mother's for this reason. Infants can learn to discriminate their mother's and father's voice from all others within the first 2 weeks of life and have, at that time, a distinct reaction pattern established to the voice they hear.

Speech Strategies. Although slightly more sensitive to the low-frequency male voice, newborn behavior sug-

gests a preference for the female voice. The gleeful response to the female voice is based primarily on the pitch, tone, and inflection pattern women demonstrate when speaking to infants. Women tend to exhibit cooing behaviors, which are various-pitched musical sounds. Instinctual maternal speech uses exaggerated intonation. Higher-pitched sounds are attention-getting sounds, while low, bass sounds are consoling and quieting. Monotonous speech and monotone sounds are boring to the newborn, who prefers modulating auditory input.[45] The infant accustoms to monotone quickly and does not attend to it. Some fathers have a tendency to speak in bass, monotone speech patterns and should be encouraged to use more inflection and exaggerated tone. Slow speech, 55 words per minute or less, is easier for the infant to discern than faster speech.[46] Talking to infants is very important. The more speech they hear, the sooner they will learn language. The more speech they are exposed to, the more likely they are to reach their potential for mental skills. Gorski and coworkers have suggested that maternal speech is the single most important aspect of the newborn's sensory environment,

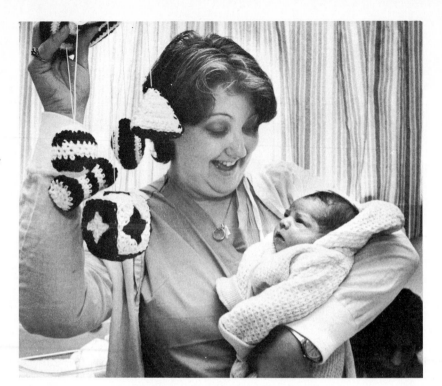

■ *Figure 31–2*
The nurse holds a mobile of black and white geometric-shaped objects that appeal to newborn visual preferences. Notice that the infant is upright, and the mobile is presented midline, 10 to 13 inches from his eyes. (Copyright 1982, Infant Development Education Association)

and desirable maternal speech can ameliorate anticipated delays and handicaps in risk infants.[47] The presence of approving parental sounds increases infant visual looking, whereas disapproving sounds inhibit visual exploration of the environment.[48]

Three qualities of desirable maternal speech are face-to-face orientation, use of questions, and speaking in turn. Talking in a face-to-face orientation is especially important. This position conveys nonverbal cues and facial expressions that relate emotion to the infant.[3] Further, in this position, infants as young as 4 months can recognize that a sequence of lip, tongue, and jaw movements corresponds to sounds they hear, facilitating sound imitation.[49] Another study found that by 3 months of age, only those infants who were exposed to simultaneous auditory and visual information were observed to imitate the vowels.[50] Because the use of vision to supplement hearing is common in everyday life, giving the infant opportunities to lip read facilitates verbal understanding.

During a face-to-face orientation, demonstrate a "listening loop." The listening loop, derived from Barnard's "learning loop,"[33] supports emerging reciprocity and interaction capabilities in the infant (see box).

Encourage parents to ask the infant questions rather than making statements or demands. For example, one can say, "Do you want to eat now?" rather than, "You're going to be fed now," or "Now, eat!" Use of questions has been positively related to early language acquisition, and a sense of importance because the elevated pitch

denoting a question leads the infant to understand that a response is requested. Speaking in turn refers to amount and timing of speech. If a parent does all the talking, the infant has no opportunity to contribute. Conversely, when maternal input is limited, infants are not incited to vocalize. A happy mix of maternal and infant vocalization can be achieved by having the mother vocalize about 25% of the time and using the listening loop described earlier.

Sound Strategies. Speech stimulates the development of the left hemisphere of the brain; music stimulates the right hemisphere.[46] Therefore, parents may provide musical stimulation for their infant also. Newborns have demonstrated less agitation in the presence of classical music than rock and roll music.[51] However, individual preference may very well be for the music the neonate was exposed to while in utero.[52] If mother played jazz

---

Listening Loop

Give the child attention—then listen to the child's response to the attention, ask the child for more information or to demonstrate what he or she is talking about—then give positive feedback to the child (which is also more attention—completing the loop).

during her pregnancy, her newborn will probably enjoy jazz more than unfamiliar classical music. Mothers have much latitude in choice of music, but true, pure tones are preferred to synthesized music.

Tactile Interventions

Tactile Capabilities. The skin is the largest sense organ in the infant. Infants are very sensitive to touch, especially around the mouth, in the palms, over the soles of the feet, and around the genitals. Tactile stimulation, or touching, is instrumental in helping the neonate adjust to life outside the womb. Skin-to-skin touch in a rhythmic, stroking pattern has been found to reduce the birth weight loss from 10% of birth weight to 3% of birth weight.[53] This is accomplished because skin-to-skin stroking stimulates the haptic nerve pathways, which in turn stimulate gastrointestinal and genitourinary system function. As a result, feces and urine are passed through the system more quickly and with better utilization of digested food.[54]

Tactile Strategies. Skin-to-skin touch is to be encouraged at all times. Newborns cannot be spoiled by too much caressing. The closer they are held and the more often they are patted, the more secure they become. Observe the power of touch on newborns: it can make them either quiescent or aroused. Reassuring parental touch makes crying subside, extremities flex, and the eyes open—if the infant doesn't fall asleep.

Skin-to-skin stroking can be provided in any number of ways and directions. Some babies prefer being stroked in the head-to-toe direction—a pattern reminiscent of the process of nerve myelinization. Stroking at a slow pace, such as 12 to 16 times per minute, has been associated with reductions in apnea and irregular breathing in the neonate.[55] As one strokes, it is wise to give extra strokes of slightly more pressure to the most sensitive tactile areas, outlined above. Stroking that is begun on the right should continue on the infant's left, to encourage midline awareness.[56] Stroking the head is very comforting to neonates, especially if the hand proceeds from the forehead to the occiput. Slow repetitive strokes over the top of the head can calm colicky infants, as do finger strokes across the forehead.

Many infants become quite fond of stroking and never tire of it. For these infants, it becomes a relaxation technique and is widely used as such in Australia and India. Touch is believed to help relieve the unspent tensions infants accumulate throughout the day, as well as accelerate neuromuscular development.[56] Two tools are available for mothers who desire to continue with a stroking treatment. *Loving Hands*, by Frederick Leboyer, has many pictures and is found in most book-

stores. A scientifically validated stroking protocol called *Loving Touch*, which is accompanied by a tape that contains appropriate music stimulation, is also available.*

Many mothers collect swatches of different textures with which to stroke the infant. These tactile experiences will be especially valuable if the texture is experienced within context (e.g., fur on a panda bear, rough on daddy's face, smooth on the mirror, etc.). Caution should be exercised so that the infant is not assaulted by multiple sensations.

Vestibular Interventions

Vestibular Capabilities. *Vestibular stimulation* refers to movement, and the term is derived from the vestibule of the ear, which perceives alterations in fluid pressure as movement occurs. Movement stimulation begins in utero as the fetus moves about in weightless space, stretching and rotating. The sucking that originates around the 8th to 11th week of gestation is a form of movement stimulation that is necessary if the fetus's chin and buccal pads are to develop sufficiently for suckling. All babies exhibit individual patterns of spontaneous activity, some quite active and others calm. Activity patterns may be an early index of a child's temperament, but we are not yet able to say with accuracy what active babies will be like when they are older.[57]

Movement stimulation, especially rotary movements, has been associated with enhanced motor development.[58]

Vestibular Strategies. Following delivery, it is important for infants to have opportunities to move about and stretch and pull and push. These activities are best facilitated by "tummy time," being placed on the tummy in a safe place for self-initiated, unstructured movement. If infants are accustomed to always sleeping on their side or back, tummy time may be upsetting. Having a parent on the floor, in a face-to-face orientation, may alleviate some of the stress of this new position. It is important to try to get a baby to enjoy this position, because the freedom of movement afforded by it enables the child to crawl within normal time limits rather than significantly later.[59]

Rocking is the most common vestibular stimulation that is passively given, providing excellent opportunities for vestibular sensations that aid in weight gain[60] and neuromuscular coordination. There is no recommended rate of rocking or frequency, but a little each day can be encouraged. Parents may prefer to provide vestibular stimulation by carrying infants in chest wraps. No det-

---

* Cradle Care, Inc., 6455 Meadow Road, Dallas, TX 75230.

rimental effects have resulted from this. In fact, infants who accompany their mother in a pouch appear to fall into deep levels of sleep more smoothly, awaken less irritable,[61] and show more secure attachment at 7 months of age.[62]

Baby exercises provide opportunities for vestibular stimulation. Extension and flexion of all extremities followed by tummy tickles, pressure against the kicking foot, circular swinging of the well-supported infant, and relaxation techniques are possibilities. Levy's book is a useful resource for additional motor games.[63] Some parents may inquire about the efficacy of gym classes for motor stimulation of infants. The American Academy of Pediatrics issued a policy statement indicating that exercise and swim classes had no known benefits and could overstress ligaments and immune systems, respectively, in the first year of life.

Olfactory Interventions

Olfactory Capabilities. Olfaction in the newborn is quite sensitive. Shortly after birth, newborns will change their breathing and activity rates in response to strong artificial odors.[64] At 5 days of age, the infant can differentiate the odor of the mother's breast pad from that of a stranger's. If mother's nipples have been smeared with petroleum jelly, the neonate will violently refuse approaching the noxiously scented nipple. This ability to perceive maternal odor originates at birth, when the infant is held close. By 2 weeks of age, infants are able to recognize their mother's axillary odors.[65] At this time, their olfactory sensitivity is instrumental to the bonding–parental-recognition process and emotional development in infants.[66] The importance of olfactory markers for emotional development is revealed when one considers that olfaction is the only sense that is not mediated by the reticular activating system, going instead directly to the limbic center of the brain. The limbic center is the seat of emotions.

Olfactory Strategies. The most potent stimulus is breast milk, followed only by the body scents of both parents. Actively providing various smells such as cherry juice, nutmeg, cinnamon, and honey is not really necessary, but may be enjoyable. The newborn detects these scents when in the kitchen environment without special attention to them for the first 6 months of life. After that, smelling can become a stimulating game. Various "scratch and sniff" books are available in toy stores.

Gustatory Interventions

Gustatory Capabilities. The fetus demonstrates a preference for sweet fluids as early as 20 weeks' gestation. When glucose water is injected into the amniotic fluid, the fetus accelerates the swallowing actions. This preference would not be manifested if gustatory sensitivity were not possible. It is known that the nerve tracts for taste sensation are operational by the 20th week of gestation and that the entire oral cavity is covered with taste receptors during gestation. Just before birth, some of these receptors are lost, leaving the tongue as the only source for taste sensitivity.

Gustatory Strategies. The most prevalent taste sensation the newborn is exposed to is breast milk (or formula). As the nipple is compressed against the hard palate, the milk spurts onto the bitter receptors in the back of the tongue. With repetitive stimulation of the bitter receptors, the infant grows quite fond of the bitter-tasting foods. Yet infants always like sweet tastes as well and can smile with sweet and frown with sour tastes. When infants require blood sampling and painful procedures such as circumcision, administration of 12% sugar water immediately before the procedure acts as a powerful analgesic agent and cuts crying by half.[67]

Breast milk is the referred gustatory stimulus for newborns. Mothers should be encouraged to avoid giving the infant sour tastes (e.g., lemon juice, cranberry juice) so that the newborn does not associate the caregiver with unpleasant stimuli. During the first year of life, infants should not be given honey because of the high likelihood of developing botulism from this source.

■ EVALUATION

The goal of sensory enrichment is a happy, secure, well-rounded infant, one who is loved by caregivers and lives in a reciprocal environment. The first signs of goal achievement may be visible before discharge, but final evaluation is many months, maybe even years, down the road.

■ RESOURCES FOR SENSORY ENRICHMENT

Family-centered maternity care recommends involvement of all family members in the care of the newborn. Siblings are eager to make simple designs to show to the newcomer, and fathers can set aside 5 minutes each day of special time with the infant to help develop a positive father–infant relationship. All nursing interventions (except breast-feeding) are suitable for the infant's various caregivers, so grandparents should be allowed an opportunity to demonstrate their sensory enrichment skills, too. In addition to the strategies already discussed, spending time with and being available to the infant are potent strategies. The value of quality time is acknowledged by all. Only recently have child developmentalists come to recognize the importance of "body time" (being near to and available to the child even though one is not interacting with the child). An example of this is having the infant remain in the same room as the mother converses with visitors, and in later years, having the parent stay in the same room as the young child watches television or reads a book.

As parents become involved with their amazing newborn, additional knowledge and support services may be sought. In addition to numerous consumer publications (a list is available from the Infant Development Education Association [IDEA]* and the Center for Parent Education),* infant stimulation classes and support groups are conducted around the nation by certified infant development instructors (a directory is maintained by IDEA). Many educational materials, such as videotapes, films, care plans, and posters, are available to health professionals and parents through the national clearinghouse for infant sensory enrichment, the IDEA.

The parents of premature and sick infants undergoing neonatal intensive care can also foster the development of their infants, but approaches and interventions with these fragile infants require special considerations that are too numerous to discuss in this chapter. The following references will provide the information needed:

1. Expected outcomes of sensory enrichment
   • Infant Health and Development Program: Enhancing the outcomes of low-birth-weight, premature infants. JAMA 263(22):3035–3042, 1990
   • Richmond J: Low-birth-weight infants: Can we enhance their development? JAMA 263(22): 3069–3070, 1990
   • Resnick MB, Eyler FD, Nelson RM, et al: Developmental intervention for low birth weight infants: Improved early developmental outcome. Pediatrics 80(1):68–74, 1987
2. Guidelines for sensory enrichment programs
   • Krywanio ML, Jones LC: Developing an early intervention program for infants at risk. J Pediatr Nurs 3(6):375–382, 1988
   • Wilson T, Broome ME: Promoting the young child's development in the intensive care unit. Heart and Lung 18(3):274–281, 1989

3. Postural positioning
   • Piper MC, Kunos I, Willis DM, et al: Early physical therapy effects on the high-risk infant: A randomized controlled trial. Pediatrics 78(2): 216–224, 1986
4. Environmental modifications—changes in the NICU
   • Lott JW: Developmental care of the preterm infant. Neonat Network 7(4):21–28, 1989
5. Sensory strategies
   • Barb SA, Lemons PK: The premature infant: Toward improving neurodevelopmental outcome. Neonat Network 7(6):7–15, 1989

■ REFERENCES

1. Segal J, Segal Z: The infant: Ready and able to learn. Child Today 19–22, April 1985
2. Zabielski MT, Guring T: Giving and receiving in the neomaternal period: A case of distributive inequity. MCN 13:19–45, 1984
3. Tronick E, Als H, Brazelton TB: Monadic phases: A structural descriptive analysis of infant-mother face-to-face interaction. Merrill-Palmer Q 26:3–24, 1980
4. Trevarthen C: Communication and cooperation in early infancy: A description of primary inter-subjectivity. In Bullowa M (ed): Before Speech: The Beginnings of Interpersonal Communication. New York, Cambridge University Press, 1979
5. Belsky J: Experimenting with the family in the newborn period. Child Dev 56:407–414, April 1985
6. Magnusson D, Allen VL: An interactional perspective for human development. In Magnusson D, Allen VL (eds): Human Development: An Interactional Perspective, pp 3–27. New York, Academic Press, 1983
7. Parmelee AH, Beckwith L, Cohen SE, et al: Early intervention and experience with preterm infants. In Brazelton TB, Lester BM (eds): New Approaches to Developmental Screening of Infants, pp 77–85. New York, Elsevier, 1983
8. Barnard KE, Bee HL, Hammond MA: Developmental changes in maternal interactions with term and preterm infants. Infant Behav Dev 7:101–113, 1984
9. Fineman JB, Boris M: Outcome of early intervention: A summary of an on-going follow-up study. In Call JD, Galenson E, Tyson RL (eds): Frontiers of Infant Psychiatry, pp 231–234. New York, Basic Books, 1983
10. Barnard K, Eyres S, Lobo M, et al: An ecological paradigm for assessment and intervention. In Brazelton TB, Lester BM (eds): New Approaches to Developmental Screening of Infants, pp 199–218. New York, Elsevier, 1983
11. Brazelton TB: Early intervention: What does it mean? In Fitzgerald HE, Lester BM, Yogman MW (eds): Theory and Research in Behavioral Pediatrics, pp 1–15. New York, Plenum Press, 1984

---

* Infant Development Education Association, C/O Mrs. Catherine Thompson, 112 Braehead Drive, Fredericksburg, VA 22401; (703) 899-1565.
* Center for Parent Education, 55 Chapel Street, Newton, MA 02150; (617) 964-2442.

12. Lipsitt L: Learning and memory in infants. Merrill-Palmer Q 36(1):53–66, 1990
13. Crnic LS: Effects of nutrition and environment on brain biochemistry and behavior. Dev Psychol 16(32):129–145, 1983
14. Bedi KS, Bhide PG: Effects of environmental diversity on brain morphology. Early Human Dev 17:107–143, 1988
15. Diamond M: Cortical change in response to environmental enrichment and impoverishment. In Brown CC (ed): The Many Facets of Touch, pp 22–28. New Brunswick, NJ, Johnson & Johnson, Roundtable No. 10, 1984
16. Ludington-Hoe SM: What can newborns really see? Am J Nurs 1286–1289, September 1983
17. Apostolakis E, Cha C: Visual preference of preterm and term neonates. J Calif Perinatal Assoc 11(1):62, May 1982
18. Ludington-Hoe SM, Golant S: How to Have a Smarter Baby. New York, Bantam Books, 1988
19. Gluck L: The cutting edge. Calif J Perinatol 50–55, Fall 1983
20. Brazelton TB: Behavioral competence of the newborn infant. In Avery GB (ed): Neonatology: Pathophysiology and Management of the Newborn, 3rd ed. Philadelphia, JB Lippincott, 1986
21. White B: Missouri's new parents as teachers project: Report on the final evaluation. Cent Parent Educat Newsl 7(6):1–5, 1985
22. Derevensky JL, Wasser-Kastner E: The Effects of an interdisciplinary stimulation-parent intervention program upon infant development. Infant Mental Health J 5(1):3–13, 1984
23. Koniak DK, Ludington-Hoe SM: Paradoxical effects of stimulation on normal neonates. Infant Behav Dev 10:261–277, 1987
24. Koniak DK, Ludington-Hoe: Developmental and temperament outcomes of sensory stimulation in healthy infants. Nurs Res 37(2):70–76, 1988
25. Barnard KE, Bee HL, Hammond MH: Home environment and cognitive development in a healthy low-risk sample: The Seattle study. In Gottfried AW (ed): Home Environment and Early Cognitive Development, pp 117–147. New York, Academic Press, 1984
26. Brazelton TB: Do you really want a super baby? Family Circle Magazine, pp 74, 76, 77, December 1985
27. Zigler E, Lang ME: The emergence of "super baby": A good thing? Pediatr Nurs 11:337–340, 1985
28. Adamson LB, Baheman R: Affect and attention: Infants observed with mothers and peers. Child Dev 56(3):582–593, 1985
29. Springer LW, Boyce WT, Gaines JA: Family-infant congruence: Routines and rhythmicity in family adaptations to a young infant. Child Dev 56(3):564–572, 1985
30. Anderson JC: Enhancing reciprocity between mother and neonate. Nurs Res 30(2):89–93, 1981
31. Bornstein MH, Benasich AA: Infant habituation: Assessments of individual differences and short term reliability at five months. Child Dev 57(3):1–10, 1986
32. Power TG, Hildebrandt KA, Fitzgerald HE: Adults' responses to infants varying in facial expression and perceived attractiveness. Infant Behav Dev 5:33–44, 1982
33. Barnard K: NCAST Learning Resource Manual, pp 50–59. Seattle, University of Washington, 1979
34. Temeles MS: The infant: A socially competent individual. In Call JD, Galenson E, Tyson RL (eds): Frontiers of Infant Psychiatry, pp 178–187. New York, Basic Books, 1983
35. Day S: Mother-infant activities as providers of sensory stimulation. Am J Occup Ther 36(9):579–585, 1982
36. Goren CG, Sarty M, Wu PYK: Visual following and preterm discrimination of facelike stimuli by newborn infants. Pediatrics 56:544–549, 1976
37. Gottlieb SJ, Sloane ME: Memory in human neonates. Society for Research in Child Development Abstracts of the April 1989 Biennial Convention, Kansas City, MO, p 251A.
38. Maurer D, Maurer C: Newborn babies see better than you think. Psychology Today, pp 85–88, October 1976
39. Morton J, Johnson MH, Maurer D: On the reasons for newborns' responses to faces. Infant Behav Dev 13:99–103, 1990
40. Haith MM: The response of the human newborn to movement. J Exp Child Psychol 31:235–243, 1980
41. Fantz RL, Miranda SB: Newborn infant attention to contour. Child Dev 46:224, 1975
42. Fantz RL, Fagan JF: Visual attention to size and number of pattern details during the first 6 months. Child Dev 46(1):3–18, 1975
43. Dunkle T: The sound of silence. Science 82:48–51, April 1982
44. Werner LA, Gillenwater JM: Pure-tone sensitivity of 2- to 5- week-old infants. Infant Behav Dev 13:355–375, 1990
45. Eimas PD: The perception of speech in early infancy. Sci Am 25(2):46–52, 1985
46. Morse PA: The discrimination of speech and non-speech stimuli in early infancy. J Exp Child Psychol 14:477–492, 1972
47. Gorski PA, Davison MF, Brazelton TB: Neurobehavioral organization of the high risk neonate. Semin Perinatol 3(1):61–72, 1979
48. Papousek M, Bornstein MH, Nuzzo C, et al: Infant responses to prototypical melodic contours in parental speech. Infant Behav Dev 13:539–545, 1990
49. Kuhl P, Meltzoff A: Sophisticated babies. The University Report 2(3):2, University of Washington, Seattle, 1988
50. Legerstee M: Infants use multimodal information to imitate speech sounds. Infant Behav Dev 13:343–354, 1990
51. Klaus MM, Fanaroff AA: Bach, Beethoven, or rock—and how much. J Pediatr 88:300, 1976
52. DeCasper AJ, Spence MJ: Prenatal maternal speech influences newborns' perception of speech sounds. Infant Behav Dev 9:133–150, 1986
53. Ludington SM: Vaginal and cesarean infants' responses to extra tactile stimulation [dissertation], p 74. Denton, Texas Woman's University, 1976
54. Rausch P: Effects of tactile and kinesthetic stimulation on premature infants. JOGN Nurs 10:34–40, 1981
55. Kattwinkel J, Nearman H, Mars H, et al: Apnea of prematurity and effects on CPAP, cutaneous stimulation

and levels of urinary biogenic amines. Pediatr Res 8: 468, April 1974

56. Rice RD: The effects of sensorimotor infant stimulation treatment on the development of high risk infants. Birth Defects 15:7–26, 1979

57. Korner AF: Individual differences in neonatal activity. In Call JD, Galenson E, Tyson RL (eds): Frontiers of Infant Psychiatry, pp 379–387. New York, Basic Books, 1983

58. Ottenbacher KJ, Petersen P: The efficacy of vestibular stimulation as a form of specific sensory enrichment: Quantitative review of the literature. Clin Pediatr 23(8): 428–433, 1983

59. Menzies A: Effect of infant temperament and prone position on motor development. Aust J Adv Nurs 2(1):24–29, 1981

60. Freeman DG, et al: Effects of kinesthetic stimulation on weight gain and on smiling in premature infants. Paper presented at the Annual Meeting of the American Orthopsychiatric Association, San Francisco, April 15, 1979

61. Kennell JH, Klaus MH: Early events: Later effects on the infant. In Call JD, Galenson E, Tyson RL: Frontiers of Infant Psychiatry, pp 7–16. New York, Basic Books, 1983

62. Anisfeld E, Wagner D, Casper V, et al: The effects of a carrying intervention on the development of attachment in infants. Society for Research in Child Development Abstracts of the April 1989 Biennial Convention, Kansas City, MO, p 126A

63. Levy J: The Baby Exercise Book. New York, Pantheon Books, 1975

64. Engen T: The Perception of Odors. New York, Academic Press, 1982

65. Cernoch JM, Porter RH: Recognition of maternal axillary odors by infants. Child Dev 56:1593–1598, 1985

66. Porter RH, Cernoch JM, Perry S: The importance of odors in mother-infant interactions. Matern Child Nurs J 12(3):147–154, 1983

67. Blass EM, Hoffmeyer LB: Sucrose is an analgesic agent in 1–3-day-old human infants. Society for Research in Child Development Abstracts of the April 1989 Biennial Convention, Kansas City, MO, April 1989, p 129A

■ SUGGESTED READING

Aslin RN, Pisoni DB, Jasczyk PW: Auditory development and speech perception in infancy. Hearing 20:573–670, October 23, 1985

Brazelton TB: Introduction: Many Facets of Touch, p vii. Skillman, NJ, Johnson & Johnson, Roundtable No. 10, 1984

Burns KA, Hatcher RP: Developmental intervention with preterm infants. In Burn WJ, Lavigne JV (eds): Progress in Pediatric Psychology, pp 47–78. New York, Grune & Stratton, 1984

Donate-Bartfield E, Passman RH: Attentiveness of mothers and fathers to their baby's cries. Infant Behav Dev 8: 385–393, 1985

Frye D, Rawling P, Moore C, et al: Object-person discrimination and communication at 3 to 10 months. Dev Psychol 19(3):383–389, 1983

Lester BM, Hoffman J, Brazelton TB: The rhythmic structure of mother-infant interaction in term and preterm infants. Child Dev 56:15–27, 1985

Yogman MW: Development of the father-infant relationship. In Fitzgerald HE, Lester BM, Yogman MW (eds): Theory and Research in Behavioral Pediatrics, pp 221–280. New York, Plenum Press, 1984

32

Nutritional Care of the Infant

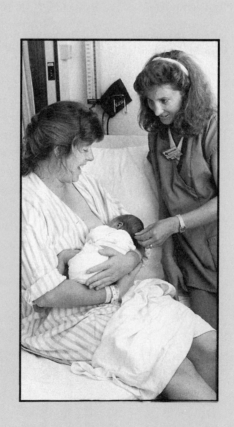

Nutrition is important in preserving health throughout the life cycle. It is particularly important during the rapid growth phase of infancy. The long-term effects of feeding practices in early infancy are gaining increased recognition. According to Neumann and Jelliffe, infant feeding is more than just "nutrient refueling"; it is also a "social, psychological and educational interaction between caretaker and baby."[1]

■ THE NEWBORN'S ABILITY TO HANDLE FOOD

Up until the time of birth, the nutritional needs of the fetus have been met through placental circulation. One of the major physiological adaptations that the infant must make in the transition from intrauterine to extrauterine life is to adjust to the change in the source of nourishment and to take food into the body orally, digest it, and assimilate it.

After birth, the infant must begin to suck and swallow as a means of taking food into the stomach. The sucking and swallowing reflexes are already present at birth and are normally strong. In fact, the swallowing reflex, as well as peristaltic movements in the stomach, becomes active during the last 2 months of fetal development, as noted by the bits of vernix caseosa and lanugo that are found with other debris in the meconium stool. In the delivery room, the infant often swallows mucus or sucks on anything that gets near his mouth.

Another important instinctive reaction is the rooting reflex, which enables the newborn to find food. Although the human infant does not have to search for its food, it does turn toward anything that touches its cheeks or lips. This is a help in latching onto the bottle or breast.

The newborn's gastrointestinal tract must suddenly begin to process a relatively large amount of food. Although the system is functional at birth and the necessary enzymes and digestive juices are present, the mucosa and musculature are somewhat immature.[2] At the time of birth, the infant's stomach is small, but it can dilate considerably and may stretch to three or four times its resting capacity. The stomach may be distended not only by the food taken in but also by air swallowed when the infant is sucking or crying.

Studies on gastric motility have demonstrated wide individual differences in the emptying time of the stomachs of newborns. The major portion of the feeding usually leaves the stomach in less than 3 or 4 hours; however, in some instances, the emptying time is more than 8 hours.

The time required for gastric emptying has been found to depend on the infant's condition and state, the type and volume of the feeding, and also on his position when fed. Delayed emptying occurs when the formula contains more fat and larger protein molecules, which probably accounts for the faster emptying in infants fed breast milk. The supine position also delays emptying time, with more rapid emptying found in the prone position.[3]

■ CHOOSING THE METHOD OF FEEDING

Choosing the method of infant feeding is an important decision for parents to make. Their ultimate choice is influenced by a variety of factors, physical and psychological as well as social. Ideally, the subject of infant feeding is raised during the antepartal period, thereby providing an opportunity to guide the parents in making a decision that is most suitable for them. The nurse should explore with the mother (and the father, if possible) attitudes concerning this subject.

In the past, breast-feeding, by the mother or a "wet nurse," was essential for the survival of the infant. This is still true to some extent in underdeveloped countries, but in most of the world modern methods of artificial feeding have offered women an alternative. Although the production of infant formulas has become a big business and the choice of artificial feeding is safe for the infant and convenient for the mother, there are still many advantages to breast-feeding.

One should avoid being so overzealously in favor of breast-feeding that it is forced on a reluctant mother. Those women who do not want to breast-feed their infants should not be made to feel guilty about their choice. On the other hand, the nurse should not hesitate to inform expectant parents of the differences between the various milks available (including human) and of the advantages of breast-feeding to both mother and infant (Table 32-1). Many women are uninformed about the differences in the available methods and may base their decision on how their mothers fed them or what a friend has said. For these women, information can be useful in helping them to make a decision based on facts.

Advantages of Breast-Feeding

For many years, the saying "breast is best" has been used when talking about the relative merits of breast- or bottle-feeding. At the same time, reassurances have been given that formula is also fine for babies.

Research Highlight

Breast engorgement in the early postpartum period has been thought to be associated with a number of breast-feeding problems including nipple trauma, breast infection, and early termination of breast-feeding. The purpose of this study was to investigate factors possibly related to engorgement, and to identify nursing implications for minimizing or preventing engorgement.

Fifty-four mothers of full-term healthy infants, born by either vaginal or cesarean delivery, were asked to rate their breasts for changes every 6 hours for the first 78 hours postpartum, on a four-point scale. Frequency of feeding during the first 48 hours was significantly correlated with amount of breast engorgement at 54 hours for primiparas. Duration of feeding time for primiparas was significantly less than that of multiparas. The authors suggest, therefore, that milk production may be stimulated by early, frequent feedings of short duration, but that the breasts may not be adequately emptied and engorgement may occur. Primiparas may be more likely to follow instructions to limit sucking time, than multiparas who are more experienced with breast-feeding.

Estimation of milk maturation, using the maturation index of colostrum and milk (MICAM), indicated that early milk maturation was associated with less engorgement at 36 hours. This finding also is consistent with previous findings that increased duration of feeding is predictive of early milk maturation.

This study lends further evidence to the suggestion that suckling time should not be limited in early breast-feeding. Encourageing mothers to breast-feed long enough to promote adequate milk removal may prevent stasis and engorgement.

Moon JL, Humenick SS: Breast engorgement: Contributing variables and variables amenable to nursing intervention. JOGNN 18(4):309–315, July/August 1989)

Research studies from many disciplines have focused attention on favorable aspects of breast-feeding, including the uniqueness of human milk and its appropriateness for human infants. Although knowledge is still incomplete, many advantages of breast-feeding have been identified.

BIOCHEMICAL AND NUTRITIONAL CONSIDERATIONS

The constituents of cow's milk and human milk are dissimilar in almost every way except for water and lactose.[4] For example, human milk contains only 1% protein whereas cow's milk contains approximately 3.3%, and whey protein, which accounts for more than 60% of the total protein in human milk, constitutes only 20% of the protein in cow's milk.[5] Companies promoting commercially prepared formula stress the modifications made in the formulas to increase their similarities to the composition of human milk and often state that modern formula is "almost like mother's milk." In reality, even when the formula has been "modified" or "humanized" by altering the protein, and vitamins and minerals are added in "appropriate" amounts, there are still many differences. Recent studies have shown that the whey-predominant formulas still result in altered protein utilization indices when compared to human milk feeding.[5]

There are also differences in the bioavailability of nutrients from human milk and infant formula. Substances, such as zinc, that are found in approximately the same amounts in both milks, may have different absorption rates. The human infant absorbs zinc more effectively from human milk because human milk has a different zinc-binding factor than is found in cow's milk. Formulas vary in other ways, such as the addition of emulsifiers, thickening agents, pH adjusters and antitoxidants, the effects of which are unknown and which are "not found in the original product for human infants."[4]

Another difference of unknown consequence is the rigidly consistent composition of formula compared with the variability of mother's milk. Besides the changes that occur in the progression from colostrum to mature milk, there is variation in the composition of mother's milk within each nursing period. The foremilk, which accumulates in the alveoli between nursings, is relatively dilute and low in fat, whereas the hindmilk, which is secreted during the nursing period is higher in fat and protein.[6] There are also differences in composition of breast milk according to the time of day of the nursing period, and long-term changes as the infant gets older.

IMMUNOLOGICAL AND ANTIALLERGENIC FACTORS

Human milk and colostrum have been shown by many studies to be rich in defense factors, such as immuno-

TABLE 32-1. COMPOSITION OF MATURE BREAST MILK, COW'S MILK, AND A ROUTINE INFANT FORMULA*

Composition/dl	Mature Breast Milk	Cow's Milk	Routine Formula with Iron†
Calories	75.0	69.0	67.0
Protein (g)	1.1	3.5	1.5
Lactalbumin (%)	80	18	
Casein (%)	20	82	
Water (ml)	87.1	87.3	
Fat (g)	4.0	3.5	3.7
CHO (g)	9.5	4.9	7.0
Ash (g)	0.21	0.72	0.34
Minerals			
Na (mg)	16.0	50.0	25.0
K (mg)	51.0	144.0	74.0
Ca (mg)	33.0	118.0	55.0
P (mg)	14.0	93.0	43.0
Mg (mg)	4.0	12.0	9.0
Fe (mg)	0.1	Tr.	1.2
Zn (mg)	0.15	0.1	0.42
Vitamins			
A (IU)	240.0	140.0	158.6
C (mg)	5.0	1.0	5.3
D (IU)	2.2	1.4	42.3
E (IU)	0.18	0.04	0.83
Thiamine (mg)	0.01	0.03	0.04
Riboflavin (mg)	0.04	0.17	0.06
Niacin (mg)	0.2	0.1	0.7
Curd size	Soft	Firm	Mod. firm
	Flocculent	Large	Mod. large
pH	Alkaline	Acid	Acid
Anti-infective properties	+	±	−
Bacterial content	Sterile	Nonsterile	Sterile
Emptying time	More rapid		

* Composite of a number of sources.
† Enfamil.
(Avery GB, Fletcher AB: Nutrition. In Avery GB (ed): Neonatology, 3rd ed. Philadelphia, JB Lippincott, 1987)

globulins, lactoferrin, enzymes, macrophages, lymphocytes, and *Lactobacillus bifidus* (a growth enhancer of lactobacilli).[6] Research in a variety of populations has indicated that breast-feeding offers effective protection against diarrhea. This protection is apparently related to the difference in intestinal flora of breast-fed infants compared to those on formula. The gut flora of breast-fed babies consists mainly of lactobacilli and bifidobacteria, which are nonpathogenic and produce feces with a pH of 5 to 6, due to fermentation of sugars and production of acetic acid. This low pH inhibits growth of bacteria such as *Escherichia coli* and *Streptococcus faecalis*, which are the predominant flora of formula-fed infants who have a higher fecal pH.[7] In addition to

antibacterial activity, human colostrum and milk also have antiviral, antiprotozoan, and anti-inflammatory properties.[6]

One known advantage of the immunoglobulin secretory IgA, which is present in human milk, is the protective antiabsorptive effect it has in keeping protein molecules from passing through the intestinal walls. During the first 6 months of life, foreign proteins are more likely to be absorbed through the intestinal wall than they are in later life, which can lead to allergies. The protein in cow's milk is one of the most common food allergens encountered in infancy. Human milk proteins, on the other hand, are virtually nonallergenic to humans.[6]

PSYCHOLOGICAL FACTORS

The psychological advantages of breast-feeding are not as easily documented as the physical aspects. Professionals often offer reassurance that bottle-feeding and breast-feeding are interchangeable for the emotional well-being of mother and child; however, breast-feeding, by establishing a more direct and intimate biological relationship between infant and mother, may influence the quality of the mother–child interaction.[4] Some studies have demonstrated that the increase in oxytocin and prolactin levels during lactation play a role in inducing mothering behavior. Also, the delay in return of the menstrual cycle that occurs with unrestricted breast-feeding has been shown to result in a more even mood cycle for the lactating woman.[6]

OTHER ASPECTS

For the baby, breast milk can be safer because it is not subject to incorrect mixing or contamination. The baby does not have to wait to eat—if mother is nearby, the milk is always available and at the right temperature. The action of sucking at breast is different from sucking on a bottle and may promote better development of the mouth and jaw (see Fig. 32-7).

For the mother, an early benefit is promotion of uterine involution stimulated by the release of oxytocin when the infant sucks. The mother also has the convenience of not having to prepare bottles or incur the added expense of buying formula. When a woman breast-feeds her infant, she is less likely to conceive again during the first 8 to 10 months of lactation. As a means of birth control, this, of course, is not as reliable as modern contraceptive measures, but it can be helpful for those who cannot afford or accept artificial contraception.[8] (See References and Suggested Readings for a more complete discussion of advantages of breast-feeding.)

Choosing to Bottle-Feed

Throughout recorded history, women have sought alternatives to breast-feeding their infants. Although the most popular alternative was the use of a wet nurse, attempts at artificial feeding were widespread, as can be seen from the remains of spouted feeding pots, artificial teats, and other mechanical feeding devices. Historical writings show that women were often urged to breast-feed their own children, but many ignored these admonitions for various reasons.[6]

PERSONAL REASONS

Women still give a variety of reasons for choosing artificial feeding. Some feel that breast-feeding is too tiring or confining or is simply distasteful; others may be afraid that it will disfigure their breasts; and still others fear that they will fail at breast-feeding, especially if previous attempts to breast-feed a child were unsuccessful.

The mores and pressures of the mother's socioeconomic class and peer group are also important in the choice of feeding method. Bottle-feeding may be the accepted practice in the community or neighborhood. Relatives, friends, and others who are against breast-feeding can sway the mother's choice, or, conversely, pressure from those who are overly enthusiastic about breast-feeding can turn the mother against it. Plans for early return to employment can be a significant factor in choosing to bottle-feed, especially if the mother perceives that too much effort is required to continue breast-feeding after going back to work.

CONTRAINDICATIONS TO BREAST-FEEDING

Certain conditions in both the mother and the infant can have a bearing on the decision to bottle-feed. There are few absolute contraindications to breast-feeding. Galactosemia in the infant is one, because it is imperative for these infants to have a lactose-free diet and breast milk is rich in lactose.[9] Other conditions and infections in the infant might also preclude breast-feeding, at least temporarily. Mothers with certain diseases or infections, such as active untreated pulmonary tuberculosis, cytomegalovirus (CMV) infection, chronic carriers of hepatitis B virus, and those infected with the human immunodeficiency virus (HIV), should be counseled not to breast-feed their infants.[10] Active herpes simplex virus infections are not contraindications to breast-feeding unless there are vesicular lesions in the breast area.[10] Certain maternal medications that are known to be detrimental to breast-feeding infants may lead to recommendations to avoid breast-feeding either temporarily or permanently (see Appendix B).

Generally when any of the above conditions are present, the decision about feeding method can be made on an individual basis. In many cases, if the mother is determined to breast-feed, she can pump her breasts and keep up her milk supply until it is possible for her to begin nursing the baby.

Breast infection or painful, cracked, or fissured nipples might require changes in the breast-feeding routine and discontinuance of sucking on the affected breast for a while, but the breast should continue to be emptied by some means. Becoming pregnant is usually an indication for weaning because of the physiological strain that it places on the mother, although some women have breast-fed through a subsequent pregnancy.

■ BREAST-FEEDING

If breast-feeding is the method of choice for a new mother, the degree to which she perseveres in this endeavor is often influenced by her care in the hospital. A consistent approach to assisting with breast-feeding is important. The development of breast-feeding protocols in hospital settings can help to standardize teaching and minimize contradictory information.

Studies have shown that many breast-feeding mothers do not perceive nurses as being helpful in either making the decision or getting started with breast-feeding.[11] This perception could keep them from asking nurses for assistance in the breast-feeding process. Because most women leave the hospital soon after giving birth, before they have time to establish lactation, it is important for nurses to gain their trust and give them anticipatory guidance about initiation of breast-feeding and ways to prevent or deal with possible problems. Support from knowledgeable nursing personnel, permissive hospital policies, and anticipatory teaching can do much to make breast-feeding a more pleasant and successful experience for mother and infant.

Mechanisms of Lactation

A working knowledge of how the breasts function in the lactation process can help the nurse with the guidance given to the new mother. The anatomy of the breasts and the physiology of lactation have been discussed previously in Chapter 26 but are reviewed briefly here. The student is referred to Chapter 26 for a renewal of background understanding of the subject. Figure 32-1 reviews the anatomical structures of the breast. Two major mechanisms are involved in lactation: the secretion of milk and the milk-ejection reflex. Figure 26-4 illustrates these mechanisms.

SECRETION OF MILK

The secretion of milk is a prerequisite for successful breast-feeding. During pregnancy, major changes occur in the mammary glands in preparation for milk production. From the second trimester on, a secretion with fairly stable composition (precolostrum) can be found in the breasts. With the birth of the baby and the expulsion of the placenta, the secretion enters a transitional phase, which begins with colostrum and changes, over the following 10 days to a month, to mature milk. It is believed that increased levels of the hormone prolactin and decreased levels of estrogen and progesterone are at least partly responsible for the changes in the mammary secretion after birth, which includes an increase in both the volume of milk secreted and the total output of nutrients.[12] The release of prolactin from the anterior pituitary is enhanced by the stimulation of afferent nerves in the nipple when the infant suckles at the breast.[13]

Colostrum is higher in protein and lower in fat and lactose than mature milk. It also contains greater amounts of other substances, such as sodium chloride and zinc, and is rich in antibodies. Besides its nutrient purpose and anti-infective function, colostrum also may act as a laxative in facilitating the passage of meconium.[6] As the prolactin levels continue to increase and the estrogen and progesterone levels drop, newly secreted milk is progressively mixed with the colostrum until the mature milk stage is reached. During this time, there is a decrease in the concentration of immunoglobulins and total protein and an increase in lactose, fat, and total calories.[6]

In the early stages of lactation, milk secretion can be stimulated by having the infant nurse from both

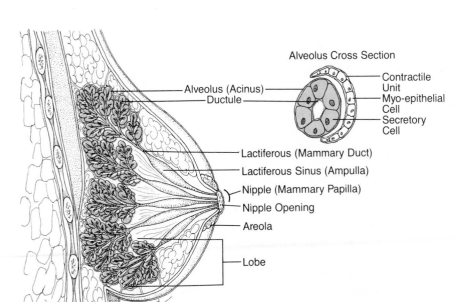

■ *Figure 32–1*
Schematic diagram of the breast. (Redrawn from Riordan J, Countryman BA: Basics of breast-feeding, part II: The anatomy and psychophysiology of lactation. JOGN Nurs 9(4):210, July/ August 1980)

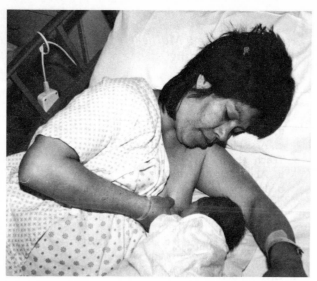

■ *Figure 32–3*
The mother who breast-feeds her newborn while lying down turns her baby toward her and curves her arm around the baby.

same position at each feeding. The area of the nipple in line with the infant's nose and chin is subjected to the greatest stress. Varying the nursing positions from one feeding to the next can be helpful because it changes the position of the infant's mouth on the nipple. This allows the breast to empty more completely and prevents the nipples from becoming tender and the ducts from becoming plugged.[17]

If the mother is lying down (Fig. 32-3), the nurse can suggest that she be on her side with her arm raised and her head comfortably supported. The baby lies on his side, flat on the bed or supported so that he can grasp the breast easily. Tucking the baby's feet close to

the mother's body helps give him room to breathe. If the mother prefers to sit up to nurse, she may be most comfortable in a chair, with a stool to support her feet, if necessary (Fig. 32-4). If she stays in bed, the high Fowler's position is probably best. For the mother after a cesarean delivery, it is usually more comfortable if the knees are bent and abducted, with pillows to support them on each side and something, such as an overturned washbasin, at the end of the bed for her to brace her feet against.[18] It is often helpful to place a pillow under the arm that is supporting the infant, to reduce the tension on the muscles, or to place a pillow under the baby to raise him to a sufficient height to reach the breast easily. An alternate position for the baby is facing the breast with his body supported on a pillow along the mother's side and under her arm in the "football hold" (Fig. 32-5). This is especially helpful for the mother who has delivered by cesarean section or the mother who wants to nurse twins simultaneously.

Some mothers improvise positions that work well for them and their baby, but the nurse may have to work with other mothers to be sure they find a comfortable position. Often, in their eagerness to get the baby on the breast, mothers become tense and assume uncomfortable positions (although they assure the nurse they are "comfortable"). Patience and gentle reminding on the part of the nurse encourage these mothers to relax more readily.

POSITIONING THE INFANT

After the mother is comfortable, the nurse can assist her in positioning the infant so that he can "latch on" to the breast correctly (Fig. 32-6).

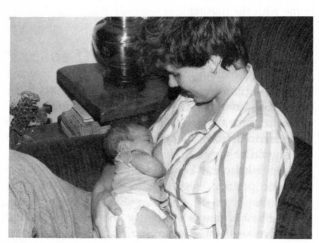

■ *Figure 32–4*
The mother may prefer to assume a sitting position while nursing. She should prop her feet or legs so she is comfortable and can comfortably hold the baby.

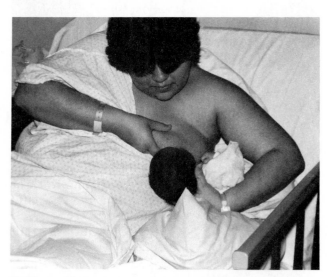

■ *Figure 32–5*
The mother may position the newborn in a football hold. The baby is supported by a pillow. The side rail is up for added security.

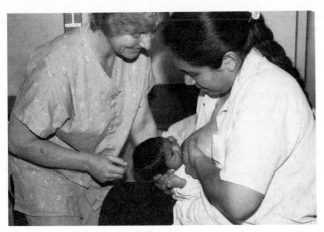

■ *Figure 32-6*
The nurse assists the mother in positioning the newborn.

Client Education

Positioning the Infant on the Breast

- Assume a comfortable position.
- Turn the infant's body toward you.
- Keep the infant's shoulder and hip in alignment.
- Support your breast with your hand, with four fingers below and thumb above.
- Tickle the infant's mouth with your breast until the infant's mouth is wide open.
- Pull the infant in close toward you against your body and your breast. (Bring the baby to the breast and not the breast to the baby.)

To nurse satisfactorily, the infant needs to be held properly by the mother. Although some mothers seem to know how to support a baby at the breast, many are awkward at first and need definite instructions. The following are some helpful teaching points:

- The mother and baby must be comfortable.
- The baby should be at the level of the breast so his weight does not pull on the breast.
- The baby must be able to grasp the nipple and most of the areola. If only the nipple is grasped, the baby is not able to draw out the milk because the milk sinuses are not compressed. Possible damage to the nipple may occur, along with pain to the mother.

If the mother is in the sitting position, cradling the infant in her arms, the following steps described by Frantz[19] have proven to be helpful in positioning the baby and preventing or decreasing nipple soreness:

- The baby's head should be in the bend of the mother's arm with her hand holding onto his buttocks or leg, turning his body completely toward her with his mouth at the level of the nipple. His lower arm should be around the mother's waist.
- The mother can help the baby grasp the nipple by supporting her breast with her hand, four fingers below and thumb above, with all fingers behind the areola.
- The mother tickles the baby's lips gently with the nipple, waits for him to open his mouth *wide*, centers the nipple, and brings him in close to her body so that his nose and chin just touch her breast and the nipple is in his mouth, past the gums.

Critical points seem to be that the infant is well over on his side facing the mother, so he doesn't have to turn his head to grasp the nipple, and that his whole body is pulled tightly against her with his shoulder and hip in alignment. These points also apply when the mother chooses the side-lying or football position.

Use of the second and third fingers to "shape" and introduce the nipple into the infant's mouth is an alternate technique that has been advocated for several years. Using this technique has often been counterproductive because the mother's fingers are frequently placed on the areola, where the infant's gums should be, and prevent the infant from getting enough of the areola into his mouth. Also, depression of the breast by the mother's index finger to allow breathing space may inadvertently result in removing the nipple from the baby's mouth.

Advice to get "all of the areola" into the baby's mouth is misleading and often impossible to follow, because many areolae are large. The important thing to remember is that the baby needs to get enough of the areola into his mouth so that his jaws can compress the sinuses, which are behind the nipple and under the areola.

INSTRUCTIONS ABOUT SUCKING BEHAVIOR

It is difficult to determine what goes on in an infant's mouth while he is sucking at the breast, because the inside of the mouth can not be visualized directly. The sucking behavior of infants has been the subject of a number of studies over the last three or four decades through the use of observation, x-rays, and more recently ultrasound.[20] Although there is still not complete agreement on the description of what happens during the process, we have a better idea of how the infant's mouth interacts with the mother's breast to obtain milk.

Breast-Feeding Aids

Breast Cups

(Sometimes called breast shells.) For treatment of inverted nipples, keeping milk from leaking onto clothing, relieving engorgement, and protecting the sore nipple from sticking to bra or bra pad. Vary in size, shape, ability to be sterilized and comfort. Prices range from $4.98 to $11.50 a pair.

Nipple Shields

(Sometimes called breast shields.) Designed to protect sore nipples or help baby who won't accept the breast easily. *Use with extreme caution.* Many potential problems: (1) may cause preference for nipple over soft breast; (2) no stimulation of breast by baby's mouth to stimulate milk production; (3) little or no areolar compression is possible to help baby extract milk efficiently so baby may have poor weight gain; (4) if a silicone shield is cut down, it may cut baby's mouth; (5) mother using shield should be advised to have infant's weight checked frequently for safety. Prices range from $0.89 to $3.80 each or from $3.00 to $6.95 a pair.

Breast Pads

To aid in stopping milk from wetting clothes. (*Caution:* Plastic or waterproof lining may contribute to nipple soreness or cutaneous monilial infection of the breasts if baby has thrush.) New mothers may want to use the all paper or all cotton pads as they start breast-feeding, and the working mother may need the pads with a barrier but should use great caution to change them often. Disposable pads are made from paper and come with or without plastic liners. They range in price from $2.50 to $6.00 for 48. Washable pads are made from cotton, and some are backed with nylon, plastic, taffeta, or polyester/rayon. They range in price from $4.22 for 6 to $3.50 for 2. Men's handkerchiefs or cut-up prefolded cloth diapers work well, can be washed and reused. Some women do not need pads at all.

Breast Pumps

Used to aid in the expression of milk. Success with pumps is highly individual; some brands or models work better for some women than others. Two different breast-pumping styles have been noted: 1. "Draw and hold" method in which the pump is used to increase the pressure to a certain point and then held there while the milk flow continues. When the milk flow slows, the pump pressure is released and built up again the same as before, 2. "One pump per second" method in which there is a continuous rhythm of pump, release, pump, release, at 1-second intervals. Babies nurse at one suckle per second intervals so "one pump per second" pumping has often been termed "physiological" pumping in action. Pumping involves creating a negative or pulling pressure at the breast as the let-down of milk occurs. Pump discomfort can interfere with the let-down. Some women let-down so abundantly that any pump will do.

Electric Pumps

SEMI-AUTOMATIC—Woman must control suction intervals and resultant pressure with her finger over an opening. *AUTOMATIC*—Automatic pressure interval built in without the danger of too much suction occurring. The automatic pumps tend to be used as "draw and hold" pumps, taking several seconds to reach a maximum pressure. Large electric pumps cost $800 to $900 but can usually be rented for about $2.00 a day, or less if rented for over 120 days. Collection units and hand pump conversions add to the cost. Mid-size electric pumps are slightly less expensive.

Battery-Operated Pumps

Not known for longevity or consistent performance. A good one lasts about eight months. Nonrechargeable pumps have the added cost of battery replacement as often as daily if pumping is done around the clock. These are all "draw and hold" pumps. They cost $30 to $50, and some include electric plug adapters or rechargeable packs.

Manual Pumps

Cylinder type pumps create negative pressure by drawing a piston through a cylinder. The amount of pressure can be controlled, but pulling too hard on the cylinder can cause too high a pressure. These cost between $12 and $24. Other manual pumps include those that create suction with bulbs, trigger handles, running water from a faucet, or the mother sucking on a tube. Costs range from a few dollars to $50.

(continued)

Feeding Tube Devices

The device delivers milk to the suckling baby at the breast by way of thin flexible tubing taped to woman's breast. These are used in adoptive nursing, relactation, reluctant nursers, suckling problems, and sick or handicapped infants. These consist of a plastic bag or bottle, which is suspended around the neck, and thin flexible tubing, which when placed in the infant's mouth with the mother's nipple carries the milk to the infant. Cost is about $32.

(Adapted from Frantz K: International Sources for Breastfeeding Aids. Lactation Educator Training Program, Los Angeles, UCLA Extension, 1990)

To extract milk from the breast, the infant needs to use more than just suction. He must draw the nipple well back in his mouth, close his lips to form a seal around the areola, compress and empty the sinuses under the areola by moving his jaws up and down, and sweep the milk into the back of his mouth with regular undulations of his tongue. Creation of a vacuum may also be involved in drawing the milk from the breast.[21] Swallowing occurs when enough milk has been obtained to induce the reflex. This activity is carried on rhythmically, at about one suck per second, interspaced with periods of rest, until the infant is satisfied (Fig. 32-7).

Sometimes the let-down reflex is so active that the milk literally streams out of the nipple. The baby may almost have to stop sucking and may have difficulty in swallowing fast enough to keep up with the stream. Placing the baby in a more upright position temporarily may help him handle the milk and prevent choking. He may have to nurse a bit, stop, and continue as he learns to cope with the increased flow.

The mother may need assistance in determining whether the infant's mouth is correctly positioned on the breast and that he is sucking effectively. When the infant latches on correctly, his mouth is opened wide and his lips are flared outward. His tongue forms a trough under the nipple and areola and extends beyond the lower gum. If there is a question about tongue placement, it can be observed by gently pulling down on the infant's lower lip.[15] Incorrect placement of tongue or lips can cause nipple damage as well as ineffective sucking. If he has a good grasp, his jaws move up and down regularly and swallowing movements can be seen in his throat. The mother can also be instructed to listen for quiet swallowing sounds.[15] If his grasp is poor, he may make clicking or smacking sounds and his cheeks may draw in with each suck. Ineffective sucking should not be allowed to continue. The infant should be removed from the breast and repositioned to start again with a better grasp.

Any time the infant needs to be removed from the breast, the mother needs to break the suction first. Failure to do this can result in pain or trauma to the nipple.

To break the suction, a clean little finger can be placed in the corner of the infant's mouth or the infant's chin can be pulled down. Sometimes the mother needs to pull away a little at the same time so the infant does not grasp the nipple again.

Breast tissue pressing against the infant's nose may obstruct his breathing and cause him to stop sucking. Pulling his buttocks and legs in closer to the mother's body may help by changing his head position slightly and allowing more air space. Lifting the breast slightly to allow more air space is another suggestion. Depressing the breast tissue with the thumb is more likely to dislodge the breast from the mouth.[22]

Individual Differences. Babies exhibit a wide variety of sucking behaviors. Some, after finding the nipple, suck vigorously without stopping until they are satisfied. Others may suck vigorously for a time, appear to sleep or to rest, and then resume sucking. Still others mouth the nipple before actually sucking, but eventually nurse well. Others seem rather disinterested in the whole thing and dawdle throughout the nursing period. When the milk comes in, however, a change usually is noted, and even the seemingly disinterested infants begin to nurse more in earnest.

The important point here is that individual differences do exist in infants, apparently from birth; hence, care must be taken to allow for these differences. To try to force the infant into a style or speed that is not natural for him only results in screaming, resistance, and refusal; the nursing period should be adapted to the infant and not the infant to the nursing period.

Mothers, especially, are appreciative of learning about this; often they think there is "a way to nurse" and do not realize that infants have different eating behaviors. Giving mothers anticipatory guidance and instruction in this aspect of nursing a baby is an important component of nursing care.

"Disinterested" Baby. Usually, getting the nipple into the mouth and tasting the milk seem to increase the baby's interest and ability to nurse. If the infant does not seem too interested or adept, moistening the nipple

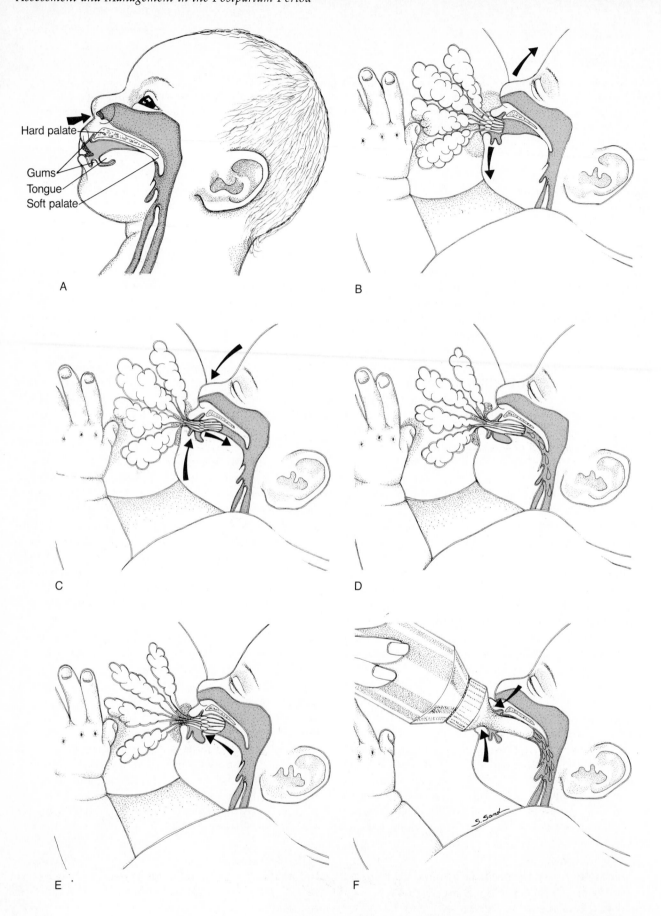

Hard palate

Gums
Tongue
Soft palate

A

B

C

D

E

F

by expressing a few drops of colostrum or milk often encourages sucking.

Sometimes a baby falls asleep instead of sucking. If the mother unwraps him, plays with his hands, sings to him, or uses some other type of loving stimulation, it may be enough to arouse him and get him started. If it does not, the mother should be reassured that the baby will nurse when he is hungry. The nurse should make sure that the baby is brought to the mother as soon as he awakens and is not given any feeding in the nursery. If possible, the infant should be left at the mother's bedside, so that she is available when the baby is ready to eat.

Nipple Confusion. If breast-feeding has not begun early and the infant has had experience with a rubber nipple, he may be "nipple confused." The sucking behavior required to obtain milk from the bottle is different from that of breast-feeding, described previously. The milk from the bottle comes into the infant's mouth with little effort on his part, and instead of using his tongue to help extract the milk, he has to thrust his tongue forward to control the flow of milk (see Fig. 32-7F). It is not surprising that many infants have some difficulty in switching from bottle to breast, but with a little time they usually do well. It is helpful for the mother to know about these sucking differences so she doesn't become frustrated.

GIVING SUPPORT AND SUPERVISION

Once the infant has taken the breast without difficulty and has been sucking well for several minutes, the nurse probably does not need to remain in constant attendance at the bedside. The mother needs some opportunity to feel that she can manage on her own. Letting her have reasonable periods of managing breast-feeding by herself helps to instill some confidence. However, she should never be left without adequate instruction and reassurance that the nurse is readily available.

When an infant has some initial difficulties with latching on to the breast, the nurse may need to remind the mother that the first few days are a learning period for both mother and baby.

Many mothers feel that all infants are born knowing how to suck and that if their infant does not latch on immediately, it must be because of something the mother is doing wrong. Some mothers even have a feeling of being rejected, stating, "The baby doesn't like me," or "The baby doesn't want my milk." Actually, taking milk from the breast is more than just a simple act of sucking, and some infants do need help in learning how. If the mother is helped to understand this, she will be less inclined to blame herself and more able to enjoy the nursing experience.

Because short hospital stays allow less time for nurses to provide assistance to the breast-feeding mother, most women need some support after leaving the hospital. The father or other family members may fill this need, but due to absence or lack of information, additional support is often needed. Sources of support include nursing mothers' groups, which have been started in most communities. One well-known group is La Leche League International, which holds breast-feeding classes for women before and after the baby is born and publishes books and pamphlets about breast-feeding. In many communities, there are 24-hour phone numbers that nursing mothers may call if they are having problems with breast-feeding.

Another source of help for the nursing mother is the lactation educator or consultant. These people have special training and experience in the area of assisting mothers with breast-feeding. The lactation educator presents prenatal classes specifically on breast-feeding and is available to the mother for counseling and advice after the baby is born. The lactation consultant is a health professional who has additional training and experience, is prepared to assist mothers with more serious breast-feeding problems, and usually works in a clinic setting or in private practice.

■ *Figure 32–7*

(A) Normal breathing for a young infant is through the nose; the back of the mouth is closed by contact of tongue and palate. (B) Infant opens mouth wide to receive the breast, the tongue comes forward over the lower gum to form a trough under the nipple and areola, and the nipple is pulled far back into the mouth. (C) Undulations of the tongue from front to back press nipple against hard palate, squeezing milk out of sinuses. Note how lips form a seal around areola. (D) When milk reaches the back of the throat, the swallowing reflex is initiated. (E) The gums open allowing sinuses to refill, followed by closure of the gums, and the cycle is repeated. Enough suction is maintained to keep nipple back in the mouth, and the infant continues to breathe through the nose, one breath to one or two swallows. (F) Rubber nipple is less pliable, maintains its shape, and may strike soft palate, interfering with normal tongue action and sometimes causing gagging. Milk comes more freely, and tongue may be thrust against gums to control overflow.

The mother may also be referred to a public-health agency if necessary. Some hospitals encourage mothers to call the nursery or obstetric unit if they need support or help with problems. Although many mothers are reluctant to call, they welcome the chance to ask questions if the nurse makes the call or a home visit. Some hospitals and some private doctors hire nurses to make follow-up visits after the woman leaves the hospital.

FEEDING SCHEDULE

A self-regulatory or self-demand schedule is the usual accepted practice today, especially for breast-fed babies (i.e., the baby is fed when he indicates hunger). When a set schedule is used and the infant is made to wait until it is "time" for a feeding, he may not nurse well. He may be over-hungry and exhibit frantic behavior that interferes with nursing, be exhausted from crying, or have lost his feeling of hunger by the time he is fed. Similarly, an infant in a deep sleep state will be difficult to arouse and will probably not feed well. Mothers can be taught to observe their infant for behavioral feeding cues.[16] Clues to a lighter sleep state would include rapid eye movements under closed eye lids, startles, and sucking movements (see Chap. 29). When mothers and babies are together most of the time as in a rooming-in situation, problems can be avoided because the mother knows when the baby is awake and can feed him as needed. She also has the opportunity to learn to recognize the cry and behavior that indicate that her baby is hungry.

Self-demand feeding does not mean that a newborn should be allowed to go for long periods of time without eating. Most breast-fed babies want to nurse every 2 to 3 hours at first and may go as long as 5 hours for one period each day. Some babies, however, who cry little and do not give the usual hunger cues, may go much longer between feedings, and the mother may need to be encouraged to feed them before they actually seem hungry. Frequent nursing is helpful in stimulating milk production, ensuring adequate intake, and in satisfying the infant's sucking needs. Each time the infant has a growth spurt he wants to nurse more frequently for a few days until the supply catches up with his increased demand. Infants do gradually go longer between feedings, and their eating patterns become less varied. This is encouraging news for the new mother who may feel at first that the baby is nursing all the time.

LENGTH OF NURSING TIME

Limitation of sucking time during the initial stages of breast-feeding, as a means of preventing sore nipples, is an idea that is still practiced in many hospitals. Most recent studies, however, have shown that this is not the case. If positioning and attachment are correct, unlimited nursing has not been found to increase nipple soreness.[23]

Time limitations can actually cause some problems for the breast-feeding mother. With severe limitation, such as starting with 1 or 2 minutes on each breast at each feeding, the let-down reflex does not have a chance to function before the baby is removed from the breast. Even with 4 or 5 minutes per side, there may be increased incidence of breast engorgement and reduction in the infant's fluid intake. Another disadvantage is that the mother may become too involved in clock watching to have a pleasant, relaxed time with her baby.[24]

It is best to offer both breasts at each feeding to provide maximum stimulation for the mother and an adequate supply of milk for the infant. The infant should be encouraged to nurse for at least 5 to 7 minutes on each side to allow time for the let-down reflex to occur and the ducts to be emptied. As the infant's thirst and hunger increase he may want to nurse 10 to 15 minutes on the first breast and a little less on the second. If the mother does develop severe nipple problems, she might need to shorten the time on the affected breast and to complete the emptying by expressing the milk.

When the breasts are full and the let-down reflex is functioning well, the baby usually gets most of the milk in the first 5 to 10 minutes of sucking. Therefore, the mother need not worry that the baby is not getting enough milk if she has to limit nursing time for a short period due to nipple soreness. Nursing should begin on the side used last at the previous feeding. A safety pin on the bra strap helps the mother remember which breast to start with.

SUPPLEMENTARY FEEDINGS

The subject of whether or not to give supplementary feedings to newborns has long been controversial. Many proponents of breast-feeding feel that giving the infant any artificial feedings is detrimental to establishing and maintaining lactation and interferes with breast-feeding success. Others feel that there are legitimate indications for occasional or regular artificial feedings. These supplementary feedings may consist of plain water, glucose water, or dilute or full-strength formula. Most of the time these are given by bottle either after a breast-feeding or instead of a feeding. Expressed breast milk can also be given by bottle when the mother is unable to feed the baby herself.

To avoid nipple confusion and encourage proper sucking even when supplements are needed, alternates to use of a bottle have been devised. Feedings can be placed in the infant's mouth by dropper, syringe, or spoon. If the mother can put the infant to breast, but needs to supplement her milk or encourage the infant to suck, a device for supplementation can be used. This consists of a pouch of milk that delivers milk to the infant through a tubing that enters the infant's mouth next to the mother's nipple (Fig. 32-8).[25,26]

If the mother is to use supplemental feedings when she returns home, the nurse should make sure that the mother understands how to prepare these feedings, the kind and the amount of feedings, and the indications for their use.

CARE OF THE NIPPLES

To facilitate breast-feeding, it is important to discuss nipple care with the new mother. Cleanliness is important in breast-feeding, but it is the hands that need washing, not the nipples. There is a natural antisepsis provided in the oils secreted by the nipple and by enzymes in the milk.[17] Washing the breasts with plain water at the time of the daily bath or shower is thought to be enough. The use of soap should be avoided because it is drying and can lead to cracking.

Keeping the nipples dry is another important aspect of their care. Air drying after each nursing period and leaving the bra flaps down for 15 to 30 minutes several times a day are recommended. The warm air from an electric hair dryer, on low setting, held 6 to 8 inches away is often helpful.[6] Milk left around the nipple after the baby nurses should be allowed to dry on the breast rather than being wiped away, because it has been found to be soothing and healing.[6] Plastic liners of any kind in the bra should be removed because they hold the moisture in. In case of some milk leakage, especially in the first days after the milk comes in, something absorbent, such as a breast pad or a clean, folded, man's handkerchief, can be used to keep the nipple drier and prevent the outer clothing from getting wet. They should, of course, be changed frequently when they get damp.

Routine use of nipple ointments and creams is not advisable. If used, the substance should be safe for both mother and baby, and not have to be washed off before the baby is fed. Some commercial products contain irritants, and lanolin may contain pesticides or may cause problems for anyone who is allergic to wool.[6,27] If the mother has extremely dry skin or application of some substance is recommended for a specific reason, it should be used after breast-feeding, applied in small amounts, and rubbed in well, so air circulation is not obstructed and the ducts in the nipple and areola do not become plugged.

ADDRESSING COMMON CONCERNS AND PROBLEMS

Painful Nipples. Nipple pain is frequently a reason mothers give for discontinuing breast-feeding. Although it may not be possible to prevent or eliminate this problem completely, it can be minimized with good care. Measures to prevent nipple trauma include the following:

1. Make sure the infant's mouth is positioned correctly on the breast so he is not chewing on the nipple.
2. Change nursing positions with each feeding so that different areas of the nipple are subjected to the greatest stress from sucking.
3. Do not allow the breasts to become engorged so that the infant has difficulty grasping the breast.
4. Feed the infant on demand so that he does not become overly hungry, causing him to suck the nipple too vigorously.
5. Start each feeding on alternate breasts so that both breasts are subjected to the vigorous sucking that occurs at the beginning of the feeding.

The mother should also avoid allowing the infant to suck on empty ducts. Before the let-down reflex is established, she can manually express a few drops of colostrum or milk to fill the ducts before allowing the baby to begin nursing.

The mother can probably benefit from some anticipatory guidance about nipple soreness. She needs to know that it is not unusual and is usually self-limiting. The discomfort is often most noticeable as the baby begins to suck but diminishes rapidly as the let-down reflex occurs. The discomfort with the first few sucks

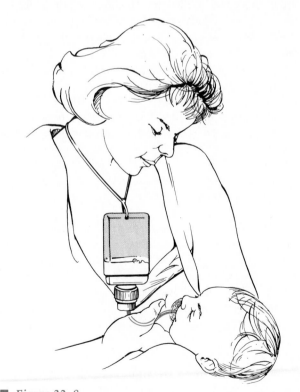

■ *Figure 32–8*
The supplemental nutrition system allows the mother to continue breast-feeding while providing supplementary formula to the infant through a tube placed next to her nipple.

can last for several days or weeks and does not mean that there is anything wrong.

It is possible, of course, for the nipples to develop fissures, erosions, or blisters, which can serve as entryways for bacteria and possible infection. If any of these do develop, the nurse should check with the mother to be sure she is carrying out proper nipple care. The nipples may be exposed to a lamp with a 40-watt bulb for 15 to 20 minutes.

If symptoms of mastitis or breast abscess develop, such as localized increased warmth, tenderness, or redness, the physician should be consulted so that treatment can be started immediately. Because these problems usually occur after the woman has left the hospital, she should be given some guidance before discharge and instructed to observe her breasts for signs of infection. Antibiotics are usually the treatment of choice. Most physicians feel that it is best for the woman to continue breast-feeding even when these difficulties develop[6] (see Chap. 40).

Engorgement. When the milk "comes in," the breasts suddenly become larger, firmer, and more tender. New mothers experience varying degrees of discomfort at this time. Two factors thought to be involved in causing this discomfort are venous and lymphatic congestion and the filling of the alveolar cells with milk. The lymphatic and venous engorgement is usually transitory. Ideally, with early, frequent sucking by the infant, establishment of the let-down reflex, and periodic emptying of the alveoli, painful engorgement does not occur.

In some women, probably at least partly due to delayed emptying, the breasts do become distended or "engorged," sometimes so much so that the skin appears shiny. The tissue surrounding the nipple may also become taut to the extent that it actually retracts the nipple, making it extremely difficult for the baby to grasp the nipple and the areola adequately. The breasts may be reddened and warm to the touch, but engorgement is *not* an inflammatory process, so if fever occurs, some other cause should be suspected. With severe engorgement, the breasts can become painful, especially when touched or moved, and throbbing pains sometimes extend into the axilla.

Although this condition is transitory and usually disappears in 24 to 48 hours, prompt treatment is important, not only for the mother's comfort but also to prevent the condition from progressing. If engorgement is allowed to become marked, emptying of the breasts (which is the basis of treatment) becomes difficult because the ducts become occluded by the surrounding congested tissues and the thick and tenacious character of the retained secretions. Secondary lymphatic and venous stasis may occur because the milk cannot be emptied.

Prevention of engorgement is preferable to treatment and is generally possible with good management. Early and regular nursing is considered by many to be the best preventive measure. When the mother and infant are together around the clock as in rooming-in, engorgement tends to occur less often because the baby can nurse in response to the mother's needs as well as his own. If rooming-in is not available, the infant can be taken to the mother as soon as her breasts begin to fill and as often thereafter as is necessary to maintain her comfort.

If engorgement does occur, management is directed toward removing the milk and relieving the discomfort. To assist in moving the milk from the alveoli to the sinuses where the baby can obtain it, it is suggested that the breasts be massaged before nursing.[22] This helps to open the lacteal ducts and relieve breast tightness by increasing circulation, thus making the breast softer and the nipple area easier to grasp. The mother can be instructed to place both hands at the upper part of the breast near the clavicle. With continuous downward pressure the fingers move out and around on opposite sides of the breast until they encircle it, then slide smoothly over the tip. Some lubrication, such as lotion, should probably be used for this procedure. When the breasts begin to soften, the infant can be placed at the breast.

The use of an oxytocin nasal spray by the mother before the baby nurses may facilitate the removal of milk by encouraging the let-down reflex.[6] Some mothers find that the use of hot packs or a hot shower before nursing also improves the flow of milk.

Another aid to emptying the breast and further relieving engorgement is alternate massage. To do this, the infant's sucking movements should be observed during nursing. When they become short and choppy instead of long and rhythmic, it indicates that the milk is no longer flowing as freely. Without removing the infant from the breast, the mother can alternately massage different areas of the breast to bring more milk down into the ducts where the infant can remove it by sucking.

For relief of discomfort, ice packs applied between nursing periods may be useful. The use of a bra for good uplift support should be stressed. Analgesics such as aspirin, acetaminophen, or codeine may be needed for pain relief. They should be given in adequate dosage and with appropriate timing so that the mother can be relatively comfortable during nursing.

Not Enough Milk. Many mothers worry that they do not have enough milk. The mother can be assured that the baby is probably getting an adequate amount of milk if he is wetting at least six to eight diapers a day, having at least one stool, sleeping fairly well, and gaining weight at a steady rate. Audible swallowing during nursing is another indication that the infant is getting milk. Crying and weight gain are not the most reliable indicators, because "colicky" babies cry for reasons other than hunger and usually gain well, and some breast-fed babies are slow weight gainers even when the milk supply is adequate.

If the mother thinks her baby is not getting enough milk, putting the baby to breast more often and not limiting the sucking time usually increase the supply. The concept of supply and demand, that the more milk the baby takes from the breast the more the mother produces, is important for the mother to remember. Sometimes women mistakenly think that they can "save" their milk and have more for the next feeding if they give the baby a bottle at one feeding. Getting more rest and increasing fluid and protein intake may also help increase the milk supply.

Some mothers fear that they are losing their milk at the time when engorgement subsides because their breasts go back to a more normal size and feel less full. An explanation that this might happen and that it is just the swelling that has gone down, not the milk supply, helps prevent worry.

If the mother's breasts seem full but the infant does not seem to be getting enough, there could be a problem with the let-down reflex. It may be helpful to the mother to learn how to recognize when the let-down reflex is occurring. Mothers usually feel the let-down as a kind of tingling or drawing sensation in the nipple, followed by a fuller, heavier feeling of the breasts. Because let-down occurs bilaterally, another sign is dripping of milk from one breast while the infant is sucking on the other. Also there is often a change in the infant's sucking as the milk begins to flow more freely and he doesn't have to work as hard.

The let-down reflex can be influenced profoundly by psychic factors and the mother's emotions. If let-down is not occurring, the nurse can help the mother determine and eliminate disturbing factors. The mother may need to lie down, have a warm drink, or discover other ways of relaxing before the feeding time. A relaxed atmosphere, adequate assistance, effective pain relief, and a supportive attitude on the part of the nurse and family are important to the establishment of the let-down reflex.

Sometimes mothers are concerned that their milk isn't "rich enough" because they compare the thin, bluish white color of breast milk with the creamy color of cow's milk. They need to know that human milk is naturally different from cow's milk in many ways, including color. They may be interested in the fact that the milk of each animal species has a characteristic color. For example, buffalo's milk is completely white and kangaroo's milk is pink.[28]

In some cases, the mother may actually have an insufficient milk supply. This can occur for a number of reasons. If the mother is receiving good guidance and support, has tried all of the usual ways to increase the milk supply, and the baby is still showing signs of not doing well, other causes for the problem should be sought and supplementation may need to begin.

Maternal risk factors for insufficient lactation include women who have had augmentation or reduction mammoplasty, and those who had minimal breast enlargement during pregnancy.[29] Infant factors can include anything that causes the infant to provide an inadequate, irregular, or ineffective sucking stimulus.[25] Early intervention in cases of lactation insufficiency is important before the infant loses too much weight and the mother gets too discouraged. Depending on the cause of the problem, the supplementation may be temporary or the mother may be able to continue partial breast-feeding with supplementation.

EXPRESSION OF MILK

There are some instances in which the mother wishes to breast-feed, but for certain reasons the infant cannot be "put to breast." There are also situations in which the breast-fed infant is not able to empty the breast completely. At such times, it becomes necessary to empty the breasts of milk by artificial means. Otherwise, if this condition is allowed to persist for several days, lacteal secretion is inhibited, and the future milk supply may be jeopardized. Before attempting to empty the breast by hand or pump, the mother may find it helpful to use measures to facilitate the let-down reflex, such as taking a warm shower, having a warm drink, or gently massaging the breasts.

Manual Expression. It is helpful if a woman can learn the technique of manual expression before the baby is born, but it can be taught afterward if necessary. The mother should have the opportunity to try it in the hospital, where she can have guided practice under the supervision of the nurse, so that she is able to do it with more confidence when she returns home.

A sterile glass or wide-mouthed container should be ready before beginning, and if the milk is to be fed to the infant, a sterile bottle and cap also are needed. It may be desirable first to massage the breast for a few seconds to stimulate the flow of milk, as described in the section entitled "Engorgement."

The hands of the person expressing the milk should be washed thoroughly with warm water and soap and dried with a clean towel. Because the daily care of the breast is designed to maintain cleanliness, the same cleansing ritual required before putting the baby to breast should be used here.

1. One hand is used to support the breast and to express the milk; the other is used to hold the container that receives the milk. Although some authorities advocate that the right hand be used to milk the left breast, the decision as to which hand is used should depend on how the mother can accomplish this with the greatest ease.
2. The forefinger is placed below and the thumb above the outer edge of the areola. The first action is gentle but firm pressure toward the chest wall and the second is movement of the finger and thumb toward each other, drawing forward with a slight milking motion. The forefinger is kept straight so that pressure can be exerted between the middle of this finger and the ball of the thumb. As the finger and thumb are alternately brought together and released, compressing the area of the lactiferous sinuses between them, milk is forced out in a stream (Fig. 32-9).
3. The fingers should not slide forward on the areola or the nipple during the milking process. It is of paramount importance to avoid pulling, pinching, or squeezing movements, because these can possibly bruise and damage the breast tissue.
4. The position of the thumb and forefinger should be changed as the sinuses are emptied, moving in a clockwise direction, so that milk can be removed from all the sinuses.

Many authorities advocate this method of emptying the breast rather than using the breast pump, because the action more nearly simulates the action of the infant's jaws as he nurses. Furthermore, because no mechanical equipment is required, it is a method that can be readily used when necessary after the mother is discharged from the hospital.

Breast Pump Expression. For many women, a breast pump is the preferred way to express milk. Many types of pumps are available, including electric, battery-operated, and hand pumps. Which pump to use, and whether to buy or rent, depends on a number of factors such as the length of time it will be needed and the reason for its use. When a pump is used, there is always the potential danger of traumatizing the breast tissue. Average sucking pressure for the normal newborn has been found to range from -50 to -155 mm Hg, with a maximum of up to -220 mm Hg.[6] Some pumps can exert pressure greater than this and are more likely to cause damage. Information about maximum pressure of specific pumps should be checked with the manufacturer.

When assisting a new mother to use an electric breast pump in the hospital, the mother should be given explanations about why the pump is used, how it works, and how to use it. This helps reduce the mother's anxiety, which could interfere with the milk-ejection reflex.

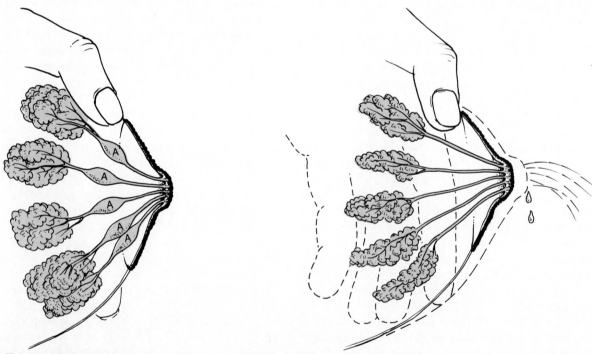

■ *Figure 32–9*

A lateral view of the left breast showing the method of expressing milk from the breast. The thumb and forefinger are placed on opposite sides of the breast just behind the areola. The lactiferous sinuses (ampulla, A) are compressed, and milk is forced out as the thumb and forefinger are brought together. See text for complete explanation.

The nurse should stay with the mother and assist her the first few times until she feels confident enough to use the pump alone. Measuring and recording the amount of breast milk obtained gives the mother evidence that she is increasing or keeping up her milk supply. If the milk is to be fed to the infant, it can be poured into a sterile nursing bottle; labeled with the infant's name, the time, and date; and refrigerated immediately. After use, the pump should be washed with soap or detergent, and the removable parts, such as the bottle and cap, the breast funnel, and the rubber connection tubing, should be washed thoroughly, wrapped, and autoclaved.

Electric pumps (Fig. 32-10*A*) may also be the choice for home use if there will be long-term separation from the baby or if the baby cannot nurse. Although expensive to purchase, these pumps can be rented, and insurance may cover this expense. *Battery-operated pumps* (see Fig. 32-10*B*), some with electric plug adapters, are less expensive and more portable, but may not be long-lasting or consistent. Without an adapter, purchasing batteries can be costly. *Manual pumps* (Fig. 32-11) are least expensive and most portable, but take more effort and both hands to operate. When choosing a pump, mothers should also consider safety (UL Approval), ease of cleaning, and how the breast cup fits or can be adapted to their breast size. Childbirth educators, the La Leche League, lactation educators, or lactation consultants are good sources for information about breast pump features and availability.

INSTRUCTIONS FOR MOTHER'S SELF-CARE

Rest. Rest is one of the most important considerations for the lactating mother. The detrimental effects of fa-

tigue and worry already have been discussed. In the hospital, the nurse is able to act as a buffer between the mother and some of these problems. In addition, the mother is relieved of household responsibilities and is able to have meals served to her. When she leaves the hospital, she no longer has this somewhat protected environment. Thus, it is important for the nurse to make sure that the parents understand the importance of rest for the mother and that they have made adequate plans to provide for it. If it is at all possible, the mother should have help at home. Her main energies can be directed to the care of the infant and other family members. Housekeeping chores have to be simplified, and the mother's activity must be restricted so she gets sufficient rest. Because her sleep is broken at night, naps during the day become particularly *essential*—they should not be considered a luxury. Without adequate rest, the milk supply soon decreases. Active women may need help to realize the importance of naps and rest periods. It is helpful, also, if visitors (including relatives) are restricted at first. They can become fatiguing to the mother, and they may be a source of potential infection to the newborn.

Diet. The daily diet of the lactating mother should be similar to that recommended during pregnancy (see Chap. 18) except that, according to the Food and Nutrition Board of the National Research Council, the need for calories, vitamin A, vitamin C, niacin, riboflavin, and iodine is greater than during pregnancy. It is hoped that the new mother has become more aware of good nutrition during her pregnancy and is able to incorporate the proper foods into her diet to meet these increased needs. The nurse should discuss the recommendations with her, assess her knowledge, and give instruction as necessary.

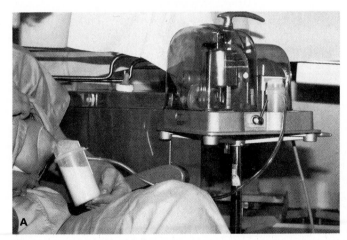
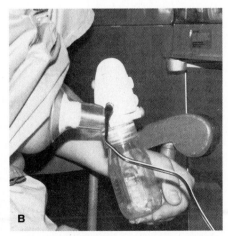

■ *Figure 32–10*
(A) *The electric pump extracts milk efficiently and can be operated with one hand. It is gentle, with a suction pattern similar to the infant's. (B) This battery-operated pump is being used with a plug-in adapter. It also requires only one hand for operation.*

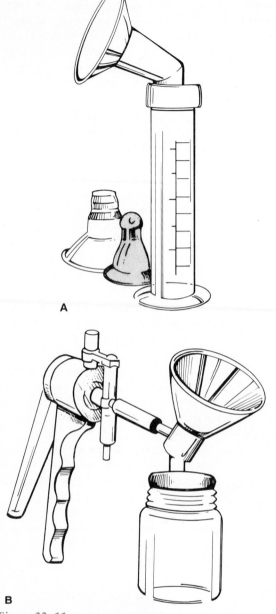

A

B

■ *Figure 32–11*
There are several types of hand-operated pumps including cylinder pumps and trigger-handle pumps. They need no batteries or electrical outlets, but they do require two hands for operation, and the pumping hand sometimes gets tired.

If the mother's diet was adequate during pregnancy, additions rather than changes are all that is necessary. Often nursing mothers, not realizing that their nutritional needs increase even over the needs of pregnancy, go back to their prepregnant diet or limit their intake in the hope of losing weight. Dieting should be discouraged during lactation. Any limitation of maternal nutrient intake during lactation can interfere with the quantity of milk produced and, if the limitation is severe, with the composition of the milk.

Individual caloric needs vary with the body size of the woman and with the quantity of breast milk produced. According to the Recommended Dietary Allowances (RDAs), 10th edition,[30] approximately 85 Kcal are required for each 100 ml of milk produced. The average milk secretion is 750 ml/day during the first 6 months and 600 ml/day during the second 6 months. Based on this, they calculate that the average lactating woman requires 500 additional Kcal per day over that recommended for a nonpregnant woman. Fat stores from pregnancy are assumed to provide some calories for the woman during the first few months. Additional calories would be needed for women whose pregnancy weight gain was below normal or whose weight during lactation falls below the standard for their age and height.[30] Women who were producing more milk, for example mothers of large babies or twins, would be likely to require additional calories. The mother's weight is one of the best criteria in determining adequate caloric intake; it should remain relatively stationary. Wide fluctuations require that the diet be adjusted, most likely in the amount of carbohydrates and fats consumed, assuming that protein intake is adequate.

Increasing the milk intake to at least 1½ qt daily fulfills the additional protein, thiamine, riboflavin, calcium, phosphorus, and niacin needs. Supplementing the citrus fruit recommendations in pregnancy with generous servings of other fruits and vegetables fulfills the vitamin C requirements. To further ensure optimum vitamin and mineral intake, many physicians prescribe that the vitamin supplement capsules taken during pregnancy be continued.

A high fluid intake also is necessary for milk production. Intake between 2500 and 3000 ml is recommended for the mother engaged in usual activity under pleasant environmental conditions. More may be required in hot weather or with physical exertion. This fluid intake should include a good deal of water as well as other beverages. Many mothers find that taking a beverage before nursing facilitates the let-down reflex. Concentrated urine or constipation may be indications of inadequate fluid intake.

Mothers have often heard that there are foods that should be avoided during lactation. Although some babies are bothered by certain foods that their mothers eat, this is not universally true. Most mothers can eat any nutritious food without causing the baby any distress. However, because many babies do seem to be upset after the mother eats large quantities of certain foods, such as chocolate or cabbage, moderation should be the rule when eating these foods. If the mother is bothered by a particular food, she would be wise to avoid it because it could have an effect on the baby also. In addition, some babies seem to have more sensitive taste buds and object to certain flavors that come through in the milk by being reluctant to nurse.

Drugs. Most drugs ingested by the mother while she is lactating are secreted in the milk, but in varying amounts and with differing effects on the infant. Concentration of the drug in the breast milk depends on several factors, including the concentration in the mother's blood, the lipid solubility of the drug, the degree of ionization, and the composition of the milk. Usually the amount of drug in the milk is small, but the cumulative effect over a 24-hour period may give the infant a fairly large dose. Some drugs seem to have highest concentrations shortly after they are ingested; therefore, taking them after breast-feeding rather than before might help to minimize the infant's exposure.[6] Delayed excretion or inactivation of drugs due to the immaturity of the infant's renal and hepatic functions can be a factor in the concentration of the drug in the infant's body. Decreased renal function in the mother can also lead to increased concentrations of drugs in the milk.

Interpreting the data concerning concentration of drugs in breast milk is hampered by the fragmentary and contradictory nature of the information available. Most drug companies state in their inserts that "safety in pregnancy and lactation has not been established and the benefits of the drug must be weighed against possible risks." When drugs are prescribed for a nursing mother, she should remind the physician that she is breast-feeding. If she is taking drugs for a chronic condition, she should discuss their possible effects with the physician during pregnancy, before she decides on the method of feeding her infant.

Certain drugs that have been shown to have adverse effects on the nursing infant are considered to be contraindicated during lactation. Other drugs are recommended to be used with caution. (See Appendix B for further information on drugs in breast-milk.) If these drugs are given to the mother, the infant should be observed closely for signs of reactions to the drugs. Many drugs that are considered safe when taken in single doses can cause problems in the infant if taken regularly and frequently. Long-acting forms of drugs should be avoided.[6]

Some nonprescription medications also contain drugs that can be harmful to the infant when passed through the breast milk. Mothers need to be warned to read the labels of any medications they plan to take, to determine the presence of potentially harmful components. Examples include Bromo-Seltzer and some over-the-counter sleeping aids containing bromides, and migraine headache remedies containing ergot. Bromides and ergot are contraindicated during breast-feeding. Also, some laxatives such as cascara can cause diarrhea in the infant.

Contaminants in Breast Milk. Ever since investigators first discovered DDT in breast milk in the 1950s, people have been asking if breast milk is still safe for babies.

A variety of contaminants are known to be present in breast milk, including other pesticides, and toxic chemicals such as PCB (polychlorinated biphenyls) and PBB (polybrominated biphenyls). These contaminants are stored in maternal body fat from which they are mobilized and transferred to the infant through the milk fat. Damaging effects of these chemicals in human infants, as a result of ingestion from mother's milk, has not been shown, although there is evidence from animal studies that heavy dosage can adversely affect the nursling. Prenatal effects of PCBs were shown in Japanese infants born to mothers with heavy contamination during pregnancy.[9]

Lead, another contaminant of human milk, is found in larger amounts in other forms of milk. More research is needed to determine the possible long-term effects of contaminated breast milk. The benefits of breast-feeding still seem to outweigh the possible dangers in most cases. Women who have had excessive exposure to contaminants should be encouraged to have their milk analyzed to aid them in making a decision about the method of feeding. Nurses should join with others in attempts to rid the environment of pollutants as a more permanent solution to the problem.

COUNSELING CONCERNING WEANING

When it comes to initiating breast-feeding, many mothers receive advice and counseling. However, frequently, little is said about how or when they should stop nursing. Although stopping abruptly at a time set by the physician has sometimes been the accepted method of weaning, this can be uncomfortable and distressing to both mother and baby. Most recent professional advice advocates that the infant be weaned slowly at a time chosen by either mother or infant. The mother should be helped, from the beginning, to feel comfortable with any length of time she chooses, even if it is considerably longer or shorter than usual.

The mother can begin to wean her infant by omitting either the feeding the infant is least interested in or the one that is least convenient for her. Another comforting experience the baby enjoys, such as rocking, cuddling or going for a walk, or something good to drink from a bottle or cup may be substituted for the feeding.[31]

Anywhere from a week to a month later, when both mother and baby are ready, another feeding may be dropped. This can be continued with periodic omissions until the child is completely off the breast. Additional omissions should be avoided when there are stressful situations in the family, such as illness, traveling, or guests. The child can be weaned to a cup or to a bottle depending on age and sucking needs.

Weaning is as likely to be traumatic to the mother as it is to the baby, especially if nursing has been a satisfying experience. Support from the father or another significant person may help guide her through this difficult time.

Sudden weaning is seldom necessary because the mother can express milk for a short time if she and the baby must be separated due to illness or absence for some other reason. If weaning does become necessary, a good supportive bra and mild analgesics for discomfort will probably be helpful for the mother. The medications that are given to inhibit lactation during the early puerperium are not used for weaning because they are not effective if started after lactation has begun.

GUIDANCE FOR WORKING MOTHERS

An increasing number of women are choosing to breast-feed even though they plan to return to work. The new mother may ask the nurse for an opinion of whether it is possible to breast-feed if she must return to work soon after the baby is born. Many factors are involved in this decision and its outcome for the individual mother. Answers to the following questions can help the nurse assess what information the mother needs to help her in the decision-making process:

1. How soon will she start working? Waiting at least 6 weeks until breast-feeding is well established is preferable.
2. How flexible is her job? Can she come home to feed during the day or have the baby brought to her? If not, is there time and a place to pump her breasts at work? The answers to these questions determine the arrangements she needs to make before starting work.
3. How much support does she have? Are family and friends supportive? Is her employer or supervisor supportive? Support from those around her will make it easier for her to continue with her dual roles.

The average working mother probably needs to be away from the baby during the entire working day. Her breasts will continue to fill at the regular feeding times when she first goes back to work. She can empty them each day by hand expression, manual pump, or electric pump to keep up the supply and have breast milk to be fed to the baby when she isn't there, or she can allow the daytime milk supply to dwindle by not pumping and have the baby receive formula during the day. Before going back to work, she needs to make these decisions and practice the method of expression she chooses. She also needs to arrange for refrigeration facilities for the breast milk at work.

Employers vary in the amount of support offered to breast-feeding mothers. In some cases, employers provide an electric breast pump, as well as a place to pump and facilities for storage, but the majority still do not have any policy to actively support the lactating woman.[32]

Some mothers find that their milk supply diminishes when they first return to work. Factors involved here may be inadequate rest, reduction of intake of food and fluids, and temporary inhibition of the let-down reflex related to the tension involved with starting back to work.[33] The working, breast-feeding mother has to pay particular attention to obtaining enough food and rest. She also should be aware that those who pump their breasts during the day can usually keep the milk supply at a higher level than those whose breasts are only emptied by the baby in the morning and evening.[34]

Studies have shown that most mothers who have breast-fed babies after returning to work have felt it was worthwhile and would do it again. They often reported how much they enjoyed the special closeness that breast-feeding promoted between them and the baby, even though they didn't have a lot of time to spend with the baby.[34]

Evaluation

The nurse's interest and assistance can play a major role in the successful outcome of the breast-feeding experience for the new mother and baby. To increase the effectiveness of her interventions, it is important for the nurse to evaluate these outcomes and to implement additional interventions when indicated. After a teaching session, the nurse evaluates whether or not the mother (1) verbalizes understanding of the breast-feeding process, (2) assumes a comfortable position, and (3) uses the suggested techniques for positioning the infant on the breast.

The infant's weight and hydration may also be used as criteria for evaluation. The infant (1) has at least four to six wet diapers a day, (2) has good skin turgor, and (3) begins to regain birth weight by 1 week of age. Other evaluations would be made depending on the situation. If the criteria are not met, the nurse might need to assess for further problems or provide the mother with additional information or demonstrations.

■ ARTIFICIAL FEEDING

The mother who chooses to bottle-feed her infant may have as many concerns about feeding as the breast-feeding mother, especially if this is her first child. She may not know how to feed an infant or prepare the formula. She may also feel a little uncertain about her choice of feeding method and wonder if the formula will agree with her infant. By keeping up to date on the

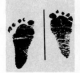

Nursing Care Plan

Infant and Mother Who Are Breast-Feeding

Patient Goals

1. Mother verbalizes understanding of:
   - Breast-feeding processes
   - Positioning of self and infant
   - Self-care during lactation
2. Mother demonstrates appropriate positioning of self and baby, and handling of baby.
3. Mother does not develop nipple or breast problems.
4. Infant "latches on" to breast, sucks, and swallows milk.
5. Infant maintains hydration and good nutritional status.

Assessment	Potential Nursing Diagnosis	Planning and Intervention	Evaluation

Mother's past experiences with breast-feeding	Knowledge deficit about breast-feeding related to lack of experience and prior information	Review with mother her prenatal preparation for breast-feeding
		
		Provide information as needed regarding:
		  Lactation process
		  Let-down reflex
		  Nutrition for lactation
			Mother expresses understanding of breast-feeding process

Mother's knowledge of self-care			

Mother's position during breast-feeding
 	
Mother's handling and positioning of infant
 	
Maternal–infant interaction
		Assist mother with breast-feeding:
		  Comfortable positiong of mother
		  Positioning of infant
		  Verify correct position of nipple in infant's mouth
		  Terminating feedings
		  Burping
			Mother assumes comfortable position and infant "latches on" to breast without difficulty
			
			Mother and infant experience satisfaction from the breast-feeding experience

Infant's reflexes (rooting, sucking, swallowing) and responsiveness		Demonstrate newborn reflexes	
Infant's sleeping and elimination patterns	Alteration in nutrition, less than body requirements, related to infant's lack of effective sucking technique or lack of responsiveness Fluid volume deficit related to inadequate fluid intake	Encourage frequent (every 2–3 h) feeding Provide further information: Determination of adequate amount of milk (4–6 wet diapers/day, sleeping well, gaining weight)	Infant experiences minimal weight loss Infant remains well hydrated

(continued)

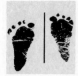

Nursing Care Plan   (continued)

Assessment	Potential Nursing Diagnosis	Planning and Intervention	Evaluation
Mother's nipples and breasts: tenderness, cracks, engorgement	Alteration in comfort, pain related to nipple tenderness	Breast and nipple care Manual expression or use of pumps Answer questions Refer to support groups or lactation counselor as appropriate Provide literature	Mother avoids tender or cracked nipples and breast engorgement

latest information about infant nutrition, the nurse can help allay the mother's fears about the adequacy of formulas, instruct her in safe preparation, and give guidance about when to seek medical assistance.

Comparison of Formulas

Formula is available in various sized cans in ready-to-use, concentrated, or powdered form. In the hospital nursery, the infant receives ready-to-feed formula in a disposable bottle. However, because formula in disposable bottles is expensive, one of the other packaging methods will probably be recommended for home use (Table 32-2). The model usually used in the composition

TABLE 32-2. TYPES OF FORMULA

Type	Packaging Available	Comments
Ready-to-feed	Small cans, large cans, bottles	Most convenient; most expensive; should not be diluted
Concentrate	Large or small cans	Less expensive; must be diluted 1:1 with water from safe source
Powder	Large cans	Least expensive; simple to prepare individual bottles with warm water from safe source; sometimes difficult to dissolve

of a formula is human milk. Companies that manufacture infant formula make frequent adjustments to match new discoveries concerning the composition of human milk (Table 32-3).

To provide adequate nutrition for an infant, a formula must meet the following criteria: it must have an appropriate distribution of calories from protein, fat, and carbohydrate; it must meet the infant's need for water, energy, vitamins, and minerals; and it must be readily digestible. Recommended standards for calories, protein, fat, vitamins, and minerals in formulas have been published by the Committee on Nutrition of the American Academy of Pediatrics.[35]

Cow's milk has more protein, sodium, and calcium and less carbohydrate than human milk, but is about the same in fat, calories, and the ratio of water to solids. The protein in cow's milk is different from that in human milk and contains much more casein and less whey protein. The approximate whey/casein ratios are 20:80 in cow's milk and 60:40 in human milk. The increased casein leads to a tougher curd, which is more difficult to digest.

Boiling or pasteurizing fresh milk, and processing evaporated milk softens the curd and makes it more digestible. Before commercially prepared formulas became widely available, evaporated milk formulas were most commonly used. Although less expensive than the commercial formulas, their composition is less like breast milk and they are no longer recommended for infant feeding in this country. Evaporated milk contains adequate amounts of vitamins A, B, and K and is usually fortified with vitamin D, but, along with fresh whole milk, it fails to meet current recommendations for vitamin C, vitamin E, and essential fatty acids.

Many ingredients and processes are used in an effort

TABLE 32–3. COMPOSITION OF FREQUENTLY USED MILKS AND FORMULAS

Milk or Formula	Cal/ dl	Percentage Composition			mmol/dl		mg/dl		Type of Carbohydrate	Type of Protein	Remarks
		Pro	Fat	CHO	Na	K	Ca	P			
Human milk	74	1.1	4.5	6.8	0.7	1.3	34	121	Lactose	Human	
Cow's milk	67	3.5	3.7	4.9	2.2	3.5	117	92	Lactose	Cow	
Goat's milk	67	3.2	4.0	4.6	1.5	4.5	129	106	Lactose	Goat	Insufficient folate
Enfamil	67	1.5	3.7	7.0	1.2	1.8	55	56	Lactose	Cow	
Enfamil With Iron	67	1.5	3.7	7.0	1.2	1.8	55	46	Lactose	Cow	
Similac	67	1.6	3.6	7.2	1.1*	2.0*	51	39	Lactose	Cow	
Similac With Iron	67	1.6	3.6	7.2	1.1*	2.0*	51	39	Lactose	Cow	
Similac PM 60/40	67	1.6	3.5	7.6	0.7	1.5	40	20	Lactose	Casein, whey	60/40 lactalbumin; casein
S-M-A	67	1.5	3.6	7.2	0.6	1.4	44	33	Lactose	Whey from cow, cow	60/40 lactalbumin; casein
Advance	54	2.0	2.7	5.5	1.3	2.2	51	39	Corn syrup, lactose	Cow, soy	16 cal/oz
Isomil	67	2.0	3.6	6.8	1.3	1.8	70	50	Corn syrup, sucrose, corn starch	Soy, methionine	
Soyalac-i	67	2.1	3.8	6.7	1.4	1.9	63	52	Sucrose, tapioca	Soy, methionine	
Nursoy	67	2.3	3.6	6.8	0.9	1.9	64	44	Sucrose	Soy, methionine	
ProSobee	67	2.5	3.4	6.8	1.8	1.9	79	53	Corn syrup solids	Soy, methionine	
Soyalac	69	2.2	3.8	6.6	1.5	2.0	63	52	Dextrose, maltose, sucrose	Soy, methionine	
Meat base	67	2.8	3.3	6.3	0.8	1.0	99	66	Sucrose, tapioca	Beef	High protein, low sodium
Nutramigen	67	2.2	2.6	8.8	1.4	1.7	63	47	Corn syrup solids	Casein hydrolysate	
Pregestimil	67	1.9	2.7	9.1	1.4	1.8	63	42	Corn syrup, tapioca	Casein hydrolysate, cystine, tyrosine, tryptophan	

* Slightly higher if made from powder.
(After Avery GB (ed): Neonatology, 3rd ed. Philadelphia, JB Lippincott, 1987)

to make commercial formulas meet the recommended nutritional standards and come as close as possible to the composition of human milk. Formulas generally use a nonfat cow's milk base with added vegetable oil and carbohydrate. Another type of formula, called "humanized," attempts to duplicate the 60:40 whey/casein ratio of human milk by using dialyzed whey. The dialysis removes electrolytes, bringing the formula closer to the lower-electrolyte human milk. Similac, Enfamil, and S-M-A all have formulas with the 60:40 ratio.

Some infants are not able to tolerate formulas based on cow's milk. Many formulas have been developed to try to meet the nutritional needs of these infants. Some of these, such as meat-based formulas, may be difficult for the mother to accept because they do not look like milk. Soybean-derived products are commonly used as the protein source in these artificial formulas. Soy protein isolate has a lower biological value than casein and whey, so slightly larger amounts are needed to meet the infant's nutritional needs. Soy protein can also cause sensitization in some infants. Formulas, such as Nutramigen and Pregestimil, that use casein hydrolysate as a protein source are expensive but are recommended for infants with true milk allergy.[2]

For the nonbreast-fed baby, formula is the recommended food for at least the first 6 months and preferably for the first year of life. In our weight-conscious society, it might seem that *nonfat milk* would be a good choice for an infant who was gaining weight too rapidly. Or nonfat dry milk may seem desirable for economic reasons. But nonfat milk is not recommended for infants under 1 year because it provides an excessive intake of protein with inadequate calories. To meet energy requirements and growth needs, body fat is mobilized. The infant may look healthy but have little reserve for illness. Nonfat milk also lacks an adequate content of iron, ascorbic acid, and essential fatty acids. *Low-fat* (2%) milk is midway between nonfat and whole milk in fat content, but probably would not meet all the infant's energy needs.[36]

Commercial milk substitutes such as *filled milk* and *imitation milk* also do not meet the infant's nutritional requirements and are not recommended for infant feeding.

Assessment

Assessing maternal concerns and knowledge about infant feeding techniques and formula is an important part of nursing care, especially for the first-time mother. If these concerns have not been addressed antepartally, the nurse needs to help her adjust in the postpartum period. The nurse should talk with the mother to assess her level of knowledge and her previous experience with infant feeding. The nurse should also observe the mother and infant during feeding to assess the mother's handling of the infant and the infant's feeding reflexes, responsiveness, and amount of intake.

Nursing Diagnosis

A possible nursing diagnosis might be "maternal knowledge deficit related to lack of information or experience with infant feeding." For the infant who is taking too little formula at a feeding or who is feeding infrequently, the nursing diagnosis might be "alteration in nutrition, less than body requirements, related to inadequate caloric intake" or "high risk for fluid volume deficit related to inadequate fluid intake." The infant

who is taking more formula than expected would have high risk for "alteration in nutrition, more than body requirements, related to excessive caloric intake."

Planning and Intervention

FEEDING IN THE HOSPITAL

Most hospitals have a routine for when the bottle-fed baby receives the first water feeding and when the formula feedings start. In some hospitals, it is the rule that the first water is given by the nurse in the nursery. Other hospitals are more permissive and allow the mother to give the first water. If this is the case, the nurse should show the mother how to use the bulb syringe because the water often causes the infant to bring up mucus. The nurse should also stay nearby to observe the infant's responses to the water.

The first feeding experiences can be important for mother and infant. The mother begins to learn how the infant communicates his wants and needs, while the infant, besides learning to coordinate his feeding behaviors, begins to find out how the discomfort from hunger is relieved and who provides the relief. The nurse can help the mother and infant with these tasks by being available during initial feeding periods to observe their behaviors, assess the interaction, and intervene with suggestions or demonstrations as necessary. When intervening, the nurse should be careful not to make the mother feel as though she is incompetent or inadequate.

Before feeding begins, the mother should be helped to get into a comfortable position. She may want to sit up in a chair instead of in the bed. Holding the baby in a semireclining position allows any air that is swallowed to rise to the top of the infant's stomach, where it is more easily expelled. To minimize the amount of air swallowed, the bottle should be tilted enough to keep the nipple filled with milk (Fig. 32-12).

The mother may need some help in getting the infant started on the bottle. If the infant does not open his mouth readily, gently stroking the lips with the nipple might help. Some babies elevate their tongue when opening their mouths, and an inexperienced mother may not recognize that the nipple is under the tongue. Stimulating the baby to open his mouth wide enough so that the tongue can be seen usually helps in placing the nipple in the right position. Also, care should be taken that the nipple is not pushed too far into the mouth, because it may cause gagging if it strikes the soft palate.

As the baby sucks, air bubbles rise in the bottle, indicating that the baby is getting milk. If air bubbles do not appear, the nipple should be checked to see if

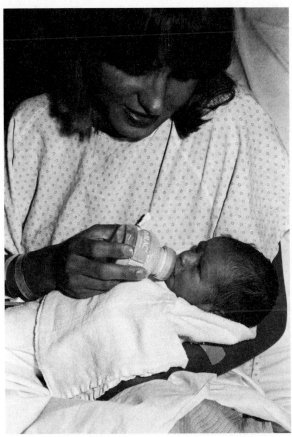

■ *Figure 32–12*
When bottle-feeding her infant, the mother tilts the bottle in such a way that the nipple is filled with milk.

ANTICIPATORY GUIDANCE

Before the mother and baby leave the hospital, the mother should be given some anticipatory guidance in how much formula the infant may take and how to prepare it.

According to the Recommended Dietary Allowances established by the Food and Nutrition Board of the National Academy of Sciences in 1973, infants from birth to 5 months need approximately 117 calories/kg (51 calories/lb) each day. From 6 months to a year, the need decreases to 108 calories/kg (47 calories/lb).[37] Using this as a guide, the nurse can help the mother calculate the infant's daily caloric needs. Most formula contains 20 calories per ounce, so a 7-lb baby would need about 17½ oz a day, or a little less than 3 oz at each of six feedings. As the infant grows, he increases his consumption. At times of particularly fast growth, he wants to eat more at each feeding or more frequently. Again, the reminder should be given that each baby is an individual and that babies of the same age and weight may have different needs.

COUNSELING CONCERNING PREPARATION OF FORMULA AT HOME

Bottles and Nipples. With the wide variety of bottles and nipples available, selection depends on the parents' preference. Some prefer glass bottles with plastic nipple caps; others opt for the boilable plastic bottles that are nonbreakable. There are also kits that have a hollow plastic holder in which a disposable plastic bag containing the milk is suspended. Supposedly less air is swallowed with this method because the bag collapses rather than filling with air when the milk is sucked out.

the hole is clogged or too small. If the milk is coming too fast, the nipple holes may be too large. Nipple holes can be checked by holding the bottle upside down. The milk should drop freely but not run in a stream. If milk is coming at the right speed, a feeding should take 15 to 20 minutes. If it takes much longer, the infant may get too tired, but if it is much shorter, the infant may not meet his sucking needs.

Babies have many different feeding behaviors, some of which may not correspond to the mother's expectations. Identifying the infant's individual behavior patterns and interpreting the baby's individuality to the mother can help to avert potential problems.

If the mother is concerned that the baby is not taking enough milk, it may help her to know that babies are often sleepy the first few days after birth but that they are born with reserves of fat and water and do not really need many calories until the second or third day.[36] The bottle-fed baby, like the breast-fed baby, should have the opportunity to be on a self-demand schedule.

Although bottle-fed babies average a longer period between feedings than breast-fed babies due to the larger curd of the formula, some are hungry every 2 to 3 hours. Others wait 4 or more hours between feedings.

However, the infant can still swallow air around the nipple.

Nipples also come in several shapes and sizes. One supposedly resembles the mother's breast in appearance; another (Nuk) is supposed to elicit sucking responses more like the breast. The standard nipple of one brand comes in three thicknesses that are color-coded to be used for milk, water or juice. The number of bottles and nipples needed depends on the method of preparation. (See Fig. 32-13 for examples of bottles and nipples.)

Methods of Preparation. Strict sterilization procedures for preparing formulas have been considered a must in the past. Most physicians are no longer insisting that bottles or formulas be sterilized if there is an uncontaminated water source and good refrigeration, and if hands and equipment are cleaned properly, because this clean technique is proving to be as safe as sterilization. There was no higher incidence of illness or infection when infants were fed formula prepared by the clean technique than when infants were fed formula prepared by terminal sterilization.[38]

There are four basic methods of formula preparation (Table 32-4). Points common to all methods of preparation are the following:

1. Hands should be washed well before starting.
2. If canned milk is used, the top of the can should be washed with soap and water using friction and rinsed thoroughly. Hot water can be poured over the top just before opening.
3. All equipment should be washed thoroughly in warm soapy water. A bottle and nipple brush should be used, and water should be squeezed through the nipple to make sure no milk particles or residue remains. Equipment should be rinsed thoroughly so all soap or detergent is gone.
4. Opened cans of formula or milk should be covered with fresh foil or plastic wrap, placed in the refrigerator, and used within 48 hours.

ONE BOTTLE METHOD. After completion of steps 1, 2, and 3, a feeding can be prepared right in the bottle. When using a concentrated prepared formula, one half of the total amount of formula desired is measured into the bottle. For example, if 4 oz of formula are needed, 2 oz of concentrated formula would be used. Assuming a safe water supply, an equal amount of fresh tap water is added. With ready-to-feed formula, the desired amount is poured into the bottle. Powdered formula can also be used by mixing one bottle at a time. Once prepared, formula should be fed to the infant within 30 minutes or be refrigerated. If not refrigerated, or used within an hour, it should be discarded.

CLEAN METHOD. This method differs from the previous one only in that the whole day's formula is prepared at one time. The bottles should be refrigerated immediately after preparation.

Because some physicians still recommend sterilization and because some people still live under conditions in which sterilization is necessary, the aseptic method and terminal sterilization are included in this discussion.

ASEPTIC METHOD. In this method, the bottles, nipples, nipple caps, and equipment used in making the formula, including a glass or enamel pitcher in which to mix the formula, are sterilized before the formula is prepared. The formula is made according to directions,

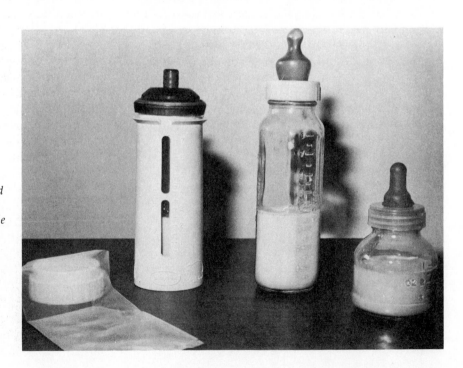

■ *Figure 32–13*

Types of bottles and nipples. (From left to right) A disposable bag and nipple cover; the bottle and nipple that are used with the disposable bag; regular bottle with Nuk nipple; and ready-to-feed bottle with standard nipple.

TABLE 32–4. FORMULA PREPARATION USING CONCENTRATED FORMULA

One Bottle Method	Clean Method	Aseptic Method	Terminal Sterilization
1. Open can of concentrated formula, pour ½ of total amount desired into bottle.	1. Same as one bottle method, but prepare day's supply at one time.	1. Equipment includes glass or enamel pitcher, measuring cup and spoons, mixing spoons, funnel, can opener, tongs.	1. Prepare as in clean method.
2. Add equal amount of fresh tap water from safe source.	2. Refrigerate immediately after preparation	2. Sterilize bottles, nipples, nipple caps, and equipment by boiling for 10 min in pan or sterilizer half full of water.	2. Apply nipples and caps loosely.
3. Feed within 30 min of preparation.		3. Mix formula in pitcher	3. Place in sterilizer with water in bottom and cover with tight-fitting lid.
4. Discard if not used within 1 h.		4. Pour into bottles.	4. Boil for 25 min.
		5. Put on nipples and caps. Refrigerate until needed.	5. Tighten nipple collars.
			6. Refrigerate until needed.

For all methods start by washing hands, formula can top, bottles, nipples, and equipment well.
Ready-to-feed and powdered formula can be prepared by any of the above methods.
Ready-to-feed formula needs no water or mixing.
For powdered formula, follow directions on can for proportions.

using aseptic technique. The desired amount of formula is put into each bottle. The bottles are nippled, capped, and refrigerated.

TERMINAL STERILIZATION. In this method, the formula is prepared under a clean but not aseptic technique. The equipment, bottles, nipples, and nipple caps are washed thoroughly but are not sterilized. The formula is prepared and poured into the bottles, and the nipples and the caps are applied loosely. They are placed in the sterilizer, covered with a tight-fitting lid, and sterilized by having the water boil rapidly in the bottom of the sterilizer for 25 minutes. In this method, formula, bottles, nipples, and protectors are all sterilized in one operation. Before the formula is refrigerated, the screw collar should be made secure.

Evaluation

To evaluate nursing care of the formula-fed infant, the nurse might ask the mother to verbalize her understanding of the infant feeding process. The nurse would observe whether the mother holds the infant for feeding and assumes a comfortable position. The nurse should also evaluate the infant's response to feeding and verify that the infant receives an appropriate amount at an appropriate rate without swallowing a large amount of air.

■ NURSING CARE RELATED TO COMMON CONCERNS IN INFANT FEEDING

Several topics related to infant feeding are of concern to the new mother regardless of the method of feeding.

Hunger

The mother may wonder how she can tell if her infant is getting enough to eat. She can be told that most babies when awakened from sleep by hunger "pains" fuss and cry and make sucking movements with their mouths, but that at first the infant may have difficulty distinguishing between hunger and other discomforts. If the baby awakens a short time after a feeding, the mother should try other comfort measures, such as holding, changing the diaper, and bubbling, before assuming he is hungry. Occasionally, a baby appears hungry when in reality he is only thirsty and is satisfied with a small amount of water. The baby who is obviously hungry and crying, refuses water with apparent disgust, and when a feeding is offered seizes the nipple ravenously and nurses with great vigor, may need to eat more fre-

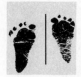

Nursing Care Plan

Infant and Mother Who Are Bottle-Feeding

Patient Goals

1. Mother verbalizes understanding of:
   - Feeding process
   - Positioning of infant while feeding
2. Mother demonstrates appropriate positioning and handling of baby.
3. Infant receives appropriate amount of formula.
4. Infant maintains hydration and good nutritional status.

Assessment	Potential Nursing Diagnosis	Planning and Intervention	Evaluation

Mother's past infant feeding experiences	Knowledge deficit about infant feeding related to lack of information and experience	Provide information as needed regarding:
		  Newborn sucking reflexes
		  Handling infant during feeding
			Mother expresses understanding of infant feeding process

Decision to bottle-feed			
Mother's handling of infant			
Infant's feeding reflexes and responsiveness		Assist mother with feeding processes:	
	Alteration in nutrition, less than body requirements related to inadequate caloric intake	Comfortable positioning of mother and infant Placing nipple in baby's mouth	Infant receives appropriate amount of formula at appropriate rate with minimal amount of air
	Alteration in nutrition, more than body requirements related to excess caloric intake	Check flow of milk Keeping nipple full Provide anticipatory guidance:	

	High risk for fluid volume deficit related to inadequate fluid intake	How much formula infant needs
		  Types of formula, bottles, nipples
		  Preparation of formula
			Infant's weight gain is appropriate

		Answer mother's questions regarding:
		  Hunger cries
		  Burping
		  Regurgitation
		  Hiccups
		  Constipation
		  Introduction of solid foods
			Infant is well hydrated and well nourished

		Distribute literature as appropriate	

quently for a while if he is breast-fed or be offered more in his bottle at each feeding if he is bottle-fed.

Bubbling (Burping)

After 5 minutes or so, or in the middle and at the end of each feeding, the infant should be held in an upright position and his back should be *gently* patted or stroked (Fig. 32-14). Pounding the baby on the back vigorously is neither effective for bubbling him nor conducive to his well-being. The change in position (from semireclining to upright) is an important factor in eliciting a bubble. Often holding the infant upright and pressing him against the breast is all that is necessary.

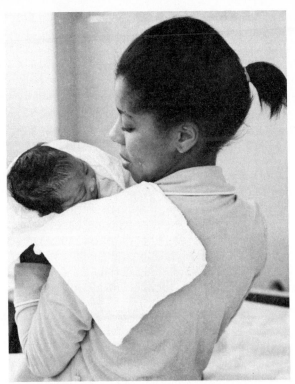

■ *Figure 32–14*
One method of bubbling or burping an infant is to place him in an upright position over the shoulder where he can be pressed against the breast.

An alternate position is for the mother to sit the infant up on her lap, with his chest resting on her hand and his chin supported by her thumb and index finger, while she pats him with her other hand. A third position is to place the infant prone over her knees with the knee

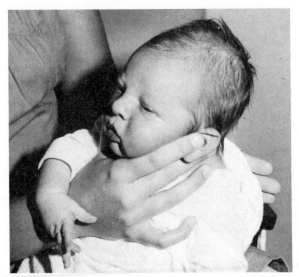

■ *Figure 32–15*
When bubbling the infant in the nursery, the nurse sits the infant up in his or her lap, with the baby's chest resting on the nurse's hand and the baby's chin supported by thumb and index finger.

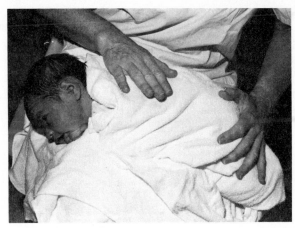

■ *Figure 32–16*
For an alternate method of bubbling, the infant is placed over the knees while his back is gently rubbed.

nearest the infant's head elevated slightly. The last two positions are sometimes preferred by nurses in the newborn nursery because they keep the infant away from the nurse's face and hair (Figs. 32-15 and 32-16).

Because the new infant's gastrointestinal tract is labile, milk may be eructated with the gas bubbles. A diaper is usually kept in front of the infant while he is being bubbled, in case this occurs (see Fig. 32-14). If there is doubt about whether the infant has brought up all the air when he is placed in his crib, putting him on his right side or in a prone position helps bring up the air and also prevents the infant from choking on any milk that might be regurgitated with the air.

Regurgitation

Regurgitation, which is merely an overflow and often occurs after nursing, should not be confused with vomiting, which may occur at any time, is accompanied by other symptoms, and usually involves a more complete emptying of the stomach. This regurgitation is the means of relieving the distended stomach and usually indicates that the baby either has taken too much food or has taken it too rapidly.

Hiccups

Some mothers need reassurance that hiccups are not unusual for infants and really do not seem to bother them. If the mother is disturbed, she can try giving the infant a few sips of water, but the hiccups go away without treatment.

Constipation

Constipation is almost nonexistent in breast-fed babies and is uncommon in those fed commercially prepared formulas, but mothers frequently express concern about possible constipation. Many parents believe that an infant is constipated if he misses having a bowel movement one day. The nurse can explain that it is quality not frequency of the stool that indicates the presence of constipation. An infant is considered to be constipated when the stools are hard, formed, and difficult to pass.

■ NUTRITIONAL CONSIDERATIONS DURING THE FIRST YEAR

Diets for infants are sometimes based on temporary scientific fashions or local customs. Long-term effects of infant diets are not known. Standards for formulas and baby foods are based on infant growth, but it is not known whether a diet that is optimum for growth in infancy offers freedom from allergy, obesity, arterial disease, or cancer later in adult life.

During the first year of life, the infant's growth exceeds that of any future period. In the first 4 months, he usually doubles his birth weight and may triple it by 1 year. Watching the infant grow is pleasing to the parents, and they often see the chubbiness of the infant as evidence of good health and their good parenting. This attitude can lead to overfeeding.

The infant's caloric needs per unit of body weight are relatively constant during the first year. This is because as he becomes more physically active from the fourth month on, his rate of growth is slowing down, and energy is relocated from growth to activity.

Introduction of Solid Foods

The time for adding solid foods is an area in which recommendations in the literature and actual practice often differ markedly. Although an adequate amount of all essential nutrients can be provided during the first 6 months without the addition of solids, many babies in the United States receive solid foods at an earlier age. This early feeding often occurs because the parents request it, thinking it helps the baby sleep through the night or considering it a sign that he is more advanced than infants who are "only taking milk."

There are many reasons suggested for delaying the introduction of solids until the infant is 4 to 6 months old. First, the baby is not developmentally ready to deal with nonliquid foods until about the end of the third month, and his tongue usually pushes them out of the mouth. Also, the large protein molecules from the foods may pass through the mucosa of the infant's immature gastrointestinal tract and become antigens, sensitizing the infant and causing allergic reactions. After 6 months, the gastrointestinal system is more mature and the infant's antibody production has reached a more desirable level. In the breast-fed infant, early introduction of solids may interfere with the desire for breast milk, decreasing the infant's sucking, and subsequently decreasing the milk supply. Other drawbacks to early feeding of solids are the potential for not supplying the infant's nutritional needs, the relatively high cost of the food, and the possibility of overfeeding.

Infantile obesity has become a growing concern in recent years because of its possible relation to adult obesity. Growth during infancy is mostly due to cell hyperplasia (tissue growth involving increases in the number of cells). It is felt that the obese infant will have more fat cells than normal throughout life and therefore be more prone to continuing obesity.[39]

Some suggestions for avoiding infant obesity are as follows:

1. Help parents use factors other than weight gain to evaluate their role as parents.
2. Help mothers discover the infant's satiety behavior and avoid encouraging the infant to get down the last drop or bite.
3. Encourage practices that promote more physical activities in infants.
4. Avoid early introduction of solids.

Nutritional Supplements

VITAMINS

Many believe that both breast milk and commercial formulas contain adequate vitamins for normal infants and that routine supplementation is unnecessary.[6] However, some sources still recommend vitamin D supplements for breast-fed infants with dark skin or those with little possibility of significant exposure to sunlight.[10] If the infant is fed a formula made of fresh or evaporated cow's milk, a vitamin C supplement might be necessary.

IRON

Iron deficiency anemia is the most common specific nutritional deficiency encountered. Infants and children between the ages of 6 and 30 months, especially those from lower socioeconomic groups, are particularly vulnerable. Breast-fed infants rarely have iron deficiency anemia, and most authorities do not recommend iron supplementation until 4 to 6 month of age. At this age, iron-fortified infant cereal can be added to the infant's diet.[6] For bottle-fed infants, formula fortified at a level of 10 mg to 12 mg/dl of elemental iron is recommended beginning at birth or by 4 to 6 months of age.[10]

These sources of iron would probably be adequate,

but they may not continue to be available to the infant as he grows older. By the age of 6 months, many infants are switched to fresh cow's milk. This causes two problems. First, cow's milk is low in iron. Second, there is increasing evidence that drinking fresh cow's milk during infancy is associated with occult blood loss from the intestine, resulting in iron deficiency anemia. The latter is less likely if the milk is boiled. Prepared formulas fortified with iron are recommended for the nonbreast-fed baby for the first 12 months of life.[36]

FLUORIDE

Some sources recommend supplementation with fluoride for all breast-fed infants because fluoride is found in only trace amounts in human milk.[40] Others suggest basing the decision on individual determinants such as family dental history and level of fluoride in the water supply.[6]

Bottle-fed infants probably receive adequate amounts of fluoride if the formula is mixed with water containing fluoride at an adequate level.[40]

■ REFERENCES

1. Neumann CC, Jelliffe DB: Foreword: Symposium on Nutrition in Pediatrics. Pediatr Clin North Am 24(1):1, February 1977
2. Avery GB, Fletcher AB: Nutrition. In Avery GB (ed): Neonatology—Pathophysiology and Management of the Newborn, 3rd ed, pp 1173–1229. Philadelphia, JB Lippincott, 1987
3. Fanaroff AA, Klaus MH: Feeding and selected disorders of the gastrointestinal tract. In Klaus MH, Fanaroff AA (eds): Care of the High-Risk Neonate, 3rd ed, pp 113–146. Philadelphia, WB Saunders, 1986
4. Nichols BL, Nichols VN: The biologic basis of lactation. Compr Ther 4(10):63–70, October 1978
5. Picciano MF: Nutrient needs of infants. Nutrition Today, January/February 1987, pp 8–13
6. Lawrence RA: Breastfeeding—A Guide for the Medical Profession, 3rd ed. St Louis, CV Mosby, 1989
7. Hayward AR: The immunology of breast milk. In Neville MC, Neifert MR (eds): Lactation-Physiology, Nutrition, and Breast-Feeding, pp 249–266. New York, Plenum Press, 1983
8. Lethbridge DJ: The use of breastfeeding as a contraceptive. JOGN 17(1):31–37, January/February 1988
9. Worthington-Roberts BS, Williams SR (eds): Nutrition in Pregnancy and Lactation, 4th ed. St Louis, CV Mosby, 1989
10. Frigoletto FD, Little GA (eds): Guidelines for Perinatal Care, 2nd ed. Elk Grove, IL, and Washington, DC, American Academy of Pediatrics and American College of Obstetricians and Gynecologists, 1988
11. Cronenwett LR, Reinhardt R: Support and breastfeeding: A Review. Birth 14(4):199–203, December 1987
12. Nevill MC, Allen JC, Watters C: The mechanisms of milk secretion. In Neville MC, Neifert MR (eds): Lactation-Physiology, Nutrition, and Breast-Feeding, pp 49–92. New York, Plenum Press, 1983
13. Neville MC: Regulation of mammary development and lactation. In Neville MC, Neifert MR (eds): Lactation-Physiology, Nutrition, and Breast-Feeding, pp 103–133. New York, Plenum Press, 1983
14. Brans YW: Neonatology in Obstetrical Practice. Philadelphia, JB Lippincott, 1987
15. Shrago L, Bocar D: The infant's contribution to breastfeeding. JOGNN 19(3):209–215, May/June 1990
16. Walker M: Functional assessment of infant breastfeeding patterns. Birth 16(3):140–147, September 1989
17. Nichols MG: Effective help for the nursing mother. JOGN 7(2):22–30, March/April 1975
18. Frantz KB, Kalmen BA: Breastfeeding Works for Cesareans, Too. RN, pp 39–47, December 1979
19. Frantz KB: Managing Nipple Problems. LaLeche League International, Reprint No. 11, March 1982
20. Minchin MK: Positioning for breastfeeding. Birth 16(2): 67–73, 76–80, June 1989
21. Smith WL, Erenberg A, Nowak A: Imaging evaluation of the human nipple during breast-feeding. AJDC 142: 76–78, 1988
22. Storr G: Prevention of nipple tenderness and breast engorgement in the postpartum period. JOGNN 17:203–209, May/June 1988
23. Moon JL, Humenick SS: Breast engorgement: Contributing variables and variables amenable to nursing intervention. JOGNN 18:309–315, July/August 1989
24. L'Esperance C, Frantz K: Time limitation for early breastfeeding. JOGNN 14(2):114–118, March/April 1985
25. Neifert MR, Seacat JM: Lactation insufficiency: A rational approach. Birth 14(4):182–190, December 1987
26. Walker M: Management of selected early breastfeeding problems seen in clinical practice. Birth 16(3):148–158, September 1989
27. Auerbach KG: Breastfeeding fallacies: Their relationship to understanding lactation. Birth 17(1):44–49, March 1990
28. Jelliffe DB, Jelliffe EFP: Human Milk in the Modern World, p 30. Oxford University Press, 1978
29. Neifert M, DeMarzo S, Seacat J et al: The influence of breast surgery, breast appearance, and pregnancy-induced breast changes on lactation sufficiency as measured by infant weight gain. Birth 17(1):31–38, March 1990
30. National Research Council, Subcommittee on the Tenth Edition of the RDAs: Recommended Dietary Allowances. Washington, DC, National Academy Press, 1989
31. Gaskin IM: Babies, breastfeeding and bonding. Massachusetts, Bergin & Garvey Publishers, 1987
32. Moore JF, Jansa N: A survey of policies and practices in support of breastfeeding mothers in the workplace. Birth 14(4):191–195, December 1987
33. Broome ME: Breastfeeding and the working mother. JOGNN 10(3):201–202, May/June 1985
34. Auerbach KG: Employed breastfeeding mothers: Problems they encounter. Birth 11(1):17–20, Spring 1984
35. American Academy of Pediatrics, Committee on Nutri-

tion: Commentary on breast feeding and infant formulas, including proposed standards for formulas. Pediatrics 57:278–285, February 1976

36. Woodruff C: The science of infant nutrition and the art of infant feeding. JAMA 240(7):657–661, August 18, 1978

37. Slattery J: Nutrition for the normal healthy infant. MCN 2(2):105–112, March/April 1977

38. Hughes RB, Sauvain KJ, Blanton LH et al: Outcome of teaching clean vs terminal methods of formula preparation. Pediatric Nursing 13(4):275–276, 1987

39. Parham E: The effect of early feeding on the development of obesity. JOGN 3(3):58–61, May/June 1975

40. Ream S, Murray S, Nath C et al: Infant nutrition and supplements. JOGNN 14(5):371–376, September/October 1985

■ SUGGESTED READINGS

Beall MH: Drugs and breastfeeding. In Petrie RH (ed): Perinatal Pharmacology, pp 419–425. Oradell, NJ, Medical Economics Company, 1989

Chandra RK: Long-term health implications of mode of infant feeding. Nutrition Research 9:1–3, 1989

Hamosh M: Breast milk jaundice (editorial). J Pediatr Gastroenterol Nutr 11:145–149, 1990

Hawkins LM, Nichols FH, Tanner JL: Predictors of the duration of breastfeeding in low-income women. Birth 14(4);204–209, December 1987

Hewat RJ, Ellis DJ: A comparison of the effectiveness of two methods of nipple care. Birth 14(1):41–45, March 1987

Humenick SS: The clinical significance of breastmilk maturation rates. Birth 14(4):174–181, December 1987

Kearney MH, Cronenwett LR, Barrett JA: Breast-feeding problems in the first week postpartum. Nurs Res 39(2): 90–95, 1990

Lawrence RA: Breastfeeding—A Guide for the Medical Profession, 3rd ed. St Louis, CV Mosby, 1989

Marmet C, Shell E: Training neonates to suck correctly. MCN 9(6):401–407, November/December 1984

Minchin M: Infant formula: A mass, uncontrolled trial in perinatal care. Birth 14(1):25–35, March 1987

Page-Goertz S: Discharge planning for the breastfeeding dyad. Pediatric Nursing 15(5):543–544, September/October 1989

Walker M, Driscoll JW: Sore nipples: The new mother's nemesis. MCN 14:260–265, July/August 1989

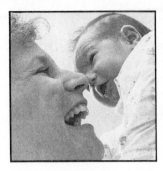

Unit VI
Assessment and Management in the Postpartum Period

CONFERENCE MATERIAL

1. Discuss in detail the mechanisms by which lactation occurs, including hormonal preparation of the breasts, neurohormonal control of milk secretion and ejection, effects of noxious stimuli, and approaches to the suppression of lactation. What implications for nursing care can be found by understanding the physiology of this delicate mechanism?

2. Describe the patterns of return of menstruation and ovulation in nonlactating and lactating women. Include in your discussion anovulatory versus ovulatory menses, the influence of breast-feeding on both ovulation and menstruation, and the risk of pregnancy with unprotected intercourse. How would you counsel a postpartum patient who was (a) not breast-feeding, and (b) one who was breastfeeding about what to expect regarding first menstruation and return of fertility?

3. A mother experienced a sudden postpartum hemorrhage after delivery and the infant had to be taken to the nursery immediately after birth. What assessments and interventions might you plan to aid in reinstituting the bonding process?

4. Rita R. delivered her second baby 3 days ago and is to be discharged this afternoon. Mother and infant are healthy and have adapted well to each other during their hospital stay. Rita is breast-feeding and her milk just began to come in today. Her husband, who will take her home later, has been able to take 1 week off from work. Their child at home is 2½ years of age. You have set aside 30 minutes to counsel Rita about the first few weeks at home. What topics will you include in this discussion, and what key points will you make concerning each? How did you set priorities for these topics?

5. Elizabeth S. is an 18-year-old primipara who underwent a long but normal labor and delivery. She and her 20-year-old husband are fascinated with their new son, although neither have experience caring for children. On her second postpartum day, Elizabeth experiences severe discomfort from her large mediolateral episiotomy, to the point of not wanting to care for the baby. What measures will you initiate to promote her comfort? What will be the primary focus of your nursing care plans for the remainder of her hospital stay?

6. What approach would you use to help a mother who was undecided about whether or not to breast-feed her infant?

7. A mother tells the nurse that she wants to breast-feed her infant for 6 months to 8 months because she knows she cannot become pregnant as long as she is nursing. What information should the nurse include in her reply?

8. A mother who is bottle-feeding tells the nurse she does not know anything about preparing formula so she thinks she will buy "ready-to-feed" formula that comes in bottles. What do you think about this plan? How can the nurse help her in choosing the type of formula to use and the method of preparation?

9. What criteria would you use to assess whether or not new parents are making a successful role transition to parenthood?

MULTIPLE CHOICE

Read through the entire question and place your answer on the line to the right.

1. Vital areas in the transition to parenthood for the couple are
   A. The early events the parents experience in the pregnancy
   B. The needs of the parents as a couple
   C. The presence of reliable supports such as grandparents
   D. The needs of each person in the system as an individual
   E. The unconscious motivation of the couple for the pregnancy
   F. The influence of the parent-child interaction over time
   G. The content of the parent-child relationship only
   H. Mainly the quality of the parents' own childhood relationships

Select the number corresponding to the correct letter or letters.
   1. All but A
   2. B, C, D, H
   3. B, D, F

4. All but G
5. A, C, D, E _____

2. Engrossment refers to
    A. The behavior noted in fathers when they are interacting with their infants
    B. The infant becoming interested in moving objects and smiling faces
    C. The behavior noted in mothers when they are interacting with their infants
    D. The behavior noted in family members when they are interacting with the infant

Select the number corresponding to the correct letter or letters.
    1. A only
    2. B only
    3. C only
    4. C and D
    5. A and C
    6. All but B _____

3. The most useful way(s) to view how individuals assume the parental role is/are
    A. Becoming a parent is a role transition.
    B. Becoming a parent is a crisis situation.
    C. Becoming a parent is both a crisis and a transition.
    D. Becoming a parent depends primarily on the ability of the individuals to totally redefine their relationship.

Select the number corresponding to the correct letter or letters
    1. A only
    2. B only
    3. C only
    4. C and D _____

4. Factors associated with positive attachment and bonding include
    A. Preconditions of emotional health, trust, social supports, infant proximity, competent communication, temperament "fit"
    B. Mutuality of interaction
    C. Claiming behaviors leading to identification of the infant
    D. Positive reciprocal feedback
    E. A strong social support system
    F. A reasonably good tempered infant

Select the number corresponding to the correct letter or letters.
    1. A, E, F
    2. B, C, D, F
    3. A, B, F
    4. All but E and F
    5. All but A
    6. All but A and F _____

5. To keep the nipples in good condition for breast-feeding, which of the following should be included in their daily care?

A. Wash with plain water once a day.
B. Air dry after each nursing period.
C. Wash with mild antiseptic solution before each feeding period.
D. Cover the nipples with clean plastic squares to avoid contamination.
E. If nipple is sore, discontinue breast-feeding until tenderness subsides.

Select the number corresponding to the correct letters.
    1. A and B
    2. A, C, and D
    3. B, D, and E
    4. All of the above _____

6. The young mother asks how she will know when her baby is hungry. Which of the following responses would be most appropriate for the nurse to give?
    A. "All crying indicates hunger."
    B. "Feed the baby whenever he is awake."
    C. "He will cry, fret, and suck on anything in contact with his lips."
    D. "Offer him water first; if he refuses the water, feed him." _____

7. How does the composition of mother's milk compare with cow's milk?
    A. Human milk contains more whey protein.
    B. Human milk contains more casein.
    C. Human milk forms a tougher curd.
    D. Human milk contains more carbohydrates.
    E. Human milk contains less sodium.

Select the number corresponding to the correct letters.
    1. A and C
    2. A, D, and E
    3. B, C, and D
    4. All of the above _____

8. Which of the following is true of the let-down reflex?
    A. It occurs unilaterally.
    B. It is under voluntary control.
    C. It is usually felt by the mother as a tingling or drawing sensation in the nipple.
    D. It is not affected by external stimuli. _____

9. What is the principle underlying the concept of demand feedings for the newborn infant?
    A. Maintaining a regular 4-hour schedule to establish eating habits
    B. Feeding the infant every 2 to 3 hours to stimulate digestion
    C. Fitting individual feedings to individual needs
    D. Permissive feeding schedule causes less conflict with the mother's household activities.
    E. More frequent feedings ensure an adequate nutritional intake. _____

10. Identify the statement that *best* describes taste perception in the newborn.
    A. Newborns possess fine taste acuity, which develops *in utero*.

B. Newborns possess an innate preference for sweet substances.

C. Newborns are unable to differentiate sweet taste from bitter taste. _____

11. The proliferation of human brain cells occurs during the

A. First half of pregnancy
B. Second half of pregnancy
C. First 6 months of life
D. Second 6 months of life _____

12. The most important benefit of vestibular stimulation in the normal newborn is improvement of

A. Sucking capability
B. Tactile sensitivity
C. Motor coordination
D. Attention span _____

13. The nurse is conducting a parenting class in the postpartum unit. Based on an understanding of the newborn's sensory needs, mothers could be advised to

A. Continuously rock their newborns during feeding
B. Stroke their newborns from toe to head daily
C. Provide auditory stimulation for 10 minutes each hour
D. Sing to infants in the *en face* position _____

DISCUSSION

14. The removal of the inhibitory effect of which two hormones, in the presence of continued secretion of which other hormone, are keys to the initiation of lactation?

15. Why is it important for mother, father, and newborn to spend some time together privately during the first hour after birth?

UNIT VII

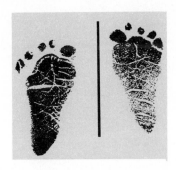

*Assessment
and
Management
of High Risk
Maternal
Conditions*

33

Pregnancy-Related Complications

HEMORRHAGIC COMPLICATIONS OF EARLY PREGNANCY
Abortion
Incompetent Cervical Os
Ectopic Pregnancy
Hydatidiform Mole

Choriocarcinoma
Hyperemesis Gravidarum
HEMORRHAGIC COMPLICATIONS OF LATE PREGNANCY
Placenta Previa
Abruptio Placentae

Other Problems Associated with Bleeding
    Hypofibrinogenemia
    Disseminated Intravascular Coagulation
HYPERTENSIVE DISORDERS OF PREGNANCY
Classification

Etiology and Pathophysiology of PIH
Preeclampsia
Eclampsia
Chronic Hypertension (With and Without Superimposed Preeclampsia)

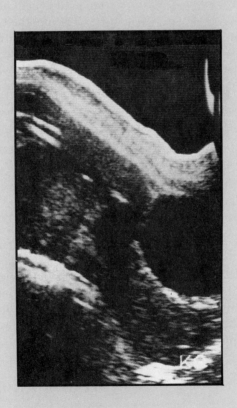

Although childbearing is considered a normal process, a number of physiological adaptations occur during the course of pregnancy that make the boundaries between health and illness less distinct. The well-being of mother and unborn child is enhanced by the existence of a healthy maternal condition prior to conception and the early and continued provision of health supervision during pregnancy. Regular prenatal care is of paramount importance in achieving a good perinatal outcome. It facilitates early detection of the warning signals of potential, unexpected alterations from the normal course of pregnancy. Serious problems can be averted or controlled by preventive care, client education, and implementation of appropriate interventions.

Pregnancy-related maternal disorders are divided into two broad categories: (1) complications related to pregnancy and not seen at other times; and (2) diseases that are not pregnancy related but occur coincidentally. The latter may arise in the nonpregnant woman as well, but when they occur during pregnancy, they may complicate the pregnancy and influence its course or may be aggravated by the pregnancy. Such conditions are considered in Chapter 34.

There are only a few major complications that result from pregnancy, but these may present serious health hazards. These complications, which will be considered here, include the following: hemorrhagic conditions of early pregnancy, hyperemesis gravidarum, hemorrhagic complications of placental origin in late pregnancy, and hypertensive disorders of pregnancy.

■ HEMORRHAGIC COMPLICATIONS OF EARLY PREGNANCY

The causes of bleeding in pregnancy are usually considered in relation to the stage of gestation in which they are most likely to cause complications. Frequent causes of bleeding during the first half of pregnancy are abortion, ectopic pregnancy, and hydatidiform mole. The two most common causes of hemorrhage in the latter half of pregnancy are placenta previa and abruptio placentae.

Abortion

DEFINITIONS

Abortion is the termination of pregnancy at any time before the fetus has attained a stage of viability (i.e.,

before it is capable of extrauterine existence). The term *miscarriage* is commonly used by lay persons to denote an abortion that has occurred spontaneously rather than one that has been induced. Spontaneous abortions occur in about 10% to 20% of all pregnancies.

Fetal weight is an important criterion often used to distinguish an abortion from a *preterm delivery*. A preterm infant is one born after the stage of viability has been reached but before it has the same chance for survival as a full-term infant. By general consensus, an infant that weights 2500 g or less at birth is termed *preterm*; one that weighs 2501 g (5½ lb) or more is regarded as *full term*. Because modern advances in the management and care of preterm infants have made it possible for smaller and smaller infants to survive, it is not uncommon for infants weighing less than 750 g (1 lb, 10½ oz) to survive. For this reason, many authorities now maintain that fetal weight of 1000 g or less but more than 500 g is classified as *immature* and that fetal weight of 500 g (about 20 weeks' gestation) or less constitutes an *abortion*. In many states, a birth certificate is prepared for any pregnancy terminating beyond the 20th week of gestation or when the fetus weighs 500 g or more. The classification of how a pregnancy is terminated in different hospitals depends on the interpretation to which they subscribe.

It is important to remember that preterm labor does not refer to abortion. *Preterm labor* is the termination of pregnancy after the fetus is viable but before it has attained full term. Although the cause of many preterm labors cannot be explained, the condition can be brought on by maternal diseases such as chronic hypertensive vascular disease, abruptio placentae, placenta previa, untreated syphilis, congenital uterine anomalies, or mechanical defects in the cervix.

TYPES OF ABORTIONS

The term *abortion* includes many varieties of termination of pregnancy prior to viability but may be subdivided into two main groups: spontaneous and induced. *Spontaneous abortion* is one in which the process starts of its own accord through natural causes. *Induced abortion* is one that is artificially induced, whether for therapeutic or other reasons. Induced abortion has been considered in Chapter 12. The diagnosis of the abortion a woman is undergoing is determined by the signs and symptoms present (see Box on page 774).

MANIFESTATIONS AND CAUSES

Clinical Picture. About 80% of all spontaneous abortions occur during the first 12 weeks of pregnancy.[1] The condition is very common; it is estimated that 15% to 20% of all pregnancies terminate in spontaneous abortion.[2] Spontaneous abortions generally occur 1 to 3

Research Highlight

Lack of accuracy in estimations of blood loss may lead to a lack of consistency in patient assessment and documentation. Luegenbiehl et al explored whether the introduction of a standard for estimating blood loss would increase accuracy and consistency among nurses.

A sample of 42 staff members and student nurse volunteers from the obstetric, gynecologic, and neonatal units were asked to estimate blood loss from predetermined measured amounts on 24 peripads, 12 from brand C and 12 from brand G. Each participant completed a data sheet with demographic information, a list of common blood loss descriptors, and a section to record a descriptive term and cubic centimeter amount for each blood-saturated peripad. On the second test day, an educational program was given to the participants regarding guidelines to describe and estimate amounts of blood loss consistently. Following the program, the participants were asked to estimate the amount of blood loss on the same 24 peripads. Accuracy and consistency increased when using cubic centimeters to estimate blood loss on peripads. Consistency increased but accuracy did not when estimations were given using descriptive terms. The researchers also found that accuracy was influenced by the pad brand or type.

These results suggest that nursing can improve the validity of statements regarding blood loss by using a consistent standard for estimation. By accurately estimating blood loss, assessments will improve leading to timely intervention for the bleeder. Consistency among the nursing staff in estimating blood loss should enable each nurse to assess the total blood loss and report accurate findings to the physician. Valid nursing assessment leads to optimal patient care and increases trust between nurses and physicians.

Luegenbiehl DL, Brophy GH, Artique GS, et al: Standardized assessment of blood loss. MCN 15:241–244, July/August 1990.

weeks after the death of the embryo or fetus. Almost invariably the first symptom is bleeding due to the separation of the fertilized ovum from its uterine attachment. The bleeding is often slight at the beginning and may persist for days before uterine cramps occur, or the bleeding may be followed at once by cramps. Occasionally, slight hemorrhage may persist for weeks. The uterine contractions bring about softening and dilatation of the cervix and either complete or incomplete expulsion of the products of conception.

Causes. The etiology of spontaneous abortion is varied and often is nature's way of extinguishing imperfect embryos. Microscopic study of the material passed in these cases shows that the most common cause of spontaneous abortion is an inherent defect in the products of conception. This defect may express itself in an abnormal embryo, an abnormal trophoblast, or both abnormalities.

In first-trimester abortions, 80% are associated with some defect of the embryo or trophoblast that is either incompatible with life or would result in a grossly deformed child.[3] The incidence of abnormalities due to chromosomal errors in the second trimester is about 53%.[3] It is usually difficult, if not impossible, to determine whether the germ plasma of the spermatozoon or the ovum is at fault in these cases.

Abortions of this sort are obviously not preventable;

however, even though they are often bitterly disappointing to the parents, they do serve a useful purpose.

Spontaneous abortions may result from causes other than defects in the products of conception. Severe acute infections, such as pneumonia, pyelitis, and typhoid fever, often lead to abortion. Endocrine disorders affecting progesterone and estrogen levels may alter the endometrial lining of the uterus and result in abortion. Occasionally, abnormalities of the generative tract, such as a congenitally short cervix or uterine malformations, produce the accident. Abortion is common in women whose mothers were treated with diethylstilbestrol during pregnancy. Retroposition of the uterus rarely causes abortion, as was formerly believed. Many women tend to explain abortion as a result of an injury or excessive activity. Women exhibit the greatest variation in this respect. In some women, the pregnancy may go blithely on despite falls, automobile accidents, and different trauma. In others, a trivial fall, anxiety, or overfatigue may appear to be related to abortion, but there is obviously no way to determine a cause–effect relationship.

MEDICAL DIAGNOSIS AND PROGNOSIS

Determination of the cause of vaginal bleeding in early pregnancy is essential for accurate diagnosis. The vagina and cervix are carefully inspected to ascertain possible

Types of Abortions and Related Symptoms

Threatened Abortion	Vaginal bleeding or spotting occurring in early pregnancy that may or may not be associated with mild cramps; closed cervix; the process may abate or result in an abortion.
Inevitable Abortion	The above process has progressed such that termination of the pregnancy cannot be prevented; bleeding is moderate to copious; uterine cramping is moderate to severe; the membranes may or may not have ruptured; the cervical canal is dilating.
Incomplete Abortion	Part of the products of conception has been passed, but part (usually the placenta) is retained in the uterus; heavy bleeding usually persists until the retained products of conception have been passed; uterine cramping is severe; the cervix is open, with tissue present.
Complete Abortion	All of the products of conception have been expelled; bleeding is slight; uterine cramping is mild.
Missed Abortion	The fetus dies in utero but is retained; regression in uterine growth and breast changes is present; if 6 weeks or more elapse between fetal death and expulsion, degenerative changes occur, e.g., maceration (general softening), mummification (drying up into a leatherlike structure) and, rarely, lithopedion formation (stony material); symptoms, except for amenorrhea, are usually lacking; malaise, headache, and anorexia are occasionally present; hypofibrinogenemia may result; the condition may be discovered because fundal height fails to increase and/or fetal heart tones are absent.
Habitual Abortion	Spontaneous abortion occurs in successive pregnancies (three or more).
Illegal Abortion	Termination of pregnancy outside of appropriate medical facilities (e.g., hospitals or clinics), generally by nonphysician abortionists; the frequency of such abortions is not precisely known but has dropped precipitously in the United States because of legalized abortion; the method may involve ingestion of drugs, such as quinine or castor oil, or the placement of a foreign body, such as a urethral catheter, into the uterus with or without the instillation of toxic substances; severe infection, often with shock and renal failure, may result.

causes of the bleeding and to determine if the cervix is dilated.

Ultrasound techniques are used to differentiate between a live fetus and a pregnancy that will end inevitably in spontaneous abortion. Prognosis is evaluated by ultrasound markers that can explain bleeding and distinguish between harmless and ominous blood loss. The accompanying clinical symptoms of pelvic cramping and low back pain are suggestive of spontaneous abortion.

In women in whom bleeding is scant and does not extend beyond 3 days and when the ultrasound scan is normal, the risk of pregnancy failure is lower than in women who bleed for 3 days or more and have at least one abnormality on ultrasound examination.[4] Epidemiologic studies have revealed that the risk of spontaneous premature birth or the term delivery of a low-birth-weight infant is significantly correlated with threatened abortion.[5] Additional associated maternal complications include preeclampsia, placenta previa, abruptio placentae, and breech delivery.

MEDICAL MANAGEMENT

The pregnant woman should be instructed to contact her physician or midwife whenever bleeding occurs during pregnancy. The client may be kept at home, and bedrest and sexual abstinence are prescribed. Occasionally, sedatives are ordered to promote relaxation. If bleeding becomes copious and is accompanied by cramps or uterine contractions, hospitalization may be recommended. Intravenous (IV) therapy for fluid replacement or blood transfusions is prescribed as necessary.

In cases of incomplete abortion, efforts are ordinarily made to aid the uterus in emptying its contents. Because there is a danger of maternal hemorrhage, oxytocin may be administered, but if this is ineffectual, surgical removal of the retained products of conception should be done promptly. Active bleeding may make this urgently necessary. Many times the tissue is loose in the cervical canal and can simply be lifted out with ovum forceps; otherwise, dilatation and curettage of the uterine cavity or vacuum extraction may be necessary.

In cases of missed abortion, the products of conception are often spontaneously expelled within 4 to 5 weeks of fetal death. If this does not occur, surgical removal of the abortus is necessary. The administration of RhoD immune globulin (RhoGAM) within 72 hours after the abortion is indicated for Rh-negative women who have not been previously sensitized.

If evidence of infection is present (e.g., fever, foul discharge), evacuation of the uterus should be delayed only long enough to obtain appropriate studies (especially smears and cultures) and to initiate antibiotic therapy. Such prompt and aggressive management of the woman with an infected abortion effectively reduces the incidence of more serious complications, such as septic shock, thrombophlebitis, and renal failure, as well as the morbidity rate and hospital stay.

NURSING ASSESSMENT

Bleeding in the first half of pregnancy, no matter how slight, always must be considered as threatened abortion. The nurse must first obtain a detailed, accurate history, including length of gestation, source of prenatal supervision, and the onset, duration, and intensity of the bleeding episode. The client should be asked to describe the quantity of bleeding in amounts that she can relate to (e.g., a teaspoon, one-half cup). The nature of the blood loss must similarly be assessed (e.g., bright red or dark brown, with or without tissue fragments or mucus, malodorous, steady trickling of blood or intermittent spotting). The presence, nature, and location of accompanying discomforts such as cramping, dull or sharp pain, and dizziness are evaluated.

Assessment of blood loss for hospitalized women often includes weighing perineal pads before and after use and then subtracting to find the difference (see Research Highlight). When tissue is present on the pad, it is useful to examine the products of conception to ascertain whether the abortion is complete.

NURSING DIAGNOSIS

As a result of the comprehensive assessment of the woman with hemorrhagic complications of early pregnancy, nursing diagnoses are formulated. The classification of diagnostic labels will vary, depending on the presenting nursing problems, and is likely to focus on the unexpected physiological alterations occurring in the reproductive system during the first trimester. An example of this type of potential or actual diagnosis is knowledge deficit related to physiological alterations occurring in the reproductive system. Other related diagnoses may include fluid volume deficit related to bleeding complication of early pregnancy; high risk for infection related to excessive fluid volume deficit; and

grieving about actual or threatened loss of pregnancy. Additional diagnoses may be identified as new information about the client is gathered or as the client's condition changes owing to progressive alterations in physiological status or recovery.

NURSING INTERVENTION

Interventions are planned based on the type of abortion, prognosis, and nursing diagnoses. The client at home is generally on restricted activity. If she is having only slight vaginal bleeding or even spotting without pain, she should be instructed to stay in bed and eat a well-balanced diet. Some midwives and physicians may not recommend restricted activity, based on the concept that the uterus is well insulated from outside influences. The client should be counseled to save all perineal pads, as well as all tissue and clots passed, for inspection. In cases in which bedrest has been prescribed, if the bleeding disappears within 48 hours, the woman may get out of bed but should limit her activities for the next several days. The nurse should counsel the client to avoid coitus for 2 weeks following the last evidence of bleeding or as otherwise recommended by the physician.

Psychosocial support is of prime importance because bleeding episodes are frightening and anxiety provoking for all pregnant women. Emotional reactions of shock and disbelief are normal responses experienced regardless of the category of abortion. The woman often searches for answers regarding the cause of her condition. She may express guilt and blame herself for behaviors that contributed to the situation. Verbalizations of feelings should be encouraged among all family members. The nurse should respond to concerns by offering accurate information on the cause of most spontaneous abortions and any facts specifically related to the actual case. False reassurance that "everything will be all right" should be avoided because in fact the client may lose her pregnancy.

Particular consideration is given to the special needs of the habitual aborter. Her prognosis for carrying a pregnancy to term decreases with each successive abortion. A complete diagnostic workup is necessary to determine the cause and treatments indicated.

NURSING EVALUATION

The expected outcomes of nursing intervention, as follows, are that the woman with a hemorrhagic complication of early pregnancy:

- Understands the physiological alterations occurring with her condition and related treatment
- Has her fluid volume deficit corrected

- Has complications prevented (e.g., infection) because of careful assessment and management
- Appropriately progresses through the grieving process

Incompetent Cervical Os

An incompetent cervical os is a mechanical defect in the cervix that causes it to dilate prematurely during the midtrimester of pregnancy, resulting in late habitual abortion or preterm labor. This relatively uncommon condition may be caused by congenital anomalies of the uterus or the cervix or prior trauma. The symptoms include painless dilatation, presence of bloody show, and premature rupture of the membranes.

When repeated termination of pregnancy in the second trimester is due to an anatomical factor, a surgical treatment known as *cervical cerclage* may be performed to prevent relaxation and dilation of the cervix. A modified *Shirodkar technique* or the *McDonald technique* is most commonly used in this procedure. In the former technique, the vaginal mucous membrane is elevated, a band of homologous fascia or a narrow strip of some material such as Mersilene is carried around the internal os and tied, and then the vaginal mucosa is restored to its original position and sutured. The McDonald technique is a simpler procedure involving placement of a nonabsorbable suture around the cervix high on the cervical mucosa. Cerclage may be done at approximately 12 to 14 weeks' gestation. Success rates with both the McDonald and the Shirodkar procedure are now approaching 80% to 90%.[2]

Postoperatively, the main concerns are monitoring fetal heart rate and observing for signs of rupture of the membranes or uterine contractions. If the membranes rupture, the suture must be removed and the uterus emptied because of the risk of infection. If contractions ensue, the client should be placed on bedrest and a pharmacologic agent such as ritodrine hydrochloride may be given in an effort to control the contractions.

The cerclage is frequently removed after week 37 of gestation. This is often followed by the onset of labor and a relatively rapid delivery. In some situations, cesarean delivery may be elected to preserve the suture for future pregnancies.

Ectopic Pregnancy

An ectopic pregnancy is any gestation located outside the uterine cavity. Most ectopic pregnancies are tubal gestations located most frequently in the ampullar portion of the fallopian tube; the isthmus portion is the next most frequent site (Fig. 33-1). Other types, which make up about 5% of all ectopic pregnancies, are interstitial (in the interstitial portion of the tube), cornual (in a rudimentary horn of a uterus), cervical, abdominal, and ovarian gestations.

The rate of ectopic pregnancy in the United States increased fourfold between 1970 and 1987, from 4.5 to 16.8 per 1000 pregnancies in women between 15 and 44 years of age.[6] Although the actual number of deaths from ectopic pregnancies has declined during this period, the percentage of all maternal deaths attributed to this condition has increased. Ectopic pregnancies are now the second leading cause of maternal mortality in this country.[3] Reported rates of ectopic pregnancies are 40% higher among women of African-American and other minority races than among white women.[6] The incidence of the disease is particularly high in women between 35 and 44 years of age. The chances of a woman having a repeat ectopic pregnancy are reported to be between 5% and 20%.[7,8]

About once in every 200 pregnancies, the fertilized ovum, instead of traversing the length of the fallopian tube to reach the uterine cavity, becomes implanted within the walls of the fallopian tube. Because the wall of the tube is not sufficiently elastic to allow the fertilized ovum to grow and develop there, rupture of the tubal wall is the inevitable result. Rupture most frequently occurs into the tubal lumen, with the passage of the products of conception, together with much blood, out the fimbriated end of the tube and into the peritoneal cavity, a so-called tubal abortion. Rupture may occur through the peritoneal surface of the tube directly into the peritoneal cavity; again, there is an outpouring of blood into the abdomen from vessels at the site of rupture. In either case, rupture usually occurs within the first 12 weeks of pregnancy.

Occasionally, an ectopic pregnancy may develop in that portion of the tube that passes through the uterine wall, a type known as *interstitial pregnancy*. In very rare instances, the products of conception, after rupturing through the tubal wall, may become implanted on the peritoneum. This extraordinary occurrence, known as an *abdominal pregnancy*, may in some cases result in delivery of a live infant via an abdominal incision.

MANIFESTATIONS AND CAUSES

Clinical Picture. The clinical symptoms of ectopic pregnancy are likely to vary, depending on the site of implantation. In cases of unruptured ectopic pregnancy, vague and variable discomforts may develop. At first, the woman exhibits the usual early signs of pregnancy and, as a rule, regards herself as being normally pregnant. Vaginal bleeding often appears scant and dark brown. Within 3 to 5 weeks after a missed menstrual period, abdominal pain often develops. The nature, duration, and intensity of pain vary considerably with the length of gestation, site of implantation, and extent of

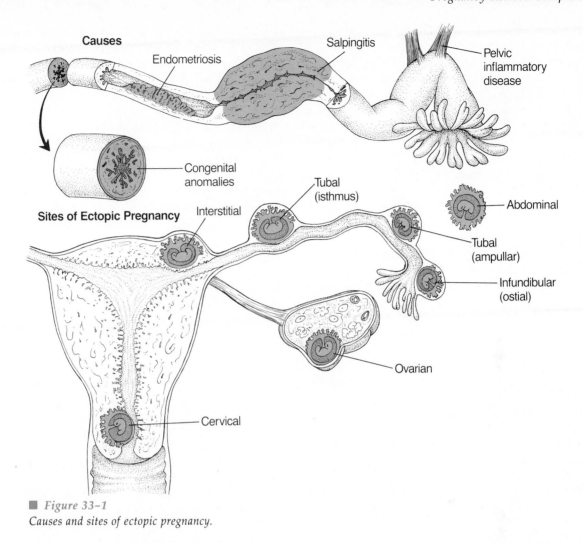

■ *Figure 33–1*
Causes and sites of ectopic pregnancy.

blood loss. Pain is the predominant symptom of tubal rupture and may be localized on one side or felt over the entire abdomen. The woman may complain of cramping or sharp, sudden, knifelike pain, often of extreme severity. Shoulder-tip pain may be present when intraperitoneal bleeding has extended to the diaphragm (phrenic nerve). Depending on the amount of blood loss, the woman may or may not manifest syncope, hypotension, tachycardia, and other symptoms of shock.

Causes. A tubal ectopic pregnancy may be caused by any condition that narrows the tube or brings about some constriction within it. Under such circumstances, the tubal lumen is large enough to allow spermatozoa to ascend the tube but not big enough to permit the downward passage of the fertilized ovum (see Fig. 33-1). Among the conditions that may produce such a narrowing of the fallopian tube are (1) previous pelvic inflammatory disease involving the tubal mucosa and producing partial agglutination of opposing surfaces, for example, chlamydia, gonorrheal salpingitis; (2) previous inflammatory processes of the external peritoneal surfaces of the tube, for example, puerperal and postabortal infections; (3) endometriosis of the tubal wall and lumen; (4) developmental abnormalities resulting in a segmental narrowing of the tubes or excessive length or kinking; and (5) previous abdominal or tubal surgery with resultant scarring and adhesions. Other factors that may potentially contribute to the incidence of ectopic pregnancies include smoking, previous tubal sterilization, and the use of low-dose progestogen oral contraceptives.[9-13] A woman who becomes pregnant with an intrauterine device (IUD) inserted has a tenfold greater chance that the pregnancy will be ectopic than if the device were not being used.[14] Although an association between prior induced abortions and increased risk of ectopic pregnancies has been suggested, little evidence exists to support this claim in women without postabortion complications.[15,16]

MEDICAL MANAGEMENT

The therapeutic goal of medical management is early diagnosis of ectopic pregnancy based on a detailed health history, physical examination, and selected diagnostic tests. The diagnostic procedures include tests for human chorionic gonadotropin (hCG), culdocentesis, curettage, colpotomy, laparoscopy, and ultrasonography. Hormonal levels of hCG are usually lower in ectopic pregnancies than in uterine pregnancies of the same gestational period.[3] The absence of ultrasonic evidence of an intrauterine pregnancy accompanied by a positive pregnancy test, with fluid in the cul-de-sac or an abnormal pelvic mass, are often diagnostic of an ectopic pregnancy.[3]

In the past, treatment of tubal pregnancy most often was salpingectomy with or without ipsilateral oophorectomy. Medical procedures that favor tubal conservation are being applied more frequently in current practice. Earlier diagnosis of ectopic pregnancy through improved techniques has made this type of conservative management possible. If the woman has no history of infertility and no gross evidence of previous salpingitis, a salpingotomy, salpingostomy, or segmental resection and anastomosis may be performed. A salpingostomy is done to remove a small pregnancy via a linear incision on the antimesenteric border over the ectopic site. The procedure for salpingotomy involves making a longitudinal incision and removing the products of conception via forceps or suction.

Postoperative management is directed toward maintaining homeostasis. In cases of ruptured ectopic pregnancy, intervention is aimed at combating shock. RhoGAM should be prescribed to protect against isoimmunization in the unsensitized Rho-negative woman.

NURSING ASSESSMENT

The initial assessment should focus on the classic three symptoms of an ectopic pregnancy: *missed menstruation* followed by *abdominal pain* and *vaginal spotting*. Abdominal pain, the most common sign of ectopic pregnancy, is often described as "crampy," "dull," or "restricting to the shoulder and back." The patient should be questioned on contraceptive method, particularly the current use of an IUD. A history of previous tubal damage caused by disease or developmental problems further supports the likelihood of a tubal pregnancy.

Vital signs are assessed; however, these may not differ markedly from normal values unless tubal rupture and internal bleeding have occurred. During the pelvic examination, the patient is assessed for fullness in the cul-de-sac, cervical pain, and adnexal tenderness. The uterus is generally not enlarged beyond the 8 weeks' gestational size. Laboratory analysis frequently reveals falling hematocrit and hemoglobin levels and leukocytosis.

The amount of bleeding evident may be a poor indicator of the severity of the situation, because blood loss may be concealed in the pelvic cavity. Extensive

blood loss leading to hypovolemic shock may be revealed through a rapid, thready pulse; tachypnea; and hypotension. The umbilicus may display a blue tinge (Cullen's sign), indicating bleeding in the peritoneal cavity.

NURSING DIAGNOSIS

Based on the nursing assessment and differential medical findings, nursing diagnoses are identified. These are most likely to relate to the presenting problem of fluid-volume deficit secondary to rupture at the implantation site. The high risk for infection secondary to this hemorrhagic disorder is another nursing problem that should be given careful consideration. Similar to the woman experiencing a spontaneous abortion, the client with an ectopic pregnancy is also in a state of grieving related to her actual or anticipated loss of the pregnancy.

NURSING INTERVENTION

The nurse explains the various diagnostic tests and provides support for the patient with a suspected ectopic pregnancy. When acute rupture of a fallopian tube occurs, the situation presents a surgical emergency requiring nursing care aimed at combating shock. An IV infusion is maintained so that blood or plasma expanders can be administered as needed to replace losses from the hemorrhage and surgery.

During the postoperative period, vital signs are carefully monitored, fluid replacement is continued, and intake and output are recorded. Oral intake of foods and fluids should be avoided until bowel function has returned to normal. Early ambulation is encouraged. The nurse must accurately record the perineal pad count. The surgical site may require special care and dressings. Patients are often given broad-spectrum antibiotics prophylactically. Steroids are administered to decrease the postoperative inflammation that can contribute to the development of adhesions.

Emotional care is directed toward facilitating effective coping by encouraging the patient and her family to verbalize their feelings, allowing them privacy to grieve the death of the fetus, and listening to their concerns about future chances for a successful pregnancy.[10] Information about the causes of ectopic pregnancy may assist them in resolving feelings of guilt and self-blame.

NURSING EVALUATION

Anticipated outcomes of nursing care, as follows, are that the woman with an ectopic pregnancy:

- Understands the pathophysiology of her condition and treatment alternatives
- Has complications (e.g., fluid volume deficit and

infection) prevented because of careful assessment and management
- Appropriately progresses through the grieving process and accepts the loss of her child

Hydatidiform Mole

Hydatidiform mole is a gestational trophoblastic neoplasm that arises from the chorion. Two types of molar growth, *partial* and *complete*, exist that have distinct cytogenic origins, pathologic characteristics, and clinical manifestations. The *partial mole* is characterized by normal villi intermingled with hydropic villi and some fetal material or an amnionic sac. It is usually associated with one haploid maternal and two haploid paternal sets of chromosomes (triploid karyotype). The *complete* mole is characterized by a large amount of edematous enlarged villi without a fetus or fetal membranes. The genetic composition is almost uniformly diploid with paternal chromosomal markers; most are 46,XX; however, a small percentage have a 46,XY karyotype.[17] The mole has a grapelike appearance with clusters of vesicles on all of part of the decidual lining of the uterus (Fig. 33-2).

Hydatidiform mole is rather an uncommon condition, occurring about once in every 1500 to 2000 pregnancies in the United States and Europe. The ratio of partial to complete moles is approximately 2:1.[18] The incidence of this complication is much higher among Asian women.

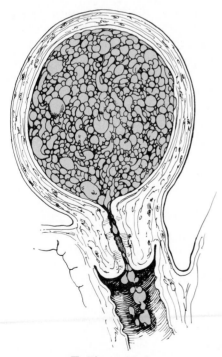

■ *Figure 33–2*
Hydatidiform mole.

MANIFESTATIONS AND CAUSES

Clinical Picture. The pregnancy appears to be normal at first, although in about one third to one half of women with complete moles, the uterus is larger than expected for gestational dates. Initial hCG levels are lower in patients with a partial mole than those with a complete mole. Bleeding is a common symptom and may vary from brownish-red spotting to heavy bright red. Vomiting in a rather severe form may appear early. Fetal heart tones are absent in the presence of other signs of pregnancy. Preeclampsia may appear before the 20th week of gestation. Women with partial moles typically have a clinical diagnosis of spontaneous or missed abortion. Vesicles may be evident in the vaginal discharge of the abortus.

Causes. The exact cause of molar pregnancies is unknown. Partial moles are believed to originate from dispermic fertilization of a haploid ovum or fertilization of a haploid ovum with a diploid sperm. Complete moles most often result from fertilization of an empty egg by haploid sperm that reduplicates. Age, multiparity, and dietary factors appear to be associated with hydatidiform mole.

MEDICAL DIAGNOSIS AND PROGNOSIS

Ultrasonography is used to establish the diagnosis in patients with suspected hydatidiform mole. A characteristic image of multiple echogenic regions within the uterus corresponding to hydropic villi and focal intrauterine hemorrhage is seen (Fig. 33-3). With appropriate therapy, hydatidiform mole is generally not associated with maternal mortality. Patients with complete hydatidiform moles have a higher incidence of malignant sequelae (10% to 30%), compared with patients with partial moles (less than 10%).[2] Other complications associated with moles include theca-lutein cysts, trophoblastic embolization of the lung, and disseminated intravascular coagulation (DIC). Blood loss commonly leads to iron deficiency anemia.

MEDICAL MANAGEMENT

The first phase of medical management for hydatidiform mole consists in emptying the uterus. Dilatation and curettage (D&C) is the usual procedure in almost all patients. Primary hysterectomy is an alternative treatment in patients who have completed childbearing and desire sterilization. The tissue obtained must be carefully evaluated by the pathologist, because, although a mole is a benign process, choriocarcinoma, an extremely malignant tumor, sometimes complicates the picture.

The second phase of medical management is hCG level surveillance by radioimmunoassay to detect any

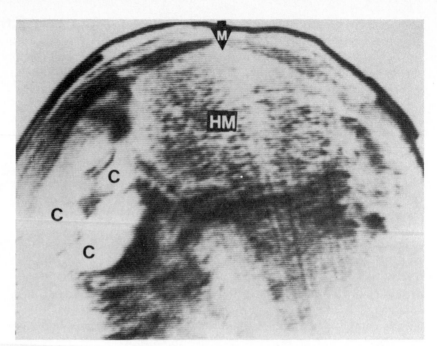

■ *Figure 33–3*
Ultrasound scan of hydatidiform mole.

changes suggestive of trophoblastic malignancy. Chorionic gonadotropin values are evaluated for about 1 year. The usual protocol consists of weekly measurements of hCG levels until they are normal for 3 weeks, then monthly measurement until they are normal for 6 months, followed by measurements every 2 months for the next 6 months. Negative hCG levels should be evident within 6 weeks after evacuation. Physical and pelvic examinations are performed at 2-week intervals until complete remission has occurred, and a chest x-ray is obtained to detect metastases. Avoidance of pregnancy is recommended during the period of postmolar follow-up.

Because the use of prophylactic chemotherapy is controversial and may produce several adverse effects, it is generally not recommended in women with uncomplicated hydatidiform mole. Women receiving chemotherapy should be observed closely for blood dyscrasias and renal complications.

NURSING ASSESSMENT

Assessment of fundal height provides basic data about expected gestational age, which in the case of hydatidiform mole is beyond that expected by menstrual history but may be suggestive of multiple gestation. Careful auscultation for fetal heart sounds reveals no findings, whereas the pregnancy tests remain highly positive (owing to unusually high levels of hCG) beyond the time of usual decline in hCG levels. The client may also report intense nausea and vomiting.

Vital signs and blood pressure (BP) evaluation may reveal hypertension before the 20th week of pregnancy.

Bleeding often develops during the second trimester. The blood should be carefully assessed by the nurse for clear, filled vesicles. Results of laboratory studies often reveal falling hemoglobin and hematocrit levels, as well as proteinuria.

NURSING DIAGNOSIS

Several of the nursing diagnoses are similar to those of other hemorrhagic complications of early pregnancy; these include knowledge deficit of pathophysiological changes in the reproductive system, fluid volume deficit related to uterine bleeding, and grieving related to loss of pregnancy. There are several other nursing problems specific to hydatidiform mole, such as alteration in tissue perfusion related to pregnancy-induced hypertension (PIH); alteration in nutritional status secondary to nausea and vomiting; and anxiety about potential malignancy.

NURSING INTERVENTION

Once the diagnoses are made, the nurse plans interventions to prepare the client for evacuation of the uterus. Preoperative nursing care will vary, depending on the type of medical procedure required.

In providing client education, it is of paramount importance that the nurse emphasize that every women who has had a hydatidiform mole must submit a urine specimen or have her serum tested for hCG each month for the course of an entire year. In addition, family planning counseling should be offered to assist the women in selecting a desirable contraceptive. Pregnancy should be avoided for at least 1 year, after which time conception is permitted.

Psychosocial support is also an important component of nursing care for the woman with a hydatidiform mole. Although the woman may never have experienced a "true pregnancy," her reactions after treatment frequently closely resemble those of women who have had a spontaneous abortion or an ectopic pregnancy. Further anxiety and despair may be created by the lengthy delay needed for future pregnancies and the risk of potential neoplasms. Opportunities should be provided by the nurse for the client to express her varying reactions to the situation, including extreme remorse, anger, and fear. Much understanding and guidance are required by the client and her family to work through grief reactions and assess future plans (see Nursing Care Plan: The Woman With Hemorrhagic Complications of Early Pregnancy).

NURSING EVALUATION

Anticipated outcomes of nursing care, as follows, are that the woman with a hydatidiform mole:

- Understands the pathophysiological changes occurring in her reproductive system and the need for immediate treatment and follow-up procedures
- Has complications prevented (e.g., fluid volume deficit, hypertension, infection) because of careful assessment and management
- Quickly recovers from the operative procedure (mole evacuation)
- Appropriately progresses through the grieving process and accepts the loss of her pregnancy

Choriocarcinoma

Choriocarcinoma is a highly malignant trophoblastic neoplasm that develops during or shortly after some forms of pregnancy. Approximately one third to one half of choriocarcinomas are preceded by hydatidiform mole. The characteristic progression of this disease involves a rapidly growing mass invading both uterine muscle and blood vessels, causing hemorrhage and necrosis. The chorionic villi of hydatidiform moles are absent. Metastases to the lungs, vagina, brain, and blood vessels are early complications, often occurring before the presentation of the primary disease symptoms.

Trophoblastic neoplasia is suspected in the presence of persistent or rising titers of gonadotropin when pregnancy is absent. Modern treatment of choriocarcinoma has greatly improved the prognosis. In the past, hysterectomy offered the only possible curative treatment. Currently, drugs such as methotrexate and dactino-mycin offer much promise as successful chemotherapeutic agents that may be used alone or in combination with irradiation. If the disease is treated early, an overall cure rate of about 85% can be achieved.[2]

■ HYPEREMESIS GRAVIDARUM

Mild nausea and vomiting is a common and normal complaint of women in early pregnancy; however, when these symptoms become exaggerated, pathological effects may result. The systemic effects may include fluid and electrolyte imbalance, marked weight loss, acetonuria, and nutritional deficits. This rare complication of pregnancy is known as *hyperemesis gravidarum* or *pernicious vomiting*. The disease affects approximately 3.5 pregnant women per 1000 pregnancies.[19]

Manifestations and Causes

Clinical Picture. The clinical picture of the pregnant woman suffering from pernicious vomiting varies in relation to the severity and the duration of the condition. The first symptom the woman experiences is a feeling of nausea, which may be most pronounced on arising in the morning or may occur at other times of the day. This pattern persists for a few weeks and then suddenly ceases in most women with hyperemesis gravidarum.

A small number of women who have morning sickness develop persistent vomiting that lasts for 4 to 8 weeks or longer. These women vomit several times a day and may be unable to retain any liquid or solid foods, with the result that marked symptoms of dehydration and starvation occur. Diminished urinary output and dryness of the skin are manifestations of dehydration. Hypovolemia with associated hypotension may result if dehydration is not corrected.

Starvation, which is regularly present, manifests itself in a number of ways. Weight loss may vary from 5 lb to as much as 20 or 30 lb. In these clinical situations, digestion and the absorption of carbohydrates and other nutrients have been so inadequate that the body has been forced to burn its reserve stores of fat to maintain body heat and energy. When fat is burned without carbohydrates being present, the process of combustion does not go on to completion. Consequently, certain incompletely burned products of fat metabolism appear in the blood and the urine (e.g., acetone and diacetic acid). In severe cases, considerable changes associated with starvation and dehydration become evident in the blood chemistry (e.g., an increase in the nonprotein nitrogen, uric acid, and urea and a moderate decrease in the chlorides). Vitamin starvation is regularly present,

(Text continues on page 785)

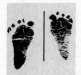

Nursing Care Plan

The Woman With Hemorrhagic Complications of Early Pregnancy

Nursing Goals

The woman with hemorrhagic complications of early pregnancy will carry fetus to term or terminate the pregnancy without complications as evidenced by:
1. Identifying signs of early antepartal bleeding.
2. Seeking appropriate medical interventions to support/terminate pregnancy.
3. Complying with restrictions prescribed to save the pregnancy.
4. Maintaining health without signs of hypovolemic shock and/or infection.
5. Expressing feelings of fear, grief, and anger to effectively cope with threatened/actual loss.

Assessment	Potential Nursing Diagnosis	Planning and Interventions	Evaluation

History
  Previous spontaneous abortions
  Multiple therapeutic abortions
  Pelvic inflammatory disease or previous tubal damage
  Previous ectopic pregnancy
  Current pregnancy confirmed
  Nausea and vomiting
  Lower abdominal pain or knifelike pain in lower quadrant (suggestive of ectopic pregnancy)
  Uterine cramping or contractions
  Previous bleeding coagulation problems
  Contraceptive use, especially IUD
	Knowledge deficit related to physiological alterations in the reproductive system	Instruct client about "danger signals" in early pregnancy and appropriate actions indicated	Client repeats danger signals in early pregnancy and what actions to take

		Maintain bedrest or limited physical activity	Client complies with limited activity
		Monitor vital signs and fetal heart tones if indicated	Client's vital signs remain stable
		Explain diagnostic ultrasound (or other prescribed procedures) and prepare for testing	Client acknowledges understanding of procedures
		Provide client education on pathophysiology of condition and management	Client repeats accurate description of her condition

Physical examination
  Spotting or active bleeding (color, quantity, consistency)
  Relaxed or dilated cervix
  Fundal height (higher than expected with hydatidiform mole)
  Tenderness in adnexa
  Lower abdominal pain (right or left side)
  Blood pressure (elevated with hydatidiform mole)
  Vital signs
		Instruct client to increase fluid intake and to eat a well-balanced diet	Client increases fluid intake and eats a well-balanced diet

(continued)

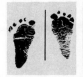

Nursing Care Plan *(continued)*

Assessment	Potential Nursing Diagnosis	Planning and Interventions	Evaluation
Laboratory Complete blood count Rh factor Hemoglobin, hematocrit			
Ultrasound to determine cause of bleeding Ectopic pregnancy Threatened abortion Incomplete abortion Hydatidiform mole			
Signs and symptoms of shock Rapid, thready pulse Tachypnea Pallor, clammy skin Decreased blood pressure Restlessness Decreased urine output Decreased level of consciousness	Fluid-volume deficit related to bleeding complications of early pregnancy	Draw blood, type and crossmatch	
		Observe, record, and report blood loss	
Laboratory screening for coagulation defect		Record pad count; note quantity, quality, and constituents of drainage	
		Start and maintain IV infusion for administration of blood, antibiotics, or other medications as prescribed (use large-bore cannula)	Client receives IV infusions and medications as ordered
		Replace IV fluids as prescribed	Client's fluid and electrolyte balance is maintained
		Monitor intake and output (insert Foley catheter, if necessary)	Client has her intake and output monitored
		Observe for signs and symptoms of shock; frequently assess vital functions, state of consciousness	Client does not show signs of hypovolemic shock
		Replace fibrinogen, if indicated	
		Institute nursing interventions for treatment of shock, if necessary; administer oxygen	Client is stabilized
		Explain potential medical or surgical procedures that may be necessary (e.g., dilation and curettage, laparoscopy, salpingectomy, induction)	Client demonstrates her knowledge of potential medical and surgical procedures in discussions

(continued)

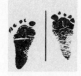

Nursing Care Plan   (continued)

Assessment	Potential Nursing Diagnosis	Planning and Interventions	Evaluation
		Administer RhoGAM to Rh-negative client who aborts pregnancy	Client receives RhoGAM if Rh negative
Physical examination 　Fever 　Local tenderness 　Malodorous vaginal discharge 　Pain in lower abdomen, adnexa	High risk for infection related to excessive fluid-volume deficit	Provide client education on 　Perineal hygiene (e.g., wipe perineal area from front to back after voiding 　Avoidance of tampons to control bleeding	Client demonstrates proper cleansing technique after voiding
History 　Large amount of antepartal bleeding 　Illegal abortion		Observe for symptoms of infection 　Tenderness 　Swelling 　Redness 　Pain	Client remains free of signs and symptoms of infection
		Encourage fluid intake or administer parental fluids as ordered	Client takes adequate amounts of fluids
		Administer antibiotics and pain medication as prescribed	Client receives antibiotics and pain medications as prescribed
Signs and symptoms of anxiety 　Jitteriness 　Restlessness 　Crying 　Nail biting	Grieving related to actual or threatened loss of pregnancy	Provide opportunities for expressions of grief, anger, self-blame	Client expresses feelings of grief, anger, and self-blame
		Allow client to be with supportive family members	Family members offer each other mutual support
Expresses 　"Why me" 　Fear of losing baby 　Anger		Accept client's feeling of grief	Client verbalizes fears related to future reproductive abilities
		Provide factual information about abortion (or ectopic pregnancy, hydatidiform mole) and possible future reproductive capacities	Client demonstrates understanding of potential loss of pregnancy
		Initiate referral for genetic counseling if appropriate	Client complies with referral suggestions
		Initiate referral for religious support services if desired	

and in extreme cases, when marked vitamin B deficiency exists, polyneuritis occasionally develops and disturbances of the peripheral nerves result.

Causes. The exact cause of hyperemesis gravidarum is unknown; however, certain organic processes are known to underlie all cases of vomiting, regardless of whether the symptoms are mild or severe. The endocrine imbalance created by a high level of chorionic gonadotropins and estrogens, metabolic changes of normal gestation, fragments of chorionic villi entering the maternal circulation, and the diminished motility of the stomach are believed to give rise to clinical symptoms.[20,21]

Because of the absence of a demonstrable pathologic explanation for the symptoms, some theorists have proposed that hyperemesis gravidarum is related to the woman's difficulty in psychologically adjusting to pregnancy and the mothering role.

Medical Diagnosis and Prognosis

Appropriate diagnostic testing should be performed to detect underlying causes of nausea and vomiting, such as gastroenteritis, hepatitis, cholecystitis, or peptic ulcer, which may contribute to the hyperemetic status of the pregnant woman.

Perinatal outcome may be improved through early treatment to prevent significant weight loss. Gross et al found that the incidence of fetal growth retardation was significantly greater in patients with hyperemesis who had lost more than 5% of their prepregnant weight.[22] Serious cases of hyperemesis gravidarum are rare, and recovery is usually rapid once fluid and electrolyte balance are restored.

Medical Management

Medical management is directed toward preventing significant weight loss, correcting fluid and electrolyte imbalance, and treating acidosis or alkalosis. Hospitalization may be recommended for pregnant women who are unable to remedy the symptoms and hyperemesis effectively at home by frequent, small feedings, avoidance of symptom-provoking stimuli, and prescribed medications (e.g., pyridoxine 10–30 mg/day, chlorpromazine 10–25 mg every 4 to 6 hours).

The goals of intervention are (1) to treat the dehydration by liberal administration of parenteral fluids (approximately 3000 ml in 24 hours); (2) to reverse the starvation by administering glucose IV and thiamine chloride subcutaneously and, if necessary, by feeding a high-caloric, high-vitamin fluid diet through a nasal tube or hyperalimentation method; and (3) to treat the emotional component with an understanding attitude (supportive measures). Oral intake of fluids is restricted until the nausea and vomiting subside. Occasionally, the hyperemetic woman may be unable to respond successfully to treatment. In such rare circumstances, total parenteral nutrition may be prescribed through a subclavian line to restore a positive nitrogen balance.

Nursing Assessment

During the initial contact with the hyperemetic woman, the nurse should assess the particular pattern of nausea and vomiting experienced by the client (e.g., onset, duration, frequency, predictability). Results of laboratory studies are carefully reviewed for evidence of hemoconcentration (elevated hemoglobin and hematocrit), fluid and electrolyte imbalance (decreased sodium, potassium, and chloride), and vitamin deficiency (B folate). The client's current weight is measured and compared with her nonpregnant weight. Selected questions are asked about activities for daily living, the client's lifestyle, and attitudes about herself and the pregnancy. Nutritional habits are evaluated in detail and then compared with findings on physical examination (e.g., skin turgor, energy level, color of mucous membranes).

Nursing Diagnosis

Assessment of the client with signs and symptoms of hyperemesis gravidarum may lead the nurse to some of the following nursing diagnoses: alteration in nutrition related to pernicious vomiting; high risk for impairment in skin integrity related to excessive vomiting and dehydration; and ineffective individual coping with the psychological tasks of pregnancy and motherhood. In addition, the fetus is at risk for alteration in nutrition secondary to maternal malnourishment.

Nursing Intervention

The nurse must monitor carefully the client's intake and output during the course of hospitalization. Generally, oral intake is restricted; however, once vomiting ceases, oral feedings are started. Various approaches are used to restore oral intake. Small quantities of dry food (e.g., crackers or toast) may be given hourly, alternating with small quantities (1 oz) of water. This is followed by a progression of clear liquids. If clear liquids and dry food are tolerated well, the client may advance slowly to a soft diet and, finally, a normal diet. In preparing solid foods, the nurse should arrange the portions attractively and in small amounts. A positive approach should be displayed when serving food. The nurse should also be aware of the effects that food odors have on the mother.

It is most important for the nurse to provide a hygienic environment for the client. Quick removal of emesis from the client's room and use of room deodorizers will decrease noxious odors that may disturb appetite and diminish food appeal.

Psychological support is most effectively provided by the nurse who demonstrates an understanding and empathetic manner. A calm and nonjudgmental attitude may facilitate the client's verbalizations of any psychological conflicts concerning family, financial, or social difficulties. Visitors may have to be restricted or limited if they have an adverse effect on the client (see Nursing Care Plan: The Woman With Pernicious Vomiting [Hyperemesis Gravidarum]).

Nursing Evaluation

Anticipated outcomes of nursing care, as follows, are that the woman with hyperemesis gravidarum:

- Understands the effects of hyperemesis gravidarum on perinatal outcome and treatment to prevent complications
- Responds to oral, IV, or total parenteral nutrition and ceases vomiting
- Regains weight lost
- Maintains her skin integrity

■ HEMORRHAGIC COMPLICATIONS OF LATE PREGNANCY

Placental disorders causing bleeding and possible hemorrhage during late pregnancy may seriously jeopardize fetal well-being and maternal health. Problems that develop may have originated either early or late in pregnancy as the placenta matures and becomes more vascular. The most common cause of bleeding and hemorrhage (blood loss of 500 ml or more) during the later months of pregnancy is placenta previa. Premature separation of the placenta (abruptio placentae) is another potentially serious condition associated with third-trimester bleeding. An overview comparison of these conditions is presented in Table 33-1.

Placenta Previa

Placenta previa is the development of the placenta in the lower uterine segment (instead of high up in the uterus as usual) so that it either wholly or partially covers the region of the cervix.

There are three types, differentiated according to the degree to which the condition is present (Figs. 33-4 and 33-5). *Total placenta previa* occurs when the placenta completely covers the internal os. *Partial placenta previa* occurs when the placenta partially covers the internal os. *Low implantation of the placenta* occurs when the placenta encroaches on the region of the internal os, so that it can be palpated by the physician on digital exploration about the cervix, but does not extend beyond the margin of the internal os.

MANIFESTATIONS AND CAUSES

Clinical Picture. Changes occurring in the lower uterine segment during the later months of pregnancy cause varying degrees of placental separation from its site of attachment. This separation opens up the underlying blood sinuses of the uterus from which the bleeding occurs. Painless, bright-red vaginal bleeding during the second or third trimester is the main sign in the woman presenting with placenta previa. The bleeding may begin as mere spotting, or it may start with profuse hemorrhage. Most commonly, uncontrolled bleeding does not occur with the first episode. In fact, there may be several episodes of bleeding before there is sufficient blood loss to necessitate aggressive intervention and pregnancy termination. The uterus usually remains soft in women with placenta previa.

Causes. There is no known cause of placenta previa. Multiparity, advancing maternal age, multiple gestation, previous cesarean birth, and uterine incisions increase the risk of occurrence.

MEDICAL DIAGNOSIS AND PROGNOSIS

The possibility of placenta previa should always be suspected in women with uterine bleeding during the latter half of pregnancy. Diagnosis can be established clearly and simply by using sonographic techniques to locate the placenta (Fig. 33-6). Placental localization by ultrasound "B" or "real-time" scanning offers 95% accuracy. Patients found to have low-lying placenta or placenta previa are now being followed by serial ultrasound examinations to observe changes in placental position. Many of the early placenta previas appear to migrate away from the cervix as pregnancy progresses because of formation of the lower uterine segment.[23]

In unusual circumstances when the diagnosis of placenta previa cannot be confirmed with ultrasound, a physical examination of the cervix may be performed in the operating room under a *double set-up*. This means preparations for an immediate cesarean section are available should severe hemorrhage result from mild manipulation.

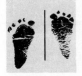

Nursing Care Plan

The Woman With Pernicious Vomiting (Hyperemesis Gravidarum)

Nursing Goals

The woman with pernicious vomiting (hyperemesis gravidarum) will maintain nutritional health of self and fetus throughout pregnancy as evidenced by:
1. Reducing and eliminating nausea and vomiting.
2. Restoring circulatory volume and fluid and electrolyte balance.
3. Preserving skin integrity.
4. Coping with the psychological tasks of pregnancy and motherhood.
5. Continuing fetal growth and development.

Assessment	Potential Nursing Diagnosis	Planning and Intervention	Evaluation
History Onset, duration, and frequency of vomiting episodes Prepregnancy weight Current weight Previous eating disorder	Alteration in nutrition: less than body requirements related to pernicious vomiting	Restrict or limit oral intake until vomiting ceases	Client responds to restricted intake by ending her vomiting
Laboratory Blood Electrolytes (decreased) Hemoglobin and hematocrit (elevated) *p*H (acidosis, alkalosis) BUN (increased) SGOT (elevated) Urine Ketones (present) Specific gravity (elevated)		Initiate and maintain IV therapy to correct hypovolemia and electrolyte imbalance Glucose Vitamins Sodium Chloride Potassium Bicarbonate Lactate	Client's electrolyte imbalances and hypovolemia are corrected
		Record intake and output, including emesis	Client's urine output remains greater than 30 ml/h
		Record daily weights	Client ceases weight loss and begins to gain weight
		Begin alternatively giving water or dry food (e.g., toast) in small quantities after vomiting has stopped	Client retains food and liquid
Other diagnostic tests Liver function Renal function Gastric function		Initiate total parenteral nutrition (TPN) if unable to establish oral feedings for prolonged period	Client receives TPN as needed
		Advance diet slowly to clear liquids, soft foods, and solid foods, respectively (if client tolerates oral feedings); arrange food attractively in small quantities	Client consumes diet that adequately meets nutritional demands of pregnancy
Personal hygiene	High risk for impairment	Encourage ambulation (if	Client ambulates or

(continued)

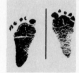

Nursing Care Plan   (continued)

Assessment	Potential Nursing Diagnosis	Planning and Intervention	Evaluation
Skin care Mouth care	in skin integrity related to excessive vomiting and dehydration	appropriate) or frequent change in position	changes positions frequently

Integrity of skin
  Pressure sores
  Turgor
  Color (jaundice, pallor)
  Dryness
  Thinness
Integrity of oral cavity
  Tenderness
  Redness
  Lesions
		Inspect mouth for irritation or lesions
		
		Assist with oral hygiene and offer frequent mouth-washes
		
		Maintain personal hygiene using mild soap and avoiding excessive moisture
		
		Explain effects of condition on skin integrity and oral cavity; emphasize importance of preventive intervention
			Client's mouth remains free of irritation and lesions
			
			Client maintains good personal and oral hygiene
			
			Client's skin retains its integrity

History
  Planned vs. unplanned pregnancy
  Financial difficulties
  Interpersonal conflicts in family
Communication patterns
  Ability to verbalize feelings
  Maintenance of eye contact
  Nonverbal behaviors
Achievement of the psychological tasks of pregnancy
  Denial
  Ambivalence
  Acceptance
  Future plans
	Ineffective coping with the psychological tasks of pregnancy and motherhood	Control environment by restricting or limiting visitors as necessary
		
		Demonstrate a calm and relaxed manner
		
		Assist client in achieving the psychological tasks of pregnancy
		
		Offer psychological support
		
		Reduce anxiety by explaining all procedures necessary for diagnosis and treatment
		
		Provide positive reinforcement for concerns expressed about pregnancy and fetal well-being
		
		Maintain good ventilation in client's room and reduce odors from vomitus, food
		
		Refer for mental health services if necessary
		
		Refer to social worker for socioeconomic assistance if necessary
			Client relaxes and remains calm
			
			Client begins achieving the psychological tasks of pregnancy
			
			Client indicates her trust in the nurse
			
			Client understands all diagnostic and treatment procedures
			
			Client verbalizes feeling about pregnancy and fetal well-being
			
			Client accepts referral sources of assistance

(continued)

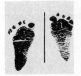

Nursing Care Plan (continued)

Assessment	Potential Nursing Diagnosis	Planning and Intervention	Evaluation
Pregnancy test positive High level of hCG Fetal heart tones (Doppler) Fundal height	Alteration in fetal nutrition related to maternal malnourishment	Explain purposes and prepare for diagnostic tests as indicated (e.g., sonography)	Client indicates her understanding of diagnostic tests and follows instructions
		Monitor fetal heart tones with Doppler	Fetus retains normal fetal heart tones
		Monitor fetal movement (if present)	Fetal movement is present
		Assess fundal height and compare measurements for growth	Client shows growth in fundal height

Until recent years, placenta previa was associated with a maternal mortality rate of approximately 10%. Early diagnosis and modern methods of management have reduced this figure considerably. The presence of this condition creates two main problems for the mother: bleeding and obstruction of the birth canal. For the baby, the most significant concern is prematurity. In utero, the fetus may be compromised because of hypoxia created by the decreased oxygen supply with placental separation. Intrauterine growth retardation may occur as a consequence of decreased circulation to the fetus.

MEDICAL MANAGEMENT

Medical interventions are planned based on the location of the placenta, the amount of bleeding, and the gestational age of the fetus. Conservative management is appropriate when the fetus is premature (by weight or dates) and the bleeding is not excessive. Under such circumstances, bedrest and observation often result in cessation of the bleeding and provide valuable days for the maturation of the fetus. Another recently reported intervention for prolonging gestation in patients with third trimester bleeding and preterm labor is tocolysis with magnesium sulfate, terbutaline, or ritodrine.[24] To confirm fetal maturity, amniocentesis is often performed prior to planned delivery. An active approach is indicated if the fetus is at term by size and dates, if labor has begun, or if bleeding is sufficient to threaten the well-being of mother or fetus. Delivery must be performed irrespective of gestational age under emergency situations.

In all instances of total or greater than 30% partial placenta previa, cesarean birth is the approach of choice for delivery. The procedure is preferably performed under light, general inhalation anesthesia. Vaginal delivery may sometimes be accomplished with low implantation of the placenta, especially if the baby is small and the cervix is partially dilated. Under these circumstances, the obstetrician may elect to rupture the membranes in the hope that the presenting part may enter the pelvis and control the bleeding by compressing the area of placenta that has separated.

NURSING ASSESSMENT

Assessment of the woman with placenta previa is similar in many ways to the approach employed for the woman with a spontaneous abortion, discussed earlier in the chapter.

Initial evaluation of the client by the nurse should include (1) baseline vital signs; (2) bleeding; (3) uterine activity and condition (size, contour, irritability, relaxation); (4) pain or tenderness, especially in the abdomen; (5) fetal heart tones and activity; and (6) level of consciousness. The client must be typed and crossmatched so that necessary transfusions may be administered. She should be instructed to save all perineal pads; these are carefully examined by the nurse for blood loss. The client is also instructed to report if she feels any fluid

TABLE 33–1. A COMPARATIVE OVERVIEW OF PLACENTA PREVIA AND ABRUPTIO PLACENTAE

	Placenta Previa	Abruptio Placentae
Etiology	Unknown	Unknown
Associated risk factors	Multiparity, multiple gestation, advancing age (especially over age 35), uterine incisions, previous cesarean birth, breech presentation	Maternal hypertension, grand multiparity, multiple gestation, hydramnios, external trauma (rare), short umbilical cord (rare)
Incidence	1:167 deliveries	1:77–1:200 deliveries
Symptoms	Painless bleeding appearing at the end of the second trimester or in the third trimester, minimal to severe (usually bright-red)	Bleeding—may or may not be external (often dark brown)
	Uterus is soft, normal tone	Uterus is rigid and tender; tetanic, persistent uterine contractions (severe abruptio)
	Observed blood loss comparable to signs of shock	Shock out of proportion to blood loss
Prognosis	Maternal mortality 0.1%	Maternal mortality 0.5%–5%
	Major problem: prematurity	Major problem: prematurity
		Perinatal mortality 15%
Ultrasonographic findings	Abnormal placental implantation—lower uterine segment	Normal placental implantation—upper uterine segment
Recurrence	1:17	1:6–1:18
Complications	Hemorrhage	Hemorrhage
	Hypovolemic shock	Hypovolemic shock
	Thrombocytopenia	Coagulation defects (e.g., hypofibrinogenemia)
	Anemia	Renal failure
	Premature rupture of membranes and labor	Anemia
	Fetal malposition	
	Air embolism	
	Postpartum hemorrhage	
	Uterine rupture	

escaping from her vulva. It is important to periodically palpate the uterus gently to detect contractions suggesting the onset of labor.

Because bleeding is from the uterine decidua, the amount of actual visible blood loss may be deceiving. Assessment should be performed for signs of shock (pallor, coldness, tachycardia) and fetal hypoxia secondary to inadequate oxygenation. Fetal heart tones and pattern are often evaluated continuously through application of an external monitoring system. Daily measurements of hemoglobin and hematocrit also may be done to assess blood loss.

NURSING DIAGNOSIS

From the assessment, the nurse formulates nursing diagnoses for the woman with placenta previa. Some of the potential nursing diagnoses may include fluid-volume deficit (hypovolemia) related to bleeding secondary to abnormal placental implantation; alteration in tissue perfusion related to hypovolemic shock; high risk for infection related to excessive blood loss; alteration in placental tissue perfusion; and ineffective maternal attachment related to disease.

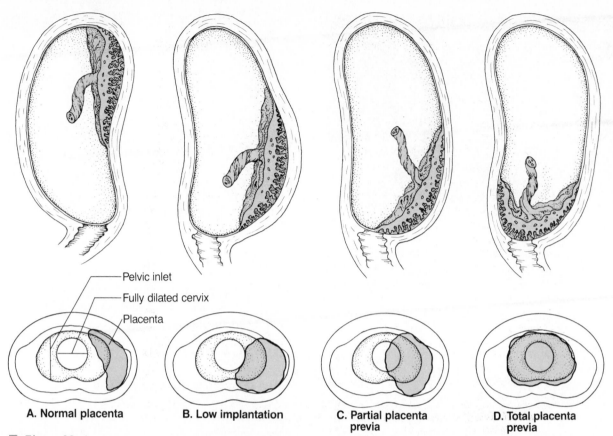

■ *Figure 33–4*

Placenta previa. (A) Normal placenta. (B) Low implantation. (C) Partial placenta previa. (D) Total placenta previa. (Redrawn from Benson RC: Handbook of Obstetrics and Gynecology, 6th ed. Los Altos, CA, Lange Medical Publications, 1977)

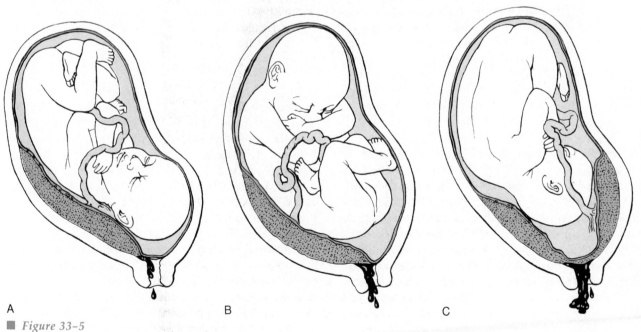

■ *Figure 33–5*

Placenta previa. (A) Low implantation. (B) Partial placenta previa. (C) Central (total) placenta previa.

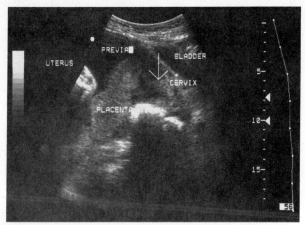

■ *Figure 33–6*
Ultrasonogram of 33 weeks' gestation and prior cesarean section showing placenta previa. The placenta is located on the posterior wall of the uterine segment and extends anteriorly to cover the cervix. The bladder and uterus are outlined. (Courtesy of Val A. Catanzarite, MD, PhD, and Cindy Maida, BS, RDMS, Sharp Perinatal Center, San Diego, California.)

NURSING INTERVENTION

Plans for nursing intervention will vary, depending on whether conservative or active medical management is prescribed. The client who is being managed at home or who is being discharged after an initial bleeding episode may require a referral for homemaking services and child care. Assistance in these areas is likely to facilitate client compliance with bedrest or restricted activities. In addition, ongoing assessments for changes in perinatal status may be performed by the community health nurse. Client education should focus on preoperative teaching to prepare the woman for a probable cesarean delivery and preparation of the family for a possible premature infant with special-care needs.

The client experiencing an excessive blood loss prior to or during delivery often requires the loss to be replaced. Because of the great cost and the danger of transfusions contaminated by acquired immunodeficiency syndrome and hepatitis, blood is not usually given unless actually needed.[25] Packed red blood cells, fresh frozen plasma, platelets, and cryoprecipitate are the most commonly used blood products. Packed red blood cell transfusions increase oxygen delivery, whereas fresh frozen plasma may be given to replace clotting factor deficiencies.[25] It may also be necessary to administer oxygen to prevent maternal and fetal hypoxia. The nurse should help the woman with a diagnosis of placenta previa to maintain her self-esteem by listening to her concerns and offering clear explanations about the situation and management approach. It is only natural for the woman and her family to have many fears about the infant's well-being, maternal

dangers, and a possible cesarean delivery. Listening to fetal heart tones with a Doppler device may provide the prenatal client with some reassurance and reduce her anxiety.

NURSING EVALUATION

Anticipated outcomes of nursing care, as follows, are that the woman with placenta previa:

- Understands the effects of placenta previa on perinatal outcome and treatment to prevent complications
- Follows the prescribed treatment protocols
- Maintains adequate tissue perfusion and oxygen to the maternal-fetal unit
- Delivers a healthy infant at or near term
- Recovers from the delivery (generally cesarean section) without complications

Abruptio Placentae

Abruptio placentae (meaning that the placenta is torn from its bed) is a serious complication of the last half of pregnancy in which a normally located placenta undergoes separation from its uterine attachment. The condition is frequently called *premature separation* of the normally implanted placenta; other synonymous terms, such as *accidental hemorrhage* (meaning that it takes place unexpectedly) and *ablatio placentae* (ablatio meaning a carrying away), are sometimes used. The incidence is about 1 in every 77 to 200 pregnancies.

MANIFESTATIONS AND CAUSES

Clinical Picture. The clinical picture will vary, depending on the type of premature separation present (Fig. 33–7). *Covert* or *severe* abruptio placentae is characterized by central separation that entraps lost blood between the uterine wall and the placenta. In this situation, there is a *concealed* hemorrhage, which often masks the seriousness of the problem. When a separation occurs at the margin, blood passes between the uterine wall and fetal membranes, creating an *external* hemorrhage. This type of abruptio is called *overt* or *partial*. Situations involving complete or almost total separation are known as *placental prolapse* and are associated with massive vaginal bleeding.

The symptoms of an abruption are vaginal bleeding that is dark, abdominal pain (often sudden and severe—"knifelike"), and a firm, tender uterus. The pain is produced by the accumulation of blood behind the placenta, with subsequent distention of the uterus. Because of the almost woody hardness of the uterine wall, fetal parts may be difficult to palpate. Shock is often out of

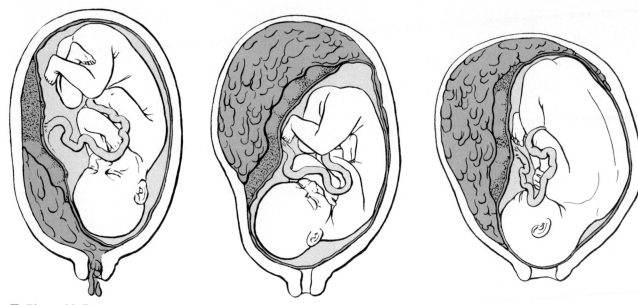

■ *Figure 33–7*
Abruptio placentae at various separation sites. (Left) External hemorrhage. (Center) Internal or concealed hemorrhage. (Right) Complete separation.

proportion to blood loss, as manifested by a rapid pulse, dyspnea, yawning, restlessness, pallor, syncope, and cold, clammy perspiration.

Although 20% to 25% of the placenta may be infarcted without fetal compromise, fetal distress is common and may be the first symptom of an abruption.[2,26] The contraction pattern typical of an abruptio placentae is frequent, low-amplitude contractions with an increase in resting tone.

Pathologic findings of placental abruption may vary and include placental infarction, decidual necrosis, polymorphonuclear infiltration, marginal thrombosis, and retroplacental blood clot.[26]

Causes. Although the precise cause of the condition is unknown, it is frequently associated with maternal hypertension, grand multiparity (five or more pregnancies), short umbilical cord, and, occasionally, automobile accidents and trauma. Other possible contributing factors include multiple gestation and hydramnios.

MEDICAL DIAGNOSIS AND PROGNOSIS

The physical signs and symptoms of placental abruption may vary greatly. Ultrasonography is often helpful in establishing the diagnosis; however, negative sonography does not exclude life-threatening degrees of placental abruption. CAT scans also may be used to differentially diagnose this condition (Fig. 33-8).

Abruptio placentae may be classified according to the degree of placental separation (see box on page 794).

Perinatal mortality rates vary greatly with the type of abruptio, ranging from 15% to approaching 100% for infants experiencing nearly total or complete abruptions. Assuming fetal survival, infant maturity at the time of delivery will also influence prognosis. Maternal mortality from abruptions has declined significantly and is now uncommon, although morbidity may be severe in some cases.[3] Some of the complications of an abruption that a woman may experience include hypovolemic shock, coagulopathy, and DIC.

MEDICAL MANAGEMENT

Treatment is dependent on the condition of the fetus and the mother at the time the diagnosis is made. If the fetus is alive and at or near term, prompt delivery is in order for moderate to severe abruptions and should be by cesarean birth, unless vaginal delivery can be accomplished quickly. If the fetus has already succumbed, this is usually an indication of an extensive placental separation. Vaginal delivery is preferred with fetal death except if hemorrhage cannot be successfully handled through blood replacement or if other complications arise. The risk of serious coagulation defects, to be described subsequently, is likely to be greater when delivery is performed transabdominally. In circumstances in which the fetus is immature and blood loss is occurring at a slow rate, delivery may be delayed. Ongoing assessment of fetal viability should be performed with ultrasonic Doppler devices to hear the fetal heart and

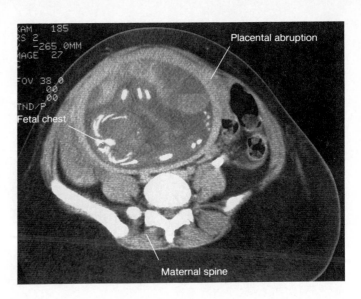

■ *Figure 33–8*
CAT scan of placental abruption at 28 weeks with fetal demise resulting from an automobile accident. The maternal spine and fetal chest are visible. (Courtesy of V A. Catanzarite, MD, PhD, and Cindy Maida, BS, RDMS, Sharp Perinatal Center, San Diego, California.)

with real-time ultrasound, which allows visualization of the heart movements.

Maternal hypovolemia and anemia may be corrected by administration of fresh whole blood plus electrolyte solution either prior to or during labor and delivery. Packed red cells and lactated Ringer's solution offer alternative replacements that may minimize transfusion requirements while increasing oxygen delivery and circulating volume.

A central venous pressure (CVP) line or arterial line is maintained for hemodynamic monitoring of critically ill women. An indwelling bladder catheter is inserted for accurate assessment of urinary output and proteinuria.

Classification of Abruptio Placentae According to Placental Separation

Grade 0 No symptoms; diagnosed after delivery when placenta is examined and found to have a dark, adherent clot on its surface

Grade 1 Some external bleeding; uterine tetany and tenderness may not be noted; no signs of shock or fetal distress

Grade 2 External bleeding; uterine tetany and tenderness; fetal distress

Grade 3 Bleeding may be external or internal; uterine tetany; maternal shock and fetal death; complicating DIC

NURSING ASSESSMENT

The nursing assessment of the woman with abruptio placentae includes all of the components described for patients with spontaneous abortion and placenta previa. In addition, the nurse must carefully assess for changes in fundal height because an increase is associated with concealed bleeding. Initial laboratory studies should include hemoglobin, hematocrit, fibrinogen levels, fibrin degradation products (FDP), thrombin time, prothrombin time, and partial thromboplastin time. These patients should be typed and crossmatched for several units of packed red blood cells because of the potential for a serious hemorrhage.

NURSING DIAGNOSIS

Assessment of the client for signs and symptoms of abruptio placentae may lead the nurse to some of the previously described nursing diagnoses for placenta previa. It should be noted that the identified problems of fluid-volume deficit and alteration in placental tissue perfusion in this clinical condition are secondary to premature separation of the normally implanted placenta. The client is likely to experience fear and anxiety related to concern about bleeding as a life-threatening situation for herself and the fetus.

NURSING INTERVENTION

Nursing interventions are planned based on the identified nursing diagnoses and on the medical plan of treatment. If the abruption is mild and the fetus is immature, careful and continuous nursing observation is necessary to detect evidence of progressive maternal blood loss or changes in fetal status (e.g., ominous decelerations, bradycardia). The patient should be placed in the left lateral recumbent position in order to increase venous return, enabling more blood to return to the lungs to be reoxygenated. This position also increases the blood available to perfuse the placenta.

In more acute situations, intake and output are recorded hourly and oxygen may be administered by mask or nasal cannula to prevent or minimize fetal hypoxia. If a CVP line is in place, readings must be carefully obtained, recorded, and reported. Occasionally, CVP monitoring may be replaced by pulmonary artery wedge pressure monitoring with the Swan-Ganz catheter. Observations should be made for signs and symptoms of hypovolemia, such as cough, abnormal respiratory sounds, and shortness of breath. It is also essential for the nurse to assess the client for adverse reactions to blood transfusions.

In cases of moderate to severe abruption and a live fetus, the nurse should provide preoperative teaching about the possibility of a cesarean delivery and birth of a preterm infant. A realistic attitude about the client's health situation and factual reassurances are important aspects of the psychological support offered by the nurse to the family.

Following delivery, the nurse should continue assessing fluid-volume balance and vital signs. The uterus should be palpated frequently for atony and excessive blood loss (see Nursing Care Plan: The Woman With Hemorrhagic Complications of Late Pregnancy).

NURSING EVALUATION

Anticipated outcomes of nursing care for the woman with abruptio placentae are similar to the woman with placenta previa. Additionally, as follows, the woman with abruptio placentae:

- Has signs of fetal distress identified early and treated before severe hypoxia occurs
- Experiencing a fetal or neonatal demise, appropriately progresses through the grieving process

Other Problems Associated With Bleeding

Bleeding may lead to hypovolemia and hemorrhagic shock unless vigorous treatment is implemented to control bleeding and replace lost blood. In most emergency situations, the uterus must be expeditiously emptied of all contents. Delay may result in complications such as *hypofibrinogenemia* and *DIC*.

HYPOFIBRINOGENEMIA

Fibrinogenopenia occurs in the childbearing woman who has depleted her blood fibrinogen in an attempt to control bleeding by clot formation. Following an abruptio placentae, thromboplastin enters the circulation, causing small fibrin clots to form in the capillaries. As the level of fibrinogen decreases in the circulating blood, normal clotting mechanisms are impaired. This complication is also seen in other entities, such as amniotic fluid embolus, prolonged retention of a dead fetus, and septic abortion. Because of the danger of this complication, the client with abruptio placentae should receive laboratory analysis for fibrinogen levels (normal, 300 to 500 mg/dl). The nurse can also perform a simple *clot observation test* by placing a small amount of fresh blood in a test tube and watching how quickly a clot is formed. A firm clot should rapidly form (normal time, 4 to 12 min).

Treatment for hypofibrinogenemia involves replacement of blood and fibrinogen and termination of the pregnancy. The administration of cryoprecipitate generally is effective in raising the fibrinogen concentration of plasma.

Another complication of impaired coagulation associated with severe abruption is *Couvelaire uterus* (uteroplacental apoplexy). In this condition, the uterine muscle fills with blood and is therefore unable to contract well after delivery. The uterus feels hard and boardlike on palpation. Treatment consists in complete evacuation of the uterus and stimulation of contractions with IV oxytocin.

DISSEMINATED INTRAVASCULAR COAGULATION

DIC is a paradoxical disorder with anticoagulation and procoagulation effects existing simultaneously.[27] In DIC, clotting is overstimulated throughout the circulatory system. The most frequently initiating event is an abruption; however, other obstetric complications, such as PIH, retained products of conception, infection, or amniotic fluid embolism may be causative factors. These pathologic conditions act on either the intrinsic or the extrinsic pathways, creating increased formation of thrombin. The thrombin interacts with fibrinogen, resulting in formation of clots.

Figure 33-9 displays how the rapid and extensive formation of clots causes platelets and clotting factors to be depleted in clients with DIC. Concurrently, thrombin stimulates the fibrinolytic system to dissolve clots of fibrin, leading to the formation of FDPs, which have an anticoagulant effect. The overall result is bleeding diathesis and potential vascular occlusion of organs due to the formation of thromboemboli. The
(Text continues on page 798)

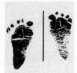

Nursing Care Plan

The Woman With Hemorrhagic Complications of Late Pregnancy

Nursing Goals

The woman with hemorrhagic complications of late pregnancy will deliver a live and stable neonate at or near term and maintain homeostasis as evidenced by:
1. Recognizing hemorrhagic disorder and seeking appropriate medical assistance.
2. Maintaining adequate fluid volume.
3. Maintaining tissue perfusion and oxygen to the maternal-fetal unit.
4. Verbalizing and understanding grief response.

Assessment	Potential Nursing Diagnosis	Planning and Intervention	Evaluation

Predisposing factors
  Grand multiparity
  Advanced maternal age
  Multiple gestation
  Hydramnios
  Hypertensive disorders of pregnancy
  History of previous bleeding disorder, blood coagulopathy
  Previous cesarean section
	Fluid-volume deficit (hypovolemia) related to bleeding complication of late pregnancy	Assess maternal blood loss and vital signs q 15 min to q1 h	Client's blood loss is controlled
			
			Client's vital signs remain stable

		Maintain bedrest in flat, lateral position	Client remains in flat lateral position
Estimated gestational age		Initiate and monitor IV-fluids to restore circulating volume (use at least 18-gauge needle)	Client receives adequate fluid replacement
Blood loss (color, quantity, consistency)		Type and crossmatch 2 or more units of whole blood	
Laboratory Complete blood count (CBC), hematocrit, hemoglobin, electrolytes		Monitor and record intake and output	Client maintains normal urine output or returns to normal urine output
		Count and weigh perineal pads, inspect contents for tissue	

		Assess for futher blood loss and integrity of maternal system
		  Serial CBC, hemoglobin, hematocrit
		  Arterial blood gases prn
			Client's arterial blood gases and other laboratory tests remain within normal limits or are restored to within normal limits

		Administer iron supplements as prescribed	Client receives iron supplements as prescribed

Vital signs and blood pressure
  Hypotension
  Tachycardia
  Tachypnea
	Alteration in tissue perfusion related to hypovolemic shock	Assess for signs of shock q15 min to q1 h
		  Pallor
		  Clamminess
		  Irritability
		  Decreased blood pressure
		  Tachycardia
			Client is comfortable and free of signs of shock

Uterus
  Pain
  Tenderness
  Rigidity
  Contour
  Height
  Contractions
		Assess for abdominal tenderness, rigidity, pain (abruption) q30 min q1 h	Client has no abdominal tenderness or rigidity

(continued)

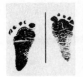

Nursing Care Plan (continued)

Assessment	Potential Nursing Diagnosis	Planning and Intervention	Evaluation
		Administer oxygen as necessary (6–8 L/min) to maintain adequate perfusion	Client receives oxygen as needed
Arterial pulse quality (decreased or absent)			
Skin (color, pallor, moistness)		Monitor vital signs q15 min to q1 h until stable	Client's vital signs remain stable
Nausea and vomiting		Assess level of consciousness and peripheral perfusion	Client remains alert and well oriented; her extremities remain warm and pink
Restlessness or irritability			
Shortness of breath		Color	
Level of consciousness (confusion)		Warmth	
		Pulses	
Urinary output and fluid intake		Prevent further bleeding by prohibiting vaginal and rectal exams, enemas	
Laboratory			
Blood type and cross-match		Administer transfusion as prescribed and observe for reaction (whole blood, frozen plasma, cryoprecipitate, as indicated)	Client receives transfusion without adverse reaction
Clotting time			
Thrombin time			
Prothrombin time			
Partial thromboplastin time			
Fibrinogen level			
Platelets		Monitor CVP line or pulmonary artery wedge pressure for vital functioning	Client maintains adequate blood return to the heart
FDP			
		Assess for sudden increase in fundal height (abruption)	Fundal height does not suddenly increase
		Assess for associated blood coagulation problems (hypofibrinogenemia and DIC)	Client remains free of blood coagulation complications
		Clot observation test	
		Coagulation studies	
		Prepare for emergency delivery (vaginal or cesarean section, as indicated)	
		NPO	Client verbalizes understanding of need for possible emergency delivery and potential method to be used
		Double-setup operating room (placenta previa only)	
		Preoperative teaching	

(continued)

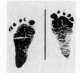

Nursing Care Plan (continued)

Assessment	Potential Nursing Diagnosis	Planning and Intervention	Evaluation
Understanding of hemorrhagic complication	Ineffective maternal attachment related to disease	Encourage client to verbalize anxieties, fears, and possible guilt feelings	Client verbalizes concerns about situation and expresses grief
Grieving response Crying Grimacing Verbalizations of anger, denial, sorrow		Demonstrate a caring and empathetic attitude	
Feelings about pregnancy		Support maternal-fetal bonding by Allowing mother to listen to normal fetal heart tones if present Maintaining a positive but realistic attitude Providing factual information on condition of fetus (or neonate)	Mother listens to normal fetal heart tones (FHT)
		Remain with mother at frequent intervals	
		Involve supportive family members in discussions and provide them with information about problems	Family members offer each other mutual support
Fetal heart tones (FHTs) Rate (120–160 beat/min) Variability (good) Reactivity (present)	High risk for injury to fetus related to alteration in utero placental tissue perfusion	Monitor fetal heart rate, activity, and response to contractions by external monitor	Fetus remains reactive with normal FHTs
Uterine activity Frequency of contractions Length of contractions Irritability		Assess uterine activity for signs of labor	
		Turn on left side and administer oxygen if signs of fetal distress are present	Client turns onto left side and restores normal FHT and rhythm
Palpation of fetal parts and movement		Prepare client for and assist with amniocentesis if ordered	Client is prepared for amniocentesis, as ordered
		Assist with emergency delivery if indicated for fetal distress	Client has successful emergency delivery, if indicated

kidneys are frequently affected, developing acute tubular necrosis and subsequent renal failure.[25]

It is imperative that the nurse perform careful assessment of women at risk for early signs of DIC. Clinical manifestations may be difficult to assess in the early stage but become more obvious as the severity of the disease progresses. Symptoms include bleeding from the gums and injection sites, petechiae and purpura on the skin, restlessness, anxiety, and tachycardia. The results of laboratory assessment reveal several abnormalities; these are presented in Table 32-2. Plasma fibrinogen and platelets are decreased; whereas FDPs, thrombin time, prothrombin time, and partial thromboplastin time are increased.

Intervention for DIC is directed toward correcting causative factors, including termination of pregnancy

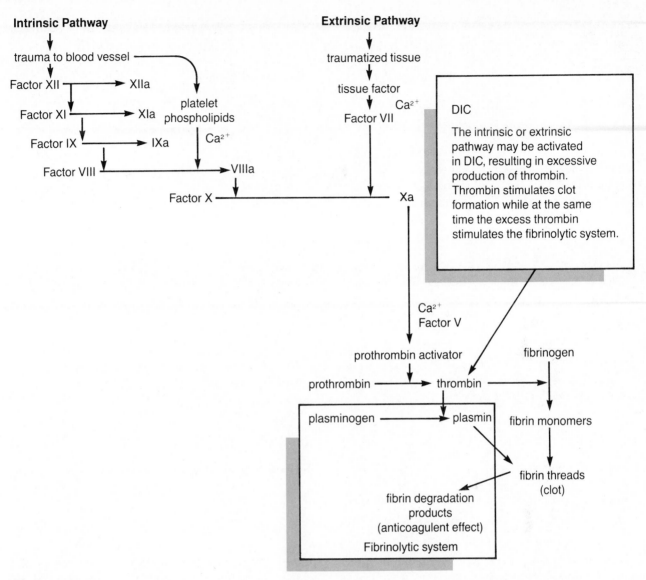

Intrinsic Pathway

trauma to blood vessel

Factor XII → XIIa

Factor XI → XIa

platelet phospholipids

Factor IX → IXa

Ca^{2+}

Factor VIII → VIIIa

Factor X → Xa

Extrinsic Pathway

traumatized tissue

tissue factor

Ca^{2+}

Factor VII

DIC

The intrinsic or extrinsic pathway may be activated in DIC, resulting in excessive production of thrombin. Thrombin stimulates clot formation while at the same time the excess thrombin stimulates the fibrinolytic system.

Ca^{2+}
Factor V

prothrombin activator

fibrinogen

prothrombin → thrombin →

plasminogen → plasmin

fibrin monomers

fibrin threads (clot)

fibrin degradation products (anticoagulent effect)

Fibrinolytic system

■ *Figure 33–9*
Normal blood coagulation pathways, the fibrinolytic system, and DIC.

if there is a placental abruption or fetal demise, and treating infection, amniotic fluid embolism, or PIH. The need for further intervention may be unnecessary once the cause of DIC is removed. If physiological support is indicated, it may be provided by (1) maintaining fluid and electrolyte balance with appropriate parenteral solutions (e.g., lactated Ringer's); (2) administering oxygen to prevent or treat hypoxia; (3) replacing whole blood or its constituents (e.g., frozen plasma and platelet concentrates often provide effective replacement therapy, cryoprecipitate may be administered to replace fibrinogen); and (4) carefully and continuously assessing vital functions through CVP monitoring or a pulmonary artery catheter. Additionally, fetal heart rate and uterine activity are closely observed through an electronic monitoring device. An indwelling bladder catheter is inserted to evaluate urinary output carefully. Output

should be maintained at 30 ml/h to assure adequate renal perfusion.

The infusion of heparin to block DIC is controversial, because heparin has the potential to aggravate hemorrhage when there has been severe disruption of the vasculature.[3]

■ HYPERTENSIVE DISORDERS OF PREGNANCY

Hypertensive disorders include a variety of vascular disturbances that either antedate pregnancy or occur as a complication during gestation or the early puerperium.

TABLE 33-2. LABORATORY TESTS FOR DISSEMINATED INTRAVASCULAR COAGULATION (DIC)

Test	Nonpregnant Values	Normal Pregnancy	Result in DIC
Clotting time	6–12 min	Normal	Normal
Clot retraction	Good	Good	Poor (lyses in 15–60 min)
Fibrinogen	200–400 mg/dl	300–500 mg/dl	Usually depressed
Thrombin time	12–18 sec	Shortened	Usually prolonged
Prothrombin time	11–13 sec	Shortened	Usually prolonged
Partial thromboplastin time or activated partial thromboplastin time	40–60 sec 25–45 sec	Shortened Shortened	Usually prolonged Usually prolonged
Factor assays		Normal	V, VIII, XIII reduced
Platelets	150,000–400,000/mm³	Normal	Usually decreased
Red blood cell morphology		Normal	Often abnormal (schistocytes, etc.)
Fibrin split products		Usually absent	Present
Euglobulin clot lysis		Normal	Usually shortened
Plasminogen		Normal	Usually depressed
Plasma protamine paracoagulation		Fibrin monomer absent	Fibrin monomer present
Ethanol gelation		Fibrin monomer absent	Fibrin monomer present
Protamine sulfate precipitation		Fibrin monomer absent	Fibrin monomer present
Staphylococcal clumping		Fibrin monomer absent	Fibrin monomer present

(Cavanagh D, et al: Obstetric Emergencies, Philadelphia, Harper & Row, 1982.)

Because of the many cardiovascular alterations, pregnancy may induce hypertension in women who have been normotensive prior to gestation or may aggravate existing hypertensive conditions. Until recently, *toxemia* was the term used to describe hypertension with an onset during pregnancy. This condition was believed to be caused by toxins derived from the products of conception circulating in the blood. In 1972, the American College of Obstetricians and Gynecologists introduced a classification system for hypertensive disorders of pregnancy that excluded the diagnosis of toxemia. The term *pregnancy-induced hypertension* is the current diagnostic label being used to describe the syndrome of hypertension, edema, and proteinuria evident in certain pregnant women. Preeclampsia and eclampsia are two categories of PIH that represent one and the same process, but the term *eclampsia* is used when the woman's clinical course has advanced to generalized convulsions or coma.

PIH is a common complication; it is seen in 5% or 7% of all gravidas. The prevalence of the disease may be much higher among certain groups, including young primigravidas, women with chronic hypertension, and women from low socioeconomic backgrounds. PIH also tends to recur in up to one third of the women, and some clients have hypertension persisting indefinitely after pregnancy.[2]

In the United States, PIH is a major cause of maternal deaths, responsible for approximately 17% of cases each year.[28,29] As a cause of fetal death, PIH is even more significant. Approximately 10% to 20% of stillbirths and neonatal deaths occur each year in the United States from hypertensive diseases of pregnancy, and those newborns who survive may suffer impairments that affect the quality of their lives.[3] Most perinatal deaths are related to prematurity.

Classification

The classification system and definition of the hypertensive disorders of pregnancy, originally developed by Chesley[30] and later modified by Gant and Worley,[31] are presented in the box that follows.

Hypertensive Disorders of Pregnancy

A. Pregnancy-induced hypertension (PIH)
   1. Preeclampsia—hypertension with proteinuria and/or edema developing after the 20th week of gestation
      a. Symptoms may occur earlier with hydatidiform mole
      b. Occurs almost exclusively in primigravidas
      c. Affects women at extremes of reproductive age (less than 20 yr or more than 35 yr)
      d. May be seen in multigravidas with the following:
         (1) Uterine overdistention as with twins or hydramnios
         (2) Vascular disease, including essential chronic hypertension and diabetes mellitus
         (3) Chronic renal disease
      Hypertension: 140/90 or an increase of 30 mm Hg systolic or 15 mm Hg diastolic over baseline; observation of these criteria on at least two occasions 6 h or more apart

      Edema: a weight gain of 5 lb or greater in 1 week or an accumulation of fluid greater than 1+ pitting edema after 12 h of bedrest

      Proteinuria: 1 g/L or greater of protein in a 24-h urine collection (2+ by dipstick)

      Severe preeclampsia:
      When one or more of the following are present:
      • Systolic blood pressure of 160 mm Hg or diastolic of 110 mm Hg on two occasions at least 6 h apart while the client is on bedrest
      • Proteinuria of at least 5 g/24 h or 3+ to 4+ by semiquantitative analysis
      • Cerebral or visual disturbances such as altered consciousness, headache, scotomata, or blurred vision
      • Pulmonary edema or cyanosis

   Signs of advancing disease:
   • Epigastric or upper quadrant pain
   • Thrombocytopenia or impaired liver function
   2. Eclampsia—extension of preeclampsia with grand mal seizure
      • One half the cases occur before labor
      • One fourth of the cases occur during labor
      • One fourth of the cases occur within 48 h postpartum

B. Chronic hypertension
   1. Blood pressure of 140/90 before pregnancy
   2. Blood pressure of 140/90 before 20th week gestation and/or persisting indefinitely following delivery
   3. For differential diagnosis after the 20th week of gestation:
      a. Hemorrhage and exudates seen on funduscopic examination
      b. Plasma urea nitrogen: 20 mg/dl
      c. Plasma creatinine levels: 1 mg/dl
      d. Presence of chronic disease, such as diabetes mellitus or connective tissue diseases

C. Chronic hypertension with superimposed preeclampsia—often a quick progression to eclampsia, which may develop before the 30th week of gestation
   1. Documented evidence of chronic hypertension
   2. Evidence of a superimposed, acute process
      a. Elevation of systolic blood pressure 30 mm Hg or of diastolic blood pressure 15–20 mm Hg above baseline on two occasions at least 6 h apart
      b. Development of proteinuria
      c. Edema as observed in women with preeclampsia

D. Late or transient hypertension—transient elevations of blood pressure are observed during labor or in early postpartum period, returning to normal within 10 days postpartum

(Gant NF, Worley RJ: Hypertension in Pregnancy: Concepts and Management, pp 2–9. New York, Appleton Century Crofts, 1980.)

The term *pregnancy-induced hypertension* covers those specific conditions that develop as a direct result of pregnancy (e.g., preeclampsia and eclampsia). If hypertension develops without edema or proteinuria during labor or in the early postpartum period and then returns to normal within 10 days following delivery, it is described as *late or transient hypertension*. The term *chronic hypertension* is used when the client has a concurrent hypertensive vascular disorder that is unrelated to pregnancy and was evident prior to gestation. If the pregnant patient with chronic hypertension or renal disease develops the complication of preeclampsia or eclampsia, the condition is referred to as *superimposed* *preeclampsia* or *eclampsia*. *Hypertensive crisis* in pregnancy exists when the maternal BP reaches 160/110 mm Hg on two occasions at least 6 hours apart. It is associated with PIH and chronic hypertension with superimposed PIH.

Etiology and Pathophysiology of PIH

Although the exact mechanism underlying PIH remains unknown, several theories exist to explain the etiology.

Because PIH is a multisystem disease, it is obvious that no single alteration or disturbance can explain the condition. A popular theory suggests that alterations in prostaglandin metabolism may be responsible for the hypertension and coagulopathy in this disorder.[32] PIH appears to be associated with increased production of thromboxane A_2. This hormone is a potent vasoconstrictor and stimulator of platelet aggregation and is believed to be an etiologic factor for the vasoconstriction, platelet hyperactivity, and uteroplacental arterial thrombosis that characterize PIH.[33]

PIH is characterized by an increase in arterial BP and an increase in peripheral vascular resistance. Arterial circulation is disrupted by alternating segments of constriction and dilation.[3,28] The vasospastic action causes damage to the blood vessels by decreasing their blood supply and by stretching them in those areas where segment dilation is occurring.[34] The endothelium is injured; platelets and fibrinogen and other blood products may be released into the interendothelium.[3,35]

There is an overall fluid shift from the intravascular space to the intracellular space. Consequently, plasma volume expansion is decreased or absent compared with normal pregnancy. Hematocrit and hemoglobin are increased as a result of vasoconstriction and the decreased intravascular fluid. Proteins and electrolytes similarly move into the intracellular space (Fig. 33-10).

The vasospasm existing in women with PIH is attributed to the extreme sensitivity of the vasculature to vasopressors. Unlike the healthy, pregnant woman who is resistant to the pressor effects of infused angiotensin II, women who will subsequently develop preeclampsia show an increased pressor responsiveness to angiotensin II several weeks prior to the appearance of clinical symptoms.[36] A similar receptivity is found in women who have chronic hypertension preceding the development of superimposed PIH.[37]

There is also a lower level of plasma renin activity, aldosterone, and angiotensin II in women with preeclampsia as compared with healthy, pregnant women. Catecholamines, prolactin, vasopressin, and prostaglandins have all been cited as humoral substances having a possible role in the pathogenesis or maintenance of PIH. A hypothesized association of circulating antigen-antibody complexes with the development of PIH is currently being investigated.[2,3]

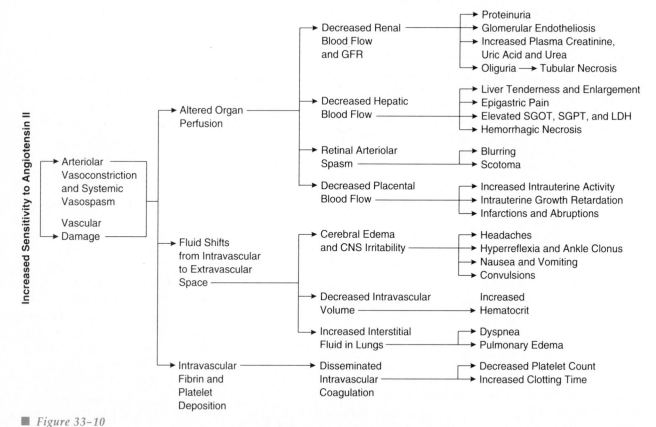

■ *Figure 33–10*

Pathophysiologic alterations occurring in SPIH. Key: SPIH, severe pregnancy-induced hypertension; CNS, central nervous system; GFR, glomerular filtration rate; SGOT, serum glutamic-oxaloacetic transaminase; SGPT, serum glutamic-pyruvic transaminase; LDH, lactate dehydrogenase. (Modified from Gilbert ES, Harmon JS. High-risk Pregnancy and Delivery: Nursing Perspectives, p 272. St. Louis, CV Mosby, 1986)

Glomerular endotheliosis often develops in the kidneys of women experiencing proteinuria of PIH. This disturbance causes partial obstruction of capillary lumina and may be related to the release of placenta thromboplastin, which initiates intravascular coagulation and formation of fibrin deposits.[38] Other PIH-associated renal alterations that are atypical of pregnancy include a decrease in the plasma renal flow and glomerular filtration rate and increased serum uric acid, serum creatinine, and urea levels. The proteinuria that usually accompanies PIH is believed to be correlated with the severity of kidney involvement as the disease advances. Related changes in the clotting mechanism (thrombocytopenia and DIC) have also been postulated as causative factors of PIH; however, it is not clearly established whether these alterations are an effect of PIH or a contributing etiologic factor.

Hepatic damage may result secondary to vasospasm, ischemia, and necrosis in the PIH client.[34] Hemorrhage necrosis may be evident along the edge of the liver, resulting in a subcapsular hematoma and possible rupture.

The uteroplacental manifestations of PIH include increased peripheral vascular resistance in the spiral and basal arteries with associated hypertensive lesions, poor placental perfusion resulting from decreased blood flow and vasospasm, and occasional decreased amniotic fluid volume. The effects of these changes can cause placental-fetal anoxia,[39] intrauterine growth retardation, and fetal death.[40] Uterine activity is increased both spontaneously and in response to oxytocin in women with PIH.

Preeclampsia

MANIFESTATIONS

Preeclampsia is characterized by elevation in BP, proteinuria, or edema after the 20th week of pregnancy in a gravida who previously has been normal in these respects. It is a forerunner or prodromal stage of eclampsia; in other words, unless the preeclamptic process is halted by treatment or by delivery, it is likely that eclampsia will ensue.

The development of hypertension may occur suddenly, or it may be gradual and insidious. The absolute BP level is probably of less significance than the relationship it bears to previous determinations and the time in gestation when these determinations were recorded. The healthy client often exhibits a lower than normal BP in the midtrimester of pregnancy, and hence a baseline reading in midpregnancy may be misleading. For example, a pressure of 120/80 mm Hg may actually indicate hypertension in a client whose midpregnancy pressure has been in the range of 100/70 mm Hg.

The next most constant sign of preeclampsia is *sudden excessive weight gain*, which is largely due to an accumulation of water in the tissues. Such weight gains represent occult edema and almost always precede the visible face and finger edema that is characteristic of the advanced stages of the disease.

The sudden appearance of *protein in the urine*, with or without other findings, should always be regarded as a sign of preeclampsia. A complete urinalysis, including a microscopic examination, helps to exclude infection as a cause of proteinuria. Because proteinuria usually develops later than the hypertension and the gain in weight, it may indicate progression of the disease process.

There are several other clinical manifestations of PIH that, when recognized by the client or health-team member, necessitate immediate attention; these include the following:

- Severe, continuous headache, often frontal or occipital
- Swelling of the face or the fingers
- Dimness or blurring of vision
- Persistent vomiting
- Decrease in the amount of urine excreted
- Epigastric pain (a late symptom)

It should be emphasized that the three early and important signs of preeclampsia—namely, hypertension, weight gain, and proteinuria—are changes of which the client is usually unaware. All three may be present in substantial degree and yet she may feel quite well. Only by regular and careful antepartal examination can these warning signs be detected. By the time the preeclamptic client has developed symptoms and signs that she herself can detect, such as headache, blurred vision, and puffiness of the eyelids and the fingers, she is usually in an advanced stage of the disease and much valuable time has been lost.

Headaches are rarely observed in the milder cases but are encountered more frequently as the disease progresses. In general, clients who develop eclampsia often have a severe headache as a forerunner of the first convulsion. The visual disturbances range from a slight blurring of vision to various degrees of temporary blindness. Although convulsions are less likely to occur in cases of mild preeclampsia, the possibility cannot be entirely eliminated. Clients with severe preeclampsia should always be considered as being on the verge of having a convulsion.

Preeclampsia can rapidly progress to a syndrome characterized by hemolysis, marked signs of liver dysfunction, as well as coagulation changes, which, within 24 to 48 hours, can reach life-threatening proportions.[41,42] This variant of the disease preeclampsia, known as *HELLP* (*h*emolysis, *e*levated *l*iver enzymes,

34

Metabolic, Cardiac, and Hematologic Diseases in Pregnancy

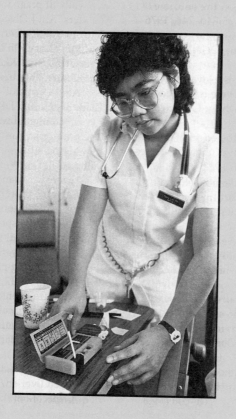

The pregnant woman can have any disease that the nonpregnant woman can have, except infertility. Many disease states are modified by the physiological changes of pregnancy. Pregnancy may alter the classic clinical picture of a disease, and some of the normal physiological changes of pregnancy mimic disease. Therapeutic approaches to diseases must be altered in some instances, especially with regard to possible effects on the fetus. For most coincidental diseases, the effects of pregnancy on the disease and of the disease on pregnancy are negligible and do not influence the management of either. Some diseases, however, have profound fetal effects, as discussed in Chapter 42; others have a predominantly maternal effect; and some, such as diabetes, affect both. The most common diseases in the latter two categories are discussed in this chapter.

■ DIABETES MELLITUS

Diabetes mellitus is a major complication of pregnancy and illustrates the interplay between the altered physiology of pregnancy and the pathophysiology of disease. There is a significant change in the course of diabetes when pregnancy supervenes, and diabetes profoundly affects the course of pregnancy and the fetus. Care of the pregnant diabetic woman involves an interdisciplinary team effort and necessitates cooperation among obstetrician, endocrinologist, pediatrician, nurse, social worker, and nutritionist.

Diabetes mellitus is an endocrine disorder of carbohydrate metabolism that results from a deficiency in insulin production by the cells of the islets of Langerhans in the pancreas. Insulin is an essential hormone required for glucose transfer into the muscle and adipose tissue cells. When glucose is unable to enter body cells because of deficient or inadequate quantities of insulin, fat and protein metabolism are altered. Protein catabolism, ketosis, and a negative nitrogen balance may result. As blood glucose levels steadily rise, cellular water is lost

---

Signs of Diabetes

Polyuria (frequent urination)

Polydipsia (excessive thirst)

Polyphagia (excessive hunger)

Orthostatic dizziness

Blurred vision

Weight loss

---

and glycosuria appears. Extracellular dehydration develops because of the high osmotic pressure and increased amount of glucose in the urine. As a result of these pathophysiological adaptations, the classic symptoms of diabetes manifest (see box below). Degenerative vascular changes, such as nephropathy (persistent proteinuria $\geq$ 300 mg/24 h prior to the 20th week of pregnancy) and retinopathy, are associated with long-term, poorly controlled carbohydrate metabolism and improper care during pregnancy.

In recent years, the incidence of diabetes during pregnancy has increased to approximately 180,000 pregnancies per year.[1] This is partly because with modern management, diabetics are now able to conceive and maintain pregnancies and partly because there is presently an increased recognition of the milder forms of gestational diabetes. Gestational, or pregnancy-induced, diabetes occurs in 1% to 2% of pregnancies; and pregestational diabetes, in 0.1% to 0.2%.[2] Approximately 25% to 50% of women with gestational diabetes initially diagnosed during pregnancy will later develop insulin-dependent diabetes.[1,3]

Effect of Pregnancy on Diabetes

During the course of pregnancy, the placenta produces human placental lactogen (HPL), which is a powerful insulin antagonist. This hormone acts by promoting lipolysis and increasing maternal utilization of fats, presumably sparing glucose for fetal use.[4] The rate of secretion is proportionate to the placental mass. The estrogen and progesterone produced by the placenta alter the maternal pancreatic response to insulin, also counteracting its influence, albeit to a lesser degree. Insulin requirements during pregnancy are further increased by the production of placental insulinase, an enzyme that accelerates the degradation of insulin. The glomerular filtration rate of glucose in the kidneys is increased, and tubular glucose reabsorption is decreased. Consequently, the renal threshold for glucose is reduced from normal nonpregnant levels. These physiological alterations occurring in insulin and carbohydrate metabolism render pregnancy a *diabetogenic* condition.

During the course of normal pregnancy, there is a lower fasting blood sugar level. There is, however, no difference between the pregnant and nonpregnant intravenous glucose tolerance test (GTT), and the degree of induced hyperglycemia is the same during the course of this test in both pregnant and nonpregnant states. When the oral GTT test is used, the hyperglycemia persists somewhat longer in pregnancy because of slower and more prolonged absorption of glucose from the gastrointestinal tract.

In the first trimester, the caloric intake may be decreased because of diminished appetite, anorexia, or

Research Highlight

A variety of screening methods to detect glucose intolerance have been described in the literature. Helton et al investigated the difference in using a 100 g carbohydrate meal or glucose loading before the postprandial blood glucose PPBG in order to recommend an inexpensive, accurate assessment for diabetes mellitus.

All patients <24 wk gestation without a history of diabetes mellitus were asked to participate in the 3-month investigation. On the second prenatal visit, all participants with an even hospital number were given a PPBG following ingestion of a 100 g carbohydrate meal and all participants with odd hospital numbers were tested after ingestion of 50 g Glucola. On the third prenatal visit, the groups were reversed and retested. Sixty-six patients completed the study. Glucose values following each type of carbohydrate loading showed: (1) 30 Glucola > meal values, (2) 34 meal > Glucola values; and (3) 2 meal = Glucola values; these findings inferred no significant difference between the Glucola loading and the meal. Further, eight of the patients experienced nausea and subsequent emesis after Glucola. In contrast, none of the patients ingesting a 100 g carbohydrate meal experienced complications. The researchers also emphasized the increase in cost of Glucola use due to repeat testing when vomiting occurs. Helton et al concluded that using the 2-h PPBG after consuming a 100 g carbohydrate meal was as accurate and more cost- and time-effective than ingestion of Glucola.

Nurses should be aware of the side effects of Glucola and possible need to repeat the test. Offering the 100 g carbohydrate meal may be an accurate alternative in screening for diabetes mellitus in pregnancy. Cost effectiveness and possible time saved with the meal should be emphasized to the physicians ordering the 2-h PPBG.

Helton DG, Martin RW, Martin JN, et al: Detection of glucose intolerance in pregnancy. J Perinatol 9(3):259–261, 1989.

vomiting. Concomitantly, there is a significant transfer of glucose and glucogenic amino acids to the embryo-fetus. These factors place the pregnant diabetic at risk for hypoglycemia or starvation *ketosis*.

During the second half of pregnancy, due to the previously described progressively increasing insulin antagonist factors and rising insulin requirements, the client is prone to develop hyperglycemia, which can lead to diabetic *ketoacidosis*. Development of diabetic ketoacidosis also has been associated with the use of beta-agonist preparations for treatment of preterm labor.[5]

Insulin demands drop dramatically in the intrapartum and early postpartum periods because of the rapid clearance of HPL and the cessation of its production, as well as the temporary suppression of pituitary growth hormone. Insulin administration must be discontinued or greatly reduced in prescribed dosage to prevent hypoglycemia following delivery.

Another potential effect of pregnancy on diabetes is to accelerate the progress of vascular diseases that are secondary to diabetes. Careful management of gestation may prevent or minimize the development of diabetic nephropathy and retinopathy.

Effect of Diabetes on Pregnancy

Despite great gains achieved in modern obstetric management, perinatal mortality and morbidity remain significantly higher in diabetic pregnancies than in normal pregnancies. Reported mortality rates for the perinatal infant vary from as high as 10% to 30% to as low as 2% to 4% in major treatment centers.[6] The risk factor for maternal-fetal complications is increased for women with a longer duration of diabetes, especially if there is a history of poor control prior to conception. The major factors affecting pregnancy outcome appear to be the degree of glycemic control and the severity of underlying vascular disease.[7]

Diabetes can have a deleterious effect on pregnancy in the following ways:

1. Infection, especially genitourinary tract infection, is more common and more serious. The presence of glycosuria places the pregnant diabetic at particular risk for monilial vaginitis, which may in some cases become intractable.
2. The fetus is often larger (macrosomia) owing to prolonged fetal hyperinsulinism and hyperglycemia, and if this occurs, the possibility of a difficult vaginal delivery and postpartum hemorrhage is increased.
3. There is a fourfold greater overall incidence of preeclampsia or eclampsia, with an increase even when there is no associated preexisting vascular disease.[8]
4. The incidence of hydramnios is increased, and if this is coupled with fetal macrosomia, it can cause cardiopulmonary symptoms.

5. The rate of cesarean section deliveries is increased (45% incidence) primarily due to fetal compromise and dystocias.[9,10]
6. Postpartum hemorrhage is more common than in the general obstetric population.
7. The incidence of congenital anomalies among infants of diabetic mothers is increased twofold to fourfold.[4,8] Mounting evidence suggests that uncontrolled diabetes during early pregnancy is a cause of fetal malformation. The frequency of malformations among women with good glycemic control in early gestation is about 3% but increases to as high as 22% in those with poor glycemic control.[11]

Other neonatal problems encountered include intrauterine growth retardation, prematurity, hypoglycemia, hypocalcemia, hyperbilirubinemia, and respiratory distress syndrome. The infant of the diabetic mother inherits a predisposition to diabetes. These and other conditions are discussed in Chapter 44.

Medical Diagnosis

During the course of normal pregnancy, glucose may appear in the urine with blood sugars as low as 100 mg/dl because of a lowered renal threshold to glucose excretion. Although the presence of glucose in the urine does not necessarily indicate high blood glucose levels, any client exhibiting glucosuria should be suspected of having diabetes. The diagnosis should be established or ruled out by evaluation of blood glucose levels.

There is lack of consensus in the literature about the type of diabetes screening test, when and how often to screen, and whom to screen.[7] A 1- or 2-hour postprandial blood glucose test may be employed for primary screening of pregnant women with known risk factors for diabetes (see Research Highlight). This test offers the advantage of being simpler to administer than the GTT; however, definitive diagnosis for the disease

cannot be established without further evaluation. A blood glucose value of 145 mg/dl or above on the postprandial test is suggestive of diabetes and necessitates follow-up with a full GTT. When a suspected diabetic obtains a normal value on the 2-hour postprandial blood glucose, the test should be repeated in the second or third trimester (Table 34-1).

The GTT may be administered orally (50 or 100 g) or intravenously (25 g). If a woman has already been identified as being diabetic prior to pregnancy, diagnostic GTTs are not required. In preparation for the GTT, the client is requested to fast overnight. A fasting blood glucose is drawn the next morning. The client is then given a carbohydrate load and 1-, 2-, and 3-hour postprandial venous blood samples are taken for glucose. O'Sullivan and Mahan have established criteria for comparative interpretations of GTTs in pregnant and nonpregnant women (see Table 34-1).[3] It should be noted that the initial peak values are higher during pregnancy and remain elevated for the entire test. An oral GTT is considered abnormal if two of the client's blood glucose values are elevated or if one blood glucose value is exceeded in two successive tests.

A client initially diagnosed for diabetes during pregnancy may regress completely following delivery. In these circumstances, the condition is referred to as *gestational diabetes*. It should be suspected on the basis of the risk factors presented in the box below. When prenatal problems develop (e.g., fetal size greater than indicated by estimated date of confinement, with ultrasound evidence of macrosomia, hydramnios, or glycosuria), the diagnosis of gestational diabetes may also be suspected.

A special diagnostic problem occurs when a client is not suspected of being diabetic until after delivery, as might be the case if she has delivered an unusually large baby or an unexplained stillborn. Because the diabetogenic effects of pregnancy disappear quickly following delivery, a normal GTT 48 to 72 hours postpartum is not necessarily reassuring. The so-called

TABLE 34-1. ORAL GLUCOSE TOLERANCE TEST

	Nonpregnant Glucose (mg/dl)		Pregnant Glucose (mg/dl)	
	Whole Blood	*Plasma*	*Whole Blood*	*Plasma*
Fasting	110	130	90	105
1 hour	170	195	165	190
2 hours	120	140	145	165
3 hours	110	120	125	145

(Data from O'Sullivan JB, Mahan CM: Criteria for the oral glucose tolerance test in pregnancy. Diabetes 13(3):278–285, 1964)

Risk Factors for Development of Gestational Diabetes

- Previous large infants (9 lb or more)
- Family history of diabetes mellitus
- Glucosuria on two successive occasions
- Obesity—weight >200 lb
- Unexplained pregnancy wastage (spontaneous abortions, stillbirths)
- Multiparity
- Presence of hydramnios
- Previous infant with a congenital anomaly

steroid enforced GTT, in which cortisone is administered prior to the testing, may elicit the abnormality.

CLASSIFICATION

Several methods for classifying diabetes are available in clinical practice. The National Diabetes Data Group[12] has developed the system in Table 34-2.

Another widely used classification scheme specific for pregnant women with diabetes was originally developed and modified by White.[13] The progressively severe categories A through T are represented in Table 34-2; in general, perinatal wastage can be related to class. The pregnancy outcome is invariably poor in those clients with vascular disease (classes D through T), and better in classes A through C. It should also be noted that mothers with significant vascular involvement often have small-for-date rather than large-for-date babies.

Nursing Process

The nursing process is designed to accomplish the following major objectives of nursing care:

1. Identification of women at risk for diabetes and provision of appropriate perinatal care.

2. Maintenance of blood glucose levels that mimic physiological levels in pregnant diabetic women (e.g., fasting blood sugar less than 90 mg/dl and 2-hour postprandial less than 145 mg/dl).

3. Provision of adequate client education and counseling for safe self-management of mother and the fetus / newborn.

4. Prevention or early detection of potential complications of diabetes during the entire childbearing cycle.

5. Promotion of a positive psychosocial adjustment to childbearing through understanding and acceptance of pregnancy and diabetes.

The plan of nursing care is developed in cooperation with the client. Evidence suggests that intensive diabetic care prior to and during pregnancy may substantially reduce perinatal morbidity and mortality.[1] All diabetic women of reproductive age should receive preconceptual counseling regarding (1) the effects of diabetes on pregnancy and the fetus, and (2) the effects of pregnancy on diabetic control and complications. Until recently, short-term hospitalization for the purpose of evaluation and regulation of disease state was recommended for diagnosed diabetic women who became pregnant. Improvements in ambulatory self-monitoring and care have reduced the need for hospitalizations without

---

TABLE 34–2. TWO METHODS OF CLASSIFICATION OF DIABETES

Classification of Diabetes by the National Diabetes Data Group*	White's Revised Classification of Diabetes in Pregnant Women†
A. Insulin-dependent diabetes (type I)	A Chemical diabetes; abnormal glucose tolerance test; initial onset during pregnancy
1. Early onset (juvenile) in most cases	B Maturity onset (age over 20 yr); duration under 10 years; no vascular disease
2. Little or no insulin produced by pancreas	C_1 Age at onset 10 to 19 years
B. Non-insulin-dependent diabetes (type II)	D_1 Under age 10 years at onset
1. Mature onset most cases	D_2 Over 10 years' duration
2. Nonobese group	D_3 Benign retinopathy
3. Obese group	D_4 Calcified vessels of legs
4. Diet control	D_5 Hypertension
C. Other types (secondary diabetes)	E Calcified pelvic arteries; no longer sought
1. Pancreatic disease	F Nephropathy
2. Hormonally induced (e.g., acromegaly or Cushing syndrome)	G Many failures
3. Chemically induced (e.g., steroids)	H Cardiomyopathy
4. Insulin receptor abnormalities	R Proliferating retinopathy
5. Certain genetic syndromes	T Renal transplant
6. Others	
D. Impaired glucose tolerance (subclinical diabetes)	
1. Fasting plasma glucose level normal or slightly elevated	
2. Glucose tolerance test abnormal levels	
E. Gestational diabetes (pregnancy-induced glucose intolerance)	

* National Diabetes Data Group: Classification of diabetes mellitus and other categories of glucose intolerance. Diabetes 28:1039, 1979.
† White P: Classification of obstetric diabetes. Am J Obstet Gynecol 130:229, 1978.

compromising maternal and neonatal outcomes.[14] Class A diabetics should receive antepartum visits with the health care team every 2 weeks until 33 to 34 weeks, then should be assessed weekly.[4] More frequent contact is often necessary for class B through T diabetics.

NURSING ASSESSMENT

Prenatal assessment should include observations for the previously identified signs and symptoms of diabetes in all pregnant women. The client's family and prenatal history should be carefully obtained and reviewed for predisposing factors.

There is some controversy as to whether all pregnant women or only those with known risk factors should receive screening for gestational diabetes (see Medical Diagnosis section). Substantial evidence suggests that as many as 50% of all gestational diabetic mothers may be undetected and therefore untreated without universal screening.[1] For all pregnant women with known risk factors, screening should occur at the first prenatal visit. The period of optimum identification and intervention in other pregnant women is between the 24th and 28th gestational week.[1] Knowledge of diabetes and the normal physiological–psychological adaptations of pregnancy are assessed.

Baseline vital signs, blood pressure, and fetal heart rate should be recorded and subsequently compared with later readings. A steady rise in blood pressure or a sudden increase in weight may be a sign of pregnancy-related hypertension, a frequent complication of diabetes. All pregnant diabetics should have a serum alpha-fetoprotein (AFP) screen performed between 16 and 18 weeks' gestation. The results of this test need to be interpreted with consideration given to the lower median AFP values in these pregnancies and the higher risk for neural tube defects.[9,15]

Measurements of glycosylated hemoglobin (A_1 or A_{1c}) are obtained because these values reflect average serum glucose concentrations over the last 4 to 12 weeks. In healthy women 6% to 8% of hemoglobin is glycosylated; however, levels are likely to be elevated in diabetes. The magnitude of the increase generally correlates inversely with the degree of long-term control of plasma glucose concentration that has been achieved.[10] Results of studies have shown that an elevation of glycohemoglobin in pregnancy is associated with an increased incidence of spontaneous abortions, congenital anomalies, neonatal macrosomia, and hyperbilirubinemia.[16]

The optic fundi should be examined to detect vascular disease at the time of the initial encounter with the pregnant diabetic and subsequently at least once per trimester. Urine analysis, culture, and sensitivity are important for detection of asymptomatic bacilluria, a precursor to overt pyelonephritis to which the diabetic is especially prone.

At each antenatal visit, results of blood glucose monitoring should be assessed to determine if hyperglycemia or hypoglycemia exists. Although urine testing is not an adequate determinant for management, most women with diabetes test their urine daily for glucose and ketones. Therefore, their knowledge of the basic testing procedures must be determined. Testape and Diastix are methods of choice for urine testing because they are specific to glucose and do not react to the presence of lactose or fructose. Urine is tested for ketones using the Ketostix, which is specific for acetoacetic acid, whereas, the Acetest is used for checking acetone and acetoacetic acid.

Accurate assessment of gestational age is especially important for managing pregnancy and planning the timing and method of delivery. Uterine size, fetal activity, and fetal heart rate sounds provide valuable information. To determine fetal size, well-being, and exact gestational age, a variety of prenatal assessments may be performed. An ultrasound examination is often done at 18 weeks' gestation to confirm gestational age and to survey the fetus for congenital abnormalities. Serial ultrasounds are performed subsequently during the second and third trimester. Weekly nonstress tests (NST) are administered beginning at approximately 32 weeks' gestation, and the frequency of testing is increased to two times per week at about 36 weeks' gestation. Additional fetal assessment techniques include contraction stress tests (CTS), fetal movement counts, biophysical profiles, amniocentesis for lecithin–sphingomyelin ratio and phosphatidylglycerol, and estriol levels (see Chap. 42).

Psychosocioeconomic factors are appraised, with special consideration given to the potential stress evoked by the high-risk pregnancy and high costs of antepartum testing procedures and possible hospitalizations. Research has shown that gestational diabetics experience more stressful responses than chronic diabetics for all aspects of the medical regimen during gestation.[17] Blood tests, amniocentesis, and particularly insulin administration are reportedly areas of greater stress for this group. The nurse should assess whether the diabetic woman has adequate resources available for social, emotional, and economic support in the home and community. Future needs for additional assistance with household chores and child care are also evaluated as they relate to the prescribed management plan.

NURSING DIAGNOSIS

As a result of the nursing assessment, several potential nursing diagnoses may be identified that focus on alterations in the life processes of the pregnant diabetic. These include (1) alteration in carbohydrate metabolism related to diabetes; (2) knowledge deficit related to diabetic self-care during pregnancy; (3) disturbance in self-concept related to complications of pregnancy; (4) alteration in tissue perfusion: uteroplacental; (5) high risk for infection: vaginal related to monilial infection; and (6) high risk for impairment in skin integrity related to skin stretching secondary to hydramnios.

NURSING INTERVENTION

Adequate control of the pregnant diabetic is of primary concern in planning nursing interventions to prevent or lessen the incidence or perinatal mortality and morbidity. Major components of direct nursing care and client education relate to nutrition management, insulin administration, blood and urine glucose monitoring, and exercise. There are several obstetric considerations of which the nurse must also be aware in implementing care.

Nutrition. Ideally, diabetic women who anticipate pregnancy will follow a well-balanced prescribed dietary regimen before conception and will be in a state of good metabolic control. The caloric requirement for the normal-weight client is approximately 2200 to 2500 cal; at least 45% of the total calories are in the form of carbohydrates (200 to 300 g), 30% are in the form of fat (70 to 80 g), and 25% are in the form of protein (100 to 125 g). At least 30 g/day more protein is recommended in the second and third trimesters than in the nonpregnant state. Clients with nephropathy and proteinuria require additional protein. The caloric requirement should be evenly distributed (three meals and three snacks), with no less than 2000 cal consumed daily. The exact caloric intake is determined based on the client's prepregnant weight and daily activities. A weight gain of 22 to 27 lb at term is most desirable.

The diabetic pregnant woman should be specifically instructed to include complex carbohydrates in each meal to delay absorption of glucose. Similarly, adequate fat consumption delays gastric emptying and prevents hyperglycemia. An evening snack consisting of a complex carbohydrate and protein is effective in preventing hypoglycemic episodes during the night. Concentrated sweets should be avoided because they are likely to produce marked swings in blood glucose.

It is difficult to decrease caloric intake below 1800 cal and maintain adequate protein and carbohydrate intake with a palatable formulation; therefore, weight reduction even for overweight women is generally not recommended. Diabetic women with deficient intake of carbohydrates are at risk for acidosis and ketonemia.

Insulin Administration. The goal of treatment with insulin is to keep blood glucose levels as near the normal range as possible. Maintaining optimal blood glucose levels requires meticulous regulation of medication, adherence to the prescribed diet, and carefully planned activity. Progressive insulin resistance is characteristic of pregnancy, and it is not unusual for insulin requirements to increase as much as fourfold. During the latter half of pregnancy, the effective half-life of insulin is reduced owing to increased placenta degradation. This commonly necessitates the use of evening as well as morning doses of insulin to achieve good control. Adjustment of insulin dosage is individualized according to the clinical picture and the results of blood glucose analysis. It is recommended that all pregnant clients requiring insulin use purified porcine or human-derived insulin.[18] The daily dosage of insulin is frequently split, with about two thirds being administered in the morning and about one third after dinner. A small amount of fast-acting insulin (regular or semilente) is often added to each dose of intermediate-acting insulin (isophane) to control the 4- to 6-hour interval before the intermediate insulin begins to have a significant effect on blood glucose level. The combined insulins are administered approximately one-half hour before meals. In some clients, more frequent, small dosages of regular insulin may have to be administered throughout the day in response to fasting and postprandial blood sugar levels.[19] It is essential that the nurse teach the client about time interval peaks for insulin. As this information is discussed, it should be related to the signs and symptoms of hypoglycemia and hyperglycemia.

The gestational diabetic may occasionally require insulin therapy despite nutritional management. Oral hypoglycemics are not recommended for use during pregnancy. Client education for the insulin-dependent gestational diabetic encompasses proper technique for injection, rotation of sites, storage of medication, and skin care.

The overt diabetic (classes B through T) should be counseled about changes in her insulin demands because of pregnancy. Counseling sessions provide excellent opportunities to reinforce the client's acquired skills in self-management and to allay fears concerning new interventions.

In an effort to improve metabolic control, some medical centers are advising pregnant diabetics to use *portable insulin pumps.* These electromechanical devices are implanted into the subcutaneous tissue of the woman's abdomen by way of a small-gauge needle, which continuously delivers a fixed small amount of insulin. A bolus of insulin may be self-administered by the client before meals. The dosage of insulin delivered by the pump is based on capillary blood sample levels drawn by the client or nurse. This type of system does not include an integral glucose sensor or feedback mechanism and is called an *open-loop system.*

Blood and Urine Glucose Monitoring. Until recent years, control of diabetes was primarily monitored by the use of preprandial determinations of the percentage of glucose in the urine. Glucosuria is a poor indicator of the diabetic's metabolic regulation because there is an alteration in the renal threshold for glucose during pregnancy. An alternative and effective means being used to accomplish the normalization of maternal glucose levels during pregnancy is home blood glucose monitoring (HBGM).[20] There are now a variety of machines such as the Dextrometer available for use with blood glucose reagent strips. Recent advances in technology allow devices to store 2 weeks to 3 months of glucose data which can be rapidly analyzed by computer to measure control by hour, day, week, and month. Clients are instructed on how to use the device. Measurements of blood glucose levels are usually obtained four times a day (upon rising in the morning, then again before lunch and dinner and at bedtime)[10] or more frequently, as indicated by metabolic control. Some physicians recommend that daily determinations include a blood glucose reading 1 hour after a major meal. All blood glucose levels should be entered by the client in her home record keeping system, which also includes insulin doses, weight, and diet. The goals of therapy are fasting glucose levels of less than 95 mg/dl and postprandial levels less than 120 mg/dl; however, this degree of rigid control should not be demanded in clients having frequent hypoglycemic reactions.[7]

Exercise. Pregnancy is not an optimum time to begin vigorous exercise. During exercise, glucose is absorbed into the muscle and the blood glucose level is lowered. The effect of exercise may last up to 12 hours.

Well-controlled diabetic women who regularly engage in exercise may continue and should be reminded to eat a snack consisting of carbohydrate or protein before activity. A consistent and structured program of activity should be followed rather than an irregular and unpredictable schedule. If signs of hypertensive complications arise, exercise programs should be discontinued.

Obstetric Considerations. The timing of delivery is probably much more critical than the method, which depends on fetal condition, cervical condition, and, to a lesser extent, maternal medical stability.[2] Because the major target of diabetes is the small blood vessels, it is not surprising that the placenta may also be involved, and therefore placental insufficiency and even fetal death may occur. This result is far less common in gestational diabetics than in prepregnancy diabetics and has been the basis for delivering diabetic mothers 3 to 4 weeks prior to the expected date of confinement. Today, this practice is often unnecessary if one can identify the fetus at risk and accurately establish gestational age and well-being through antenatal testing techniques, careful surveillance, and glucose self-monitoring. Early delivery may still be necessary for large fetal size relative to gestational age, maternal vascular disease, hypertension, and previous stillbirth.

The method of delivery is a matter of obstetric judgment at the time. Vaginal delivery is carried out whenever possible. Cesarean section is indicated for cases of fetal compromise, macrosomia, or an unfavorable cervix. Cousins recently examined the results of 24 investigations on pregnancy complications among diabetics.[5] His findings revealed that primary, repeat, and total cesarean section rates increase in a step-wise fashion from nondiabetic to gestational, to class B and C, to class D, F, and R diabetics.[5]

In situations where a planned delivery is scheduled for an insulin-dependent diabetic, an intravenous infusion with regular insulin may be started 24 to 48 hours before the induction or cesarean section. The purpose of this infusion is to titrate blood glucose levels accurately. A heparin lock is often inserted as a means of avoiding the repetitive venipunctures required for close blood glucose surveillance. The laboring client may receive a continuous insulin infusion using a calibrated pump if glucose levels are over 120 mg/dl. Capillary blood glucose should be assessed every 1 to 2 hours. Uterine activity and fetal heart rate are monitored continuously. Following delivery, insulin is administered as indicated by blood glucose monitoring and the client is closely observed for insulin reactions. The nurse should provide family planning counseling to the postpartum diabetic woman. Special areas for consideration include (1) the need to use safe barrier methods of contraception (conflicting opinions exist about the safety of oral contraceptives for diabetics); (2) family size and spacing in relation to disease progression; and (3) the risk of developing gestational or overt diabetes in the future.

NURSING EVALUATION

Anticipated outcomes of nursing care are that the pregnant woman with diabetes does the following:

- Understands the effects of her disease on pregnancy, labor and delivery, and perinatal outcomes
- Recognizes symptoms of disease progression and reports them promptly
- Implements the prescribed treatment plan of self-care activities and prevents potential complications
- Maintains adequate tissue perfusion and oxygenation to the maternal-fetal unit
- Delivers a healthy infant at or near term

(Text continues on page 831)

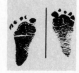

Nursing Care Plan

The Pregnant Diabetic Woman

Nursing Goals

The pregnant diabetic woman will successfully maintain pregnancy without perinatal complications as evidenced by:

1. Maintaining blood glucose levels of fasting blood sugar <90 mg/dl and 2-h postprandial <145 mg/dl.
2. Complying with self-management instructions (e.g., diet, exercise, monitoring blood sugar, insulin management) as ordered.
3. Expressing fears, griefs, and concerns regarding self-care and effects on the fetus.
4. Delivering a healthy term infant without signs of distress and/or hypoglycemia.

Assessment	Potential Nursing Diagnosis	Planning/Intervention	Evaluation

Maternal factors
  Previous large infant (9 lb or greater)
  Family history of diabetes mellitus
  Glucosuria
  Obesity
  Unexplained pregnancy wastage (previous habitual spontaneous abortions or unexplained stillbirth)
  Previous birth of infant with congenital abnormality
  Multiparity
	Alteration in carbohydrate metabolism related to diabetes	Screen for predisposing factors for diabetes
		
		Determine blood glucose levels by Dextrostix or Chemstik
		
		Check urine specimens for glucose and acetone as ordered
		
		Observe for signs and symptoms of hypoglycemia or hyperglycemia
		
		Administer 4 oz orange juice for symptomatic hypoglycemia
			Client at risk for diabetes is identified
			
			Client has no signs and symptoms of hypoglycemia or hyperglycemia
			
			Client maintains normal blood glucose level or restores normal level after administration of orange juice

Fetal–newborn factors
  Hydramnios
  Low-gestation-age infant
Signs of diabetes
  Polyuria
  Polydipsia
  Polyphagia
  Weight loss
 	
Signs and symptoms of hypoglycemia (hunger, weakness, nausea, agitation, pallor, perspiration) and hyperglycemia (nausea and vomiting, flushed skin, deep rapid respirations, restlessness, thirst, acetone odor to breath)
		Chart blood glucose levels, treatments, and insulin administration
		
		Assist in preparing for 2-h postprandial or oral glucose tolerance test
		
		Administer insulin as ordered
		
		Refer to community health nurse for home follow-up and additional teaching as needed
			
			Client repeats instructions to indicate understanding the purpose of testing and follows instructions
			
			Client displays no insulin reaction
			
			Client cooperates with follow-up referrals

(continued)

Nursing Care Plan *(continued)*

Assessment	Potential Nursing Diagnosis	Planning/Intervention	Evaluation
Physical examination, including assessment of optic fundi, cardiovascular system, vital signs, blood pressure, fundal height			
Glucose tolerance test Fasting 90 mg/dl 1 h 165 mg/dl 2 h 145 mg/dl 3 h 125 mg/dl			
Knowledge of carbohydrate metabolism	Knowledge deficit related to diabetic self-care during pregnancy	Review normal carbohydrate and fat metabolism	Client repeats explanation of effects of diabetes on pregnancy and effects of pregnancy on diabetes
Knowledge about pathophysiology of diabetes during pregnancy		Discuss pathophysiology of diabetes during pregnancy	
24-h diet recall		Explain changes in insulin regulation throughout childbearing cycle	
Past experience managing diabetes (e.g., self-administration of insulin)		Request nutritional consultation	Client understands changes in insulin demand throughout pregnancy
Exercise schedule (predictability, length)			
Knowledge of complications of diabetes		Review prescribed dietary plan (exchange lists)	Client follows prescribed diet based on knowledge of nutritional needs
		Record dietary intake on appropriate record	Client records dietary intake
		Teach newly diagnosed insulin-dependent diabetic the techniques for insulin preparation, administration and storage	Client demonstrates safe procedure in preparation, self-administration and storage of insulin
		Instruct in regulation and care of insulin pump prn	Client correctly regulates and cares for insulin pump
		Instruct in blood glucose monitoring and importance of maintaining fasting blood sugar between 60 and 120 mg/dl	Client shows proper technique in return demonstration of blood glucose monitoring
		Instruct in fractional urine	Client correctly checks

(continued)

Nursing Care Plan *(continued)*

Assessment	Potential Nursing Diagnosis	Planning/Intervention	Evaluation
		testing for glucose and acetone levels by TesTape or Diastix	urine for glucose levels and acetone levels
		Provide specific information on signs and symptoms of diabetic complications (e.g., ketoacidosis, insulin shock, hypertensive disorders of pregnancy, urinary tract infection)	Client identifies signs and symptoms of diabetic complications during pregnancy
		Discuss activities for daily living and exercise schedule (prn)	Client maintains safe level of activities and avoids hypoglycemia
Response to diabetes Expectations about pregnancy	Self-concept disturbance related to complication of pregnancy	Discuss family adaptation to pregnancy and alterations necessitated by diabetes	Client expresses fears, griefs, and concerns
Achievement of maternal tasks of pregnancy		Define possible stressors and resources in family community	Client identifies possible stressors and resources in family community
		Involve supportive family member(s) in education about complication	Family member(s) provide appropriate support
		Develop strategies for adjusting to complication	Family demonstrates effective problem-solving skills

Fetal factors
  Heart rate
  Activity (e.g., kicking)
  Periodic changes, variability on electronic fetal monitor
	Alteration in tissue perfusion: uteroplacental related to diabetes in pregnancy	Frequent monitoring of fetal heart rate (q2–4 h if stable); report any periodic changes or decreased variability	Fetal heart rate remains within normal limits, without signs of distress

Prenatal diagnostic tests
  Lecithin-sphingomyelin ratio
  Nonstress test
  Oxytocin challenge test
  Sonography
  Estriol levels
		Instruct client to maintain fetal activity record (kick counts) and report any significant changes in fetal activity	Fetus remains active

		Discuss importance of frequent prenatal evaluations during entire pregnancy	Client keeps scheduled prenatal and testing appointments
		Explain rationales and prepare for prenatal diagnostic tests (e.g., amniocentesis, sonography, nonstress test) and provide support during procedures	Client remains relaxed for testing

■ CARDIAC DISEASE

Approximately 1% of all pregnant women have some type of cardiac disorder. In the past, rheumatic heart disease was the most common type of heart disease seen in pregnancy. The mitral valve is most often affected by this disease, with stenosis resulting. Recognition of the role of streptococcal infection and its appropriate therapy has greatly reduced the frequency of rheumatic fever and its cardiac consequences. Congenital heart disease is now becoming the most common cardiac problem encountered in pregnancy. Another new population of women has been added by cardiac surgeons. Surgically treated women, some with valve replacements, now often proceed through pregnancy uneventfully.

About 6% to 10% of women of childbearing age are affected by a cardiac condition known as *mitral valve prolapse* (MVP).[21] The underlying pathology involves prolapse of the mitral valve leaflets into the left atrium during ventricular systole, causing some backflow of blood. A midsystolic click and late systolic murmur are characteristic of the syndrome. Most women with MVP are asymptomatic and are able to tolerate pregnancy well.

A relatively rare condition that may cause devastating problems is *peripartum cardiomyopathy*. This disease manifests between the last trimester of pregnancy and 5 postpartum months without obvious cause or history of cardiac disease.[22] The main pathological features are reduction of the ejection fraction of the left ventricle and impairment of ventricular contractile power. The prognosis of this disease is directly related to the duration of the illness. Clinical manifestations include breathlessness, tachycardia, arrhythmias, cardiomegaly, and edema.

The risks of perinatal mortality, maternal morbidity, and maternal mortality for pregnant women with a cardiac disorder depend on three factors: (1) the underlying cardiac lesion; (2) the functional derangement produced by the lesion; and (3) the development of pregnancy-related complications such as pregnancy-induced hypertension (PIH), hemorrhage, and infection. The quality of health services rendered and the client's psychosocial capabilities may also influence outcome.[10] For most types of heart disease, the major threat imposed by pregnancy is that the increasing blood volume will precipitate congestive heart failure.[23] Overall, maternal-fetal prognosis for pregnancies complicated by cardiac disease is steadily improving.

Effect of Pregnancy on the Cardiovascular System

The cardiovascular adaptations normally occurring in pregnancy were comprehensively described in Chapter 15. As background for discussion on the perinatal effects of heart disease, a brief review is presented here. Cardiac output progressively rises during pregnancy, with maximum output (30% to 50%) reached between 28 and 32 weeks.[24] Increases in both stroke volume and heart rate (10 beats per minute) contribute to the change. Blood volume expands approximately 40% by the 30th week of pregnancy and then remains fairly constant. Most of the increase in plasma volume occurs in the second trimester. Vascular resistance and blood pressure decrease during the course of pregnancy.

In normal pregnancy, functional systolic murmurs are rather common. Upward displacement of the diaphragm and heart by the enlarging uterus moves the apex of the heart laterally. This may create a false impression of cardiac enlargement. Progesterone stimulates the respiratory center, accentuating breathing effort, which is reminiscent of the dyspnea sometimes seen in heart disease. Edema of the lower extremities that is commonly encountered in normal pregnancy is also a sign of cardiac failure. The normal changes must be considered when the cardiac status of the pregnant woman is evaluated.

The first stage of labor is associated with a modest increase in cardiac output, and there is an appreciable change related to the expulsive efforts of the second stage. The healthy woman has the ability to adapt to the stresses that pregnancy superimposes on the cardiovascular system; however, the woman with heart disease may not have the cardiac reserve to adjust to these new demands.

Effect of Cardiac Disease on Pregnancy

The pathophysiology of disease evident in pregnancy depends on the type of cardiac disorder present. For most types of heart disease, the major threat imposed by pregnancy is that the increasing blood volume will precipitate congestive heart failure. If maternal blood flow is severely compromised, signs and symptoms of right-sided, left-sided, or total failure may develop in the mother and placental circulation may diminish, resulting in a higher risk of prematurity and low birth weight.[25] Pregnant women who have successfully undergone surgical repair and have no residual effects of heart disease generally may experience pregnancy without complication. Unlike these women, clients with cyanotic heart disease are at greater risk for perinatal morbidity and mortality. The incidence of congestive heart failure increases over the age of 30 and is further aggravated by parity.

A major problem in managing clients with artificial cardiac valves (e.g., ball valves, tilted disk valves, and bileaflet valves) is that of coagulation. Clients with biosynthetic tissue valves (e.g., porcine valves) usually do not require anticoagulants, unless they are experiencing other cardiac complications. Reports have revealed that such pregnancies are relatively uneventful; however, in women who are anticoagulated because of artificial heart valves, the rate of fetal loss is 33%.[26] This finding may be partially related to the fact that gravidae with a prosthetic heart valve have a cardiac output that is relatively fixed. They demonstrate a suboptimal increase in cardiac output and stroke volume in comparison to that usually seen during pregnancy and particularly in labor.[27] Newer mechanical valves have reduced this problem to some extent. Pregnancy exposes women who have had previous valvuloplasty to three most common complications: thromboembolism, infective endocarditis, and myocardial decompensation. Several factors contribute to the risk of thromboembolism from either the valve site or the periphery: thrombogenicity of the valve, trauma to the formed elements of blood, increased clotting factors, and venous stasis.[28] The danger is increased if the pregnant woman discontinues anticoagulants to protect the fetus from teratogenic effects (as experienced with sodium warfarin and related drugs).

Other conditions that contribute to the severity of the effects imposed by cardiac disease during pregnancy include obesity, smoking, and anemia. The incidence of spontaneous abortion, preterm labor, and intrauterine growth retardation is higher in this obstetric population.

Medical Diagnosis

The most useful criteria in establishing a diagnosis of heart disease in pregnancy include a diastolic, presystolic, or continuous heart murmur; unequivocal cardiac enlargement; a harsh systolic murmur associated with a thrill; or a significant cardiac arrhythmia.[29] Serious heart disease is usually absent in pregnant women who do not fulfill the above criteria.

CLASSIFICATION

The American Heart Association has developed a classification system for heart disease based on the woman's functional capacity (Table 34-3). This taxonomy is used as a guide for therapy by members of the health care team. With appropriate management, women in classes I and II generally are able to experience a normal pregnancy with no or few problems, whereas women in classes III and IV are at much greater risk for decompensation and other complications. Whenever possible, class III and IV women with correctable lesions should be counseled to undergo cardiac surgery before conception. It is now the very rare cardiac client (class IV) who should be considered for therapeutic abortion on medical grounds.

TABLE 34–3. CLASSIFICATION OF HEART DISEASE

Class	Description
I	Cardiac disease with *no* limitation of physical activity. Absence of symptoms of cardiac insufficiency and anginal pain.
II	Cardiac disease with *slight* limitation of physical activity. Comfortable at rest. Experience fatigue, palpitation, dyspnea, or anginal pain with *ordinary* physical activity.
III	Cardiac disease with *moderate* to *marked* limitation of physical activity. Comfortable at rest. Experience excessive fatigue, palpitation, dyspnea, or anginal pain with *less* than ordinary physical activity.
IV	Cardiac disease with *inability* to perform any physical activity without discomfort. Symptoms of cardiac insufficiency or of the anginal syndrome may occur *at rest* and with *any* physical activity.

(Criteria Committee of New York State Heart Association: Nomenclature and Criteria for Diagnosis of Diseases of the Heart and Blood Vessels, 6th ed. Boston, Little, Brown, 1964)

Nursing Process

An interdisciplinary team effort is needed for appropriate management of the pregnant woman with cardiac disease. The nurse may be closely collaborating with the obstetrician, cardiologist, nutritionist, and social worker. Nursing care is determined to a considerable extent by the functional capacity of the client.

NURSING ASSESSMENT

A thorough history is obtained on all women with heart disease. Questions should be asked about the client's ability to perform various types of physical activity before pregnancy and during pregnancy and the associated cardiovascular effects (e.g., dyspnea on exertion, palpitations, coughing). A complete physical examination is performed, with special attention given to auscultation of heart and breath sounds. The extremities and more central body surfaces are carefully palpated for edema and tenderness. Baseline maternal vital signs, blood pressure, and fetal heart rate are determined at the initial assessment and then frequently compared with subsequent readings. Capillary filling time is assessed, and observations are made for venous distention.

The pattern of weight gain, discomforts of pregnancy, and side effects and interactions of any prescribed medications are assessed continuously. The nurse should observe carefully for symptoms of *cardiac decompensation* that may be evidenced with congestive

---

Signs of Cardiac Decompensation

Dyspnea

Palpitations

Chest pain

Cough

Pulse irregularity

Sweating

Orthopnea

Weakness

Progressive, generalized edema

Rales at the base of the lungs

Pallor

---

heart failure and other complications; these symptoms may appear suddenly or develop gradually and are presented in the box above. Observations must also be made for arrhythmias. The onset of atrial fibrillation in pregnancy or the puerperium is particularly ominous, because the condition is often associated with various types of heart failure and pulmonary emboli.

Results of an electrocardiogram, chest x-ray, and other prescribed tests are reviewed by the nurse, as are laboratory findings. Hemoglobin and hematocrit are carefully assessed because anemia places an increased stress on the heart. Possible infection may be revealed by results of the urinalysis and white blood cell count. If the client is receiving anticoagulant therapy, the nurse should check prothrombin, partial thromboplastin, thrombin clotting times, and heparin assay, as appropriate.

Hemodynamic monitoring provides valuable information about the cardiac status of the acutely ill pregnant woman (predominantly functional classes III or IV) and may be implemented during the intrapartum period. The Swan-Ganz flow-directed pulmonary artery catheter allows continuous measurement of right atrial pressure, pulmonary artery pressure, pulmonary capillary wedge pressure, and central venous pressure. It can be used effectively to assess cardiac output as well as to administer fluids or drugs. In clients without hemodynamic monitoring, vital signs may be assessed as frequently as every 10 to 30 minutes during labor. If the pulse rate increases above 100 beats per minute, the physician should be notified.

NURSING DIAGNOSIS

As is true of all concurrent diseases of pregnancy, nursing assessment is an essential step in formulating nursing diagnoses. Examples of nursing diagnoses that specifically appertain to the woman with a pregnancy complicated by heart disease are activity intolerance related to increased metabolic requirements (pregnancy) in the presence of impaired cardiac function; risk of clotting disorder secondary to venous stasis; alteration in cardiac output and circulation related to cardiac decompensation; infection related to bacterial invasion; and anxiety related to fears concerning perinatal outcome. The patient may also have a knowledge deficit related to the effects of cardiac disease on pregnancy and signs and symptoms of complications; self-care deficit related to dyspnea, fatigue, and discomforts of pregnancy; and high risk for fetal distress related to intrauterine hypoxia secondary to maternal cardiac decompensation.

NURSING INTERVENTION

Nursing intervention is directed toward assisting the client in minimizing the work load on the cardiovascular system and reducing the risks of complications developing during pregnancy and the postpartum period. The nurse should review the signs and symptoms of cardiac decompensation as well as other complications (e.g., PIH, preterm labor) with all clients.

Stress, Rest, and Activity. Regardless of cardiac classification level, all women with heart disease should be exposed to a minimum of stress and obtain additional rest during pregnancy. A minimum of 10 hours of sleep per night plus additional morning and afternoon rest periods are recommended. Based on knowledge of the client's functional capacity, the nurse and client should explore the need for modification of and adjustments in activity level during pregnancy (e.g., limiting housework, shopping). Some women may need to terminate employment. Complete bedrest in the second half of pregnancy is necessitated by certain cardiac disorders and is required for all class IV women. Elastic support stockings should be applied to bedridden women and are probably beneficial to all cardiac clients in the latter half of pregnancy. They reduce hemodynamic fluctuations that accompany changes in maternal posture and increase venous return.[27]

Nutrition. Pregnant woman with cardiac disease should eat a well-balanced nutritional diet (approximately 2200 cal), with large amounts of high-quality protein and iron. Salt should not be added to food (2 g sodium per day) and may need to be restricted (1 to 1.5 g/day) if complications arise or the disease is severe. All women should be instructed to avoid foods rich in sodium. Supplementary iron is often prescribed to prevent anemia. Foods and beverages containing caffeine should be limited or avoided. Women receiving heparin need to be advised to eliminate foods high in vitamin K (e.g., raw, deep-green, leafy vegetables). A weight gain between 22 and 27 lb is desirable. Excess weight gain places additional strain on the heart and circulatory system. The lateral recumbent position is recommended for clients on bedrest or in labor.

Medications. Women who were receiving *digitalis* prior to pregnancy must continue use of the drug throughout the childbearing cycle. Changes in the cardiovascular system may also necessitate the initiation of digitalis treatment for previously nonmedicated women. Maternal and fetal heart rate are both slowed by the administration of digitalis, which crosses the placental barrier. If arrhythmias should develop during pregnancy, cardioversion may be safely accomplished through the use of *quinidine.*

Diuretic therapy is generally not recommended for class I and II women during pregnancy; however, it may be prescribed for class III and IV women. *Thiazides* are the commonly prescribed diuretics (e.g., chlorothiazide, hydrochlorothiazide). The woman on diuretic therapy should be observed for potassium depletion and postural hypotension. Neonatal thrombocytopenia has been observed in infants whose mothers used thiazide diuretics in the third trimester.[30]

Propranolol (Inderal) may occasionally be administered to clients who develop symptoms (e.g., palpitations, chest pain, dyspnea) with conditions such as mitral valve prolapse.

Just prior to delivery, some physicians prescribe prophylactic antibiotic for women with valvular heart disease and congenital defects because of their high susceptibility to subacute bacterial endocarditis.

The use of *sodium warfarin* (Coumadin) as an anticoagulant for women who have had valve replacements is associated with an increased risk of congenital anomalies (nasal hypoplasia, stippling of bones, intrauterine growth retardation, and ophthalmologic abnormalities) in the first trimester and questionable safety factors in later pregnancy.[31-33]

Heparin, an alternative anticoagulant that does not cross the placental barrier, may be prescribed prior to conception and during early pregnancy. The drug is administered in two to three subcutaneous boluses or continuous via an infusion pump.[23] Specific information about the actions, side effects, and self-administration of heparin is provided by the nurse to all women beginning therapy. The nurse should be aware that use of this drug increases the risk for maternal hemorrhage, preterm birth, and stillbirth.[10]

Prevention of Infection. Febrile episodes increase the cardiac demands and are often associated with tachycardia. Spread of the infectious organism may cause direct damage to the heart. Therefore, the nurse should caution the pregnant woman with cardiac disease against contact with people suffering from respiratory infections or other contagious diseases. An early dental examination and treatment of all caries (with antibiotic prophylaxis) is encouraged. The importance of using proper perineal care should be emphasized as a means of preventing urinary tract infections (UTIs) and pyelonephritis. Emphasis is placed on the need to report signs of potential infections immediately and to follow prescribed treatment protocols.

Obstetric Considerations. Prior to conception, the client with cardiac disease should be counseled as to the risks she and her fetus may experience during pregnancy. Additionally, those with congenital heart disease must be advised as to the danger of their child inheriting a congenital lesion. Most of these lesions follow a polygenic–multifactorial mode of inheritance with a 2% to 5% risk of recurrence.[23]

During the antepartum period, many clients with cardiac disease are monitored more frequently than healthy, pregnant women. Prenatal visits may be scheduled as often as every 2 weeks in the first half of pregnancy and every week thereafter. The nurse should assist the client and her family to understand the disease process and its relationship to pregnancy. Because the risk for premature labor and delivery is increased, pregnant women with cardiac disease should be instructed on the presenting symptoms. Serial ultrasound examinations may be recommended for clients with heart conditions that reduce cardiac output (mitral valvular disease) because of the increased risk for intrauterine growth retardation. Other types of antepartum fetal surveillance that may be undergone include NSTs, CSTs and amniocentesis with lung maturation studies.

The diagnosis of cardiac disease is not an indication for early induction of labor. Clients are usually allowed to go into spontaneous labor. Hospitalization for a short period prior to the expected onset of labor is occasionally recommended. It is essential that the laboring woman with heart disease be relieved of discomfort and anxiety. Effective intrapartum pain relief may reduce cardiac workload by as much as 20%.[34] Systemic analgesics combined with sedatives may be administered early in the first stage of labor. Caudal or epidural anesthesia may be initiated as labor advances or for delivery. The nurse can help the client and her family to relax by maintaining a calm manner and keeping them informed about intrapartum progress. To improve cardiac circulation and maximize oxygenation, the client is placed in a side-lying position, with her head and shoulders elevated. Oxygen may be administered if pulmonary complications arise. Continuous fetal heart rate monitoring is performed.

Many laboring clients with cardiac disease require continuous electrocardiogram surveillance and some also need hemodynamic monitoring with a central venous or arterial line. The degree of intrapartum monitoring necessary is determined individually, based on the client's functional status, underlying disease, and secondary complications.

Clients with prosthetic valves should have anticoagulation discontinued during labor and delivery and resumed 6 to 12 hours after delivery.[27] The administration of antibiotic prophylaxis for those undergoing cesarean section, induction of labor, or forceps delivery is an important part of their intrapartum care. Risk of intrapartum hemorrhage is related to the coagulation status of the mother and fetus.[27]

Controlled vaginal deliveries are preferable to cesarean births. In the second stage of labor, forceps or a vacuum extractor are commonly applied to avoid the stress of increased abdominal pressure created by maternal pushing. Delivery may be accomplished in the lateral position or in a supine position with the client tilted to the left to decrease the risk of supine hypotension. The use of high stirrups is inappropriate for women with cardiac disease. Drugs containing ergot should not be administered because of increases in blood pressure that result. Broad-spectrum antibiotics may be administered during the intrapartum and postpartum periods to prevent development of bacterial endocarditis and bacteremia.

Nursing care in the postpartum period is similar to that for other clients, with special consideration given to the possible need for limited activity and additional rest. Stool softeners may be prescribed to prevent stressful elimination. Discharge planning is particularly important for clients with cardiac disease. The nurse should refer the family to community agencies if assistance is needed with infant care or household responsibilities.

NURSING EVALUATION

Anticipated outcomes of nursing care are that the pregnant woman with cardiac disease does the following:

- Understands the effects of her disease on pregnancy, labor and delivery, and perinatal outcome
- Recognizes signs and symptoms of cardiac decompensation and obstetric complications and reports them promptly
- Implements the established treatment plan (e.g., limited activity and rest, prescribed diet and medications, avoidance of contact with infected persons) and prevents potential complications
- Maintains adequate tissue perfusion and oxygenation to the maternal-fetal unit
- Delivers a healthy infant at or near term

- Secures the needed additional resources to assist with child care, household and other responsibilities

■ HEMATOLOGIC DISORDERS

Although a variety of hematologic disorders may affect the pregnant woman, about 90% of the diagnosed cases are classified as iron deficiency anemia. The remaining 10% of cases encompass a variety of acquired and hereditary anemias, such as folic acid deficiency and the hemoglobinopathies (sickle cell disorders). The existence of a hematologic abnormality increases the pregnant woman's risk for developing other complications, such as infection.

Iron Deficiency Anemia

Iron deficiency anemia is the most common hematologic disorder in pregnancy, affecting approximately 20% of pregnant women. Several physiological alterations occurring in pregnancy contribute to the risk for this type of anemia. There is a pronounced increase in maternal plasma volume and a relatively lower increase in total red blood cells. These alterations increase the nutrient-carrying capacity of the plasma but reduce the viscosity of whole blood. The disproportionate rise in blood constituents causes hemodilution with a resultant fall in hemoglobin concentration unless the need is met by augmented hematopoiesis. These blood changes are unrelated to the pregnant woman's iron status; they occur whether the client is or is not receiving iron supplementation.

In addition, the fetus has a requirement for iron that must be secured from the mother. Because many women have depleted iron stores as a result of regular menstrual blood loss, these added demands often result in the total depletion of storage iron and the development of overt anemia during pregnancy. The socioeconomically deprived woman with poor general nutrition is more susceptible to this condition.

MEDICAL DIAGNOSIS

A hemoglobin level below 11 g/dl or a hematocrit of less than 35% is generally considered suggestive of anemia, and further evaluation is indicated to determine the reasons for the condition. Erythrocyte indexes aid in assessing the cause of the low hemoglobin level. The red blood cells are characteristically found to be microcytic and hypochromic. There is a decrease in the mean

(Text continues on page 839)

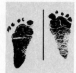

Nursing Care Plan

The Antepartum Woman with Heart Disease

Nursing Goals

The antepartum woman with heart disease will carry fetus to term without perinatal complications as evidenced by:
1. Maintaining cardiac functioning throughout the childbearing cycle.
2. Decreasing risks of complications by complying with medical management (e.g., rest, diet, medications, use of referral agencies).
3. Reporting all signs and symptoms of infections or cardiac problems to appropriate medical personnel.
4. Delivering a healthy newborn at or near term.
5. Displaying positive feelings toward infant.

Assessment	Potential Nursing Diagnosis	Planning/Intervention	Evaluation

Physical examination
  Heart rhythm
  Bradycardia
  Tachycardia
  Murmurs
  Hypotension/hypertension
  Skin color
  Venous distention
  Edema
  Rales
  Cough
History
  Fatigue
  Vertigo
  Angina
  Dyspnea
  Activity level
  Age
  Parity
  Duration of heart disease
  Complications of heart disease
  Medications (digoxin, warfarin, diuretics, antibiotics)
Dietary history
  Weight
  Sodium and fluid intake
ECG and x-ray results
Laboratory
  Hemoglobin, hematocrit
	Activity intolerance related to increased metabolic requirements secondary to pregnancy in the presence of impaired cardiac function	Recommend 10 h of sleep per night and frequent rest periods during the day as necessary
		
		Assist in modifying schedule to allow rest
		
		Instruct to record a 24-h dietary history
		
		Provide nutritional counseling
		  Well-balanced, high-protein diet with no added salt
		  Identify foods high in sodium that should be avoided
		
		Administer iron supplement as ordered
		
		Discuss normal cardiovascular changes in pregnancy and how these interact with heart disease
		
		Counsel to avoid strenous work (e.g., heavy housekeeping)
		
		Review actions, side effects, and administration of each prescribed medication
		
		Initiate referral to community agency for household
			Client sleeps a minimum of 10 h per night and rests in morning and afternoon
			
			Client records 24-h diet
			
			Client avoids foods with high sodium content; consumes 2200-cal diet with 125 g protein per day
			
			Client indicates her understanding in discussion of extra demands placed on cardiovascular system during pregnancy
			
			Client limits her work activities
			
			Client discusses actions, use, and side effects of medications
			
			Family follows through on referral

(continued)

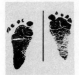

Nursing Care Plan   (continued)

Assessment	Potential Nursing Diagnosis	Planning/Intervention	Evaluation
Complete blood count Electrolytes Cholesterol Phospholipids		help or assistance with child care	

Physical Examination
Extremities (swelling, redness, numbness)
Laboratory
Prothrombin time
Partial thromboplastin time
Thromboplastin generation test
Bleeding time
Platelet count
Fibrinogen level
	Tissue perfusion, altered, peripheral related to venous stasis during pregnancy*	Observe for signs and symptoms of thromboemboli and identify these for client
		  Numbness
		  Tingling
		  Color change of legs
		  Chest pain
		  Abdominal discomfort
			Client identifies absent or early signs and symptoms of clotting disorder

		Apply antiemboli stockings	
		Administer anticoagulants as prescribed	

		Explain anticoagulant therapy and provide rationale for any medication changes
		  Actions
		  Adverse effects
		  Interactions:
		    Warfarin: hematuria, epistaxis, gingival bleeding, hematomas
		    Heparin: thrombocytopenia, alopecia, fever, osteoporosis
		    Note: Therapy is discontinued prior to delivery
		  Discuss importance of avoiding salicylates with heparin and verifying use of any medication before self-administering
			Client discusses the actions, adverse effects, and precautions of prescribed anticoagulants

		Demonstrate heparin administration (if prescribed), including preparation, injection procedure, rotation of sites	Client demonstrates correct administration of heparin
		Observe for adverse effects of anticoagulation	Client shows no adverse effects of anticoagulation

(continued)

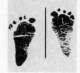

Nursing Care Plan (continued)

Assessment	Potential Nursing Diagnosis	Planning/Intervention	Evaluation
		Maintain schedule of regular anticoagulant studies during pregnancy (1–3-wk intervals)	Client regularly returns to laboratory for blood studies
		Avoid intramuscular injections	

		Secure and store specific antidotes for anticoagulants
		  Vitamin K—heparin
		  Protamine sulfate—warfarin	

Physical examination (signs of cardiac decompensation—heart failure)
  Tachycardia (≥100 beats per min)
  S3
  Peripheral edema
  Dyspnea
  Orthopnea
  Tachypnea (>24 per min)
  Cough unrelated to respiratory disease
  Hemoptysis
  Rales at base of lung
  Excessive weight gain
  Hepatomegaly
Laboratory studies
  Electrolytes
	Cardiac output, altered: decreased related to cardiac decompensation during pregnancy	Maintain bed rest	Client remains on bed rest

		Assist with physical care and personal hygiene as necessary	
		Administer digoxin and diuretics as prescribed	Client takes medication as prescribed
		Restrict sodium in diet as prescribed (0.5–2 g/day)	Client restricts sodium intake

		Observe for side effects of diuretic therapy
		  Electrolyte imbalance
		  Water depletion
			Client remains well hydrated and electrolytes within normal limits

		Discuss "warning signals"
		  Shortness of breath, dyspnea
		  Sudden change in ability to do activities
		  Extreme fatigue
		  Swelling
			Client understands warning signals

		Monitor fetal well-being
		  Fetal heart rate, activity level
		  Nonstress tests, sonography
			Fetus shows no signs of distress

History
  Valve replacement (duration and procedure)
  Rheumatic fever
Laboratory studies
  Culture and sensitivity of ordered specimens
	Infection, high risk for: related to bacterial invasion of the myocardium	Review signs and symptoms of infective bacterial endocarditis, urinary tract infection, and other complicating infections	Client identifies signs and symptoms of bacterial endocarditis and other complicating infections

		Advise to immediately report signs and symptoms	Client reports all signs of possible infections

(continued)

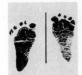

Nursing Care Plan *(continued)*

Assessment	Potential Nursing Diagnosis	Planning/Intervention	Evaluation
Platelets Anemia Leukocytes Erythrocyte sedimentation rate		of *any* infection, including urinary tract, respiratory, (cold)	
		Instruct about administration of prescribed prophylactic antibiotics	Client correctly self-administers antibiotics
		Discuss importance of regular and frequent antepartial supervision	Client attends clinic or visits physician as recommended
		Teach principles and techniques of perineal hygiene	Client uses proper hygiene when voiding
		Caution against contact with "sick" people (with colds, fever, etc.)	Client avoids interaction with people experiencing colds, fever, etc.
Expectations of pregnancy Past obstetric history Support systems in home or community Knowledge about labor and delivery	Anxiety related to fears concerning perinatal outcome	Demonstrate acceptance of expressed concerns about pregnancy outcome	Client verbalizes concerns about stressors of pregnancy
		Clearly explain purpose of all treatments and antepartal diagnostic tests	Client demonstrates decreased anxiety about treatments
		Reinforce positive aspects of pregnancy (e.g., normal fetal heart rate and activity level)	Client displays positive reaction to fetal movement
		Offer reassurance for progress being made (e.g., ability to tolerate activities and to manage components of self-care)	
		Involve family members or other supportive people in discussions, whenever possible and acceptable	Family demonstrates understanding of client's fears and offers support appropriately

* Prosthetic valves also contribute to risk

corpuscular volume (MCV; size of the erythrocyte) and mean corpuscular hemoglobin (quantity of hemoglobin in the erythrocyte).

EFFECT OF IRON DEFICIENCY ANEMIA ON PREGNANCY

In most clients with mild to moderate anemia, the signs and symptoms (fatigue) are few and often indistin-guishable from the normal symptoms of pregnancy. Such women are detected by frequent antepartal hemoglobin or hematocrit determinations. Iron deficiency anemia renders the pregnant woman particularly susceptible to infection and increases her risk of postpartum hemorrhage. Severely anemic women (hemoglobin < 8 g/dl) are symptomatic and, in the most severe cases, can even develop heart failure as a result of the anemia. Chronic anemia limits the amount of oxygen available for fetal exchange. There is an increased risk for abortion and premature birth. Severe anemia is associated with increased frequency of neonates in the small-for-gestational-age (SGA) category.

NURSING PROCESS

All pregnant women should have a complete blood count, including hemoglobin, hematocrit, and red blood cell indices, early in the prenatal period. Oral administration of iron is commonly prescribed to prevent or cure iron deficiency. It should be noted that the prophylactic use of iron during pregnancy is somewhat controversial. Approximately 3 to 5 mg iron per day is needed to supply the needs of mother and fetus, with demands for iron increasing in the last 5 months of pregnancy to as much as 3 to 7.5 mg/day.[10] A number of oral preparations of organic and inorganic iron are available for treatment; the most common compounds include ferrous sulfate (200 to 300 mg three times daily) or ferrous gluconate (320 mg three times daily). These drugs should be ingested with meals to decrease gastrointestinal side effects. The absorption of iron and the metabolism of folic acid are enhanced by vitamin C (ascorbic acid). Injectable iron therapy is rarely required because absorption is generally not a limiting factor. More often a failure to respond to oral iron therapy is the result of failure to take the medication (iron tends to produce gastrointestinal symptoms) or a concurrent folic acid deficiency. It is important to assess the existence of side effects in all pregnant women receiving iron supplementation. Constipation may be a particularly troublesome side effect; it can be relieved by prescribing stool softeners such as dioctyl sodium sulfosuccinate (Colace).

An iron-rich diet is recommended for all pregnant women. Ideally, an extra 1000 mg iron intake should be added to the daily diet.

Folic Acid Deficiency

Folic acid deficiency can produce severe anemia of the megaloblastic type in pregnancy. Megaloblastic anemia is much less common than iron deficiency anemia, occurring in fewer than 3% of gravidae and with a higher prevalence in twin gestations. In its fullblown form, hemoglobin may be as low as 3 to 5 g/dl, white blood cells and platelets are reduced, and the MCV is elevated. Symptoms of this type of anemia include glossitis, sore tongue, and anorexia. Perinatal outcome may be seriously threatened by folic acid deficiency, which is reportedly associated with a higher incidence of early abortion, UTIs, and abruptio placentae.

Treatment consists of oral administration of 1 mg folic acid daily and ingestion of a diet that contains foods high in folic acid (fresh vegetables, especially of the uncooked green leafy variety, red meats, fish, legumes, and poultry). Preparing vegetables by steaming them in small quantities of water will decrease folic acid loss. Prevention is achieved by the inclusion of 0.4 mg folic acid in prenatal vitamin-mineral supplements.

Hemoglobinopathies

Hemoglobinopathies present special problems in pregnancy. The most commonly encountered of the hemoglobinopathies are sickle cell anemia (SS disease), sickle cell–hemoglobin C disease (SC disease), and sickle cell–β-thalassemia disease (S-thalassemia disease). These are recessively inherited diseases that are seen principally in the African-American population and are invariably associated with an increased perinatal morbidity and mortality (e.g., increased rate of spontaneous abortion). Susceptibility to some infections is increased because of impaired immune system function.

Detailed counseling is required in the management of hemoglobinopathies. Important considerations include (1) the impact of pregnancy in precipitating crises; (2) the genetic implications of childbearing; and (3) the limited life expectancy of women with certain conditions such as SS disease. Women with SS disease should decide carefully whether to limit childbearing or even avoid pregnancy completely.

SICKLE CELL ANEMIA (SS DISEASE)

Sickle cell anemia occurs when the gene for the production of S hemoglobin is inherited from both parents. When S hemoglobin is transmitted from one parent but not the other, the person does not exhibit frank anemia but has *sickle cell trait*. Between 8% and 10% of the African-American population have the sickling trait only or are heterozygous.[35] Pregnant women with sickle cell trait have a predisposition to UTIs and hematuria but are otherwise normal. About 1 in 12 African-Americans has sickle cell trait, whereas 1 in every 576 African-American women has the disease.[36] The actual incidence of sickle cell anemia in pregnancy is about one third as high as in the general population, probably because many affected people do not survive to childbearing age or elect not to carry their pregnancies to term.

People affected by sickle cell anemia have inherited a defect in the hemoglobin molecule that causes erythrocytes to become elongated and crescent shaped (sickle), particularly when they are exposed to temperature variations, lowered blood pH, or increased blood viscosity. Decreases in circulating oxygen levels resulting from exercise, anesthesia, high altitudes, and air pollution may also cause sickling.[37]

Sickle cell anemia has great impact throughout the childbearing cycle. The anemia is exacerbated during pregnancy, and life-threatening hemolytic crises can occur, especially during the intrapartum period. Maternal mortality rates are high (10% to 20%) owing to the risk of pulmonary complications, infection, congestive heart failure, and hypertension. Other problems encountered by pregnant women with sickle cell disease are severe anemia, pyelonephritis, pneumonia, and PIH. About one half of the pregnancies end in spontaneous abortion, neonatal death, or stillbirth. The risk for intrauterine growth retardation and spontaneous premature labor is similarly high.

All African-American pregnant women not previously tested should be screened for sickle cell anemia at the time of their first prenatal visit. Women with diagnosed sickle cell anemia require the most meticulous of prenatal care. The main goal of therapy is to prevent conditions that cause sickling and to minimize the complications of sickling when it occurs. Antepartal diagnostic procedures are frequently performed to assess uteroplacental functioning and fetal well-being. Nonstress testing is particularly useful for identifying problems of placental dysfunction associated with placental infarction.[38]

Throughout pregnancy, the diet of women with sickle cell anemia should be supplemented with folic acid because of the rapid turnover of red blood cells. Fluid intake should be well maintained to prevent dehydration. Regular screening of urine is recommended for early diagnosis of asymptomatic bacteriuria. Hemoglobin levels are frequently assessed for rapid decreases in value, which are suggestive of sickle cell crisis. It is not unusual for pregnant women with sickle cell disease to have hemoglobin levels in the range of 6 to 9 g/dl. Multiple prophylactic transfusions of packed red cells are sometimes used to suppress the client's bone marrow from forming abnormal cells while at the same time permitting her to exist on transfused cells during the period of risk. All clients with sickle cell disease should be advised to avoid contact with people suffering from infectious diseases. Intrapartum management is similar to that for cardiac disease.

SICKLE CELL–HEMOGLOBIN C DISEASE (SC DISEASE)

Sickle cell–hemoglobin C disease occurs when the gene for the production of hemoglobin C is inherited along with that for hemoglobin S. It is much less common and certainly less serious in the nonpregnant state. During pregnancy and the puerperium, however, mortality and morbidity are greatly increased, with a maternal mortality reported in some series as high as 2%.[10] In contrast to sickle cell anemia, the perinatal mortality is increased only slightly.

SICKLE CELL–β-THALASSEMIA DISEASE (S-THALASSEMIA DISEASE)

Sickle cell–β-thalassemia disease results from the inheritance of the gene for hemoglobin S from one parent and the allelic gene for β-thalassemia from the other parent. Perinatal mortality and morbidity of this disease are similar to sickle cell–hemoglobin C disease.[10] Although β-thalassemia has been reported among all populations, it is most common in people from the Mediterranean region, with a significant prevalence among Africans and among Southeast Asians from Cambodia, Laos, and Vietnam.

■ URINARY TRACT AND RENAL DISEASE

Almost all forms of acute and chronic renal disease have been reported in association with pregnancy. Not infrequently, specific diagnosis is difficult during pregnancy because proteinuria and hypertension may mimic preeclampsia and also because definitive studies such as renal biopsy and intravenous urography are generally contraindicated.

The most common medical and renal complication of pregnancy is UTI. Anatomical changes as well as hormonal effects cause narrowing of the lower ureter and renal pelvis, with dilation of the upper ureter. These changes result in stasis of urine, delayed emptying, backward urine flow, and an increased risk of infection. The risk increases as pregnancy progresses and continues into the puerperium.

Approximately 2.5% to 9.7% of all pregnant women have *asymptomatic bacteriuria* (ASB), depending on parity, race, and socioeconomic factors.[39] Recurrent episodes of ASB are common and seem to be independent of the use of antibiotic therapy.[40] In pregnancy, this condition is significant because of its high association with subsequent lower UTI (*cystitis*) and upper UTI (*pyelonephritis*), preeclampsia, and hypertension.[40–42] Association with other obstetric problems, such as prematurity and congenital abnormality, has been suggested, but it has not been clearly established.

The presence of 100,000 (10^5/ml) organisms in a urine culture is diagnostic of bacteriuria. *Escherichia coli* (E. coli) is the most common causative agent of UTIs. Other causative organisms include *Chlamydia trachomatis*, *Klebsiella*, and *Proteus*. ASB should be treated promptly with an appropriate antibiotic drug and forced fluids because 30% to 40% of clients will progress to symptomatic UTIs if untreated.[41–44]

Pregnant women with sickle cell trait, multiparity, multiple sex partners, or a past history of renal disease are at greater risk for bacteriuria and therefore must be frequently screened. Manifestations of cystitis include dysuria, pyuria (>10 white blood cells per high-power field in a spun urine specimen), frequency, urgency, chills, low-grade fever, hematuria, and lower abdominal pain.

Acute pyelonephritis may be characterized by the previously described symptoms of cystitis plus pain in the lumbar area (usually right side but may be bilateral), costovertebral angle tenderness, malaise, high fever, backache, and gastrointestinal disturbances. Diastolic blood pressure is increased, and creatinine clearance is decreased. Because uterine irritability is a complication of pyelonephritis, clients with premature labor should be assessed for renal disease.

Hospitalization is generally recommended for treatment of acute pyelonephritis, because intravenous therapy and bedrest in the left lateral position are prescribed. Although this condition is the most common nonobstetric indication for hospital admission of the pregnant client, outpatient management is now being attempted in some cases.[45,46]

Antibiotic therapy is indicated for the treatment of women with all types of UTIs. The penicillins and cephalosporins are considered safe for use during pregnancy and are commonly administered. Other antimicrobial agents must be used with caution (sulfonamides and nitrofurantoin) or are contraindicated (e.g., tetracycline, chloramphenicol [Chloromycetin], trimethoprim-sulfamethoxazole [Bactrim, Comoxol, Septra, and others]). The nurse should carefully review the actions, side effects, and administration of the prescribed drug, as well as stress the importance of maintaining good fluid intake (3 to 4 L/24 h) orally or parenterally, as indicated. Temperature elevation is controlled by antipyretics (acetaminophen), analgesics, and cool sponge baths. It is also necessary to reculture urine 1 week after completion of the 7- to 10-day antimicrobial therapy. Recurrences are common, causing some authorities to recommend long-term suppressive antimicrobial therapy.

Women with chronic renal disease and renal transplants are now living long enough to bear children. A potentially deleterious effect of pregnancy in women with underlying renal disease is the tendency of pregnancy to cause hypertension, which can further decrease renal function by causing an increase in glomerular capillary pressure.[47] Renal disease and hypertension in combination may be associated with fetal growth retardation and increased perinatal mortality. Therefore, an important goal of management is to prevent elevations in blood pressure. Pregnant women who have renal transplants may be treated with corticosteroids such as prednisone. The prognosis for pregnancy after transplantation is good if the woman's general health is optimum, blood pressure is normal, and there are no signs of graft reaction. Hemodialysis may be performed for failing renal function during pregnancy. Infants born to mothers on immunosuppressive therapy are prone to hyperglycemia at birth owing to suppression of fetal insulin activity by corticosteroids.

As part of the prenatal education, the nurse should instruct all pregnant women to recognize the signs of a UTI and to use selective preventive measures. Emphasis must be placed on the importance of personal hygiene practices (e.g., wiping from front to back), because most UTIs result from bacteria ascending through the urethra. Urinary stasis can be prevented through frequent voiding. This is particularly important before and after sexual intercourse. Daily consumption of cranberry juice, in addition to plenty of water, is recommended because it helps to acidify the urine. Clients with a history of UTIs should avoid bladder irritants such as caffeine products, carbonated beverages, and alcohol.

Screening for renal disease during pregnancy is performed by carefully collecting a midstream clean-catch urine specimen at the time of the first prenatal visit. To ensure an adequate specimen, the nurse should instruct the client as to the proper method of collecting the sample. An examination of the urinary sediment as well as culture and antibiotic sensitivity studies should be carried out.

■ CHORIOAMNIONITIS

Chorioamnionitis is an intrauterine infection involving mononuclear and polymorphonuclear leukocytic infiltration of the fetal membranes and amniotic fluid. Symptoms of the disease are maternal fever and fetal tachycardia. Premature rupture of the membranes (PROM) is believed to be the most common cause of the disease; however, some studies have suggested that chorioamnionitis may be the precursor to PROM.

The danger of chorioamnionitis is increased by repeated vaginal examinations and intrauterine manipulation. In many hospitals it has become common practice to give antibiotics prophylactically to women with PROM. When membranes are ruptured more than 24 hours, the incidence of chorioamnionitis rises dramatically.

Interventions include culturing of the amniotic fluid and maternal blood for causative organisms (most often *E. coli*, anaerobic and aerobic streptococci and staphylococci), administering appropriate intravenous antibiotic therapy, and carefully monitoring the fetus.

Labor is induced in cases of mild infection if delivery may be accomplished within 6 to 8 hours. In severe cases or when the fetus is distressed, cesarean delivery is elected.

■ THYROID DISEASE

Hyperthyroidism (Maternal Thyrotoxicosis)

Hyperthyroidism is probably the second most significant endocrinopathy in pregnancy, second only to diabetes mellitus. Approximately 0.04 to 0.075% of pregnancies are complicated by hyperthyroid disease.[34] Most commonly, hyperthyroidism during pregnancy is caused by *Graves' disease*. Although a woman with uncontrolled hyperthyroidism is likely to be anovulatory and thus unable to conceive, many women with milder disease do conceive. In some cases the hyperthyroidism is first diagnosed during pregnancy. If the condition is not detected and treated properly, maternal complications may occur such as spontaneous abortion, PIH, perinatal death, premature labor, and postpartum hemorrhage. There is a greater risk for delivering an SGA infant and for neonatal thyrotoxicosis.

Signs of hyperthyroidism during pregnancy are tachycardia that exceeds the increase caused by normal pregnancy, a high pulse rate while sleeping, an enlarged thyroid gland, exophthalmos, weakness, sweating, and failure to gain weight normally.[10]

Findings of diagnostic laboratory studies may be confusing, especially in milder cases, because pregnancy and hyperthyroidism are both hypermetabolic states with increased protein binding of thyroid hormone.[48] This results in higher values for studies such as the protein-bound iodine and total thyroxine, with lower triiodothyronine uptake. Multiple thyroid function studies and the use of newer supersensitive immunoradiometric assays for thyroid stimulating hormone may prove useful in diagnosis.

Surgical treatment (subtotal thyroidectomy) was once a treatment option that is seldom considered now, except in special cases (e.g., reaction to the antithyroid drugs, unusually large dosage requirements). The problem with medical therapy is that the preferred antithyroid drug (propylthiouracil [PTU]) crosses the placenta, and if doses are excessive, the fetal thyroid can be suppressed, leading to fetal goiter or even cretinism. This is best avoided if the mother is maintained in a euthyroid or very mildly hyperthyroid state using the lowest possible dose of PTU.[49]

Women with exophthalmic goiter produce a long-acting thyroid stimulator, which is an immunoglobulin G (IgG). This crosses the placenta and, if present, can cause hyperthyroidism in the newborn.

A major complication of hyperthyroidism is the rare occurrence of *thyroid storm* during pregnancy and the puerperium. This condition is manifested by high fever, tachycardia, sweating, severe dehydration, and occasional cardiac decompensation. Treatment consists of early recognition followed by in-hospital intense therapy with large doses of PTU and potassium iodide and possibly intravenous administration of steroids.

Severe Hypothyroidism

Severe hypothyroidism is rare during pregnancy because the condition is usually associated with amenorrhea and anovulation. Women with mild hypothyroidism may conceive but are at greater risk for spontaneous abortion. Infants of hypothyroid mothers with mild disease generally appear healthy; those born to more severely hypothyroid mothers have an increased risk of congenital goiter and other anomalies, cretinism, and transient hypothyroidism.

Hypothyroidism is characterized by easy fatigability, cold intolerance, lethargy, constipation, dry skin, headache, thin nails, and delayed deep-tendon reflexes. *L-thyroxine* replacement (0.15 to 0.30 mg/day) is usually required to treat this condition.[34]

■ SYSTEMIC LUPUS ERYTHEMATOSUS

Systemic lupus erythematosus (SLE) is a chronic, multisystem disorder that primarily affects the connective tissue. Among childbearing women, the disease can be mistaken for preeclampsia and eclampsia.[50] African-American women are disproportionately affected by SLE, with one in 200 women having the disease.[51] The clinical manifestations are numerous and may vary widely among individuals. The revised criteria for the diagnosis of SLE established by the American Rheumatism Association include the presence of four or more of the following criteria: (1) malar rash (fixed erythema, flat or raised); (2) discoid rash (raised erythematous patches with scales); (3) photosensitivity; (4) oral or nasal ulcers; (5) arthritis; (6) serositis; (7) renal disorder (persistent proteinuria); (8) neurological disorder (seizures or psychotic symptoms); (9) hematologic disorder (hemolysis, leukopenia, or thrombocytopenia); (10) immunologic disorder (positive LE preparation, anti-DNA, anti-SM, or false-positive serologic tests for syphilis; and (11) antinuclear antibody.[52] SLE is believed to have a multifactorial etiology.[50] The prognosis is related to the systems involved. Studies examining the effects of SLE on pregnancy reveal inconsistent findings.[53,54] Pregnancy does not appear to influence the long-term prognosis of clients with SLE; however, short-term effects may be seen in exacerbations of the disease during pregnancy.[55] It has been suggested that most exacerbations of lupus nephropathy during pregnancy represent the adverse effect of hypertension or superimposed PIH.[47] Clients who have been in complete remission for 6 months before conception have the least complicated pregnancies and best perinatal outcomes.[55] The overall risk of abortion in clients with SLE is increased (25% to 35% incidence), with recurrent abortions common. The placenta vasculature may be affected by lesions and immunoglobin depositions, which can lead to stillbirths, intrauterine growth retardation, and other perinatal complications. Treatment of the disease involves corticosteroids and immunosuppressive agents. Additional supplementation with low-dose aspirin (about 75 mg) has been found to improve perinatal outcomes in women who have suffered excessive reproductive losses associated with the lupus anticoagulant (an IgG or IgM immunoglobin).[34] Infection control is particularly important during steroid therapy. Because exacerbations of the disease commonly occur after delivery, careful observation during the postpartum period is critical.[50]

■ REFERENCES

1. Langer O: Critical issues in diabetes and pregnancy: Early identification, metabolic control, and prevention of adverse outcome. In Merkatz IR, Thompson JE, Mullen PD, et al (eds): New Perspectives on Prenatal Care, pp 445–459. New York, Elsevier, 1990
2. Brown ZA: Diabetes in pregnancy. FCH/Perinat Health Promot 1:43–45, 1978
3. O'Sullivan JB, Mahan CM: Criteria for the oral glucose tolerance test in pregnancy. Diabetes 13:278–285, 1964
4. Jones P: Evaluating and managing diabetes mellitus in pregnancy. J Perinatol 5:71–74, 1985
5. Cousins L: Pregnancy complications among diabetic women: Review 1965–1985. Obstet Gynecol Survey 42: 140–149, 1987
6. Hollander P, Maeder EC: Diabetes in pregnancy: No longer a barrier to successful outcome. Postgrad Med 77:132–146, 1985
7. Barss VA: Diabetes and pregnancy. Med Clin North Am 73:685–700, 1989
8. Nuwayhid BS, Brinkman CR, Lieb M: Management of the Diabetic Pregnancy. New York, Elsevier, 1987
9. Simpson JL, Elias S, Mantor AO, et al: Diabetes in pregnancy, Northwestern University series (1977–1981.) Am J Obstet Gynecol 146:263–210, 1983
10. Cunningham FG, MacDonald PC, Gant NF: Williams Obstetrics, 18th ed. Norwalk, CT, Appleton & Lange, 1989
11. Miller E, Hare JW, Cloherty JP, et al: Elevated maternal hemoglobin A_{1c} in early pregnancy and major congenital anomalies in infants of diabetic mothers. N Engl J Med 304(22):1331–1334, 1981
12. National Diabetes Data Group: Classification of diabetes mellitus and other categories of glucose intolerance. Diabetes 28:1039, 1979
13. White PL: Classification of obstetric diabetes. Am J Obstet Gynecol 130:229, 1978
14. Diamond MP, Vaughn WK, Salyer SL, et al: Efficacy of outpatient management of insulin-dependent diabetic pregnancies. J Perinatol 5:2–8, 1985
15. Milunsky A, Alpert E, Kitzmiller JL, et al: Prenatal diagnosis of neural tube defects: VIII. The importance of serum alpha-fetoprotein screening in diabetic pregnant women. Am J Obstet Gynecol 142(8):1030–1032, 1982
16. Jovanovic L, Peterson CM, Fuhrman K: Diabetes in Pregnancy, pp 235–236. New York, Praeger, 1986
17. Zigrossi ST, Riga-Ziegler M: The stress of medical management on pregnant diabetics. MCN 11:320–323, 1986
18. Gargiulo P, Di Mario U, Zuccarini O, et al: Treatment of diabetic pregnant women with monocomponent insulins. Acta Endocrinol (Suppl) 227:60–74, 1986
19. Engel NS: Insulin therapy in pregnancy. MCN 14:19, 1989
20. Good-Anderson B: Home blood glucose monitoring in the pregnant diabetic. JOGNN 12:89–92, 1983
21. Cruikshank DP: Cardiovascular, pulmonary, renal, and hematologic diseases in pregnancy. In Scott JR, DiSaia PJ, Hammond CB, et al (eds): Danforth's Obstetrics and Gynecology, 6th ed. Philadelphia, JB Lippincott, 1990
22. Schmidt J, Boilanger M, Abbott S: Peripartum cardiomyopathy. JOGNN 18(6):65–472, 1989
23. Gianopoulos JG: Cardiac disease in pregnancy. Med Clin North Am 73:639–651, 1989
24. DeSwiet M: The cardiovascular system. In Hytten FE, Chamberlain GVP (eds): Clinical Physiology in Obstetrics, pp 3–42. Oxford, Blackwell Scientific, 1980
25. Ueland K: Pregnancy and cardiovascular disease. Med Clin North Am 61:17–41, 1977
26. DeSwiet M: Pregnancy and heart valve replacement. Int J Cardiol 5:741–743, 1984
27. McColgin SW, Martin JN, Morrison JC: Pregnant women with prosthetic heart valves. Clin Obstet Gynecol 32:76–88, 1989
28. Chyun DA: Pregnancy and cardiac valvular prostheses. JOGNN 14:38–44, 1985
29. Burwell CS, Metcalfe J: Heart Disease and Pregnancy. Boston, Little, Brown, 1958
30. Little BB, Gilstrap LC: Cardiovascular drugs during pregnancy. Clin Obstet Gynecol 32:13–20, 1989
31. Shaul WL, Hall JG: Multiple congenital abnormalities associated with oral anticoagulants. Am J Obstet Gynecol 127:191–198, 1977
32. Carson M, Reed M: Warfarin and fetal abnormality. Lancet 1:1127, 1976
33. Sherman S, Hall BD: Warfarin and fetal abnormality. Lancet 1:692, 1976
34. Scott JR, DiSaie PJ, Hammond CB, et al: Danforth's Obstetrics and Gynecology, 6th ed. Philadelphia, JB Lippincott, 1990

35. Kneut C: Sickle-cell anemia. Issue Compr Pediatr Nurse 4:19–27, 1980
36. Ship-Horowitz T: Nursing care of the sickle cell anemic patient in labor. JOGNN 12:381–386, 1983
37. Anionwu E: Sickle-cell disease. Health Visitor 55:336–341, 1982
38. Richardson EA, Milne RS: Sickle cell disease and the childbearing family: An update. MCN 8:417–422, 1983
39. Martens MG: Pyelonephritis. Obstet Gynecol Clin North Am 16(2):305–315, 1989
40. Rosenfeld JA: Renal disease and pregnancy. Am Fam Physician 39:209–212, 1989
41. Hill JA, Devoe LD, Bryans CI Jr: Frequency of asymptomatic bacteriuria in preeclampsia. Obstet Gynecol 67:529–32, 1986
42. Krieger JN: Complications and treatment of urinary tract infections during pregnancy. Urol Clin North Am 13:685–693, 1986
43. Diokno AC, Compton A, Seski J, et al: Urologic evaluation of urinary tract infection in pregnancy. J Reprod Med 31:23–26, 1986
44. Van Dorsten JP, Bannister ER: Office diagnosis of asymptomatic bacteriuria in pregnant women. Am J Obstet Gynecol 155:777–780, 1986
45. Angel JL, O'Brien WF, Finan MA, et al: Acute pyelonephritis in pregnancy: A prospective study of oral versus intravenous antibiotic therapy. Obstet Gynecol 76:28–32, 1990
46. Harris RE: Acute urinary tract infections and subsequent problems. Clin Obstet Gynecol 27:874–90, 1984
47. Ferris TF: Pregnancy complicated by hypertension and renal disease. Adv Intern Med 35:269–288, 1990
48. Wang KW, Sum CF: Management of thyroid disease in pregnancy. Sing Med J 30:476–478, 1989
49. Burr W: Thyroid disease. Clin Obstet Gynecol 13:277–290, 1986
50. Sala DJ, Lentz JR: Pregnant women with systemic lupus erythematosus. MCN 11:382–387, 1986
51. Dubois E, et al: Systemic lupus erythematosus: "Wolf" in sheep's clothing. Patient Care 18(6):134–136, 145, 174, March 1984
52. Tan Em, Cohen AS, Fries JF, et al: The 1982 revised criteria for the classification of systemic lupus erythematosus. Arthritis Rheum 25(11):1271–1277, 1982
53. Hayslett JP, Lynn RI: Effect of pregnancy in patients with lupus nephropathy. Kidney Int 16:207–220, 1980
54. Lockshin MD, Harpel PC, Druzin ML, et al: Lupus pregnancy: II. Unusual pattern of hypocomplementemia and thrombocytopenia in the pregnant patient. Arthritis Rheum 28(1):58–66, 1985
55. Michael J: The management of renal disease in pregnancy. Clin Obstet Gynecol 13:319–334, 1986

■ SUGGESTED READING

Balen AH, Kurtz AB: Successful outcome of pregnancy with severe hypothyroidism: Case report & literature review. Br J Obstet Gynaecol 97(6):536–539, 1990

Burrow GN, Ferris TF: Medical Complications During Pregnancy. Philadelphia, WB Saunders, 1988

Clark SL: Labor and delivery in the patient with structural cardiac disease. Clin Perinatol 13(4):695–703, 1986

Hankins GDV, Wendel GD, Levano KJ, et al: Myocardial infarction during pregnancy: A review. Obstet Gynecol 65:139, 1985

Katz VL, Dotter DJ, Droegemueller W: Low dose dopamine in the treatment of persistent oliguria in pre-eclampsia. Int J Gynaecol Obstet 31(1):57–59, January 1990

Lowenstein BR, Vain NW, Derrane SV, Wright DR, et al: Successful pregnancy and vaginal delivery after heart transplantation. Am J Obstet Gynecol 158(3):589–590, March 1988

Marchbanks PA, Annegers JF, Coulam CB, et al: Risk factors for ectopic pregnancy: A population-based study. JAMA 259(12):1823–1827, 1988

O'Brien ME, Gibson G: Detection and management of gestational diabetes in an out-of-hospital birth center. J Nurse–Midwif 32(2):79–84, 1987

Tamaki H, Amino N, Takeoka K, et al: Thyroxine requirement during pregnancy for replacement therapy of hypothyroidism. Obstet Gynecol 76(2):230–233, August 1990

35

Infectious Diseases in Pregnancy

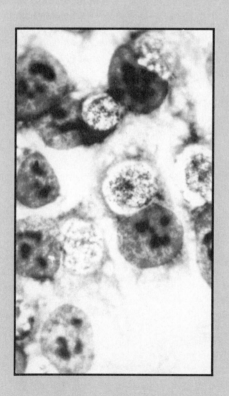

nfectious diseases can pose a wide range of health risks to both mother and fetus, ranging from simple discomfort and pain experienced by the mother in the case of vaginitis to diseases causing much more serious complications in mother and infant, such as blindness and birth defects with untreated syphilis, and sometimes death as is seen with acquired immunodeficiency syndrome (AIDS). Many infectious diseases can be prevented, either by immunizations or by use of safe sex practices; education is often the key to prevention. The nurse can play a crucial role in both the prevention and successful treatment of infectious diseases in pregnant women and their partners by participating in patient education and public health promotion, such as immunizations and increasing public awareness of risk-increasing behaviors. This chapter examines the most common infectious diseases and nursing care for each of three broad categories of infectious diseases: sexually transmitted diseases, urinary tract infections, and other miscellaneous infectious diseases.

■ SEXUALLY TRANSMITTED DISEASES (STD)

Sexually transmitted diseases are those that are predominantly or exclusively spread through sexual contact. Some of these diseases can be treated successfully if detected early, whereas others are incurable or cause recurrent episodes. The detection of many of these diseases in pregnancy automatically places the pregnancy in the high-risk category, which calls for special monitoring and treatment throughout the course of the pregnancy. Public education, especially for childbearing families and adolescents at risk for pregnancy, must emphasize the importance of preventing infectious diseases to reduce the burden of suffering to patients and the cost to the health-care system.

Nursing Assessment for STD

The nurse should be knowledgeable about the symptoms of these diseases and their associated risk factors. Symptoms of STD include increased or foul-smelling vaginal discharge, itching or burning for vaginitis. Lesions of the vulva or labia may be reported, and the woman may have noticed enlarged lymph nodes in the groin, axilla, or neck. Pain or burning on urination can be associated with urethral irritation or vulval lesions. Rash and oral lesions may be present with syphilis, AIDS, or gonorrhea. More general symptoms of infection may be present when the STD has systemic effects. Fever, malaise, fatigue, anorexia, or abdominal discomfort may be associated with hepatitis B or HIV infections. Changes in menstrual patterns or symptoms in connection with the menstrual cycle may be reported with some STD.

Beginning at the first prenatal visit and periodically throughout the pregnancy, while taking the mother's history, the nurse should evaluate for the presence of STD and for factors that increase the risk of such infections. It is important that the nurse inquire about the symptoms in the sexual partner because the woman may be asymptomatic but her sexual partner may have symptoms signaling the presence of the disease. The nurse also assesses for specific risk factors for exposure to HIV infection.

Physical examination includes vital signs, with particular attention to temperature, general appearance and affect, and signs of infection. The skin is observed for rashes and lesions and evidence of IV drug use such as needle tracks, usually on forearms but possibly on legs and feet. The nurse may assist the physician during the abdominal and pelvic examination to assess the condition of abdominal organs, the vulva and vagina, cervix, uterus, and ovaries.

On the first prenatal visit, a series of standard laboratory tests are performed to screen for the more common infectious diseases in pregnancy (syphilis, gonorrhea, *Chlamydia*, urinary tract infection, and rubella). Other specimens may be taken or blood may be drawn for other tests as indicated (see Table 35-1 for a complete list).

Nursing Diagnoses Relating to STD

Pregnant women with risk factors for infectious diseases can be diagnosed as *high risk for infection*, related to the

---

High-Risk Groups for Sexually Transmitted Diseases

Younger than 20 years old

Sexually active

Multiple sexual partners

Sexual partner who has multiple sexual contacts

Prior history of STD

Sexual partner diagnosed with STD

Prostitutes

(From Willson JR, Carrington, ER: Obstetrics and Gynecology, 8th ed. St. Louis, CV Mosby, 1987; and Centers for Disease Control: Sexually Transmitted Diseases Treatment Guidelines, September, 1989. DHHS/PHS, Center for Preventive Services, Division of STD/HIV Prevention. Atlanta, GA, 1989.)

Research Highlight

Condom Use After AIDS Education and Publicity

After the report on AIDS by the U.S. Surgeon General (1986), an extensive public health campaign promoted condom use, particularly latex condoms containing spermicide, unless in a mutually monogamous relationship. To examine the effects of this campaign, condom sales were counted at about 550 drug stores across the United States from 1984 to 1988. A national probability sample of drug stores was used stratified by size, geographic region, and relative urbanization. Condom sales at the drug stores were audited every 2 months from 1984 to 1988 and compared to the same period a year earlier to control for seasonal variation. Publicity over this time period was monitored by counting the number of articles regarding condom use using three different indexes to newspapers across the country.

Drug store condom sales grew slowly from 1984 to 1988, except for a 20% increase in 1987. Between 1986 and 1987, sales of all latex condoms increased 25% and those with spermicide increased 116%. Natural membrane condom sales increased 7.8%. Sales of condoms in areas with high incidence of AIDS were growing vitrually throughout the study period. Sales increases in other areas did not begin until early 1987 and stopped increasing in summer of 1988. In both high-risk and other areas of the United States, condom sales grew rapidly throughout 1987 and early 1988 after the release of the Surgeon General's report in November 1986. Newspaper publicity about condoms (which were rarely mentioned before the report) increased to a peak in February 1987, with 182 items appearing in 19 newspapers. Newspaper items continued through 1988, but slowly diminished.

The 20% increase in drug store condom sales during the year after the Surgeon General's report indicates that Americans responded to his message about AIDS prevention. The greatest increase was in latex condoms with spermicide, which cost more but may provide additional protection against HIV transmission. The overall increase in drug store condom sales between 1984 and 1988 was 26%, most of which probably reflected concerns about AIDS prevention.

(Moran JS, Janes HR, Peterman TA et al: Increase in condom sales following AIDS education and publicity, United States. Am J Public Health 80:607–608, May 1990)

Assessment Tool

Assessing Women's Risk for HIV Exposure

Nurses can use these questions as part of the prenatal interview to assess the woman's risk for exposure to HIV infection:

How many sexual partners have you had in the past 10 years?

Have your sexual partners had several sexual partners in the past 10 years?

Have you had a sexual partner who is bisexual or who had homosexual contact since 1978?

Do you have anal intercourse?

Have any of your sexual partners had a positive HIV test or become sick with AIDS?

Have you had a blood transfusion in the United States between 1978 and 1985, or in another country since 1978?

Have you had artificial insemination using untested donor semen since 1978?

Have you or your sexual partners used IV street drugs since 1978?

Have you been exposed to blood or body fluids in your work (e.g., nurse, physician, dentist, dental hygienist)?

Assessment Tool

Physical Examination for STD

Pelvic examination
    Inspection of vulva and perineum for lesions, erythema, discharge, edema
    Speculum examination of vagina and cervix; note:
        Vaginal discharge (color, amount, odor, other characteristics)
        Vaginal mucosa (erythema, edema, ulcerations, lesions)
        Cervical discharge (color, amount, odor, other characteristics)
        Cervical mucosa (erythema, edema, lesions, ulcerations, ectropion, erosion, petechiae)
    Bimanual examination; note:
        Cervical tenderness, irregularity
        Uterine tenderness, enlargement, irregularity
        Adenexal tenderness, enlargement, fullness; masses of ovaries, tubes, or in cul-de-sac
        Rectovaginal examination for condition of posterior uterine wall, rectovaginal septum, cul-de-sac,
        uterosacral ligaments
Specimens
    Pap smear (cervix, herpetic lesions)
    Saline mount (*Candida, Trichomonas, Gardnerella, Chlamydia*, PID)
    KOH mount (*Candida, Gardnerella*)
    Gonorrhea culture (Thayer-Martin)
    Herpes simplex type 2 culture (if media and procedures available)
    Chlamydia culture (if media and procedures available)
Abdominal examination
    Superficial and deep palpation for condition of organs, tenderness, masses
    Palpation of groin lymph nodes
    Auscultation of bowel sounds
Vital signs
    Temperature
    Pulse
    Respiration
    Blood pressure
Skin
    Rashes (characteristics and distribution)
    Lesions (ulcers, nodules, warts, scars, tracks)
    Color (jaundice, pallor, erythema)
    Texture (hydration, scaling, wasting)
Lymph nodes
    Size, number, location
    Tenderness
    Heat
    Erythema

specific risk factors in each instance. For example, an adolescent with multiple sexual partners would have High Risk for STD Infection, related to age and sexual practices. A woman whose sexual partner is an IV drug user would have high risk for HIV infection, related to situational relationship factors. Once an infectious disease has occurred, the nursing diagnosis is High Risk for Infection Transmission, in which the woman is at risk for transferring the infectious agent to others. Transmission of STD occurs through sexual contact, IV drug use, blood products, and lack of knowledge about how to reduce the risk of exposure. Lack of knowledge of reducing the risk of transmitting AIDS virus is a specific cause of high risk for infection transmission. The

TABLE 35–1. LABORATORY TESTS FOR INFECTIOUS DISEASES

Laboratory Test	Source/Site	Infectious Disease
VDRL/RPR	Blood	Syphilis
Gonorrhea culture	Cervix, rectum	Gonorrhea
Chlamydia culture	Cervix	*Chlamydia trachomatis*
Hemagglutination-inhibition antibodies	Blood	Rubella
Urinalysis, urine culture	Urine	Urinary tract infection
Tuberculin skin test	Skin	Tuberculosis
Hepatitis B surface antigen (HBsAg)	Blood	Hepatitis B
Toxoplasmosis antibody	Blood	Toxoplasmosis
Cervical/vaginal culture	Cervix, vagina	Group B streptococcus
Viral culture	Cervix, genital lesions	Herpes simplex I and II
Enzyme-linked immunosorbent assay (ELISA), Western blot test	Blood	HIV infection/AIDS

fetus and newborn are at risk for infection transmission from the mother, either transplacentally or through the birth canal.

Knowledge deficits are often present related to the progress and effects of infection, treatment requirements, and risks of communicability. The woman may experience Anxiety or Fear, related to effects of the infectious process and its treatment. There is a perceived threat to biological integrity from the disease, possible hospitalization if the disease is severe, and invasive procedures may be required during treatment. The woman's status and prestige may be adversely affected, especially by an STD or HIV infection. Altered Comfort may result from the pathophysiological effects of illness or from diagnostic tests and treatments. There may be Altered Family Processes related to the woman's illness, particularly the effects of STD on sexual and emotional relations. Breach of trust between partners may be an issue, involving dishonesty, adultery, or moral conflicts. The woman may experience Body Image Disturbance related to perceived changes in structure or function due to the infection, or Self-Concept Disturbance with decreased self-esteem, diminished role performance, and negative effects on personal identity.

Nursing Planning and Intervention for STD

The primary goal of nursing care is to prevent the occurrence of STD. Client education is the major strategy in prevention, and the nurse helps women and families to identify factors that increase the risk of these infections and methods of preventing them. Because many of these diseases are treated more effectively if detected early, the education of clients should include the early signs and symptoms of STD and the importance of seeking medical attention as soon as such symptoms occur.

As part of preventive education, nurses should instruct clients in general health measures that promote overall good health and enhance immune system function. Nurses should stress the importance of the benefits of balanced diet, adequate rest and exercise, engaging in satisfying life work and activities, developing a support network, and avoiding harmful and toxic substances, such as alcohol and cigarettes.

When the client has already contracted an infection, nursing care focuses on facilitating effective treatment, reducing complications and progression of the disease, and preventing potential further spread of the infection. Many STD can be treated with antibiotics or other medications. If treatment includes taking medications, the nurse should stress the importance of taking the medications as directed, completing the course of treatment, and following other directions, such as refraining from alcohol intake when taking some medications. The nurse can facilitate the client's compliance with medication regimens by reviewing expected minor side-effects, such as diarrhea and gastric upset, and advising remedies to ease these effects. Nurses must inform clients clearly of all potential allergic reactions, such as hives and respiratory distress. If nonprescription medications are advised by the physician, the nurse can review correct use and explain the expected symptomatic relief.

Many STD cause local vulvar inflammation and pain, and the client may experience discomfort or pain during intercourse (dyspareunia) or during urination (dysuria). The nurse can instruct the client about measures that can help alleviate these conditions such as sitz baths or use of topical steroid creams. In some cases, it is necessary for the client to refrain from intercourse for 2 to 3 days and for the client's sexual partner(s) to receive simultaneous treatment. Such special instructions should be emphasized.

The nurse explains the purposes and procedures for diagnostic tests that are required, answers questions, and provides reassurance. Nurses often help in collecting and processing specimens.

THE NURSE AS COUNSELOR

The woman who contracts an STD often feels anxious or fearful about the outcome for her and her baby. She may also experience body image or self-concept disturbances. The nurse can provide support and opportunities for clients to discuss and express such feelings and expectations to help alleviate them. In providing care related to the emotional responses of the client and her partner, the nurse must demonstrate a nonjudgmental and accepting attitude, as well as an empathic manner. Most clients have great concern about the effects of infectious disease on the fetus. The nurse, in conjunction with the physician and other health team members, provides an assessment of risk to the fetus and allows the client the opportunity to express fear, guilt, and other emotions. When infections occur early in pregnancy and there is a high probability of fetal damage, options including abortion are discussed.

Counseling regarding modification of sexual practices is often indicated. If the couple practices high-risk sexual behaviors, the nurse educates the client about ways to reduce risky behaviors and how to practice safer sex, such as limiting the number of partners and using condoms in risky situations (see Chap. 11). The nurse must make sure the client understands that she could become reinfected even after successful medical treatment if her sexual partner(s) remains untreated and still has the disease. Therefore, with many STD, sexual partner(s) must receive treatment simultaneously if the woman is to continue free of infection.

Because of the severe complications and eventual fatal outcome for those who contract HIV infection and the extreme importance of halting transmission of this disease to others, there are special considerations for the nurse in counseling clients. Nurses must instruct clients clearly about the modes of transmission and how to prevent transfer of the virus, and must dispel common myths regarding transmission. Client education also includes the expected progression of the disease, how it affects the immune system and symptomatic effects, and

Client Education

Preventing Transmission of STD

Limit the number of sexual partners; preferably have only one.

Abstain from sexual contact whenever genital or oral lesions are present.

Use condoms and spermicides whenever with new partner, if partner is not well known, or if partner has other sexual contacts.

Observe sexual partner for lesions or discharge, or ask about symptoms, and be prepared to say no if these are present.

Be responsible with sexual partner(s): advise about history of STD and avoid contact if symptoms and signs are present.

methods of treatment. In addition, nurses often refer clients for long-term management and to HIV and AIDS support groups that can help them cope with this serious disease and offer strategies for living as fully as possible.

Evaluation

The most desired outcome criterion for nursing intervention in sexually transmitted diseases is *prevention*, so that clients never contract these infections. The goals for the client include that she demonstrates an understanding of how these diseases are transmitted, specific measures to avoid unsafe sex practices and reduce exposure to these infections, and how to maintain a health-promoting lifestyle. Nursing interventions for early detection are considered effective if nurses and clients recognize symptoms of STD early, and clients seek medical care promptly. Successful nursing interventions can be evaluated by how well the disease resolves within the expected time without complications or sequelae for mother or infant.

Client education is considered effective if the woman and family can demonstrate knowledge of the signs and symptoms of STD and take steps to prevent transmission to others. Additional indications of effective client teaching are when clients comply with treatment regimens, including completion of medications and using measures for symptom relief. The nurse can conclude that intervention for emotional needs is successful when the clients and families can express their feelings, receive and provide support, and take necessary actions with confidence and hope. If a client decides to terminate a pregnancy, the client should be able to accept her choice without guilt or remorse.

■ SIGNS, SYMPTOMS, AND MEDICAL THERAPY

Candida (Monilia) Vaginitis

Candidal infections are often not sexually transmitted, although they can be. This common vaginal infection is caused by the fungus *Candida albicans*, which is widely distributed in nature and often found on the skin and mucous membranes. Because it thrives well in vaginal tissue that is well-estrogenized and has high glycogen content, it occurs more frequently in women who are pregnant, women who have diabetes, and those who take higher estrogen oral contraceptives. Women who are taking systemic antibiotics are more susceptible to *Candida* because of suppression of the normal vaginal flora and changes in pH and enzymes. Stress and decreased resistance may contribute to *Candida* vaginitis, as may hygiene practices such as douching, using perfumed or medicated sprays and soaps, or nylon underwear. Although there has been little research to support the effectiveness of some widely used natural remedies,

Client Education

Natural Remedies for Vaginitis

Women are increasingly interested in self-care that includes preventing or minimizing vaginitis, and they are using natural remedies for therapy. The following natural remedies have been suggested or used by women. Little research supports these approaches, and effectiveness is variably reported. However, such approaches are compatible with the life-style and philosophy of growing numbers of women.

Candida (Monilia) Vaginitis

Douche with white vinegar, 1 tablespoon/pint water, one to two times each day for 1 week.

Douche with acidophilus culture, 2 tablespoons/pint water, one to two times each day for 1 week.

Apply acidophilus yogurt or buttermilk to labia, to vulva, or intravaginally every 2 to 3 hours, as needed, for relief of itching and burning (may assist growth of normal flora).

Take sitz baths every 2 to 4 hours, as needed, for relief of itching, burning, and swelling of labia and vulva.

Make tea of equal parts of uva ursi, parsley root, dandelion root, and burdock root; use 1 oz of herbs per pint of water in decoction. Drink ½ to 1 cup tea every 2 hours.

Douche with solution of equal parts of goldenseal, chaparral, comfrey root, and kava kava; use 1 oz herbs per pint water, simmer gently for 30 minutes, strain, cool, and add 1 tablespoon vinegar per pint. Douche once daily for 1 to 3 days.

Trichomonas Vaginitis

Douche with solution of equal parts of chaparral and chamomile; use 1 oz of herbs per pint water, steep for 20 minutes, strain, and cool. Douche two to three times each day for 1 or 2 weeks.

*Combine powders of *Echinacea*, goldenseal, chaparral, and squawvine in equal parts; fill gelatin capsules. Take 2 capsules three times each day before meals; also take 1 teaspoon garlic oil with meals.

Bacterial Vaginitis

Douche with white vinegar, 1 tablespoon/pint water, once each day for 1 week.

Douche with solution of 1 teaspoon goldenseal and 1 clove minced garlic steeped in 1 quart boiling water, strained and cooled. Use daily for 1 week.

Insert Betadine gel or solution intravaginally two times each day for 1 week.

* For use in bacterial vaginitis also.

many clients find these remedies beneficial in helping to relieve some of the irritating and uncomfortable symptoms of vaginitis.

The discharge in *Candida* vaginitis is typically white, thick, curdy, and adherent to the cervix and vaginal walls. However, thin, milky, and more confluent whitish discharge is not uncommon. Itching is moderate to severe, especially on the vulva and perineum. The labia and vulva may be bright red, swollen, sensitive to touch, and painful during intercourse. The extent of symptoms varies, but if the labia are involved and white discharge is present, this is a good area for taking a specimen. Usually saline and KOH mounts are prepared from vaginal or labial secretions. Microscopic examination shows the hyphae and spores of *Candida albicans* (Fig. 35-1). On saline mount, the vaginal epithelial cells appear normal and there are numerous lactobacilli (normal flora) and few white blood cells (WBC).

Vaginal tablets or creams, such as mycostatin (Nystatin), miconazole (Monistat), and chlordantoin (Sporostacin), are prescribed for insertion twice daily for 10 to 14 days.

The nurse instructs the client on insertion and can advise wearing a minipad during the day to absorb the drainage these medicines cause. Clients should be advised not to use tampons because they absorb the medication. Douching should be avoided, and intercourse is preferably stopped during the course of treatment, or a condom is used. If vulvar inflammation and itching are problems, antifungal or steroidal creams can be applied for several days. If *Candida* vaginitis is recurrent, the male partner should be examined and skin scrapings should be taken if inflammation is found at the base of the penis or perineum; antifungal treatment is prescribed if indicated.

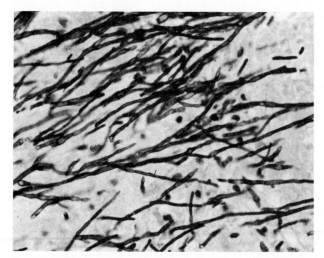

■ *Figure 35-1*
Candida albicans growing as hyphae and pseudohyphae within infected tissue. (Monif GRG: Infectious Diseases in Obstetrics & Gynecology. Hagerstown, Harper & Row, 1974; PAS, original magnification ×320)

Trichomonas Vaginalis

A unicellular protozoan flagellate, *Trichomonas vaginalis* is nearly always transmitted through sexual intercourse. In women, it usually infects the vagina and Skene's ducts; in men, it can be present in the lower genitourinary tract and may cause prostatitis.

The vaginal discharge in *Trichomonas* vaginitis is typically yellow green, frothy or bubbly, and copious and has a strong, foul odor. The cervix and upper vagina often have tiny petechiae due to inflammation. With severe inflammation, the vaginal wall, cervix, and vulva may be edematous and erythematous. Small, irregular erosions may be found on the labia. Moderate to severe itching is common, and some women have dysuria or dyspareunia secondary to inflammation. *Trichomonas* infections can be milder, with great variation in symptoms. Discharge can be thin, slight, whitish yellow, and without the typical foul odor.

Routine Pap smears not infrequently indicate the presence of trichomonads. Even in the absence of cytological changes (inflammation, atypia), treatment is needed because trichomonads are vaginal pathogens and may have recently colonized the vagina. During pelvic examination, a saline mount (Fig. 35-2) is taken and examined microscopically as soon as possible. Motile trichomonads are usually seen; under high power, these organisms are about two to three times the size of WBC and their flagella can be seen moving. Lactobacilli are usually absent, many WBC are present, and a range of vaginal intermediate and parabasal epithelial cells are present (Fig. 35-3).

Medical treatment for *Trichomonas* vaginitis consists of metronidazole (Flagyl), 2 g orally in a single dose, or 250 mg tid for 5 to 7 days. The single dose may not be as effective as longer treatment, but it facilitates compliance. The client's sexual partner also should be treated simultaneously with the same dosage. They are cautioned to avoid alcohol during the course of treatment because in combination with metronidazole it may cause abdominal cramps, nausea, vomiting, headaches, and flushing. Lactating women can be treated with 2 g metronidazole but should take the baby off the breast for 24 hours after therapy. Metronidazole is contraindicated during the first trimester of pregnancy and preferably should be avoided throughout. Clotrimazole (Gyne-Lotrimin) vaginal cream or tablets at bedtime for 7 days can provide symptomatic relief for pregnant women.[1]

Local vulvar inflammation can be treated with sitz baths or steroid creams. If intercourse is painful owing to inflammation, it should be avoided for 2 to 3 days to permit healing. Dysuria related to urethral inflammation responds to these treatments also. Again, some clients find natural remedies helpful in relieving uncomfortable symptoms (see box entitled "Natural Remedies for Vaginitis").

Client Education

Preventing Vaginitis

Personal hygiene
Wash labia and vulva with mild soap (not antiseptic) daily.
Dry external genitals and perineum thoroughly.
Wipe front-to-back after voiding and bowel movements.
Wash hands before inserting tampons, diaphragm, and contraceptive creams or sponges.
Avoid or minimize douching (once per week, use water or mild solutions).
Avoid deodorants, perfumed sprays or lotions, powders, antiseptic soaps, perfumed toilet paper.
Change tampons and pads every 1 to 4 hours, depending on flow.
Avoid using superabsorbent tampons, or use only during heaviest flow.
Wear cotton underclothing; avoid tight-fitting clothing in genital area.

Sexual practices
Limit the number of sexual partners or have one partner.
Ask or check sexual partner for symptoms (penile discharge, lesions, dysuria); avoid sex or use condom with spermicide if present.
Know the sexual partner (history of genital infections or STD, other sexual contacts).
Avoid intercourse when you have symptoms (increased discharge, itching or burning, lesions, pain).
Avoid oral–genital contact if vulvar or mouth lesions are present in either partner.
Avoid anal–vaginal penetration or use different condoms for each.

General health status
Eat well-balanced, nutritious meals and avoid less-healthful foods (sweets, red meats, salty foods, saturated fats).
Get regular exercise.
Get enough sleep (6–8 hours per night).
Find time each week for personal interests and hobbies.
Recognize sources of stress at home and work, and find methods to reduce stress (progressive relaxation, autogenic training, yoga, biofeedback, meditation, imagery, quiet time).
Maintain satisfying relationships and friendship networks.

Bacterial Vaginosis

Bacterial vaginosis is caused by *Gardnerella vaginalis,* a short, gram-negative rod (coccobacillus) that is transmitted sexually. The organism is a surface parasite and does not invade deeper tissue; thus there may be fewer symptoms of inflammation such as itching, burning, dysuria, or dyspareunia (Table 35-2).

The vaginal discharge is typically thin, gray white, and homogeneous; it is infrequently frothy. There is a fishy odor to the discharge, particularly after sexual intercourse. In many instances, the symptoms are minimal and women are uncertain whether they should be concerned about having a vaginal infection. A common presentation might be a woman with variable slight increase in vaginal discharge that has a bad odor. Many women with *Gardnerella* infections have no symptoms.

Few changes are noted on pelvic examination. If discharge is typical, this assists diagnosis. Adding 10% KOH to the discharge may produce an evanescent fishy odor owing to production of two malodorous amines, putrescine and cadaverine. A saline mount (see Fig. 35-2) is taken and examined microscopically. Diagnosis is made when clue cells are present; there are vaginal epithelial cells that appear stippled due to growth of *Gardnerella* organisms. Lactobacilli usually are absent; vaginal epithelial cells are mature forms.

Medical treatment is with metronidazole (Flagyl), 250 mg orally three times daily for 7 days. Ampicillin, 500 mg orally four times a day for 7 days, is an alternate treatment, recommended for use during pregnancy. When metronidazole is used, advice is given about avoiding alcohol during the course of treatment. The woman's sexual partner(s) should also be treated simultaneously with the above dosage of metronidazole. Often male sexual partners have some symptoms, and *Gardnerella* is a common cause of urethritis in men.[2]

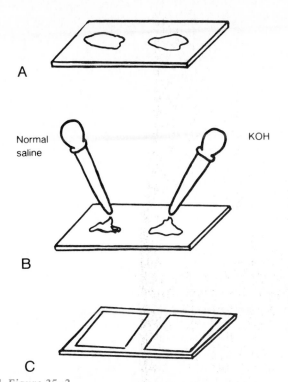

A

Normal
saline   KOH

B

C

■ *Figure 35–2*
Preparation of wet mount of vaginal discharge for microscopic examination. (A) Using a cotton-tipped applicator or Pap stick, two separate drops of the vaginal discharge are placed on a glass slide and spread thinly. (B) One drop of normal saline is added to one specimen for microscopic examination for Trichomonas vaginalis. One drop of 10% to 20% potassium hydroxide (KOH) is added to the other specimen for microscopic examination for Candida albicans. (C) Separate coverslips are placed over each specimen, and excess moisture is blotted with a paper towel. Slides are examined under high- and low-power lenses of microscope. (Nursing Services Manual, Newton, MA, Preterm Institute, 1976)

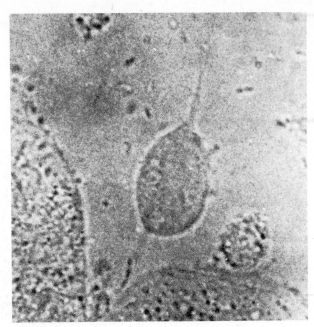

■ *Figure 35–3*
Characteristic configuration of a trichomonad seen in wet smear at high-power magnification. (Monif GRG: Infectious Diseases in Obstetrics & Gynecology. Hagerstown, Harper & Row, 1974)

Condyloma (Papillomavirus)

Condyloma (genital warts) are skin lesions caused by human papillomavirus (HPV) and are sexually transmitted. About 67% of exposed sexual partners develop condyloma.[3] The lesions may be large, cauliflowerlike clusters or tiny, single closely grouped or widely dispersed bumps. Condyloma are usually multiple, although single lesions can occur, and are usually found on the vulva, vagina, cervix, and rectum. About 15 varieties of HPV are known to infect the genital tract, but the most common are HPV-6 and HPV-11. Cervical neoplasia has been associated with HPV-16 and 18.[4,5]

The incidence of condyloma in the United States has been increasing rapidly since the 1960s. Risk factors are young age, multiple sexual partners, and pregnancy. About 30% of pregnant women have been found to harbor HPV in the genital tract.[6] Cervical, vaginal, and vulval lesions may increase in size during pregnancy, and occasionally become so large that they interfere with vaginal delivery. Condyloma frequently regress after pregnancy and may become subclinical. Infants exposed perinatally to condyloma may develop laryngeal papillomatosis, with most cases occurring between the ages of 2 and 4. About one fourth of cases occur during infancy. The presenting symptoms are hoarseness and a croupy cough. Laryngeal papillomas are treated by incision.

Diagnosis of condyloma during pregnancy is by visualization of the lesions, colposcopy, biopsy, and occasionally by Pap smears, which identify nuclear abnormalities in cervical epithelium. The standard treatment of 25% podophyllin application is contraindicated in pregnancy, because it is teratogenic and both maternal and fetal deaths have been reported.[7] Cryosurgery is most commonly used during pregnancy, although occasionally 5-FU in 5% cream (a highly effective cytotoxic agent with few systemic effects) or trichloroacetic acid 50% solution are also used. Repeated treatments are often necessary for multiple or resistant lesions.

Hepatitis B

Hepatitis B virus (HBV) is most frequently transmitted in the United States by sexual contact and is also transmitted in body fluids (blood, saliva, breast milk, vaginal

TABLE 35–2. COMMON TYPES OF VAGINITIS: CHARACTERISTICS AND TREATMENT

Type of Vaginitis	Erythema and Itching	Discharge	Saline Mount	Potassium Hydroxide Mount	Culture or Other	Medication or Other Treatment
Candida albicans (Monilia)	Vulva, labia, perineum, thighs Mild to severe	Mild to moderate Curdy white	Hyphae or spores Many lactobacilli	Hyphae or spores	Nickerson's grows brown or black colonies	Vaginal tablets or cream: Mycostatin, miconazole, chlordantoin
Trichomonas vaginalis	Severe vulval itching, ±erythema Petechiae of cervix and vagina	Copious Yellow-green frothy	Trichomonads Few lactobacilli Many WBC	Negative	None	Clotrimazole vaginal tablets Metronidazole (Flagyl) orally* (treat sexual partner)
Bacterial vaginosis	Mild to moderate	Mild to moderate Homogeneous Gray, foul	Clue cells Small rods Many WBC Few lactobacilli	Negative	Blood agar ± colonies	Ampicillin orally Metronidazole (Fagyl orally* (treat sexual partner)
Chlamydia trachomatis	None to mild	Slight to moderate, varies	Many WBC Few lactobacilli	Negative	Pap smear with inclusion bodies *Chlamydia* culture	Erythromycin, ceftriaxone or amphicilin (treat sexual partner)
Allergic or irritative	Mild to severe	Varied	Unremarkable	Negative	No growth	Remove source of allergy or irritation Topical steroid if severe inflammation
Foreign body	Mild or absent	Serous, purulent, fetid	Many WBC	Negative	+Specific organism if secondary infection	Remove foreign body Treat secondary infection with specific antibiotic

* Metronidazole is contraindicated during the first trimester of pregnancy; use in later pregnancy is controversial and should preferably be avoided.

fluid, and semen). The risk of contracting hepatitis B increases with the number of sexual partners, use of IV drugs, and frequent exposure to body fluids. Groups with high prevalence of hepatitis B include prison inmates, hemodialysis patients, users of homeless shelters, Asians, Pacific Islanders, Alaskan Eskimos, and women from Haiti or sub-Saharan Africa.[8]

Infection with HBV results in hepatitis (liver infection) with a wide range of clinical manifestations. Most cases of acute viral hepatitis are asymptomatic, or the client may have vague flulike symptoms. Classic symptoms include fatigue, nausea, anorexia, abdominal pain, low-grade fever and, in 25% of cases, jaundice. Hepatitis B infection can become chronic, ranging from an asymptomatic carrier state to persistent hepatitis, cirrhosis, or hepatocellular carcinoma. About 5% to 10% of infected adults develop persistent hepatitis.[9] There is no effective treatment for HBV infection; immunization is the only protection against the disease.

Perinatal HBV transmission generally occurs during passage through the birth canal, although 6% of cases are acquired transplacentally. Seventy to 90% of infants born to mothers infected with HBV are at risk for becoming congenitally infected. Infected infants who are not treated can become chronic carriers (80%–90%), and of these, 25% develop cirrhosis or hepatocellular carcinoma.[10] The risk of becoming carriers is higher in children than adults, and female carriers can transmit the infection to their sexual partners, family members, and children. Prevention of HBV infection in the newborn is extremely important.

Hepatitis B is diagnosed by serological testing to identify antigen and antibody systems. Hepatitis B surface antigen (HBsAg) is found on the surface of the virus, appears 30 to 60 days after exposure, and persists for an indefinite period. All HBsAg-positive people are potentially infectious. An HBV carrier is HBsAg-positive on at least two tests a minimum of 6 months apart. Several other antigen and antibody tests are used to evaluate the stage and progression of the infection. Anti-HBs (antibody to surface antigen) indicates past infection and immunity to HBV or immune response to HBV vaccine.

Screening for HBsAg is done on all high-risk pregnant women, but some authorities recommend routine prenatal screening for all women.[11,12] Active immunization with hepatitis B vaccine is recommended for all people with multiple sex partners, IV drug users, residents of correctional and long-term care facilities, people seeking treatment for STD, prostitutes,[12] and others with high-risk factors. Health-care workers at risk for exposure to body fluids should also seek immunization. HB vaccine is administered in three doses, the first two are given 1 month apart and the third is given in 6 months. After exposure to HBV infection, prophylactic treatment with hepatitis B immune globulin (HBIG) within 14 days of exposure is recommended. This is followed by hepatitis B vaccine to provide active immunity.[8]

Information about pregnant clients with positive HBsAg results should be communicated to obstetric and pediatric staffs, so the newborn can receive prompt treatment and health workers can take appropriate precautions. HBV infection can be prevented in the newborn by administering HBIG as soon as possible after birth, preferably within the first 12 hours, along with the first dose of HB vaccine. This is followed by doses of HB vaccine at 1 and 6 months of age. Immunization is promoted for all infants of women from areas with high endemic rates of HBV infection (Haiti, Africa, East Asia)[8] and women in shelters and prisons (see Table 35-2).

Chlamydia

Infections caused by *Chlamydia trachomatis* are the most prevalent of the STD in the United States.

Chlamydia is an obligatory intracellular organism that selects the lower genital tract of both women and men. *Chlamydia* cervicitis occurs in about 30% of pregnant women. Risk factors include being age 24 or younger, new sexual partner in the past 2 months, mucopurulent cervical discharge, friable cervix, and non-barrier method of contraception or no contraception.[11] Among women with gonorrhea, 25% to 50% also have *Chlamydia*. In the woman, chlamydial infections often cause salpingitis and pelvic inflammatory disease (PID), and increase the incidence of infertility and ectopic pregnancies. There is increased risk of late onset endometritis after vaginal delivery.

Infants delivered vaginally by infected mothers have a 60% to 70% risk of acquiring infection during passage through the birth canal. Inclusion conjunctivitis of the newborn is the most common infection, occurring in up to 50% of exposed infants, and often resulting in conjunctival scarring and corneal vascularization. Chlamydial neonatal ophthalmia is several times more frequent than gonorrheal. Pneumonia occurs in about 10% to 20% of infected neonates.[1]

Chlamydia tissue cultures are used for definitive diagnosis, but are expensive and take up to 1 week to obtain results. Antigen detection tests offer more rapid identification (Microtrak, a direct immunofluorescent test, requires 30 minutes; Chlamydiazyme, an enzyme-linked immunosorbent assay, requires 4 hours). Treatment is with erythromycin 500 mg qid for 7 days. Sexual partners should receive the same treatment regimen. Another approach is ceftriaxone, or amoxicillin with probenecid, initially followed by erythromycin in the pregnant woman. Silver nitrate eye prophylaxis in the newborn does not prevent chlamydial infections, and the Centers for Disease Control and the American Academy of Pediatrics support using erythromycin or tetracycline ophthalmic ointment.[13]

High-Risk Factors for Hepatitis B

IV drug users

Recipients of blood products

Prostitutes

Women with multiple sex partners

Women with history of liver disease

Woman who have occupational exposure to blood and blood products (health-care workers, lab technicians, and so forth)

Indochinese refugees

Women of Asian descent or women born in Haiti or South Africa

(From Lemon SM: Viral hepatitis. In Holmes KK, Mardh P, Sparling PF, Wiesner PJ (eds): Sexually Transmitted Diseases. New York, McGraw-Hill, 1984; and Centers for Disease Control: Sexually Transmitted Diseases Treatment Guidelines, September, 1989.)

Genital Herpes

Two types of herpes viruses that are immunologically and clinically distinct may involve the genital tract. Type I herpes hominis is mainly associated with nongenital lesions, but may also involve the genital tract. Type II herpes hominis is almost entirely genital and is generally sexually transmitted. Herpes type II is one of the most rapidly spreading STD, with between 5 and 20 million American adults infected.

Approximately 1% to 2% of pregnancies are complicated by herpesvirus infection. The incubation period is 3 to 14 days for the primary infection and 7 to 10 days for the secondary infection. The lesions are characterized by painful vesicles in the vulva and perineal areas that commonly rupture and become secondarily infected (Fig. 35-4). The cervix and vagina are also commonly infected with lesions that are asymptomatic and may shed for several months. The infected woman may experience flulike symptoms. Inguinal adenopathy may be severe. Cytological smears reveal large multinucleate cells with eosinophilic inclusion bodies, and unsuspected herpes is frequently diagnosed as an incidental finding by Pap smear. The initial herpes symptoms usually disappear within 3 weeks; however, recurrences are frequent and associated with stress or illness.

The maternal infection is only rarely transmitted transplacentally to the fetus, but when this occurs in the first trimester, spontaneous abortion or severe fetal abnormalities may result. After the 20th week of gestation, infection increases the risk for premature birth but not for fetal abnormalities. The fetus is most likely to be infected after rupture of the membranes or during the course of delivery, because the virus can be transmitted through lesions in the genital tract. Detection of active herpes infections before delivery is most important, because disseminated neonatal herpes has a 50% mortality rate and ocular and central nervous system damage occurs in about two thirds of the survivors (see Chap. 46).[1]

There is no effective treatment for herpes. The main goal of care is to prevent neonatally acquired herpes infection. Pregnant women with a history of herpes or with infected partners are monitored carefully in the third trimester to detect active infection. Serial viral cultures of the cervix and external genital area are taken. About 50% of neonatal infections occur with no or minimal maternal genital symptoms at birth. In the presence of active maternal genital lesions or positive cultures, cesarean delivery should be performed.

Acyclovir (Zovirax) has not been tested in pregnancy and therefore is not recommended except in life-threatening situations.[14]

Topical application of acyclovir has been used to modify the symptomatology and shorten healing time of lesions, but the benefits of its use during pregnancy must justify the potential risk to the fetus. Broad-spectrum antibiotic therapy is often prescribed to treat secondary infection. Perineal comfort may be promoted by taking sitz baths two to three times per day and keeping the infected region clean and dry.

When an uninfected pregnant woman has a sexual partner with a history of genital herpes, condoms should be used to reduce the possibility of transmission, even in asymptomatic phases of the disease. In addition, women with a history of genital herpes should be advised to have Pap smears performed annually, because there is evidence suggesting that herpes type II may have a causal role in cervical carcinoma.[15]

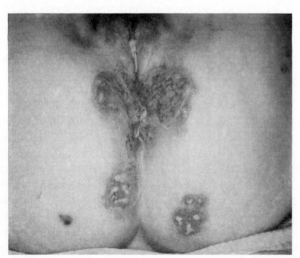

■ *Figure 35-4*
Herpes genitalis lesions are characterized by painful vesicles in the vulva and perineal areas.

Syphilis

Syphilis can be transmitted through exposure to infected exudate during sexual contact, by contact with open wounds or infected blood, and can be acquired congenitally through transplacental inoculation. Syphilis is caused by the spirochete *Treponema pallidum*. An increased incidence of primary and secondary syphilis occurred in 1987, particularly in New York, California, and Florida.[11] Congenital syphilis began increasing around 1983 to 1985 when 300 cases were reported in the United States.

Syphilis can occur at any stage during pregnancy. The primary stage, which lasts 1 to 6 weeks, is characterized by classic lesions (chancres), which are deep and painless ulcers often found on the genitalia, lips, or rectal area. In the secondary stage of syphilis, which lasts 2 to 10 weeks, a macular rash appears on the entire body. In latent syphilis, the diagnosis is based on a positive serology, and the infection is usually subclinical. The early latent stage is 1 year from onset of the infection, and the late latent stage occurs after 1 year and may last the rest of the person's life. About one third of cases progress to late latency. Cardiovascular, neurological, cutaneous, and visceral tissue damage may occur during late syphilis.

The rate of acquisition of syphilis from an infected partner is about 30%. The disease is rarely transmitted sexually after 2 years but can be acquired by the fetus of an infected mother when transmitted through the placenta as early as the 6th week of pregnancy, although clinical manifestations of disease in the fetus usually do not occur unless infection is present after 16 weeks gestation. The risk of prematurity, perinatal death, and congenital syphilis depends on the mother's stage, ranging from 70% to 100% in primary syphilis to 30% in latent syphilis.[11]

Congenital syphilis is a systemic infection with a wide range of presentations. At birth, there may be no sign of disease, or the infant may be severely affected with hepatosplenomegaly, hemolytic anemia, osteochondritis, bullous skin eruptions containing spirochetes, and "snuffles" (rhinitis due to nasal mucosal involvement).

Diagnosis of primary and secondary syphilis is made by darkfield microscope identification of spirochetes in samples from a chancre or skin lesion. Serological tests are also used, including nontreponemal tests (VDRL, RPR), which are quantifiable but less accurate in primary and late syphilis, and treponemal tests for specific antibody (FTA-ABS, HATTS), which are sensitive. A small number of pregnant women have a biological false-positive test, requiring serology titers.

Treatment is with 2.4 million units of benzathine penicillin administered intramuscularly weekly for 3 weeks. Erythromycin is used when there is a penicillin allergy, but the fetus may not be adequately treated because of poor placental transfer. Both mother and baby are followed postpartally with monthly VDRL titers to assess effectiveness of treatment. Sexual contacts must also be treated, and the infant may need additional treatment depending on titers.

Gonorrhea

Gonorrhea is caused by the gram-negative coccus *Neisseria gonorrhoeae*, an organism that may attack the mucous membrane but most commonly affects the mucosa of the lower genital tract. The endocervical glands and urethra are common foci, but for complete detection, the anus and oropharynx should be cultured.

Gonorrhea is spread by sexual contact and in the majority of women remains asymptomatic except for a nonspecific vaginal discharge. This is particularly the case in pregnancy, in which the normal route of spread through the endometrial cavity to the tubes is occluded by the pregnancy.

Women of lower socioeconomic status are at increased risk for gonorrhea in pregnancy. Prevalence ranges from 0.6% to 7.6% and is higher in California, New York, and Florida.[11] Reinfections occur in 11% to 30% of women with a history of gonorrhea.

Although gonorrhea causes few problems for the client during pregnancy, it can produce serious puerperal infection if present in the cervix at the time of delivery. Routine gonorrhea cultures are recommended in early pregnancy.

Gonorrhea infection during pregnancy increases the risk of chorioamnionitis, premature delivery, premature rupture of membranes, and intrauterine growth retardation. When the mother is infected at delivery, 30% to 35% of infants contract gonorrhea during passage through the birth canal. Risk is increased with prolonged rupture of membranes, and infection can be transmitted through the amniotic fluid. The major effect of gonorrhea in the infant is ophthalmic infections, but infections of the nasopharyngeal passages, vagina, anus, ear canals, and scalp abscesses (from fetal monitoring electrodes) may also result.

Treatment during pregnancy consists of 4.8 million units of aqueous procaine penicillin intramuscularly in two sites, plus 1 g of oral probenicid to increase penicillin blood levels. In areas with a high rate of penicillinase producing *Neisseria gonorrhoeae*, ceftriaxone 125 to 250 mg IM or spectinomycin 2 g IM is used. Some clinics are using ampicillin or amoxicillin to treat gonorrhea. Cure should be proven by reculture. Sexual partners must be identified and treated. In the neonate, prophylaxis against gonococcal ophthalmia is accomplished by topical application of silver nitrate, erythromycin, or tetracycline. Infants who are infected perinatally need treatment with parenteral antibiotics.[16]

Human Immunodeficiency Virus (HIV)

Infection with human immunodeficiency virus (HIV) causes a progressive disruption of immune system functioning, the last stage of which is AIDS (acquired immunodeficiency syndrome; Table 35-3). AIDS was first identified among homosexual men in 1981, and within the decade spread to epidemic proportions among both homosexual and heterosexual populations in the United States. About one million people were estimated by the Centers for Disease Control (CDC) to be HIV infected in 1991, with 60,000 to 90,000 new cases expected annually.[17] The number of cases of AIDS has grown from over 83,000 in 1988 to over 224,000

TABLE 35-3. CENTERS FOR DISEASE CONTROL CLASSIFICATION SYSTEM FOR HIV INFECTION

Group	Description
I	Acute HIV infection (mononucleosislike syndrome) with documented seroconversion for HIV antibody
II	Asymptomatic infection, seropositive but no signs or symptoms of infection
III	Persistent generalized lymphadenopathy, defined as ≥1-cm nodes at ≥2 extrainguinal sites, persisting for >3 months
IV	Other AIDS-related diseases
A	Constitutional disease: unexplained fever, diarrhea, weight loss
B	Neurological disease: unexplained dementia, neuropathy, or myelopathy
C	Opportunistic infections: viral, fungal, parasitic, bacterial, other
D	Opportunistic neoplasms: Kaposi's sarcoma, lymphoma
E	Other conditions (including chronic lymphocytic interstitial pneumonitis)

cases in 1991.[18,19] AIDS cases are expected to continue to increase at least through 1993, reaching a total of over 300,000.[18] AIDS is the second leading cause of death in men age 25 to 44 and is among the top five killers of women in this age group.[20]

HIV infection carries a serious prognosis, because most (if not all) infections progress gradually to end-stage disease and premature death. A retrovirus, HIV substitutes its own RNA/DNA for a portion of the T4 cell DNA. T4 cell replication produces new infected cells, and eventually these cells release additional virus that in turn infects more T4 cells. After exposure to HIV, some people experience a flu or mononucleosislike syndrome, but others have no symptoms. From 6 weeks to a year after exposure, HIV antibodies appear in the serum and can be detected by enzyme-linked immunosorbent assay (ELISA), which is usually confirmed by a Western blot test. The appearance of HIV antibodies is called seroconversion. People who test positive for HIV are able to transmit the infection to others.

Although producing no symptoms, the virus continues to destroy T4 cells and slowly alters immune system functioning. Usually within 6 months to a year, chronically swollen lymph nodes develop as the body attempts to combat the HIV through overproduction of B cells (abundant in the lymph nodes). In about 3 to 5 years, there is a persistent drop of T4 cells to less than $400/mm^3$. This is the harbinger of decline in immune functioning. The person begins to lose the ability to mount an effective cellular immune response to patho-

gens and neoplasia. Usually within another 2 to 5 years, the breakdown of cell-mediated immunity is evident by opportunistic infections caused by *Candida albicans*, herpes simplex, cytomegalovirus, papovavirus, *Histoplasma*, *Toxoplasma*, *Pneumocystis carinii*, and others. Oral hairy leukoplakia and neoplasms such as Kaposi's sarcoma and lymphoma often occur. People in later stages of HIV infection are susceptible to tuberculosis and other bacterial infections including *Legionella* and *Salmonella*. When the T4 cell count drops to $100/mm^3$ or less, death usually ensues within 2 years (Fig. 35-5).[21]

There is no curative treatment, although some drugs such as zidovudine (Retrovir), formerly called AZT (azidothymidine) appear to delay progression. Research is focused on finding a vaccine to provide immunity against HIV infection. Prevention of HIV transmission is critical to reduce the incidence and spread of AIDS. HIV is transmitted through blood and body fluids, transplacentally and through breast milk. The primary mode of transmission is sexual, with greater risk from anal than from vaginal intercourse. Oral–genital contact probably has a lower risk than does vaginal intercourse. HIV also is transmitted by blood transfusions, sharing of needles used for IV drugs, and occasionally by needle prick or accidental blood and fluid contact with mucous membranes of health workers.

HIV INFECTION IN WOMEN

The risk to women of sexually spread HIV infection is rising. About 10% of all AIDS cases occur in women, but the rate of increase is greater among women than men. Nearly 30% of AIDS cases in women are caused by heterosexual transmission. The risk is especially severe among minority groups, with over 70% of AIDS cases occurring in African-American and Hispanic women. African-American women have 13.6 times and Hispanic women have 10.2 times the risk of contracting AIDS as white women. This is related partly to greater IV drug use among both minority women and their sexual partners.[18] The proportion of women with AIDS contracted from sexual partners in high HIV risk groups appears to be increasing. As part of the prenatal interview for women in the high-risk category, the nurse should ask certain questions to screen the woman for exposure to HIV (see Assessment Tool entitled "Assessing Women's Risk for HIV Exposure").

Heterosexual transmission of HIV is an escalating problem. In 1985, heterosexuals represented only 1.4% of all AIDS cases; this increased to 4% in 1988 and is expected to be 10% by 1991.[22] More than 100,000 women in the United States are estimated to be HIV-infected. Studies of the seroprevalence of HIV (presence of HIV antibodies in the serum) have shown some surprisingly high rates, especially in New York, New Jersey, and Florida. Seroprevalence rates of 2% to 4% were

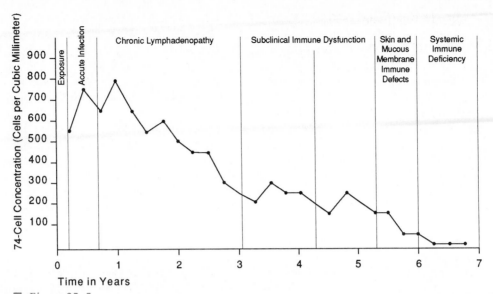

■ *Figure 35–5*

Decline in T4 cells in HIV/AIDS disease progression. Seroconversion occurs about 3 months after exposure to HIV, with a drop in T4 cells, then a rebound. Chronic lymphadenopathy develops around 9 months and a long, slow decline of T4 cells occurs. As the T4 cell count falls below 400/mm³ at about 3 years, delayed hypersensitivity occurs. Gradually, the ability to mount a cellular immune response fails, with early signs such as thrush and oral hairy leukoplakia. When the T4 count falls below 100/mm³ (shortly before 6 years), opportunistic infections and neoplasms occur, leading to death usually within a few years.

found among women in hospital screening programs in Newark and Brooklyn.[23,24] In other large-scale studies, seroprevalences for women were reported as 0 to 0.4% in premarital screenings[25] and 1.1% in the military.[26] Minority women have higher rates of HIV infection than either white women or men, and African-American and Hispanic men appear to have three to four times greater risk of being infected with HIV than white men.[26]

The AIDS epidemic is spreading into the heterosexual population, especially among minority women. Parts of rural America are about to experience the impact of the AIDS epidemic. There has been a 37% increase in AIDS cases in rural areas within a 1-year period, compared to a 5% increase in large urban areas. In many rural areas, there is little information about HIV infection and overwhelming fear of people infected with HIV or AIDS victims. This ignorance and fear can seriously hamper efforts to treat people with HIV and AIDS and works against prevention.[27]

HIV INFECTION AND PREGNANCY

Most women infected with HIV are in the reproductive years. Perinatal transmission is an increasingly important mode of HIV infection and can result in birth of severely ill infants who die early from AIDS and often are abandoned in the hospital nursery. Studies have not demonstrated conclusively that HIV infection adversely affects the course of pregnancy, although there may be an association with premature rupture of membranes, preterm birth, and low birth weight.[24]

Perinatal transmission occurs frequently when the mother is HIV infected, with between 35% and 50% of infants testing positive for HIV antibodies. Because maternal IgG (anti-HIV antibody) crosses the placenta, diagnosis of infant infection is difficult before 15 months of age, unless signs of AIDS are present. Transmission from an infected mother can occur by three routes:

1. Transmission of HIV virus across the placenta in utero
2. Transmission of HIV virus by way of exposure to maternal blood and body fluids during passage through the birth canal
3. Transmission of HIV virus through the breast milk

Symptoms of Fetal AIDS Syndrome

Growth failure	Prominent eyes
Microcephaly	Blue sclerae
Prominent forehead	Oblique eyes
Flattened nasal bridge	Triangular philtrum
	Patulous lips

The use of scalp electrodes and scalp or percutaneous umbilical blood sampling should be avoided when the mother is HIV positive. These procedures may increase the infant's risk of exposure to the HIV virus. Cesarean delivery does not appear to have a protective effect against perinatal transmission.[28]

The risk of HIV transmission in utero has not been related to the trimester during which exposure occurred. The absence of maternal symptoms does not seem to reduce risk of HIV infection for the infant. There is some evidence that children whose mothers had symptoms before delivery are more likely to develop AIDS symptoms earlier. A characteristic syndrome in the infant has been described and attributed to in-utero HIV infection. The severity of the syndrome correlated with the age at diagnosis of immunodeficiency in the child.[28]

HIV infection and AIDS in children follow the pattern found among women; most cases occur in African-American (53%) and Hispanic (23%) children and were acquired perinatally from infected mothers.[18] AIDS has become a leading cause of death among children less than 4 years old in these populations, exceeding deaths from accidental injuries and other infectious diseases.[19] About 20% of pediatric HIV infections are from blood transfusions and blood products used to treat hemophilia.

Maternal risk factors that increase the likelihood of perinatal HIV infection include IV drug use and sexual partner who is an IV drug user or has other risk factors for HIV infection. The proportion of perinatally infected children whose mothers had sexual partners infected with or at risk for HIV infection has been rising.[18] Many women are unaware of their risk for HIV and become infected as teenagers, remaining undiagnosed until a perinatally infected child becomes ill.[29]

CLINICAL MANAGEMENT

Pregnant women who are at risk for HIV infection should be screened in early pregnancy. In addition, women in high-risk categories for HIV infection should be screened again in the third trimester.[30] This includes women with STD during the current pregnancy (gonorrhea, syphilis, *Chlamydia,* hepatitis B, prolonged herpes), and with oropharyngeal or chronic vaginal candidiasis, tuberculosis, cytomegalovirus, and toxoplasmosis.

The Institute of Medicine has recommended that HIV screening should be offered to all pregnant women, but that the test should be voluntary. Routine screening of newborns was not recommended because of antibody transfer from the mother. Women must have the right to consent to or refuse HIV testing, because the diagnosis has powerful psychological and social consequences.[31] Routine maternal screening remains controversial because of the low population prevalence rates (less than 0.1% in most parts of the United States) and the impact of false-positive tests with such a devastating diagnosis.[24]

When a pregnant women is HIV positive, counseling includes instruction in safe sex practices and information on both sexual and perinatal transmission. Abortion and sterilization services are offered when appropriate. Because HIV infection is frequently associated with other STD, the mother who is HIV positive is screened for syphilis, gonorrhea, *Chlamydia,* and hepatitis B. Baseline antibody titers are drawn for rubella, chickenpox, cytomegalovirus, and toxoplasmosis, because these infections are common in HIV patients and can cause serious illness. Tuberculin skin testing is done (PPD), and vaccination status is determined.

Because many women infected with HIV are IV drug users, the issue of substance abuse must be assessed and treatment and counseling must be provided. The nurse carefully evaluates symptoms and discomforts of pregnancy (i.e., anorexia, fatigue, weight loss, vaginitis) because these may also be evidence of HIV disease progression. Opportunistic infections can occur during pregnancy and are generally treated with the recommended drugs, although little is known about the adverse effects of these drugs on either mother or fetus. Nutritional counseling is important to promote health, and the woman is counseled about getting adequate sleep, rest, and exercise and stress reduction to support immune system functioning. The use of alcohol and cigarettes is discouraged because these may interfere with medical treatments and may further stress the immune system. Family and sexual counseling are often

---

High-Risk Groups for HIV Infection and AIDS

History of IV drug use or current use

Long-term residence or birth in area with high prevalence of HIV infection or AIDS

Received blood transfusion between 1978 and 1985 (before HIV screening was standard practice)

Diagnosed with another sexually transmitted disease

History of frequent sexual partners or prostitutes

Past or present sexual partner who is IV drug user, bisexual, or HIV infected; has signs or symptoms of AIDS; has frequent sexual partners; or who has received a blood transfusion between 1978 and 1985

(From Centers for Disease Control: HIV prevalence estimates and AIDS case projections for The United States: Report based upon a workshop. MMWR 39(16):1–15, 1990; and Centers for Disease Control: Update: Acquired immune deficiency syndrome—United States, 1981–1988. MMWR 38:229–236, 1989)

necessary, and the woman may be referred to HIV and AIDS support groups. Although the risk of HIV transmission through breast milk is not well known, the woman is advised not to breast-feed because the virus has been isolated from breast milk.[32]

■ URINARY TRACT INFECTIONS

The most common urinary tract problem in pregnancy is urinary tract infection (UTI). Anatomical changes as well as hormonal effects cause narrowing of the lower ureter and renal pelvis, with dilation of the upper ureter. These changes result in stasis of urine, delayed emptying, and an increased risk of infection. The risk increases as pregnancy progresses and continues into the puerperium.

Assessment

The nurse obtains a history regarding urinary tract symptoms. Women with UTI usually report pain or burning on urination (dysuria), urgency, and frequency. They may have noticed discolored urine that may be darker than normal, cloudy, or bloody. Suprapubic cramping with cystitis and lower to mid-back pain with pyelonephritis may also occur. Fever, chills, anorexia, nausea, and vomiting are more common with acute pyelonephritis. Nursing assessment includes information about voiding practices, changes in sexual partners or activities, genital hygiene practices, and use of topical soaps, sprays, or lotions.

Physical examination includes vital signs, particularly temperature, as indicators of infection. The nurse obtains a clean catch, midstream urine specimen for chemical and microscopic analysis and culture if indicated.

Nursing Diagnosis

Alteration in comfort: pain related to urinary tract inflammation is a frequent nursing diagnosis with UTI, because women often experience considerable discomfort. Altered patterns of urinary elimination may be diagnosed, when the woman experiences urgency, frequency, hesitancy, or dribbling associated with a UTI. A self-care deficit may exist, because the women may not know how to relieve or prevent urinary infections. The client may experience anxiety or have knowledge deficits related to the causes and treatment of her symptoms and may have fears about the effects of the urinary infection on her body.

Planning and Intervention

Nursing care focuses on promoting effective treatment of UTI and preventing recurrences. Careful instructions are provided about taking medications correctly and completing the course of treatment. Women are counseled to increase fluid intake to 8 to 10 glasses of liquids daily, and to void promptly and thoroughly. Good bladder hygiene is emphasized with proper front-to-back wiping techniques. Factors that may predispose the women to urinary infections are identified and eliminated, such as perfumed soaps and sprays. The woman is counseled to avoid sexual practices that traumatize the urethra or may spread intestinal bacteria toward the vagina and urinary meatus.

Evaluation

Nursing care can be evaluated as effective when the UTI is successfully treated and symptoms resolve, when the women understands the contributing factors and eliminates these, and when good bladder hygiene is followed. The client reports her anxieties or fears are relieved, and she is able to implement appropriate self-care.

Asymptomatic Bacteruria (ASB)

Approximately 2% to 10% of all pregnant women have significant asymptomatic bacteruria during pregnancy. The probability of developing ASB is related to parity, race, and socioeconomic status. White, primigravid, private clients have the lowest incidence; the highest incidence is found among African-American multiparas with sickle cell trait.[7] ASB is identified by urine culture with more than 100,000 colonies/ml of a single organism in a clean catch urine specimen. With elevated counts less than 100,000/ml, repeated cultures demonstrating the same organism are necessary to diagnose ASB. The most common causative organisms are *Escherichia coli*, *Enterobacter* species, and *Klebsiella*.

ASB is important because over 30% of affected women develop symptomatic UTI later in pregnancy or postpartum. Bacteruria usually is present during the first trimester and persists until after delivery in about 80% of untreated women. About 4% of these clients develop pyelonephritis.[7] It has been suggested that premature labor is more common in women with ASB, but this is not well-demonstrated by research. The major risk to the woman and fetus is the subsequent development of cystitis or pyelonephritis.

Routine screening for ASB in all pregnant women is recommended. Urine cultures early in the second trimester detect nearly all women with bacteruria. ASB in pregnancy is treated with antibiotics, including sulfisoxazole (Gantrisin) 1 g four times a day, ampicillin 1 g/day, nitrofurantoin 50 to 100 mg four times a day, or cephalexin 250 to 500 mg four times daily; all for 10 days. Repeat urine cultures are obtained monthly, with continued antibiotic suppression for persistent infections, during pregnancy and after delivery.[33]

Cystitis and Urethritis

Acute lower urinary tract infections (cystitis, urethritis) occur in 1% to 2% of women during pregnancy. One third of these women have had ASB, which if detected and treated would have prevented acute lower UTI from developing. The symptoms of UTI include frequency, urgency, dysuria, and suprapubic pain. Occasionally, the pregnant women have hemorrhagic cystitis with hematuria. Urinalysis shows many WBC, RBC, and bacteria; urine culture is positive for the same organisms that cause bacteruria.

Treatment is with antibiotics, including sulfisoxazole, nitrofurantoin, ampicillin, or cephalexin in the doses described above. Treatment is continued for 10 days. Clients are taught good bladder hygiene, including voiding every 2 hours, drinking 8 to 10 glasses of water daily, and proper wiping techniques. Allowing the bladder to become overdistended by holding urine predisposes women to infections. Repeat cultures are performed as a test of cure and to detect recurrent infections.

Management of Asymptomatic Bacteria (ASB) in Pregnancy

Screening

Urine culture and sensitivity on initial prenatal visit or early in second trimester

Antibiotic Treatment

Sulfisoxazole

Nitrofurantoin

Ampicillin

Cephalexin

Follow-Up

Monthly urine culture and sensitivity tests

Monitoring for symptoms of infection affecting lower or upper urinary tracts

Antibiotic suppression for persistent or recurrent infection

Teaching bladder hygiene and prevention of infection

Pyelonephritis

Acute upper urinary tract infection (pyelonephritis) occurs in 1% to 3% of women during pregnancy, usually in the late second or early third trimesters, or postpartally. Approximately 66% of pregnant women with acute pyelonephritis had ASB early in pregnancy.[7] Characteristic signs and symptoms of pyelonephritis include fever, chills, nausea and vomiting, dysuria, and flank pain (costovertebral angle [CVA] tenderness). Temperature often swings from high levels (104–106°F) to subnormally low levels (93–97°F). Dehydration and the inability to tolerate oral fluids are common, and the patient looks acutely ill. Marked tenderness is found over the kidney area, with the right kidney most often involved, but both kidneys are frequently infected.

Urine culture shows many WBC (as high as 20,000–30,000/ml), RBC, and bacteria. Sensitivities are performed to identify appropriate antibiotic treatment. Pregnant women with pyelonephritis are best treated in the hospital with parenteral antibiotics and hydration. With effective antibiotics, temperature usually returns to normal in 3 to 5 days. Medication is continued for 14 days, with repeat urine cultures to follow progress. Hydration includes at least 3000 ml of fluids daily; this may need to be supplied intravenously if the patient is vomiting. Urinary output is monitored because renal function is significantly reduced during the acute phase of infection.

Women with pyelonephritis are at increased risk for premature labor and septic shock. Control of the infection reduces the likelihood of these complications. Recurrences of infection usually mean treatment was discontinued before eradication of the organism, or that there is another underlying cause such as renal abnormalities or systemic disease. Persistent infection requires continuous antibiotic treatment until after delivery. Recurrences occur in about 33% of cases.[33]

Management of Acute Pyelonephritis in Pregnancy

Hospitalization

IV hydration

IV antibiotic therapy

Monitoring vital signs and urinary output

Urine and blood cultures

Monitoring for multisystem dysfunction

Follow-up urine cultures, continuing after discharge

Continuous suppressive antibiotic therapy for persistent or recurrent infections

CHRONIC PYELONEPHRITIS

If acute pyelonephritis is not treated adequately, the infection persists although the woman may become asymptomatic. Over time, tissue damage may occur, which impairs kidney function and can lead to hypertension and renal insufficiency. Women with chronic pyelonephritis who become pregnant often suffer acute attacks of infection and have inadequate renal function to respond to the demands of pregnancy. Prophylactic antibiotic treatment during pregnancy may prevent acute recurrences of pyelonephritis.

■ OTHER INFECTIOUS DISEASES

A number of other infectious diseases, primarily viral and bacterial, may affect the mother or fetus during pregnancy. These effects range from inconsequential to life-threatening, and many diseases, particularly viral infections, can cause significant congenital abnormalities in the infant. Immunizations are available for many of the common contagious diseases, and this mode of primary prevention is often the only approach to avoiding the consequences of infection.

Assessment

As part of prenatal care, the nurse assesses the immunization status of the client. Although most women have had the common childhood communicable diseases (rubella, rubeola, mumps, chickenpox) or have been immunized as children, a small percentage remain susceptible to infections as adults. Rubella (German measles) infections during early pregnancy pose significant risks of fetal abnormalities. Other viral and bacterial diseases have variable degrees of teratogenic effects or may cause serious perinatal infections.

Many pregnant women are unaware that they have been exposed to a communicable disease. When symptoms develop, the nurse assesses possible sources of exposure, such as contact with ill children or known epidemics in the community. The common symptoms of communicable diseases include fever, nasal discharge, sore throat, cough, malaise, anorexia, and occasionally nausea and vomiting. The women may notice a skin rash or enlarged lymph nodes.

Physical examination includes vital signs, with particular attention to elevated temperature. The nasal mucosa, pharynx, and tympanic membranes are examined for signs of infection (redness, swelling, discharge). When the client has a cough and expectoration, the lungs are auscultated for adventitious sounds. The skin is inspected for rash; if present, its color, characteristics, and distribution are noted. The examination also includes the degree and location of lymphadenopathy.

Nursing Diagnosis

When the pregnant woman is not immune to communicable diseases, the nursing diagnosis is high risk for infection related to nonimmunity. The woman is at risk for invasion by viral, bacterial, protozoan, or fungal agents that may cause an infectious disease. When the woman has been exposed to, or has developed symptoms of an infectious disease, the nursing diagnosis is high risk for infection transmission. Communicable diseases usually are spread by droplet or airborne transmission, although some have water or vectorborne transmission. Direct contact may spread some infections. The woman may have knowledge deficits related to the causes, consequences, and treatment of the infection. She may have anxiety or fear about the effects of the infection on the fetus. There may be potential altered health maintenance, related to lack of knowledge about prevention of infectious diseases.

Planning and Intervention

The nurse identifies women at risk for communicable diseases and other infections during pregnancy, and provides education and counseling about risk reduction. Many vaccines cannot be administered during pregnancy because of risk to the fetus, but the client can be alerted to her nonimmune status and advised to avoid situations in which she may be exposed to communicable diseases. The importance of immunizations after delivery is emphasized. Often the only effective treatment is prior immunization; many communicable diseases cannot be treated once contracted.

When the pregnant woman has developed a communicable disease, the nurse informs her about the expected course and effects of the disease. The length of communicability is carefully described, and the woman is taught how to avoid exposing other people. If the potential effects on the fetus are serious, the nurse provides opportunity for the woman to express her fears and concerns in a caring supportive environment. Options for terminating the pregnancy are discussed when fetal anomalies are probable or have been identified. The woman is supported in making her own decision and feeling satisfied with her choice.

Symptomatic relief during the course of the illness is discussed by the nurse, including adequate rest and fluids. Natural remedies for relieving a stuffy nose, sore throat, and nausea may be suggested (see Chap. 19). Medications are avoided or minimized during pregnancy; however, if the physician prescribes antibiotics or advises over-the-counter medications for symptom relief, the nurse reviews with the client how to take the medications and stresses completing the course of treatment.

Evaluation

Nursing care is most effective when communicable diseases are prevented or their spread is minimized. Teaching and counseling are effective when the client is able to describe her risks for communicable diseases and knows ways to reduce risk and avoid exposure. She expresses her anxieties or fears and reports an understanding of the disease process and its potential effects. She obtains symptomatic relief or completes the course of prescribed medications. When decisions about termination of pregnancy must be made, the client feels satisfied and accepting of her decision.

Influenza

The occurrence of influenza infection during pregnancy poses serious risks of maternal and fetal morbidity and has been correlated with higher premature labor and abortion rates. Symptoms of influenza include high fever, muscle aches and back pain, sore throat, and prostration.

Although the pregnant woman is not more likely to contract influenza, she is more prone to the development of complicating pneumonia, especially if she is in the third trimester, during which time the diaphragm is elevated and respiration is compromised. The development of pneumonia represents a serious threat to the gravida, because maternal mortality increases significantly when this complication occurs.

In the face of an epidemic involving a specific strain of influenza virus, immunization with a killed or attenuated virus vaccine is indicated. Nonspecific polyvalent vaccines are probably ineffective.

Measles (Rubeola)

Ill effects are not commonly noted in pregnancy, but pregnant women who contract measles are said to be more likely to have spontaneous abortions and premature labor. No congenital defects are reported, although the typical skin rash has been noted on infants at birth, and premature infants are particularly prone to adverse sequelae from measles infection.

Many areas of the United States experienced measles epidemics in the late 1980s and early 1990s. Underimmunization is believed to be a major factor in these outbreaks. Guidelines issued by the Centers for Disease Control for areas experiencing epidemics include revaccination of students whose most recent vaccination was before 1980, and administration of immune globulin within 6 days of exposure to pregnant women with no firm history of the disease or of immunization. People who received the measles, mumps, and rubella (MMR) vaccine before 15 months of age were probably not adequately immunized and should receive another vaccination.[34]

Rubella

Approximately 10% of women in the United States of childbearing age are susceptible to rubella (German measles). There is a high incidence (74%) of congenital abnormalities in infants whose mothers contract rubella during the first 4 months of pregnancy.[7] The most common defects include heart disease, hearing loss, cataracts, and psychomotor retardation (see Chap. 46). Other effects of infection in early pregnancy include abortion, premature delivery, and intrauterine fetal death. There is evidence that rubella infection late in the second trimester also causes congenital abnormalities.

Abortion is usually recommended when rubella is contracted in early pregnancy. It is extremely important to verify rubella infection, which is done on the basis of hemagglutination-inhibition (HI) antibodies, complement-fixing antibodies, and rubella-specific IgM antibodies. Each of these follows a typical pattern, which in combination allows an accurate diagnosis. If rubella infection during pregnancy is verified, gamma globulin is not recommended because this does not appear to prevent viremia and fetal involvement.

Rubella antibody titer is done routinely as part of the prenatal panel. A titer of 1:8 or more indicates that the woman is immune. When the titer is less, the woman is susceptible and is advised to avoid contact with ill people and to seek medical care at once if she develops a viral syndrome with a rash. Rubella vaccination is not recommended during pregnancy, because virus has been recovered from fetal tissues after vaccination. Although the vaccine virus is less teratogenic than the wild virus, abnormalities have occurred with vaccination during pregnancy. A nonpregnant woman who is vaccinated for rubella should not become pregnant for at least 3 months.[7]

Chickenpox (Varicella)

Varicella during pregnancy is rare; however, when it does occur, it is likely to be severe. If varicella pneumonia or necrotizing angitis develop as complications, the infection is often fatal. Treatment includes maintaining adequate oxygenation, controlling bacterial superinfection, and administering acyclovir. Herpes zoster (shingles) is another manifestation of the infection in mothers.

Maternal chickenpox during the first trimester may be associated with congenital malformations such as limb defects, skin scars, Horner's syndrome, and low birth weight. Exposure of the fetus to the virus just before delivery poses serious risk for disseminated visceral and central nervous system disease. Specific varicella-zoster globulin (VZIG) administered to the mother may be life-saving for the fetus.

Mumps

Infection with the mumps virus (parotitis) during pregnancy can cause abortion or premature labor. Fetal death and abnormalities such as endocardial fibroelastosis have been reported. Evidence of diffuse necrotic villitis and viral inclusions in both chorionic and fetal tissues verify that the mumps virus does cross the placenta. In nonimmune pregnant women during a mumps epidemic, administration of hyperimmune mumps gamma globulin may be protective.

Malaria

A serious disease of worldwide proportions, malaria is caused by the mosquitoborne protozoan, *Plasmodium falciparum*. No vaccine has yet been developed to prevent malaria infection. Pregnant women with malaria may experience exacerbations of the disease cycle, with recurrent fever and chills. Abortion, premature labor, and long, difficult labor have been associated with malaria in pregnancy. The placenta often is extensively affected, and the infant may be stillborn or small for gestational age. About 10% of newborns acquire malaria from their infected mothers. Treatment for malaria is with chloroquine phosphate (quinine), which can be toxic to the fetus. In severe maternal disease, it may be necessary to treat with chloroquine despite fetal effects.

Typhoid Fever

Typhoid fever, which is rare in the United States, in former years caused serious complications in pregnancy, resulting in abortion, prematurity, and infant mortality. Treatment with ampicillin is effective in arresting the disease. Immunization is not contraindicated during pregnancy, and antityphoid vaccine should be administered when necessary.

Tuberculosis

Tuberculosis remains a significant cause of morbidity and mortality, with increased prevalence among immigrants and refugees from countries where tuberculosis is common (Asia, Africa, Latin America). The disease is more common in crowded semi-industrialized societies and among the poor or those who experience nutritional deprivation.[35]

Pulmonary tuberculosis, caused by a mycobacterium, has little effect on the course of pregnancy, because it rarely predisposes to abortion, premature labor, or stillbirth. The disease is seldom acquired congenitally. Pregnancy does not exert an adverse effect on tuberculosis when properly managed. Only a woman whose tuberculosis is arrested should consider becoming pregnant. Pregnancy is undertaken with some risk, for although tuberculosis lesions may remain latent for an indefinite time, pregnancy may overtax resistance sufficiently to convert latent, inactive lesions into active ones. Maintenance of proper nutrition and rest helps to prevent activity in latent lesions.

Treatment with the antituberculosis drugs, streptomycin, isoniazid (INH), ethambutol hydrochloride, and para-aminosalicylic acid (PAS), usually provides good control of the disease. Streptomycin may cause congenital nerve deafness in the infant. Women with active tuberculosis are advised not to become pregnant. Conception should be delayed until the woman has been disease-free, or arrested, for about 2 years.

Screening of all pregnant women for tuberculosis using the tine test or PPD (purified protein derivative) is recommended. In high-risk groups or if there is clinical indication of disease, testing should be repeated later in pregnancy. Infants born to mothers with active tuberculosis infection are isolated from the mother and others who may be contagious, until the disease is controlled. For the effectively treated mother, breast-feeding is acceptable.

Poliomyelitis

Poliomyelitis generally does not complicate pregnancy or delivery, except in the unusual cases in which respiratory paralysis develops; in these rare cases, cesarean birth has given satisfactory results. Fortunately, as a result of immunization, the disease has virtually disappeared in the United States. It is still prevalent in parts of Asia and Africa, however.

Maternal infection with polio during the first trimester may result in abortion, intrauterine growth retardation, and congenital abnormalities. Infection of the infant during passage through the birth canal is possible. Pregnant women can be immunized with Salk vaccine (killed virus), which confers immunity for about

2 years. Immunization with Sabin's vaccine (attenuated live virus) is contraindicated during pregnancy.

Cytomegalovirus (CMV)

Approximately 60% of the general population have antibodies to CMV by age 35 to 40. Transmission occurs by close contact and through sexual intercourse. CMV has been isolated in the cervical secretions of 5% of pregnant women. Virus has also been recovered from breast milk, urine, tears, and saliva. Most infections in adults are mild and go unnoticed. Seropositivity for CMV is associated with low socioeconomic status, older age, multigravidity, multiple sexual partners, early age at first pregnancy, abnormal cervical cytology, and STD.[7,11]

The risk of congenital CMV infection is 1.2% to 1.8%. Nearly all congenitally infected infants who do not have symptoms appear to develop normally. Symptoms of infection occur in 1 of every 100 infants, and the most serious resulting effects include microcephaly, hydrocephaly, cerebral calcification, deafness, chorioretinitis, hepatosplenomegaly, jaundice, hemolytic anemia, and convulsions. Infants with mild or unrecognized initial infections have later been found with impaired intelligence and hearing defects.[36]

The rate of seroconversion during pregnancy (acquiring a primary infection) is probably less than 1%.[7] Having a primary infection in pregnancy is thought to increase infant risk of congenital CMV. The infection is transmitted to the fetus at a rate of 20% to 40%, and it is not clear whether risk is related to time of exposure during pregnancy.[37] Because acute CMV infection in adults causes few if any symptoms, it is nearly impossible to predict birth of an affected infant. There is no effective treatment for either mother or infant.

Toxoplasmosis

Toxoplasmosis is caused by the protozoan *Toxoplasma gondii*, which is transmitted to humans in raw meat or from cat feces. In adults, the symptoms of acute infection resemble influenza, but this is accompanied by lymphadenopathy. There are no symptoms of infection in 90% of adults who are exposed to toxoplasmosis. Fetal infection occurs as a result of maternal parasitemia during the initial acute attack. Chronic maternal infection does not result in fetal infection.

When toxoplasmosis is acquired in early pregnancy, abortion occurs frequently. In later pregnancy, about half of the fetuses are affected with increased perinatal mortality, encephalitis, microcephaly, hydrocephaly, chorioretinitis, convulsions, hepatosplenomegaly, jaundice, and mental retardation.

Antibody titers for toxoplasmosis and complement-fixation tests are used to diagnose the disease. Abortion is provided as an option to women with acute infections occurring in early pregnancy. There is no vaccine or treatment for toxoplasmosis. Pregnant women should avoid eating raw meat and exposure to infected cats.

Group B *Streptococcus* (GBS)

Group B beta-hemolytic *Streptococcus* is a common bacterial infection that can have serious effects in both mother and infant. Approximately 14% to 20% of pregnant women and 12% of neonates are colonized by GBS, but few of those colonized develop clinical disease.[38] Although the rate of significant neonatal infection with GBS is only 3.3 per 1000 live births, up to 15,000 cases of neonatal sepsis per year result from these infections with a 50% mortality rate.[11]

Colonization with GBS in women can be chronic or intermittent. Transmission of infection to the infant is more common among chronic carriers. No differences in colonization have been found related to age, race, or parity. Maternal perinatal morbidity from GBS includes abortion, premature rupture of membranes, premature delivery, prolonged labor, endometritis, chorioamnionitis, septicemia, cellulitis, impetigo, and scarlet fever.[39]

Neonatal infection usually begins in utero from ingestion of infected amniotic fluid. Factors associated with early onset (before 7 days after birth) of infant disease include prolonged labor, premature delivery, premature rupture of membranes, and overt maternal infection with fever. Infant sepsis may be apparent at birth or 48 hours, or may not appear until after a week. Infections may lead to meningitis with residual neurological or developmental deficits, or to death. GBS is treated with antibiotics (penicillin, ampicillin).

Routine culture of prenatal women for GBS is not recommended, because accurate and cost-effective screening is not available. Prophylactic treatment of pregnant women with chronic GBS (repeated positive cultures) has been suggested.[11]

TORCH Infections

A group of infections that the infant may contract are known by the acronym TORCH. These have been discussed here relative to maternal effects. (See Chap. 46 for discussion of neonatal effects.) TORCH stands for:

T—Toxoplasmosis
O—Other (Hepatitis B, HIV, syphilis, GBS, *Chlamydia*, varicella)

R—Rubella
C—Cytomegalovirus
H—Herpes simplex

■ REFERENCES

1. Hacker NF, Moore JG: Essentials of Obstetrics and Gynecology. Philadelphia, WB Saunders, 1986
2. Hatcher RA, Stewart F, Trussell J et al: Contraceptive Technology 1990–1992, 15th ed. New York, Irvington Publishers, 1990
3. Margolis S: Genital warts and molluscum contagiosum. Urol Clin North Am 11(1):163–170, 1984
4. Bourcier KM, Seidler AJ: *Chlamydia* and condylomata accuminata: An update for the nurse practitioner. JOGN Nursing 16(1):17, 1987
5. Garry R, Jones R: Relationship between cervical condylomata, pregnancy and subclinical papillomavirus infection. J Reprod Med 30(5):393–399, 1985
6. Ferenczy A (moderator): Symposium: Treating condylomata. Contemp Obstet Gynecol 30(3):158, 1987
7. Willson JR, Carrington ER: Obstetrics and Gynecology, 8th ed. St Louis, CV Mosby, 1987
8. Centers for Disease Control: Protection against viral hepatitis—Recommendations of the Immunization Practices Advisory Committee (ACIP). MMWR 39(2):16–19, 1990
9. Lemon SM: Viral hepatitis. In Holmes KK, Mardh P, Sparling PF, Wiesner PJ (eds): Sexually Transmitted Diseases. New York, McGraw-Hill, 1984
10. DePotter CR, Robberech E, Laureys G et al: Hepatitis B related childhood hepatocellular carcinoma. Cancer 60(3):414–418, 1987
11. Wilson D: An overview of sexually transmitted diseases in the perinatal period. J Nurse Midwifery (33):115–128, 1988
12. Centers for Disease Control: Sexually Transmitted Diseases Treatment Guidelines, September 1989. DHHS/PHS, Center for Preventive Services, Division of STD/HIV Prevention. Atlanta, GA, 1989
13. Guide to Clinical Preventive Services. Report of the US Preventive Services Task Force. Baltimore, Williams & Wilkins, 1989
14. Baker DA, Milch PO: Acyclovir for genital herpes simplex infections. J Reprod Med 31(5 Suppl):433–438, 1986
15. Brown ZA, Vontuer LA, Benedetti J et al: Genital herpes in pregnancy: Risk factors associated with recurrences and asymptomatic viral shedding. Am J Obstet Gynecol 153(1):24–30, 1985
16. Laga M, Naamara W, Brunham RC et al: Single dose therapy of gonorrhea ophthalmia neonatorum with ceftriaxone. N Engl J Med 315(22):1382–1385, 1986
17. Centers for Disease Control: HIV prevalence estimates and AIDS case projections for the United States: Report based upon a workshop. MMWR 39(16):1–15, 1990
18. Centers for Disease Control: Update: Acquired immune deficiency syndrome—United States, 1981–1988. MMWR 38:229–236, 1989
19. Cummings D: Caring for the HIV-infected adult. Nurs Pract 13(11):28–48, 1988
20. Centers for Disease Control: Mortality attributable to HIV infection/AIDS—United States, 1981–1990. MMWR 40(3):41–55, 1991
21. Redford RR, Burke DS: HIV infection: The clinical picture. In The Science of AIDS: Readings from Scientific American Magazine, pp 63–74. New York, WH Freeman & Co, 1989
22. Laurence J: HIV infection and the female genital tract. PA—Physicians Assist (42–47), 1988
23. Centers for Disease Control: AIDS and human immunodeficiency virus infection in the United States: 1988 update. MMWR 38:8–9, 1988
24. Dinsmoor MJ: HIV infection and pregnancy. Med Clin North Am 73(3):701–711, 1989
25. Petersen LR, White CR et al: Premarital screening for antibodies to human immunodeficiency virus type 1 in the United States. Am J Public Health 80(9):1087–1090, 1990
26. Kelley PW, Miller RN, Pomerantz R et al: Human immunodeficiency virus seropositivity among members of the active duty United States Army 1985–89. Am J Public Health 80(4):405–409, 1990
27. AIDS Commission raises alarm on epidemic in rural areas. The Nation's Health 22(9):1, 12, 1990
28. Minkoff HL, Nanda D, Menez R et al: Pregnancies resulting in infants with acquired immune deficiency syndrome or AIDS-related complex. Obstet Gynecol 69:285, 1987
29. Centers for Disease Control: AIDS in women—United States. MMWR 39(47):845–846, 1990
30. Minkoff HL: Pregnant women with HIV. JAMA 258(19):2714, 1987
31. IOM: Offer pregnant women test for HIV antibodies. The Nation's Health XXI(3):2, March 1991
32. Ziegler JB, Johnson RO, Cooper DA et al: Postnatal transmission of AIDS-associated retrovirus from mother to infant. Lancet 1:896, 1985
33. Gilstrap LC, Wendel GD: Urinary tract infections in pregnancy: Presentations and approaches. PA—Physicians Assist (107–112), 1988
34. Centers for Disease Control: Recommendations of the Immunization Practices Advisory Committee. Measles prevention: Supplementary statement. MMWR 38(1):11–14, 1989
35. Kohl S, Pickering L: Infectious diseases. In Behrman RE and Kliegman R (eds): Essentials of Pediatrics, pp 320–324. Philadelphia, WB Saunders, 1990
36. Kumar ML, Nankervis GA, Jacobs IB et al: Congenital and postnatally acquired cytomegalovirus infections. J Pediatr 104(5):674–679, 1984
37. Preece PM, Blount JM, Glover J et al: The consequences of primary cytomegalovirus infection in pregnancy. Arch Dis Child 58(12):970–975, 1983
38. Dillon HC, Khare S, Gray BM: Group B streptococcal

	Why Do You Smoke?				
	Always	Frequently	Occasionally	Seldom	Never
A. I smoke cigarettes to keep from slowing down.	5	4	3	2	1
B. Handling a cigarette is part of the enjoyment of smoking it.	5	4	3	2	1
C. Smoking cigarettes is pleasant and relaxing.	5	4	3	2	1
D. I light up a cigarette when I feel angry about something.	5	4	3	2	1
E. When I run out of cigarettes I find it almost unbearable until I can get them.	5	4	3	2	1
F. I smoke cigarettes automatically without even being aware of it.	5	4	3	2	1
G. I smoke cigarettes to stimulate me, to perk myself up.	5	4	3	2	1
H. Part of the enjoyment of smoking a cigarette comes from the steps I take to light up.	5	4	3	2	1
I. I find cigarettes pleasurable.	5	4	3	2	1
J. When I feel uncomfortable or upset about something, I light up a cigarette.	5	4	3	2	1
K. I am very much aware of the fact when I am not smoking a cigarette.	5	4	3	2	1
L. I light up a cigarette without realizing I still have one burning in the ashtray.	5	4	3	2	1
M. I smoke cigarettes to give me a "lift."	5	4	3	2	1
N. When I smoke a cigarette, part of the enjoyment is watching the smoke as I exhale it.	5	4	3	2	1
O. I want a cigarette most when I am comfortable and relaxed.	5	4	3	2	1
P. When I feel "blue" or want to take my mind off cares and worries, I smoke cigarettes.	5	4	3	2	1
Q. I get a real gnawing hunger for a cigarette when I haven't smoked for a while.	5	4	3	2	1
R. I've found a cigarette in my mouth and didn't remember putting it there.	5	4	3	2	1

How to Score

1. Write the number you have circled after each statement in the corresponding space below.
2. Total the scores in each column. For example, the sum of your scores A, G, M gives you your score for the first column.

A _____ B _____ C _____ D _____ E _____ F _____

G _____ H _____ I _____ J _____ K _____ L _____

M _____ N _____ O _____ P _____ Q _____ R _____

Column Totals   (1) _____ (2) _____ (3) _____ (4) _____ (5) _____ (6) _____

In this test examining reasons why you smoke, a score of 11 or above on any factor indicates that it is an important source of satisfaction for you. The higher you score (15 is the highest), the more important a particular factor is in your smoking. A low score on all the factors usually indicates that you do not smoke much or have not been smoking for many years. If so, giving up smoking—and staying off— should be easier.

1. Stimulation:

If you score high or fairly high on this factor, it means that you are one of those smokers who is stimulated by the cigarette—you feel that it helps wake you up, organize your energies, and keep you going. If you try to give up smoking, you may want a safe substitute, a brisk walk or moderate exercise, for example, when you feel the urge to smoke.

2. Handling:

Handling things can be satisfying, but there are many ways to keep hands busy without lighting up or playing with a cigarette. Substitute a favorite pen, piece of jewelry, or some other harmless object.

■ *Figure 36–1*
Analysis of smoking behavior.

How to Score

3. Accentuation of Pleasure—Pleasurable Relaxation:

Those who do get real pleasure out of smoking often find that an honest consideration of the harmful effects of their habit is enough to help them quit. They substitute social and physical activities and find that they do not seriously miss their cigarettes.

4. Reduction of Negative Feelings, or "Crutch":

Many smokers use the cigarette as a kind of "crutch" in moments of stress or discomfort. But the heavy smoker, the person who tries to handle severe personal problems by smoking many times a day, is apt to discover that cigarettes do not help in dealing with problems effectively. Stress management strategies are often helpful for this type of smoker, as are physical exertion and social activities.

5. Craving or Dependence:

Quitting smoking is difficult for the person who scores high on this factor. Going "cold turkey" usually works better for this type of smoker. Aversion strategies are often helpful for they serve to create negative mental images of smoking.

6. Habit:

If you are smoking out of habit, you no longer get much satisfaction from your cigarettes. Gradual reduction may be an effective strategy. The key to success is becoming aware of each cigarette smoked and asking, "Do I really want this cigarette?"

Government document. Reprinted with permission from U.S. Department of Health and Human Services. Oct. 1983 (revised). *A Self-Test for Smokers.* DHEW Publication No. (CDC) 75-8716. Washington, DC: U.S. Government Printing Office.

■ *Figure 36–1*
Continued

experimental studies on the topic. Although it is unclear exactly the minimum dose required to produce FAS or specifically when alcohol causes its havoc, the body of findings has shown that ethanol and its metabolites have the potential to alter the growth and development of the embryo and fetus.[26,27] As research evidence continues to grow, the terms *fetal alcohol effects* (FAE) and *alcohol-related birth defects* (ARBD) have been coined to differentiate the syndromes more specifically.[28]

There is little conclusive evidence regarding the effects of paternal drinking on childbearing; the evidence is also inconclusive for other types of drug use.

Effects on the Maternal-Placental-Fetal System

EFFECTS ON THE MOTHER

The effects of ethanol on the human organism are well known. Taken in small to moderate amounts, for those who are not alcoholic, there is a feeling of general CNS stimulation, relaxation, mild euphoria, vasodilation, and well-being. However, alcohol is a CNS depressant, and these initial effects soon wear off and can be replaced with symptoms associated with CNS depression. Judgment is impaired even in the euphoria stage and, if drinking continues, motor responses and other physiological responses such as loss of concentration, mood alteration, nausea, headache, and sleepiness can occur. Stupor, coma, and death occur if dosage is sufficient.[29–]

[31] For chronic alcoholics and even those for whom moderate drinking is a daily affair, there can be adverse nutritional effects, impulsive behavior, impaired judgment, and family, occupational, and social problems.[29–31]

A woman does not necessarily have to be an alcoholic to place her infant at risk for FAS. Defining what constitutes alcoholism and an alcoholic is often a problem because amount and frequency of drinking are not the

---

Standard Minimal Criteria for the Diagnosis of Fetal Alcohol Syndrome

One or more signs should be present in *each* of the following categories:

- Prenatal or postnatal growth retardation (weight, length, or head circumference below the tenth percentile)
- CNS involvement (signs of neurological abnormality, developmental delay, or intellectual impairment)
- Characteristic facial dysmorphology with *at least two* of the following signs:
    Microcephaly
    Microphthalmos or short palpebral fissures
    Poorly developed philtrum, thin upper lip, or
        flattening of the maxillary area

(Rosett HL: Alcohol and the Fetus: A Clinical Perspective. New York, Oxford University Press, 1984)

Ten Question Drinking History (TQDH)

Beer	How many times per week?
	How many cans each time?
	Ever drink more?
Wine	How many times per week?
	How many cans each time?
	Ever drink more?
Liquor	How many times per week?
	How many cans each time?
	Ever drink more?

Has your drinking habit changed during the past year?

(Weiner L, Morse BA: Fetal alcohol syndrome: Clinical perspectives and prevention. In Chasnoff IJ (ed): Drugs, Alcohol, Pregnancy and Parenting. Boston, Kluwer Academic Publishers, 1988)

as the Indicators for Alcohol Abuse or Dependence (Table 36-1), which provides signs and symptoms for the nurse to observe, can form the backbone of thorough assessment and basis for diagnoses. Jessup suggests the latter tool can be useful also in helping make the mother aware of some of her own behaviors.[28]

Weiner and Morse recommend that separate, direct questions be asked about the consumption of the three categories (TQDH). When the questions are asked in a direct, nonjudgmental fashion, most patients accept the nurse's concern and respond as honestly as they can. Patients who answer evasively should be calmly and firmly engaged in further discussion. Defensive reactions often indicate alcohol problems. The TQDH takes about 5 minutes to administer when the patient is not drinking at risk levels.[26]

Planning and Intervention. Intervention for the problem drinker and alcoholic can be conceptualized as a

TABLE 36–1. INDICATORS OF ALCOHOL ABUSE AND/OR DEPENDENCE

Medical Indicators	Historical Indicators	Behavioral Indicators
Liver disease	Depressive disorder	Smell of alcohol on breath
Pancreatitis	Psychiatric treatment or hospitalization	Mood swings
Hypertension	Reference to alcohol (or other drug) abusing partner	Memory lapses or losses
Gastritis; esophagitis		Difficulty concentrating
Hematological disorders	Physician prescription or other procurement of psychoactive drugs	Blackouts
Poor nutritional status		Inappropriateness
Cardiac arrythmias; other cardiac disease	Multiple emergency room visits	Irritability or agitation
	Complicated perinatal history	Depression
Alcoholic myopathy	Low birth weight	Slurry speech
Ketoacidosis	Prematurity	Staggering gait
Neurological disorders	FAS or FAE	Bizarre behavior
Intrauterine growth retardation	Foster or other caretaker placement of another child	Loss of job
		Decreased job performance
	Learning disability or hyperactivity in another child	Suicidal feelings; gestures, or attempts
		Sexual dysfunction
		Conflicts with spouse; family or friends
		Domestic violence
		Child abuse and neglect
		Autotmobile accidents or citation arrests
		Children with scholastic or behavioral problems
		Secretiveness or vagueness about personal or medical history

(Jessup M, Green J: Treatment of the pregnant alcohol-dependent woman. J Psychoactive Drugs 19(2):16, April–June 1987)

Intervention Process for Problem Drinking and Dependence

1. Expression of concern
   - Discuss concern about continued drinking in a nonjudgmental manner.
2. Presentation of consequences
   - Make use of the powerful motivator of mother's sense of responsibility for a new life.
   - Present consequences of drinking and options open to the mother in as positive terms as possible. Women respond positively to a hopeful message of potential benefits of drinking cessation. Avoid provoking guilt and self-criticism because these can result in increased alcohol consumption.
3. Referral for treatment
   - Utilize inpatient and outpatient detox and rehabilitation programs.
   - Utilize self-help, 12-step programs: Alcoholics Anonymous, Al Anon.

Classification of Problem Drinking

Social problem drinking: an essential ingredient in marriage and social life. Social networks pressure to drink. Alcohol used to alleviate boredom. Brief, supportive counseling and information help stop drinking at least for pregnancy. Referral to agencies and self-help 12-step groups most important.

Symptom problem drinking: alcohol used to relieve wide range of psychological symptoms (fear, anger, depression, confusion, self-blame) and to alter mood and perception. Pregnancy activates fears, conflicts, and ambivalence about self and ability to mother. Realistic discussion of fears and conflicts with repetition of information about pregnancy and the birth process is needed. These women need extensive counseling and support regarding social problems and pregnancy as well as referral to self-help 12-step programs.

Alcohol dependence (alcoholism): physiological and psychological tolerance and dependence has developed (addiction). Medical complications are apparent. Extensive assistance needed with medical problems as well as child care and social problems. Alcohol treatment centers, halfway houses, and Alcoholics Anonymous are absolutely essential for therapy and support.

(Weiner L, Morse BA: Fetal alcohol syndrome: Clinical perspectives and prevention. In Chasnoff IJ (ed): Drugs, Alcohol, Pregnancy and Parenting. Boston, Kluwer Academic Publishers, 1988)

---

process whereby the drinking woman is no longer supported to drink, but is instead supported to begin the recovery process. When open and honest discussion of the alcohol problem occurs between the nurse and patient, the "conspiracy of silence" is challenged and the patient and clinical team can address the problem appropriately.[28]

CLASSIFICATION OF PROBLEM DRINKING. Weiner and Morse suggest a three-phase classification of problem drinking, which has been found to be helpful in designing treatment strategies. The classification is based on motivating factors rather than on quantity or frequency of drinking.[26] It is important to note that, although the phases are not invariably progressive, most clients move from one to the next if help is not received because alcohol addiction is progressive. Moreover, not all clinicians, particularly those whose specialty is treatment of addictive behaviors, would classify the problem drinker differently from the alcoholic. However, for treatment strategies to help the nurse refer and counsel, these have been found useful.

TREATMENT AND REHABILITATION PROGRAMS. Treatment of alcoholism and problem drinking consists of extensive assessment, counseling, and participation in an outpatient, inpatient, or residential program and involvement in self-help, 12-step programs (Alcoholics Anonymous). Women alcoholics usually appear depressed and tend to drink in isolation. Involvement in self-help, 12-step programs can create a sober support system for the recovering mother and provide her with ongoing role models, particularly after she has received institutional and professional help.[26,32]

Evaluation. When the woman returns for subsequent visits, the nurse can question and determine by the TQDH or similar tool and the Indicators of Alcohol Abuse and/or Dependence chart how the woman is progressing. Abstinence indicates successful counseling. If the woman does not return, this is a strong indication that she may be drinking. She may, however, be influenced in her drinking patterns if she attends Alcoholics Anonymous and is able to become sober eventually. The nurse should employ whatever means available for follow-up.

■ DRUG ABUSE

Problems associated with drug use in pregnancy have become endemic; cocaine has become the illicit drug of choice for millions of Americans, including pregnant women. Although AIDS has become more prevalent in women and infants due to drug use and legal cases raise the question of fetal abuse, no professional group has become the known advocate for this special population of substance abusers. Nurses are in an ideal position to assume this role. All health professionals, social service and public health agencies are inundated with infants showing the effects of their mother's drug use.[37] Health professionals must keep in mind that when dealing with a drug-addicted mother they will also eventually be dealing with a drug-addicted infant.

Over-the-Counter and Prescription Drugs

Studies in the late 1970s evaluating drug use by women during pregnancy revealed that as much as 50% to 60% of women used some analgesic and around 25% used sedative drugs during pregnancy. These women were receiving prenatal care, and the use of illicit drugs was rarely considered.[38,39] However, in 1982, Chasnoff and Schnoll found that 3% of their maternity patients at Prentice Women's Hospital and Maternity Center, screened for routine prenatal care, had sedative-hypnotics in their urine. With the propensity for mixing licit and illicit drugs, it is difficult to get true prevalence figures.[39] Moreover, among those who use drugs liberally, even prescribed and over-the-counter (OTC) drugs, there is substantially more use of cigarettes, alcohol, and caffeine, all of which have known noxious effects on the mother and the fetus.[5,40] The nurse should remember that many women feel that taking their "prescribed" drugs is really not abuse even though they may shop physicians, hoard medications, and self-medicate because "the doctor gave them to me."[41]

The teratogenic effects are unclear with many of the OTC and prescribed drugs most frequently used by pregnant women.[42] Appendix E lists drugs and chemicals known to have a teratogenic effect.[43]

Illicit and Street Drugs

Street drug use often means that the person has no idea of the drug being taken. Drugs purchased on the street are often adulterated with various substitute substances. Caffeine, pseudoephedrine, and phenylpropanolamine are sold as amphetamine. Valium is passed off as Quaalude, and street tetrahydrocannabinol (THC) is almost always phencyclidine (PCP). Contaminants pose another hazard because the drugs are often cut with sugar, talcum powder, and other inert substances. PCP is a common contaminant and adulterator because it is

---

Drugs and Chemicals Commonly Used by Pregnant Women

Antibiotics	Hair cosmetics	Sugar substitutes
Analgesic and anti-inflammatories	Antihistamines	Anthelmintics
Paints or solvents	Pediculocides	Laxatives
Cold medications	Psychotropics	Antiemetics
Pesticides	Corticosteriods	
	Contraceptives	

(Koran G: Teratogenic drugs and chemicals in humans. In Koran G (ed): Maternal-Fetal Toxicology: A Clinician's Guide, New York, Marcel Dekker, 1990)

---

widespread and inexpensive. These substances are often teratogenic in their own right or cause teratogenic interactions and pose difficult problems in getting accurate drug histories.[44]

In the following discussion, cocaine is used as a benchmark drug in describing many effects on the mother and fetus. It would be impossible to describe all of the effects of all of the drugs in use because of space limitations. Cocaine has similar effects as other street drugs, and users appear to have similar characteristics. In a study comparing cocaine and heroin users, Hasin and colleagues found that cocaine dependence indicators did not differ from heroin dependence indicators among regular users. These abusers tended to be poly-abusers of drugs in addition to alcohol, caffeine, and cigarettes, and many pharmacological, physiological, and social effects were the same.[45] Moreover, cocaine and its derivative, "crack," have become the nation's top concern, particularly for the pregnant woman.

Effects on the Maternal-Placental-Fetal System

EFFECTS ON THE MOTHER

Pregnancy is associated with a plethora of physiological changes, which may affect the natural course of diseases, the way the body handles drugs, or both. The woman who is pregnant is at particular risk for herself as well as her fetus when she uses drugs.

Physiological Effects. Two principal groups of changes characterize pregnancy and drug disposition. These are (1) alterations in kinetics due to maternal changes and (2) the effects of the placental-fetal compartment. Other important determinants of drug transport across the placenta are water and lipid solubility, molecular weight of the drug, and the surface available for diffusion. The increase in maternal renal function and blood volume results in a decrease in protein binding because of the decrease in serum albumin concentration. This allows for easier passage of drugs across the placental-fetal compartment.[46]

COCAINE. The alkaloid cocaine, an odorless, crystalline powder, is illustrative of the mechanism and effects of many drugs. It is readily absorbed through the mucous membranes, although it is smoked, and injected, and is a powerful short-acting CNS stimulant similar to amphetamines. Cocaine reaches the brain and the neurons of the sympathetic nervous system in 3 minutes after being snorted, 15 seconds after intravenous administration, and 7 seconds after being smoked in a free base form (crack). Euphoria is rapid but short-lived (30 minutes).[47]

Cocaine blocks presynaptic reuptake of norepinephrine and dopamine, producing an excess of these neurotransmitters at the postsynaptic receptor sites. This flood of neurotransmitters, combined with reduced reuptake in the cerebrocortex, hypothalamus, and cerebellum, results in a hyperaroused, extremely euphoric state equivalent to electric stimulation of the reward centers of the brain. Thus, cocaine is highly addictive and dependence is extremely difficult to break because the stimulation is so pleasurable. Because there is little physiological withdrawal, there are many misconceptions about the drug, especially among young people. The initial euphoric rush soon tapers off to be replaced by dysphoria, irritability, impatience, pessimism, fatigue and a strong desire for additional use of cocaine and other drugs.[47]

Figure 36-3 summarizes the process by which cocaine affects the mother and fetus. Many other drugs utilize the same process with similar actions and effects. Cocaine's extreme euphoric effect, however, surpasses other substances.[47-49]

Pregnancy Outcomes. There are a variety of pregnancy complications for mothers who use drugs, even those that are prescribed. As mentioned previously, many abusers are poly-abusers, hence specific outcomes for specific drugs may be difficult to determine even if the research is directed toward users of a specific substance. In general, research has shown a significant incidence in spontaneous abortion, maternal anorexia, with consequent fetal malnutrition, uteroplacental insufficiency, intrauterine growth retardation, premature separation of the placenta and other placental abnormalities, hyperirritability of the uterus leading to premature labor, and chorioamnionitis.[49] Figure 36-4 illustrates the outcomes of cocaine and other substance abuse on the mother, fetus, and infant.[48]

EFFECTS ON THE INFANT

As with the mother, poly-abuse results in a variety of poor fetal outcomes. The mother's use affects multiple organ systems and consequent growth and development including intellectual and learning ability. Low birth weight, CNS dysfunction, hyperirritability, developmental delay, SIDS, and learning disabilities are all associated with drug use by the mother.[45,49,50]

Figure 36-4 illustrates the effects on the fetus and infant.

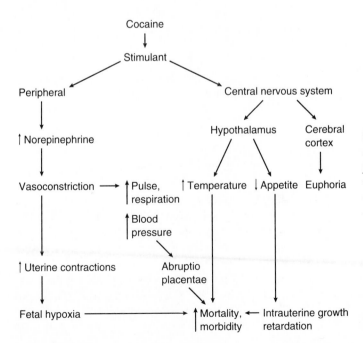

■ *Figure 36–3*
Physiological effects of cocaine on the maternal-placental-fetal system. (Weiner L, Morse BA: Fetal alcohol syndrome. Clinical perspectives and prevention. In Chasnoff IJ (ed): Drugs, Alcohol, Pregnancy and Parenting. Boston, Kluwer Academic Publishers, 1988, 138)

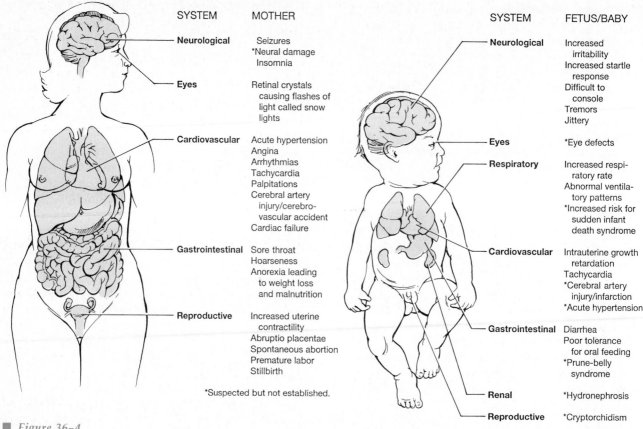

■ *Figure 36–4*
Outcomes of substance abuse on mother, fetus, and infant.

Assessment and Management

Besides doing physical and psychological harm to the mother and her fetus, substance use in pregnancy raises difficult ethical and legal questions. How can health professionals and society provide a safe intrauterine environment for the fetus and simultaneously respect the mother's right to privacy? Should infants and children be allowed to live with known substance users?

Recently in Illinois, two cocaine-using mothers were held responsible for their infants' demise and morbidity, respectively. The one whose infant died due to cocaine-induced oxygen deprivation was charged with involuntary manslaughter. The other infant was removed from the mother's custody, and the mother was charged with child abuse and neglect. These cases represent a turn from the trend to protect the person's privacy to protection of the fetus. The issues are volatile and are reviewed in most settings on a case-by-case basis. Nursing interventions require cautious, cooperative decision making.[47–49] (The article by Pollitt listed in the Suggested Readings section at the end of this chapter provides an interesting perspective to these emerging dilemmas.)

Perinatal nurses need to work with their institution's legal departments to develop policies that delineate each health provider's responsibilities when caring for women involved in substance abuse. Communication networks among health providers, especially nurses, need to be established so that expertise in dealing with these clients can be kept current and at maximum efficiency.[47]

NURSING PROCESS

Assessment and Diagnosis. As with the addicted smoker and the alcoholic patient, it is essential that the assessment and diagnosis stages be done carefully and thoroughly. The steps outlined for care of the alcoholic pertain to the drug user as well because both are in the throes of an addictive, progressive disease. In the assessment and diagnosis phase, care should be taken to

TABLE 36–2. IDENTIFYING CHARACTERISTICS OF THE SUBSTANCE ABUSER

Physical Appearance and Demeanor

Patient looks physically exhausted

Pupils are extremely dilated or constricted

Appearance of pregnancy fails to coincide with stated gestational age

Track marks, abscesses, or edema are visible in upper or lower extremities

Nasal mucosae are inflamed or indurated

Patient is not well oriented

Medical History

Acquired immunodeficiency syndrome

Cellulitis

Cirrhosis

Endocarditis

Hepatitis

Pancreatitis

Pneumonia

Obstetric History in Prior Pregnancies, History of

Abruptio placentae

Fetal death

Low-birth-weight infant

Meconium staining

Premature labor

Premature rupture of membranes

Sexually transmitted disease

Spontaneous abortion

In Current Pregnancy, History or Evidence of

Early contractions

Inactive or hyperactive fetus

Poor weight gain

Sexually transmitted disease

Spotting or vaginal bleeding

(Lynch M, McKeon VA: Cocaine Use During Pregnancy. JOGN Nursing 19:285–289, July/August 1990)

TABLE 36–3. LABORATORY SCREENING OF THE PREGNANT ADDICT

Blood Work

Complete blood count with indices

α-Fetoprotein (if between 16 and 18 weeks' gestation)

Rubella titer

Blood type

Rh determination

Coombs' test

Sickle-cell preparation, if indicated

Urine Tests

Urinalysis

Culture

Toxicology

Screening for Infection

Chest x-ray

Tuberculin skin test

Hepatitis B antigen and antibody

Serology

Venereal disease reaction level (VDRL)

Fluorescent treponemal antibody (lues) test (FTA)

Cervical culture for *Chlamydia trachomatis*

Human immunodeficiency virus (HIV) antibody screen

Cervical-rectal cultures for *Neisseria gonorrhoeae*

Obstetric Screening

Ultrasound scan to confirm pregnancy after 6 weeks' gestation and serial scans for fetal measurement between 20 and 38 weeks' gestation

Cervical Pap smear

(Chasnoff IJ. [Ed.]: Drug Use in Pregnancy, pp. 7–16. Boston, MIP Press Limited, 1986))

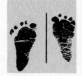

Nursing Care Plan

The Pregnant Substance Abuser

Nursing Goals

The pregnant substance abuser completely stops all substance use for the duration of the pregnancy and thereafter as evidenced by:
1. Performing self-help activities to stop substance use
2. Securing needed resources for meeting support needs
3. Keeping medical appointments throughout pregnancy and for infant after delivery
4. Delivering a healthy term infant without perinatal complications
5. Maintaining her own health and health of infant

Assessment	Potential Nursing Diagnosis	Planning and Intervention	Evaluation
Physical appearance and demeanor (see Table 36-2)	Knowledge deficit related to effects of substance abuse on self, fetus, and infant	Establish a trusting, therapeutic relationship with the client, remaining nonjudgmental	Client discloses drug use and keeps medical appointments
Medical history for opportunistic diseases (see Table 36-2)		Counsel regarding the benefits to the fetus, infant, and self with cessation of substance abuse	Client states benefits of cessation of substance abuse for fetus/infant/self and takes steps to stop substance abuse
Prior obstetric history (see Table 36-2)			
Current problems of contractions, spotting, bleeding		Instruct regarding the effects of substance abuse on health	Client states effects of substance abuse on health
Weight gain/loss			
Sexually transmitted diseases		Refer to 12-step program	Client attends 12-step program
Drinking history utilizing TQDH			
Medications taken		Refer to inpatient and outpatient detox and rehabilitation programs as needed	Client admits herself to inpatient or outpatient detox or rehabilitation programs as needed
Illicit drug use			
Support systems, including spouse, family, and friends		Encourage use of positive support systems to assist the client to stop substance abuse	Client utilizes positive support systems to stop substance abuse
			Toxicology screens remain negative
History of substance abuse (See Table 36-2 and TQDH)	Parenting, altered related to substance abuse	Refer to 12-step program or other rehabilitation group	Client attends and continues to participate in self-help programs
Involvement and success of self-help programs		Involve spouse/family/friends in infant care	Support systems are actively involved in infant care
Toxicology screening results			
Spousal/family/friends support		Encourage attendance at childbirth and infant care classes	Client attends childbirth and infant care classes

(continued)

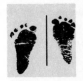

Nursing Care Plan *(continued)*

Assessment	Potential Nursing Diagnosis	Planning and Intervention	Evaluation
Current physical and emotional state		Counsel regarding withdrawal behaviors of infants and comfort measures to be employed	Client recognizes withdrawal behaviors in infant and takes appropriate measures to comfort
Involvement in prenatal care and childbirth classes		Discuss passage of drugs/alcohol through breast milk	Client remains drug/alcohol free
Perception of parenting role		Instruct regarding infant care	
Desire for having and keeping the infant			Client gives appropriate care for the infant
Knowledge of infant care		Refer to home health nurse for follow-up visits after birth	Home health nurse finds infant well cared for
History of substance abuse (see Table 36-2 and TQDH)	Injury, high risk for fetus related to substance abuse effects	Refer to 12-step program	Client paticipates in self-help program
Involvement and success of self-help programs		Record fetal heart tones	Fetal heart tones remain within normal limits
Toxicology screening results		Administer non-stress test/biophysical profile as ordered	Non-stress test results remain reactive and biophysical profile score is 8–10
Fetal heart tones/reactivity			
Presence of pre-term uterine contractions		Counsel regarding signs and symptoms of: (1) spontaneous abortion, (2) preterm labor, (3) premature rupture of membranes, (4) abruptio placentae and placenta previa	Client describes signs and symptoms of: (1) spontaneous abortion, (2) preterm labor, (3) premature rupture of membranes, (4) abruptio placentae and placenta previa
Vaginal bleeding or leaking fluid			
Fetal activity			
Results of ultrasound		Use written handouts to teach client: (1) fetal movement counting, (2) palpation and timing of uterine contractions, (3) determining leaking membranes or vaginal bleeding, (4) when to call the doctor	Client: (1) counts fetal movements, (2) palpates and times contractions, (3) observes for leaking membranes or vaginal bleeding, (4) calls the doctor when appropriate

obtain a detailed drug use history as well as an alcohol use history even if the mother does not exhibit the gross signs of substance abuse. Table 36-2 illustrates characteristics indicative of moderate to heavy substance abuse. Again, a concerned, nonjudgmental approach brings better information.

The nurse should remember that the mother does not have to be using "street drugs" to inflict harm on her infant. The patient who is dependent on OTC and prescription drugs is also an addict; her use can have harmful effects on the maternal-placental-fetal system as well.

Issues of codependency for the nurse are applicable here also. Because the use of illicit drugs is a legal problem, the nurse may have more problems with a judgmental attitude for these patients. The suggestions for

National Resources for Drug Treatment

American Council for Drug Education
204 Monroe Street
Rockville, MD 20850

National Association for Perinatal Addiction Research
    and Education
11 E. Hubbard Street, Suite 200
Chicago, IL 60611

National Council for Drug and Alcohol Information
P.O. Box 2340
Rockville, MD 20857

National Institute on Drug Abuse
5600 Fishers Lane
Rockville, MD 20857

National Perinatal Association
101 1/2 South Union Street
Alexandria, VA 22314-3323

Office for Substance Abuse Prevention
Parklawn/Rockwall II
5600 Fishers Lane, 9th Floor
Rockville, MD 20857

Parent Care, Inc.
101 1/2 South Union Street
Alexandria, VA 22314-3323

the nurse's utilizing Al Anon in the care of the alcoholic patients pertain also for the nurse caring for the drug-addicted mother.

Planning and Intervention. Most drug-using clients are latecomers for prenatal care. Indeed, most of these clients delay until they feel that they are ready for delivery to avoid a long labor without drugs and to satisfy their need for a last "fix" before submitting to the confinement of the hospital. As a result, there is evidence that a substantial proportion of deliveries to this population occurs at home, in the ambulance, or on the stretcher. Also, addicts make considerable efforts to nourish their addiction during enforced periods of confinement in a hospital. Such clients either hide their drugs or obtain them from others in or outside the hospital. A portion of these clients supplement their supply with barbiturates, tranquilizers, or cocaine.[51–53] If the mother is delivering in the hospital, however, the nurse should prepare immediately for high-risk conditions because the labor, birth, and infant are all considered high risk. Management of the labor, birth, and infant is discussed in detail in subsequent chapters.

The nurse should remember that many of these women are truly addicts and deteriorated; they may have lost nearly all, if not all material necessities. In addition, their moral sense, judgment, and cognitive functioning are often blunted or nonoperational; care of these patients requires a multidisciplinary team, including a member who is skilled in identifying and treating the medical problems frequently found in substance-abusing women.[47,51]

As for the alcoholic, therapy entails a process of supporting the mother to start the recovery process (see box). The nurse should meet with the mother on an ongoing basis prenatally whenever possible and help plan concretely for labor and delivery. Written material should be used liberally because memory is often impaired and advice and instructions soon may be forgotten. Every effort should be made to determine, support, enhance, and teach parenting skills. Clear, concrete directions are necessary, and as with the alcoholic, reinforcement and reiteration regarding all phases of child care are necessary.

TREATMENT AND REHABILITATION PROGRAMS. Withdrawal medication may be needed, and the patient needs to be referred to appropriate inpatient and detoxification units. Table 36-3 summarizes the laboratory screens that are ordered for the mother. Many tertiary care hospitals have alcohol and drug abuse units. However, many are reluctant to take pregnant women because there are no perinatal care experts on staff routinely. Hence, the nurse must be thorough in her referral, and the perinatal team must be aware of all options. It is important to remember that referral to a 12-step program is as crucial for the drug addict as for the alcoholic. Alcoholics Anonymous accepts drug-addicted patients, and many recovering alcoholics had a drug addiction problem as well.

If the mother is laboring and drug use is recent, the goal is to stabilize the mother and fetus. The mother is placed in the left lateral recumbent position, administered oxygen, and closely monitored. Seizure precautions and neurological assessments are required if the woman is experiencing a cocaine-induced hypertensive episode. The nurse should maintain ongoing assessment of vital signs to detect any respiratory or cardiovascular impairment.[47,48,54] The use of the fetal monitor is imperative for these patients because they are extremely high-risk. As stated previously, a high-risk addicted infant is expected, and all necessary precautions are taken for its safety.

Appendix C illustrates a Perinatal Protocol developed by the Obstetric Advisory Committee of the Perinatal Advisory Council of Los Angeles Communities (PACLAC) for use when substance abuse is suspected or known.[55] It delineates the responsibilities of the health team, the procedures to be followed, and the tests to be ordered.

Evaluation. Reduction and cessation of drug use would be indicators of success of intervention. For the addict particularly, however, recovery is a long process and

Video Resources

This list of video resources is a sample of the many excellent videos available for education of professionals, patients, and the general public. These videos have been recommended highly by practitioners. Whenever possible, the name and phone number of the producer/distributor have been included.

Substance Abuse and Pregnancy: A Health Professional's Guide

RT: 30 min

Polymorph Films
University of Minnesota Film and Video
612-627-4270

Reviews issues of substance abuse during pregnancy including alcohol, nicotine, illicit substances, and over-the-counter medications. Demonstrates interview technique for life-style assessment.

Staying Off Cocaine: Avoiding Relapse

RT: 38 min

Reelizations
914-679-8363

Features Dr. Arnold Washton and is designed for patient viewing. Especially useful for facilitating discussion in patient education sessions and groups. Identifies eight common trouble spots in cocaine recovery and three positive changes that must be made for long-term recovery to occur.

Sex and Drugs: The Intimate Connection

RT: 30 min

Reelizations
914-679-8368

Features Dr. Arnold Washton and Nannette Stone-Washton. Describes the dual-addiction to sex and drugs. Includes personal testimony by recovering addicts and presents information for patient education and staff training.

Recovery from Cocaine Addiction ("The Wall")

RT: 35 min

Sierra-Tucson, Consolidated Media Service
415-680-0651

A step-by-step presentation of the stages of recovery from cocaine addiction. Includes an analysis of various justifications for relapse. Deals with the main obstacle in the recovery process: "The Wall." Includes personal statements from recovering addicts.

The Haight-Ashbury Cocaine Film: Physiology, Compulsion, Recovery

RT: 35 min

Cinemed
213-545-6536

Teaching film that details what cocaine is and how it manipulates brain chemicals. Demonstrates how cocaine inhibits the natural balance of the brain's chemistry and can replace basic survival mechanisms such as sleeping, eating, drinking, and the sex drive with the compulsive use of cocaine.

Smokeable Cocaine: The Haight-Ashbury Crack Film

RT: 28 min

Cinemed
213-545-6536

This film examines the danger of smokeable cocaine to the fetus of a crack-using mother-to-be. Details how free base and crack manipulate brain chemistry. Demonstrates how the effects as well as the compulsion to use are enforced by the nature of this new form of cocaine. Describes the use of alcohol and other drugs in combination with crack.

A Love Story for My Unborn Child

RT: 8 min

University Health Associates, Inc.
202-429-9506

Designed for client education and appropriate for use in the clinic setting. Appropriate for use with adolescents.

Cry for Help

RT: 30 min

Combined Services, Inc.
612-871-5503

Produced in Minnesota by A. Kronick, this film highlights Minnesota programs that provide services to women who abuse substances. It deals specifically with the problem of cocaine addiction and the impact on women and the family. The effect of cocaine on infants exposed prenatally is described. The video is in two parts. Part 1, "The Fetal Drug and Alcohol Crisis," is meant for providers from a variety of disciplines. Part 2, "Drugs, Alcohol and Pregnancy," is for client viewing.

(continued)

Women, Drugs, and the Unborn Child

RT: 58 min (2 parts)

Pyramid Film and Video
213-828-7577

"Treating the Chemically Dependent Woman and Her Child," Part 1 of this series is designed for professionals and describes strategies for treating pregnant women. It includes personal stories.

"Innocent Addicts," Part 2, is designed for use by clients and illustrates the impact of drug abuse on the unborn child.

A Pregnant Woman Never Drinks Alone

RT: 8 min

University Health Associates, Inc.
202-429-9506

Excellent teaching video for use in a clinic setting. Describes the dangers of alcohol use during pregnancy.

48 Hours on Crack Street

RT: 1 hour, 45 min

CBS

Portrays crack addicts in their own environment. Describes the problem of infants exposed to cocaine in utero including the "border baby" phenomenon. Includes review of treatment approaches and policy alternatives.

Cocaine: Beyond the Looking Glass

RT: 28 min

Hazelden
1-800-328-9000 (US)
1-800-257-0070 (MN)

Advocates recovery through the 12-step process and describes the support received from Narcotics Anonymous. Suitable for adolescents and families. This video highlights recovering addicts who describe their struggle to quit cocaine.

Crack

RT: 30 min

Hazelden
1-800-328-9000 (US)
1-800-257-0070 (MN)

Taped on location in and around New York City, this documentary reveals how crack is one of the most dangerous, most addictive, most destructive drugs to ever threaten communities. Presents personal stories of crack users, those affected by crack use, and those fighting crack use.

Soft is the Heart of the Child

RT: 30 min

Hazelden
1-800-328-9000 (US)
1-800-257-0070 (MN)

This award-winning film deals with the subject of how children are affected by alcoholism in the family. It illustrates a classic alcoholic family situation.

spectacular results are not readily seen. Often just the keeping of prenatal appointments is an excellent indicator that the nurse is making an impact. The nurse should not be discouraged if patients do not seem to respond dramatically. Often, it takes a critical "bottoming out" before the addict can accept her disease and begin recovery. Continued referral to 12-step programs as well as inpatient treatment when indicated is crucial.

The far-reaching impact of the addictive disorders of smoking, drinking, and drug abuse is staggering in terms of wasted human potential. Nurses need to develop methodologies and protocols to identify all substance abuse in the pregnant patient and to establish protocols for primary, secondary, and tertiary intervention for the mother and her infant. Evaluation of these protocols is a fertile and challenging field for nursing research.[47,48,54]

■ REFERENCES

1. Adams EH, Gfroerer JC, Rouse BA: Epidemiology of substance abuse including alcohol and cigarette smoking. In Hutchings DE (ed): Ann NY Acad Sci 562:14–20, June 30, 1988
2. Hamilton D: Crack's children grow up. Los Angeles Times, pp 1A ff, August 24, 1990
3. Warner KE: Smoking and health. AJPH 79:141–143, February 1989
4. Kleinman J, Kopstein A: Smoking during pregnancy. AJPH 77(7):823–825, 1987
5. Aaronson LS, MacNee CL: Tobacco, alcohol and caffeine use during pregnancy. JOGN Nurs 18:279–287, July/August 1989
6. Fingerhut L, Kleinman JC, Kendrick JS: Smoking before, during and after pregnancy. AJPH 80:541–544, May 1990

7. United States Public Health Service: Smoking and Health, A Report of the Surgeon General, US Department of Health, Education and Welfare. Publication No. (PHS) 79-50066, Washington, DC, Public Health Service, Office of Smoking and Health, 1979

8. Zuckerman B: Marijuana and cigarette smoking during pregnancy: Neonatal effects. In Chasnoff IJ (ed): Drugs, Alcohol, Pregnancy and Parenting. Boston, Kluwar Academic Publishing, 1988

9. Finnegan LP: Smoking and its effect in pregnancy and the newborn. In Harel S, Anaastasiow N (eds): The At Risk Infant: Psycho/Socio/Medical Aspects, pp 127–136. Baltimore, Paul H Brookes Publishing, 1985

10. Alexander L: The pregnant smoker: Nursing implications. JOGN Nurs 16:167–173, September/October 1987

11. Sandahl B: A prospective study of drug use, contraceptives and smoking. Acta Obstet Gynecol Scand 64:381–386, 1985

12. Mochizuki MT, Mauro T, Masuko K et al: Effects of smoking on the fetoplacental-maternal system during pregnancy. Am J Obstet Gynecol 149:413–420, 1984

13. Anderson KY, Hermann J: Placenta flow reduction in pregnant smokers. Acta Obstet Gynecol Scand 63:707–709, 1984

14. Meyer MB, Tonascia JA: Maternal smoking, pregnancy complications and perinatal mortality. Am J Obstet Gynecol 128:492–502, 1977

15. Stein Z, Kline J: Smoking, alcohol and reproduction. AJPH 75:593–625, October 1983

16. Fox NL, Sexton M, Hebel JR: Prenatal exposure to tobacco: I & II: Effects on physical growth at age three. Int J Epidemiol 19:66–77, March 1990

17. Haglund B, Cnattingius S: Cigarette smoking as a risk factor for sudden infant death syndrome: A population based study. AJPH 80:29–32, 1990

18. Fried PA, Watkinson B: 36 and 48 month neurobehavioral follow up of children prenatally exposed to marijuana, cigarettes and alcohol. Dev and Behav Pediatrics 2:49–58, April 1990

19. Rush D, Callahan KR: Exposure to passive cigarette smoking and child development. In Hutchings DE (ed): Ann NY Acad Sci 562:74–100, June 30, 1989

20. Neuspiel DR, Cereen S, Andrews P et al: Parental smoking and post-infancy wheezing in children: A prospective cohort study. AJPH 79:168–171, February 1989

21. Moessinger AA: Mothers who smoke and the lungs of their offspring. In Hutchings DE (ed): Ann NY Acad Sci 562:101–104, June 30, 1989

22. Gillies PA, Madeley RJ, Power FL: Why do pregnant women smoke? Public Health Rep 103:337–343, September 1989

23. Gritz ER, Marcus AC, Berman BA et al: Evaluation of a worksite self-help smoking cessation program for registered nurses. Am J Health Promotion 3:26–35, Fall 1988

24. Windsor RA, Cutter G, Morris J et al: Effectiveness of smoking cessation methods for smokers in a public health maternity clinic: A randomized trial. AJPH 75:1389–1392, December 1985

25. Burton R: Causes of melancholy, Vol I, Part I, Section

2. The Anatomy of Melancholy. London, William Tegg, 1906 (orig 1621)

26. Weiner L, Morse BA: FAS: Clinical perspectives and prevention. In Chasnoff IJ (ed): Drugs, Alcohol, Pregnancy and Parenting. Boston, Kluwer Academic Publishers, 1988

27. Jones KL, Smith DW: Recognition of the fetal alcohol syndrome in early infancy. Lancet 2:999–1001, 1973

28. Jessup M: Fetal alcohol syndrome: Prevention and intervention for the nurse. California Nurse 84:12–13, February 1990

29. Healy JM: Reducing the destructive impact of alcohol: The search for acceptable strategies continues. AJPH 76:749–750, July 1986

30. Eward AM, Wolfe R, Moll P et al: Psychosocial and behavioral factors differentiating past drinkers and lifelong abstainers. AJPH 76:68–70, January 1986

31. Chasnoff IJ: Alcohol use in pregnancy. In Chasnoff IJ (ed): Drug Use in Pregnancy, pp 75–80. Boston, MTP Press Limited, 1986

32. Weiner L, Rosett HL: Alcohol effects of pregnancy: The experience of the Boston City Hospital. Currents 1(1): 4–7, 1985

33. Kaminski M, Rumeau C, Schwartz D: Alcohol consumption in pregnant women and the outcome of pregnancy. Alcoholism (NY) 2(2):155–163, 1978

34. Abel EL: Fetal alcohol syndrome in families. Neurotoxicol Teratol 10:1–2, 1988

35. Hill RM, Hegemeir S, Tennyson LM: The fetal alcohol syndrome: A multihandicapped child. Neurotoxicology 10:585–596, 1989

36. Weinberg J: Effects of ethanol and maternal nutritional status on fetal development. Alcoholism (NY) 9(1): 1063–1067, 1985

37. Chasnoff IJ: The interfaces of perinatal addiction. In Chasnoff IJ (ed): Drugs, Alcohol, Pregnancy and Parenting. Boston, Kluwer Academic Publishers, 1988

38. Kaul AF, Harsfield JC et al: A retrospective analysis of analgesics and sedative hypnotics in hospitalized obstetric and gynecologic patients. Drug Intell Clin Pharm 12:95–99, 1978

39. Chasnoff IJ, Schnoll SH et al: Maternal substance abuse during pregnancy: Effects on infant development. Toxicology Teratol 6:277–280, 1984

40. Sobatka TJ: Neurobehavioral effects of prenatal caffeine. In Hutchings DE (ed): Ann NY Acad Sci 562: 327–339, June 30, 1989

41. Isacson D, Smedby B: Defining heavy use of prescription drugs. Med Care 26:1103–1110, November 1988

42. Bologna M, Koren G, Jones M et al: Drugs and chemicals most commonly used by pregnant women. In Koren G (ed): Maternal-Fetal Toxicology: A Clinician's Guide. New York, Marcel Dekker, 1990

43. Koran G: Teratogenic drugs and chemicals in humans. In Koran G (ed): Maternal-Fetal Toxicology: A Clinician's Guide. New York, Marcel Dekker, 1990

44. Schnoll SH: Pharmacologic basis of perinatal addiction. In Chasnoff IJ (ed): Drug Use in Pregnancy, pp 7–16. Boston, MTP Press Limited, 1986

45. Hasin DS, Grant BF et al: Cocaine and heroin dependence compound in poly-abusers. AJPH 78:567–573, May 1988

46. Koran G: Changes in drug disposition in pregnancy and their clinical implications. In Koran G (ed): Maternal-Fetal Toxicology: A Clinicians Guide, pp 3–13. New York, Marcel Dekker, 1990

47. Lynch M, McKeon VA: Cocaine use during pregnancy. JOGN Nurs 19:285–289, July/August 1990

48. Smith J: The dangers of prenatal cocaine use. MCN 13:174–179, May/June 1988

49. Keith LG, McGregor S, Frank A et al: Substance abuse in pregnant women: Recent experience at the Perinatal Center for Chemical-Dependence of Northwestern Memorial Hospital. Obstet Gynecol 73:715–720, May 1989

50. Wilson GS: Clinical studies of infants and children exposed prenatally to heroin. In Hutchings DE (ed): Ann NY Acad Sci 562:183–193, June 30, 1989

51. Silver H, Wapner R, Lorz-Vega M et al: Addiction in pregnancy: High risk intrapartum management and outcome. J Perinatol 7:178–184, Summer 1987

52. von Windeguth BJ, Urbano MT: Cocaine abusing mothers and their infants: A new morbidity brings challenges for nursing care. J Community Health Nursing 6:147–153, 1989

53. Reichett S, Christensen B: Reflections during a study on family therapy with drug addicts. Family Process 29:273–287, September 1990

54. Michaels B, Noonan M, Hoffman S et al: A treatment model and nursing care for pregnant chemical abusers. In Chasnoff IJ: Drugs, Alcohol, Pregnancy and Parenting, pp 47–57. Boston, Kluwer Academic Publishers, 1988

55. Obstetric Advisory Committee of PACLAC: Perinatal protocol: Maternal substance use and neonatal drug withdrawal. J Perinatol 8:387–392, Fall 1988

■ SUGGESTED READINGS

Burd L, Martsolf JT: Fetal alcohol syndrome: Diagnosis and syndromal variability. Physiol Behav 46:39–43, 1989

Eliason MJ, Williams JK: Fetal alcohol syndrome and the neonate. Journal of Perinatal and Neonatal Nursing 3(4):64–72, 1990

Fost N: Maternal-fetal conflicts: Ethical and legal considerations. In Hutchings DE (ed): Ann NY Acad Sci 562:248–254, June 30, 1989

Hickner J, Cousineau A, Messimer S: Smoking cessation during pregnancy: Strategies used by Michigan family physicians. J Am Board of Family Pract 3:39–42, January–March 1990

House MA: Cocaine. Am J Nurs 90:41–45, April 1990

Kelley RD: The path to addiction—and recovery. Am J Nurs 87:176–179, 1987

McCormick MC, Brooks-Gunn J, Shorter T et al: Factors associated with smoking in low-income pregnant women: Relationship to birth weight, stressful life events, social support, health behaviors and mental distress. J Clin Epidemiol 43:441–448, 1990

Michaels B, Noonan M, Hoffman S et al: A treatment model of nursing care for pregnant chemical abusers. In Chasnoff IJ (ed): Drugs, Alcohol, Pregnancy and Parenting, pp 47–57. Boston, Kluwer Academic Publishers, 1988

Naegle MA: Targets for change in alcohol and drug education for nursing roles. Alcohol Health & Research World 13(1):52–55, 1989

Pollitt K: A new assault on feminism. The Nation 250(12):409–418, March 26, 1990

37

Adolescent Sexuality, Pregnancy, and Childrearing

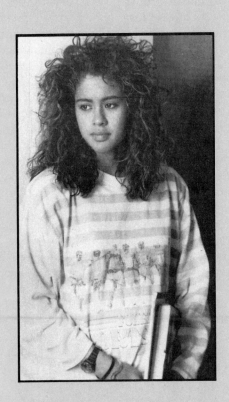

Adolescence is the developmental period that bridges the gap between childhood and adulthood. It is the stage in which the person is required to adapt and adjust childhood behaviors to the culturally acceptable norms of society. Important in this process are the tasks of ego (identity) development, achievement of personal independence, and attainment of higher cognitive skills. Biological changes rapidly occur during this period. Primary and secondary changes in sexual characteristics are described in Chapter 8. As a result of these biological changes, others' expectations for the adolescent's behavior change, and the adolescent's self-image may be modified. All of these changes impact on the person's cognitive, social, and personal development.

During adolescence, boys and girls experiment with a variety of adult roles and attempt to develop a realistic sense of self.[1,2] The stage of adolescence provides the person with a legitimate time to acquire the education, training, and skills necessary to function in our complex society, as well as to learn other, non-work-related adult activities and skills. Adolescent behavior frequently involves experimenting with a variety of new activities, many potentially harmful, such as unsafe sexual encounters, substance abuse, and violence. The increasing mortality of adolescents during the past 25 years, as compared to other age groups in this country, is a reflection of adolescent risk-taking behavior.[3] Violence is the leading cause of adolescent deaths, with accidents, suicides, and homicides contributing to more than 75% of adolescent mortality.[4]

Substance abuse while driving partially accounts for the high automobile fatality rate among adolescents. Adolescents are also the victims of violence, exploitation, and abuse. Sexual experimentation may lead to unplanned pregnancy or occurrence of sexually transmitted diseases (STDs). Most adolescent pregnancies are unintentional and result from a combination of risk-taking behavior, inadequate reproductive knowledge, and general belief of invulnerability that "it would not happen to me."[5]

This chapter introduces the student to the developmental process of adolescence; trends and issues in adolescent sexuality, pregnancy, and childbearing; and the antecedents and consequences of these phenomena. Approaches to nursing care are described as they relate to primary, secondary, and tertiary prevention. The importance of directing intervention toward the goal of preventing unintended adolescent pregnancy is emphasized. Applications of the nursing process are identified that promote optimum health, social, and developmental outcomes for childbearing and childrearing adolescents and their offspring.

■ THEORETICAL CONSIDERATIONS

According to Erikson's theory of psychosocial development, adolescence is a particularly decisive period for forming an identity. Adolescents must become persons in their own right—individuals who are in charge of their lives, who know who they are. The major developmental task of adolescence is to resolve the conflict between identity achievement and identity diffusion. The person's personality formation during adolescence is influenced by how the previous stages of development were completed.[6] For example, adolescents who failed to establish a sense of trust during the stage of early childhood may continue to display distrusting attitudes toward others. Similarly, adolescents who do not develop a sense of initiative during the preschool years may subsequently lack the confidence needed to experiment with different identities and to become comfortable with their own individuality.

During adolescence, the person faces the challenge of developing a vocational and sexual identity necessary for establishing intimate relationships in adulthood. If the identity confusion crisis is resolved with reasonable success during adolescence, the person advances into the adult stages of development and their corresponding crises with a firm identity. If the person does not solve the adolescent ego-identity crisis successfully, maldevelopment of the ego occurs and the person is less likely to resolve the crises of adulthood.

Marcia refined Erikson's conceptualization of adolescent identity formation by viewing identity as a continually changing organization of one's own attitudes, values, and beliefs. A well-developed identity enables the person to be aware of personal strengths and uniqueness. A less well-developed identity results in the person's not being able to define strengths and weaknesses, and not possessing a well-articulated sense of self. Four identity statuses are described by Marcia: *identity achievement, foreclosure, identity diffusion,* and *moratorium*; these are individual styles of coping with the identity crisis. *Identity achievers* have experienced a period of decision making and are now committed to an occupation and to a set of ideological values, all of which are primarily self-chosen. These people have strength in their belief system and are adaptive and well-adjusted. People in the *foreclosure* status are similar to identity achievers, but some of their choices have been determined by parents or others and are not self-selected. People with the status of *identity diffusion* demonstrate no commitment to an occupation or ideological system. Those classified as *moratoriums* are char-

Research Highlight

Developmental studies have shown that the task of adolescence is to formulate identity, the task of young adults is to search for intimacy, and the task of adults is to create the next generation. Unresolved tasks of an earlier stage may interfere with one's ability to achieve tasks at a later stage. Maternal role adaptation and the child's adjustment may be affected by the developmental stage of the mother. Research has suggested that a secure sense of self may influence mothering behavior. Mercer's study explored the relationship between developmental variables and maternal behavior.

The 294 women studied were divided into three groups: 15 to 19 years old, 20 to 29 years old, and 30 to 42 years old. The subjects were interviewed and completed a battery of instruments during postpartum hospitalization and again at 1, 4, 8, and 12 months after birth. Flexibility of childbearing attitudes, maternal empathy, maternal temperament, self-concept, and maternal behavior were measured.

The major findings were: (1) older women had greater flexibility in parenting; (2) teenagers had less empathy for their infants; (3) women between 20 and 42 years were higher in adaptability, were lower in intensity, and had a more positive mood state regarding parenting than the teenagers; (4) women between 20 and 42 years scored significantly higher in self-concept and personality integration than the teenage group; and (5) a positive correlation existed between age and competent maternal behavior: the older the woman, the more competent the maternal behavior.

Nurses need to assess the developmental level of mothers to determine age and competency of maternal behavior and assist them in adapting to the mothering role. Adolescent mothers need to be closely assessed for self-concept disturbance and altered parenting and assisted in improving self-concept and adaptation to parenting.

(Mercer RT: The relationship of developmental variables to maternal behavior. Res Nurs Health 9:25–33, 1986)

acterized by the presence of struggle and attempts to make commitments about occupational or ideological decisions.[1,7,8]

Piaget contends that adolescence is a qualitatively unique period of life, set apart from childhood by the person's expanding cognitive abilities.[9] Young adolescents have not cognitively entered the stage of formal operations. This stage is attained by most adolescents between 15 and 20 years of age but is individually influenced by social and school experiences and neurological development. The thought processes of adolescents in the stage of concrete operations or only partial formal operation are somewhat egocentric. Consequently, they may have difficulty planning for the future and implementing behavior change. Older adolescents are capable of abstract thinking (formal operational thought), which enables them to understand the thought processes of others and to interact with the environment in new and different ways.

Havighurst proposed eight developmental tasks for the adolescent years (see box).[2] It should be noted that the first four tasks assume central importance during early adolescence. They are more dependent on physical maturity and biological changes than the other tasks that characterize later adolescence. According to Havighurst, the developmental tasks through which the

person must proceed may differ from culture to culture; however, *biologically determined tasks* (e.g., tasks 1 through 3) are more likely to be culturally universal

---

Developmental Tasks of Adolescence

Task 1   Achieving more mature relations with age-mates of both sexes

Task 2   Achieving a masculine or feminine social role

Task 3   Accepting one's physique and using the body effectively

Task 4   Achieving emotinoal independence from parents and other adults

Task 5   Preparing for marriage and family life

Task 6   Prepaing for an economic career

Task 7   Acquiring a set of values and an ethical system as a guide to behavior: Developing an ideology

Task 8   Desiring and achieving socially responsible behavior.

(Havighurst RJ: Developmental Tasks and Education. New York, David McKay, 1972)

than are *tasks that have a strong cultural component* (e.g., tasks 5 through 8).[2] Successful mastery of the developmental tasks promotes the adolescent's emergence into adulthood as a well-adjusted person who should be competent and capable of adapting to future demands of development.

Growth during adolescence is divided into three substages: early, middle, and late adolescence. Early adolescence occurs between pubescence and age 15 years and is characterized by rapid physical growth and development, beginning assertion of independence with movement away from parents, increasing emphasis on close peer relationships, concrete thinking with some effort toward abstract problem solving, egocentricism, and present orientation. Middle adolescence spans from ages 16 to 17 and is distinguished by development of formal abstract thinking abilities, introspection, increasing future orientation, preoccupation with sexual exploration, and more formal separation from parents. Testing of limits and a preference for peer activities are evident in this stage. Late adolescence extends from 18 to 20 years of age and is characterized by establishment of a secure body image and gender identity, maintenance of stable relationships, behaviors oriented toward others and self, and realistic problem-solving skills. Emotional intimacy and career planning are major concerns.

Pregnancy during any substage of adolescence makes the normal developmental issues of this period more difficult to resolve. Concerns over changing body image, increasing dependence on family members for emotional and financial support, and the normal physiological and psychological changes of pregnancy create internal stress, which the adolescent is often unprepared to cope with. To further complicate this situation, the adolescent faces many potential conflicts between the developmental tasks of adolescence and the tasks of parenthood. Sadler and Catrone identified five major areas of conflict (Table 37-1).

An unplanned and early pregnancy requires the adolescent to shift her energies from the task of internalizing an identity to generativity in rearing the next generation, often without having mastered a true sense of intimacy. As a parent, the adolescent must attempt to meet the daily care needs of an infant by providing a safe environment, adequate caregiving, and nurturing. The infant's sense of trust is fostered through mothering behaviors that encompass providing consistent and developmentally appropriate care. Because the adolescent mother must prematurely assume an adult role, she may be forced to remain in the developmental stage of foreclosure.[10]

Similar psychological risks may exist for the adolescent father. His developmental tasks are likely to be interrupted by an early, unplanned pregnancy. The young father may feel isolated, alone, and overwhelmed. A variety of stressors may impact his life and influence his future plans (e.g., potential interruption of education, lack of family support, and financial difficulties).

TABLE 37–1. DEVELOPMENTAL TASKS OF ADOLESCENCE AND PARENTHOOD, AND RELATED CONFLICTING BEHAVIORS

Adolescence	Parenthood	Conflicting Behaviors
Narcissism and egocentrism; focus on self and needs	Forming an empathic and mutualistic relationship with infant	Competition between adolescent and infant for attention of mate, family, friends; unable to differentiate own feelings from infant
Identity formation: develop peer relationships, participate in role experimentation, need for period of moratorium	Maternal identification and role differentiation	Reluctance to assume parenting responsibilities; resentment toward infant
Body image formation and sexual identity formation	Acceptance of body image changes of pregnancy, labor and delivery, and postpartum	Rejection of body image changes; refusal to breast-feed
Emancipation from family	Family role reassignments	Resentment of dependence on family for support and financial assistance; conflict with mother about childrearing
Cognitive development: transition from concrete to formal operations	Decision making and future planning regarding childrearing	Difficulty understanding general principles of child development, infant play, and safety

(Modified from Sadler LS, Catrone C: The adolescent parent: A dual developmental crisis. J Adol Health Care 4:100–105, 1983)

TABLE 37-2. DECISION POINTS LEADING TO PARENTHOOD

Decision 1	Sexual activity	To become sexually active or to remain sexually inactive
Decision 2	Contraception	To use or not to use contraceptives appropriately
Decision 3	Pregnancy resolution	To deliver or to abort
Decision 4	Parenthood	To rear the child or to place the child formally or informally for adoption

(Modified from Flick LH: Paths to adolescent parenthood: Implications for prevention. Public Health Rep 101(2): 132–147, 1986)

■ PATHWAYS TO ADOLESCENT PREGNANCY

The pathway to adolescent pregnancy and childbearing encompasses a series of choices the adolescent makes in the area of sexuality. Flick identified four steps or decisions the adolescent consciously or unconsciously makes that lead to parenthood (Table 37-2).

National survey data suggest that adolescent sexual behavior has risen dramatically. By age 20, most unmarried young males and over 70% of females report that they have engaged in sexual intercourse.[11] The change in attitudes toward adolescent sexuality that became evident in the 1960s has resulted in the gap between males' and females' sexual behavior narrowing as more and more girls became sexually active.[12] Because an increasing number of unmarried females in all segments of society in the United States are having intercourse at an earlier age, the period of exposure to unintended adolescent pregnancy has expanded. The younger the adolescent, the more sporadic and infrequent is the level of sexual activity.

Research findings indicate that many factors are associated with increased levels of adolescent sexual activity (e.g., low socioeconomic status [SES], poor educational achievement, large family size or a single-parent household, and lack of sex education).[12–17] Sexually active girls tend to be those who are susceptible to pressure from their boyfriends and are influenced by perceived sexual activity of their peer group.[14,15,17]

Adolescents considering becoming sexually active and those engaged in sexual activity face decisions regarding contraception. The use of contraceptive techniques among adolescents tends to be erratic and is limited. Nonuse or inadequate use of contraceptives by sexually active adolescents has been found to be associated with low SES, low educational achievement, little communication with parents, and lack of knowledge of their siblings' or their parents' birth control experience.[14,16–19] Peer influences include having friends who are parents. A positive relationship has been found between age at first intercourse and effective contraceptive use.[14,17,19] Older adolescents are much more likely to use contraceptives than are younger adolescents. Sachs demonstrated that cognitive development in adolescents is a predictor of contraceptive choices.[20] Although some data suggest that knowledge of contraceptive methods increases adolescents' use of contraceptives, case studies by the Alan Guttmacher Institute indicate that adolescents are exposed to mixed messages about contraception.[14,16,17,19,21] Furthermore, birth control services are not effectively delivered to American youth.[16,22,23]

About one half of all adolescents do not use contraceptives the first time they have sexual relations, and a substantial number use birth control occasionally or not at all during subsequent sexual encounters.[17,24] Because one half of all first pregnancies occur in the 6 months after the first intercourse, and one fifth in the first month, these delays in contraceptive use may have serious consequences for adolescents.[25–27]

Adolescents who become pregnant because of ineffective use or nonuse of contraceptive methods face the decision of whether or not to terminate voluntarily their pregnancies. Approximately 40% of pregnant adolescents elect to terminate their pregnancies by abortion.[28] Results of some studies indicate that the decision to deliver an infant rather than to abort is more likely for older adolescents, for high school dropouts and those with poor school performance, for members of large families and those in single-parent households, and for girls who had a sister who was pregnant as an adolescent.[17–19] The adolescents most likely to terminate an unwanted pregnancy are the affluent, the white, and the well educated.[28–30] The adolescent's abortion decision is apt to be influenced by the values of her mother, boyfriend, and female friends who may provide advice; the significance of other people's opinions does not appear to be a constant or predictable variable.[30]

Fewer data are available about adolescents who

choose adoption, because approximately 96% of those who do deliver choose to rear their child.[28] The limited published studies suggest that adolescents who make adoption plans are more similar to those who choose abortion than to those who become parents.[31,32] Few negative consequences have been found for adolescents who relinquish their children compared with those who keep them.[32] Several factors reportedly influence the decision as to whether to keep or to relinquish a child; these include: (1) maternal age—parents tend to be younger than those who relinquish their child; (2) SES and family constellation—adolescents who relinquish their child tend to belong to a higher SES, whereas parents are more likely to be members of single-parent families; and (3) possession of a traditional value system about abortion and family life—parents tend to have traditional views about family and express less approval of abortion as an alternative to childbirth.

Responsible decision making regarding sexual activity and parenthood requires certain skills that adolescents often lack (Fig. 37-1). These include the ability to (1) understand the factual information that applies to them (cognition); (2) incorporate their sexual identity into their evolving value structure in the presence of peer pressure (socialization); and (3) evaluate the many variables that influence them on a daily basis and change from day to day (situation-specific behavior).[33]

■ INCIDENCE OF ADOLESCENT PREGNANCY, ABORTION, AND BIRTH

Each year over a million teenagers become pregnant and approximately 500,000 of them give birth.[34] The rate of births has declined only slightly among adolescents aged 15 to 19 years during the past decade; the rate has stayed nearly unchanged among those younger than 15 years. Each year approximately 11% of females 15 to 19 years of age become pregnant.[35] The incidence of nonmarital childbearing is twice as high among African-Americans as among whites, although in the past 15 years the occurrence of adolescent childbearing has risen more rapidly among young unmarried whites.[36] The large majority of pregnant adolescents are single and have an unplanned pregnancy.

The United States has a higher rate of unintended adolescent pregnancy, abortion, and childbearing than any other developed country.[22] A comparison of the rates of pregnancy, abortion, and birth between 1980 and 1985 for 10 states is displayed in Table 37-3.

An ethnic and age comparison of pregnancy, abortion, and birth rates for all adolescents in the United States is presented in Table 37-4. The statistics record the age at the time of the pregnancy outcome rather than the age at which the pregnancy occurred.

The rate of abortion among adolescents has remained level during the 1980s, with 9% to 11% of sexually active adolescent females having an abortion each year. Four in ten pregnancies among adolescents 15 to 19 years of age end in abortion.[35] One quarter of all U.S. abortions performed in 1987 were to women 19 years of age or younger.[37] Proportionately, more abortions occur among younger than older adolescents. The least urbanized states tend to have the lowest rates of abortion, probably partly due to the lack of accessible abortion services for women.[38]

■ IMPACT OF ADOLESCENT PREGNANCY AND CHILDREARING ON SOCIETY, THE FAMILY, AND THE INDIVIDUAL

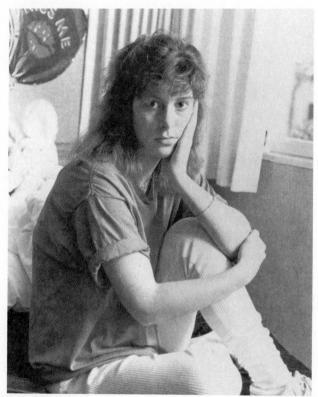

■ *Figure 37-1*
It is often difficult for adolescents to make responsible decisions because they lack the required skills. (Photo courtesy of St. Anne's Maternity Home.)

Despite the increasing effort to reduce its incidence, adolescent pregnancy and parenthood remain major na-

TABLE 37–3. RATES OF ADOLESCENT PREGNANCY, ABORTION, AND BIRTH IN 1985 AND 1980*†

	Pregnancies per 1000 Females Age 15–19		Abortions per 1000 Females Age 15–19		Births per 1000 Females Age 15–19	
	1985	1980	1985	1980	1985	1980
District of Columbia	211	200	113	114	72	62
California†	151	140	79	69	54	53
Alaska†	144	124	59	43	66	64
Georgia	132	131	44	41	70	72
Texas†	131	137	39	44	73	74
Arizona	128	123	43	41	67	65
Florida†	126	131	51	55	58	59
Nevada	125	144	57	67	53	59
Hawaii	125	106	61	41	48	51
Maryland	121	123	59	64	47	43

* Ten states with highest incidences of adolescent pregnancy in 1985.

† Abortion estimates are based on the proportion of abortions obtained by Women of the same age in neighboring or similar states.

(Modified from Henshaw S, Van Vort J, et al.: Teenage Pregnancy in the United States. New York, The Alan Guttmacher Institute, 1989)

tional concerns because of the potentially adverse consequences for society, the family, and the individual. The National Research Council's Panel on Adolescent Pregnancy and Childbearing published an extensive review of the literature that documents the public and private costs of early childbearing. Since the report's publication, additional data on the association between adolescent parenthood and long-term welfare dependence have indicated that early childbearing may be an important mechanism in understanding the intergenerational transmission of disadvantage.[39,40] Approximately half of the money spent on Aid to Families with Dependent Children (AFDC) is given to adult women who first became mothers as adolescents.[41]

The results of a major study entitled *Estimates of Public Costs for Teenage Childbearing* indicate that the cost of adolescent childbearing in the United States in 1985 was estimated at $16.65 billion.[42] This figure was derived based on the costs of AFDC, Medicaid, and food stamp payments and excluded special education, child protective services, day care, and other special service programs.

The family of the adolescent is greatly affected by an unplanned pregnancy. Many parents initially react with anger and hurt to the news of their child's conception; however, they may become more supportive at the birth of a grandchild and offer assistance to their daughter in need. The majority of pregnant and parenting adolescents choose to remain single and live within the context of their nuclear or extended family. Furstenberg and Crawford found that 88% of adolescents remained in this arrangement 1 year after birth, and 5 years later 70% of never married mothers still lived with their families of origin.[43] The roles of family members shift in situations where grandparents and significant others assume additional financial and childcare responsibilities. The developmental stage of the adolescent mother influences her level of dependence on family members and the family adaptation required. Economic and social support increase the adolescent's potential for psychological development and emotional satisfaction in the role of "mother."[44]

Maternal age at the time of conception often affects the life course of the adolescent. An unplanned pregnancy has different implications for the 18- or 19-year-old high school student than for the 13- or 14-year-old junior high school student. In general, adolescent parents are less likely to complete high school, attend college, find stable employment, or be self-supporting than later childbearers[11,12,45] (Fig. 37-2). Adolescents who become mothers are disproportionately poor and dependent on public assistance for their economic support.[45] Additionally, they are likely to have more children, closer spacing of births, and to be single parents than women who begin childbearing in their twenties.[41]

Although few adolescent mothers marry the fathers of their infants, many may maintain regular or sporadic contact with their mates. Early marriage to the child's

TABLE 37-4. ABORTION, BIRTH AND PREGNANCY RATES, AND ABORTION RATIO PER 1,000 WOMEN, BY AGE AND RACE*

Measure	Total	White	Nonwhite
Pregnancy Rate‡			
<15 y	16.6	8.8	50.8
15–19 y	109.8	92.9	185.8
15–17 y	71.1	57.1	134.0
18–19 y	166.2	145.1	261.3
Abortion Rate			
<15 y	9.1	5.0	27.0
15–19 y	43.8	37.8	71.1
15–17 y	30.7	25.7	53.2
18–19 y	63.0	55.4	97.1
Birthrate			
<15 y	5.5	2.7	17.6
15–19 y	51.3	42.8	89.7
15–17 y	31.1	24.0	62.9
18–19 y	80.8	70.1	128.7
Abortion Ratio†			
<15 y	45.6	46.0	45.5
<20 y	42.1	42.3	41.7
15–17 y	43.2	44.5	40.6
18–19 y	41.0	40.6	42.1

* United States, 1985.

† The denominator is number of abortions plus live births 6 months later (to match times of conception for pregnancies ending in births and pregnancies ending in abortions), both adjusted to age of woman at time of conception.

‡ Pregnancy rates include estimated number of pregnancies ending in miscarriage and stillbirths.

(Henshaw SK, Van Vort, J: Teenage abortion, birth and pregnancy statistics: An update. Fam Plann Perspect 21(2):85, 1989)

father does not seem to improve the course of events as reflected in the fact that adolescent mothers who stay single are more likely than those who marry to finish high school and to avoid another pregnancy. The divorce rate for young mothers is three times that of couples who delay childbearing until their twenties.[41]

In general, adolescent fathers tend to be less adversely affected by early parenthood than adolescent mothers; however, they are at risk for lower educational achievement and associated decreased vocational and economic attainment.[27,46] High school dropout rates are higher for adolescent fathers than other young men and are not influenced by marital status. The results of studies suggest that the effects of adolescent parenthood on school completion are graver for whites and Hispanics than for African-Americans.[27,47]

■ RISKS OF PREGNANCY AND CHILDBEARING DURING ADOLESCENCE

Perinatal Risks

Childbearing at any age is a momentous event. For the adolescent, however, it is often accompanied by a different set of problems from those experienced by adult mothers. Older adolescent mothers and their expected child face minimal biomedical risk in comparison to younger adolescents who experience disproportionately high rates of both maternal and neonatal deaths.[48] The population that is particularly at risk for adverse outcomes is nonwhite adolescents. For the young mother under the age of 15, there is a greater probability that her infant will be stillborn or premature, will have a low birth weight (LBW), or will die soon after birth. In addition, the mother is at greater risk for decreased weight gain, urinary tract infections, STDs, pregnancy-induced hypertension (PIH), iron deficiency anemia, cephalopelvic disproportion (CPD), and prolonged labor. Although more evidence is needed, the available information suggests that early childbearing may adversely affect linear growth of young adolescent girls because the circulating estrogens of pregnancy irreversibly accelerate epiphyseal closure.[49,50]

It is difficult to isolate and to identify the independent effect of maternal age on perinatal complications because the majority of adolescents who become pregnant are poor, have limited access to and use of health care, and display a variety of behaviors known to have a negative influence on pregnancy outcomes.[50] Available data indicate that early and regular, comprehensive prenatal care plus adequate nutrition decrease the risks of perinatal complications for pregnant adolescents and their children.[50,51]

Sexually Transmitted Diseases

The incidence of sexually transmitted diseases (STDs), especially acquired immune deficiency syndrome (AIDS), among adolescents has risen dramatically in recent years. According to the Centers for Disease Control, 2.5 million adolescents are estimated to be affected by STDs annually.[35] Female adolescents have the highest rates of STDs (e.g., gonorrhea, cytomegalovirus, chlamydia cervicitis, and pelvic inflammatory disease) of any age group, excluding homosexual men and prostitutes.[52] The rising incidence of AIDS in the 20- to 29-year-old age range is of major concern because many of these cases are likely to have originated in the late adolescent years.[53] If the proportion of reported cases increases in the heterosexual population as projected in the years ahead, adolescents will be at even higher

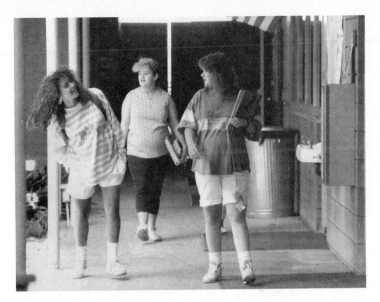

■ Figure 37-2
Although many adolescent mothers do not complete high school, some are able to continue and complete their education. (Photo courtesy of St. Anne's Maternity Home.)

risk for the infection.[54] (For further information, see Chap. 35.)

Low Birth Weight

The increased risk of low birth weight is one of the most important medical aspects of adolescent pregnancy. In considering this neonatal risk, it is important to recognize that findings from studies adjusting for socioeconomic factors and prenatal care indicate that the percentages of low birth weight and rates of infant mortality are fairly similar for the infants of adults and adolescents.[55] There are apparent linkages between low birth weight and other sequelae: epilepsy, cerebral palsy, mental retardation, a variety of learning disabilities, and a higher risk of deafness and blindness.[56] (Low birth weight is discussed further in Chap. 44.)

Infant Health Risks

McCormick and coworkers found high levels of health problems among infants of two groups of mothers, primiparas who were 17 years old or younger and multiparas who were 18 to 19 years old and who began their childbearing under the age of 18. They observed that despite decreases over the period of the study, neonatal mortality remained over one and a half times higher for infants of adolescent mothers than for those of other mothers. This was due largely to the relatively high proportion of low-birth-weight infants born to adolescent mothers. The adolescents had limited resources available to help them cope with their own and their infant's health problems.[57]

A variety of health problems have been found to contribute to increased infant mortality and morbidity, particularly in offspring of African-American adolescent mothers; these include hypoglycemia, respiratory distress syndrome, pneumonia, seizures and apnea, and necrotizing enterocolitis.[28,58] Additionally, infants of adolescent mothers experience an increased mortality in the postneonatal period from external events such as accidents, violence, and infection.[59] Infants born to younger adolescents have a higher rate of mortality by their second birthday than those born to older adolescents and adults.[60] The causes of this increased mortality and morbidity in infants of adolescent mothers are believed to be multifactorial, including client factors such as child spacing, SES, race, educational attainment, prenatal health care (availability and utilization), health habits (smoking, alcohol use, drug use, personal hygiene), low gynecological age, and acute and chronic medical problems. Utilization of early prenatal health care and avoidance of detrimental health habits are the most significant factors in limiting mortality, low birth weight, and prematurity.[49]

Psychosocial Risks for the Adolescent Parent and Child

The psychosocial consequences of premature parenting may be disturbing and appear to increase with socioeconomic disadvantage and decreasing age of adolescent parents. The findings of several recent studies suggest that adolescent mothers have poorer patterns of interaction with their infants and toddlers, spend less time talking to them, maintain less eye contact, and use less praise and more punishment than adult women.[50,61,62] Older adolescents often are able to view childrearing problems more realistically than younger adolescents because of their more advanced cognitive skills, greater psychosocial assets, and larger support networks. Young adolescent mothers tend to show aggressive behaviors toward the baby (jealous sibling), to use teasing, and to relate to the child like a plaything to meet their needs. Inconsistencies in parenting behaviors are often displayed by middle adolescents who sometimes are able to respond appropriately to their baby's needs and at other times are not interested.

Although the literature is inconclusive, there appears to be more neglectful parenting and a higher incidence of poor intellectual, developmental, and educational outcomes in children of adolescent mothers compared with children of older mothers.[40,62] Many of these differences become more pronounced as the children develop, with boys being more affected by adolescent childbearing than are girls, at least in the early years. By the high school years, educational failure and juvenile delinquency become major problems for the offspring of adolescent parents.[63]

The results of many studies suggest that low SES, poor education of the parents, and higher incidence of family instability with multiple caregivers are associated factors, rather than the specific age of the mother.[50,51,64] Changes in maternal life course (e.g., moving off welfare after the child's preschool years, entrance into a stable marriage) may significantly influence the child's outcome in the years after birth.

Sugar and others observed that to the extent that becoming an adolescent parent constrains or prohibits freedom of choice in a variety of areas (e.g., education, occupation, marriage), it inhibits the development of feelings of individual autonomy.[65,66] The occurrence of a first birth by age 18 has also been associated with a decrease in perceived personal efficacy among equally educated women from equivalent socioeconomic backgrounds.[66]

■ THE NURSING PROCESS AND THE WELL ADOLESCENT (PRIMARY PREVENTION)

Nursing care of the well adolescent is directed toward optimizing health status, preventing illness, and interrupting the sequence of steps leading to parenthood.[14] Although this section focuses on the latter area, secondary emphasis must be placed on the importance of appraising where the adolescent is physically, cognitively, and psychosocially along the developmental scale.[15,17,67] Particular consideration is given to assessment of health history, physical examination, and identification of health risks related to growth during adolescence (e.g., eating disorders, iron deficiency anemia, STDs, skin lesions, sports-related trauma, and dental caries). (See "Assessment Tool: Physical Examination for STDs" in Chap. 35.) Development of secondary sex

characteristics, menstrual history, and concerns about body image should be carefully assessed. Specific laboratory tests are often included in the health evaluation (e.g., hemoglobin and hematocrit, urinalysis, sickle cell screening for African-American adolescents, VDRL, and so forth).

One of the major nursing goals in primary prevention is to avert conception through either promotion of abstinence or with regular use of medically prescribed, effective methods of birth control.

Nurses employed in hospitals, community agencies, and schools have the opportunity to provide education, counseling, and family planning services that can prevent premature parenthood. A particularly important area for nursing involvement is in active outreach activities, especially to young, sexually active adolescents. To effectively provide care, the nurse must create an environment in which adolescents feel comfortable in seeking help with their health concerns. Adolescents are particularly interested in the issue of confidentiality, which, if not carefully considered, may serve as a significant access barrier to health care.[68] Providers, adolescents, and their parents need to be aware of the nature and effect of laws and regulations in their jurisdictions requiring notification or consent that may place constraints on relationships.

Family Life and Sex Education

The need for family life and sex education is foremost in the area of primary prevention because many adolescents do not comprehend the potential consequences of their sexual activity or, specifically, the risks of pregnancy with unprotected intercourse. The principal theme of the "Just Say Later" model is abstinence from sexual activity during adolescence. The "Safe Sex" model advocates prevention strategies on the assumption that most adolescents are going to be sexually active. Both models incorporate family life and sex education and counseling designed to increase the adolescent's knowledge and decision-making skills.[23] Results of many sex education studies indicate that increasing an adolescent's sexual knowledge does not increase his or her sexual activity and that adolescents acquire little information regarding sexuality from reliable sources.[15–17,26,27]

Family life and sex education should begin as soon as the child expresses curiosity about sex and related matters and can comprehend accurate explanations. Hayes and Crovitz recommend introduction of simple material as early as the third grade, with the content becoming more complex and detailed as the child grows.[69] The overriding object is to ensure that by the time the child is an adolescent, he or she has a clear understanding of how fertilization occurs and the events from fertilization through delivery and the postpartum periods, including both the biological and the social consequences of pregnancy. A variety of other topics may be included in family life and sex education programs such as the types of contraception available (see section entitled "Contraceptive Methods" in Chap. 11), the effects of childbearing on the adolescent's present life and future life course, and rational decision making. The importance of making conscious decisions regarding life options needs to be emphasized because many adolescents have difficulty delaying gratification and planning for the future. By strengthening the value of competing goals (such as school achievement and employment opportunities) and by providing alternative means of achieving goals (such as intimacy without sexual behavior or with regular contraceptive use), the adolescent's motivational constructs may be changed.[17] Adolescents often require assistance to recognize when they want to say no and to develop the skills to do so effectively.

The exact nature and scope of family life and sex education courses is partially determined by the sponsoring organization, the age of participants, the community involved, and available resources. Teaching methods need to be concrete, with frequent reinforcement of content provided because of the wide variation in abstract thinking abilities among adolescents. Role play may be employed as a method for assisting adolescents to cope with issues related to peer pressure and to explore individual decision making.

An increasingly important component of sex education and family life programs is teaching and counseling directed toward reducing the incidence of STDs, especially AIDS. Adolescents need to be aware of the many types of STDs for which they may be at risk. (See "Client Education: Preventing Transmission of STDs" in Chap. 35.) Specific methods for decreasing risk must be identified by the nurse (e.g., increasing the use of condoms, advocating the practice of less risky sexual behaviors, minimizing the sharing of needles among IV drug users, and decreasing and eliminating the use of intravenous drugs). Family life and sex education programs should be conducted by professionals who are knowledgeable and skilled group leaders. Parents need to be encouraged to participate in these programs, as well as to discuss sex and contraception with their children on an individual basis.

Contraception

Family planning services that provide education, counseling, contraceptives, and basic laboratory testing need to be accessible and available to adolescents. Three quarters of adolescent girls using contraception utilize prescription methods, primarily oral contraceptives.[17] The birth control pill appears to be the contraceptive method of choice for many adolescents because it may not be directly associated with planned sexual intercourse. In contrast, a barrier method, such as the diaphragm, may be rejected because adolescents perceive the technique as being messy and involving self-manipulation of the genitals. A comprehensive history and physical examination should precede the recommendation or prescription of contraception. (Further information on specific contraceptive methods is found in Chap. 11.)

Because contraceptive behavior may be influenced by many factors, it is important to identify and discuss the adolescent's concerns over side-effects of various techniques. Individual counseling about the actions, effectiveness, and safety of selected methods helps allay anxieties and ensure matching of the adolescent and an appropriate contraceptive method. Consideration must be given to the fact that actual behavior may not always be predicted by personal attitudes toward contraception.[70] The adolescent's motivation to control fertility must also be appraised. The sexually active adolescent who is not using or is ineffectively using contraceptives must be aided in recognizing a compelling reason for use of contraception, or there will be no change in behavior. For the adolescent who is not sexually active, counseling is directed toward reinforcing the choice of abstinence and supporting feelings of comfort with that decision.

■ THE NURSING PROCESS AND THE PREGNANT ADOLESCENT (SECONDARY PREVENTION)

Nursing care in the area of secondary prevention encompasses assessment, diagnosis, planning and intervention, and evaluation directed at supporting the adolescent and her family from conception through childbirth. The scope of secondary prevention differs depending on whether the decision is made to abort or to carry the fetus to term. The essential components of intervention programs for pregnant and childbearing adolescents, their families, and male partners have been identified by the Office of Adolescent Pregnancy Programs (OAPP) in the Department of Health and Human Services; these include pregnancy testing; maternity counseling; family planning counseling and services; primary and preventive health care; nutrition counseling, education, and services; venereal disease counseling, testing, and treatment; family life education; adop-

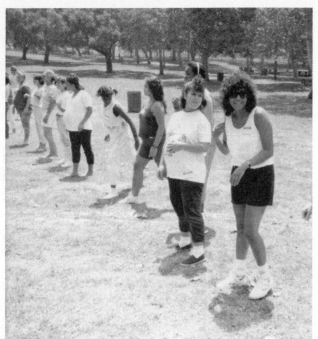

■ *Figure 37-3*
Intervention programs for pregnant and childbearing adolescents can have great impact on their well-being and quality of life. (Photo courtesy of St. Anne's Maternity Home.)

tion counseling and referral; and pediatric care. A well-planned and coordinated interdisciplinary effort is necessary to meet effectively the health-care needs of pregnant and parenting adolescents (Fig. 37-3). The nurse functions as an essential member of the multidisciplinary team, which is often comprised of physicians, social workers, nutritionists, psychologists, and other health professionals.

Early entry of the pregnant adolescent into the health-care system is of crucial importance in secondary prevention because a delayed onset of prenatal care or a decreased number of prenatal visits increases the risk for poor obstetric outcome. A variety of reasons may contribute to the pregnant adolescent's failure to seek adequate prenatal care; among these are lack of knowledge, lack of motivation, lack of financial resources, fear of exposure of the pregnancy and embarrassment, and fear of the health-care delivery system.

Assessment

The goal of assessment is to obtain the necessary data to plan interventions directed at promoting optimal health and development for the pregnant and parenting adolescent, her child, and family. The nurse's assessment of the adolescent includes both direct questions and clinical observations. Demonstration of genuine interest in the adolescent and the ability to be a good listener are essential for an accurate nursing assessment. Mercer identified four major areas of nursing assessment: (1) the adolescent's developmental level, (2) her health status, (3) her knowledge base, and (4) her social support system.[71]

DEVELOPMENTAL LEVEL

The adolescent's developmental level is assessed carefully by the nurse because it may differ from her chronological age. Examples of questions that may be presented in the assessment include: Have the major developmental tasks of adolescence been achieved? What personal values does the adolescent express? Does the adolescent demonstrate increasing independence from her parents and development of a strong sense of personal identity? Is the adolescent attending school or employed? How does she spend her free time and with whom? Does the adolescent keep her scheduled appointments for prenatal care and arrive on time? Is she able to express herself freely to members of the health team? What are her major goals and plans for the future? Is the adolescent in the cognitive stage of concrete thinking or formal operations? If she is able to present her situation logically and to consider her problems in the situation realistically, she is at the formal operations level of cognitive functioning.[9] Younger adolescents functioning at the concrete level are not capable of solving complex problems or understanding abstractions.

The adolescent's reaction to the psychological changes of pregnancy is a particularly important area of assessment. Does the adolescent's verbal expressions reflect a positive or negative attitude about being pregnant? Is she depressed over the pregnancy? Does she feel frightened or alone? What does this pregnancy represent to the adolescent? Does she verbally or nonverbally express negative feelings about her changing body image? What does the nurse observe about the adolescent's appearance (appropriateness of dress, posture, eye contact).

The adolescent's prenatal and postnatal feelings about the infant, and the quality of mother–infant interactions are influenced by her developmental level. What does the adolescent verbally and emotionally express about her child during the prenatal and postnatal periods (positive or negative statements, complaining remarks, facial gestures)? Are her self-care activities consistent with these expressions? Does the infant meet the adolescent's expectations about the fantasized child? Who does she think the baby looks like? How does the adolescent handle her infant (use of touch, stroking, verbalizations)? Does she avoid eye contact with her infant or seem tense during interaction? What is the adolescent's response to her infant's cries?

HEALTH STATUS

The nurse's assessment of the pregnant adolescent's health status includes a comprehensive nursing history, physical examination, and selected laboratory tests (Fig. 37-4). (A detailed discussion of the health status assessment and examples of prenatal assessment tools are contained in Chap. 19.) It is important for the nurse to devote particular attention to selected components of the assessment when caring for pregnant adolescents; these include the sexual history, substance abuse history, nutritional status, immunization status, and the pelvic examination.

Many adolescents are sensitive about their sexual history and may show embarrassment in responding to selected questions. The nurse should demonstrate a nonjudgmental attitude and reassure the adolescent that information related to initiation of coital activity and frequency, sexual partners, previous use of contraceptive methods, prior conceptions and abortions, and history of STDs will be kept confidential. The history of substance abuse includes questions related to past and current use of caffeine, nicotine, alcohol, and over-the-counter and recreational drugs.

The adequacy of the adolescent's dietary intake is determined using a comprehensive nutritional assessment tool (see Chap. 18). In assessing nutritional status,

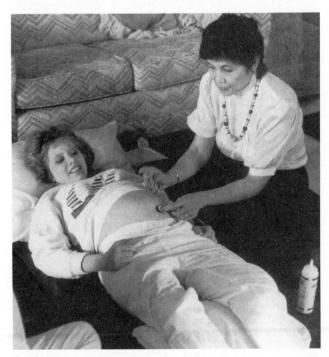

the nurse should understand that young adolescents are at higher risk for nutritional deprivation during pregnancy because they often have lower nutrient stores at the time of conception.[72] Their nutrition during pregnancy may not accommodate their own growth needs plus those of the fetus. In addition to assessing diet history (dietary habits, likes, and dislikes), the nurse must assess who in the adolescent's family is responsible for making major dietary choices (selecting, purchasing, preparing, and serving food). Because the adolescent is at risk for anemia, hemoglobin and hematocrit values are assessed.

Baseline weight and blood pressure measurements are determined. These two components of the physical assessment are significant because pregnancy-induced hypertension is the most prevalent medical complication of adolescent pregnancy.[49] Currency of immunizations is assessed (diphtheria, tetanus, polio, measles, mumps, and rubella), and tuberculosis screening is performed. Vision and dental evaluations may be given, if necessary.

Because the pelvic examination may be anxiety-inducing for the adolescent, the nurse prepares her for this assessment by carefully explaining each step of the procedure in relation to reproductive anatomy. Demonstration of relaxation techniques may be helpful. Some adolescents benefit from observing the examination by way of a mirror or by assisting in insertion of the speculum. Clinical pelvimetry is performed using a gentle technique to determine spatial capacity and risk for CPD. Cervical cytology is done to rule out dysplasia and carcinoma in situ. Additional gonococcal cultures and wet preps for *Candida, Chlamydia, Trichomonas,* and *Gardnerella* may be collected because of the increased incidence of STDs in adolescents. (See section entitled "Sexually Transmitted Diseases" in Chap. 35.)

In assessing health status, consideration must also be given to the influence of cultural and religious practices on the belief system of the pregnant adolescent. For example, many immigrants of Haiti living in areas such as New York and Miami are followers of voodoo.[73] Their belief system may include consultation with the root doctor and certain prescribed healing ceremonies. Hispanic pregnant adolescents may seek health care from Curanderas who reside in their communities. These people may offer information about folk remedies and general advice.[74]

KNOWLEDGE BASE

The nurse identifies the learning needs of the adolescent by assessing her knowledge base and determining her immediate and future concerns. Several important areas for assessment are described in the box entitled Assessment: Adolescent's Knowledge and Attitude.

Assessment: Adolescent's Knowledge and Attitude

Knowledge

- Sexual functioning
- Reproduction
- Pregnancy and childbirth
  Anatomy and physiology of pregnancy, labor and delivery, and postpartum
  Medications and anesthesia
  Breathing and relaxation techniques
- Infant growth and development
  Nutritional needs
  Developmental milestones
  Behavioral cues
- Parenting Skills
  Bathing
  Diapering
  Feeding
  Mother–infant communication
- Family planning
  Past experiences and preferences

Attitude and Feelings

- Preparations for infant
- Level of interest in learning about infant
- Discipline techniques and strategies
- Mother–infant interaction (during feeding and caretaking)

SOCIAL SUPPORT

The assessment of social support encompasses four types of supportive acts as defined by House: emotional support (empathy, caring, love, and trust), instrumental support (assistance with finances, child care, and so forth), informational support (information for problem solving), and appraisal support (information for self-evaluation).[75] The following specific questions may be asked by the nurse:

Who does the adolescent live with?
How does she feel about these people?
Does the SES of the family place the pregnant adolescent at risk?
What is the nature of her relationship with the infant's father and his family (marital or nonmarital relationship and quality of relationship)?
What types of support does the pregnant adolescent receive from family members, her partner, and friends (information, financial, and so forth)?
Other than the pregnancy, are there significant family or marital problems in the adolescent's life?

Who will help the adolescent care for her baby when she returns to school or work?
How long will this assistance be available?
Are agencies available in the adolescent's community to assist her with financial problems, child care, and educational and vocational needs?

If opportunity is available for interaction with other family members such as the adolescent's mother, the nurse should assess how they feel about the adolescent's pregnancy and capability for parenting and for adequacy of the home environment, asking such questions as:

Do they plan to provide the aid the adolescent expects?
How does the adolescent interact with members of the family?
Are the living conditions safe for a pregnant adolescent and infant (overcrowding, violence in neighborhood, pollutants)? Is transportation available to and from the prenatal care setting?

The specific needs of the adolescent father should be assessed by the nurse. Panzarine and Elster identified areas of potential psychosocial stresses that may be experienced by prospective adolescent fathers; these relate to (1) the role and responsibilities of fatherhood; (2) the relationship with his partner; (3) changes in usual sources of support; (4) the health of both mother and baby; and (5) anxiety regarding labor and delivery.[76]

The following are examples of specific questions that may be posed:

What are the young man's concerns regarding his role as father?
Is he experiencing any self-doubts about his capabilities to be a parent?
Does he express feelings of "being trapped," or does he feel committed to the relationship and the new baby?
What is the reaction of the adolescent father's family and friends to the pregnancy?
Is he interested in learning more about childbirth and child care?
What are his anxieties about labor and delivery and his role during this event?

Financial responsibilities and anticipated changes in vocational or educational plans may be of particular concern. Although many adolescent fathers do not have the skills necessary for securing a well-paying job, they may feel obligated to compromise school plans because of financial necessities.[76] The adolescent father's perceptions about his relationship with his partner may differ from those of the pregnant adolescent.

Diagnosis

The nursing diagnoses are based largely on psychosocial and physical data obtained during assessment. Adolescents are likely to possess knowledge deficits in several areas. Initially, these deficits may be related to pregnancy options available and related care needs. Later, knowledge deficits are related to physiological, psychological, and social implications of early childbearing, self-care needs during pregnancy, signs and symptoms of pregnancy complications, preparation for childbirth, infant growth and development, parenting skills, and family planning. Examples of specific diagnoses include:

- Altered nutrition: less than body requirement (related to lack of knowledge of adequate nutrition or availability of quality food)
- Body image disturbance related to pregnancy weight gain and altered body dimensions
- Altered comfort related to physiological changes of pregnancy
- Altered family processes related to the stress of adolescent pregnancy and parenting
- Self-concept disturbance related to conflict between the maternal role and identity formation
- Altered parenting related to impaired parent–infant attachment (bonding), adolescent egocentrism, inadequate support systems, or unrealistic expectations of the infant

Planning and Intervention

The adolescent's specific health-care plan depends on the stage of adolescence, her level of cognitive development, and ability to achieve the tasks of adolescence.[71] In general, nursing interventions are directed toward the following goals:

- Establishing a trusting relationship with the client. To achieve this goal, the nurse must be knowledgeable about normal adolescent growth and development and be aware of personal feelings about adolescent sexuality and pregnancy. Additionally, the nurse must demonstrate a nonjudgmental attitude and effective interpersonal communication skills.
- Securing a safe pregnancy outcome for the adolescent and her unborn child or a safe termination of pregnancy
- Promoting the adolescent's self-care activities during pregnancy, labor and delivery, and the puerperium (e.g., personal hygiene, exercise, nutrition, postpartum family planning, and follow-up)
- Assisting the adolescent to secure resources for meeting her support needs (emotional support, instrumental support, informational support, and appraisal support)
- Facilitating the adolescent's attainment of the maternal role, which includes demonstration of effective parenting skills and attachment behaviors
- Enhancing the adolescent's self-esteem and maturation

PREGNANCY

To meet the previously described goals most effectively, the adolescent should be assigned to a primary care nurse who is regularly responsible for her prenatal nursing care follow-up. The nurse must emphasize the importance of initiating care early in pregnancy, keeping prenatal appointments, and communicating significant symptoms and problems to members of the health-care team. Use of a nonauthoritarian manner in relating information is likely to improve nurse–client communications and to increase satisfaction with services and client compliance. Active involvement of the adolescent in the various components of her prenatal care (such as self-care activities and prenatal education) should be encouraged as an approach to promoting personal responsibility and autonomy. The adolescent's sense of control may be enhanced if she is allowed to test her urine, weigh herself, plan her diet, and listen to fetal heart tones.[71]

One of the most important aspects of nursing care is prenatal education. Instructional programs for pregnant adolescents may include information on the basic anatomy and physiology of pregnancy, labor and delivery and the postpartum; body mechanics and exercise during pregnancy; nutritional intake for pregnancy and lactation; signs of true versus false labor; breathing and relaxation techniques; breast-feeding; and family planning. To promote maternal role acquisition, anticipatory guidance should be provided about normal infant growth and development, child care, and mother–infant communication styles.

Prenatal classes may be offered in a variety of settings such as hospitals, churches, and other community agencies. Instructional programs are frequently divided into weekly sessions that vary in length from 30 minutes to 2 hours. Several teaching methods may be used, including lecture, discussion, demonstration, and role play. Active participation in activities such as role play helps the adolescent to integrate her personal experiences with theoretical knowledge.[77] Examples of situations appropriate for role play include (1) how to schedule follow-up well-baby care; (2) what to do when a child has a fever or diarrhea or a diaper rash; and (3) what to do when an infant doesn't stop crying in the middle of the night.

The nurse is likely to discover that giving demonstrations and having the adolescent perform selected

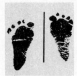

Nursing Care Plan

The Pregnant Adolescent

Nursing Objectives   The pregnant adolescent will demonstrate physiologicial and psychological adaptation to the stressors of adolescence and pregnancy as evidenced by:
1. Establishing a trusting relationship with the health-care team.
2. Performing self-care activities during pregnancy, labor and delivery, and the puerperium
3. Delivering a healthy term infant without perinatal complications
4. Securing needed resources for meeting support needs
5. Demonstrating attainment of the maternal role
6. Manifesting increased self-esteem and maturation

Assessment	Potential Nursing Diagnosis	Planning and Intervention	Outcome Criteria
Developmental and cognitive level	Self-concept disturbance related to conflict between the maternal role and identity formation	Assist in development of problem-solving techniques and provide positive reinforcement of problem-solving skills	Client demonstrates ability to problem solve effectively.
Relationship with peers and family			
Planned versus unplanned pregnancy			
Attitude towards pregnancy		Assist in achievement of the psychological tasks of pregnancy	Client progressively achieves the tasks of pregnancy
Achievement of the psychological tasks of pregnancy		Discuss potential areas of conflict between pregnancy and adolescence while offering psychological support regarding these conflicts (e.g., peer and family relationships, educational and personal goals)	Client expresses less conflict about maternal role and positive feelings about self and develops future plans for self and infant (e.g., child care, continued education, and employment).
Problem-solving skills			
Goals and values			
		Counsel regarding developmental versus pregnancy related psychological adaptation	Client identifies and differentiates normal psychological adaptations of adolescence and pregnancy
		Refer client to adolescent pregnancy support group	Client participates in an adolescent pregnancy support group
Concerns with body image	Body image disturbance related to body changes in pregnancy	Counsel client regarding normal body changes during pregnancy	Client verbalizes concerns about body changes during pregnancy. Client accepts body changes
Prepregnancy weight and weight gain during pregnancy			
Reactions of family and friends to body changes		Counsel client regarding ways to promote a posi-	Client dresses neatly, maintains a groomed ap-

(continued)

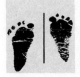

Nursing Care Plan *(continued)*

Assessment	Potential Nursing Diagnosis	Planning and Intervention	Outcome Criteria
Self-concept Developmental level		tive self-image (dressing neatly, grooming, and good posture)	pearance and good posture
Baseline weight and weight gain or loss during pregnancy HGB and HCT	Altered nutrition: Less than the body requirement related to lack of knowledge of adequate nutrition	Discuss relationship between weight gain, nutritional intake, and infant development Discuss foods to eat and to avoid to ensure nutritional intake	Client gains adequate weight (24–30 lb) Client follows adequate nutritional diet utilizing the four basic food groups. HGB and HCT levels remain within normal limits
Nutritional intake Nausea, vomiting, anorexia		Instruct client regarding the use of a 24-hour food diary and encourage its utilization	Client records dietary intake for 24 hours
Who is the primary meal preparer?		Collaborate with the primary meal provider to ensure nutritional foods are being prepared	Primary meal provider prepares nutritional foods.
Use of prescribed vitamins and iron		Instruct the client regarding the purpose, side-effects, and administration of prenatal vitamins and iron	Client takes prenatal vitamins and iron as prescribed
Financial constraints influencing dietary intake		Discuss financial management and refer to social services	Client effectively budgets for purchasing nutritional food
Maternal–infant attachment	Altered parenting related to impaired parent–infant attachment, adolescent egocentrism, inadequate support systems or unrealistic expectations of the infant	Discuss parenting skills and infant care Refer client to parenting and infant care classes	Client demonstrates appropriate parenting skills Client attends classes on parenting and infant care.
Clients expectations of infant behavior Developmental level		Discuss expectations of infant behavior and parenting role	Client states expectations and responsibilities of parenting role and infant behavior.
		Provide role-playing opportunities of parent–infant interactions	Client enacts appropriate parenting role.
		Explain importance of parent–infant attachment. Provide information to enhance bonding	Client seeks interactions with infant.

(continued)

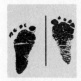

Nursing Care Plan   (continued)

Assessment	Potential Nursing Diagnosis	Planning and Intervention	Outcome Criteria
		Instruct client regarding bonding opportunities after delivery	Client seeks bonding opportunities after delivery.
Peer and family support systems		Discuss use of support systems as coping mechanisms for new parents	Client utilizes peer and family social support.
Client's relationship with family members, especially mother	Altered family processes related to the stress of adolescent pregnancy and parenting	Encourage communication of expectations between family members and client	Client and family communicate expectations
		Encourage discussion of future plans for client, infant, and family	Client makes future plans for self, infant, and family.
Extent of involvement of the baby's father		Encourage the involvement of the infant's father if both partners agree	Baby's father is present and supportive if agreeable
Role expectations of family members		Discuss importance of support from the family	Client is supported throughout pregnancy.

caretaking tasks (such as taking the infant's temperature, cleaning the cord, and burping) are more effective than didactic approaches in increasing knowledge. Audiovisual presentations and written materials should be used whenever possible to stimulate interest and to reinforce learning. Opportunities should be available for exploration of individual concerns and discussion of conflicts between information taught in class and practices in the home.

Nutritional counseling is provided on an individual basis. The four food groups should be reviewed in relation to fetal growth and development. The nurse should provide examples of food rich in iron and folate, because inadequate intake of these nutrients contributes to the high prevalence of anemia in adolescent pregnancy.[78,79] The distribution of additional weight to the baby, placenta, breasts, and body fluids should be fully explained to allay possible anxieties that the adolescent may have about excessive weight gain during pregnancy. Opportunities are provided for the adolescent to plan meals with consideration given to age-related and cultural preferences.

The nurse should initiate a referral to the nutritionist for follow-up services of the adolescent who is at nutritional risk because of poor weight gain, eating disorders, iron deficiency anemia, or slow fundal growth.

The Special Supplemental Food Program for Women, Infants, and Children (WIC) serves as an additional source of nutritional assistance for some pregnant adolescents (see Chap. 18).

Nursing intervention is also designed to assist the adolescent in developing problem-solving skills. To solve problems effectively, the adolescent must learn how to (1) identify the problem and the goal; (2) obtain appropriate data; (3) generate and weigh options; (4) decide on one option; and (5) implement the option and evaluate potential outcomes. Sachs recommends that adolescents be assisted with practice decision making in groups possessing similar cognitive skills.[20]

The family system of the pregnant adolescent must be considered in planning and implementing nursing care. A variety of family forms may exist; however, pregnant adolescents most frequently live with one or both parents or with another member of the family. The father of the infant also may be considered an important member of the unmarried or married adolescent's family. The nurse should facilitate effective family communications whenever possible by encouraging the adolescent to involve her family in the childbearing experience (e.g., attendance at prenatal classes and birth). Parental support is particularly important because it has been found to increase the potential for dealing with the adolescent's problems on a continuing basis.[80] Because the adolescent may have difficulty in accepting help from others and trusting that others will help her, the nurse may need to provide counseling on how to secure a supportive environment.

Consideration by the nurse of the adolescent father is also important because his needs are often ignored by health-care professionals. Before interacting with adolescent fathers, the nurse must carefully appraise whether any biased attitudes exist toward these young men. It is commonly assumed that adolescent fathers are uninterested in becoming involved in their partner's pregnancies or the rearing of their children; however, the results of several studies indicate that many young fathers become deeply involved when permitted.[81-83] The nurse can assist the prospective adolescent father to cope with the stresses of pregnancy by several interventions. Including him in the decision-making process is particularly helpful because it may allay his fears, decrease his sense of helplessness and alienation, and provide an opportunity to function in an adult role.[84] Counseling is provided early in the prenatal period, whenever possible, regarding the psychological and physiological changes occurring during pregnancy and how these may impact on the couple's relationship. Accurate information about the childbirth process and health-care services should be included. The prospective father should be invited to attend routine prenatal visits and to participate by listening to fetal heart tones and palpating fetal movements. Anticipatory guidance is offered regarding issues specific to adolescent fatherhood (e.g., the father's role in labor and delivery, future financial responsibilities, sources of support, and legal rights). The couple should be encouraged to verbalize their feelings about the pregnancy and expectations of each other during the phases of childbearing and childrearing.

LABOR AND DELIVERY

Optimal intrapartum care for adolescents should include all of the features of nursing care described in Chapter 22. Adolescents have a particularly great need for adequate support during labor because they may be afraid of the hospital and have fears related to lack of accurate knowledge of the birthing process. Adequate intrapartum support is also important because it has been associated with a decreased need for analgesia and anesthesia, lower pain, more enjoyment, and greater satisfaction with the birth experience.[85] Unfortunately, many adolescents do not have supportive family members, mates, or friends present during the intrapartum period. Therefore, supportive nursing interventions are particularly needed and beneficial; these may include information about the labor and delivery process, demonstration of relaxation and breathing techniques to cope with contractions, provision of physical comfort measures, and encouragement and reassurance. Continuous primary care from the same nurse is highly desirable whenever possible.

If the infant's father is present and interested in supporting the laboring adolescent, his active participation in the birth process should be encouraged. The nurse may need to support the father in his efforts to assist his partner, to interact with the infant after delivery, and to cope with his new parenting role. The initiation and maintenance of early infant contact after delivery is especially important for adolescent parents (Fig. 37-5). The nurse may assist the adolescent mother and father in getting acquainted with their infant by encouraging touch, verbalization, proximity, and caretaking behaviors.

PUERPERIUM

The adolescent mother requires the same physical nursing care in the postpartum period as the adult woman (see Chap. 28). However, her developmental and cognitive level may necessitate further focus on self-care (perineal and breast care, sleep and rest, comfort measures) and selected psychosocial aspects of the puerperium. In particular, emphasis needs to be placed on planning and implementing nursing care to promote the adolescent's maternal role acquisition. The nurse should provide:

- Opportunities for extended contact with the infant. Rooming-in or mother–baby units are bene-

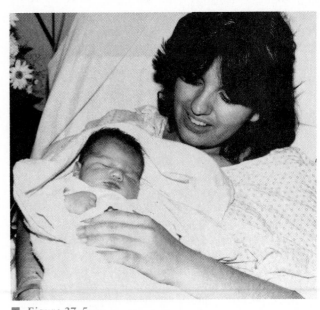

■ *Figure 37-5*
The initiation of early infant contact helps the adolescent adjust to her new role as mother. (Photo courtesy of St. Anne's Maternity Home.)

ficial because these care options allow the adolescent mother to receive more patient teaching, promote satisfaction with care, and may increase attachment to the infant.[86]

- Instruction and counseling regarding safe and effective parenting skills such as infant feeding (techniques, timing, positioning, intake), bathing, diapering, and dressing. Content on "how to care for the sick baby" and " protecting the infant from accidents" should also be presented. The latter two informational needs were identified as most important in a survey of postpartum adolescents.[87] Other instructional areas include the stages of infant and child growth and development, methods to enhance the child's cognitive and social development through maternal verbalizations and sensory stimulation (see Chap. 31), infant supplies, alternative methods of child care, and immunizations.
- Positive reinforcement of self-care activities and effective mothering skills. Whenever desired maternal behaviors are demonstrated, the nurse should praise the client, because this reinforcement can enhance her self-esteem and promote learning.

The developmental level and cognitive abilities of the adolescent must be considered in client teaching and counseling. Younger adolescent mothers may prefer short sessions of individualized instruction rather than formal hospital classes that remind them of school. "Hands-on" teaching sessions are particularly effective with adolescents whose thinking is still fairly concrete.[88] To maximize learning with group instruction, classes should be short in length, small in size, and conducted among peers. Media such as videocassettes, film, and closed circuit hospital television may be useful for instruction because many adolescents are familiar and comfortable with these techniques. If written materials are distributed, they should be appropriate for the adolescent's developmental and reading level.

The nurse may assist the adolescent to make decisions about family planning by first asking her about her knowledge of contraception and her experience with various methods. Misconceptions about actions and side-effects of specific contraceptive methods should be clarified. Regardless of the preferred method of contraception, the nurse must determine how the adolescent will obtain and pay for the contraceptive. If medical supervision is required, the adolescent should be aware of sources of follow-up health care.

In providing postpartum care, it is important to remember that the adolescent's normal egocentrism may require the nurse first to concentrate care on the mother and her immediate concerns. Feelings about the labor and delivery experience and her current physical status

often need to be discussed before infant caretaking. Some young mothers appear excessively demanding of the nurse's attention and time because of fears related to their lack of experience with child care and hospitalization. Others seem passive and afraid to initiate interactions with their infant until the nurse or a close family member is present. Older adolescents may demonstrate effective problem-solving skills and the ability to communicate their needs clearly to the nurse.

Several interventions may facilitate interpersonal communications with adolescent mothers who often have difficulty spontaneously speaking with adults.[88] The nurse should avoid open-ended questions and long silences because they may increase the adolescent's anxiety. Gentle inquiries and supportive statements may help to relax the adolescent (e.g., "young mothers are often concerned about"). A checklist approach to assessment should be avoided.

Early discharge planning is of prime importance in the care of postpartum adolescents, their infants and families. Optimally, plans for follow-up care are begun during pregnancy and are a component of the comprehensive adolescent health-care service. In situations where this type of assistance is unavailable or the adolescent has received no prenatal care, the nurse may need to initiate a referral to the social worker for additional support (such as housing, financial aid, temporary foster care for the infant, WIC, alternative schools with child care). The adolescent should be referred to the community health nurse if continued assessment and instruction are required for self-care or educational needs. Research indicates that most adolescent mothers and fathers benefit from parenting education programs offered during early childrearing.[89,90] A variety of programs may be available in local schools and community facilities. The nurse may provide valuable assistance by discussing the advantages of these programs and giving the adolescent mother current information on the types and locations of adolescent parenting groups.

ABORTION CARE

The physical and psychosocial nursing care needs of adolescents considering clinical interruption of pregnancy are similar to those of adult women (see Chap. 12). The procedure to be used for an abortion is determined by the length of pregnancy. Before counseling a pregnant adolescent about abortion as an alternative option to childbearing, the nurse must be knowledgeable about state law regarding minors' abortion. A minor woman has a constitutional right to consent to an abortion; however, states may impose parental notification requirements consistent with constitutional principles. Parental approval or notification is not required unless the state has enacted such a requirement.[91] In states having no legal requirement for parental notification, informing a parent, without the adolescent's permission, of her intent to have an abortion, may subject the nurse to liability for breach of client confidentiality.

The adolescent receiving abortion counseling is likely to have had little or no experience with an unplanned pregnancy or abortion decision. She may experience feelings of fear related to being judged by health-care professionals, confusion, and isolation. Multiple or conflicting goals may make the decision to abort complex (e.g., the desire to please her parents and her partner, affirm her own values and ethics, and balance a career and motherhood goals).[92] Through reflective listening, the nurse can help the adolescent to clarify the conflicts she may be experiencing between the needs of self and the needs of her partner and family. Other issues surrounding the adolescent's abortion decision that may need to be addressed by the nurse in counseling include how to (1) inform her partner and parents about the pregnancy; (2) secure funds for the abortion procedure; and (3) explain absence from school or work.

Evaluation

Evaluation of nursing care is conducted through a variety of techniques. Records are maintained on the adolescent's attendance at prenatal visits. Learning outcomes in prenatal classes may be evaluated by written multiple choice tests, verbal questions, and problem-solving exercises. Logs containing descriptions of the adolescent's behavior observed by nurses in the labor and delivery and postpartum units are also helpful. The health and growth of the infant may be evaluated by progression of height and weight, immunization status, incidence of illness, emergency room visits, and hospitalizations.

Other examples of specific criteria for evaluating nursing care are described below. The adolescent:

- Initiates early prenatal care and returns for regular prenatal care
- Implements appropriate self-care activities during pregnancy (adequate nutrition, exercise, personal hygiene, attendance at prenatal classes)
- Establishes and maintains a positive relationship with a support person during pregnancy, labor and delivery, and the puerperium
- Demonstrates an increase in self-esteem and maturity level during pregnancy
- Effectively copes with labor and delivery.
- Delivers a healthy, term infant of birth weight within normal limits
- Acquires appropriate maternal role behaviors (affection for baby; appropriate and safe feeding, bathing, and diapering techniques; effective communications, recognition of illness)
- Returns for scheduled family planning follow-up care and well-baby care.
- Expresses gratification in the maternal role
- Secures needed assistance for continued schooling or employment and other needs through appropriate utilization of community resources

■ THE NURSING PROCESS AND THE CHILDREARING ADOLESCENT (TERTIARY PREVENTION)

The objectives of tertiary prevention are (1) to enhance the ability of the adolescent mother and her family to assume useful, satisfying, and self-sufficient roles in society; (2) to optimize the physical, psychosocial, and intellectual development of the adolescent's child; and (3) to prevent recidivism (rapid, repeat, unplanned pregnancy). Most repeat adolescent pregnancies are unplanned and unwanted. The younger the adolescent at the time of her first pregnancy, the more likely she will conceive again as an adolescent. Two major studies have reported a 30% to 40% incidence for second pregnancies by 24 months after birth.[93,94] Repeat pregnancies during adolescence are of concern because there is greater morbidity and mortality for the subsequent children born to adolescents, as well as spiraling psychosocial problems.[95] Factors associated with a decrease in repeat pregnancies include return to school after delivery, and extending comprehensive health and social services beyond the immediate postpartum period.[96]

Tertiary prevention programs employ a multidisciplinary team that may consist of nurses, case managers, nutritionists, counselors, physicians, social workers, and teachers. Services available are individualized for the needs and stage of development of each parent, the infant, and family. A variety of specialized services may be offered, such as (1) family planning and reproductive health services; (2) pediatric care—well-baby care and emergency care for young children; (3) parenting education; (4) life skills training (consumer education, budgeting, household financial management, homemaking skills); (5) alternative school programs; (6) employment training and counseling; and (7) referral to community support services (WIC, Aid for Dependent Children [ADC], child care, and so forth).

The role of the nurse in tertiary prevention programs varies greatly. In some programs, the nurse assumes broad responsibilities as the case manager accountable for coordination of services; in other programs, the nurse's role is narrower in scope (e.g., family planning nurse, parenting class instructor, support group leader).

Opportunities exist in many tertiary prevention programs for an ongoing relationship between the nurse and the adolescent mother. The nurse should encourage involvement of the adolescent's family system in supporting her efforts to gain the education and skills that optimize her life choices and to rear her infant in a nurturing and stimulating environment. Research findings indicate that African-American grandmothers, in particular, provide valuable support which ensures that adolescents develop in their mothering roles and prepares them for the full responsibility of infant care.[97] The infant's father may also have an important impact on how the adolescent mother adapts to parenthood. The nurse may assist the father by helping him to perceive his parental role realistically and by facilitating communications with his child's mother. Promoting mutual responsibility for the well-being of the child is one of the major challenges nurses face in caring for adolescent parents.

■ REFERENCES

1. Marcia JE: Identity in adolescence. In Adelson J (ed): Handbook of Adolescent Psychology, pp 159–187. New York, Wiley & Sons, 1980
2. Havighurst RJ: Developmental Tasks and Education. New York, D McKay Co, 1972
3. Greydanus DE: Risk-taking behaviors in adolescence. JAMA 258(15):2110, October 1987
4. Blum R: Contemporary threat to adolescent health in the United States. JAMA 257:3390–3395, 1987
5. Howe CL: Developmental theory and adolescent sexual behavior. Nurse Practitioner 11(2):65–71, February 1986
6. Erikson EH: Identity and the life cycle (monograph). Psychol Issues 1(1):1–171, 1959
7. Marcia JE: Development and validation of ego identity status. J Pers Soc Psychol 3:551–558, 1966
8. Marcia JE: Ego identity status: Relationship to change in self-esteem, "general maladjustment," and authoritarianism. J Pers 35:119–133, 1967
9. Piaget J: The theory of stages in cognitive development. In Green D (ed): Measurement and Piaget. New York, McGraw-Hill, 1971
10. Sadler LS, Catrone C: The adolescent parent: A dual developmental crisis. J Adol Health Care 4:100–105, 1983
11. Hayes CD (ed): Risking the Future: Adolescent Sexuality, Pregnancy and Childbearing, Vol I. Washington, DC, National Academy Press, 1987
12. Hofferth SL, Hayes CD (eds): Risking the Future: Adolescent Sexuality, Pregnancy, and Childbearing, Vol II. Washington, DC, National Academy Press, 1987
13. Hogan P, Kitagawa E: The impact of social status, family structure and neighborhood on the fertility of black adolescents. Am J Sociology 90:825–855, 1985

14. Flick LH: Paths to adolescent parenthood: Implications for prevention. Public Health Rep 101(2):132–147, 1986
15. Howard M, McCabe JB: Helping teenagers postpone sexual involvement. Fam Plann Perspect 22(4):21–26, January/February 1990
16. Trussele J: Teenage pregnancy in the United States. Fam Plann Perspect 20(6):262–271, November/December 1988
17. Brooks-Gunn J, Furstenberg FF: Adolescent sexual behavior. Am Psychol 44(2):249–257, February 1989
18. Friede AF, Hogue CJR, Doyle LL et al: Do the sisters of childbearing teenagers have increased rates of childbearing? Am J Public Health 76(10):1221–1224, October 1986
19. Abrahamse AF, Morrison PA, Waite LJ: Beyond Stereotypes: Who Becomes a Single Teenage Mother? New York, Rand, 1988
20. Sachs B: Reproductive decisions in adolescence. Image J Nurs Sch 18(2):69–72, Summer 1986
21. Alan Guttmacher Institute: Factbook on Teenage Pregnancy. New York, Alan Guttmacher Institute, 1981
22. Jones EF, Forrest JD, Goldman N et al: Teenage pregnancy in developed countries: Determinants and policy implications. Fam Plann Perspect 17(2):53–63, 1985
23. Macdonald DI: An approach to the problem of teenage pregnancy. Public Health Rep 102(4):377–385, July/August 1987
24. Zelnik M, Shah FK: First intercourse among young Americans. Fam Plann Perspect 14(3):117–126, May/June 1983
25. Orr DP, Wilbrandt ML, Brack CS et al: Reported sexual behaviors and self-esteem among young adolescents. Am J Dis Child 143:86–90, January 1989
26. Zabin LS, Kanter JF, Zelnik M: The risk of adolescent pregnancy in the first months of intercourse. Fam Plann Perspect 11(4):215–222, July/August 1979
27. Marsiglio W, Mott FL: Impact of sex education on sexual activity, contraceptive use and premarital pregnancy. Fam Plann Perspect 18(4):151–162, July/August 1986
28. Alan Guttmacher Institute: Teenage Pregnancy: The Problem That Hasn't Gone Away. New York, Alan Guttmacher Institute, 1981
29. Kafka D (ed): NYC teenagers who are young, white or unmarried are the most likely to end unwanted pregnancies. Fam Plann Perspect 20(5):240–241, September/October 1988
30. Neilsen L: Adolescent Psychology: A Contemporary View. New York, Holt Rinehart & Winston, 1987
31. Resnick M: Adoption decision-making project. Washington, DC, Office of Adolescent Pregnancy Prevention, US Department of Health and Human Services, 1984
32. McLaughlin SD, Manninen DL, Winges LD: Do adolescents who relinquish their children fare better or worse than those who raise them? Fam Plann Perspect 20(1):25–32, January/February 1988
33. Juhasz AM, Sonnenshein-Schneider M: Adolescent sexual decision-making: Components and skills. Adolescence 15:743–750, 1980

34. Henshaw SK, Van Vort J: Teenage abortion, birth and pregnancy statistics: An update. Fam Plann Perspect 21(2):85–88, 1989

35. Facts at a Glance. Washington, DC, Child Trends Inc, 1989

36. National Center for Health Statistics (NCHS): Advance Report of Final Natality Statistics, 1986. Monthly Vital Statistics Report, 37(3)(suppl), 1988

37. MMWR: CDC Surveillance Summaries 38(38):664. Atlanta, GA, US Dept of Health and Human Services, September 29, 1989

38. Henshaw SK, Forrest JD, Van Vort J: Abortion services in the United States, 1987 and 1988. Fam Plann Perspect 22(3):102–108, 142, 1990

39. Duncan GJ, Hoffman SD: Teenage welfare receipt and subsequent dependence among black adolescent mothers. Fam Plann Perspect 22:16–20, 1990

40. Furstenberg FF, Levine JA, Brooks-Gunn J: The children of teenage mothers: Patterns of early childbearing in two generations. Fam Plann Perspect 22(2):54–61, 1990

41. Alan Guttmacher Institute: US and Crossnational Trends in Teenage Sexuality. New York, Alan Guttmacher Institute, 1984

42. Center for Population Options: Adolescent Abortion and Parental Involvement Laws: Encouraging Communication or Conflict? Washington, DC, Center for Population Options, 1989

43. Furstenberg FF, Crawford A: Family support, helping teenage mothers to cope. Fam Plann Perspect 8:148–164, 1978

44. Friedman SB, Phillips S: Psychosocial risk to mother and child as a consequence of adolescent pregnancy. In McAnarney ER (ed): Premature Adolescent Pregnancy and Parenthood, pp 269–277. New York, Grune & Stratton, 1983

45. Moore KA, Burt MR: Private Crisis, Public Cost: Policy Perspectives on Teenage Childbearing. Washington, DC, Urban Institute, 1982

46. Elster AB, Lamb ME, Tavare J: Association between behavioral and school problems and fatherhood in a national sample of adolescent youths. J Pediatr 111(6):932–936, December 1987

47. Hardy JB, Duggan AK: Teenage fathers and the fathers of infants of urban, teenage mothers. Am J Public Health 78(8):919–922, August 1988

48. Committee on Adolescence: Care of adolescent parents and their children. Pediatrics 83(1):138–140, 1989

49. Zuckerman B, Walker DK, Frank DA et al: Adolescent pregnancy and parenting. Advances Dev Behav Peds 7:275–311, 1986

50. Spivak H, Weitzman M: Social barriers faced by adolescent parents and their children. JAMA 258(11):1500–1504, September 1987

51. Gale R, Seidman DS, Dollberg S et al: Is teenage pregnancy a neonatal risk factor? J Adol Health Care 10(5):404–408, September 1989

52. Cates W, Rauh JL: Adolescents and sexually transmitted diseases: An expanding problem. Introduction. J Adol Health Care 6(4):257–261, 1985

53. Curran JW, Jaffe HW, Hardy AM et al: Epidemiology of HIV infection and AIDS in the United States. Science 239:610–616, 1988

54. Brooks-Gunn J, Boyers CB, Hein K: Preventing HIV infection and AIDS in children and adolescents: Behavioral research and intervention strategies. Am Psychol 43:958–964, 1988

55. McAnarney E: Young maternal age and adverse neonatal outcome. Am J Dis Child 141:1053–1059, 1987

56. Phipps-Yonas S: Teenage pregnancy and motherhood. Am J Orthopsychiatry 50(3):403–431, 1980

57. McCormick L, Shapiro S, Starfield G: High-risk young mothers: Infant mortality and morbidity in four areas in the United States, 1973–1978. Am J Public Health 74(1):18–23, 1984

58. Miller KA, Field CS: Adolescent pregnancy: Critical review for the clinician. Semin Adolesc Med 1(3):195–211, 1985

59. Babson G, Clarke N: Relationship between infant death and maternal age. J Pediatr 103:391–393, 1983

60. Lawrence RA, Merritt TA: Infants of adolescent mothers: Perinatal, neonatal and infancy outcome. Semin Perinatol 5:19–32, 1981

61. Osofsky JD, Culp AM, Ware LM: Intervention challenges with adolescent mothers and their infants. Psychiatry 51:236–241, 1988

62. Brooks-Gunn J, Furstenberg FF: The children of adolescent mothers: Physical, academic, and psychological outcomes. Developmental Review 6:224–251, 1986

63. Furstenberg FF, Brooks-Gunn J, Morgan P: Adolescent Mothers in Later Life. New York, Cambridge University Press, 1987

64. Coll CG, Vohr BR, Hoffman J et al: Maternal and environmental factors affecting developmental outcome of infants of adolescent mothers. Dev Beh Pediatr 7(4):230–236, August 1986

65. Sugar M: Developmental issues in adolescent motherhood. In Sugar M (ed): Female Adolescent Development, pp 330–343. New York, Brunner/Mazel, 1979

66. McLaughlin SD, Micklin M: The timing of the first birth and changes in personal efficacy. J Marriage Fam 45(1):47–55, February 1983

67. Daniel WA, Brown RT, Garrison CL: Adolescence: The clinical encounter and common health problems. In Mercer RT (ed): Perspectives on Adolescent Health Care, pp 147–171. Philadelphia, JB Lippincott, 1979

68. Thompson HA: Consent requirements for treatment of minors. Tex Med 85(8):56–59, August 1989

69. Hayes L, Crovitz E: Adolescent pregnancy. South Med J 72(7):869–874, 1979

70. Gispert M, Brinich P, Wheeler K et al: Predictors of repeat pregnancies among low-income adolescents. Hosp Community Psychiatry 35(7):719–723, 1984

71. Mercer RT: Assessing and counseling teenage mothers during the perinatal period. Nurs Clin North Am 18(2):293–301, June 1983

72. Frisancho AR, Matos J, Flegel P: Maternal nutritional status and adolescent pregnancy outcome. Am J Clin Nutr 38(5):739–746, 1983

73. Gustafson MB: Western voodoo: Providing mental health care to Haitian refugees. J Psychosoc Nurs Ment Health Serv 27(12):22–25, 1989

74. Clark AL: Culture/Childbearing/Health Professionals. Philadelphia, FA Davis, 1979

75. House JS: Work Stress and Social Support. Reading, MA, Addison-Wesley, 1981

76. Panzarine S, Elster AB: Prospective adolescent fathers: Stresses during pregnancy and implications for nursing interventions. J Psychosoc Nurs Ment Health Serv 20(7):21–24, 1982

77. Ruszala-Herbst H: Providing primary care to adolescent mothers and their babies. In Robinson J, Sachs B (eds): Nursing Care Models for Adolescent Families, pp 29–31. Kansas City, MO, American Nurses' Association, 1984

78. Bailey LB, Mahan CS, Dimperio D: Folate and iron status in low-income pregnant adolescents and mature women. Am J Clin Nutr 33:1997–2001, 1980

79. Kaminetsky HA, Langer A, Baker H: The effect of nutrition in teenage pravidas on pregnancy and status of the neonate. Am J Obstet Gynecol 29:1276–1383, 1976

80. Hartman K (ed): Joint statement on adolescent health care. NAACOG Newsletter 16(4):5–16, April 1989

81. Hardy JB, Duggan AK, Masnyk K et al: Fathers of children born to young urban mothers. Fam Plann Perspect 21(4):159–163, 187, 1989

82. Redmond MA: Attitudes of adolescent males toward adolescent pregnancy and fatherhood. Family Relations 34:337–342, 1985

83. Robinson BE, Barret RL: The developing father: Emerging trends in contemporary society. New York, Guilford Press, 1986

84. Barret RL, Robinson BE: Adolescent fathers: Often forgotten parents. Pediatric Nursing 12:273–277, 1986

85. Hodnett DE, Osborn RW: A randomized trial of the effects of montrice support during labor: Mothers' views two to four weeks postpartum. Birth 16(4):177–183, December 1989

86. Winkelstein ML, Carson VJ: Adolescents and rooming-in. Matern Child Nurs J 16(1):75–88, Spring 1987

87. Howard JS, Sater J: Adolescent mothers: Self-perceived health education needs. J Obstet Gynecol Neonatal Nurs 14:399–404, 1985

88. Fullar SA: Care of postpartum adolescents. MCN 11:398–403, 1986

89. Glanville CL, Tiller CM: Implementing negotiating strategies into teen parenting programs. J Natl Black Nurses Assoc 4(1):45–54, Fall/Winter 1990

90. Heifer RE: The perinatal period, a window of opportunity for enhancing parent–infant communication: An approach to prevention. Child Abuse Negl 11(4):565–579, 1987

91. Rhodes AM: MCN focus on legal issues: Options and issues for pregnant adolescents. MCN 13:427, 1988

92. Brown MA: Adolescent and abortion: A theoretical framework for decision making. J Obstet Gynecol Neonatal Nurs 12:241–247, 1983

93. Zelnik M: Second pregnancies to premarital pregnant teenagers. Fam Plann Perspect 12:69–76, 1980

94. Mott EL: The pace of repeat childbearing among young American mothers. Fam Plann Perspect 18(1):5–12, January/February 1986

95. McAnarney E, Thiede HA: Adolescent pregnancy and childbearing: What we learned during the 1970s and what remains to be learned. In McAnarney E (ed): Premature Adolescent Pregnancy and Parenthood, pp 375–395. New York, Grune & Stratton, 1983

96. Stevens-Simon C, Parsons J, Montgomery C: What is the relationship between postpartum withdrawal from school and repeat pregnancy among adolescent mothers? J Adol Health Care 7:191–194, 1986

97. Flaherty MJ: Seven caring functions of black grandmothers in adolescent mothering. Matern Child Nurs J 17(3):191–207, 1988

■ SUGGESTED READING

Barret RL: Adolescent fathers: Often forgotten fathers. Pediatr Nurs 12(4):273–277, 1986

Burt M, Haffner D: Teenage Child Bearing: How Much Does It Cost? Washington, DC, Center for Population Control, 1986

CDF's Adolescent Pregnancy Prevention Clearing House: Adolescent Pregnancy: An Anatomy of a Social Problem in Search of Comprehensive Solutions. Washington, DC, Children's Defense Fund, 1987

Clewell BC, Brooks-Gunn J, Benasich AA: Evaluating child related outcomes of teenage parenting programs. Family Relations 38:201–209, 1989

Corbett M, Meyer JH: The Adolescent and Pregnancy. Boston, Blackwell Scientific, 1987

Dash L: When Children Want Children. New York, William Morrow, 1989

Furstenberg FF Jr, Brooks-Gunn J, Morgan SP: Adolescent Mothers in Later Life. Cambridge, Cambridge University Press, 1988

McAnarney ER (ed): Premature Adolescent Pregnancy and Parenthood. New York, Grune & Stratton, 1983

Mercer RT: First-Time Motherhood: Experiences from Teens to Forties. New York, Springer, 1986

Osofsky JD, Culp AM, Ware LM: Intervention challenges with adolescent mothers and their infants. Psychiatry 51:236–241, 1988

Weatherley RA, Perlman SB, Levine MH et al: Comprehensive programs for pregnant teenagers and teenage parents: How successful have they been? Fam Plann Perspect 18(2):73–78, March/April 1986

Whitman TL, Borkowski JG, Schellenbach CJ et al: Predicting and understanding developmental delay of children of adolescent mothers: A multidimensional approach. Am J Ment Defic 92(1):40–56, 1987

Yoos L: Perspectives on adolescent parenting: Effect of adolescent egocentrism on the maternal–child interaction. Pediatr Nurs 2(3):193–200, 1987

38

Complications of Labor

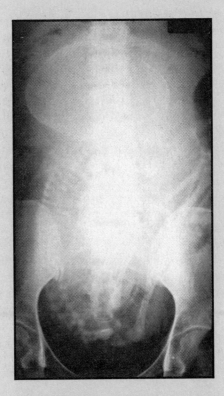

Acomplicated labor requires sensitive and astute nursing care, because it represents a period of great stress for the laboring woman, her partner, nurses, and physicians. The principles of nursing care during normal labor (see Chap. 22) also apply when the labor is complicated, with certain modifications depending on the nature of the problems. The nurse's ability to use clinical judgment is crucial, because the nursing diagnoses and care deriving from such judgments may be of lifesaving significance to both the mother and the infant. Assessment skills including observation, interviewing, and physical examination provide important data on the nature and extent of the problem. Reporting, recording, and professional intercommunication promote accurate decision making and implementation of appropriate treatment. Physical and emotional supportive measures assist the mother and father to understand and cope with the unusual events in the labor experience, which is often prolonged and painful.

■ DYSTOCIA

Dystocia, or difficult labor, is a term usually used to refer to a labor that is made longer or more painful by problems with the mechanics of the labor, involving the "three Ps," the powers, passageway, and passenger (discussed in Chaps. 20 and 21). A fourth "P," the person or psyche, is often added to the list because certain aspects of maternal response to labor can also affect the length of labor. These problems in mechanics of labor may include any or a combination of the following:

Powers. The uterine contractions may not be sufficiently strong or appropriately coordinated during the first stage of labor to effect cervical dilatation and effacement, or during the second stage, voluntary pushing combined with uterine contractions may not be sufficient to effect descent and expulsion of the fetus.

Passageway. There may be variations in the size and shape of the bony pelvis or other abnormalities of the reproductive tract that interfere with engagement, descent, or expulsion of the fetus.

Passenger. There may be faulty presentation or position, unusual size, or abnormal development of the fetus that prevents entrance into or passage through the birth canal.

Psyche. Maternal factors such as anxiety, lack of preparation, and fear can interact with the other factors, or sometimes operate alone, to cause prolongation of the labor.

Therefore, for progress in labor to be made and the birth to occur, the forces or *powers,* including uterine contractions and maternal "bearing down" in second stage, must be coordinated and of adequate strength to propel an irregular object, the fetus, or *passenger,* through the birth canal, or *passageway.* The passenger must be of appropriate size and shape and able to undergo the necessary maneuvers to pass through the different dimensions of the birth canal. The passageway must also be of normal size and configuration and not present undue obstacles to the descent, rotation, and expulsion of the baby.

Problems With the Powers— Uterine Dysfunction

CLASSIFICATION AND RESEARCH

Many attempts have been made to classify labors that do not follow the usual pattern, so that the problems may be more easily identified and managed. One method is classification according to the *quality* of uterine contractions. Ineffectual contractions can be described as hypotonic, hypertonic, or incoordinate.[1] A second classification is by *time of onset.* Primary inertia (dysfunction) occurs at the beginning of labor. Secondary inertia develops after labor is established.

Dysfunctional labor may also be classified by the *pattern and timing* of the disruption of progress. Friedman has plotted cervical dilatation and degree of descent against lapsed time on a graph, demonstrating the normal labor pattern as an S-shaped curve (see Fig. 21-1). Categories of delayed progression according to Friedman are prolonged latent phase, protraction disorders, and arrest disorders (Fig. 38-1).[2]

There is some overlapping between these classifications. Hypertonic uterine dysfunction, primary inertia, and prolonged latent phase all occur in early labor and are most common in the nullipara. Hypotonic uterine dysfunction, secondary inertia, and protraction or arrest of the active phase all occur later in labor and tend to be more common in the multipara.

A number of researchers have contributed to the understanding and measurement of uterine contractions. Larks described the stimulus of a contraction as starting in one cornu and developing several milliseconds later in the other cornu, then joining and descending down over the fundus and upper uterine segment, resulting in a pulling up of the isthmus and cervix.[3] Caldeyro-Barcia and associates in Montevideo determined that the pressure of a contraction necessary to dilate the cervix is at least 15 mm Hg. Measurement of contractions in terms of Montevideo units, the average intensity of the uterine contractions multiplied by the number of contractions in a 10-minute period, also

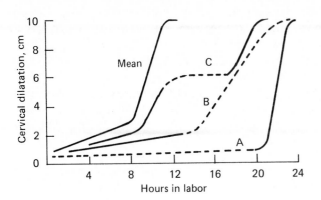

■ *Figure 38–1*
The major labor aberrations shown in comparison with the mean cervical dilatation time curve for nulliparas. A = prolonged latent phase, B = protracted active phase dilation, and C = secondary arrest of dilation. (Friedman E: Greenhill Obstetrics, 13th ed. Philadelphia, WB Saunders, 1965)

comes from the work of this group.[1] In normal labor, the intensity or amplitude of the contractions is usually between 30 and 50 mm Hg, and the frequency is usually two to five contractions in 10 minutes.[4]

Friedman's division of the first *stage* of labor into two *phases*, the latent phase and the active phase, and his use of curves to plot both dilatation and descent have been found to be useful in detecting and estimating the severity of dysfunctional labor.[5] There are those who feel, however, that the latent phase is the end of several weeks of "prelabor," which is a preparatory period for labor.

As defined by Friedman, the *latent phase* is a period of effacement and beginning dilatation of the cervix, lasting an average of 8½ hours in a nullipara and a somewhat shorter time in the multipara. During this phase, 3 to 4 cm of dilation are accomplished. The *active phase*, or clinically apparent labor, is briefer and consists of an acceleration phase, a phase of maximum slope, and a deceleration phase before full dilatation is accomplished. This phase of labor lasts approximately 3½ to 4 hours in the primigravid patient.

Friedman classifies dysfunction by the length of the phases of labor rather than by the quality of the contractions. However, his prolonged latent phase occurs during the onset and first phase of labor and hence can be associated with hypertonic dysfunction. By definition, the latent phase is prolonged if it lasts longer than 20 hours in the primigravida or 14 hours in the multigravida. In practice, however, the diagnosis should be suspected and treatment should be instituted many hours before these time intervals have elapsed.[1]

Friedman describes two types of dysfunction that can occur during the active phase of the first stage of labor: protraction disorders and arrest disorders.[2] Protraction disorders are characterized by a slower than

normal rate of cervical dilation and by delayed descent of the fetal head in the active phase of labor. The expected rate of cervical dilation is 1.2 cm or more per hour for nulliparas and 1.5 cm or more for multiparas. The rate of descent for the fetal head should be approximately 1.0 cm/h for nulliparas and 2.0 cm/h for multiparas.[6] Although a slowing of progress can be an indication of cephalopelvic disproportion, especially in a nullipara, most of the patients with protraction disorders, given supportive fluids, reassurance, and minimum sedation, go on to dilate fully, although more slowly than usual.[7]

Arrest disorders are diagnosed when cervical dilation or descent of the fetal head has ceased for more than 2 hours in the active phase of labor. These disorders may follow protraction disorders, or a normally progressing labor may suddenly stop. Arrest disorders are frequently associated with cephalopelvic disproportion.[6]

Hendricks and associates have described slightly different curves for normal labor (Fig. 38-2).[8] They found in normal active labor that there is a rather constant active acceleration phase without the deceleration described by Friedman. Also, although it is often assumed that the nullipara progresses more slowly than the multipara, these investigators found that cervical dilation progressed at about the same rate in both after the cervix was dilated to 4 cm.[8] Despite variations in the description of normal labor, any significant prolongation of any of the phases described by Friedman or any significant variation from the curves presented by Hendricks and associates constitutes uterine dysfunction.[1,2,8]

When there is failure to progress in early labor despite the presence of uterine contractions, one of the first factors to consider is whether the patient is actually in labor. It is not unusual for a woman in late pregnancy to experience Braxton Hicks contractions that are so strong and regular that they can easily be mistaken for true labor. However, true labor contractions do accomplish at least some cervical effacement and dilatation; therefore, progressive cervical changes must take place to signify true labor. Appearance of bloody show assists in the diagnosis of labor, particularly when it accompanies cervical changes. Without signs of progress to confirm labor, uncomfortable uterine contractions signify false labor. For the diagnosis of dystocia, cervical changes must have occurred and progressed, only to have the progression slowed or halted at some point.

ETIOLOGICAL FACTORS

The chief factors associated with uterine dysfunction are injudicious use of analgesia (i.e., excessive or too early administration of the drugs), minor degrees of pelvic contraction, and fetal malposition of even a small degree, such as a slight extension of the head as seen

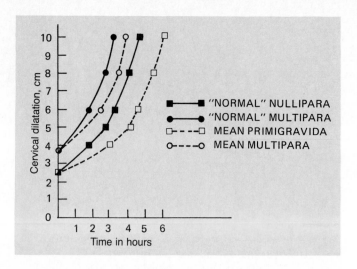

■ *Figure 38-2*
Cervical dilatation in normal nulliparous and multiparous women after the onset of true labor. (Hendricks CH, Brenner WE, Kraus G et al: The normal cervical dilatation patterns in late pregnancy and labor. Am J Obstet Gynecol 106:1065, 1970)

in some occiput posterior positions. Postmaturity and large infants have also been found to be significantly related to dysfunctional labor. These conditions may occur singly or in combination in cases of dysfunction.

Other factors associated with this condition include overdistention of the uterus, grand multiparity, excessive cervical rigidity, and maternal age. Although the latter group of factors has been shown to play some etiological role, they are less important than was once believed. In over 50% of the cases, the cause is unknown. Considering the possible role of corticosteroids in the initiation of labor, and their relation to stress states, the effects of emotional factors in dystocia cannot be overlooked when no other cause is apparent. More research at the cellular level is needed to obtain increased definitive knowledge concerning the etiological factors in this condition.

COMPLICATIONS

Uterine dysfunction with prolonged labor can result in complications for both mother and fetus. Intrauterine infection is a common maternal complication, especially if the membranes are ruptured. This can result in fetal or neonatal infection and death, even if antibiotics are used to treat the mother.[1] Exhaustion and dehydration may also occur in the mother if labor is allowed to become too prolonged.

Fortunately, the role of prolonged labor as a contributor to perinatal mortality and morbidity is fairly well understood. Careful observation of the condition of the mother and fetus usually leads to timely intervention to prevent complications. These interventions include supportive therapy with adequate intravenous fluids, the judicious use of dilute intravenous oxytocin to facilitate the progress of labor, or performance of cesarean delivery when oxytocin fails or is inappropriate for use.

HYPERTONIC DYSFUNCTION

Hypertonic dysfunction, the least common type of uterine dysfunction, generally occurs at the onset of labor.[1] The gradient of the contraction is distorted either by the midsegment contracting with more force than the fundus or by complete asynchronism of the electrical impulses originating in each cornu. There is an elevation of the resting tone of the uterus, but the contractions are of poor quality (Fig. 38-3).

Although the contractions in this type of dysfunction are ineffectual in accomplishing dilatation, the increased uterine tone usually results in maternal discomfort. These contractions are often described as "colicky" and extremely painful. The uterus may be tender to palpation, even between contractions (Table 38-1).

In cases of uterine hypertonus, it is important to rule out abruption of the placenta as a cause.[1]

Management. Treatment for this type of dysfunction usually consists of rest and administration of fluids. When medication is indicated to produce the needed rest and relaxation, an injection of 10 to 15 mg of morphine may be prescribed because it usually stops the abnormal contractions. A short-acting barbiturate may also be administered to help promote rest. Intravenous fluids are used to maintain hydration and electrolyte balance, and in most instances normal labor resumes when the client awakens. Tocolytic agents such as ritodrine have been used with some stated success, especially in other countries.[1]

Oxytocin is usually contraindicated in treating this type of dysfunction, although there is some disagreement on this point.[5,6] With the uterus in a constant state of increased muscle tone, oxytocin presents the danger of causing an even greater resting tension, which might interfere with fetal oxygenation. Also, it may not correct

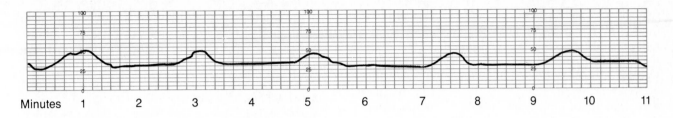

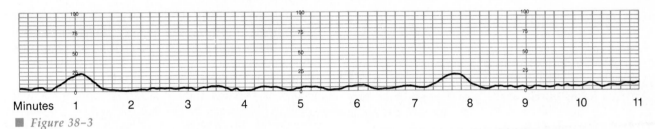

■ *Figure 38–3*

Dysfunctions of uterine motility: top, *hypertonic*; bottom, *hypotonic*

the uncoordinated action of the two segments, which underlies this problem.

Occasionally, the contractions remain uncoordinated and ineffective even after the client has rested. In these cases, cesarean delivery is usually the choice, especially if any signs of fetal distress are evident.[1]

Complications. Fetal distress tends to appear early in labor when there is hypertonic dysfunction. The constant increase in uterine tone predisposes to fetal hypoxia. Occasionally, prolonged rupture of membranes may accompany this condition and can lead to intrapartum infection.

HYPOTONIC DYSFUNCTION

When the uterine contractions decrease in strength and uterine tone is less than usual after the onset of true labor, the patient is considered to have hypotonic dysfunction. Minimum uterine tension during the resting stage is about 8 to 12 mm Hg in the normally functioning uterus, whereas normal labor contractions reach an intrauterine pressure of 50 to 60 mm Hg at the acme. These values are reduced in hypotonic dysfunction, and contractions are not strong enough to dilate the cervix. Contractions may also become farther apart and irregular (see Fig. 38-3). This condition usually occurs in the acceleration or active phase, but contractions may become hypotonic during the second stage of labor also (see Table 38-1).

Management. Possible courses of action for the management of hypotonic uterine dysfunction include simple corrective measures, amniotomy or oxytocin administration, and cesarean delivery. The decision is

usually made on the basis of the general condition of the mother and fetus and on the presence or absence of mechanical obstruction. If the mother is becoming fatigued or dehydrated, rest and fluids may be tried first. If a marked degree of disproportion is found to exist or there is an uncorrectable malposition or marked fetal distress, a cesarean section is employed to effect delivery. If these conditions are not present, stimulation of labor is generally the treatment of choice, rather than "watchful waiting" for more effective labor to resume spontaneously.

If membranes are intact and the head is engaged, initial treatment may be to rupture the membranes artificially (amniotomy). (See Chap. 39 for further discussion.) This procedure alone may stimulate effective contractions, but it must be used judiciously because it is a commitment to deliver the baby within a reasonable time. Augmentation of labor by the use of intravenous oxytocin is usually the treatment of choice when strong,

TABLE 38-1. CRITERIA FOR DIFFERENTIATING DYSFUNCTIONAL LABOR

Criteria	Hypertonic	Hypotonic
Phase of labor	Latent	Active
Symptoms	Painful	Painless
Fetal Distress	Early	Painless
Medication		
Oxytocin	Unfavorable reaction	Favorable reaction
Sedation	Helpful	Little value

(Modified from Pritchard JA, McDonald PC: Williams Obstetrics, 16th ed, p. 660. New York, Appleton-Century-Crofts, 1980)

regular contractions with progressive cervical effacement and dilatation, or fetal descent, fail to occur or
when membranes are already ruptured.

Complications. Untreated hypotonic uterine dysfunction exposes the mother to the dangers of exhaustion,
dehydration, and intrapartum infection. Signs of fetal
distress often do not appear until intrapartum infection
has developed. Although treatment of intrauterine infection with antibiotics offers protection to the mother,
it appears to be of little value in protecting the fetus.[1]

OXYTOCIN STIMULATION

Oxytocin acts on the myometrium, causing it to contract.
Natural oxytocin is produced in the body by the hypothalamus and stored in the posterior pituitary gland.
Maternal levels of oxytocin increase as gestation progresses, although the exact role of this increase in human
labor is not known. Animal extracts of oxytocin were
once used to stimulate uterine contractions. Synthetic
oxytocin is as effective as the natural substance, is
chemically pure, and eliminates the danger of reaction
to animal protein. Therefore, synthetic oxytocin is the
product used in modern obstetrics.[4] In relation to stimulation of labor, oxytocin may be used to initiate (induce)
labor contractions or to augment contractions that are
weak and ineffective, as in cases of hypotonic dysfunction. (The role of oxytocin in the postpartum period, to
contract the uterus and control bleeding, is discussed
in Chapter 22.)

Contraindications to Use of Oxytocin. The following
are usually considered to be contraindications to the
use of oxytocin for either augmentation or induction:[1,4]

- Any obstruction that would interfere with descent
  of the fetus, such as cephalopelvic disproportion
  or anomaly of the birth canal
- Conditions that would increase the danger of
  uterine rupture, such as high parity (greater than
  four), previous uterine incision (cesarean section
  or extensive myomectomy), or overdistention of
  the uterus (twins, hydramnios)
- Hypertonic or incoordinate uterine contractions,
  because oxytocin makes the condition worse and
  may lead to formation of a constriction ring
- Fetal distress, because the change in the contractions brought about by the oxytocin may add to
  the distress
- Placenta previa

Method of Oxytocin Administration. The amount and
rate of oxytocin administration must be carefully controlled, and this can be done effectively only by use of
the intravenous route. Optimally, an infusion pump is

used to administer the intravenous oxytocin, to help
provide a consistent and precise rate. Types of solution,
amount of oxytocin added, and rate of infusion vary
according to agency protocols or physician preference.
The usual choice of solution is 5% dextrose in water,
normal saline, or lactated Ringer's solution; 10 units
(10,000 mU) of oxytocin is added to 1000 ml of solution
and started at a rate of 0.5 mU to 2 mU/min.

A piggyback system, using two bottles of the same
solution, one containing oxytocin and the other without,
is recommended because this makes it possible to discontinue the oxytocin if necessary and still keep the
intravenous line open. Contractions and fetal heart rate
are carefully evaluated, and if no problems develop, the
infusion is gradually increased. The usual maximum is
20 mU/min, but levels above 10 mU/min are seldom
needed for augmentation of labor and levels of 30 mU
to 40 mU/min may be needed for some inductions.[1]
Ideally the contractions stimulated by the oxytocin
mimic natural labor as closely as possible, with uterine
contractions of moderate to strong intensity occurring
every 2 to 3 minutes, lasting no more than 45 to 60
seconds, and with at least a 30-second rest between
contractions. Signs of fetal distress must be carefully
watched for, and the infusion must be slowed or stopped
if any signs are detected. Use of external or internal
electronic monitors is mandatory when oxytocin stimulation of labor is employed. Internal monitoring of
uterine activity has the advantage of providing a more
accurate picture of the intensity of the contractions than
external monitoring.

Extreme caution is necessary, especially at the beginning of the oxytocin infusion, because of the unpre-
dictability of individual response. Sensitivity of the individual client should be assessed carefully by beginning
with small amounts. Sensitivity to oxytocin varies
widely from client to client and from time to time in
the same client depending on a variety of influencing
factors. Increased sensitivity is associated with ruptured
membranes, term gestation, high parity, favorable cervix
(soft, effacing, dilating, and anterior), and irritable
uterus.[9]

Dangers of Oxytocin Use. When oxytocin is administered to the pregnant woman it is potentially dangerous
to both mother and fetus. These dangers can be minimized by careful monitoring of the administration of
the drug, the character of the contractions, and the condition of the fetus. When the contractions increase in
frequency, strength, and length above normal levels,
the fetal and placental circulation may be impaired and
fetal distress may result. Another potential danger to
the fetus is possible birth injuries from being propelled
too rapidly through the birth canal or being forced

Nursing Guidelines for Oxytocin (Pitocin) Induction and Augmentation

Intervention	*Rationale and Comments*
1. Explain procedure and rationale to client.	1. An informed client is less anxious and fearful.
2. Apply fetal monitor and monitor the fetal heart rate (FHR) to establish a baseline tracing.	2. Ensures fetal reactivity.
3. Start an IV infusion (primary line) using an electrolyte solution.	3. An electrolyte solution minimizes the risk of water intoxication.
4. Prepare a second IV (secondary line) and add the prescribed amount of oxytocin (usually 10 U/1000 ml). The IV tubing is inserted into the infusion controller (or pump) and primed to clear air from the line.	4. Oxytocin must be administered with an infusion pump (or controller) to ensure accurate dose administration.
5. "Piggyback" the secondary line into the primary line at the port closest to the needle insertion site and then turn on at the prescribed rate of infusion.	5. The secondary line contains the oxytocin. If there is an indication to stop the oxytocin infusion, it can be done without affecting the infusion of the primary line, and fluid volume can be maintained.
6. Turn on oxytocin infusion pump at prescribed rate.	6. No other medications should be given through the oxytocin (secondary) line, because it is given at prescribed rates and may be turned off if contractions are too close, hypertonus occurs, or the FHR pattern indicates fetal distress.
7. Monitor FHR, uterine resting tone, frequency, duration and intensity of contractions, blood pressure, and pulse and record at intervals comparable to the *dosage regimen* (i.e., at 30- to 60-min intervals) when the dosage is evaluated for maintenance, increase, or decrease. Evidence of maternal and fetal surveillance should be documented. All observations and increases or decreases in oxytocin are documented on the fetal heart tracing and the mother's chart.	7. If uterus becomes hyperstimulated, blood flow to uteroplacental site is decreased and fetus will suffer from hypoxia.
8. Once the desired frequency of contractions has been reached and labor has progressed to 5 to 6 cm dilatation, oxytocin may be reduced by similar increments (or as prescribed by physician).	8. Sensitivity to oxytocin increases as labor progresses. If stable pattern is achieved, need for oxytocin decreases.
9. If hyperstimulation of the uterus occurs (less than 2 min between contractions and lasting longer than 60 s) or a nonreassuring FHR pattern occurs, the following actions are taken: a. Turn off oxytocin infusion. b. Speed up primary infusion. c. Change position, may turn to left side. d. Give oxygen 6 to 8 L/min by face mask. e. Notify charge nurse (supervisor) and physician STAT. f. Provide support to parents. g. Document on monitor strip and client's chart. h. Document effectiveness of interventions.	9. Intrauterine resuscitation is initiated when there is significant interruption of oxygenation due to decrease or cessation of uteroplacental perfusion.
10. Notify the physician of hypertonic or hypotonic contractions or failure to progress.	10. Clients may vary in their individual responsiveness to oxytocin. Some may require more; some may require less.

(continued)

11. Continue to assess client's progress, both physically and emotionally (care for the client, not the monitor).

12. Notify the physican to evaluate client when oxytocin infusion is 10 mU/min.
    Note. A client seldom requires more than 20 to 40 mU/min of oxytocin to achieve progressive cervical dilation; 90% of clients respond to 16 mU or less.

13. Accurately record fluid intake and output every 2 h.

11. Induced or augmented labor is stressful to couple. The nurse is attuned to their responses and intervenes as indicated. They need to know that progress is occurring.

12. Assesses client's response to oxytocin.

13. To ensure proper hydration and to rule out fluid retention due to antidiuretic action of oxytocin.

(Adapted from NAACOG: The nurse's role in the induction/augmentation of labor. OGN Nurs Pract Resource, January 1988)

---

through a pelvis that is too small for it. Tetanic and tumultuous contractions can result in abruptio placentae or rupture of the uterus, resulting in adverse effects on both mother and fetus. Cervical lacerations from too rapid passage of the fetus through the pelvis and amniotic fluid embolism are additional dangers for the mother when this type of contraction occurs.[4,10]

Side-effects. Oxytocin infusion may also have some maternal side-effects. Hypertension may develop, with frontal headache. Both of these effects disappear when the drug is discontinued. Oxytocin has antidiuretic properties that can lead to water intoxication when used in large amounts. The prevalence of this problem can be decreased by using an electrolyte solution for the infusion rather than dextrose in water and by avoiding infusion of a large volume of fluid.[10]

NURSING PROCESS
IN DYSFUNCTIONAL LABOR

Assessment. Ongoing nursing assessment is an essential component of the care of the client with uterine dysfunction, to aid in detecting the condition, to assist in decisions about the course of treatment, and to monitor maternal and fetal well-being during attempts to promote more effective contractions. The labor room nurse is often the one to detect the first deviations from the normal labor pattern. Either an internal or an external electronic fetal monitor is helpful to the nurse in assessing the length and frequency of contractions, but the external monitor does not accurately portray the strength of the contraction. The nurse must be able to evaluate the intensity of labor contractions by palpation, without relying exclusively on the electronic monitor. (See Chap. 22 for assessment of uterine contractions.) Subjective statements of pain and related behavior, such

as crying and moaning, are often not reliable indicators of the strength of contractions and should be evaluated in light of objective data from tactile examination and the electronic monitor, rather than be taken at face value.

Assessing the condition of the fetus is also important. The nurse needs to watch the monitor for changes in the fetal heart rate and baseline variability. The nurse should also be alert for other signs of fetal distress, such as meconium-stained amniotic fluid and increased fetal activity.

Maternal vital signs should be checked frequently. Elevation of maternal temperature and increased pulse rate are clinical signs that may alert the nurse to the onset of secondary complications such as infection. Urine should be checked for acetone. Acetonuria is a sign of exhaustion and dehydration. A record of intake and output is also helpful in assessing hydration.

Nursing Diagnosis. From the assessment the nurse assists with recognizing the medical diagnosis of dysfunctional labor. The nurse can also make a number of potential nursing diagnoses, which could become actual depending on the progress of the situation. Some of the nursing diagnoses might be High Risk for Fluid Volume Deficit related to prolonged labor and restricted fluid intake; High Risk for Infection related to prolonged rupture of membranes; Alteration in Comfort related to ineffective uterine contractions; and Anxiety or Fear related to unexpected length of labor.

Planning and Intervention. The nurse plans interventions based on the nursing diagnoses and on the medical plan of treatment. Care includes comfort measures, emotional support, and explanations of what is happening, as well as administering and monitoring effects of ordered medications.

EMOTIONAL SUPPORT. Labors of this type are extremely discouraging for the mother and the father. The diagnostic procedures as well as the therapy take a certain amount of time, and carrying out these measures requires patience and waiting on the part of everyone concerned. It is essential that the couple know and understand this fact. The physician and nurse need to spend sufficient time with the parents to explain what is happening in depth and in terms that are appropriate for them. It is possible that repeated reinforcement of the explanations about progress and so on will be needed. In stressful situations, people often do not hear all that is said. Feedback from the parents should be encouraged, so their level of understanding and acceptance can be ascertained. The normal tension and anxiety found in any labor certainly is intensified in a dysfunctional labor, and it is important that it not be compounded by fantasy or misunderstanding.

Because dysfunctional labor is so variable, it is often impossible (and unwise) to give the parents any definite reassurances as to when effective labor will commence or when the birth will occur. Yet some kind of boundaries must be placed on when this ineffective phase will end and progress will begin, so that the mother has some goal to look forward to and to work for. Therefore, it is important to reassure the client, reminding her that her case is not unique (after many hours clients think that theirs is the longest labor in obstetric history), that certain specific measures are known and can be taken to help effective labor to begin, and that competent medical and nursing care will be given throughout labor.

An explanation of the plan for treatment enables the parents to anticipate more realistically what is in store and therefore reassures them that certain definite measures are available and are being employed.

COMFORT MEASURES. Comfort measures that promote relaxation should be used. Sponge baths, various changes in position, soothing back rubs, quiet conversation, reading or other diversionary activities, and clean, dry linen, as well as a quiet, restful environment, are all appropriate. However, isolating the client in a dark room on the premise that she needs sleep or rest only contributes to her fear unless she is actually sleeping, and frequent observations are needed to see when she awakens. Human contact is one of the most important items of "treatment" in cases of complicated labor and should never be neglected. The presence of the same person, nurse, or physician is helpful for the reasons already mentioned in Chapter 22. Allowing the client to have with her a familiar person of her choice, such as husband or mother, is also important. Coaching the client in breathing patterns and relaxation techniques also can be comforting and helps to conserve her strength.

Certain comfort measures can actually aid in correction of some dysfunctional labor patterns. For example, an overdistended bladder may not be noticed by the client, but may add to her discomfort. Encouraging emptying of the bladder often speeds cervical dilatation, possibly by allowing the fetal head to descend further with better proximity to the cervix. Similarly, emptying the rectum by means of an enema has also been found to enhance uterine contractions.

Position changes may also improve uterine contractions. In general, uterine contractions come less frequently but tend to be better coordinated and more intense when the mother is in the side-lying position, as compared with the supine position. She may need some encouragement to assume the side-lying position at first, but usually will try it willingly when told that it may improve her contractions. Walking in the hall or sitting in a comfortable chair may also assist in the resumption of effective contractions in some cases. However, the client should not be allowed out of bed if the membranes have ruptured and the head is not well engaged.

OXYTOCIN MONITORING. When oxytocin stimulation of labor is used a physician is required to be available, but it is often the nurse who is actually in the client's room. It is the doctor's responsibility to specify the dosage of oxytocin and the rate of infusion; however, the nurse has the responsibility to be knowledgeable about the specific protocol for oxytocin stimulation, the effects of the drug, and pertinent information about the individual patient. The mother should, at all times, have someone in attendance who is trained to recognize and respond to hyperstimulation of the uterus or signs of fetal distress.[11]

In setting up a piggyback system for the infusion, the nurse should make sure that the bottle containing the oxytocin is clearly labeled as such and that the piggyback line is inserted in the port closest to the client.[10] Even though an infusion pump is used, the nurse should ascertain that the infusion is running at the prescribed rate because there is always the possibility of pump malfunction.

Although uterine contractions and fetal heart tones are being continuously monitored electronically, they need to be assessed by the nurse at least every 15 minutes. If there is any doubt about the accuracy of the monitor, especially if external monitors are being used, the contractions should be evaluated by palpation and the heart tones should be checked by Doppler. Any contraction lasting over 90 seconds indicates that the uterus is being overstimulated, and the rate of flow should be either decreased or temporarily discontinued. The fetal heart rate pattern should be observed for changes. Late decelerations or severe variable decelerations are an indication for discontinuation of the oxytocin infusion. With any signs of fetal distress the oxytocin should be turned off, the mother turned on her left side, oxygen started by mask, and the physician notified.

Maternal blood pressure and pulse are to be checked every half hour. Because of oxytocin's antidiuretic properties, intake and output should also be monitored carefully and decreased urinary output should be reported. Another concern is the monitoring of labor progress. With the stimulation of more effective uterine contractions, cervical dilation may occur much more rapidly, and this needs to be detected soon enough for preparations to be made for the birth.

It is important to have a method for recording the times, amount, and rate of oxytocin infused, the fetal heart tones, the maternal blood pressure and pulse, the frequency, intensity, and length of contractions, and other relevant comments. The client's labor record may be used, or there may be a specific "oxytocin record" or flow sheet that provides an easily accessible record of the client's progress during the infusion. Significant information is also written at the appropriate times on the electronic monitor strip.

Recording and reporting the physiological signs and symptoms cannot be stressed enough during these infusions. However, supportive care continues to be important, and the nurse must avoid the pitfall of "monitoring the monitor" instead of caring for the client. Because the nurse is with the client continuously over a period of time, this time can be used to establish rapport and provide adequate explanations and reassurance. Before the oxytocin infusion is started, the nurse can help prepare the client by explaining the procedure and expected changes in the uterine contractions. The often rapid change from mild to strong uterine contractions can be difficult for the client to adjust to, but anticipatory guidance and assistance with breathing and relaxation can make the adjustment easier. Although the infusion stimulates contractions, and therefore discomfort, the mother and her partner often look on this treatment optimistically, because it marks the end of a desultory, ineffective period in labor and brings with it promise of termination of a difficult time. The nurse's explanations and reassurance can reinforce this positive attitude.

Evaluation. The effectiveness of nursing interventions for the woman with dysfunctional labor is evaluated on a continuous basis, and interventions are revised as necessary to ensure maternal and fetal well-being. Maintenance of the client's fluid and electrolyte balance, absence of signs of infection or other complications, absence of fetal distress, and the progress of labor to the birth of a healthy infant all indicate successful attainment of nursing goals. Other evaluative criteria include the client's verbalizations of her fears and concerns, of her understanding of the disruption of the labor progress and planned interventions, and of her experience of minimal pain and discomfort.

OTHER PROBLEMS WITH THE EXPULSIVE FORCES

Inadequate Voluntary Expulsive Force. When the cervix is fully dilated, most women cannot resist the urge to push or bear down during a uterine contraction. The combined force of the maternal use of abdominal musculature and the contraction of the uterus helps propel the fetus down the vagina and through the vaginal outlet. The urge and ability to push can be interfered with by such factors as anesthesia and heavy sedation. Fatigue or intensification of pain during pushing can also cause the woman to push with less effectiveness. In rare instances, a physical problem such as a spinal cord injury may be the reason for insufficient expulsive efforts.[1]

Management is usually related to the cause. Careful selection and timing of analgesia and anesthesia can be helpful in preventing the problem. If continuous epidural anesthesia is used, it may be necessary to allow the effects to wear off sufficiently for the woman to be able to push. If the woman is "holding back" because of pain, analgesia may be needed. In any event, appropriate encouragement, support, instruction, and positioning can be helpful.

Precipitate Labor and Delivery. Labor that lasts less than 3 hours is called precipitate labor. It is most often the result of lack of resistance of maternal tissues, allowing the fetus to pass easily through the pelvis. It can also be due to contractions with an amplitude over 50 mm Hg, or occasionally to the mother's lack of awareness of the sensations of vigorous labor.[1] Precipitate delivery may, but does not necessarily, follow precipitate labor and may occur after a labor of normal length. Although rapid labor is sometimes associated with increased danger of maternal lacerations or fetal asphyxia from interference with the placental circulation, some recent studies have shown that the risk to mother and child is not necessarily increased greatly over that of the average labor.[4] If labor is progressing rapidly because of tetanic contractions caused by infusion of an oxytocic agent, the infusion should be stopped immediately. Spontaneous forceful contractions are difficult to modify, but tocolytic agents may be effective.[1]

Pathological Retraction and Constriction Rings. Localized rings or constrictions of the uterus sometimes

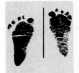

Nursing Care Plan

Woman with Dysfunctional Labor

Patient Goals:

1. Client's fluid and electrolyte balance is maintained.
2. Client experiences minimal pain and discomfort.
3. Client verbalizes fears and concerns about labor.
4. Client verbalizes understanding of disruption of labor progress and planned interventions.
5. Client does not develop infection or other complications.
6. Fetal distress does not develop.
7. Labor progresses to birth of healthy infant.

Assessment	*Potential Nursing Diagnosis*	*Planning and Intervention*	*Evaluation*
Uterine contractions for dysfunctional patterns		Monitor frequency, duration, and intensity of contractions	
Level of fatigue and ability to cope with pain	Alteration in comfort related to ineffective uterine contractions	Stay with client or have partner stay continuously; coach in breathing and relaxation techniques; record and report behavior; assist as needed with position changes, effleurage, concentration or distraction for pain management; keep linen clean and dry; provide quiet environment	Client avoids exhaustion Client attains as much comfort as possible
Emotional status	Anxiety or fear related to unexpected character or length of labor	Explain labor progress, plan of treatment, and what can be expected; reassure as appropriate	Client avoids panic and discouragement
Hydration	High risk for fluid volume deficit related to prolonged labor and restricted fluid intake	Give oral or intravenous fluids as ordered Check for dryness of lips and for decreased skin turgor	Client maintains normal fluid and electrolyte balance
Bladder		Encourage client to void frequently; catheterize as necessary	Client avoids bladder distention
Vital signs Signs of infection	High risk for infection related to prolonged rupture of membranes	Check temperature-pulse-respiration and blood pressure every 2 h or more frequently if indicated	Client remains free of infection

(continued)

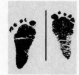

Nursing Care Plan (continued)

Assessment	Potential Nursing Diagnosis	Planning and Intervention	Evaluation
		Report and record temperature increase or other changes in vital signs	
		Use clean technique in client care with good handwashing	
Response to oxytocin (if given)		Monitor oxytocin infusion; maintain rate as ordered	Client progresses in labor
		Monitor uterine contractions and fetal heart rate carefully; report and record	Client remains free of complications
Fetal well-being	High risk for fetal distress related to prolonged labor	Monitor fetal heart rate tracing for changes in variability, reactivity, rate, or pattern or auscultate fetal heart tones frequently if fetal monitor not in use	Fetus remains in good condition
		Check for meconium staining of amniotic fluid or sudden increase in fetal activity	
		If signs of fetal distress are detected, position client on left side, start oxygen, turn off oxytocin (if in use), notify physician	

occur in association with prolonged rupture of the membranes or long labors (Fig. 38-4). The *pathological retraction ring* (Bandl's ring) is the most common. It is an exaggeration of the normal physiological retraction ring, which occurs at the junction of the upper and lower uterine segments (see Chap. 21). The uterus above the ring becomes thicker, whereas the lower uterine segment thins out and will rupture unless the obstruction is relieved or delivery is accomplished by cesarean section.[5] *Constriction rings* are rare and not well understood. They usually conform to a depression in the baby, such as the neck or abdomen, and do not go all the way around. The area of spasm is thick, but the lower uterine segment does not become stretched or thinned out.[4]

Cesarean birth, using an anesthetic that relaxes the uterus, is usually the treatment of choice.

Problems With the Passageway

The second major category of factors causing dystocia is related to variations or abnormalities of the maternal reproductive tract, especially the pelvis, that interfere with engagement, descent, or expulsion of the fetus.

CONTRACTED PELVIS

Disproportion between the size of the infant and the size of the birth canal is caused most frequently by a

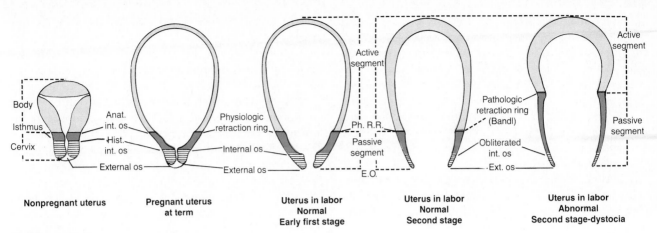

■ *Figure 38-4*
Sequence of development of the segments and rings in the uterus in pregnant women at term and in labor. Note comparison of the uterus of a nonpregnant woman, the uterus at term, and the uterus during labor. The passive lower segment of the uterine body is derived from the isthmus; the physiological retraction ring develops at the junction of the upper and lower uterine segments. The pathological retraction ring develops from the physiological ring. (Anat. Int. Os, anatomical internal os; Hist. Int. Os, histological internal os; Ph. R. R., physiological retraction ring; E.O., external os) (After Pritchard JA, MacDonald PC, Gant NF: Williams Obstetrics, 17th ed, Chap 15, p 308. New York, Appleton-Century-Crofts, 1985)

contracted pelvis. A contracted pelvis is a pelvis in which there is sufficient reduction in one or more of its major diameters to interfere with the progress of labor. The pelvis may be contracted at the inlet, the midpelvis, or the outlet.

In the case of *inlet contraction*, the anteroposterior diameter of the inlet is decreased to 10 cm or less or the greatest transverse diameter is 12 cm or less. Either of these contractions results in an increase in obstetric difficulties. The incidence of difficult labors is increased even more when both diameters are contracted.[1] Contraction of the inlet may be the result of rickets or generally poor development. A small woman is more likely to have a pelvis that is small in all dimensions, but she is also more likely to have a small baby. Effects of a contracted pelvic inlet on the fetus include failure of the presenting part to engage, increased incidence of malpositions and deflexed attitudes, and extreme molding of the presenting part. Because the presenting part does not fit the inlet well, prolapsed umbilical cord is also more likely.

Midpelvic contraction is less well defined than contraction of the inlet or outlet; however, the midpelvis is considered contracted when the distance between the ischial spines is less than 9.0 cm (normal is 10.5) or when the sum of the interspinous and the posterior sagittal distance is less than 13.5 cm (normal is 15.0–15.5 cm). Contraction of the midpelvis is a fairly frequent cause of dystocia. Because the presenting part is able to engage in the pelvis, this condition is harder to recognize than inlet contraction, making management more difficult. As labor progresses, molding and caput

formation may give the impression that the head is lower than it actually is, and a difficult forceps delivery may result. Transverse arrest of the head may also occur.

Contraction of the pelvic outlet is identified when the distance between the ischial tuberosities is less than 8 cm. Other dimensions of the outlet are also important in determining the degree of difficulty caused by the outlet contraction. The incidence of perineal tears and the need for forceps are increased, but cesarean section is rarely necessary. Severe dystocia is usually the result of an association with a midpelvic contraction.

VARIATIONS IN PELVIC SHAPE

The shape of the pelvis may be equally important or more important than its size, although these factors may complement each other. For example, large size may compensate for a shape that is not optimal. The normal female or *gynecoid* pelvis has the best dimensions in all planes for the passage of the fetus. The other three pelvic variations adversely influence the prognosis for a vaginal delivery (see Chap. 20 for discussion of pelvic types).

CEPHALOPELVIC DISPROPORTION

The term *cephalopelvic disproportion* (CPD) implies a relationship between the size of the fetal head and the size of the pelvis. This indicates that the problem could originate with either the passageway or the passenger, or a combination of the two. It involves an interplay among the factors in the preceding section and those in the following section. Cephalopelvic (or fetopelvic if the head is not the presenting part) disproportion can be either absolute or relative. When the fetus cannot pass safely through the birth canal under any circumstances, it is considered absolute. In many cases, however, whether the fetus can be delivered vaginally depends on the efficiency of the uterine contractions; the stretchability of the maternal soft tissues; the attitude, presentation, and position of the fetus; and the moldability of the fetal head.[4]

Extreme degrees of pelvic contraction or problems with the fetus can often be detected during antepartal care and a decision can be made about the advisability of cesarean delivery. In doubtful cases, the client may be given a "trial labor" of 4 to 6 hours to determine whether, with adequate contractions, the head can pass through the pelvis. For these mothers, labor may be even more anxiety provoking than usual, depending partly on the support and information they have received. If cesarean delivery is the eventual outcome, there may be a great deal of disappointment and perhaps even a feeling of failure. The warm, empathic attitude of the nurse is particularly needed for these clients. Frequent reports on the progress of labor should not be overlooked, whether or not the progress is favorable. The perinatal team does the client a disservice by avoiding the subject if progress is not made in labor.

Problems With the Passenger

The position and presentation of the fetus at the beginning of labor can greatly influence the progress of the labor. Even slight deviations can affect the uterine contractions adversely or prevent the fetus from passing through the birth canal.

PERSISTENT OCCIPUT POSTERIOR AND TRANSVERSE ARREST

The fetal head usually enters the pelvic inlet transversely and therefore must traverse an arc of 90° in the process of internal rotation to the direct occiput anterior position (see Fig. 20-2). In about a quarter of all labors, however, the head enters the pelvis with the occiput directed diagonally posterior, that is, in either the right occipitoposterior (R.O.P.) or the left occipitoposterior (L.O.P.) position. Under these circumstances, the head must rotate through an arc of 135° in the process of internal rotation (Fig. 38-5A–D).

With good contractions, adequate flexion, and a baby of average size, the great majority of these cases of occiput posterior position undergo spontaneous rotation through the 135° arc as soon as the head reaches the pelvic floor. This is a normal mechanism of labor.

In a minority of cases (approximately 10% or less),

rotation may be incomplete,[1] or the head may rotate through a 45° arc to the direct occiput posterior position, a condition known as *persistent occiput posterior* (see Fig. 38-5E,F). If rotation is incomplete, the head becomes arrested in the transverse position, a condition known as *transverse arrest.* Both transverse arrest and persistent occiput posterior position represent deviations from the normal mechanisms of labor. It is thought that narrowing of the midpelvis plays a role in the etiology.

Some controversy persists in the management of persistent occiput posterior. When labor progresses, although first and second stages tend to be prolonged in primigravidas, management is the same as for occiput anterior positions and results in no increased risk to the fetus. Premature operative intervention, particularly if the station is high, seems contraindicated. Forceps rotation on the perineum is appropriate to reduce lacerations if this can be easily accomplished.[1]

When the fetus is in an occiput posterior position, regardless of how rotation eventually occurs, the labor is usually prolonged and the mother has a great deal of discomfort in her back as the fetal head impinges against the sacrum in the course of rotating.

Nursing intervention is aimed at relieving the back pain as much as possible. Sacral pressure, back rubs, and frequent change of position from side to side can be helpful, and they should be employed to the degree that seems to be well tolerated by the client.

BREECH PRESENTATION

The breech is the presenting part in 3% to 4% of singleton deliveries and is more common when the baby is premature or there is multiple gestation. The reasons for breech presentation are not always apparent, although associated factors include great parity, twinning, hydramnios, hydrocephalus, placenta previa, and implantation of the placenta in the cornual fundal regions of the uterus. Studies have not indicated a positive correlation between breech presentation and contracted pelvis.[1]

Classification. Breech presentations are classified as follows:

Complete. The buttocks present with the feet and legs flexed on the thighs and the thighs flexed on the abdomen (Fig. 38-6A).
Frank. The buttocks present with the hips flexed and the legs extended against the abdomen and chest (see Fig. 38-6B); this is the most common type of breech presentation.
Incomplete. One or both feet or the knees extend below the buttocks (see Fig. 38-6C); this type of presentation is also known as a single or double footling breech.

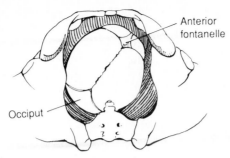

A. Right occiput posterior

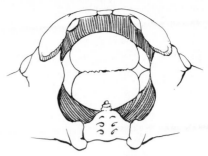

B. Internal rotation: ROP to ROT

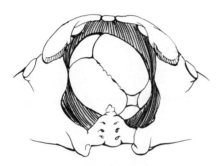

C. Internal rotation: ROT to ROA

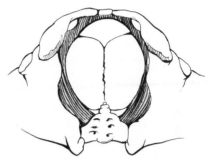

D. Internal rotation: ROA to OA

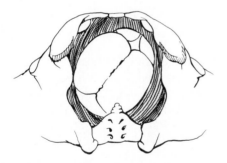

E. Right occiput posterior

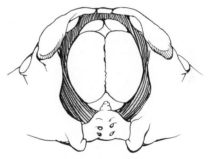

F. Internal rotation: ROP to OP

■ *Figure 38–5*
Occiput posterior. (A through D) Long arc rotation from right occipitoposterior (R.O.P.) to occipitoanterior (O.A.) position. (A) R.O.P. (B) Internal rotation: R.O.P. to right occipitotransverse (R.O.T.). (C) Internal rotation: R.O.T. to right occipitoanterior (R.O.A.). (D) Internal rotation: R.O.A. to O.A. (E and F) Short arc rotation from R.O.P. to occipitoposterior (O.P) position. (E) R.O.P. (F) Internal rotation: R.O.P. to O.P.

Compound. The buttocks present together with another part such as a hand (rare).

Delivery Methods for Breech Presentation. Choosing the route of delivery for an infant in the breech presentation is the subject of much debate. Many studies have shown that neonatal morbidity and mortality are considerably higher when infants with breech presentations are delivered vaginally as compared to the out-

come of cesarean deliveries. Therefore, the incidence of cesarean delivery for breech presentation has increased substantially in the last few decades. Several studies have found that, even with delivery by cesarean section, the infant in breech presentation is at increased risk for morbidity and mortality.[1]

There is no significantly increased danger for the life of the mother in breech presentations, although there is increased incidence of lacerations of the birth

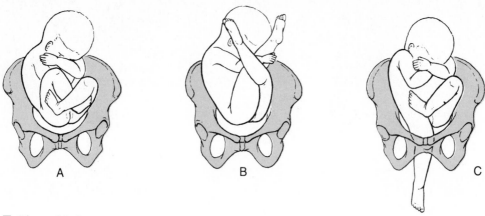

■ *Figure 38–6*
Breech presentation may be (A) complete breech, (B) frank breech, or (C) an incomplete or footling breech.

canal, episiotomy extensions, cesarean deliveries, and postpartum infections. Labor is not prolonged, contrary to previous belief.[1] For the infant, however, there is considerably increased risk of both death and injury in comparison to vertex presentations. Factors related to breech presentation, such as prematurity and congenital malformations, account for a good number of the deaths and long-term sequelae. Mortality from vaginal delivery for all preterm and term infants in breech presentation is about 5.5 times that of infants in vertex presentation. Even with preterm infants excluded, the perinatal mortality in many studies is still 3.5 times higher than for vertex.[12] In term breech births, the majority of perinatal deaths are related to cord prolapse and other cord complications or to tentorial tears and cerebral hemorrhage, which occur during delivery of the aftercoming head.

Other factors related to death or damage of the baby include asphyxia from aspiration of amniotic fluid due to breathing before the head is born, injury due to trapping of the head by the incompletely dilated cervix and

injury, such as fractures, resulting from manipulation and possible rough handling during the delivery.[4]

Although increasing the cesarean delivery rate may decrease the perinatal morbidity and mortality, it increases the maternal morbidity related to major surgery.[1,10] The question is how to select those cases in which the infant can be delivered vaginally with minimum risk, so that the cesarean delivery rate can be kept as low as possible.

Several scoring systems have been developed to evaluate the feasibility of vaginal delivery in breech presentations. The Zatuchni-Andros Prognostic Index (Table 38-2) is an example. These systems are designed to serve as a guide in deciding on the route of delivery. The effectiveness of low scores in predicting patients at risk for infant morbidity and mortality, prolonged labors, and eventual cesarean delivery has been reported. The recommendation is that a score of three or less is a good indication for a cesarean birth, a score of four requires further observation and subsequent evaluation,

TABLE 38-2. ZATUCHNI-ANDROS PROGNOSTIC INDEX

	Points		
	0	*1*	*2*
Parity	Primigravida	Multipara	
Gestational age	39 weeks or more	38 weeks	37 weeks or less
Estimated fetal weight	8 lb (3630 g)	7–7$^{15}/_{16}$ lb (3176–3629 g)	<7 lb (3173 g)
Previous breech*	0	1	2 or more
Dilation†	2 cm	3 cm	4 cm or more
Station†	−3 or higher	−2	−1 or lower

* Greater than 2500 g.
† Determined by vaginal examination on admission.
(Zatuchni GI, Andros GJ: Prognostic index for vaginal delivery in breech presentation. Am J Obstet Gynecol 98: 854, 1967)

and a score of five or more will hopefully result in a successful vaginal delivery. Some investigators have found that low scores are of great prognostic value, but that high scores are less significant and may still be associated with high morbidity and mortality.[4]

One problem with the scoring system is that it does not take into account all of the important factors that must be considered; therefore, it should not take the place of the obstetrician's clinical judgment for each individual woman.

Circumstances in association with breech presentation that are usually considered to be indications for cesarean delivery and those generally considered favorable for vaginal delivery are listed in the box below.[1,12]

Factors Used in Clinical Decisions Related to Delivery Method for Breech Presentations

Circumstances Considered Indications for Cesarean Delivery	*Circumstances Usually Favorable for Vaginal Delivery*
A large fetus >8½ lb	Gestational age between 36 and 38 weeks
Any degree of contraction or unfavorable shape of the pelvis	Estimated fetal weight between 6 and 7 lb
A hyperextended head	Presenting part at the beginning of labor at 0 station or below
Either maternal or fetal indications for delivery, but not in labor	Soft, effaced cervix, dilated to 3 cm or more
Complications of labor, such as acute fetal distress, placenta previa, abruptio placentae, prolpased cord, or uterine dysfunction	Ample pelvis with expectation of head entering in direct occiput anterior position
An apparently healthy preterm fetus of 26 or more weeks gestation; mother in active labor or in need of delivery	Prior obstetrical history of breech delivery of infant weighing greater than 7 lb, or vertex delivery of infant weighing greater than 8 lb
Severe fetal growth retardation	Frank breech presentation
Previous pregnancies resulting in perinatal death or birth trauma	
A firm request for sterilization	
Footing presentation	
Previous cesarean	
Fetal anomalies	

Of the breech presentations, frank breech is usually considered most favorable for vaginal delivery because the buttocks fits into the pelvis more evenly, helping to prevent cord prolapse and acting as a better cervical dilator than other breech presentations.[12]

It would seem that the small preterm infant might be easy to deliver vaginally. In reality, these infants are apt to have proportionately larger heads. The cervix dilates sufficiently for the breech to pass, but the head may become trapped by the cervix. The deflexed head represents another situation in which a baby's head may become trapped, but this time by the bony pelvis.

A most important consideration in the delivery decision is the obstetrician's knowledge of and skill in vaginal breech deliveries. This can be a problem because the current trend toward cesarean delivery for breech presentation does not allow opportunity for much practice in breech vaginal delivery.

EXTERNAL VERSION. With the increasing use of cesarean birth for breech presentation, many obstetricians are taking a new look at external version as a way to prevent breech deliveries. This is most likely to be attempted if the breech presentation is recognized during the third trimester. Some fetuses do return to the breech position after version, but studies have shown a significant decrease in breech deliveries when external version is used. There is a difference of opinion among obstetricians concerning the degree of risk with this procedure and whether the results are worth the risk. Researchers have reported antepartal hemorrhage, premature labor, premature rupture of membranes, and fetal death as complications. Fetal-maternal bleeds have also been reported and led to the recommendation of giving anti-D globulin to Rh-negative women before attempting external version.[4]

VAGINAL DELIVERY. The *mechanism of labor* in breech delivery, except for the reversal of polarity, is comparable to that for vertex presentations. The steps are shown in Figure 38-7. Descent is slower initially in the case of a breech but, among women of similar parity, dilatation and effacement are approximately the same for breech and vertex presentations.

Spontaneous breech deliveries sometimes occur, but usually some degree of assistance is necessary. Assistance is most often needed for delivery of the aftercoming head. This may be accomplished by the application of Piper forceps (see Chap. 39) or by one of several maneuvers, such as the Mariceau-Smellie-Veit maneuver (Fig. 38-8) Maintenance of flexion of the head is important, and suprapubic pressure by the obstetrician or an assistant is usually needed.[12]

Many physicians prefer local or pudendal anesthesia for vaginal breech deliveries because it does not interfere with labor and allows the mother to participate actively. Epidural anesthesia is also preferred for the same reasons and, additionally, it permits more com-

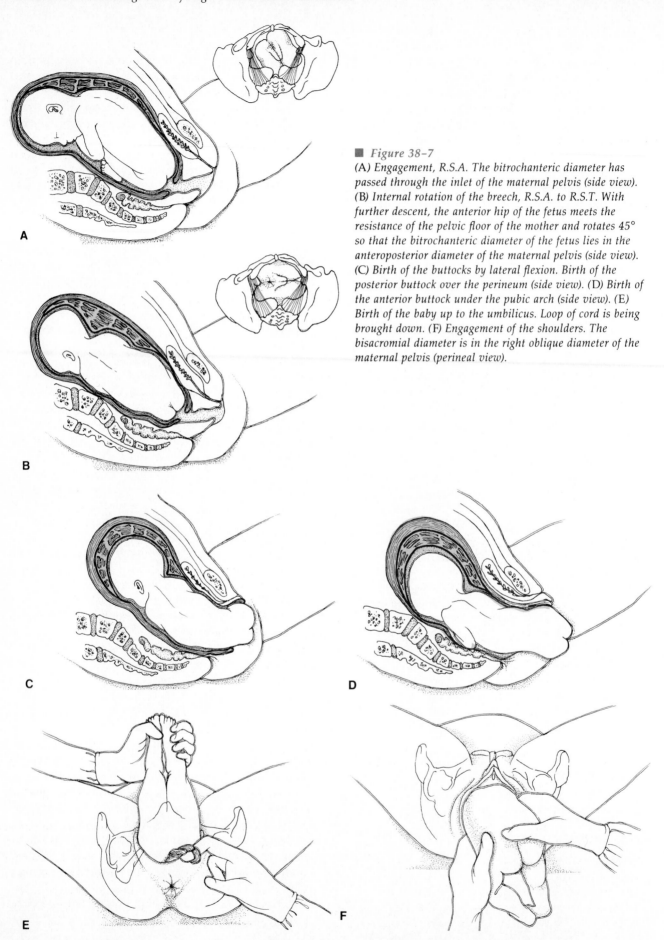

■ Figure 38–7
(A) Engagement, R.S.A. The bitrochanteric diameter has passed through the inlet of the maternal pelvis (side view). (B) Internal rotation of the breech, R.S.A. to R.S.T. With further descent, the anterior hip of the fetus meets the resistance of the pelvic floor of the mother and rotates 45° so that the bitrochanteric diameter of the fetus lies in the anteroposterior diameter of the maternal pelvis (side view). (C) Birth of the buttocks by lateral flexion. Birth of the posterior buttock over the perineum (side view). (D) Birth of the anterior buttock under the pubic arch (side view). (E) Birth of the baby up to the umbilicus. Loop of cord is being brought down. (F) Engagement of the shoulders. The bisacromial diameter is in the right oblique diameter of the maternal pelvis (perineal view).

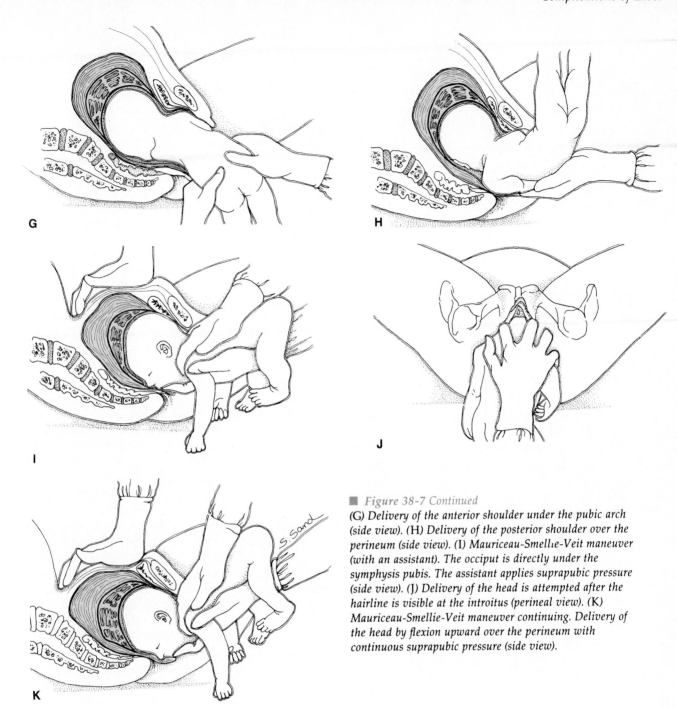

■ *Figure 38-7 Continued*
(G) Delivery of the anterior shoulder under the pubic arch (side view). (H) Delivery of the posterior shoulder over the perineum (side view). (I) Mauriceau-Smellie-Veit maneuver (with an assistant). The occiput is directly under the symphysis pubis. The assistant applies suprapubic pressure (side view). (J) Delivery of the head is attempted after the hairline is visible at the introitus (perineal view). (K) Mauriceau-Smellie-Veit maneuver continuing. Delivery of the head by flexion upward over the perineum with continuous suprapubic pressure (side view).

fortable intravaginal manipulation and extractions. For difficult breech deliveries, a general anesthetic such as halothane might be used because these agents inhibit uterine contractions and make intravaginal manipulation easier.

Assessment in Breech Presentation. Through assessment of the woman in labor, the nurse may be the one who initially identifies signs that the fetus is in a breech presentation. These signs might include palpating the head in the fundus when doing Leopold's maneuvers, locating the fetal heart tones slightly above the umbilicus, feeling the buttocks when doing a vaginal examination, and noting the passage of meconium after the membranes have ruptured.

When breech presentation is confirmed, the nurse continues to monitor the condition of both mother and fetus while the decision of delivery method is being made. Information provided by the nurse often plays an important role in this decision. Continuous assessment of fetal well-being is particularly important due to the increased possibility of cord prolapse with a

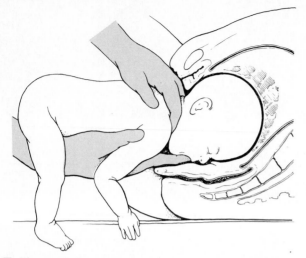

■ *Figure 38–8*
Mauriceau-Smellie-Veit maneuver for extracting the head in breech delivery.

breech presentation. Use of an electronic fetal monitor is helpful in this regard.

Nursing Diagnosis. The following nursing diagnoses might be used: High Risk for Fetal Distress related to increased risk of prolapsed cord, Anxiety and Fear related to concern about possible cesarean section, High Risk for Postpartum Hemorrhage related to interventions necessary for delivery, or Knowledge Deficit related to breech birth.

Planning and Intervention. Based on the nursing diagnoses and the medical treatment plan for the individual patient, the nurse plans her nursing interventions to meet specific goals. Interventions would include initiating monitoring techniques; reporting maternal and fetal condition and any changes in condition; preparing the patient for the selected type of delivery, whether vaginal or cesarean; and explaining to the patient and her family what is happening. Explanation and appropriate reassurance are important for mothers who have breech presentations because many have heard frightening stories of what may happen if the baby is "breech," and anxiety and fear may interfere with the woman's ability to work effectively with her labor.

Evaluation. Effective care for the mother and fetus is demonstrated by absence of fetal or maternal distress, prompt preparation for cesarean delivery, or progress in labor if vaginal delivery is selected, and the birth of an infant in good condition. Nursing interventions to promote the patient's psycho-emotional well-being can be evaluated by the patient's verbalizations that she understands the chosen method of delivery and that

she is less anxious or fearful as well as by her facial expressions and improved relaxation.

ABNORMAL PRESENTATIONS

Shoulder Presentation. Shoulder presentation, or "transverse lie," occurs when the infant lies crosswise in the uterus instead of longitudinally. The shoulder is usually the fetal part in the brim of the inlet, but sometimes it is the back, abdomen, ribs, or flank, depending on how the infant is positioned. Studies have shown this complication to occur once in 300 to 500 cases, and it is seen most often in multiparas, because of relaxation of the abdominal wall. Other common etiological factors are prematurity, placenta previa, and contracted pelvis.[1]

This is a serious complication that increases the hazards of delivery for the mother and even more so for the fetus. Frequently, an arm prolapses into the vagina, making the problem of delivery even more difficult. If neglected, this presentation results in rupture of the uterus and death of both mother and fetus.

External version in late pregnancy or early labor is occasionally successful, especially in the multipara, in converting the shoulder to a longitudinal lie. A transverse lie with the woman in active labor is generally an indication for cesarean delivery. Internal podalic version and extraction is a hazardous procedure frequently associated with rupture of the uterus (see Chap. 39). It is rarely justified except in the case of a second twin.

Face Presentation. Face presentations are seen in about one of 600 patients. Factors that favor extension of the head and prevent flexion are implicated in these presentations, a contracted pelvis being paramount among these. These infants may deliver spontaneously if labor is effective and the pelvis is adequate. The face comes through the vulva with the chin anterior.

However, if there is indication that the pelvis is contracted or that there is fetal distress, a cesarean delivery is indicated. As edema of the scalp is common in vertex presentations, facial edema is often present to the extent that the landmarks resemble a breech presentation. The edema and purplish discoloration disappear within a few days, but the infant's appearance gives the parents a great deal of concern. The nurse can be helpful in reassuring the parents that the condition is temporary and will resolve without sequelae.

Brow Presentation. Brow presentations are somewhat more rare than the other malpresentations. Because the largest diameter of the fetal head, the occipitomental, presents, the fetus is impossible to deliver as long as the brow presentation persists, unless the fetus is small and the pelvis is large. This is, however, an unstable presentation, and often spontaneously converts to an

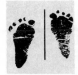

Nursing Care Plan

Woman With Breech Presentation

Patient Goals:
1. Client verbalizes understanding of breech birth and possible cesarean delivery.
2. Mother has minimal discomfort and does not develop complications.
3. Fetal distress does not develop.
4. Infant is born without complications.

Assessment	Potential Nursing Diagnosis	Planning and Intervention	Evaluation
Signs of breech presentation Leopold's maneuver: head in fundus; breech in pelvis Vaginal examination: breech presenting Passage of meconium		Check for fetal presentation and position; report and record findings	
Progress of labor	High risk for alteration in labor progress related to abnormal fetal presentation	Monitor uterine contractions Monitor changes in cervical dilatation and effacement and in fetal presentation and position	Client progresses in labor
Condition of fetus Fetal heart rate and pattern Fetal movement	High risk for fetal distress related to increased risk of prolapsed cord	Monitor fetal heart rate tracing for changes, particularly variable decelerations; check for increased fetal movement; (passage of meconium not indication of fetal distress in breech presentation)	Fetus remains free of distress
Indications for cesarean delivery Fetal distress Position other than frank breech (complete or footling breech position) Evidence of CPD	Knowledge deficit related to breech birth Anxiety and fear related to concern about possible cesarean section	Gather data to assist in decision concerning route of delivery Keep client and family informed of progress of labor and plan of treatment Reassure as appropriate Prepare for surgery, if decision made for cesarean section: have laboratory work done, shave abdomen, insert Foley, do preoperative and postoperative teaching	Client verbalizes understanding of breech birth and cesarean delivery Client verbalizes relief from anxiety and fear Infant is born in good condition

withstand. Uterine rupture may occur in pregnancy but is far more frequent in labor.[1]

Although the incidence has not changed to any degree in the past several decades, the etiology has changed, and the outcome has improved significantly. Today, the most common cause is attributed to rupture of the scar from a previous cesarean section, especially from a classical incision. Women in labor after a cesarean are observed closely for any signs of uterine rupture. The second most common etiological agent is felt to be injudicious stimulation of labor with oxytocin. Other contributing factors include previous surgery involving the myometrium, prolonged or obstructed labor, certain faulty positions or fetal abnormalities, multiparity, excessive fetal size, and traumatic delivery, such as version and extraction, or injudicious use of forceps.[13]

When rupture occurs, the clinical picture depends on a number of factors including the cause, degree (complete or incomplete), extent, and location of the rupture. Oxorn[4] classifies ruptures in four groups according to clinical signs: (1) the silent or quiet rupture, (2) the usual variety, (3) violent rupture, and (4) rupture with delayed diagnosis. The silent rupture has a slow onset and initially occurs without signs and symptoms. The rupture with delayed diagnosis is characterized by bleeding into an area that is not detectable, such as the broad ligament. They may not be detected until the patient has severely deteriorated. In the "usual variety" of uterine rupture, signs and symptoms develop over a period of several hours. These include: abdominal pain and tenderness to palpation, absence of fetal heart tones, vaginal bleeding, vomiting, and signs of developing shock, such as faintness, rapid pulse rate, and pallor.[4] Symptoms of violent rupture are the ones most usually described in relation to uterine rupture: the woman suddenly complains of a severe, sharp pain during a strong labor contraction and expresses the feeling that something has "torn" inside her; uterine contractions cease; the fetus is often expelled from the uterus and may be palpated in the uterine cavity, sometimes with the uterus palpable as a firm mass beside it.[14]

As soon as the diagnosis of rupture of the uterus is made, rapid preparations for an abdominal operation must be made so that the bleeding can be controlled as rapidly as possible. Hysterectomy is the treatment of choice in most cases, but, depending on the woman's condition, age, and desire for more children, an alternate treatment is to repair the uterine tear.[4] Additionally, blood transfusions and intravenous fluids are given to replace lost blood and alleviate shock, and antibiotics are given to prevent or combat infection.

INVERSION OF THE UTERUS

Inversion of the uterus is a highly fatal accident of labor in which, after the birth of the infant, the uterus turns inside out. Shock is profound, and hemorrhage may occur, which if not treated quickly causes the death of the mother.

Predisposing factors for this condition include certain abnormalities of the uterus and its contents such as a short umbilical cord, implantation of the placenta in the fundus of the uterus, and an adherent placenta. The most common precipitating causes, pulling on the umbilical cord and trying to express the placenta or blood clots when the uterus is relaxed, are both preventable. In the former case, the traction on the attached placenta simply pulls the uterus inside out, whereas in the latter, the hand pushes the relaxed muscular sac inside out. Thus, the umbilical cord should never have strenuous traction applied nor should the uterus be pushed downward unless it is firmly contracted.

It is imperative that several steps in treatment be taken promptly and simultaneously.[1] Two intravenous infusion systems are instituted, one with lactated Ringer's solution and one with whole blood. These are given promptly to refill the intravascular compartment and support cardiac output.[2] An anesthesiologist gives a general anesthetic, usually halothane, to relax the uterus. The placenta is left in place until the infusions are operational and uterine relaxation has been accomplished. If the placenta is removed prematurely, hemorrhage is increased. Attempts are made to replace the uterus in the vagina by placing the palm of the hand on the center of the fundus with the fingers extended to identify the cervical margins. The fundus is pushed up through the cervix. When the uterus is returned to its normal shape, anesthesia is discontinued and oxytocin is begun to help the uterus remain contracted. Bimanual compression also aids in this. Until normal tone is ensured, the uterus is monitored transvaginally to detect any possible recurrence.

If the uterus cannot be placed from below because of a constriction ring, a laparotomy is performed so that the uterus can be pulled up simultaneously from above and pushed up from below. The constriction ring may be incised. A traction suture in the fundus aids in repositioning. Treatment continues as previously described. Subsequent inversion is unlikely.[1,6]

Early Postpartum Hemorrhage

Hemorrhage during the postpartum period is the most common cause of serious blood loss associated with pregnancy, and it causes about one fourth of all maternal deaths from hemorrhagic complications. The debilitation and lowered resistance that often accompany it are related to postpartum infections, another leading cause of maternal death. To a large extent, death from postpartum hemorrhage is preventable if the condition is diagnosed early and treated aggressively.

DEFINITION AND INCIDENCE

Postpartum hemorrhage is commonly defined as loss of more than 500 ml of blood during the first 24 hours after giving birth. However, ordinary blood loss after vaginal delivery frequently is more than 500 ml by accurate measurement. Most obstetricians estimate the amount of bleeding at delivery, and studies show that estimated blood loss is usually only about one half of actual loss. Therefore, an *estimated* blood loss over 500 ml serves to alert the nurse and physician that the client has bled excessively and is in danger of postpartum hemorrhage.

With quantitative measurement of blood loss, it has been found that approximately 5% of women who deliver vaginally lose more than 1000 ml of blood, and this amount is increased for women experiencing cesarean birth. Hemorrhages of 1000 ml and over are encountered once in about every 75 cases, whereas blood losses of 1500 and 2000 ml are encountered less frequently. Postpartum hemorrhage is a fairly common complication of labor, and one with which the nurse should be intimately familiar, because nurses are expected to assume an important role in its prevention, detection, and treatment.

CAUSES

In order of frequency, the three immediate causes of postpartum hemorrhage are uterine atony, lacerations of the birth canal (perineum, vagina, and cervix), and retained placental fragments. Clotting defects, uterine tumors, and infections, as well as obstetric accidents such as inversion of the uterus, can also be classified as causes of postpartum hemorrhage, but they are less common and of a more indirect nature.

Uterine Atony. Uterine atony is by far the most common cause of postpartum hemorrhage. The uterus contains huge blood vessels within the interstices of its muscle fibers, and those at the placental site are open and gaping. It is essential that the muscle fibers contract down tightly on these arteries and veins if bleeding is to be controlled. They must *stay* contracted down, because relaxation for only a few seconds gives rise to sudden, profuse hemorrhage. They must stay *tightly* contracted down, because continuous, slight relaxation gives rise to continuous oozing of blood, one of the most treacherous forms of postpartum hemorrhage.

In a study of 56 maternal deaths from pregnancy-related hemorrhage over a 9-year period in California, 19 were due to uterine atony. The majority of these women died within 4 hours of delivery, possibly before the seriousness of their bleeding was recognized. Generally, these patients were older multiparas with spontaneous term deliveries; most of the deaths were avoid-able had the hemorrhage been diagnosed earlier and adequate treatment instituted in time.[1]

Lacerations. Lacerations of the perineum, the vagina, and the cervix are naturally more common after operative delivery. Tears of the cervix are particularly likely to cause serious hemorrhage. Bright red arterial bleeding in the presence of a hard, firmly contracted uterus (no uterine atony) suggests hemorrhage from a cervical laceration. The physician establishes the diagnosis by actual inspection of the cervix (retractors are necessary) and, after locating the source of bleeding, repairs the laceration.

Perineal and vaginal tears also contribute to postpartum blood loss. In addition, perineal tears may do great damage in destroying the integrity of the perineum and in weakening the supports of the uterus, the bladder, and the rectum. Unless these lacerations are repaired properly, the resultant weakness, as the years go by, may cause prolapse of the uterus, cystocele (a pouching downward of the bladder), or rectocele (a pouching forward of the rectum). These conditions, which often originate from perineal lacerations at childbirth, give rise to many discomforts and often necessitate operative treatment.

Lacerations of the birth canal sometimes occur during the process of normal delivery and may be unavoidable even in the most skilled hands.

Retained Placental Fragments. Small, partially separated fragments of placenta may cause postpartum hemorrhage by interfering with proper uterine contraction (Fig. 38-12). Careful inspection of the placenta to determine whether a piece is missing should be routinely carried out at delivery. If a portion is missing, exploration of the uterus is indicated to remove the placental fragment. In the case of continued postpartum bleeding, retention of placental fragments is generally ruled out by manual exploration. However, this is rarely a cause of immediate postpartum hemorrhage and is more commonly implicated in late hemorrhage in which profuse bleeding occurs suddenly a week or more after delivery.

PREDISPOSING FACTORS

Certain factors predispose to postpartum hemorrhage, so in a majority of cases it may be anticipated in advance. Hemorrhage due to uterine atony can be anticipated after labors with overdistention of the uterus (large baby, twins, hydramnios), labors in which deep anesthesia was used, and labors in which there were either vigorous contractions or hypotonic contractions. High parity or previous postpartum hemorrhage also puts the woman at increased risk for hemorrhage due to uterine atony.

■ *Figure 38–12*
Postpartum hemorrhage. Retained tissue demonstrated on sonogram. This requires surgical evacuation. (Cavanagh D, Woods RE, O'Connor TCF, Knuppel RA: Obstetric Emergencies, 3rd ed. Philadelphia, Harper & Row, 1982)

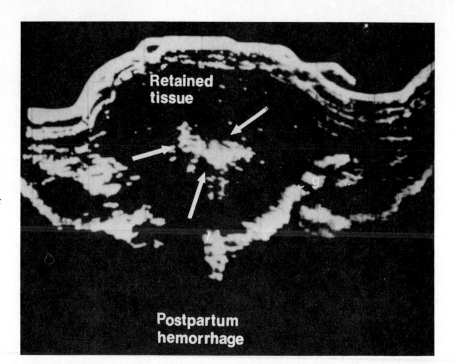

Delivery of a large baby, midforceps or forceps rotation, intrauterine manipulation, and delivery after cesarean section are examples of situations in which trauma is likely to lead to postpartum hemorrhage, probably from lacerations of the uterus or birth canal. Attempts to hasten the delivery of the placenta in the third stage of labor may also lead to hemorrhage. It should also be noted that a small woman may withstand blood loss less well than a woman of average size or larger, because she is more likely to have a smaller blood volume.[1]

CLINICAL PICTURE

Excessive bleeding resulting from trauma to the birth canal or a retained placenta may begin during the third stage of labor, but more commonly hemorrhage is noted at some point after expulsion of the placenta. Although this early hemorrhage is occasionally torrential, with large amounts of blood and clots expelled, the nurse must be aware that it may also be seen as a continuous trickle, minute by minute. These small constant trickles are not alarming in appearance and are therefore more treacherous, because they may not arouse concern and, consequently, there may be no action taken. If the bleeding continues, signs and symptoms of hypovolemic shock develop.

MEDICAL MANAGEMENT

Medical interventions for the woman experiencing a postpartum hemorrhage depend on the cause of the hemorrhage. If the bleeding is from a retained placenta, the physician may find it necessary to remove the placenta manually. Early postpartum hemorrhage due to uterine atony usually is treated with fundal massage and oxytocics. If the hemorrhage is the result of lacerations or retained placental fragments, the patient may be returned to the delivery room for repair or uterine evacuation.

If the above therapy fails to stop the bleeding, the physician may perform bimanual compression of the uterus. This provides the most efficient means of compressing the site of bleeding. Packing the uterus with gauze, a procedure once considered valuable to promote hemostasis in such cases, is seldom used today. It is considered by many to be inadequate treatment and is also conducive to infection.[4]

In cases of continued bleeding, additional pharmacological interventions might include injection of oxytocin or prostaglandin into the myometrium (Table 38-3).[4,15] In some instances, surgical intervention may become necessary. Ligation of the uterine or hypogastric arteries is often attempted before resorting to hysterectomy to prevent continuing and potentially fatal blood loss.[15] Measures to prevent and treat shock are used concurrently with efforts to control the bleeding.

Hemorrhage and Shock

The normally expanded blood volume of the pregnant woman may allow for a larger absolute blood loss to occur before the appearance of clinical evidence of

TABLE 38-3. PHARMACOLOGICAL METHODS USED TO CONTROL UTERINE ATONY

Agent	Dose	Route
Oxytocin	10–20 units	IV drip,* IM, intramyometrial (multiple sites)
Methylergonovine	0.2 mg	IM
Prostaglandin F$_{2a}$	1 mg	Intramyometrial
Prostaglandin 15 methyl	0.25 mg	IM, intramyometrial (multiple sites)

(Gonik B: Intensive care of the critically ill pregnant patient. In Creasy RK, Resnik R (eds): Maternal-Fetal Medicine, 2nd ed. Philadelphia, WB Saunders, 1989)

shock.[15] The pulse and blood pressure may not change significantly until large amounts of blood have been lost. The condition and size of the client help determine the amount of blood loss that can be tolerated, with exhaustion from prolonged labor, preexisting anemia, or chronic disease reducing the ability of the body to compensate. When hemorrhage has been profuse enough, compensatory mechanisms are activated and signs and symptoms of shock ensue.

Shock occurs when the patient's functional intravascular blood volume falls below that of the capacity of the body's vascular bed.[15] In response to this fall in pressure in the blood vessels, the adrenal glands release catecholamines, which cause blood to be shunted away from nonvital areas such as the skin, kidney, and muscles by vasoconstriction, and diverted to the brain and heart.[9] If the condition is not corrected, continuing generalized intense vasoconstriction results in cellular acidosis and hypoxia, which eventually leads to death. The degree of vasoconstriction is influenced by both the amount of blood loss and the elapsed time until the blood is replaced.[15]

Signs and symptoms of shock are related to the compensatory mechanisms. Initially, the pulse becomes rapid, the skin is pale and cool, and the respirations may be rapid and deep. In response to further vasoconstriction, the pulse rate continues to increase and become thready; the skin is cool, pale, and clammy; blood pressure falls; the respirations become more rapid and shallow; and urinary output decreases. Nausea and vomiting and increasing restlessness may also occur. As shock deepens, changes occur in level of consciousness from mental cloudiness, to lethargy, coma, and death (Table 38-4).[9,15] Acceptable ranges in various systems while managing shock are given in Table 38-5.

MANAGEMENT OF SHOCK

Identification and definitive treatment of the cause of the hemorrhage is a primary step in the prevention and treatment of hypovolemic shock. Other measures are directed toward the body's responses to the blood loss. An important aspect of the management of serious hemorrhage is *fluid replacement* to combat hypovolemia.

TABLE 38-4. SYMPTOMS OF SHOCK RELATED TO VOLUME OF BLOOD LOSS

	Mild (20%–25% Loss)	Moderate (25%–35% loss)	Severe (>35% loss)	Irreversible
Respirations	Rapid, deep	Rapid, becoming shallow	Rapid, shallow, may be irregular	Irregular or barely perceptible
Pulse	<100 beats per minute	100–120 beats per minute	>120 beats per minute	Irregular apical pulse
	Rapid; tone normal	Rapid; tone may be normal but is becoming weaker	Very rapid; easily collapsible; may be irregular	
Blood pressure	Normal or hypertensive	80–100 mm Hg systolic	<60 mm Hg systolic	None palpable
Skin	Cold and pale			
	Peripheral vasoconstriction	Cool, pale, moist; knees cyanotic	Cold, clammy; cyanosis of lips and fingernails	Cold, clammy, cyanotic
Urinary output	No change	Decreasing to 10–22 ml/h	Oliguric (<10 ml) to anuric	Anuric
Level of consciousness	Alert, oriented; diffuse anxiety	Oriented, mental cloudiness, or increasing restlessness	Lethargy; reacts to noxious stimuli; comatose	Does not respond to noxious stimuli
Central venous pressure	May be normal	3 cm H$_2$O	0–3 cm H$_2$O	

TABLE 38-5. PHYSIOLOGICAL PARAMETERS IN SHOCK MANAGEMENT

Variables	Acceptable Adult Ranges
Cardiovascular	
Pulse rate	<90 beats per minute
Arterial pulse pressure	>30 mm Hg
Central venous pressure	5–12 cm H_2O
Pulmonary arterial pressure	
Systolic	25–30 mm Hg
Diastolic	8–10 mm Hg
Pulmonary wedge pressure	8–15 mm Hg
Hematocrit	35%–45%
Hemoglobin	>11 g/dL
Respiratory-metabolic	
Respiratory rate	12–15 breaths per minute
Arterial PO_2	80–100 mm Hg
Arterial PCO_2	37–45 mm Hg
Arteriovenous O_2 extraction	40 ml/L
Arterial pH	7.35–7.45
Renal	
Urinary output	30–50 ml/h

(Court D: Maternal cardiovascular and renal disorders: Maternal shock in pregnancy. In Creasy RK, Resnik R (eds.): Maternal-Fetal Medicine. Philadelphia, WB Saunders, 1984)

It is recommended that lactated Ringer's solution be given in the amount and proportion necessary to maintain a urine flow of at least 30 ml/h and preferably 60 ml/h.[1,15] If initial vigorous fluid replacement therapy does not restore urine flow, insertion of a central venous catheter to obtain *central venous pressure* (CVP) readings, or a Swan-Ganz catheter to obtain *pulmonary wedge pressure* (PWP) provides important information about fluid balance and needs, and can aid in preventing circulatory overload.[15]

Because *blood transfusion* plays an important role in preventing serious shock, the blood groups of *all* maternity clients should be known before labor, and cross-matched blood should be available for those in whom hemorrhage is anticipated or appears imminent. Seeing that the blood typing is carried out, ordering and calling for the cross-match, and making sure that the blood is sent to the unit are usually responsibilities of the nurse. Time is of the essence for these clients; therefore, the nurse must preplan and establish priorities rapidly. For best results, sufficient blood replacement should be given to maintain the hematocrit at 30%.[15]

The body's oxygen-carrying capacity is diminished by blood loss, therefore, oxygen administration by mask is usually ordered to increase the amount of oxygen in the circulating blood. Additionally, elevating the lower extremities increases perfusion to vital organs until sufficient blood and fluid volume replacement can be ac-

complished. Some sources recommend use of Trendelenburg's position, whereas others suggest that it be avoided because it may interfere with cerebral circulation and respiratory exchange.[16]

NURSING PROCESS IN HEMORRHAGIC COMPLICATIONS

Assessment

The nurse plays a primary role in the prevention, detection, and treatment of hemorrhage, especially that caused by uterine atony. Routine nursing assessment of vital signs, condition of the uterus, and amount of bleeding in the early postpartum period is directed toward detecting uterine atony and subsequent increased bleeding (see Chaps. 22 and 28). Assessment should include review of the chart to identify any factors that would place the client at risk for hemorrhage. For the client at risk, or any client with increased bleeding, the vital signs, fundus, and amount of bleeding should be checked more frequently than routine. The client should also be monitored for other signs of impending shock, such as changes in skin color and temperature, decreased urinary output, or changes in level of consciousness.

NURSING DIAGNOSIS

Assessment of the client for signs and symptoms of hemorrhage may lead the nurse to some of the following nursing diagnoses: Fluid Volume Deficit related to excessive blood loss and manifested by increased pulse rate, decreased blood pressure, and decreased urinary output; High Risk for Infection related to decreased resistance secondary to excessive blood loss; Fear and Anxiety related to concern about bleeding as a life-threatening situation.

PLANNING AND INTERVENTION

If one suspects that a woman may be hemorrhaging, it is important that the nurse remain with her constantly. The fundus should be checked immediately. The physician needs to be notified, and emergency equipment must be easily accessible, including intravenous tray with large-bore (#18) needles, retention catheter, oxygen, suction, blood pressure, and CVP apparatus.

Massaging the Fundus. The uterus should be located immediately and massaged gently but firmly. The lower uterine segment is supported with the edge of the hand a little above the mother's symphysis, while the fundus is massaged with the other hand (see Fig. 22-19). Thus, the uterus is cupped between the two hands and is supported as it is massaged. Massage is to be continued until the uterus assumes a woody hardness; if the slightest relaxation occurs, the massage must be reinstituted. In many cases, the uterus stays contracted most of the time, but occasionally it relaxes; it is therefore obligatory to keep a hand on the fundus constantly for a full hour after bleeding has subsided. When the uterus is well contracted, care should be taken to *avoid overmassage*, because such practice contributes to muscle fatigue, which in turn further encourages uterine relaxation and excessive bleeding.

It must be remembered that relaxation sometimes occurs 2 or more hours after delivery; in these cases, the uterus may balloon with blood, with little escaping externally. Accordingly, the consistency, size, and height of the uterus should be checked frequently until several hours have elapsed. Ordinarily, the height of the fundus after delivery is about at the level of the umbilicus. If the uterus becomes distended with blood, or if the bladder becomes full and presses upward against the uterus causing it to rise in the abdomen, the fundus can be palpated several centimeters above the umbilicus. The nurse must make absolutely certain that the uterus is, in fact, being massaged, and not a roll of abdominal fat or a distended bladder. When properly contracted, the uterus should feel about the size and consistency of a small, firm grapefruit.

Frequently, a big, boggy, relaxed uterus is difficult to outline through the abdominal wall, and it may be necessary to push the hand well posteriorly toward the region of the sacral promontory to reach it. The fact that the uterus is hard to identify often means that it is relaxed, but palpation and massage usually cause it to become firm.

Allaying Anxiety. The frequent massage and deep palpation may be painful to the mother; at best, they are disturbing, because they come at a time when she wants nothing more than to rest and sleep after her great effort. If she is awake and alert, the continued attention and scrutiny may increase her anxiety. It must be remembered that apprehension is a natural concomitant of hemorrhage and shock. Quick and efficient nursing observations and appropriate explanation and reassurance help allay the concerns of both the mother and her partner.

This aspect of nursing care may be difficult to implement. If the mother or the father expresses concern and questions the activity by asking "What's wrong?" the nurse can simply say, "The uterus has a tendency to relax and must be massaged so that it contracts as it should." Usually, such a statement suffices. This indicates the reason for the continued activity without associating hemorrhage and its fearsome consequences with the actions of the attendants. If the mother drifts off to sleep between the nurse's observations, the nurse can gently rouse her by speaking her name before commencing massage, so that the mother is not awakened abruptly to the painful sensation of someone squeezing her abdomen.

Other Aspects of Care. Vital signs must be checked every 5 to 15 minutes, and any variation, however slight, is to be reported immediately. Skin condition, level of consciousness, and urinary output are also monitored.

One way that the nurse can keep a more accurate account of the blood loss is by keeping a perineal pad count. A record is kept of the number of pads saturated, how fully they are saturated, and the time it took for the saturation to occur. Thus, the nurse's notes might read: "Two pads ¾ saturated in 20 minutes." This type of report is more helpful to the physician than a more general, vague statement like, "Saturating perineal pads quickly."

EVALUATION

The effectiveness of nursing interventions related to hemorrhage and shock is evaluated first on the basis of prevention of the conditions, and if they occur, on the responsiveness to treatment. Maintenance of vital signs within normal limits, minimal amounts of blood loss, and a firm uterus in the case of a postpartum patient, all indicate successful prevention of hemorrhage and shock. For the client who experiences hemorrhage, response to treatment is evaluated on an ongoing basis. A client who hemorrhages during the intrapartum or postpartum period demonstrates appropriate response to treatment if her vital signs return to and remain within normal limits; her blood loss decreases to minimal amounts; her output is approximately equal to her intake; she remains free of infection; and she verbalizes understanding of her condition and treatment. For intrapartum hemorrhage, the condition of the fetus would also be of concern with effectiveness of treatment focusing on his well-being before and after birth. When the hemorrhage occurs postpartum, effective treatment is demonstrated by the uterus remaining contracted.

■ PRETERM LABOR AND BIRTH

Preterm labor is defined as labor that begins before 37 completed weeks of pregnancy. The lower limit is not well established. Twenty-eight weeks was most frequently used in the past, but with the increasing ability to care for the infant born before 28 weeks, 20 weeks is more frequently used as the lower limit. The infants resulting from these preterm labors account for a significant proportion of perinatal morbidity and mortality.

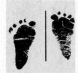

Nursing Care Plan

Woman With Postpartum Hemorrhage

Patient Goals:
1. Vital signs and urinary output are within normal limits.
2. Fundus is firm, lochia is moderate.
3. Client does not develop infection.
4. Client verbalizes understanding of her condition.

Assessment	Potential Nursing Diagnosis	Planning and Intervention	Evaluation

Risk factors for postpartum hemorrhage:
  Overdistention of uterus (large baby, twins, hydramnios)
  Abnormal uterine contractions (hypotonic, tetanic)
  Oxytocin induction or augmentation of labor
  Grandmultiparity
  Previous postpartum hemorrhage
  Difficult (traumatic) delivery
	High risk for excessive vaginal bleeding related to relaxation of uterine muscle secondary to twin pregnancy	Review chart for risk factors
		
		Identify client at risk, and monitor uterus, lochia, and vital signs closely	

Conditions of uterus
  Firmness
  Size
  Height of fundus
		Check uterus every 15 min times 4 or until it remains firm without excessive bleeding	Client has a firm fundus with return to normal lochia

Lochia
  Amount
  Color
  Presence of clots
		Massage fundus until firm, express blood and clots as necessary
		
		Estimate amount of bleeding
		
		Initiate pad count
		
		Observe for continuous trickle of blood in presence of contracted uterus
		
		Start IV line if not in place
		
		Maintain IV with oxytocin at ordered rate
		
		Administer other medications as ordered	

Vital Signs
  Temperature-pulse-respiration
  Blood pressure
	Fluid volume deficit related to excessive blood loss and manifested by increased pulse rate, de-	Check every 15 min or as ordered
		
		Report and record
			Client avoids hypovolemic shock
			
			Client's vital signs stabilize

(continued)

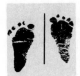

Nursing Care Plan   *(continued)*

Assessment	Potential Nursing Diagnosis	Planning and Intervention	Evaluation
CVP (if used)	creased blood pressure and decreased urinary output		
Urinary output		Keep accurate intake and output record; insert Foley catheter for more accurate output, if indicated	Client voids adequate amounts
		Encourage emptying of bladder	
Skin: color and temperature		Observe for pallor; cool, moist skin	
Level of consciousness		Check orientation of client by speaking to her frequently	
Emotional status	Fear and anxiety related to concern about excessive bleeding as life-threatening situation	Keep client and family members informed about what is happening and what is being done	Client verbalizes her confidence in recovery
		Reassure as indicated	
Laboratory values		Make sure that type and cross-match are done if indicated	
		Make sure that hemoglobin, hematocrit, other laboratory work are done, as ordered	
Need for surgical intervention		Make sure client is informed about procedure	Client repeats information she understands about procedures
		Complete surgical checklist	
	High risk for infection related to decreased resistance to pathogenic organisms secondary to excessive blood loss	Maintain aseptic technique	Client remains free of infection

Studies have shown that the rate of preterm birth varies from country to country and from institution to institution, occurring in developed countries in approximately 5% to 10% of all births.[17] In the United States, the incidence of preterm birth is about 9% overall, however in further analysis, the rate is about 8% for white women and between 16% and 17% for African-American women.[18] The prevention of preterm birth is considered to be the most important problem to be dealt with in improving the outcome of pregnancies in which there are no congenital anomalies.[17] The problem of preterm labor is the focus of many studies and pilot projects. These are directed toward several different aspects of the problem including prediction, prevention, early detection, diagnosis, and management. In the absence of conclusive data in any of these areas, interventions and protocols in different institutions or geographic areas are varied.

Prediction

Prediction of the woman who is most likely to experience spontaneous preterm labor and delivery would not be such a difficult task if the causes of preterm labor were better understood. In most cases, however, the cause of preterm labor is unknown. Factors that seem to be most clearly related to the initiation of preterm labor include conditions that cause overdistention of the uterus, uterine anomalies, surgical procedures on the uterus, previous or present early uterine activity, and fetal anomalies.[4,19]

In an effort to predict which women are at increased risk for spontaneous preterm labor and delivery, studies have identified a number of related maternal risk factors, but these are not consistent from study to study. Many of them are the same risk factors that place the expectant mother at increased risk for other pregnancy problems (see Chap. 6). Risk factors can be grouped into categories including demographic risks, past reproductive history, medical history, behavioral and environmental characteristics, obstetric factors of the present pregnancy, and psychological factors (Table 38-6).[17,18]

A number of risk scoring systems have been developed using the identified risk factors. Creasy reports a study of one such scoring system using major and minor risk factors to predict spontaneous preterm labor.[17] When one or more major factors or two or more minor factors are present, the woman is considered to be at high risk for preterm labor (Table 38-7). Although these systems are of some predictive value, many more women are identified as at risk than actually experience preterm labor. Also, risk scoring systems fail to identify approximately 50% of pregnant patients who subsequently have spontaneous preterm births.[17] It is hoped that eventually biochemical and biophysical measurements, developed to be used with the scoring systems, will improve the accuracy of predicting the woman at risk. Scoring systems may also need modifications for use with different populations.[20]

Prevention

Efforts to prevent preterm labor are directed toward prevention or detection of risk factors and treatment of these factors as appropriate. Interventions to prevent the onset of labor in women found to be at risk have not proved to be effective in most cases. Good dietary counseling and encouragement to reduce or preferably

---

TABLE 38-6. FACTORS ASSOCIATED WITH PRETERM LABOR

Demographic Factors	Medical History and Status	Obstetric Factors in Present Pregnancy
Nonwhite	Heart disease	Lack of or late prenatal care
Unmarried	Anemia	Low prepregnancy weight
Two children at home	3rd trimester urinary tract infection	Weight gain < 5 kg by 32 weeks
Low socioeconomic status	DES exposure in utero	Engagement of head at 32 weeks
Maternal age < 20 years or >40 years		Development of pregnancy complications
Single parent	**Behavioral and Environmental Characteristics**	
Height < 150 cm	Poor nutrition	**Psychological Factors**
Weight < 45 kg	Smoking	Stress
	Use of alcohol or illicit drugs	Psychic trauma
Past Reproductive History	Exposure to toxins	Negative attitude toward pregnancy
Prior induced abortions	Working outside home	
Prior low-birth-weight baby	Heavy or stressful work	
Prior preterm delivery	Long, tiring trip or commute	
Prior 2nd trimester spontaneous abortion	Unusual fatigue	
Less than 1 year since last birth		

(Adapted from Kulb NW: Preterm labor. In Buckley K, Kulb NW [eds]: High Risk Maternity Nursing Manual. Baltimore, Williams & Wilkins, 1990, and Creasy RK: Disorders of parturition: Preterm labor and delivery. In Creasy RK, Resnik R [eds]: Maternal-Fetal Medicine: Principles and Practice. Philadelphia, WB Saunders, 1984)

TABLE 38–7. MAJOR AND MINOR RISK FACTORS IN PREDICTION OF SPONTANEOUS PRETERM LABOR

Previous Medical History	Aspects of Current Pregnancy	Daily Habits
Major Risk Factors		
Previous preterm delivery	Multiple gestation	
DES exposure	Hydramnios	
Previous preterm labor, term delivery	Abdominal surgery during pregnancy	
Uterine anomaly	Cervix dilated >1 cm at 32 weeks	
History of cone biopsy	Cervical shortening: <1 cm at 32 weeks	
Second-trimester abortion ×2	Uterine irritability	
Minor Risk Factors		
Second-trimester abortion ×1	Febrile illness	Cigarettes— more than 10 per day
More than two first-trimester abortions	Bleeding after 12 weeks	
History of pyelonephritis		

Presence of one or more major factors or two or more minor factors places patient in high-risk group.
(Adapted from Creasy RK: Preterm labor and delivery. In Creasy RK, Resnik R [eds]: Maternal-Fetal Medicine: Principles and Practice, 2nd ed. Philadelphia, WB Saunders, 1989)

eliminate maternal cigarette smoking or use of unnecessary drugs are appropriate interventions for pregnant women in general, but may be particularly helpful for the woman at risk for preterm labor. Bedrest has proved useful in preventing preterm labor with multiple gestations, but its usefulness in single gestation is not known. Bacterial infection of the lower genital tract is suspected by some researchers to contribute to the onset of preterm labor. Prevention of infection might help prevent some preterm labors. Avoiding intercourse has also been suggested as a preventive measure, both for reducing the risk of infection and because the prostaglandins in seminal fluid are thought possibly to stimulate uterine contractions.[21] Cervical cerclage has sometimes been suggested as a method of preventing preterm labor and birth, but there is some evidence that placement of the cerclage may promote uterine contractions.[22]

There have been some efforts to use pharmacological methods prophylactically. Use of progesterone in preventing preterm labor has shown mixed results. Suggestions of possible teratogenic effects have resulted in a ban on the use of progestins during pregnancy by the U.S. Food and Drug Administration (FDA). The usefulness of prophylactic β-adrenergic therapy is also unclear after several studies.[19]

Early Detection and Diagnosis

Prevention of preterm birth through early detection and treatment of preterm labor has become more possible since the discovery of new, more effective tocolytic agents to arrest labor. Preterm labor must be detected early if tocolytic agents are to be used, because their effectiveness decreases with the advance of labor. Client education and frequent evaluation of the cervix for high-risk patients have proved effective in early identification of preterm labor in some studies.[19]

Home uterine activity monitoring, which has been shown to contribute to earlier detection and treatment of preterm labor, is being used as part of many preterm prevention projects and by an increasing number of private physicians.[23–25]

Diagnosis of preterm labor in time to prevent preterm birth is often difficult. Possible early signs and symptoms including abdominal, intestinal, or menstrual-like cramps, pelvic pressure, diarrhea, low backache, and increased vaginal discharge are difficult to differentiate from false labor or common discomforts of advancing pregnancy.[18] Even the presence of regular uterine contractions does not always mean true labor has begun. Rupture of the membranes accompanied by regular uterine contractions establishes the diagnosis, but attempting to stop the labor at this point is problematic. Progressive cervical effacement and dilatation can also establish the diagnosis but must be detected early because advanced dilatation is a contraindication to tocolysis. In an attempt to establish an accurate diagnosis, the following criteria are usually used when membranes are intact:

1. Documented uterine contractions (four in 20 minutes or eight in 60 minutes)
2. Documented cervical change or cervical effacement of 80% or dilatation of 2 cm[17]

Management

Until fairly recently measures available to arrest the progress of preterm labor were limited to conservative treatment such as bedrest. Today, there are a number of drugs that are used to try to inhibit preterm labor. These are referred to as *tocolytic agents.* If preterm labor begins, the question becomes whether or not to use these agents in an attempt to prevent preterm birth. Indica-

tions for use of a tocolytic drug to inhibit labor include: a diagnosis of preterm labor; gestational age greater than 20 weeks, but less than 35 weeks; cervical dilatation less than 4 cm; estimated fetal weight less than 2500 g; intact fetal membranes; a viable, nondistressed fetus and no contraindications to continuing the pregnancy or to the use of the tocolytic agent.[10,26]

Before deciding to attempt to inhibit labor, assessment of the condition of mother and fetus must be made to determine whether continuation of the pregnancy would be detrimental to the mother, and whether the fetus would have a better chance of survival inside or outside the uterus. Contraindications to tocolysis include: maternal medical complications such as uncontrolled diabetes or severe preeclampsia; active uterine bleeding; intrauterine infection (chorioamnionitis); chronic fetal distress such as intrauterine growth retardation; acute fetal distress; ruptured membranes; cervical dilatation greater than 4 to 5 cm; major fetal anomalies incompatible with life; or intrauterine fetal death.[4,27] Some of the contraindications are relative, and tocolysis may be attempted even though they are present, especially if gestation is around 25 to 27 weeks and a delay of 1 to 2 weeks might significantly improve fetal outcome (Table 38-8).[17]

If the decision is made to attempt to halt the labor, a combination of supportive and pharmacological interventions will probably be implemented.

GENERAL MEASURES

Bedrest in the left lateral position is sometimes effective in reducing the frequency and intensity of uterine contractions. Hydration, usually by intravenous infusion, is also used. It is thought to decrease release of antidiuretic hormone and oxytocin from the posterior pituitary gland.[27] If urinary tract infection is suspected, antibiotic therapy may be initiated without waiting for the results of the culture.[28] Unnecessary vaginal manipulation should be avoided.

USE OF TOCOLYTIC AGENTS

Ethyl alcohol (ethanol), administered intravenously to the mother, was the first tocolytic agent used with success and was a popular intervention in the 1960s and 1970s. However, the high levels needed to suppress uterine contractions caused intoxication in the mother and fetus; ethanol has also been found to cause metabolic problems, and with the growing concern over the effects of alcohol on the fetus, it has mostly been abandoned for use in arresting preterm labor.[1]

β-adrenergic agonists are in use as tocolytic agents. This group of drugs includes ritodrine (Yutopar), terbutaline (Brethine), isoxsuprine (Vasodilan), and others

---

TABLE 38-8. CONTRAINDICATIONS TO TOCOLYTIC INHIBITION OF PRETERM LABOR

Absolute Contraindications

Severe pregnancy-induced hypertension
Severe abruptio placentae
Severe bleeding from any cause
Chorioamnionitis
Fetal death
Fetal anomaly incompatible with life
Severe fetal growth retardation

Relative Contraindications

Mild chronic hypertension
Mild abruptio placentae
Stable placenta previa
Maternal cardiac disease
Hyperthyroidism
Uncontrolled diabetes mellitus
Fetal distress
Fetal anomaly
Mild fetal growth retardation
Cervix more than 5 cm dilated

(Creasy RK: Preterm labor and delivery. In Creasy RK, Resnik R [eds]: Maternal-Fetal Medicine: Principles and practice, 2nd ed. Philadelphia, WB Saunders, 1989)

which are used in other countries. Only ritodrine is approved by the U.S. Food and Drug Administration for use in inhibiting preterm labor, but terbutaline and isoxsuprine are also used in the United States on an experimental basis.

These drugs are primarily β_2 stimulators and lead to relaxation of bronchial, vascular, and uterine smooth muscle, but they also exhibit some β_1 effects, stimulating myocardial contractility and heart rate. Common, potentially serious side-effects of these agents include maternal and fetal tachycardia, hypotension (especially a decrease in diastolic pressure), cardiac arrhythmias, hypokalemia, and pulmonary edema. Other, less serious side-effects such as nervousness, emesis, headache, and tremulousness can be disturbing.[1]

Initial administration of these drugs is usually by the intravenous route, but some may be given intramuscularly, subcutaneously, or orally.[19] Oral administration has been most commonly used for maintenance after contractions have been stopped by intravenous administration. A portable subcutaneous terbutaline pump has been introduced and found useful for home maintenance.[26] (See Table 38-9 for further discussion of these tocolytic agents.)

Magnesium sulfate has been used with some success in arresting preterm labor, although it is not yet approved for this purpose by the FDA. The mode of action is thought to be reduction of myometrial activity by lowering the intracellular concentration of calcium.[4] Complications are rare but may include hypotension and respiratory depression in the mother and hypotonia in the infant.

Prostaglandin synthetase inhibitors are another class of drugs that have been shown to reduce uterine activity. Indomethacin and aspirin are two of the drugs in this group. Although some studies have shown indomethacin to be effective, because of the potential danger of premature closure of the ductus arteriosus in the fetus they are not advocated for use in inhibiting preterm labor at this time.[4,28]

Calcium antagonists, such as nifedipine, are among other tocolytic agents being investigated. In small studies, oral nifedipine has been shown to be effective in stopping uterine contractions with few side-effects. Further studies are needed to establish safety and effectiveness.[17,28]

USE OF STEROIDS

Although the ideal objective of the treatment of preterm labor is to prevent delivery until term when the fetus is mature, realistically this is possible only about 20% of the time with our current methods.[20] A short-term objective that is more attainable is to stop labor temporarily for 24 to 48 hours to allow time for maturation of the fetal lungs. Respiratory distress syndrome (RDS) is the most common cause of morbidity and mortality in preterm infants. This condition is related to a deficiency of surfactant in the immature lungs. Some studies have shown a decrease in RDS when betamethasone or dexamethasone is administered to the mother before delivery. Few side-effects have been demonstrated, but long-term effects are not known, so the drugs are not used indiscriminately. The treatment seems to be most effective for gestations of less than 33 weeks.[4]

PRETERM BIRTH

Not all women are candidates for arrest of preterm labor, and not all attempts to arrest labor are successful. If preterm labor continues, preparations must be made for the birth of a preterm infant. In some situations, when continuation of the labor is inevitable and a specialized health-care team and equipment are not available, the decision may be made to transport the pregnant mother (maternal–fetal transport) to a tertiary care center.

The focus of management of preterm birth is on careful, continuous observation of the status of the fetus. Systemic anagesics and anesthetics given to the mother during labor might depress the infant at birth and should be avoided. Generous episiotomies, delivery of the head between contractions, use of forceps, and cesarean sections for breech presentation, are interventions used to protect the preterm infant's head during the birth process because these infants are more susceptible to intracranial hemorrhage.[19]

NURSING PROCESS IN PRETERM LABOR

Assessment. Initial assessment of the woman who is thought to be in labor before 37 weeks' gestation includes basic information about her health and obstetric history plus evaluation of her current condition. The nurse can assist in determining the presence of true labor by monitoring the frequency, intensity, and duration of contractions, checking for cervical effacement and dilatation, and observing for other signs of labor, such as rupture of membranes and bloody show. Assessment of the fetus for approximate size, maturity, and signs of fetal distress is also important. Prenatal history, fetal monitoring, ultrasound, and determination of the lecithin/sphingomyelin ratio are all methods that might be used in the assessment.

Once treatment is begun, the nurse continues to assess the signs of labor and also assesses for side-effects of the treatment on both mother and fetus. Continuous electronic fetal and contraction monitoring is used, and the nurse assesses the monitor strip for any changes.

(Text continues on page 960)

TABLE 38-9. DRUGS USED FOR PRETERM LABOR

Tocolytic Agents

General indications for use:
- Signs of preterm labor
- Gestational age > 20 wk but <36 wk
- Estimated fetal weight > 500 g but < 2500 g
- No contraindications to continuation of pregnancy

General contraindications:
- Pregnancy < 20 wk
- Ruptured membranes, especially with signs of infection
- Active uterine bleeding
- Maternal medical complications such as diabetes mellitus or severe preeclampsia
- Acute or chronic fetal distress
- Major fetal anomalies
- Intrauterine fetal death
- Any maternal or fetal condition contraindicating the continuation of pregnancy
- Advanced labor with cervical dilatation beyond 3 cm

Drug	Action	Additional Contraindications	Side-effects and Complications	Dosage and Route	Remarks
β-Adrenergic Agonists					
Ritodrine (Yutopar)	Exerts preferential effect on β_2 receptors in smooth muscle of uterus inhibiting contractility; in blood vessels causing vasodilation	Maternal cardiac disease, renal disease, diabetes, or hyperthyroidism Known hypersensitivity to drug	Maternal: Cardiovascular: Increased heart rate Widening pulse pressure: Slightly increased systolic BP Decreased diastolic BP Increased cardiac output Hyperglycemia Hypokalemia Fluid retention Pulmonary edema Subjective reactions Palpitations Tremors Nausea and vomiting	Intravenous infusion: 150 mg ritodrine to 500 ml of solution = 0.3 mg/ml Begin at 0.05 mg to 0.1 mg/min; increase by 0.05 mg/min every 10 min until UCs stop, side-effects are unacceptable or maximum recommended dose of 0.35 mg/min is reached; continue IV 12 h after labor	Only drug approved by FDA for treatment of preterm labor Risk of pulmonary edema increased when given concurrently with corticosteroids Nurse should be alert for signs of pulmonary edema

Drug		Side Effects/Adverse Reactions	Dosage	Comments
		Headache Nervousness Restlessness Anxiety Chest tightness or pain Dyspnea Fetal: tachycardia Neonatal: hypoglycemia	ceases; 30 min before discontinuing IV, start ritodrine PO Oral: Ritodrine 10 mg every 2 h for 24 h, then 10–20 mg every 4–6 h for maintenance	
Isoxsuprine hydrochloride (Vasodilan)	Similar to ritodrine	Higher rates of cardiovascular side-effects, hypotension, fetal distress Others similar to ritodrine	Intravenous infusion: 80 mg in 500 ml solution Begin at 0.25–0.5 mg/min; increase to maximum of 0.75–1.0 mg/min; continue with: Intramuscular maintenance doses: 10 mg every 6 h for 12–24 h; continue with: Oral maintenance: 10–20 mg 4 times/day	Not approved by FDA for tocolytic use
Terbutaline (Brethine, Bricanyl)	Similar to ritodrine	Client taking terbutaline for asthma Others same as ritodrine	Intravenous infusion: 0.01 mg/min, increase to 0.085 mg/min maximum Oral maintenance dose: 2.5 mg every 4–6 h Subcutaneous injections: 0.25 mg q 20–60 min Subcutaneous pump: Basal rate 0.05–0.1 mg/h with	Not approved by FDA for tocolytic use Advantages over ritodrine: less expensive; may be given subcutaneously

(continued)

TABLE 38-9 DRUGS USED FOR PRETERM LABOR *(continued)*

Drug	Action	Additional Contraindications	Side-effects and Complications	Dosage and Route	Remarks
β-Adrenergic Agonists					
				Bolus of 0.25 mg/h (max of 7/day)	
Magnesium Sulfate	Exact mode of action unknown—depresses uterine activty when maternal serum magnesium levels 6–8 mEq/L	CNS depression Cardiac dysfunction Renal pathology	Maternal Related to increasing serum magnesium levels: hypotension, respiratory depression, hypotonus Magnesium toxicity: Respiratory arrest Circulatory collapse Cardiac arrest Fetal: distress in response to mother's symptoms Neonatal: respiratory depression, hypotonus	Intravenous infusion: Loading dose: 4 g by slow IV push or over 30 min by infusion Maintenance: 2 g/h until UCs stop or signs of toxicity appear	Not approved by FDA for tocolytic use Nursing responsibilities: Monitor VS q 5 min during loading dose and q 15 min during maintenance Stop infusion and report if: BP is ≤ 90/60, respiration is ≤ 12/min; there is no patellar reflex; urine output is ≤ 30 cc/h Keep calcium gluconate at bedside
Prostaglandin Synthetase Inhibitors					
Indomethacin Naproxen Aspirin	Interfere with synthesis of prostaglandins	Gastrointestinal lesions Coagulation defects Allergy to specific drug Epilepsy Psychiatric disturbance	Maternal: Nausea and vomiting GI bleeding Headache Drowsiness, dizziness, and vertigo Allergic reactions Postpartum hemorrhage Fetal/neonatal: Premature closure of	Route: Oral Dose: No routine dose established	Advantage: Tocolysis without hypotension Disadvantages: Potential danger to mother and fetus/infant may outweigh advantage—not recommended for use with preterm labor in United States

Calcium Antagonists

Drug	Action	Indications	Contraindications	Side-effects/Complications	Dosage and Route	Remarks
Nifedipine	Inhibits influx of calcium ions through cell membrane; Reduction in calcium concentration inhibits myometrial contractions			ductus arteriosus; Other cardiac and pulmonary changes; Hyperbilirubinemia; Hemorrhagic disorders; Flushing; Transient increased heart rate	Oral route: 30 mg initial dose then 20 mg every 8 h	Fewer side-effects; Good results in early studies; Further studies needed; Concern about effect on uteroplacental blood flow

Corticosteroids

Drug	Action	Indications	Contraindications	Side-effects/Complications	Dosage and Route	Remarks
Betamethasone (Celestone); Dexamethasone	Increased production of surfactant in fetal lungs	Preterm labor at gestational age of 28–32 wk; L/S ratio not known or <2:1; Fetal membranes intact; Possibility of delaying delivery for 48 h after initiation of therapy without undue risk to mother or fetus	Inability or contraindications to delaying delivery; Gestational age 34 wk; L/S ratio ≥2	Maternal: May increase adverse effects of diabetes or preeclampsia; Increased risk of infection; Delayed wound healing if cesarean birth; Fetal/neonatal: No reports of serious side-effects, but long-term effects not known	12 mg IM, repeat in 12–24 h × 1; 6 mg IM, repeat in 12–24 h × 1; then weekly until L/S ratio 2:1; Effects seem to be transitory, peak at 48 h and last approximately 1 wk	Not approved by FDA for this use; controversy exists about effectiveness and potential dangers; Use with tocolytic agent appears to increase risk of pulmonary edema

NURSING DIAGNOSIS

Preterm labor is an alteration in the childbearing process. The nurse is an active participant, with the physician, in making and interpreting the assessment data to make the diagnosis of preterm labor and arrive at decisions for interventions. Specific nursing diagnoses might be made during this time to guide the nurse in providing appropriate nursing care.

Possible nursing diagnoses would include:

1. Anxiety and Fear related to the unpredictable prognosis for the continuation of the pregnancy.
2. Alteration in Comfort related to uterine contractions.
3. Alteration in Comfort related to prolonged bedrest in side-lying position.
4. Alteration in Family Processes related to the effect of the mother's extended hospital stay on the family.
5. Knowledge Deficit concerning condition and treatment of preterm labor related to unexpected signs of labor before due date.

PLANNING AND INTERVENTION

The woman who is admitted in preterm labor, and her family, can be expected to have a high level of anxiety. This is understandable, because they are usually not prepared for the labor physically or emotionally and may be fearful that the baby will not survive. Support from a primary nurse who can be with them through the admission process and provide information about what is and will be happening can be helpful in allaying their anxiety.

Bedrest in the side-lying position and adequate hydration, either oral or intravenous, are interventions that are usually instituted while the decision on further treatment is being made. An intake and output record should be kept. Comfort measures should be employed as with any labor (see Chap. 22), and analgesic medications should be avoided or kept to a minimum.

Care of the Woman Receiving Tocolytic Treatment. The nurse's role is an important one in the care of the patient receiving a tocolytic agent by intravenous infusion. The nurse can help determine whether the patient understands the nature of the treatment and the possible side-effects and can provide information when needed. The patient should be helped to maintain the left lateral position in bed to minimize the risk of supine hypotension, and this is more easily accomplished when the rationale is understood. Baseline data should be obtained before the infusion is started. This includes fetal heart rate, uterine activity, and maternal vital signs. The physician also usually orders baseline laboratory studies

including complete blood count with differential, blood glucose, and serum electrolytes; urinalysis and urine culture to check for latent urinary tract infection; and a baseline electrocardiogram.[29]

The nurse may be responsible for starting the IV and mixing the medication. The protocol varies according to the hospital, the doctor's orders, and the drug to be used. A large-gauge intravenous catheter is usually used, and the solution should be administered with the use of an infusion pump so the dosage can be carefully titrated. The usual initial dosage of ritodrine is 0.1 mg/ min with the infusion rate being increased by increments of 0.05 mg/min every 10 minutes until uterine activity ceases, or significant side-effects develop. The usual effective dosage range is 0.15 to 0.35 mg/min.[30]

Although the side-effects for the different β-adrenergic agonists vary somewhat, ritodrine is fairly typical and is used in this example. While the infusion rate of the ritodrine is being increased, the pulse, respirations, and blood pressure are taken as often as every 10 minutes, and after the infusion rate is stabilized, every 30 minutes until 1 hour after the infusion is discontinued.

Significant side-effects to be reported are: maternal pulse rate greater than 140 beats per minute, chest tightness or pain, dyspnea, blood pressure less than 90/ 60 or a significant decrease from the patient's baseline, or fetal tachycardia greater than 180 beats per minute.[30] These symptoms may require decreasing the IV rate or discontinuing the therapy. Milder symptoms, such as headache, restlessness, or nausea, may respond to a slight decrease in the dosage.[25] Intake and output should be recorded, and the 24-hour intake should be limited to 1500 to 2000 ml to avoid fluid overload, which could lead to pulmonary edema.[30]

If uterine contractions are successfully inhibited, the woman may be put on oral maintenance therapy. The initial oral dose should be given 30 minutes before the intravenous ritodrine is discontinued. Vital signs should be taken every 2 hours for the first 24 hours, then every 4 hours. Uterine activity and side-effects should also be monitored. The side-effects of the oral drug can sometimes be minimized by taking it with food.

Women on tocolytic therapy need lots of emotional and physical support. Not only are they concerned about the outcome for themselves and their baby, but they may be uncomfortable from the side-effects of the drug and from the enforced bedrest. Helpful hints from a nurse who was also a patient on long-term intravenous tocolytic therapy include the following:

- Suggesting use of a mattress pad or "egg-crate" mattress to help alleviate the hip discomfort from the side-lying position
- Encouraging use of pillows from home for comfort and to brighten up the room
- Assisting with personal hygiene such as brushing teeth and washing hair

- Providing passive range of motion or isometric exercises to assist in maintaining muscle tone
- Assisting with finding activities that can be accomplished while lying in bed
- Providing comfort measures such as back rubs[31]

Home Monitoring and Care. Nurses play a significant role in the monitoring and care of the patient who is at risk for or experiencing preterm labor and is being monitored or treated at home. Studies of the effectiveness of home uterine monitoring have frequently raised the question of whether the positive results are related to the monitor or to the increased nurse–patient interaction. When a patient is being monitored at home, nursing responsibilities include daily evaluation and reporting of uterine activity, responses to treatment, and general health. The nurse also educates the patient about monitoring, pregnancy, nutrition, and stress management and is available by telephone 24 hours a day. In addition, the nurse can suggest helpful books to increase knowledge about the situation, and make referrals to support groups and other appropriate sources of assistance.[24]

When the home care includes use of a portable subcutaneous terbutaline pump, the nurse must have knowledge of the pump, the medication being used, and its side-effects. The patient is usually hospitalized at the beginning of therapy, for stabilization and for instruction in self-administration of terbutaline using the pump. When she returns home, the nurse continues assessment of her condition and her ability to use the pump effectively.[26]

EVALUATION

For the woman at risk for preterm labor, effective nursing care is demonstrated by the birth of a healthy baby at or near term. During her pregnancy, the woman should be able to recognize signs of preterm labor, initiate steps to decrease risk, and seek appropriate care if preterm labor begins. In the case of actual preterm labor, the woman should be able to verbalize understanding of her condition, should demonstrate minimal anxiety and discomfort, and should cope with the prolonged bedrest and/or hospitalization by maintaining the prescribed regimen.

■ PROLAPSE OF UMBILICAL CORD

In the course of labor, the umbilical cord sometimes prolapses alongside or in front of the presenting part.

Overall, this occurs about once in 400 births. Factors that predispose to cord prolapse by preventing proper adaptation or the presenting part to the maternal pelvis include: breech presentation (especially footling), transverse lie, unengaged presenting part, twin gestation, hydramnios, or a small fetus. When cord prolapse occurs, it is a potentially grave complication for the fetus, because the cord is compressed between the presenting part and the bony pelvis, and the fetal circulation may be shut off.

Manifestations

A fairly common time for prolapse to occur is after rupture of the membranes, either spontaneous or artificial, when the presenting part (head, breech, or shoulder) is not engaged and is therefore not sufficiently down in the pelvis to prevent the cord from being washed past it in the sudden gush of amniotic fluid. The prolapse may be apparent (Fig. 38-13C), with the cord visibly protruding from the vagina, or it may be concealed (see Fig. 38-13B), with the diagnosis being made when the cord is felt during vaginal examination. Fetal distress, detected by heart rate changes, is sometimes the first indication, especially of occult cord prolapse (see Fig. 38-13A).

Management

The immediate treatment of cord prolapse is any method that reduces the pressure of the presenting part on the umbilical cord in an effort to prevent or minimize impairment of fetal circulation. Tilting the mother's body to place her head and shoulders lower than her hips, as in Trendelenburg's position, knee—chest position, or elevating the hips with a pillow, allows the presenting part to gravitate out of the pelvis and relieve the pressure on the cord (Figs. 38-14). Alternately, or additionally, the presenting part may be pushed upward by pressure from a sterile gloved hand in the vagina (Fig. 38-15). This pressure needs to be maintained until preparations are made to deliver the infant. If the cord has prolapsed outside the vagina, no attempt should be made to reposition it in the vagina. To avoid cooling and drying of the cord, it may be covered with sterile towels, moistened with warm sterile saline.

The goal of therapy is to deliver the infant as soon as possible. If dilatation is incomplete, immediate cesarean section yields the best results for fetal salvage. In occasional, carefully selected cases, prolapsed cord in vertex presentations with nearly complete dilatation can be delivered with minimal trauma to mother and infant using vacuum extraction or forceps.

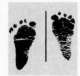

Nursing Care Plan

The Patient at Risk for Preterm Labor

Patient Goals:

1. Client is able to identify factors that put her at risk for preterm labor.
2. Client takes steps to change behavior and reduce risks.
3. Client identifies early signs of preterm labor and seeks appropriate medical care.
4. Client undergoes tocolytic treatment:
   • Verbalizes understanding of condition, treatment and instructions for self-care
   • Verbalizes concerns and subsequent reduction in fear and anxiety
   • Experiences minimal side-effects
   • Copes effectively with situation.
5. Fetus does not develop signs of distress or signs of distress are detected early and minimized.
6. Client undergoing preterm birth:
   • Verbalizes understanding of situation
   • Progresses in labor with minimal discomfort, and without complications
   • Fetus/neonate has minimal distress and is born in good condition.

Assessment	Potential Nursing Diagnosis	Planning and Intervention	Evaluation
Risk factors associated with preterm labor: Maternal age < 18 or > 40 Low socioeconomic status Poor nutritional status Employment outside of home Heavy cigarette smoking Alcohol or drug abuse Previous reproductive loss Previous low-birth-weight or preterm infant Maternal disease or infection Present pregnancy: Bleeding, overdistention of uterus, premature rupture of membranes	Knowledge deficit regarding factors related to risk of preterm labor	Take history at first antepartum visit to determine presence of risk factors; reassess at each antepartum visit	Clients at risk are identified
		Teach client to identify risk factors	Client identifies risk factors
		Teach methods of possible risk reduction: Improve nutrition Decrease or stop smoking Avoid alcohol and drugs Reduce stress	Client takes steps to reduce risks
Signs of labor Contractions q 10 min lasting 30 s or more Cervical change, Effacement = 80% Dilatation = 2 cm	Knowledge deficit regarding signs of preterm labor	Provide information about signs of preterm labor to clients at risk: menstrual-type cramps, lower abdominal tightening or pressure, intermittent back ache, bloody show, watery vaginal discharge	Client describes signs of preterm labor

(continued)

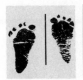

Nursing Care Plan *(continued)*

Assessment	Potential Nursing Diagnosis	Planning and Intervention	Evaluation
		Provide information about when and how to contact health-care provider and come to hospital	Client seeks medical care appropriately
Labor progress 　Continued cervical changes 　Frequency, intensity, and duration of uterine contractions 　Rupture of membranes or leaking amniotic fluid 　Bloody show	Anxiety and fear related to unexpected early labor	On admission to labor unit: observe for signs of labor and progressive changes; obtain laboratory values—CBC, urinalysis; test vaginal discharge with nitrazine paper for presence of amniotic fluid	Client responds positively to care aspects
		Encourage left side-lying position	
		Provide oral or intravenous fluids to maintain hydration—initial 200 ml to 500 ml bolus as ordered	
		Monitor and record intake and output	
Maternal emotional status		Provide appropriate, factual information to client and family about progress of labor and plan of care	Family understands client's condition and plan of care
		Allow husband or other person of client's choice to be present as desired	Client acknowledges reduction of fear
Gestational age 　EDD 　Height of fundus 　Ultrasound		Assist in estimation of gestational age to help determine choice of treatment	
Fetal well-being 　Fetal heart rate, baseline, periodic changes, variability 　Fetal movement 　Tests of fetal maturity, L/S ratio, ultrasound		Apply external fetal monitor and observe for fetal status	Fetal distress is detected early, and appropriate measures are instituted
		Prepare client for ultrasound or amniocentesis if ordered	
		Explain all procedures and their purposes	
Response to tocolytic treatment 　Uterine contractions 　Side-effects (depending on agent used):		Explain procedures to client	Client understands procedure
		Follow agency protocol for starting and monitoring infusion	

(continued)

Nursing Care Plan (continued)

Assessment	Potiential Nursing Diagnosis	Planning and Intervention	Evaluation
Maternal vital signs: changes in heart or respiratory rate, blood pressure, or temperature		Monitor vital signs, fetal heart rate, uterine activity, maternal subjective reactions	
Fetal heart rate		Report side-effects or complications	
		Provide physical and emotional support	
Maternal subjective reactions: tremors, palpitations, nausea and vomiting, restlessness, chest tightness or pain, dyspnea	Alteration in comfort related to unpleasant side-effects and prolonged bed-rest	Provide comfort measures, additional pillows for positioning, back rub, assisting, back rub, assistance with personal hygiene, restful atmosphere	Client responds to comfort measures
Boredom, discouragement	Ineffective individual coping related to prolonged hospitalization	Provide for appropriate diversions or companionship as desired	Client copes effectively
Family concerns	Alteration in family process related to the effect of extended hospital stay on family functioning	Provide opportunity to discuss concerns about family	Client verbalizes concerns for family
		Allow visits of other children when hospitalization is long-term	Children visit mother as appropriate
		Make referrals to public health nurse or social service as needed for assistance	
		Provide information about possible continuation of preterm labor; teach about labor and delivery, cesarean delivery, facilities, and care available for preterm infant	
Contraindications to tocolytic treatment: Pregnancy < 20 weeks > 36 weeks Active uterine bleeding Maternal illness Fetal distress or intrauterine death Advanced labor—cervi-	Fear for self and fetus related to imminent preterm delivery	Keep client and family informed concerning progress of labor, plan of treatment, status of fetus	Client and family are knowledgeable about situation
		Provide physical and emotional support, avoid leaving her alone	Client affirms that her fear has been minimized
		Monitor signs of progress	Infant receives prompt and efficient resuscitation as needed

(continued)

Nursing Care Plan *(continued)*

Assessment	Potiential Nursing Diagnosis	Planning and Intervention	Evaluation
cal dilatation > 3 cm Ruptured membranes		of labor and fetal well-being Prepare for preterm delivery or cesarean delivery—alert surgical team and neonatal intensive care team	

Nursing Process Related To Prolapsed Cord

ASSESSMENT

When conditions exist that predispose to cord prolapse, more frequent vaginal examinations and closer attention to fetal heart rate changes can assist in early detection. An important routine practice after rupture of the membranes is to listen to and record the fetal heart rate immediately after the rupture, and again in 10 to 15 minutes to detect decreased rate or irregularities if the cord has prolapsed. When fetal heart tones are electronically monitored, the cord compression from a cord prolapse usually is manifested by moderate to severe variable decelerations.

NURSING DIAGNOSIS

For the fetus, a potential nursing diagnosis would be: Altered Cardiac and Cerebral Tissue Perfusion related to impaired umbilical cord circulation. For the mother, the major nursing diagnosis would be: Anxiety and Fear related to danger to the fetus. Knowledge Deficit related to the condition, and Grieving related to potential loss of the infant would be additional nursing diagnoses for the mother.

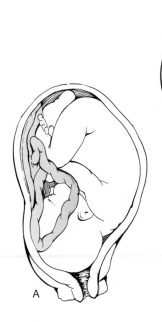
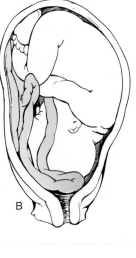
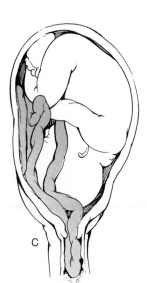

■ *Figure 38–13*
Prolapse of the cord. As the head comes down, the compression of the cord between the fetal skull and the pelvic brim will shut off its circulation completely. (A) Occult prolapse. (B) Cord prolapsed in front of head. (C) Cord prolapsed into vagina.

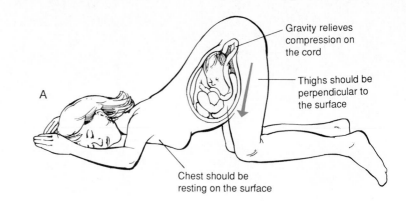

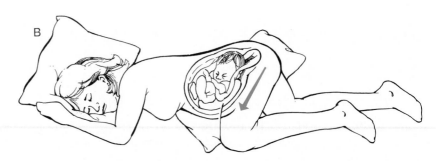

■ *Figure 38–14*
Prolapsed cord. (A) Knee–chest position and (B) lateral Sim's position reduce cord compression and help to maintain umbilical cord circulation. Positioning should be combined with administration of oxygen to the mother.

PLANNING AND INTERVENTION

The nurse is often the one who first detects signs of a prolapsed cord. The nurse needs to act quickly to institute emergency procedures, such as positioning the mother and administering oxygen; to alert the physician and other staff; and to prepare for cesarean delivery, if necessary.

Although the mother is not in physical danger or discomfort herself from the prolapsed cord, she usually senses from the heightened tension and the interven-

tions being rapidly employed that something is wrong. The calmness, warmth, and efficiency of the nurse are needed to reassure the mother that all possible measures are being taken to bring the situation under control.

It goes without saying that these women never should be left unattended, and their partners, if they are present, should be treated with consideration. It is sometimes difficult, when a crisis occurs, to deal with the relatives of the mother with appropriate thoughtfulness, because most of the energy is directed toward meeting the pressing (and often lifesaving) demands of

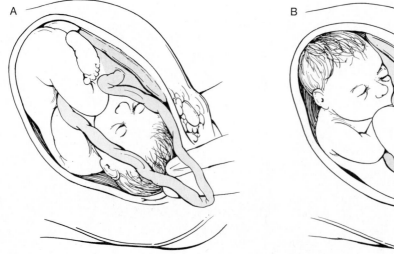

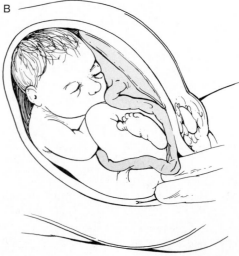

■ *Figure 38–15*
Prolapsed cord. Reduction of cord compression using gloved examiner's hand in vagina to elevate presenting part, (A) vertex or (B) breech).

the situation. However, it must be remembered that the mother and her family are considered as a unit, and a few moments spent providing the family with support and essential information enable them to help support the mother.

EVALUATION

Effectiveness of nursing interventions when a prolapsed cord occurs can be evaluated on the basis of fetal and maternal outcome. Positive outcomes of effective nursing care would include: the fetal heart rate remains within normal limits, the fetus is born in good condition, and the mother understands what is happening, has adequate support, and has minimum anxiety.

■ AMNIOTIC FLUID EMBOLISM

Although it is a rare complication of labor, amniotic fluid embolism has a high mortality rate and may be responsible for approximately 15% of overall maternal mortality.[32] This life-threatening condition develops when amniotic fluid enters the maternal circulation and subsequently reaches the pulmonary capillaries. For this to occur, there must be a tear through the amnion and chorion, an opening into the maternal circulation, and increased intrauterine pressure to force the fluid into the venous circulation. The most likely sites of entry are the endocervical veins and the uteroplacental area.

It most typically occurs during or just after the birth of the infant, after a tumultuous labor, or one in which oxytocin induction or augmentation was used. Other predisposing factors associated with amniotic fluid embolism include multiparity, advanced maternal age, large baby, intrauterine fetal death, and meconium in the amniotic fluid.

Amniotic fluid invariably contains small particles of matter, such as vernix caseosa, lanugo, and sometimes meconium, and these form multiple tiny emboli, which reach the lungs and cause occlusion of the pulmonary capillaries. Initially, there is a transient phase of intense pulmonary vasospasm leading to acute right heart failure and hypoxemia. This may account for the 25% to 50% mortality in the first few hours.[15] There may also be an anaphylactic reaction to fetal debris as matter foreign to the mother's body.[32] Hemorrhage is another major concern, with thromboplastic materials in the amniotic fluid triggering a sequence of events leading to disseminated intravascular coagulation (DIC).[33]

The *clinical characteristics* of the condition include sudden restlessness, chills, pallor, hypotension, and tachycardia accompanied by signs of acute respiratory distress: dyspnea, tachypnea, and chest pain. Hemorrhage, cardiovascular collapse, convulsions, and coma may follow.

The general aims of *medical management* are to reduce pulmonary hypertension, increase tissue perfusion, relieve bronchospasm, control hemorrhage, and provide supportive measures.[4] More specifically, treatment may include intubation and ventilation with oxygen, central venous pressure monitoring, and intravenous fluids and blood transfusions as appropriate. Pharmacological interventions, such as morphine to decrease anxiety, aminophylline to relieve bronchospasm, digoxin to prevent or treat cardiac failure, and hydrocortisone to decrease pulmonary edema and help overcome the overwhelming stress, are also used as the patient's condition indicates.[4,32]

The *nurse's role* in the event of amniotic fluid embolism includes responsibility for carrying out the doctor's emergency orders, as well as providing supportive care for the patient and her family. The patient should be placed in Fowler's position; oxygen, medication, and blood products should be administered as ordered; intake and output should be monitored; and the patient should not be left alone. If the fetus is undelivered, monitoring the fetal heart and preparing for emergency delivery are additional nursing activities.[32] Because there is such a high incidence of maternal death with this condition, the nurse may also need to help the family through the grieving process.

■ MULTIPLE PREGNANCY

When two or more embryos develop in the uterus at the same time, the condition is known as multiple pregnancy. These are considered complicated pregnancies because there is an appreciable increase in morbidity and mortality. Multiple pregnancies account for about 2% to 3% of all viable births. The frequency of identical (monozygotic or one-egg) twins is apparently relatively constant throughout the world at about 1 set in every 250 pregnancies. Moreover, their appearance is largely independent of race, heredity, maternal age, parity, infertility drugs, and environmental factors. On the other hand, fraternal (dizygotic, two-egg) twins *are* influenced by these factors. Their incidence in the white race is about 1 set in 95 and in the African-American race 1 set in 78. Twinning among Orientals is less common. Women who were a dizygotic twin tend to have more multiple pregnancies. Similarly, increased age, parity, endogenous gonadotropin, and taking infertility drugs also increase the probability of multiple pregnancy.[34]

Types of Twins

Multiple fetuses result from two basic processes. Twin fetuses more commonly result from the fertilization of two different ova. This type of twinning is known as dizygotic, or fraternal twins. About one third as often, twins arise from the fertilization of a single ovum, monozygotic or identical twins. Either or both processes may be at work in the production of larger numbers of fetuses in one birth. Quadruplets, for instance, may arise from one to four ova.[1] An interesting feature of twinning is that, although dizygotic twins are not in the strict sense true twins because they result from the union of two separate ova and sperm, if they are of the same sex, they often resemble each other as closely at birth as a pair of monozygotic twins. The process of the division of one fertilized zygote into two does not always result in an equal sharing of the protoplasm; thus, the growth of monozygotic twins is often dramatically discordant.[1]

Basically, two types of placentas exist in twins, those with monochorial (one chorion) and those with dichorial (two chorions) membranes (Fig. 38-16). Also, the placentas may be fused, separate, or a single disk, and there may be one or two amnions. However, each fetus usually has its own umbilical cord. The possible combinations thus include the following:

1. Monozygotic (identical)
   a. Diamniotic dichorionic (two amnions, two chorions), 30%
   b. Diamniotic monochorionic (two amnions, one chorion), most common
   c. Monoamniotic monochorionic (one amnion, one chorion), rare
2. Dizygotic (fraternal or nonidentical)
   a. Diamniotic dichorionic (two amnions, two chorions)

Examination of the fetal membranes is used to assist in diagnosing the zygosity of twins but is not always accurate. Only monozygotic twins can have a single chorion, which establishes identical twinning. Two chorions are always present in dizygotic twins, but are also the placentation of about 30% of monozygotic twins. If the sexes are different, the twins are obviously fraternal, but if twins are the same sex and dichorionic, the diagnosis is uncertain.[1,34] The usual twin placentations are shown in Figure 38-17. In the United States, 33% of twins are identical.

Diagnosis

Early diagnosis of multiple pregnancy is an important factor in improving the perinatal outcome. Detection late in pregnancy or at delivery correlates with increased risk for perinatal morbidity and mortality. One of the advantages of early diagnosis is that it allows time for the mother and her family to be informed of the differences involved in multiple pregnancy and what can

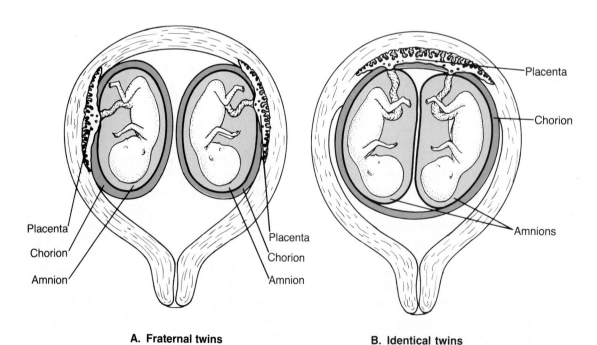

A. Fraternal twins   **B. Identical twins**

■ *Figure 38–16*

Twin pregnancy. (A) Fraternal twins with two placentas, two amnions, and two chorions. (B) Identical twins with one placenta, one chorion, and two amnions.

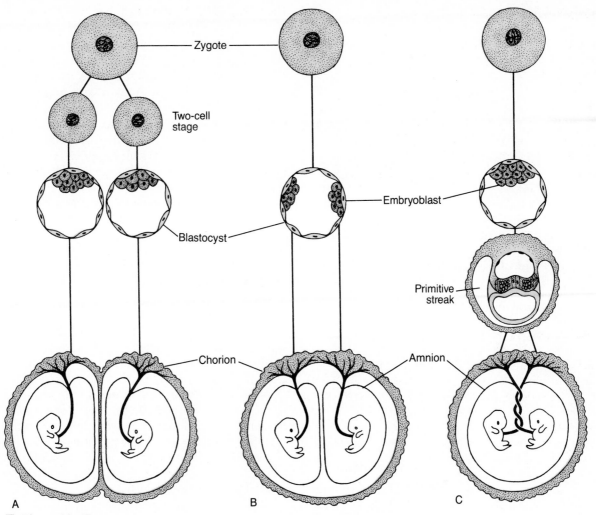

■ *Figure 38-17*

Membranes and placenta in twin pregnancies. (A) Two placentas, two amnions, two chorions (from either dizygotic twins or monozygotic twins with early cleavage of the zygote. (B and C) Single ovum twins. (B) One chorion and two amnions and one placenta. (C) One chorion and one amnion (note entanglement of cords, a danger when there is only one amnion)

be done to improve the outcome.[35] Referral to a perinatal center can also be made at a more optimum time.

Twins are suspected whenever uterine size is greater than ordinarily expected for any point in the pregnancy. In addition, the palpation of three or four large parts in the uterus, the auscultation of two fetal heart tones of differing frequencies, or the history of twins "running in the family" all serve to alert the obstetrician or nurse to the possibility of a multiple pregnancy.

Ultrasound can aid in the diagnosis of multiple pregnancy, and the use of routine ultrasound screening of all pregnancies before the 20th week is practiced in some areas. There is no biochemical test that clearly differentiates between multiple and single pregnancies, but assay of one of the hormones, such as chorionic gonadotropin or placental lactogen, that are usually elevated during multiple pregnancy has been suggested.[35]

Pathophysiology

Several high-risk conditions are associated with multiple pregnancy. These include premature delivery (50%), hemorrhage (20%), hypertensive disorders, preeclampsia and eclampsia (25%), abnormal presentation and position (10%), hydramnios (7%), and uterine dysfunction (10%). Cord compression and entanglement, intrauterine growth retardation, and operative delivery also contribute to morbidity and mortality. In addition, monozygotic twins are less hardy than dizygotic twins. Weight differences are more pronounced, and they have a higher incidence of congenital anomalies and neonatal mortality.

Some of these problems may be due to the monochorionic placenta, which is thought to be less competent than the dichorionic variety. The problems center on placental vascular disorders. The most serious of these is the shunting of blood due to vascular anastomosis, which results in a twin-to-twin transfusion syndrome (intrauterine parabiosis). The anastomosis may be artery-to-artery, artery-to-vein, or vein-to-vein. An artery-to-vein anastomosis is the most serious and accounts for the disparity in size and appearance seen in these supposedly identical infants. The *donor* twin is pallid, anemic, dehydrated, growth retarded, and hypovolemic. Hydrops and cardiac decompensation may be present, as well as hydramnios. In contrast, the *recipient* twin appears healthy, large by contrast, and ruddy. However, this appearance is due to edema, plethora, and hypertension. Kernicterus, ascites, glomerular-tubal hypertrophy, enlarged heart and liver, or congenital heart anomalies may be accompaniments. Fetal polyuria and hydramnios may also be present. These infants are at great risk for death in the first 24 hours of life.[35]

Management

Because of the antepartal and perinatal risk, the mother needs to be monitored carefully during the antepartal period. She is asked to see the obstetrician more frequently, at least every 2 weeks in the second trimester and at least weekly in the third trimester if there are no complications. Diet is regulated to allow for adequate weight gain. An increase of 300 kcal or more per day in energy sources in the diet is not too much. Protein intake is supervised, and iron, folic acid, and vitamin supplements are increased. Rest periods on the side may be prescribed, although the efficacy of complete bedrest even in the last trimester for higher socioeconomic status women seems equivocal.[1] Pritchard and associates, however, have found that women who are socioeconomically deprived seem to benefit from hospitalization with some ambulation privileges during the last trimester. In their opinion, there are better outcomes in the incidence of premature labor and preeclampsia and a generally lowered perinatal mortality.[1]

The latter weeks of a twin pregnancy are likely to be associated with heaviness of the lower abdomen, back pains, and swelling of the feet and the ankles. Abdominal distention makes sleeping difficult, and therefore the physician may prescribe a hypnotic. A well-fitting maternity girdle makes daytime more comfortable. Because of the excessive abdominal size, the mother may find that frequent small feedings are more suitable than the usual three larger meals a day. The nurse can be helpful in giving the mother anticipatory guidance regarding these matters during the antepartal period.

Travel is curtailed because labor may begin at any time without warning, and delivery in strange surroundings may be hazardous.

LABOR AND DELIVERY

If not already hospitalized, the mother is requested to come to the hospital at the first sign of labor. When labor is confirmed, a decision must be made on the route of delivery, taking into account the presentation of the twins, the presence of any maternal or fetal complications, the gestational age, and the availability of anesthesia, an experienced obstetrician, and neonatal intensive care.[35] During the labor, steps are taken to ensure a successful outcome for mother and fetuses.

First, the mother is attended at all times by a qualified perinatal team member. Here the nurse can be invaluable. Fetal heart rates must be monitored continuously, and maternal vital signs must be recorded. A combination of external and internal fetal monitoring after the membranes have ruptured usually proves satisfactory. A liter of cross-matched blood or its equivalent is to be available and in the area. In addition, an intravenous infusion system capable of delivering the blood is to be instituted. Lactated Ringer's solution alternated with a 5% dextrose solution at 60 ml to 120 ml/h has been found to be satisfactory in the absence of hemorrhage or metabolic disturbance during labor.[1]

It is recommended that two obstetricians be available and scrubbed for the delivery and an anesthesiologist be in attendance, especially for the contingency of a cesarean delivery. Moreover, *two* people, with at least one being skilled in resuscitation, are needed for *each* fetus at the time of delivery.

A local or pudendal block is preferred to minimize the effect of anesthetic on the infants. However, a combination of thiopental, nitrous oxide plus oxygen, and succinylcholine given in timed, appropriate doses has been found to be effective when cesarean section is indicated. The general anesthetic halothane also may be used when operative intervention is needed.[1]

The first twin is delivered either by vertex or assisted breech delivery. If the first infant is transverse, an external version is used to bring about a deliverable presentation.

If the twins are monozygotic, the first infant's cord must be clamped to prevent the second twin from bleeding through it. The cords should be labeled. The position of the second twin is ascertained, and it is brought into position by a combination of vaginal and abdominal manipulation. If there is a second sac, it is carefully ruptured to allow a slow loss of fluid and to guard against cord prolapse. A spontaneous or a prophylactic forceps vertex delivery is preferred. If the breech presents, the physician may have to assist in the extraction. If descent does not come about, a version and extraction may be required. These require astute management on the part of both the obstetrician and the anesthesiologist.[1]

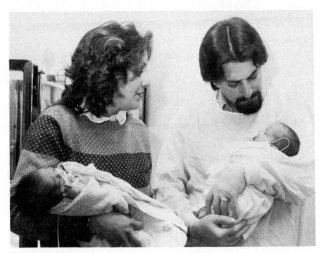

■ *Figure 38–18*
Parents of twins need support from the nursing staff, even if twins were expected. (Courtesy of The Children's Hospital of Philadelphia)

Routine use of oxytocin is delayed until after the delivery of the second twin, when it is added to the intravenous infusion. The uterus is not massaged until after the placenta(s) are expelled, then massage is continued until the uterus remains firm and contracted (15–30 minutes). Ergonovine or methergine may be given intramuscularly after expulsion of the placenta(s), if the mother is not hypertensive.

As with any delivery, the nurse has the responsibility of supportive care for the mother as well as assisting the physician in whatever activities are indicated. Because these infants are apt to be small, oxygen or resuscitative measures may be necessary. The care is similar to that for any premature baby (see Chap. 44). Sufficient supplies and equipment for resuscitation for each baby should be procured early in the delivery and kept in readiness. Maternal vital signs as well as the fetal heart rate should be checked frequently.

POSTPARTUM

Physically, the care required by the mother depends on her general condition and the type of delivery. Complications are the same as those after single births, but the frequency of complications such as uterine atony may be increased due to the overdistention of the uterus.

The birth of more than one infant can be a psychological shock to the parents, even if expected (Fig. 38-18). One additional child may be desired and acceptable; two may impose an emotional or financial burden. The parents may wonder if they can manage the care of two newborns simultaneously. Problems may be compounded in feeding, especially if the mother plans to breast-feed, and in providing two of everything.

Parents need anticipatory guidance and support during the initial adjustment period. Some may need referral to a social worker or public-health nurse to assist with plans for the unexpected new baby. Many also appreciate information about special clubs for mothers of twins, or introduction to other mothers who have successfully coped with the first few months after the birth of twins. If the infants are small, the parents need the same type of extra support given to other parents of preterm infants (see Chap. 44).

■ REFERENCES

1. Cunningham FG, MacDonald PC, Gant NF: Williams Obstetrics, 18th ed. Norwalk, CT, Appleton & Lange, 1989
2. Friedman EA: Labor, Evaluation and Management. New York, Appleton-Century-Crofts, 1978
3. Larks SD: Electrohysterography. Springfield, IL, Charles C Thomas, 1960
4. Oxorn H: Human Labor and Birth. Norwalk, CT, Appleton-Century-Crofts, 1985
5. Sokol RJ, Brindley BA: Practical diagnosis and management of abnormal labor. In Scott JR, DiSaia PJ, Hammond CB et al (eds): Danforth's Obstetrics and Gynecology, 6th ed. Philadelphia, JB Lippincott, 1990
6. Bowes WA Jr: Clinical aspects of normal and abnormal labor. In Creasy RK, Resnik R (eds): Maternal-Fetal Medicine: Principles and Practice, 2nd ed. Philadelphia, WB Saunders, 1989
7. Friedman EA: Dysfunctional labor. In Cohen W, Friedman EA (eds): Management of Labor. Baltimore, University Park Press, 1983
8. Hendricks CH, Brenner WE, Kraus G: The normal cervical dilatation patterns in late pregnancy and labor. Am J Obstet Gynecol 106:1065, 1970
9. Beischer NA, Mackay EV: Obstetrics and the Newborn, 2nd ed. Sydney, WB Saunders, 1986
10. Malinowski JS: Labor stimulation. In Malinowki JS, Pedigo CG, Phillips CR (eds): Nursing Care During the Labor Process, 3rd ed. Philadelphia, FA Davis, 1989
11. Kulb NW: Oxytocin induction/augmentation of labor. In Buckley K, Kulb NW (eds): High Risk Maternity Nursing Manual. Baltimore, Williams & Wilkins, 1990
12. Cruikshank DP: Malpresentations and umbilical cord complications. In Scott JR, DiSaia PJ, Hammond CB et al (eds): Danforth's Obstetrics and Gynecology, 6th ed. Philadelphia, JB Lippincott, 1990
13. Dunn LJ: Cesarean section and other obstetric operations. In Scott JR, DiSaia PJ, Hammond CB et al (eds): Danforth's Obstetrics and Gynecology, 6th ed. Philadelphia, JB Lippincott, 1990
14. Scott JR, Goplerud CP: Late pregnancy bleeding. In Scott JR, DiSaia PJ, Hammond CB et al (eds): Danforth's Obstetrics and Gynecology, 6th ed. Philadelphia, JB Lippincott, 1990

15. Gonik B: Intensive care monitoring of the critically ill pregnant patient. In Creasy RK, Resnik R (eds): Maternal Fetal Medicine, Principles and Practice, 2nd ed. Philadelphia, WB Saunders, 1989

16. Botoms SF, Scott JR: Transfusions and shock. In Scott JR, DiSaia PJ, Hammond CB et al (eds): Danforth's Obstetrics and Gynecology, 6th ed. Philadelphia, JB Lippincott, 1990

17. Creasy RK: Preterm labor and delivery. In Creasy RK, Resnik R (eds): Maternal-Fetal Medicine, Principles and Practice, 2nd ed. Philadelphia, WB Saunders, 1989

18. Kulb NW: Preterm labor. In Buckley K, Kulb NW (eds): High Risk Maternity Nursing Manual. Baltimore, Williams & Wilkins, 1990

19. Klein L, Goldenberg RL: Prenatal care and its effect on preterm birth and low birth weight. In Merkatz IR, Thompson JE (eds): New Perspectives on Prenatal Care. New York, Elsevier, 1990

20. Main DM, Gabbe SG, Richardson D et al: Can preterm deliveries be prevented? Am J Obstet Gynecol 151:892–898, 1985

21. Hobel CJ: Prevention of Preterm Delivery. In Beard RW, Nathanielsz PW (eds): Fetal Physiology and Medicine, 2nd ed. New York, Marcel Decker, 1984

22. Parisi VM: Cervical incompetence. In Creasy RK, Resnik R (eds): Maternal-Fetal Medicine, Principles and Practice, 2nd ed. Philadelphia, WB Saunders, 1989

23. Chhibber G, Cohen AW, Lindenbaum CR et al: Patient attitude toward home uterine activity monitoring. Obstetrics and Gynecology 76:90S–92S (Suppl), July 1990

24. Koehl L, Wheeler D: Monitoring uterine activity at home. Am J Nurs 89:200–203, February 1989

25. Morrison JC, Martin JN Jr, Martin RW et al: Prevention of preterm birth by ambulatory assessment of uterine activity: A randomized study. Am J Obstet Gynecol 156:536–543, 1987

26. Sala DJ, Moise KJ: The treatment of preterm labor using a portable subcutaneous terbutaline pump. JOGN Nursing 19:108–115, March/April 1990

27. Whitley N: A Manual of Clinical Obstetrics. Philadelphia, JB Lippincott, 1985

28. Anderson HF, Merkatz IR: Preterm labor. In Scott JR, DiSaia PJ, Hammond CB et al (eds): Danforth's Obstetrics and Gynecology, 6th ed. Philadelphia, JB Lippincott, 1990

29. Aumann GM, Blake GD: Ritodrine hydrochloride in the control of premature labor. JOGN Nursing 11:75–79, March/April 1982

30. Malinowski JS: Fetal well-being in preterm and postterm gestation. In Malinowski JS, Pedigo CG, Phillips CR (eds): Nursing Care During the Labor Process, 3rd ed. Philadelphia, FA Davis, 1989

31. Cagney EN: Nursing care during the treatment of preterm labor. In Fuchs F, Stubblefield PG (eds): Preterm Birth—Causes, Prevention and Management. New York, MacMillan, 1984

32. Buckley K: Pulmonary disorders. In Buckley K, Kulb NW (eds): High Risk Maternity Nursing Manual. Baltimore, Williams & Wilkins, 1990

33. Anderson HM: Maternal hematologic disorders. In Creasy RK, Resnik R (eds): Maternal-Fetal Medicine, Principles and Practice, 2nd ed. Philadelphia, WB Saunders, 1989

34. Benirschke K: Multiple gestation—Incidence, etiology, and inheritance. In Creasy RK, Resnik R (eds): Maternal-Fetal Medicine, Principles and Practice, 2nd ed. Philadelphia, WB Saunders, 1989

35. MacLennan AH: Multiple gestation—Clinical characteristics and management. In Creasy RK, Resnik R (eds): Maternal-Fetal Medicine, Principles and Practice, 2nd ed. Philadelphia, WB Saunders, 1989

39

Operative Obstetrics

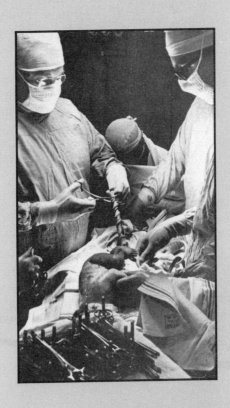

One of the primary goals of obstetric care is the safe delivery of a healthy newborn. Should circumstances arise that threaten this goal, the obstetrician has several methods to assist the delivery and prevent harm to the infant and mother. These methods are collectively called operative obstetrics and include version, induction of labor, repair of lacerations, assisted delivery using forceps or a vacuum extractor, and cesarean birth.

■ VERSION

Version consists of turning the baby in the uterus from an undesirable position to a desirable position. There are two types of version, external and internal.

External Version

External version is the external manipulation of the fetus through the abdominal and uterine walls in an attempt to change a breech or transverse presentation to a vertex presentation. It is attempted in the hope of averting the difficulties of a breech delivery. Obstetricians find the procedure most successful when performed about a month before the expected date of delivery (EDD). Some physicians prefer giving the mother a mild sedative before the attempted version to reduce anxiety and enhance muscle relaxation. External fetal monitoring (EFM) is used to monitor the fetal condition before, during, and after the procedure. When successful, the fetus remains in a vertex presentation and subsequently delivers. This procedure occasionally fails, and the fetus does not turn or reverts to a breech position within a few hours.

Internal Version

Most useful in cases of multiple gestation, internal version (also called internal podalic version) is a maneuver designed to change any fetal presentation to a breech to facilitate delivery (Fig. 39-1). It is used when the delivery of the second twin is delayed or when the fetus is in a transverse lie.

When cervical dilatation is complete, the whole hand of the operator is introduced high into the uterus and one or both of the baby's feet are grasped and pulled downward in the direction of the birth canal. With the external hand, the obstetrician may expedite the turning by pushing the head upward. The version is followed by breech extraction.

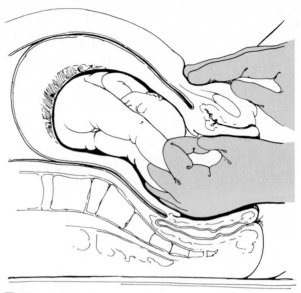

■ *Figure 39-1*
Internal podalic version.

■ INDUCTION OF LABOR

Readiness for Induction

Induction of labor means the artificial initiation of labor after the period of viability. Induction of labor is indicated when continuation of pregnancy would adversely affect maternal health or when there are conditions in the mother that would affect fetal well-being.

Complications of pregnancy that may require induction include pregnancy-induced hypertension, diabetes, hemolytic disease, and postmaturity (see Chaps. 33 and 34).

Before induction is attempted, the physiological readiness of both the mother and fetus is evaluated. Tests of fetal maturity and well-being are usually done before induction. These include gestational age assessment by ultrasound, biophysical profile, amniotic fluid volume measurements, and fetal lung maturity assessment through the analysis of amniotic fluid for lecithin/ spingomyelin ratio and phosphatidylglycerol (see Chap. 15 for additional information).[1,2]

Maternal readiness refers to the condition of the cervix and is related to the likelihood that induction will be successful. A soft, partially effaced and dilated cervix indicates the physiological readiness for labor. A well-engaged fetus also contributes to the likelihood of a successful induction.

When the cervix is found to be unfavorable for induction (unripe) and prompt delivery of the fetus is deemed necessary, an attempt may be made to prime the cervix by one of several methods.

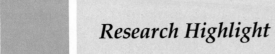

Research Highlight

VBAC: Successful Pregnancy and Labor Management by Nurse-Midwives

Vaginal birth after cesarean (VBAC) has become a common occurrence in recent years. Safety has been well documented. ACOG has set rational guidelines for the selection of VBAC patients and the safe managment of their pregnancies and labors, but makes no mention of the selection of a primary provider to monitor these pregnancies and deliver these infants.

This study, representing 5 years of research and practice, outlines the policies and protocols used by a nurse–midwifery service. Careful selection of patients and prudent managment of their pregnancies and labors yielded in 83% success rate in completion of VBAC. The number of successful VBAC rose each year of the study while morbidity and mortality were kept at a minimum. These results are comparable to outcomes described by physicians managing similar populations.

Patients with a documented low-transverse scar and sincere motivation to attempt VBAC were monitored throughout their pregnancies. They were encouraged to participate in prepared childbirth classes that focused on the VBAC experience and explained hospital policies and procedures.

When the patient was admitted in labor, an obstetrician–consultant was notified by the midwife but did not intervene unless an emergency arose. Intermittent external fetal monitoring was used. The major difference in labor management protocol for VBAC candidates was the presence of a heparin lock should IV fluids be required.

The authors conclude that nurse–midwives are capable of providing quality prenatal care, preparing women for the VBAC experience, and safely performing the subsequent vaginal deliveries. They caution that appropriate physician consultation and comprehensive emergency obstetric services should be readily available in any setting where VBAC occurs.

(Hangsleben KL, Taylor MA, Lynn NM: VBAC program in a nurse–midwifery service, five years experience. Nurse Midwifery 34(4):179–184, July/August 1989)

LAMINARIA TENTS

Laminaria tents are a specific type of seaweed that is dried, compressed, shaped, and sterilized. Synthetic laminaria are also available.[3] Laminaria are most commonly used before induced abortion and occasionally before labor induction. When inserted in the cervical os, the smooth, rounded stem absorbs moisture and swells to three to five times its original size. When inserted the night before induction, the laminaria causes gradual softening and dilatation of the cervix by morning. This dilatation can cause mild to moderate cramping, and the patient should be advised of this possibility.

PROSTAGLANDIN

Prostaglandin E_2 (PGE$_2$) in the form of vaginal suppositories or gel has been shown effective in ripening the cervix.[2,4] It is felt that this hormone stimulates biochemical changes in the cervix, resulting in cervical dilatation and stimulating uterine contractions. Although still being used on an experimental basis in this country, PGE$_2$ is gaining popularity for pre-induction treatment.

OXYTOCIN

Oxytocin may be given as an intravenous infusion for a number of hours daily over 2 to 3 days. This is sometimes referred to as serial induction. The oxytocin-induced contractions often bring the fetal head down into the pelvis and assist in ripening the cervix.[4] The infusion is usually stopped at night so the client can eat and rest.

Methods of Induction

It was once believed that intestinal peristalsis caused by a cathartic would transfer to the uterus and bring on labor. Castor oil, soap suds enemas, and strong laxatives have been employed in attempts to induce labor. Unfortunately, these remedies usually fail and serve only to increase discomfort. There are two reliable methods to initiate labor safely.

ARTIFICIAL RUPTURE OF MEMBRANES (AROM)

Even in early Roman times, the artificial rupture of membranes was used as an obstetric procedure. Soranus, a 2nd century Roman scholar and practitioner, demonstrated a sophisticated knowledge of parturition and recommended rupturing the membranes to reduce a prolonged labor.[5]

Amniotomy, or artificial rupture of the membranes, is a common method of enhancing labor and has been used to induce labor. When the client is near term and the cervix is favorable, amniotomy is almost always followed by labor within a few hours.

The intact membranes form a barrier against bacterial invasion of the uterus. For this reason, delivery should be accomplished as quickly as is safely possible. Twenty-four hours with ruptured membranes is usually considered the maximum safe time period, after which amnionitis may occur. Besides the danger of infection, amniotomy also increases the risk of cord prolapse and fetal head or cord compression. Amniotomy is contraindicated when the presenting part is high in the pelvis, or if the fetus is in the breech or transverse positions.

To perform an amniotomy, the obstetrician inserts the first two fingers of one hand into the cervix until the membranes are encountered. A long hook, usually an Allis clamp or a plastic Amnihook, is inserted into the vagina and the membranes are simply hooked and torn by the tip of the sharp instrument. The fluid may initially come out with a gush or leak out slowly. Leaking of amniotic fluid from the vagina usually continues throughout labor. The color, odor, and consistency of the amniotic fluid should be noted. It is usually clear and almost odorless, and deviations can indicate problems. For example, brownish or greenish discoloration is a sign that the infant has passed meconium in utero, and a foul odor is a sign of infection.

Nursing Process in Amniotomy. Assessment is an ongoing part of the nurse's responsibility when an amniotomy is performed. The condition of mother and fetus is assessed before, during, and after the procedure, and any changes are reported to the physician. Possible nursing diagnoses might include high risk for infection related to rupture of membranes, alteration in comfort related to increasing strength of uterine contractions, or anxiety or fear related to an unfamiliar procedure.

Nursing planning and intervention involve preparing the client for the procedure and carrying out the necessary assessments. The nurse should explain the procedure to the client, reassure her that it is no more uncomfortable than a vaginal examination, and describe the warm, wet sensations that she will probably experience. Expectations for increased strength of uterine contractions should also be explained.

Before the procedure, the nurse can assist the client in assuming a supine position, with knees flexed and relaxed. Antiseptic preparation of the vulva is accomplished according to hospital policy. Fetal heart tones should be monitored before, during, and after the procedure, or with continuous EFM. Cord compression or prolapse are clearly evident in changing EFM patterns. The time of amniotomy should be marked on the monitor strip. Time of procedures, as well as color, character, and amount of amniotic fluid are noted in the client's chart. The client's comfort is maintained by providing fresh bed linens and underpads as needed, because the amniotic fluid continues to leak during the ensuing labor.

OXYTOCIN ADMINISTRATION

An efficient and safe method of induction is by intravenous administration of oxytocin. The properties of this drug and its use in third stage labor are discussed in Chapter 22; its use in induction and augmentation of labor are discussed in Chapter 38.

■ INSTRUMENT-ASSISTED VAGINAL DELIVERY

Reasons for Assisted Delivery

During the second stage of labor, it may become necessary to use instruments to assist with the delivery. Maternal indications for instrument delivery include the inability of the mother to push due to conduction anesthesia, maternal exhaustion, heart disease, or any health condition adversely affecting the mother that is likely to be improved by delivery. The chief fetal indications for assisted delivery are fetal distress, as suggested by decreasing fetal heart rate, or disadvantageous fetal positions (such as occiput posterior or occiput transverse).

Vacuum Extraction

Increasingly, an instrument known as the vacuum extractor is used in place of the forceps. The vacuum extractor consists of a cup that is applied to the fetal head and tightly affixed there by creating a vacuum in the cup through withdrawal of the air by a pump. Cups are supplied in various sizes. The largest cup that can be applied with ease is selected for use. Vacuum is built up slowly, and the suction creates an artificial caput within the cup, providing a firm attachment to the fetal scalp. Traction can be exerted by means of a short chain attached to the cup, with a handle at its far end.

NURSING PROCESS

The nurse should briefly explain the procedure and its necessity to the mother and father. The mother feels pressure and pulling sensations, but does not feel pain with adequate regional or spinal anesthesia. Breathing techniques to prevent tensing and pushing are encouraged during application of the vacuum extraction cup. The mother is kept informed by the nurse during the procedure.

The nurse provides the physician with the vacuum extraction equipment, including the size cup requested and sterile tubing. After the physician assembles the cup and tubing, the nurse attaches the distal end to suction. With the cup applied to the fetal head, the nurse activates the suction. To avoid damaging vaginal tissues,

suction must be released if the cup slips off the fetal head. The nurse encourages the mother to push during contractions to aid birth, while traction is applied by the physician (Fig. 39-2).

The fetal heart rate should be monitored frequently by the nurse during the procedure. Infant resuscitation equipment should be available, and the pediatrician should be called if complications are expected with the infant. Parents are informed that the baby's head will have a caput (chignon) where the cup was applied, but that this disappears in a few hours.

Forceps Deliveries

TYPES OF FORCEPS

Forceps are instruments that may be used during delivery for holding, repositioning, or extracting the fetal head.

Some of the common types of obstetric forceps are illustrated in Figure 39-3. The instrument consists of two steel parts that cross each other like a pair of scissors and lock at the intersection. The lock may be of a sliding

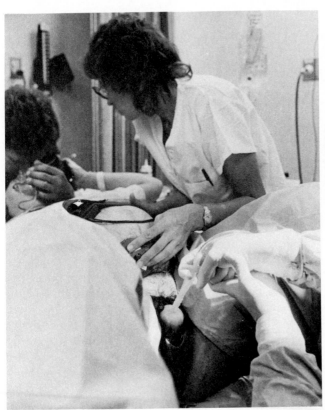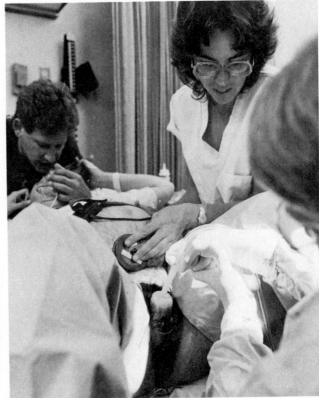

■ *Figure 39–2*
The nurse keeps the couple informed during the procedure, encourages the mother to push during the contractions, and monitors the fetus as traction continues. (Photos by Kathy Sloane)

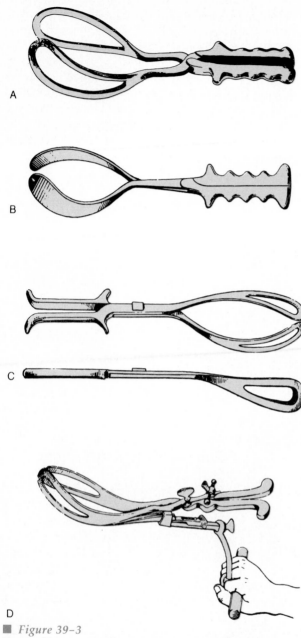

■ *Figure 39–3*
Types of forceps. (A) Simpson forceps. (B) Tucker-McLean forceps. (C, top) Kielland forceps, front view. (C, bottom) Kielland forceps, side view. (D) Tarnier axis-traction forceps.

type, as in the first three types shown, or a screw type, as in the Tarnier instrument.

Each part consists of a handle, a lock, a shank, and a blade; the blade is the curved portion designed for application to the sides of the fetal head. The blades of most forceps (the Tucker-McLean is an exception) have a large opening or window (fenestrum) to give a better grip on the head and usually consist of two curves, a cephalic curve, which conforms to the shape of the head, and a pelvic curve, to follow the curve of the birth canal. Axis-traction forceps, such as the Tarnier, have a mech-

anism attached below that permits the pulling to be done more directly in the axis of the birth canal. An axis-traction handle is also available for use on standard forceps.

The two blades of the forceps are designated as right and left. The left blade is introduced into the vagina on the client's left side; the right blade goes in on the right side.

TYPES OF FORCEPS DELIVERIES

In the vast majority of instances today, the forceps delivery is carried out at a time when the fetal head is on the perineal floor (visible or almost so) and internal rotation may have already occurred, so that the fetal head lies in a direct anteroposterior position. This is called *low forceps,* or "outlet forces." When the head is higher in the pelvis but engaged and its greatest diameter has passed the inlet, the operation is called *midforceps.* If the head has not yet engaged, the procedure is known as *high forceps.* High-forceps delivery is an exceedingly difficult and dangerous operation for both mother and baby and is rarely done. Increasingly, cesarean birth is preferred to a potentially difficult midforceps delivery.

PROCEDURE

After a decision is made to use forceps, the obstetrician selects the type of instrument to be used. Several pairs of the generally approved forceps, each encased in suitable wrappings, are autoclaved and kept in the delivery room for immediate use. The other instruments needed for a forceps delivery are the same as those required for a spontaneous delivery.

Anesthesia is recommended, but in low-forceps deliveries it may be light, and in most institutions this type of operation is performed in association with conduction anesthesia or under pudendal block anesthesia. The client is placed in the lithotomy position and prepared and draped in the usual fashion. For a midforceps delivery, the bladder should be emptied by catheterization.

After checking the exact position of the fetal head by vaginal examination, the physician introduces two or more fingers of one hand into the left side of the vagina; these fingers guide the left blade into place and at the same time protect the maternal soft parts (vagina and cervix) from injury. The other hand is used to introduce the left blade of the forceps into the left side of the vagina, gently insinuating it between the baby's head and the fingers of the hand (Fig. 39-4). The same procedure is carried out on the right side, and the blades are articulated. Traction is not continuous but intermittent (Fig. 39-5), and between traction, the blades are partially disarticulated to release pressure on the fetal head. Episiotomy is routine in these cases.

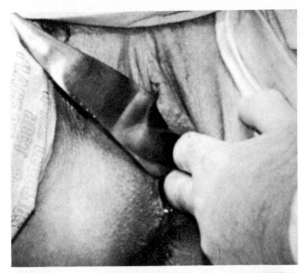

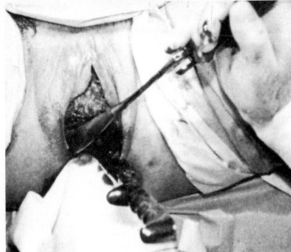

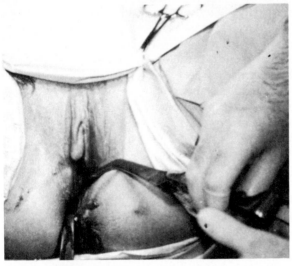

■ *Figure 39–4*
Insertion of the two blades of the forceps. (From the film
Human Birth, published by JB Lippincott, Philadelphia)

NURSING PROCESS

When forceps delivery is anticipated, the nurse can briefly explain the procedure and its necessity to the mother and father. The mother feels pressure and pulling, but does not feel pain with adequate regional or spinal anesthesia. Breathing techniques to prevent muscle tensing and pushing during application of the forceps should be encouraged, as well as other techniques used by the mother and couple to cope with labor.

The nurse provides the physician with the required type of forceps. This often can be determined in advance, and the forceps can be put on the delivery table. Once the forceps are applied, the nurse monitors contractions and advises the physician, so traction with the forceps can be coordinated with contractions. The mother is also encouraged to continue pushing as the physician applies traction.

Continuous fetal monitoring is a nursing responsibility because fetal bradycardia is common with forceps delivery. Appropriate infant resuscitation equipment should always be available, and a pediatrician should be present if fetal distress prompted the use of forceps. Bruises on the infant's head are common, and the parents should be advised and reassured that these disappear within a few days of birth.

PIPER FORCEPS FOR BREECH DELIVERY

The Piper forceps have been designed to assist in the delivery of the aftercoming head in breech presentations (Fig. 39-6). They are applied after the shoulders have been delivered and the head has been brought into the pelvis by gentle traction combined with suprapubic pressure. Suspension of the body and arms with a towel facilitates application of the blades. The left blade is introduced in an upward direction along the fetal head on the left side, and the right blade is applied in a similar fashion. The forceps are locked in place, and their position on the head is confirmed by palpation. An episiotomy is made and, as traction is applied, the chin, mouth, and nose emerge over the perineum. The Piper forceps are often used electively as a substitute for the Mauriceau-Smellie-Veit maneuver, or when the Mauriceau-Smellie-Veit maneuver for delivery of the fetal head has failed (see Chap. 38).

■ REPAIR OF LACERATIONS

Except for clamping and cutting the umbilical cord, episiotomy is the most common operative procedure performed in obstetrics. In view of the fact that this

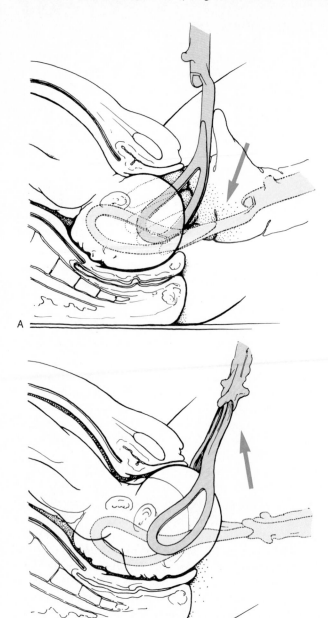

■ *Figure 39–5*
(A) *Insertion of forceps blade and* (B) *applied forceps and direction of traction.*

incision of the perineum, made to facilitate delivery, is employed almost routinely in primigravidas, the procedure has been discussed in the section on the conduct of normal labor (see Chap. 25).

Lacerations of the perineum and the vagina that occur in the process of delivery have also been discussed previously, because some tears are unavoidable, even in the most skilled hands. The suturing of spontaneous perineal lacerations is similar to that employed for the repair of an episiotomy incision, but may be more difficult because such tears often are irregular in shape with ragged, bruised edges.

The chance of lacerations increases with instrumented delivery, especially when forceps are employed.[6]

■ CESAREAN BIRTH

Cesarean birth (also called cesarean delivery or cesarean section) is the delivery of the fetus through incisions made in the abdominal wall and uterus. It is considered major abdominal surgery. The name is derived from the legend that Julius Caesar was born in this manner, but considering the dangers of surgery in his time, it is highly unlikely that he or his mother would have survived the operation. Before the advent of safe surgery, abdominal birth was reserved for instances in which the mother was dying and the child was to be saved. It was not until the late 19th century that cesarean birth was safely accomplished.[5]

Indications

The indications for cesarean birth fall into maternal and fetal categories:

Maternal reasons for cesarean birth include the following:

- Maternal disease that would adversely affect the birth process, such as heart disease, diabetes, severe preeclampsia, eclampsia, or severe infection
- Previous uterine surgery, including myomectomy, previous cesarean birth with a classical incision, or uterine reconstruction
- Obstruction of the birth canal by a tumor mass
- Placenta previa
- Premature separation of the placenta (abruption)
- Herpes simplex virus type II (HSV II or herpes genitalis) in the active phase (or within 2 weeks of active lesions)
- Failure of the labor to progress within normal parameters.[2,7,8]

Fetal indications include the following:

- Real or impending fetal distress
- Cephalopelvic disproportion (CPD; i.e., a discrepancy between the size of the fetal head and the maternal bony pelvis [contracted or small pelvis])
- Prematurity (usually less than 32 weeks' gestation)
- Multiple gestation in which the presenting twin is in the breech or transverse position
- Breech or transverse fetal position, especially in the primigravida.[2,8]

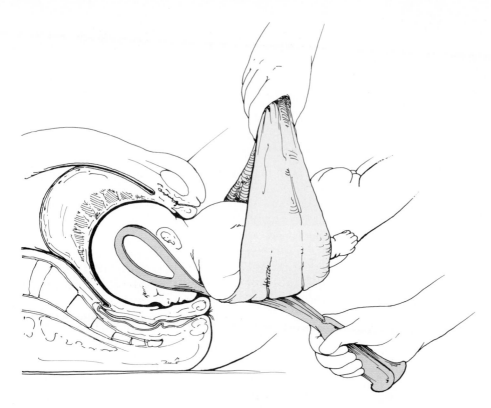

■ *Figure 39-6*
Piper forceps are used to deliver the aftercoming head in breech presentations, while the body and arms are suspended in a towel.

When a cesarean delivery is performed before the onset of labor, as the result of a prearranged plan, it is called *elective* cesarean delivery (as with elective low forceps, the obstetrician is not forced to perform the operation immediately, but elects to do it as the best procedure for mother and baby).

Prematurity is the most common fetal complication of elective cesarean birth. Assessment of fetal age has been previously discussed in this chapter.

The incidence of cesarean birth has increased dramatically in the past several years, from about 4.5% before 1965 to 22.7% in 1985, and to 24% in 1988. This increase suggests that the cesarean rate could reach 40% by the late 1990s.[8-10] This increase has fostered great controversy, and research has begun examining the reasons for the high rate of operative deliveries. This controversy is discussed later in this chapter.

Types of Cesarean Birth

Although there are four types of cesarean delivery, the low-segment section is usually the operation of choice. In this operation, the uterus is entered through an incision in the lower segment. Other types of cesarean delivery include the classical cesarean section, in which the incision is made directly into the wall of the body of the uterus; the extraperitoneal cesarean section, in which the operation is arranged anatomically, such that the incision

■ *Figure 39-7*
Cesarean birth. (A) Pfannenstiel's incision through the skin at the start of the operation. (B) The fascia has been nicked at the midline and is being opened in a smiling fashion with heavy scissors. (C) The fascia is separated from the underlying rectus muscle in a combination of blunt (shown in picture) and sharp dissection. (D) The peritoneum has been opened (hemostats on the edges), and the bladder blade has been positioned. The lower uterine segment is visible through the incision. (E) The bladder flap has been created; a low transverse uterine incision has been made, and the operator's hand is introduced in the lower uterine segment to facilitate the delivery of the fetal head. (F) The vertex has been brought to the site of the uterine incision, and the operator's right hand is guiding the delivery of the head. Fundal pressure from the right hand of the surgical assistant is facilitating the process. (G) The fetal head is gently being delivered through the uterine and abdominal incisions. (H) The fetal head has been delivered; the index finger of the assistant is being introduced into the baby's mouth to facilitate oropharyngeal suctioning of the amniotic fluid and secretions prior to the baby's first breath. (I) Nasopharyngeal and oropharyngeal suctioning are being performed by both the operator and the assistant using DeLee catheters. (J) Delivery first of the posterior shoulder through the uterine and abdominal incisions by gentle upward traction. (K) Delivery of the anterior shoulder by gentle downward traction. (L) The baby has been delivered, and the umbilical cord has been clamped with Kelly clamps and cut.

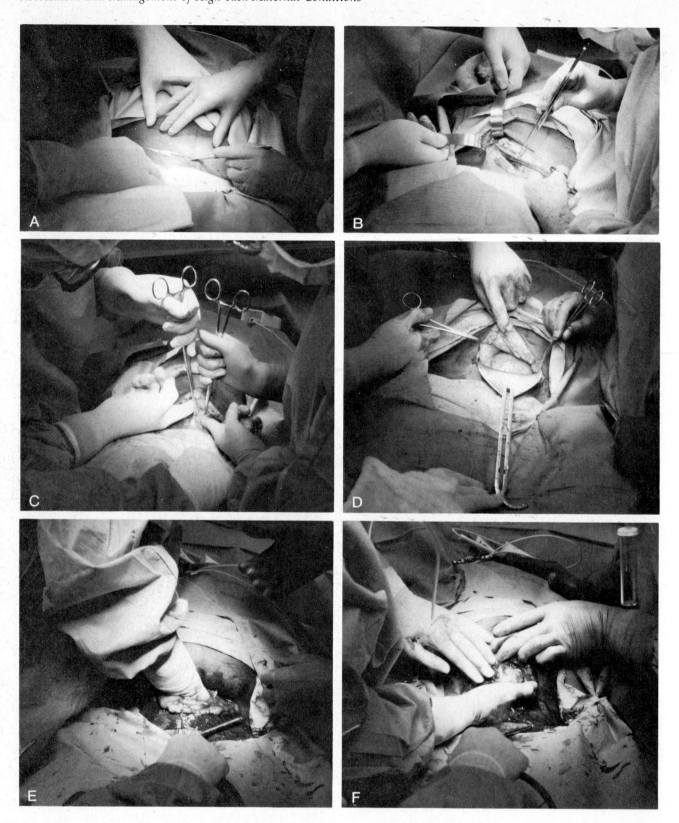

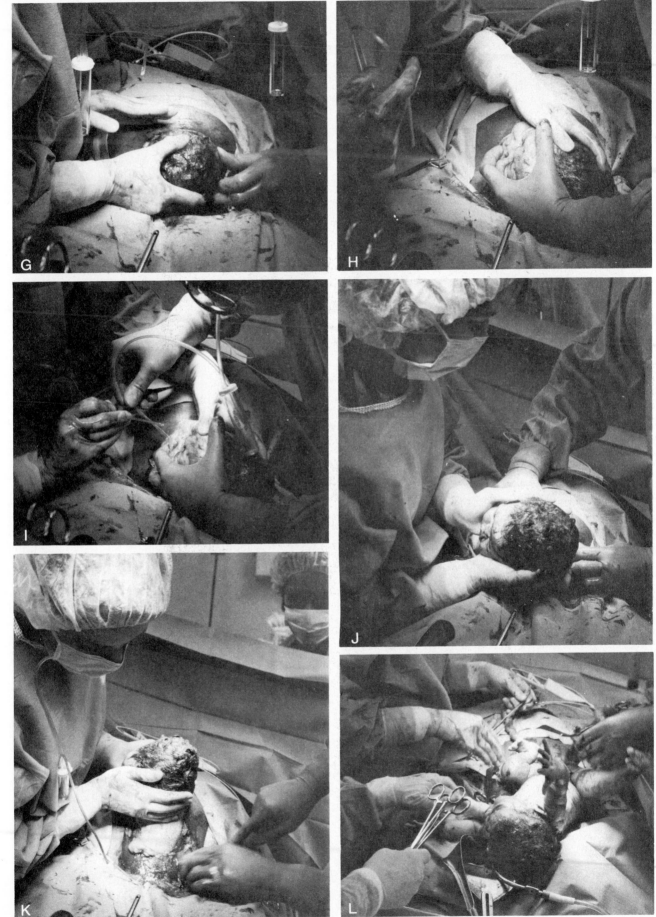

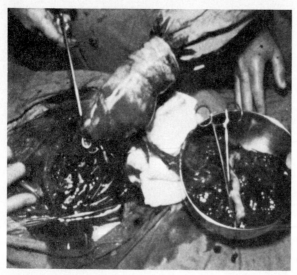
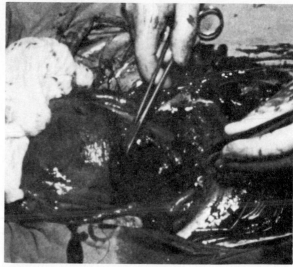

■ *Figure 39–8*
The placenta is extracted through the abdominal incision. (From the film Human Birth, published by JB Lippincott, Philadelphia)

is made into the uterus without entering the peritoneal cavity; and cesarean section-hysterectomy, which involves a cesarean section of any variety followed by removal of the uterus.

LOW-SEGMENT (LOW-TRANSVERSE) CESAREAN DELIVERY

Low-segment cesarean delivery is usually the operation of choice for a number of important reasons. Because the incision is made in the lower segment of the uterus, which is its thinnest portion, there is minimal blood loss, and the incision is easy to repair. The lower segment is also the area of least uterine activity, and thus the possibility of rupture of the scar in a subsequent pregnancy is lessened. Because the incision can be properly peritonealized, the operation is associated with a lower incidence of postoperative infection.

The initial incision (the abdominal cavity having been opened) is made transversely across the uterine peritoneum, where it is attached loosely just above the bladder. The lower peritoneal flap and the bladder are dissected from the uterus, and the uterine muscle is incised either vertically or transversely (Fig. 39-7A through D). The membranes are ruptured, and the baby is delivered (see Fig. 39-7E through L). The placenta is extracted (Figs. 39-8 and 39-9), and intravenous Pitocin is administered to contract the uterus. The uterine incision is sutured, and the lower flap is imbricated over the uterine incision. This two-flap arrangement seals off the uterine incision and is believed to prevent the egress of infectious lochia into the peritoneal cavity.

CLASSICAL CESAREAN BIRTH

A vertical incision is made directly into the wall of the body of the uterus; the baby and the placenta are extracted, and the incision is closed by three layers of absorbable sutures. Thus, this approach requires traversing the full thickness of the uterine corpus. It is still recommended in certain circumstances. It is particularly useful when the bladder and lower segment are involved in extensive adhesions resulting from a previous cesarean section and occasionally is selected when the

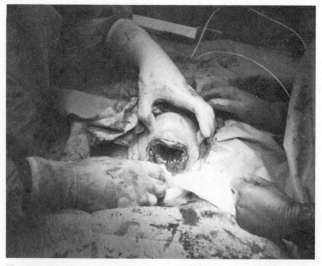

■ *Figure 39–9*
After delivery of the baby and placenta, the low transverse incision is clearly visible.

fetus is in a transverse lie or when there is an anterior placenta previa.

The classic cesarean is the method of choice when acute hemorrhage is occurring or in other emergency situations in which time is critical and the lives of the mother and baby are threatened.

EXTRAPERITONEAL CESAREAN BIRTH

Used primarily before the era of antibiotics, the extraperitoneal cesarean delivery does not require surgical entrance into the peritoneum. Access to the lower uterine segment is accomplished by dissecting the tissues around the bladder, thus avoiding the possible spill of amniotic fluid or pus into the peritoneum.

CESAREAN BIRTH WITH HYSTERECTOMY

Porro's operation, named for one of the 19th century physicians who perfected the cesarean approach,[5] combines birth with the removal of the uterus. It may be necessary after massive abruption, in cases of multiple fibroids, or when the placenta has embedded deep into the myometrium (placenta accreta). On rare occasions, and in conjunction with other gynecological disorders, this operation may be used for sterilization purposes.[2]

Increasing Cesarean Delivery Rates

The rapid increase of cesarean delivery rates has become a major concern for the health-care system. Operative delivery potentially poses more risks to the mother and her infant, yet must be balanced with the possible risks of vaginal birth.

Factors Contributing to the Increased Cesarean Birth Rate

Understanding the rise in the cesarean birth rate is a complex task because it involves many factors, including standards of care, changing diagnostic criteria, the medicolegal climate, and consumer demands. Improved fetal outcome is the goal of intervention in the birth process. In cases of maternal disease, fetal jeopardy, or labor complications, operative delivery can reduce the risk to the mother and fetus. Although operative delivery can pose its own potential dangers, the total risks and benefits must be balanced to ensure the safest outcome.

Previous cesarean birth is a leading indication for operative delivery, accounting for about 25% to 30% of cesareans. "Once a cesarean, always a cesarean" was the rule until the last decade when research began to

demonstrate that up to 85% of women could deliver vaginally after a prior cesarean.[11] When the primary cesarean was performed for reasons other that true cephalopelvic disproportion (CPD), a trial of labor and subsequent vaginal birth after cesarean (VBAC) is a feasible goal. This movement toward vaginal birth should decrease the overall rate of cesarean births, but other factors have increased the rate. VBAC is fully discussed later in this chapter.

The tremendous *increase in obstetric technology* has assisted physicians in monitoring the fetal condition and has increased their ability to diagnose potentially dangerous situations. The use of prenatal stress testing, electronic fetal monitoring (EFM), internal uterine pressure transducers, fetal scalp blood pH assessment, and other diagnostic procedures has expanded the knowledge of the condition of the fetus before birth. Although the technology has inherent risks, the information gained has enabled obstetricians to modify standards of care and improve the outcome.

Technology has changed the definition of *fetal distress,* which has shown an eightfold increase over the past decade and accounts for 10% to 15% of all cesareans. The association of fetal distress as documented by EFM and cesarean birth is complex and controversial. There is no proof that EFM is the cause for the increase in the diagnosis of fetal distress, although widespread use of EFM and the dramatic increase occurred at about the same time. This may reflect a greater reliance on technology and intervention overall. The key question is whether EFM permits more accurate identification of fetal distress than auscultation or whether fetal distress is being overdiagnosed. It is recognized that monitors malfunction, that physicians and nurses misread the tracings, and that abnormal tracings do not always correlate with low Apgar scores or low scalp pH. In addition, EFM appears involved indirectly in increasing cesarean rates for indications other than fetal distress. Some studies have found a higher incidence of dystocia in women who are monitored during labor. The stress produced by procedures used to insert monitors, by tension in the environment, and by fear of the implications of EFM could contribute to reduced uteroplacental perfusion and general muscular tension in the woman. Having to lie stationary on her back to accommodate the equipment's needs is detrimental to effective labor and the woman's ability to cope with contractions. Monitors might also lead to premature diagnosis of failure to progress, with physicians allowing less time to determine effective labor.

This reliance on EFM and the need for mothers to remain in bed has changed the working definition of *dystocia,* which includes such diagnoses as CPD, prolonged labor, uterine dysfunction, and failure to progress in labor. This accounts for 30% of the increase in the rate of primary cesareans. Obstetric management has shifted from an anatomical approach with assessment of the person to that of a functional definition of the progress of labor. Labor graphs set the parameters for normal progress in relation to time, centimeters dilated, and effectiveness of contractions. When a woman deviates from those graphic definitions, the diagnosis of dystocia can be quickly made. Management strategies such as adequate rest and hydration, appropriate ambulation or sedation, childbirth preparation, maternal choices, and a supportive environment are often forgotten in favor of the textbook definitions of the conduct of labor. Labor progress, as well as the maternal and fetal conditions, must be evaluated on an individual basis and in a timely fashion to diagnose dystocia.[7,8]

Increasingly *active labor management* with aggressive use of oxytocin and epidural anesthesia may contribute to the increased cesarean rate. As the interventions increase, the reliance on natural processes decreases. These interventions seem to interfere with the birth process, leading to an increase in the number of cesarean births.[12]

Changes in the philosophy of *breech management* have led to an increase of 10% to 15% in the cesarean rate. Although some studies have suggested that there is an increase in fetal morbidity and mortality in breech-born infants, there is no significant indication that overall perinatal mortality is lessened with cesarean birth.

The National Institutes of Health (NIH) Consensus Development Task Force on Cesarean Childbirth recommended that vaginal breech delivery continue to be an accepted practice with a full-term baby not over 8 lb, a normal pelvis, frank breech presentation without hyperextended head, and an experienced obstetrician. This last requirement is becoming more and more difficult to fulfill, however, because of the diminishing experience of resident physicians in delivering breech infants vaginally. Because of policies tending toward cesarean delivery as standard for all breech presentations, residents have less and less experience with vaginal breech deliveries. They become reluctant to do this when in practice later and are also concerned with possible lawsuits for not doing cesareans if the infant is injured by vaginal birth.

Shifts in the philosophies of *medical education and training* also contribute to the rise in cesarean birth. Obstetric residents receive less preparation and experience in the use of forceps, especially midforceps. They deliver fewer breech presentations and are taught to rely more on operative intervention. They learn values that support active and aggressive intervention rather than to wait and encourage the natural process of birth. Appropriate use of forceps, prudent management of breech presentations, and clearer research-supported definitions of dystocia and fetal distress must be reintegrated into the medical curriculum if physicians are to contribute to stabilizing or decreasing the rate of cesarean births.[10]

Directly related to medical education are the dilemmas of *economics and malpractice.* Cesareans are up to three times more costly than vaginal birth and require longer hospitalization. The potential drain on economic resources is clear. The threat of malpractice suits appears to be an enormous concern for many physicians. Awards for birth-related injuries have reached astronomical proportions, and physicians fear the economic implications as well as the potential damages to their practices and community trust and goodwill. Substantial changes in the malpractice insurance industry as well as legislation protecting physicians and hospitals are needed before physicians are willing to return to nonoperative interventions in certain situations where sound medical judgment and intervention occurred but the outcome was less than ideal. No-fault government insurance funds could provide the financial support needed for a birth-injured child.[10]

Shifts in the *demographics of medical care providers and consumers* may also contribute to the rising cesarean rate.

The proportion of nulliparous mothers has increased, and the average age of the obstetric population has risen recently. Both of these groups have higher incidences of cesarean births. A greater proportion of maternity care is being provided by obstetricians (rather than family or general practice physicians), who perform cesarean sections more frequently than nonobstetricians.

Characteristics of *hospitals* also affect the cesarean delivery rate. Hospitals with neonatal intensive care units (NICUs) are most likely to provide cesareans. Public hospitals have slightly lower, and proprietary hospitals slightly higher, cesarean rates than voluntary hospitals. Cesarean rates rise with hospital bed size. The age mix and complications of clients in various types of hospitals play important roles in the indications for surgical delivery. However, hospitals with medical school affiliations and NICUs have the most serious case mixes but are least likely to do cesareans for several types of complications.[13] The teaching function in hospitals appears to provide some control over appropriate use of technology.

Disadvantages of Cesarean Delivery

There are, of course, disadvantages to delivering by cesarean. Maternal mortality and morbidity are involved along with the discomforts occurring after any surgery. Maternal–infant bonding may be affected, including development of mothering skills and breast-feeding.

Maternal Risks in Cesarean Birth

Maternal mortality, although rare, is four times higher with cesarean delivery than with vaginal delivery. Half of this increase is due to complications leading to the cesarean or to maternal disease. The other half is due to the surgery itself.

Maternal mortality in repeat cesarean is about twice that in vaginal deliveries.

Maternal morbidity is much greater after cesarean; the major risks are from:
Infection of uterus and other genital tract structures
Infection of respiratory or urinary tract
Hemorrhage

Postoperative discomforts occur frequently, including incisional pain, gas, weakness, and difficulty in movement.

Maternal–infant bonding is interfered with through common hospital practices such as:
General anesthesia during surgery
Separation of mother and infant during recovery and first day
Analgesics given the mother for pain relief
Isolation necessary for infections

Development of mothering skills is interfered with because of:
Disorientation after anesthesia and surgery
Pain limiting activities and requiring sedation
Weakness, which limits the energy the mother can give to infant caretaking
Postoperative complications further reducing mother–infant contact
Emotional turmoil and the need to process feelings (anger, loss, confusion, fear, inadequacy, and so forth) associated with undergoing cesarean birth and operative procedures
Delay and increased difficulty gaining a sense of mastery over the mother's body

Breast-feeding is more difficult or impossible because of:
Pain, weakness, limited activities
Infections or other serious complications
Medications that may be excreted in breast milk
Sense of inadequacy related to childbearing capabilities

Education to Avoid Cesarean Delivery

Women and their partners can benefit from understanding how they can help avoid unnecessary cesarean birth. Often a series of occurrences from early pregnancy through the labor process leads to the decision for surgical delivery. Different choices by parents, or different actions in relation to health providers, might lead to a different outcome. Choice of birth attendant, locale for delivery, health practices, level of knowledge about childbearing, and participation in childbirth preparation can all affect the type of delivery.[14]

■ VAGINAL BIRTH AFTER CESAREAN (VBAC)

As previously stated, more and more women are electing to attempt labor and vaginal delivery after a prior cesarean. Safety and feasibility are being demonstrated repeatedly.[11,15] In 1980, the NIH Consensus Development Task Force on Cesarean Childbirth provided guidelines for attempting a VBAC. In 1988, the American College of Obstetricians and Gynecologists (ACOG) elaborated on these guidelines, stressing the individual assessment of candidates and the development of institutional policies for VBAC.[9] The use of oxytocin augmentation and epidural anesthesia presents no greater risk to the VBAC patient than to the patient with no history of operative delivery.[2,9,16,17]

When the previous cesarean was performed for reasons other than true CPD, VBAC is a feasible alternative to repeat surgery. Careful selection of clients and prudent monitoring of the pregnancy can enhance the chance for successful VBAC. Routine obstetric care, provided by physicians or nurse–midwives, is essential.[18] Concurrent medical conditions such as gestational diabetes must be successfully managed. In such cases, close observation of fetal weight gain by way of ultrasound can assist in the detection of a fetus who might be too large to deliver vaginally.[19]

Clients electing a trial of labor and VBAC should be encouraged to participate in childbirth education classes. Specialized classes for VBAC couples are becoming available across the country. These classes utilize information provided by the growing research on VBAC and can provide the couple with realistic expectations for the experience.

Women experiencing VBAC have similar labor patterns to those without a history of cesarean birth. In other words, prior cesarean birth does not affect the time required for the first full labor and vaginal birth. A woman whose first child was delivered by cesarean will have a labor similar to that of a primiparous woman. There seems to be no increase in the incidence of complications of labor for VBAC.[16,17]

Client Education

Avoiding Unnecessary Cesarean Birth

Cesarean births are necessary for a small proportion of women with serious conditions threatening fetal or maternal life. For many other women, a series of events takes place that, in their combined effects, leads to an inevitable decision for cesarean birth, which is usually necessary at that time, but which might have been prevented had different choices been made. Some approaches to minimizing the risk of cesarean birth follow:

- Carefully choose a birth attendant who will be most supportive of your needs and desires for the birth experience. A nurse–midwife, if available, might be more compatible with your chosen style of birth.
- Select a birth environment that provides the type of setting compatible with your objectives for the birth experience. This may be an alternate birth center or a hospital with policies permitting many choices.
- Become informed about childbearing, its potential risks, choices available at various decision points, and legal rights and responsibilities.
- Participate in childbirth-preparation classes, which increase knowledge and reduce fear, provide tools for positive management of labor and delivery, and help the mother attain optimal physical and emotional conditions for undergoing labor and birth.
- Maintain your general health throughout appropriate nutrition, exercise, weight, and activities; avoid habits or practices that increase risk such as smoking, alcohol or drug use.
- When the birth attendant is an obstetrician, discuss his or her beliefs and practices related to cesareans, such as indications for surgery, induction, or labor stimulation and the percentage of deliveries done by cesarean section (above 10% increases risk).
- Determine the hospital's policies regarding cesarean operations and fetal monitoring and what percentage of deliveries are by cesarean section (above 30% increases risk).

■ NURSING PROCESS FOR CESAREAN BIRTH

Preoperative Care

ASSESSMENT

Having an operative delivery increases the parents' anxiety, adds numerous factors that must be understood and accepted, makes postdelivery recovery more difficult, places an additional strain on the developing mother–infant relationship, and creates a need for processing and integrating the altered birth experience.

Nursing assessment in the preoperative period includes physical parameters, evaluation of the patient's readiness for and understanding of the procedure, and identification of possible risk factors. This information is gathered from the patient's prenatal records (often transferred to the hospital before the delivery date), physical assessment (vital signs, laboratory data), and by interviewing the patient and her support person at the time of admission.

NURSING DIAGNOSIS

Potential nursing diagnoses related to the preoperative period include:

1. Anxiety related to cesarean birth
2. Anxiety related to lack of knowledge of preoperative routines
3. Knowledge deficit related to cesarean birth
4. Powerlessness related to lack of choice in childbirth options
5. Self-esteem disturbance related to inability to complete a vaginal birth

PLANNING AND INTERVENTION

Nursing care should assist the mother and family to have a satisfying childbirth experience. The woman undergoing a cesarean birth is in need of the same sensitive and supportive care recommended for vaginal births by the Interprofessional Task Force on Health Care of Women and Children.

Guidelines for Vaginal Delivery After a Previous Cesarean Birth

Each hospital should develop its own protocol for management of patients who are encouraged to deliver vaginally after a previous cesarean birth. Suggested guidelines include the following:

1. The concept of routine repeat cesarean birth should be replaced by a specific indication for a subsequent abdominal delivery, and in the absence of a contraindication, a woman with one previous cesarean delivery with a low transverse incision should be counseled and encouraged to attempt labor in her current pregnancy.
2. A woman with two or more previous cesarean deliveries with low transverse incisions who wishes to attempt vaginal birth should not be discouraged from doing so in the absence of contraindications.
3. In circumstances in which specific data on risks are lacking, the question of whether to allow a trial of labor must be assessed on an individual basis.
4. A previous classical uterine incision is a contraindication to labor.
5. Professional and institutional resources must have the capacity to respond to acute intrapartum obstetric emergencies, such as performing cesarean delivery within 30 minutes from the time the decision is made until the surgical procedure is begun, as is standard for any obstetric patient in labor.
6. Normal activity should be encouraged during the latent phase of labor; there is no need for restriction to a labor bed before actual labor has begun.
7. A physician who is capable of evaluating labor and performing a cesarean delivery should be readily available.

(Guidelines for Vaginal Delivery After a Previous Cesarean Birth: ACOG Committee Opinion, 64, 1988)

Report of the NIH Consensus Development Task Force on Cesarean Childbirth

In 1979, the National Institutes of Health convened a Consensus Development Task Force to examine cesarean childbirth. A group of experts from medicine, research, law, social sciences, and the public examined all available evidence about cesareans and arrived at consensus recommendations for practice. In 1980, their report was published with these recommendations for lowering the cesarean birth rate:

1. Labor and vaginal delivery are a safe, relatively low-risk choice after a previous low-segment transverse uterine incision.
2. Trials of labor after previous cesareans should take place in facilities with the capability of a prompt emergency cesarean if necessary. Hospitals that lack such facilities should inform clients in advance and refer them to the nearest fully equipped hospital.
3. Prolonged labor (dystocia) should be treated with such measures as rest, hydration, sedation, ambulation, and oxytocin stimulation before resorting to cesarean.
4. Research should continue into means for evaluating the progress of labor, the effects of conservative treatment of dystocia, and the effects of emotional support and regional anesthesia.
5. Vaginal breech delivery should continue to be an accepted practice with a full-term baby not expected to be over 8 lb, normal pelvis, frank breech presentation without hyperextended head, and an experienced obstetrician.
6. All clients should have the choice of regional anesthesia.
7. Fathers should be allowed to be present at cesarean births.
8. Parents and infants should not be routinely separated after birth, unless indicated by the mother's or infant's condition.
9. Parent education and information about cesareans should be provided during pregnancy by childbirth educators and health professionals.

The Nurse as Counselor and Supporter. Psychoemotional factors are important for couples experiencing cesarean birth. Many describe feelings of fear, disappointment, frustration over loss of control, grief over losing their ideal birth experience, anger or victimization, or confusion over the necessity for the procedure. Mothers are particularly susceptible to decreased self-esteem. They may have disturbed body image and role expectations and may feel they have failed in reproductive functions. Worry about the scar affecting their attractiveness and the effects of the surgery on sexual processes is often present.

Women facing a repeat or elective cesarean birth, who know in advance that their birth will be operative, have time to prepare psychologically for the experience.

Other women do not know in advance and must contend with the decision for a cesarean delivery while undergoing labor. Each situation presents its particular stresses and coping demands.

The nurse must be prepared to deal with these feelings, fears, and uncertainties. Opportunity for exploration and expression of feelings and clarification of uncertainties and misunderstandings must be provided either in group or individual discussions. Working within a crisis framework, the nurse can assist women and their partners to progress through appropriate stages to achieve acceptance and a sense of readiness.

Client Education

Some Alternatives Available to Women Undergoing Cesarean Birth

- Regional (epidural) anesthesia so you can be awake during the birth
- Partner or other support person present during surgery and birth
- Hands freed from restraints for touch contact with father and baby
- Dropping the screen (which prevents view of the surgery) at the time of delivery
- Having an advocate (usually a nurse) who describes to parents what is going on during the operation and delivery
- Touching or holding the baby immediately after birth
- Delaying instillation of silver nitrate drops into the baby's eyes for the first hour after birth
- Continual contact between mother, father, and baby during first hour of life if the baby is stable
- Breast-feeding the infant immediately after birth in delivery or recovery room
- Initiation of rooming-in as soon as you desire
- Extended or unlimited visiting priviledges for the father (or support person) during the postpartum period
- Utilization of medications (when necessary) that are not secreted in significant amounts in the breast milk

---

The nurse can help create a positive context by emphasizing that cesarean birth can be a satisfying and fulfilling experience, in which both parents can mature, expand their self-concepts, and grow in self-esteem by effectively handling this experience. They can develop a nurturing relationship with the baby and increase their mutuality as a couple. The nurse plays a key role in helping the couple become well-prepared for physical and emotional events, which can be key in the couple's success.

Childbirth Classes. Childbirth classes in preparation for cesarean birth are increasing in number. Some educators feel all childbirth classes should present information about cesareans, even when vaginal delivery is anticipated. Considering that in some medical centers the cesarean rate is nearly one in four deliveries, this approach has merit.

Cesarean prenatal classes usually cover content common to all prenatal classes, including onset of labor and contact person should labor begin at home. Special emphasis is given to prenatal testing (i.e., tests of fetal condition, preoperative tests), surgical procedures, analgesia and anesthesia, technologies (sonography, intravenous fluids, urinary retention catheter), the operating room experience, and postoperative recovery.

Techniques for increasing comfort and relaxation are taught. Although labor is not anticipated, the woman will find these techniques useful during tests and examinations and to alleviate pain after surgery. Hospital policies are reviewed, including the father's presence in the operating room and after surgery. The delivery and care of the infant are detailed, including procedures in the operating and recovery rooms and normal variations in early mother–infant relations. The course of postoperative recovery, both in the hospital and at home, is related to the pacing of caretaking responsibilities and need for assistance at home.

Preoperative Preparation. Preparation for cesarean birth involves readying the mother for surgery and making the necessary preparations for care of the infant. The usual preparations of laboratory tests, physical examination, typing and cross-matching blood, abdominal shaving, and other customary procedures are carried out. The physician discusses the type of operation and anesthesia with the woman and family, and informed consent is obtained.

When the client is admitted for an elective cesarean section, nursing care includes checking fetal heart tones and being alert to prodromal signs of labor. Oral intake should be discontinued for at least 8 hours before surgery.

The lower abdomen is shaved including the pubic hair. A retention catheter may be inserted and attached to a constant drainage system to ensure that the bladder remains empty during the operation. The nurse should make certain that the catheter is draining properly before the procedure.

An intravenous infusion (commonly Ringer's lactate solution or 5% dextrose in water, 1000 ml) is started. Valuables are taken for safekeeping, and routine preoperative precautions are taken, such as removing fingernail polish, dentures, glasses, and contact lenses.

Preoperative medications (atropine and, on occasion, an analgesic or mild tranquilizer) are administered according to the physician's orders.

In addition to the preparation of the operating room for the surgical procedure, the nurse makes the necessary preparations for care of the infant. The nurse makes sure that the necessary equipment is present, including a warm crib and equipment for the resuscitation of the infant. An infant resuscitator, equipped with heat, suction, oxygen (open mask and positive pressure), and an adjustable frame to permit the proper positioning of the infant, is most useful.

Interventions for Unanticipated Cesarean Delivery. Emergency cesareans are performed when fetal or maternal complications pose serious risks. Complications may arise at any stage of labor, but often the decision for surgery is made after hours of nonprogressive labor or as a result of abnormal tracings on the fetal monitor. The woman is often discouraged, exhausted, worried about her own or the baby's condition, and possibly dehydrated with low glycogen reserves. Preoperative preparations usually must be done rapidly, leaving little time for explanations.

The nurse should provide short, simple, and concise explanations of the surgery and procedures that must be done. It is important that the nurse offer as much reassurance about the mother's and baby's conditions as can reasonably be given. However, the client's and her partner's anxiety level are high, and they may not recall much or may misunderstand. After the operation, the nurse should spend time reviewing events leading up to the surgery, what occurred in the operating room, and the baby's status to allow the parents to understand and integrate their experiences.

Care During Surgery

Nurses assist during cesarean birth by either scrubbing or circulating in the operating room. The surgical team consists of obstetrician, surgical assistant, anesthesiologist, pediatrician, and nurses. The nurse has a special role in keeping parents informed, providing calm reassurance, and interpreting events for the parents. Many cesareans are done under conduction anesthesia, so the woman is aware of events. The father, gowned appropriately, may also be in the room, sitting close to the mother's head. The surgical team must take the above into consideration in their communications with each other.

A trained person should be present at cesarean birth to give the infant initial care and to resuscitate if necessary. This person may be an experienced nurse with advanced training in infant resuscitation, a nurse anesthetist, anesthesiologist, or perinatologist.

Immediate transport to the NICU must be available, in case the infant is compromised at birth. Depending on the infant's condition and hospital policies, newborn care and evaluation may be done in the operating room.

In many hospitals, it is customary to have a pediatrician at hand to take over the care of the infant as soon as it is born and free the obstetrician to devote full attention to the mother.

The father may be given the baby to hold and show to the mother, or they may be united in the recovery room.

The nurse should encourage and foster the parent–infant bonding process by providing the mother (when she is awake) and the father the opportunity to touch and hold the newborn. When it is difficult for the mother to hold the infant, the nurse can hold the infant in an en face (face-to-face) position to facilitate the maternal–infant bonding process.

Immediate Postoperative Postpartum Care

The woman who has had a cesarean delivery has undergone both abdominal surgery and a birth. Postoperative care includes the same procedures as for any abdominal surgery with the added dimension of postpartum care.

ASSESSMENT

Blood Loss. Bleeding is assessed the same as in any delivery. The woman must be watched for hemorrhage by frequently inspecting the perineal pad and checking the fundus. Usually the abdominal dressings are not bulky, and the nurse can palpate the fundus to see if the uterus is well contracted. Skin and uterine sutures are secure, and gentle but firm pressure can be used to assess uterine consistency. This may cause some discomfort, but does not disturb the sutures. Oxytocics are usually ordered to contract the uterus and control bleeding.

The amount and character of lochia are noted, using the same guidelines as with vaginal deliveries (see Chap. 28). Some women have less lochia after cesarean birth because of operative techniques used in placenta removal and hemostasis. The skin incision is examined regularly for signs of hematoma, bleeding, or infection. Vital signs are taken every 4 hours for the first few postoperative days, or until stable. It is particularly important to watch for signs of shock or infection.

Input and Output. If the retention catheter is to remain in place until the following morning, it should remain attached to "constant drainage" and should be watched to see that it drains freely. Intravenous fluids are usually administered during the first 24 hours, although small amounts of fluids may be given by mouth after nausea has subsided. A record of the mother's intake and elimination is kept for the first several days or until the need is no longer indicated.

NURSING DIAGNOSIS

In the immediate postoperative period, the following nursing diagnoses are possible:

1. Alteration of respiratory function due to shallow breathing secondary to incisional pain
2. Alteration of tissue perfusion due to blood loss of surgery and inadequate contraction of the uterus
3. Alteration of fluid and electrolyte balance
4. Alteration of comfort, related to incisional pain and uterine involution.

PLANNING AND INTERVENTION

Analgesic drugs should be used to keep the mother comfortable and encourage her to rest. Her position in bed during the early postoperative hours may be dictated by the type of anesthesia that she received. She should be encouraged to turn from side to side every hour. Deep breathing and coughing should also be encouraged to promote good ventilation. Most mothers who deliver cesarean are allowed early ambulation. This contributes considerably to maintaining good bladder and intestinal function.

Pain after cesarean birth most often involves the incisional site, gas pain as bowel function is restored, flank pain from stretching of abdominal muscles during surgery, muscle aches from immobility, afterpains, and sometimes discomfort from bladder distention. Analgesic medication should be timed to provide maximum relief during the times the mother spends feeding and caring for the baby. She can devote her energy to the infant and avoid the distraction of postoperative pain.

Continued Postpartum Care

After the immediate postoperative period, the mother receives routine postpartum care and continued post-surgery observations. Postpartum care includes vital signs, lochia observation, fundal assessment, breast and perineal care, attention to bladder and bowel elimination, ambulation, and hygiene.

ASSESSMENT

Care related to the surgery includes observation of the skin incision, pain control, respiratory function, and increased needs for rest and restoration.

Showers may be taken on the second day if staples were used to close the incision.

Assessment and intervention in the development of mothering skills, and family adaptations to cesarean birth are of central importance. The woman's and family's response to the birth process must be carefully observed and assessed. Especially in unanticipated cesareans, the levels of anxiety, anger, disappointment, and confusion may be high. Many women feel overwhelmed by an unexpected cesarean birth and are completely unprepared for their physical and emotional responses. They express feelings of anxiety for themselves or the baby. They experience anger or depression because they expected a normal birth. They tend to feel a sense of loss over not experiencing vaginal delivery, not witnessing the birth, and not having their partner's or family's participation. There are often altered body perceptions as well as many concerns surrounding mothering the infant during their recovery from surgery.[20]

The physical discomfort of the mother after the surgery, combined with her feelings of disappointment or guilt, can interfere with her ability to bond to her infant. The long-term consequences of inadequate or delayed maternal–infant bonding can range from poor growth and development of the infant to blatant child abuse.

However, mothers who were allowed early and continuous contact with their infants after cesarean birth (with spinal anesthesia and delivery of a healthy, normal infant) were found to have significantly more positive perceptions of their infants in the early postpartum period. They also displayed more maternal behavior in caretaking at this time and when the infant was 1 month old than cesarean mothers who only had brief contact in the first 12 hours after birth.[21]

At this time, the woman finds herself burdened with an abdominal operative procedure. Her needs for physical and emotional recovery may dominate her mothering interests initially. She may need to deal with her reduced ability to care for the infant, separation from the infant (especially with maternal or neonatal complications), discomfort in holding and feeding, and concern about the infant's well-being. The father likewise may have needs to review and integrate the experience and to learn the new processes involved in recovery and procedures after cesarean birth.

NURSING DIAGNOSIS

For the postpartum, postoperative period, the following additional nursing diagnoses are possible:

1. Knowledge deficit related to the cesarean birth
2. Alteration of parenting skills
3. Alteration in body concept and self-esteem
4. Grieving related to cesarean birth or fetal demise
5. Alteration of family process.

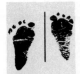

Nursing Care Plan

The Woman Experiencing Cesarean Birth

Patient Goals:
1. Mother and family indicate readiness for cesarean birth.
2. Mother and family indicate understanding of the cesarean process.
3. Normal maternal–infant bonding occurs.
4. Mother's comfort and body functions are maintained or restored.
5. Mother and family indicate integration of the cesarean birth as a positive and satisfying birth experience.

Assessment	Potential Nursing Diagnosis	Planning and Intervention	Evaluation
Preparation for cesarean birth (unanticipated, elective)	Knowledge deficit related to reasons for cesarean, procedures, relaxation, pain relief	Include cesarean birth in childbirth preparation classes	Parents recognize the potential for cesarean birth and feel prepared
	Fear related to condition of self or baby, pain, procedures, outcomes, aftermath	Provide information and explanation of reasons for cesarean, preparations for surgery, and processes to anticipate	Parents verbalize understanding, accept need and processes, cooperate in preparations
		Assist parents to express their feelings of fear, disappointment, grief, powerlessness, and so forth	Parents express feelings freely and begin to accept and prepare for cesarean delivery
		Provide information and reassurance (as much as possible) about condition of mother and baby	Parents feel reasonably reassured or able to cope with risks
Postoperative condition: Fundal contraction Bleeding Vital signs Input and output Incision Respiratory function Comfort	Potential complications: hemorrhage, uterine atony, hematomas, shock, depressed respiratory function	Monitor postoperative progress, report early signs of problems, take emergency actions as needed	
	Alteration in comfort: pain related to incision, afterpains, stretched abdominal muscles	Administer analgesics, change position, adjust bedding	Mother reports increased comfort or sleeps or rests
Early bonding with infant Mother Father	High risk for alteration in parenting related to lack of early contact, complications, pain, anesthesia, disappointment over birth, powerlessness	Provide opportunity for parents to see, hold, and explore infant in recovery area (if possible); or report on infant's condition and characteristics (sex, weight, normalcy, progress)	Parents have satisfying early contact or have their questions about the baby answered and feel well-informed
	High risk for alteration in parenting related to lack of early contact due to exclusion, condition of mother or infant, power-	Discuss parents' feelings and reactions to cesarean birth; provide information	Mother is awake and reasonably comfortable; can hold and interact with baby
			Parents express feelings freely, fit missing pieces

(continued)

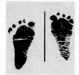

Nursing Care Plan (continued)

Assessment	Potential Nursing Diagnosis	Planning and Intervention	Evaluation
	lessness, disappointment	and explanations	together, begin to integrate the experience

Postpartum observations:
  Incision healing
  Pain
  Fluids and nutrition
  Bowel function
  Bladder function
  Respiratory function
	For general postpartum care, see Nursing Care in the Postpartum Period, Chapter 28. Observations specific to cesarean sections are included here.	Monitor condition of incision, input and output, bowel and bladder function, respiratory function	Mother takes fluids and food, moves bowels as expected, voids well after removal of catheter, and aerates lungs adequately

	High risk for complications; infection, hematoma, incisional bleeding, wound dehiscence	Identify signs of complications early; report and take action	Mother feels comfortable
	Alteration in comfort related to incision, afterpains, stretched abdominal muscles, gas	Administer analgesics, assist in positioning, teach splinting and movement to minimize pain	Mother reports increased comfort, holds and cares for infant, and interacts with partner satisfactorily
	High risk for complications: persistent nausea and vomiting, continued intravenous therapy, lack of appetite, decreased gastrointestinal functioning		
	Alteration in bowel elimination: decreased functioning related to anesthesia and surgery (decreased peristalsis and activity), gas, constipation		
	Alteration in patterns of urinary elimination related to surgery, anesthesia, indwelling catheter; high risk for urinary retention		
	High risk for complications: decreased oxygenation due to limited ventilation, pneumonia, pulmonary embolus		
Mothering skills	High risk for alteration in parenting related to discomfort following surgery, disappointment with birth, feeling incomplete or powerless, anger, inexperience	Provide pain relief, explanations and information about cesarean, opportunity to explore events surrounding cesarean birth	Mother is comfortable, expresses feelings freely, gains understanding and acceptance of cesarean birth

(continued)

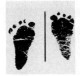

Nursing Care Plan (continued)

Assessment	Potential Nursing Diagnosis	Planning and Intervention	Evaluation
	Knowledge deficit of special needs following cesarean birth, effect of postsurgical recovery on strength and emotions, managing discomforts	Teach parents about special needs of mother for rest, recovery, and emotional processes	Parents understand and accept special needs, make provisions for these
Adjustment to cesarean birth	High risk for disturbance in self-concept related to body changes (incision), failure to have "normal" birth, insufficient "control" over childbearing, time required for recovery	Encourage mother to express feelings, support positive interpretations, reinforce normal aspects	Mother expresses feelings and identifies positive aspects of cesarean birth
	Anxiety/fear related to effects of surgery on self or infant		
Family adjustment	High risk for alteration in family processes related to disappointment, anger, powerlessness, blame seeking, coping inexperience, or lack of understanding	Encourage parents to express feelings, clear misunderstandings, process their experience, relate it to needs for home management	Parents express feelings, integrate the experiences surrounding cesarean birth, make plans for managing at home
	Impaired home maintenance management related to increased needs of mother for rest and recovery time following cesarean		
	High risk for sexual dysfunction related to misunderstandings or fears of surgery effects on sexual functioning	Discuss sexuality after cesarean birth; correct misunderstandings	Parents understand effects of cesarean birth on sexual functioning, feel prepared to accept limits, are supportive of each other

PLANNING AND INTERVENTION

In addition to caring for the mother's physical needs in the postpartum period, the nurse has a large responsibility in providing explanations of events and decisions, and in giving support through physical contact, calmness, comfort measures, verbal reassurances, and assisting the mother to gain mastery of her body and infant-care tasks.

Nursing care must provide opportunity to review events, seek understandings of what happened and why, remember responses and work these through, clear up questions and misunderstandings, and alter self-concept and expectations to be congruent with reality.

One or 2 days after the birth, a visit from the labor and delivery nurse who assisted the couple during the childbirth is often beneficial for the integration of the event into their lives. The filling in of missing pieces is important for all women who experience gaps in their memories of the labor and births of their infants.[22]

This may be more important when the woman is attempting to understand the reasons for surgical intervention in what is often expected to be a natural process. Visits such as this also provide the couple with the opportunity to discuss any feelings of failure, guilt, or anger they may be experiencing. A sensitive and responsive nurse can effectively help the couple work through such feelings by remaining open to their comments and honestly addressing their concerns. If the family unit is to be strengthened through the childbearing process, and if childbirth is to be a family-centered event, every attempt should be made by the obstetric staff to help families incorporate this experience into their lives.

Issues of sexuality can also be addressed in the postpartum period. The mother may fear pain with intercourse (when resumed) or that the surgery will affect her partner's concept of her body. Reassurance and factual information usually assist the mother in resolving these issues. Involvement of the partner in this discussion often helps the couple in their adjustment.

Grief counseling should also be available, especially in cases of fetal demise or when the infant is seriously ill and in the NICU. Chapter 45 addresses the emotional, psychological, and spiritual care of the family in this instance.

Discharge Planning

Hospitalization after cesarean birth usually lasts 3 to 5 days. Discharge preparation includes that for any postpartum patient (see Chap. 31) and also teaching specific to postoperative considerations. Mothers may be prescribed analgesics for use at home and should be reminded of their increased need for rest. Exercises may begin when abdominal pain has decreased, but lifting heavy objects should be avoided for 2 to 3 weeks. Most mothers are able to lift their infants without problem.

Instruction about complications is important, including signs of infection (fever, dysuria, flank pain), hemorrhage, thrombosis (severe chest or leg pain, leg swelling), and wound dehiscence. Guidelines for contacting physician or clinic are given. Intercourse may be resumed when lochia has ceased and there is no undue abdominal or perineal discomfort. Contraceptive information is provided as for other postpartum patients. A return visit is usually scheduled for 3 weeks after delivery, and another at 6 weeks.

A referral for follow-up by the public health nurse or home care service is appropriate if the nurse observes the mother exhibiting undue difficulty in the adaptation to her infant, in cases of teenage mothers with no support system in the home, or in other cases in which ongoing assistance may be desired.

■ REFERENCES

1. Assessment of Fetal Maturity Prior to Repeat Cesarean Delivery or Elective Induction of Labor. ACOG Committee Opinion, 77, 1990
2. Cunningham FG, MacDonald PC, Gant NF: Williams' Obstetrics, 18th ed. Norwalk, CT, Appleton and Lange, 1989
3. Blumenthal PD, Ramanauskas R: Randomized trial of Dilapan and laminaria as cervical ripening agents before induction of labor. Obstet Gynecol 75:365–368, March 1990
4. Oxorn H: Human Labor and Birth. Norwalk, CT, Appleton-Century-Crofts, 1986
5. Lyons AS, Petrucelli RJ: Medicine, An Illustrated History. New York, Abradale Press, 1987
6. Shiono P, Klebanoff MA, Carey JC: Midline episiotomies: More harm than good? Obstet Gynecol 75:765–770, May 1990
7. Kilpatrick SJ, Laros RK: Characteristics of normal labor. Obstet Gynecol 74:85–87, July 1989
8. Neuhoff D, Burke S, Porreco RP: Cesarean birth for failed progress of labor. Obstet Gynecol 73:915–920, June 1989
9. Guidelines for Vaginal Delivery After a Previous Cesarean Birth. ACOG Committee Opinion, 64, 1988
10. Seiler JS: The demise of vaginal operative obstetrics: A suggested plan for its revival. Obstet Gynecol 75:710–712, April 1990
11. Phelan JP, Ahn MO, Diaz F et al: Twice a cesarean, always a cesarean? Obstet Gynecol 73:161–165, February 1989
12. Thorp JA, Parisi VM, Boylan PC et al: The effect of continuous epidural analgesia on cesarean section for dystocia in nulliparous women. Am J Obstet Gynecol 161:670–675, September 1989
13. Goldfarb MG: Who Receives Cesareans: Patient and Hospital Characteristics. National Center for Health Services Research, Hospital Cost and Utilizations Project and Research Note. Rockville, MD, DHHS Publication No (PHS) 84-3345, September 1984
14. Young D: Unnecessary cesareans: Ways to avoid them. Birth Fam J 8(1):47+, Spring 1981
15. Aylsworth J: Vaginal birth after cesarean section: Where do we stand now? OB/GYN Nursing and Patient Counseling 1(1):6–8+, Autumn 1990
16. Chazotte C, Madden R, Cohen WR: Labor patterns in

women with previous cesareans. Obstet Gynecol 75: 353–355, March 1990

17. Harlass FE, Duff F: The duration of labor in primiparas undergoing vaginal birth after cesarean delivery. Obstet Gynecol 75:45–47, January 1990

18. Hangsleben KL, Taylor MA, Lynn NM: VBAC program in a nurse-midwifery service, five years experience. J Nurse Midwifery 34(4):179–184, July/August 1989

19. Flamm BL, Goings JR: Vaginal birth after cesarean section: Is suspected fetal macrosomia a contraindication? Obstet Gynecol 74:694–697, November 1989

20. Affonse DA, Stichler JF: Cesarean birth: Women's reactions. Am J Nurs 80(3):468–470, March 1980

21. McClellan MS, Bavianca WA: Effects of early mother–infant contact following cesarean birth. Obstet Gynecol 56(1):52–55, July 1980

22. Affonso D: "Missing pieces"—a study of postpartum feelings. Birth Fam J 4(4):159–164, Winter 1977

■ SUGGESTED READINGS

Baumann H, Alon E, Atanassoff P et al: Effect of epidural anesthesia for cesarean delivery on maternal femoral arterial and venous, uteroplacental, and umbilical flow velocities and waveforms. Obstet Gynecol 75:194–198, 1990

Blakemore KJ, Quin N, Petrie RH et al: A prospective comparison of hourly and quarter-hourly oxytocin dose increase intervals for the induction of labor at term. Obstet Gynecol 75:757–761, 1990

DeMuylder X, Thiery M: The cesarean delivery rate can be safely reduced in a developing country. Obstet Gynecol 75:360–364, 1990

O'Grady JP: Unexpected problems at cesarean section. Contemporary OB/GYN 35(3):86–100, 1990

Sakala EP, Kaye S, Murray RD et al: Oxytocin use after previous cesarean: Why a higher rate of failed labor trial? Obstet Gynecol 75:356–350, 1990

40

Postpartum Complications

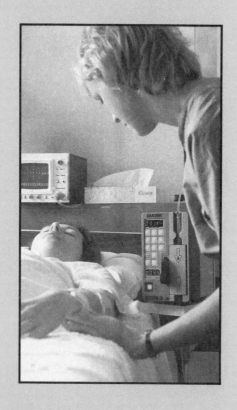

The postpartum period is a time of increased physiological stress, as well as a phase of major psychological transition. During this time, the woman's body is more vulnerable because of the energy depletion and fatigue of late pregnancy and labor, the tissue trauma of delivery, and the blood loss and propensity for anemia that frequently occur. Most women recover from the stresses of pregnancy and childbirth without significant complications. When postpartum complications do occur, the most common are infection involving the genital tract, urinary system, and breasts; hemorrhage, immediate or delayed; embolic and thrombotic disorders; and uterine subinvolution. Postpartum depression is another relatively frequent complication. The potentially critical nature of many postpartum complications; the associated pain, procedures, and medications; the frequent need to be isolated or separated from the infant; and the emotionally disruptive effects of the physiological malfunction can interfere with the maternal–infant bonding process.

■ INFECTIONS OF THE GENITAL TRACT

Postpartum infections of the birth canal usually are the result of bacterial ascension from the genital tract and are known as *puerperal infections.* These conditions often

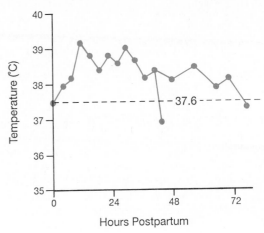

■ *Figure 40-2*
The pattern of fever (>38.4°C) in the first 3 days postpartum after either spontaneous vaginal delivery or cesarean birth. Fever may persist longer in more serious infections.

remain localized but may extend along vascular or lymphatic pathways to produce extensive pelvic infections. Febrile reactions are the principle symptom, and the course of the illness varies according to the size of the bacterial inoculum; the virulence of the organisms; the pelvic tissues affected; and the host defense mechanisms, including general health and immunologic competence. Puerperal infection is one of the most common causes of morbidity in the postpartum period and is a leading cause of death in association with childbearing.

The postpartum woman is assumed to have an infection if she has a temperature elevation of 39°C (102.2°F) at any time, or 38.5°C (101.3°F) on two occasions 4 hours apart after the first 24 hours postdelivery. Low-grade temperature elevations are not uncommon and have been attributed to such factors as dehydration, infusion of fetal protein, breast engorgement, and respiratory infection. When delivery has occurred vaginally, the spontaneous clearance of necrotic decidua and blood from the uterine cavity usually is adequate to remove bacteria. The transient temperature elevation seen in the first 24 hours after delivery represents this process. With cesarean birth, a much higher risk of postpartum infection exists. Figures 40-1 and 40-2 show febrile patterns of transient temperature elevation in the first 24 hours compared with clinically significant postpartum infection.

PATHOPHYSIOLOGY

The most frequent soft-tissue infections following vaginal delivery include endometritis, salpingitis, tuboovarian abscess, pelvic abscess, pelvic cellulitis, and surgical site infection.[1] Postpartal genital tract infections are polymicrobial, involving an average of four anaerobic and two aerobic microorganisms. Most of these

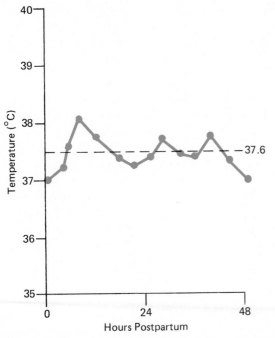

■ *Figure 40-1*
The pattern of resolving postpartum fever (single spike) after spontaneous vaginal delivery.

Research Highlight

Bacterial Vaginosis and Postcesarean Endometritis

Bacterial vaginosis is the most common vaginal infection in pregnant women. It is associated with high concentrations of microorganisms, particularly *Gardnerella vaginalis*, *Bacteroides* species, and *Peptostreptococcus* species. Organisms from these species have been found in 60% of endometrial cultures obtained from women with postpartum endometritis, whereas the prevalence of bacterial vaginosis among postpartum women is 15% to 20%.

This study assessed the influence of bacterial vaginosis and multiple obstetric variables on the development of postpartum endometritis. Vaginal Gram stains were obtained in the hospital before delivery from 462 women who delivered by cesarean; the stains were scored as normal or as indicating bacterial vaginosis. Records of women with cesarean deliveries were reviewed for selected obstetric variables, including maternal age, gestational age, insurance status, indication for cesarean, duration of labor and membrane rupture, prophylactic antibiotics, temperature in first 24 hours postpartum and during hospital stay, and other antibiotic therapy.

Postpartum endometritis was diagnosed in 69 (15%) of the subjects; 8% of these had a normal Gram stain and 31% had stains indicative of bacterial vaginosis. This difference was highly statistically significant. Obstetric variables associated by univariate analysis with postpartum endometritis were maternal age under 30 years, duration of labor longer than 12 hours, any duration of ruptured membranes, more than four vaginal examinations, use of antibiotic prophylaxis, amniotic fluid infection, and bacterial vaginosis. In multivariate analysis, the characteristics related independently to postpartum endometritis were maternal age less than 30, hours of membrane rupture, and bacterial vaginosis.

Women with bacterial vaginosis were six times more likely to develop postpartum endometritis after cesarean delivery than were women with a normal Gram stain. About one third of the women with bacterial vaginosis developed endometritis despite prophylactic antibiotics. Antenatal bacterial vaginosis has been associated with preterm labor and birth and now appears to be an important risk factor in postcesarean endometritis. Bacterial vaginosis, however, is not detected or treated routinely during pregnancy.

Results of this study indicate the need for further examination of treatment regimens for bacterial vaginosis and effects of therapy on preterm birth and postpartum infections. Nurses should be aware that new approaches may be recommended for treating bacterial vaginosis during pregnancy.

Watts JD, Krohn MA, Hillier SL, et al: Bacterial vaginosis as a risk factor for post-cesarean endometritis. Obstet Gynecol 75(1):52–58, January 1990.

microorganisms are part of the normal microflora of the vagina and cervix. A wide range of these indigenous microorganisms may be involved in postpartal genital tract infections; the most common organisms are the aerobic gram-positive cocci (such as *Streptococcus* species) and anaerobic gram-positive bacilli (such as *Bacteroides* species; Table 40-1).[1-3]

Because many of these organisms are part of the complex genital tract flora, the exact pathogenesis of infections is not completely understood. Women generally are more susceptible to infections during the postpartum period, because of soft-tissue trauma during birth, lowered resistance due to fatigue or stress, and blood loss. Tissues particularly susceptible to infection include the placental site; lacerations of the cervix, vagina, and perineum; and surgical incisions, such as an episiotomy or cesarean incision. Lochia provides a good culture medium for bacterial growth and ascension.

A number of factors are associated with increased risk of postpartal genital tract infection. Prolonged labor and prolonged rupture of membranes, with associated greater number of vaginal examinations, are among the most important factors as they increase the size of the bacterial inoculum. Cesarean delivery is probably the single greatest risk factor for developing a postpartal infection. Low socioeconomic status, with related suboptimal prenatal care and nutritional deficiencies, appears to be a key factor in host defense mechanisms (Table 40-2).[3]

Nursing Assessment

Postpartum nursing assessment focuses on identifying infections early, implementing treatment without delay, monitoring progress and physiological functions, noting with the infant, client and family responses to the complication, and relationship with the husband or partner.

TABLE 40-1. MICROORGANISMS COMMONLY INVOLVED IN POSTPARTUM GENITAL TRACT INFECTIONS

Aerobes	Anaerobes
Gram Positive	**Gram Positive**
Streptococcus	Peptostreptococcus
Group B	Peptococcus
Alpha hemolytic (A)	Clostridium
Streptococcus	
Staphylococcus	
Gram Negative	**Gram Negative**
Gardnerella vaginalis	Bacteroides
Escherichia coli	B. bivius
Klebsiella pneumoniae	B. disiens
Proteus mirabilis	B. fragilis
Enterobacter	Fusobacterium

Sexually Transmitted

Chlamydia trachomatis
Neisseria gonorrhoeae
Mycoplasma hominis
Ureaplasma urealyticum

needs for comfort and education, identifying emotional reactions and needs, and monitoring postpartum involution.

The signs and symptoms of each specific infection are noted, as well as vital signs, condition of perineum and uterus, character of lochia, condition of extremities and breasts, and status of bladder and bowel function. The mother's needs for physical comfort are assessed, including rest and sleep, nutrition and hydration, and pain relief. Psychosocial assessment covers relationship

Nursing Diagnosis

The major nursing diagnosis is high risk for injury that involves a maturational process (childbirth) and physiological deficits (decreased resistance, tissue trauma). Pathophysiological contributing factors include tissue hypoxia and trauma, pain, fatigue, and altered immune function. Injury from postpartum infections can lead to delayed healing, abscess formation, and serious sequelae such as septicemia, shock, or death.

Other nursing diagnoses include high risk for infection transmission related to contact with others, equipment-borne exposure, or lack of knowledge of preventing transmission; alterations in comfort related to pain in the infection site, procedures, or treatments; anxiety related to the illness process and its effect on recovery; altered parenting related to impaired mother-infant attachment, as a result of limited contact, pain, or inability to focus attention; and self-concept disturbance related to decreased ability to assume caretaking, discomfort, or altered body image.

Knowledge deficits often occur, related to lack of information about the infectious process and its treatment and the associated implications for caretaking of self and infant. The client may not know how to promote comfort and healing, how to prevent spread of infection or reduce further complications, or how to identify signs of illness progression. She is often concerned about how this will affect the length of hospitalization and her abilities to assume responsibilities at home.

TABLE 40-2. RISK FACTORS FOR DEVELOPING POSTPARTUM INFECTIONS

Related to General Infection Risk	Related to Labor Events	Related to Operative Risk Factors
Anemia	Prolonged labor	Cesarean delivery
Poor nutrition	Prolonged rupture of membranes	General anesthesia
Lack of prenatal care		Urgency of operation
Obesity	Chorioamnionitis	Breaks in operative technique
Low socioeconomic status	Intrauterine fetal monitoring*	
Sexual intercourse after rupture of membranes	Number of examinations during labor*	Manual placental removal
Immunosuppression	Hemorrhage	Forceps delivery
		Episiotomy
		Lacerations

* Related to longer labors and high-risk maternal status.

Nursing Planning and Intervention

Nursing care assures prompt diagnosis and treatment of postpartum infections to minimize serious sequelae and reduce their dysfunctional effects. Medical treatment regimens (antibiotic therapy, wound debridement or cleansing, analgesics) are carried out and their effects monitored (e.g., vital signs, disease progression, symptoms, specimen collection). Comfort measures for pain are provided and nutrition and fluid intake are enhanced to promote healing and well-being.

It is important to encourage maximum mother–infant contact, given the requirements for isolation and prevention of the spread of infection. Newborn infants deprived of close access to their mothers are considered at increased physiological and developmental risk.[4] Attachment can be enhanced by providing information about the infant, discussing the baby's behavior and characteristics, providing pictures of the baby, and supporting visits to the nursery. As soon as the infection allows, the mother can be assisted to hold and care for her infant as much as possible.

Explanations are provided about the infectious process and its expected course and treatment. The partner should be involved in these discussions when possible and helped to understand and provide support for the mother's emotional needs. The nurse also can respond to the mother's or family's needs for emotional support and encouragement and can assist them to work through fears of the consequences or grief about the effects of the infection on the postpartum experience (see the Nursing Care Plan).

PREVENTION OF INFECTION

The prevention of infection is important throughout the maternity cycle. Health teaching is emphasized during pregnancy and postpartally, particularly in regard to diet, rest, exercise, and stress. The client is advised to avoid possible sources of infection, especially upper respiratory tract infections. Anemia is identified and treated with diet and iron supplements.

During labor and delivery, care is exercised to limit opportunity for ascending infection from the genital tract and to reduce exposure to exogenous bacteria. Postpartally, individual care techniques reduce the chance of cross-contamination; each client should have her own equipment. Careful handwashing on the part of all personnel after contacts with each client helps to prevent the transfer of infection from one client to another. Universal precautions for exposure to blood and body fluids are followed in all maternity procedures.

Personnel with an infection of the skin or the respiratory tract should not work in the maternity department. The nasopharynx of personnel is a common exogenous source of contamination, and regular nasopharyngeal cultures of maternity personnel are often required. To be effective, masks worn during delivery and procedures must cover the nose and the mouth and be clean and dry; thus, they must be changed frequently and should not hang around the neck when not in use.

For many days following delivery, the surface of the birth canal is a vulnerable area for pathogenic bacteria. Clients are taught preventive principles of perineal care, with emphasis on not touching the labia or perineal pad with the fingers and not separating the labia as this permits the cleansing solution to enter the vagina (see Chap. 28). Breast-feeding mothers are taught to inspect nipples for redness or cracks after each nursing and to report soreness early. Clients are taught to report signs of genital tract infection promptly to their physician or primary care provider.

Evaluation

A return of temperature to normal marks recovery from a postpartum infection. Vital signs are stable, and appetite has returned. The woman is able to ambulate normally, and she is free of pain in the site of infection. Her uterus and lochia are normal for the stage of involution. She is able to rest and sleep well. She assumes self-care and infant caretaking. Her partner provides support, and she continues breast-feeding if she had been breast-feeding previously.

When alterations in self-concept or parenting, anxiety, and knowledge deficits are present, nursing care is successful when the mother (and partner) has worked through her concerns and negative perspectives, feels assured of normal functioning, has integrated the disappointments of experiencing a complication, is ready to assume self- and infant-care responsibilities, and feels knowledgeable about illness processes, treatment, and recovery.

Infections of the Perineum and Vulva

PATHOPHYSIOLOGY

Localized infections of the perineum and vulva commonly involve a repaired perineal laceration or episiotomy wound. These infections usually are not severe, involve moderate discomfort, and may only minimally affect functioning.

The usual symptoms are elevation of temperature, pain, and a sensation of heat in the affected area. The area involved is red and edematous, the skin edges separate, and there is seropurulent discharge. In some vulval infections, the entire vulva may become edematous, causing the patient considerable pain.

Nursing Care Plan

The Woman With Postpartum Complications

Nursing Goals

1. Client receives prompt diagnosis and treatment of postpartum complications to minimize risk of morbidity, mortality, and dysfunctional effects.
2. Client indicates comfort is increased by physical-care measures and pain-relief therapies.
3. Client and family indicate understanding of the complication and integration of the experience.
4. Separation of mother and infant is minimized and mother-infant relationship is enhanced through information and support.
5. Client and family indicate ability to deal with anxiety, anger, grief, and fear through self-expression and acceptance.

Assessment (For All Complications)	Potential Nursing Diagnosis	Intervention	Evaluation
Physiological Assessment			
Vital signs	High risk for complications such as hemorrhage, urinary tract infection, urinary retention, infection of the genital tract, embolism, subinvolution, vulvar hematoma, mastitis related to abnormal conditions of the puerperium	Record and report signs and symptoms	Mother's vital signs are stabilized
Patterns of temperature elevation		Administer medications and treatments	Mother voids completely
Condition of perineum and uterus		Monitor vital signs	Mother remains symptom free
Character of lochia		Monitor fluids and hydration	
Tenderness and pain		Collect specimens	
Condition of legs	High risk for injury related to physiological deficits		
Condition of breasts			
Status of bladder and voiding			
Physical Comfort			
Rest and sleep	Alteration in comfort: pain related to spread of infection, procedures, incisions, uterine contractions	Provide physical care to promote comfort (e.g., cold–heat therapy, bath, backrub, clean and dry linens, positioning)	Mother rests and sleeps well
Appetite, nutrition, and hydration			
Pain or discomfort		Enhance fluid and food intake (relaxed atmosphere, preferences)	Mother takes adequate fluids and food
		Carry out treatments promptly and efficiently (e.g., sitz baths, medications, dressings)	Mother reports relief of pain and discomfort
Psychosocial Assessment			
Relation to infant	Knowledge deficit related to cause, progress, and care of complication	Encourage maximum mother–infant contact, provide continuous information on infant	Mother assumes as much caretaking of infant as condition permits
Response to complication			
Response of partner			

(continued)

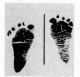

Nursing Care Plan (continued)

Assessment (For All Complications)	Potential Nursing Diagnosis	Intervention	Evaluation
	Alteration in parenting related to physical or emotional effects of complication	Explain and discuss complication, expected course and treatment	Mother maintains interest in infant
		Involve partner in education about complication, relating to infant, understanding mother's emotional needs, providing support	Mother understands treatment and expected course of complication
			Partner understands above and provides support
		Respond to needs for support and encouragement, working through grief and fear	Mother expresses grief and fear
Genital Tract Infection			
Fundal size, consistency, tenderness; lochia odor, character; temperature condition of perineum, wound, legs	Alteration in comfort: pain related to progress of infection	Obtain specimens, report findings, administer antibiotics/medications, note response, isolate as needed, monitor	Mother is pain free
	Knowledge deficit of self-care related to particular infection		Mother performs self-care and infant care
Hemorrhage			
Fundal size, consistency, tenderness; amount of lochia, clots, character; pulse and blood pressure; blood loss	High risk for injury: complications of hemorrhage (tissue damage, cerebral anoxia, death)	Massage uterus, facilitate voiding, report blood loss, prepare for IVs and transfusion, monitor for shock, administer medications and oxygen, keep family informed	Mother returns to stable condition
	Fluid-volume deficit altered tissue perfusion		Mother and family understand events and treatment
Pulmonary Embolism			
Respiratory distress and pain, hypotension, cyanosis, hemoptysis	High risk for injury: complications of pulmonary embolism (cerebral anoxia, death)	Evaluate respiratory status, report signs and symptoms and frequent vital signs, administer medications and oxygen, note response to treatment, obtain specimens, institute emergency cardiopulmonary resuscitation/therapy if needed	Mother breathes normally
			Mother returns to symptom-free condition
			Mother's vital signs and cardiopulmonary condition stabilize
Mastitis			
Temperature and pulse; swelling, pain, redness of	Alteration in comfort: pain related to infection	Obtain specimens for milk culture, report findings,	Mother's vital signs are stable

(continued)

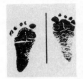

Nursing Care Plan *(continued)*

Assessment (For All Complications)	Potential Nursing Diagnosis	Intervention	Evaluation
breasts; nipple soreness, fissures; axillary nodes, tenderness	Knowledge deficit related to care of breasts Self-concept disturbance related to inability to nurse	assist at procedures (incision and drainage), change dressings, administer antibiotics/medicines, provide ice packs or hot compresses and comfort measures (support brassiere), monitor vital signs and progress of healing	Mother returns to symptom-free condition Mother continues nursing
Urinary Retention/Infections			
Frequency and amount of voiding, dysuria, hematuria, suprapubic or flank pain, temperature and pulse, height and consistency of uterine fundus	High risk for injury: complications of urinary retention, cystitis, pyelonephritis related to trauma or decreased tonus Alteration in comfort: pain related to infection	Obtain specimens, report findings, administer antibiotics/medications, insert intermittent or indwelling catheter as needed, note response to treatment, isolate as needed, monitor signs/symptoms	Mother voids normally Mother is pain free Mother's vital signs are stabilized
Thrombophlebitis			
Pain, swelling, stiffness in leg and calf, temperature, chills	Alteration in comfort: pain High risk for injury from embolism	Rest, elevate leg, analgesics, antibiotics, anticoagulents, bed cradle, heat–cold therapy, careful handling of leg, support and teaching	Mother is comfortable Signs of thrombophlebitis improve or resolve Mother able to provide self- and infant care
Postpartum Depression			
Mood, affect Interaction with spouse or partner Interaction with visitors and friends Relating to baby Caretaking of baby Feelings expressed Sleep disturbances	Ineffective individual coping related to depression Impaired social interactions	Assist expression of feelings, provide acceptance, support emotionally, help with problem solving, teach relaxation, encourage support network, refer for self-help or support groups, mental health or psychotherapy	Mother expresses feelings Identifies coping patterns, strengths Seeks and accept help from others, uses resources Mood becomes positive Mother able to provide self- and infant care Seeks therapy when needed

NURSING PLANNING AND INTERVENTION

These localized infections seldom cause severe problems, provided that good drainage is established and the patient's temperature remains below 38.4°C (101°F). To promote good drainage, the sutures are removed and the wound opened. Because the drainage is a source of contamination, precautions are taken against spread of infection. The wound must be kept clean and the perineal pads changed frequently. Sitz baths provide both pain relief and promotion of drainage. The perineal heat lamp also provides pain relief. Antibiotics are prescribed, which the nurse administers according to schedule.

The nurse evaluates the progression of wound healing, noting characteristics of drainage and condition of the wound site. The presence of fever, malaise, and decreased appetite is recorded. Additional fluid intake is promoted to 2000 ml/day. The client is instructed in proper perineal care and pad hygiene and prevention of infection transferral. She is encouraged to care for and feed her infant, and she is reassured that the risk of infection to the infant is minimal when preventive techniques are followed.

Endometritis

PATHOPHYSIOLOGY

Endometritis is a localized infection of the inner uterine wall. It frequently begins at the placental site and may spread to involve the entire endometrium (Fig. 40-3). Following vaginal delivery, about 2% to 3% of women develop endometritis. The most important risk factors include prolonged labor and ruptured membranes, which lead to increased colonization of the lower uterine segment due to numerous vaginal examinations. Amniotic fluid infection develops in about one third of women when membranes are ruptured greater than 6 hours before birth. Although internal fetal monitoring has been associated with development of endometritis, this is probably related to longer labors, prolonged ruptured membranes, and high-risk status of the women rather than the monitoring itself.[3]

When endometritis develops, it is usually manifest about 48 to 72 hours after delivery. In the milder forms, the patient may have no complaints or symptoms other than a rise in temperature above 38°C (100.4°F), which persists for several days and then subsides. More typically, infections are accompanied by lower abdominal pain, uterine tenderness, foul-smelling discharge, higher fever, tachycardia, and leukocytosis (Fig. 40-4). The patient often experiences chills, malaise, loss of appetite, headache, and backache. There may be severe and prolonged afterpains. The uterus is usually large (subinvolution) and extremely tender when palpated abdominally. The lochial discharge may be decreased in amount with red-brown appearance and foul odor. Infections caused by hemolytic streptococcus usually have odorless lochia.

NURSING PLANNING AND INTERVENTION

Medical treatment for endometritis is with parenteral antibiotics, using broad-spectrum coverage with second- and third-generation cephalosporins or semisynthetic penicillins (Table 40-3). A trend toward use of single-agent therapy rather than combination therapy has emerged, with the advantages of less toxicity and greater

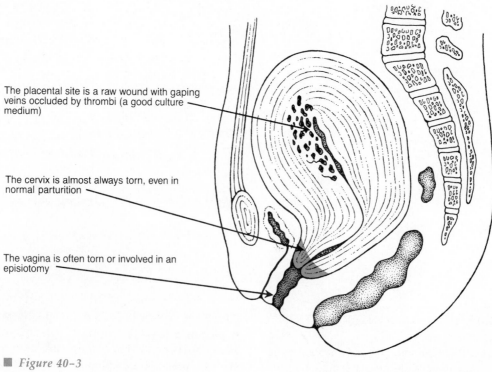

The placental site is a raw wound with gaping veins occluded by thrombi (a good culture medium)

The cervix is almost always torn, even in normal parturition

The vagina is often torn or involved in an episiotomy

■ *Figure 40-3*
Sites of common postpartum infection.

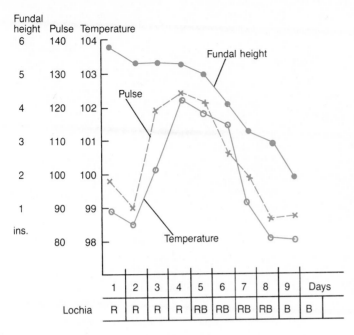

■ *Figure 40–4*
Febrile pattern in endometritis. The four classic signs of postpartum endometritis are temperature elevation to 101°F (38.4°C), increase in pulse rate (100–120), delayed involution with fundal height not decreasing, and lochia remaining red with foul odor. (R, red; B, brown)

effectiveness in administration of medications. Treatment with antibiotics is continued for 24 to 36 hours after the patient's temperature has returned to normal. At this time, she may be discharged home; continued oral antibiotics are generally unnecessary.[5] The nurse administers antibiotics as scheduled and observes for allergic reactions.

The nurse encourages the patient to assume the Fowler's position, as this facilitates lochial drainage. Oxytocic medications may be ordered (ergonovine or methylergonovine) to promote uterine contractions and aid lochial flow. The nurse monitors the progress of involution, including fundal height and firmness, tenderness, and the amount and characteristics of lochia. Fluids are increased to 3000 to 4000 ml/day, and nutritious meals are encouraged. Temperature, pulse, and blood pressure are taken every 4 hours. Isolation may be needed to prevent exposure of other patients and to afford the mother greater rest. It is unnecessary to discontinue breast-feeding, unless the infection is severe.

Nursing care includes emotional support; client teaching; and family interventions to assist with integrating the experience, working through feelings, and learning about the infection and its treatment. Assistance is provided with self-care and infant care, and any modifications needed are identified.

With prompt antibiotic treatment, the infection often is resolved and the client discharged after 3 to 4 days. The nurse provides discharge teaching, which includes drinking 8 to 10 glasses of water daily, eating a diet high in proteins and vitamins, monitoring for signs of infection, and keeping her follow-up appointment.

TABLE 40–3. ANTIMICROBIAL REGIMENS FOR TREATMENT OF GENITAL TRACT INFECTIONS

Combination Regimens	Single-Agent Regimens
Clindamycin and aminoglycoside	Cephalosporins and cephamycins
	Cefoxitin
Metronidazole and aminoglycoside	Cefotetan
	Cefmetazole
	Ceftizoxime
Clindamycin and aztreonam	Cefotaxime
	Moxalactam
Clindamycin and gentamicin	Extended-spectrum penicillins
	Mezlocillin
	Piperacillin
	Carbapenems
	Imipenem
	Beta-lactams and enzyme blocker
	Ampicillin-sulbactam
	Ticarcillin-clavulanic acid

Pelvic Cellulitis and Peritonitis

PATHOPHYSIOLOGY

Pelvic cellulitis (parametritis) is an infection that extends along the blood vessels and lymphatics to the loose connective tissue of the broad ligament or other pelvic structures. The source of infection may be cervical lacerations or endometritis. Ascending organisms from the vaginal microflora are the most common pathogens; the infection usually is polymicrobial. Pelvic cellulitis usually is unilateral but may involve both broad ligaments.

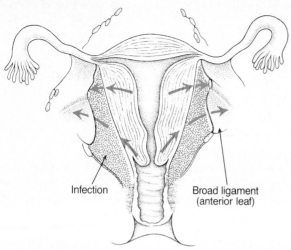

■ *Figure 40–5*

Parametritis or pelvic cellulitis. Infection may spread from the uterus, a cervical laceration, or thrombophlebitis into the loose connective tissue. It may extend retroperitoneally in any direction, commonly between leaves of the broad ligament, and around the vagina or rectum. Pelvic examination reveals a large, hard mass representing a pelvic abscess in some instances.

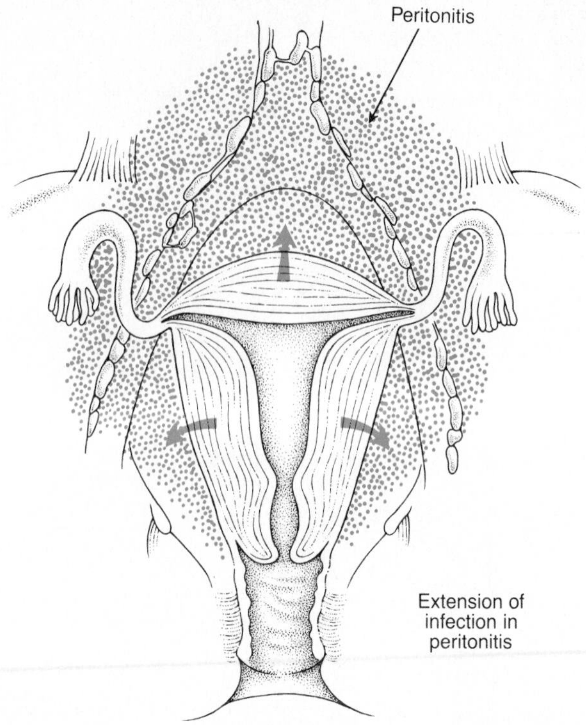

The patient has persistent fever that may reach 39.5° to 40°C (103–104°F) with chills, malaise, and lethargy. The uterus is boggy and tender, limited in mobility, and may be displaced to one side. There is marked abdominal pain on palpation. The pulse is elevated, and the white blood count may reach 30,000/mm³ or more. An abscess may develop in the center of the area of cellulitis, which may extend downward into the posterior cul-de-sac or upward to the inguinal ligament. Signs of pelvic infection become more pronounced with development of an abscess (Figs. 40-5 and 40-6).

Peritonitis almost always accompanies pelvic cellulitis, involving the peritoneum to varying degrees. In

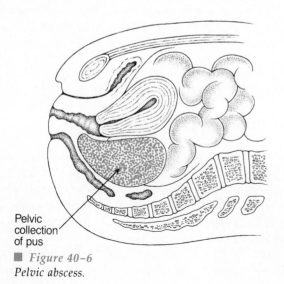

■ *Figure 40–6*
Pelvic abscess.

■ *Figure 40–7*

Postpartum peritonitis. The pelvic peritoneum may become involved in an infection in the same ways as the parametrium. Generalized peritonitis may occur with development of paralytic ileus. Although uncommon, peritonitis can be severe and life threatening.

mild peritonitis, the peritoneal covering of the broad ligaments may be the only area involved; in severe cases, there is widespread, generalized infection (Fig. 40-7). The patient appears profoundly ill with a high fever and rapid pulse. She is usually restless, anxious, and sleepless and has constant and severe abdominal pain. Hiccups, nausea and vomiting, abdominal distention, and excessive thirst often are present. Phlebitis in the pelvic and ovarian veins occurs with nearly all serious puerperal infections, producing bacteremia. This does not appear to adversely affect outcomes.[6]

NURSING PLANNING AND INTERVENTION

Aerobic cultures from the lochia are obtained for specific sensitivities; it is very difficult to obtain reliable anaerobic cultures uncontaminated by vaginal flora. Blood cultures may provide useful information, especially in patients who do not respond to standard therapy or who develop an abscess or peritonitis. The nurse assists with collection of culture specimens.

Antimicrobial therapy is prescribed with broad-spectrum, single or combination agents with activity against the principal aerobic and anaerobic bacteria that infect the upper genital tract (see Table 40-3). It is especially important that the antibiotic be effective against *Bacteroides* and *Enterobacter* species, which commonly cause peritonitis, abscess formation, and sepsis.[2] Analgesic drugs are prescribed for discomfort, and mild sedative drugs are given to relieve the client's restlessness and apprehension. If there is intestinal involvement, oral feedings are withheld until normal intestinal function is restored. The nurse administers and monitors intravenous fluids and antibiotic therapy. Intake and output and physiological signs are measured and recorded frequently.

These significant infectious complications affect the mother's ability to function, her level of awareness, and her energy. Parenting is usually disrupted during the acute course of the infection, and self-concept and coping may be adversely affected. The nurse intervenes in these problems with emotional support, client teaching, and family counseling.

Salpingitis

PATHOPHYSIOLOGY

Salpingitis, an infection of the fallopian tubes, may occur following childbirth. Bacteria may ascend from the uterine cavity or by venous spread to cause salpingitis. Symptoms often resemble peritonitis and include high fever, rapid pulse, nausea and vomiting, and abdominal pain and rigidity. Although usually bilateral, unilateral salpingitis may occur and mimic appendicitis when it occurs on the right side. The fallopian tubes become hyperemic and edematous, and purulent discharge often fills the tubal lumina. Tubal abscesses may occur, causing tender adnexal masses (Fig. 40-8). Laparoscopy may be necessary to establish the correct diagnosis. Salpingitis usually is a multibacterial infection, involving many

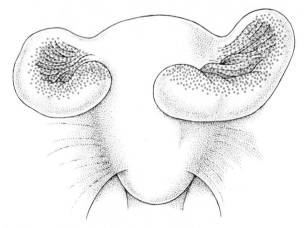

■ *Figure 40–8*
Postpartum salpingitis. Infection of the fallopian tubes leads to hyperemia, edema, and purulent discharge into the tubal lumina. The tubes are enlarged, swollen, and tender. Tubal abscesses may occur, creating tender adnexal masses.

gram-positive and gram-negative aerobes and anaerobes, in addition to *Neisseria gonorrhoeae*. Cervical cultures are taken to detect *N. gonorrhoeae*. Problems with tubal patency and subsequent infertility are frequent sequelae of salpingitis.

NURSING PLANNING AND INTERVENTION

Treatment is with broad-spectrum antibiotics, analgesics, and sedatives, as discussed above. The nurse administers medications and monitors effects, provides comfort measures, and records vital signs and physiological observations regularly. Intravenous fluids may be administered, with intake and output monitored and recorded. Depending on the severity of the infection, maternal functioning may be affected and problems with parenting and self-concept can develop. Nursing intervention for these diagnoses has been discussed above.

Infection Following Cesarean Delivery

PATHOPHYSIOLOGY

The incidence of genital tract infection is significantly increased with cesarean delivery, with endometritis occurring in 10% to 20% of patients despite the use of prophylactic antibiotics.[7] The incidence of genital tract infections after cesarean delivery is much greater in high-risk populations. Infections are consistently related to prolonged labor, prolonged ruptured membranes, and a large number of vaginal examinations.[3] Operative trauma increases the risk of infection, which is caused by mixed anaerobic and aerobic organisms indigenous to the genital tract. Bacterial vaginosis, a common vaginal infection in pregnant women associated with high concentrations of *Bacteroides*, *Peptostreptococcus*, and *Gardnerella vaginalis* organisms, is an important risk factor for postcesarean endometritis. Women with bacterial vaginosis were found to be six times more likely to develop endometritis after cesarean delivery, especially when associated with prolonged ruptured membranes and maternal age less than 20 years.[8]

Operative trauma, with tissue ischemia and collection of blood and serum in the wound, myometrium, or endometrium, plays an important role in the development of postpartum endomyometritis, pelvic abscesses, and incisional wound infections and abscesses. The incidence of wound infection following cesarean delivery is between 6% and 11%. Risk factors for development of wound infections include obesity, diabetes, number of vaginal examinations, length of labor, emergency cesarean, and duration of operation. The organisms causing wound infections are indigenous and commonly include aerobic and anaerobic gram-positive cocci, predominately *Streptococcus*, *G. vaginalis*, *Staphylococcus epidermidis*, *Bacteroides*, *Escherichia coli*, and, rarely, *Clostridium*.

The initial signs of wound infection usually begin 36 to 48 hours after surgery, with temperature elevation, pain, induration, and erythema of the incision. Areas of fluctuance often develop and may form into abscesses. Anaerobic infections are characterized by foul odor, the presence of gas in the tissue (crepitus), and necrosis of the wound area.

NURSING PLANNING AND INTERVENTION

Each client is evaluated individually for antibiotic prophylaxis when cesarean delivery is done. Risk of postcesarean infection is increased with prolonged labor, membranes ruptured 6 to 12 hours before surgery, internal fetal monitoring, obesity, anemia, and low socioeconomic status. A 1-day, three-dose regimen or a single perioperative dose of cephamycins have been found effective in providing prophylaxis.[2,9]

Treatment is by broad-spectrum antimicrobial therapy (see Table 40-3), drainage of abscesses, and extirpation of crepitant and necrotic tissue. The wound may be packed several times daily to keep it open and draining. Intravenous fluids are usually administered. The nurse initiates intravenous infusions; administers antibiotics; performs dressing changes; and monitors physiological signs, including wound characteristics and drainage, vital signs, and involution progress.

Women undergoing cesarean birth may experience problems with self-esteem, self-concept, altered parenting, anxiety, fear, altered comfort, and altered family processes. They often must grieve the deviations in the childbearing experience caused by a cesarean birth and may feel inadequate as mothers or women. The additional pain, functional limitations, and separation from the infant may affect mother-infant bonding and development of caretaking skills. Nursing intervention provides an opportunity to express and explore feelings, relieve the birth experience, and grieve the loss of a vaginal birth. Emotional support, comfort measures, assistance with infant caretaking, client teaching, and family counseling may be included in nursing care.

■ OTHER INFECTIONS

Mastitis

PATHOPHYSIOLOGY

Mastitis in the postpartum period is an acute infection of the glandular tissue of the breast and occurs mostly in breast-feeding mothers. The microorganism most frequently involved in mastitis is *Staphylococcus aureus*; occasionally it is caused by hemolytic streptococcus. The infection is usually preceded by fissures or erosions of the nipple or areola, which provide a site of entry to the subcutaneous lymphatics. Occasionally, plugged lactiferous ducts are involved in providing an opportunity for growth of microorganisms. The infant may be a source of infection, having acquired the pathogen orally from the mother's skin or in the nasopharynx from a health care provider in the nursery. The patient's hands can be a source of infection, particularly when mastitis is caused by other organisms. On occasion, epidemics of mastitis occur when organisms are transmitted by nursery personnel to many infants and by infants to mothers. Any hospital personnel having direct physical contact with infant or mother can be a source of infectious organisms.

Puerperal mastitis may occur any time during lactation. The woman usually reports a tender area in one breast that is warm, firm, and red. Engorgement of the breast may precede mastitis, although engorgement does not cause the infection. The patient experiences pain in the affected area of the breast and may have malaise, chills, and elevated temperature. The inflammation may be generalized or confined to a lobe or local area of the breast, with induration, tenderness, and erythema. Red streaks may occur along lymphatic channels, and tender, enlarged axillary nodes may be present. Mastitis is usually unilateral. Without effective treatment, local abscesses may form (Fig. 40-9).

NURSING PLANNING AND INTERVENTION

Early identification of mastitis is important to prevent complications and minimize its impact on breast-feeding. Many breast infections are caused by penicillin-resistant staphylococci; antibiotic treatment is with oxacillin or cloxacillin, cephalosporins, or vancomycin, depending on microorganism sensitivity. Cultures or gram stains may be taken of breast milk to identify the causative organism. If areas of fluctuation or abscesses develop, these must be incised and drained. The nurse administers antibiotics and applies dressings following incision and drainage. With effective antibiotic therapy, the infection can often be controlled within 24 hours.

Treatment usually includes discontinuing nursing from the affected breast and application of cold–heat therapy to the breast. There are varying opinions about discontinuing breast-feeding; this often is recommended when the client's fever is high. Breast support is provided with a firm brassiere or binder. The mother may express milk from the affected breast every few hours when pain has decreased to maintain lactation.

Mastitis usually is preventable by avoiding nipple fissures, and prompt treatment is required if these de-

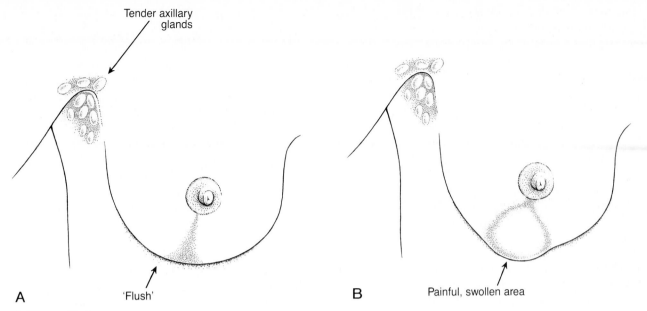

Tender axillary
glands

A

'Flush'

B

Painful, swollen area

■ *Figure 40–9*
*Mastitis. (A) Early mastitis. Fever is followed by a painful area on the breast and a "flush" that
is red and tender but not fluctuant or swollen. (B) Overt inflammation in mastitis. A swollen,
painful, red-to-brawny area develops. The purulent drainage gradually localizes into an
abscess; when fluctuant, it must be incised and drained.*

velop. Sore, tender nipples reported by the mother
should be inspected immediately. There may be a very
small break in the skin surface or a slight erosion. These
can be treated with lanolin cream and use of a nipple
shield. Once a break in the skin occurs, the chances of
infection are greatly increased.

The mother may have knowledge deficits related to
care of the breasts that the nurse helps resolve through
client teaching (see Chaps. 28 and 32). Other problems
may involve pain related to spread of infection; alteration in parenting related to the mother's inability to
continue breast-feeding; and anxiety related to infection
and its effects on breast-feeding. The nurse provides
emotional support, client teaching, family counseling,
and comfort measures. If breast-feeding is continued,
it should be resumed as soon as the temperature is normal and the signs of infection (pain, redness, edema)
have decreased. If a decision has been made to discontinue breast-feeding, assessment should be made of the
woman's acceptance of this and adjustment to formula
feeding and alterations in role and self-concept.

Urinary Tract Infections

PATHOPHYSIOLOGY

The physiological urinary stasis, dilatation of the ureters,
and vesicoureteral reflux that occur during pregnancy
persist for several months after delivery. Postpartum

urinary retention and incomplete emptying of the bladder are common because of increased bladder capacity,
decreased tone, and decreased perception of the urge
to void caused by perineal trauma. If the patient is unable to empty the bladder fully, the remaining urine
serves as a culture medium for bacterial growth, often
leading to cystitis or pyelonephritis. Urinary tract infections occur in about 5% of postpartum patients and
are usually caused by coliform bacteria (*E. coli*, entero-
cocci, *Klebsiella pneumoniae*).

Factors that increase the risk of urinary tract infection include cesarean birth, use of forceps or vacuum
extraction, epidural anesthesia, and catheterization
during labor. Only about 20% of women with bacteriuria have symptoms of lower urinary tract infection such
as dysuria, urgency, and suprapubic pain.[10] Because of
postpartum diuresis, it is common for women to void
large amounts of urine (500–1000 ml) frequently during
the first few days after delivery. Voiding less than 300
ml indicates urinary retention.

Cystitis. Symptoms of cystitis include burning or pain
on urination, urgency, frequency, suprapubic tenderness, and, occasionally, low-grade fever. Urinalysis
shows leukocytosis, red blood cells, and bacteria; urine
culture is positive with over 100,000 colonies per milliliter in a catheterized or clean-catch specimen.

Pyelonephritis. Symptoms of pyelonephritis include,
in addition to dysuria, urgency and frequency; temper-

ature elevation to 40° to 41°C (104–106°F), with spikes then drops and chills; flank pain; lower abdominal pain; and costovertebral angle tenderness. A markedly elevated white blood count (20,000–30,000/mm³) is often present. Urinalysis results are similar to those of cystitis.

NURSING PLANNING AND INTERVENTION

The patient should void within 6 hours after delivery (see Chap. 28). If she has not voided within 8 hours, depending on the degree of bladder distention, catheterization is necessary. When the mother voids small amounts (less than 300 ml) at frequent intervals, an overflow of residual urine is indicated, especially when there is some bladder fullness and suprapubic discomfort. The treatment is usually catheterization after each voiding until the residual urine becomes less than 30 ml, or an indwelling catheter may be indicated. Catheterization for residual urine, to be completely accurate, must be done within 5 minutes after the patient voids. If 60 ml or more of urine still remains in the bladder, voiding is considered incomplete.

When symptoms of cystitis or pyelonephritis are present, nursing care includes collecting urine specimens, either by clean-catch midstream voiding or catheterization. The technique for catheterization is discussed in Chapter 28. Because catheterization increases the risk of infection, a clean-catch midstream voided specimen often is preferred (see Nursing Guidelines: Clean-Catch Midstream Voided Specimen). This method often yields good results in obtaining uncontaminated specimens, if done carefully under the continued supervision of the nurse.

Postpartum screening for bacteriuria is routinely performed in many facilities, with the diagnosis made by cultures of voided midstream urine specimens. Diagnosis of urinary tract infection is confirmed by urine culture. Sensitivity studies are usually performed to identify the appropriate antibiotic for the causative organism. Commonly used antibiotics include amoxicillin or ampicillin; for penicillin allergy or resistant bacteria, cephalexin or sulfamethoxazole/nitrofurantoin are used. Medication is usually administered orally, except in acute febrile pyelonephritis, in which intravenous antibiotics are often used. Symptoms are usually relieved within 24 to 48 hours, and treatment is continued for 10 days to 2 weeks. Repeat urine cultures are performed following the course of therapy to be certain the urine is free of organisms.

When indwelling catheters are necessary because of inability to void and persistent residual urine, patients with catheters in place for longer than 4 days have a significantly higher incidence of bacteriuria. Almost all such infections are caused by *E. coli*. Patients with indwelling catheters for longer than 24 hours usually are treated with prophylactic antibiotic therapy.

> ### Nursing Guidelines: Clean-Catch Midstream Voided Specimen
>
> #### Steps in Collecting Urine Specimen:
>
> The patient is instructed not to void for 1–2 hours before the specimen will be collected.
>
> Moderate fluid intake is encouraged.
>
> When ambulatory, the patient is instructed to collect the specimen in the bathroom.
>
> Using sterile wipes, the vulva and introitus are carefully cleansed, or perineal care may be done.
>
> A large sterile cotton ball is placed over the introitus to absorb lochial flow.
>
> If not ambulatory, the patient is placed in a sitting position on a bedpan, and the nurse provides perineal care and cleansing of the vulva and introitus, placing a sterile cotton ball over the introitus.
>
> The woman is instructed to void a little urine into the toilet or bedpan but not to empty her bladder yet.
>
> After the stream of urine has been established, a sterile urine specimen bottle or sterile basin is placed under the urine stream and a specimen is collected.
>
> The specimen is labeled and sent to the laboratory for examination and culture.

The necessity of treating asymptomatic bacteriuria in nonpregnant women is controversial; among postpartum women, about 30% have persistent asymptomatic bacteriuria, which may predispose them to pyelonephritis because physiological changes that occurred during pregnancy have not yet resolved. Asymptomatic postpartum women with positive midstream-voided urine specimens should have repeat examinations. With confirmed bacteriuria, a 3-day course of antibiotic therapy should be sufficient to clear the urine of bacteria.[10]

■ HEMORRHAGIC AND THROMBOEMBOLIC COMPLICATIONS

PATHOPHYSIOLOGY

After delivery, the woman's cardiovascular system undergoes substantial changes, with reductions in cardiac output and blood volume after the first 48 hours. Most of the cardiac changes to prepregnant conditions have occurred by 2 weeks after delivery. The increase in coagulation factors typical of pregnancy continues postpartally, with several clotting factors activated extensively following delivery then returning to prepregnant levels in a few days. Fibrinogen and thromboplastin remain elevated for 3 weeks after delivery (see Chap. 26).

Postpartum women are at increased risk for hemorrhage and thromboembolic problems. Postpartum hemorrhage complicates about 5% to 10% of vaginal deliveries and is a leading cause of maternal mortality.[11] Immediate postpartum hemorrhage occurs with blood loss of more than 500 ml during the first 24 hours after delivery. It is most commonly the result of uterine atony, caused by overdistention during pregnancy or factors complicating labor and delivery (see Chap. 38). Hemorrhage may be delayed, occurring more than 24 hours after delivery and resulting from retention of placental fragments or abnormal involution. Late hemorrhage occurs most frequently between the 5th and 15th postpartal day and can occur as long as 6 weeks after delivery. Retained placental fragments are the most common cause of late hemorrhage.

Thromboembolic problems develop in about 1% of postpartum women. Venous thrombosis is the formation of a blood clot attached to the wall of a superficial or deep vein, usually in the legs or pelvis. When inflammation of the vessel wall accompanies thrombosis, the condition is called *thrombophlebitis*. There is a risk that the thrombus (clot) will break off from the vessel wall, causing an embolus. The embolus travels through the vessels until it becomes trapped in small capillaries; most frequently there are problems with pulmonary embolism in the postpartal period.

Nursing Assessment

The nurse uses data from the postpartal woman's history and physical examination to identify increased risk for hemorrhage (see Assessment Tool: Risk for Delayed or Late Postpartum Hemorrhage). Women at increased risk are observed carefully during the postpartal period. Regular observations of the condition of the fundus, the amount of bleeding, and lochial flow enable the nurse to identify hemorrhage early. Hemorrhage may be signaled by a sudden, profuse outpouring of blood from the vagina, or a very large pool of blood may be found under the mother's hips. Often hemorrhage is steady, heavier-than-usual vaginal bleeding that continues for hours. It may not be immediately recognized as hemorrhage, especially if the fundus is well contracted. As blood loss increases, signs and symptoms of hypovolemic shock become more pronounced. How rapidly these develop depends on blood volume before and during pregnancy, the amount of blood volume and hemoglobin lost during hemorrhage, and the woman's general resilience and health (see Assessment Tool: Assessing Extent of Hemorrhage).

Because of compensatory cardiovascular mechanisms, changes in pulse rate and blood pressure may not occur until a large amount of blood has been lost

Assessment Tool

Risk for Delayed/Late Postpartum Hemorrhage

Prior History

High parity (grand multipara)

Prior postpartum hemorrhage

Uterine fibroids

Systemic diseases (leukemia, idiopathic thrombocytopenia, coagulation defects)

Related to Present Pregnancy and Labor

Overdistention of the uterus (multiple pregnancy, polyhydramnios, macrosomic infant)

Bleeding problems (placenta previa, abruptio)

Labor/delivery trauma (midforceps, cesearean delivery, intrauterine manipulation)

Hypertonic–hypotonic contractions (precipitate, dysfunctional, prolonged labor)

Deep anesthesia

Pregnancy-induced hypertension

Chorioamnionitis

Subinvolution

Assessment Tool

Assessing Extent of Hemorrhage

Blood Volume Loss	Signs and Symptoms
15% to 20% reduction (750 to 1250 ml)	Uterus boggy Blood pressure normal or slightly decreased Pulse rate normal or slightly elevated Mild vasoconstriction (cool hands, feet) Normal urinary output Aware, alert, oriented, may have anxiety
25% to 35% reduction (1250 to 1750 ml)	Atonic uterus Systolic blood pressure < 90 to 100 mm Hg Moderate tachycardia 100 to 120 beats/min Moderate vasoconstriction (skin pallor, cold, moist extremities) Decreased urinary output (oliguria) Increased restlessness, may become disoriented
35% to 50% reduction (1800 to 2500 ml)	Atonic uterus Systolic blood pressure < 60 mm Hg, may be unobtainable by cuff Severe tachycardia > 120 beats/min Pronounced vasoconstriction (extreme pallor, cold, clammy, cyanotic lips and fingers) Urinary output ceases (anuria) Mental stupor, lethargy, semicomatose

(up to 1500 ml). Cardiac output remains adequate until about 15% to 20% of the woman's total blood volume has been lost. After this, pulse and blood pressure can change suddenly, as cardiac output and stroke volume decrease. By the time that significant tachycardia (100–120 beats per minute) and hypotension occur (<90–100 mm Hg systolic), the woman has lost about 25% to 35% of her blood volume.

The nurse monitors the pulse rate and blood pressure every 5 to 10 minutes when hemorrhage is suspected. Because these signs may not change in early hypovolemic shock while the client is supine, the nurse can have the client sit up. This may produce dizziness, hypotension, and tachycardia, indicating substantial blood loss and shock. Women with pregnancy-induced hypertension (PIH) may appear to have normal blood pressure in early hypovolemic shock. However, these women develop symptoms of shock earlier than nor-

motensive women because PIH causes an interstitial fluid shift that rapidly produces hypovolemia.

The presence of clots in vaginal blood indicates heavy bleeding or pooling of blood in the vagina. Restlessness, anxiety, and thirst can also indicate excessive bleeding.

Nursing Diagnosis

Women experiencing postpartum hemorrhage will have fluid-volume deficit related to excessive blood loss, which may be the result of uterine atony, retained placental fragments, or cervical-vaginal lacerations. They will have decreased cardiac output related to hypovolemia, which is caused by excessive blood loss. The potential complication of hypovolemic shock is a collaborative problem with medicine. Another collaborative problem is altered tissue perfusion (particularly cerebral, cardiopulmonary, and renal) related to hypovolemic shock, with potential complications that could include brain and kidney damage, cardiac arrest, and death. The woman often experiences fear related to the threat of disability or death. She may have alteration in comfort: pain related to uterine contractions caused by oxytocic medications, fundal massage, or other procedures. Knowledge deficits usually are present related to the course and extent of hemorrhage, the treatments and procedures used, the seriousness of the threat, and the expected course of recovery. Anxiety often occurs related to the need for blood transfusions, which place the woman at risk for human immunodeficiency virus and hepatitis exposure, separation from the infant, and long-term impact on caretaking and self-care activities.

Nursing Planning and Intervention

Postpartum hemorrhage and shock are treated with immediate intravenous fluid administration to replace circulatory volume and to serve as a quick route for intravenous medications, particularly oxytocins to contract the uterus. The nurse initiates or assists beginning the intravenous fluids and anticipates medication orders. Oxygen may be administered in severe emergencies when a large blood volume has been lost. The client is often placed in Trendelenburg position to increase venous blood return to the heart and maximize cardiac output.

The nurse monitors vital signs every 5 to 10 minutes and observes the client's color, capillary refill, skin temperature, and sensorium. The fundus is palpated for firmness and massaged frequently to restore tone when indicated. The amount of vaginal bleeding is evaluated, noting the extent of perineal pad saturation in a given time period, color and consistency of bleeding, clots, and pooling blood on the underpad.

Intravenous or intramuscular medications are administered as ordered, and their effects are monitored. Blood transfusions are administered adequate to replace blood loss. If bleeding is not controlled, surgery is necessary to determine and halt the source of bleeding. Usually a curettage is the first procedure, in which retained placental fragments are removed. Severe, uncontrolled bleeding from a uterine source may require a hysterectomy to save the woman's life. The nurse assists with preparations for these surgical procedures.

The nurse needs a calm, reassuring manner in caring for clients experiencing hemorrhage. The family or partner should be encouraged to remain with the client to the extent possible. Nursing care includes responding to the woman and family's needs for information to alleviate knowledge deficits and support and reassurance to minimize fear and anxiety. The nurse explains the physiological process of hemorrhage and interprets medical treatments and procedures. Fears and anxiety are acknowledged, and reassurance is given that all necessary measures are being taken. Once hemorrhage is controlled, the nurse assists the women and family to understand what happened and why; to anticipate what impact this complication will have on postpartal course, caretaking, and self-care activities; and to plan for special needs at home. Complications that may occur as an aftermath of hemorrhage, such as infection or persistent weakness, are discussed. The normal progression of lochia is reviewed, and the need to contact the physician if fresh bleeding recurs or fever develops is emphasized.

Evaluation

Intervention for postpartum hemorrhage is successful when the bleeding is controlled and blood replaced as necessary to maintain the client's health and strength. Vital signs will remain stable, and blood values will be normal. The woman and family express understanding of the complication and its treatment and are able to integrate this experience psychologically and emotionally. The woman resumes infant caretaking and self-care activities and returns home quickly. Pain is relieved or minimized, fears and anxiety are resolved, and the complication can be placed in an accepting perspective.

Delayed and Late Postpartum Hemorrhage

PATHOPHYSIOLOGY

Delayed postpartum hemorrhage occurs when blood loss is greater than 500 ml after the first 24 hours following delivery and within the first few days after birth. Late postpartum hemorrhage may take place between the fifth day and the sixth week postpartum. These types of hemorrhage are usually sudden in onset and may be so massive as to produce hypovolemic shock. Late postpartum hemorrhage is uncommon, occurring perhaps once in 1000 cases.

The most frequent causes of delayed and late postpartum hemorrhage are subinvolution of the placental site, retained placental tissue, and infection. Regeneration of the placental site takes longer (about 42 days) than the rest of the endometrium (about 21 days). Until the site is firmly epithelialized, sloughing of clots may cause bleeding. Certain factors are associated with clot sloughing and hemorrhage, including low-grade fever, a history of abortion, uterine bleeding during pregnancy, and not breast-feeding.

Placental fragments that have been retained may become necrosed. As fibrin is deposited and builds up, pseudopolyps can form. When pseudopolyps become detached, brisk bleeding may occur from the placental site, which has not accomplished adequate hemostasis. This leads to delayed or late postpartum hemorrhage.

NURSING PLANNING AND INTERVENTION

Treatment of late postpartum hemorrhage is to identify and correct the cause of bleeding. Oxytocic agents are often administered, with curettage if necessary, to remove retained placental tissue. Antibiotics are administered if infection is present. Fluids and blood are replaced as necessary.

During the acute phase of bleeding, the nurse assesses vital signs, blood loss, and cardiovascular function, administers medications, and assists with operative procedures, such as curettage. Informing the family of the client's condition and progress is important. The nurse assists with arrangements for care of the infant, especially if hospitalization will involve several days. Measures to support breast-feeding (if appropriate), such as emptying the mother's breasts and providing the breast milk to family members for infant feeding, can be instituted.

Intervention includes allaying anxiety about the effects on parenting by allowing expression of concerns, providing accurate information about condition and progress, correcting misconceptions, giving reasonable encouragement, and assisting the client and family to put the experience in perspective. Knowledge deficits about the complication and its causes, consequences, and treatment can be alleviated by client teaching.

When the mother must return to the hospital, the beginning relationship with the newborn is upset to some degree. Much of the mother's anxiety or desire to return home as quickly as possible may arise from the often abrupt and temporary arrangements that she has had to make. Understanding and counseling the mother about these concerns and helping with planning can relieve much anxiety. Arrangements for the mother to get adequate rest after her return home are helpful.

Early postpartum hemorrhage, occurring within the first 24 hours of delivery, is discussed in Chapter 38.

Pulmonary Embolism

PATHOPHYSIOLOGY

Pulmonary embolism is usually caused by a thrombus fragment (embolus) carried by venous circulation to the right heart. It occurs once in every 2500 to 3000 deliveries. The thrombus usually originates in a uterine or a pelvic vein. When the embolus occludes the pulmonary artery, it obstructs the passage of blood into the lungs, either wholly or in part, and the patient may die of asphyxia within a few minutes. If the clot is small, the initial episode may not be fatal, but recurrent emboli increase the mortality risk. Emboli may follow infection, thrombosis, severe hemorrhage, or shock.

Symptoms associated with smaller pulmonary emboli include sudden onset of chest pain, cough or throat clearing, and expectoration of blood-streaked mucus. Larger pulmonary emboli cause sudden, intense chest pain, severe dyspnea, air hunger, apprehension, syncope, hemoptysis, tachypnea, pallor, cyanosis, and irregular or faint pulse. Fever, tachycardia, diaphoresis, and hypotension may occur. The client often reports headache, lethargy or confusion, restlessness, and anxiety. Respiratory or cardiac arrest may occur. With severe pulmonary obstruction, death may result within a few minutes or hours.

NURSING PLANNING AND INTERVENTION

When embolism occurs, rapid emergency measures to combat anoxia and shock must be carried out promptly. Institution of cardiopulmonary resuscitation may be necessary, with oxygen administration following. Diagnostic tests include chest x-ray, electrocardiogram, arterial blood gasses, lung scan, and pulmonary angiography. Shock and acid-base imbalances are treated, and anticoagulants are often administered. Intravenous morphine or meperidine (Demerol) may be given to help relieve the patient's apprehension and pain.

During the acute, life-threatening phase, the nurse monitors blood pressure, pulse, and respirations every 5 minutes. An intravenous infusion is initiated, and medications are administered. Skin color, breathing difficulty, and neck vein engorgement are observed. The chest is auscultated for rales, friction rub, or atelectasis. The nurse prepares the client and assists with collection of specimens and performance of procedures. The client and family are kept informed about progress of the complication and the diagnostic and treatment processes. Support, encouragement, and reassurance are provided as must as possible to allay anxiety and apprehension.

Once the crisis phase and need for hospitalization are over, anticoagulant therapy is continued from 6 weeks to 6 months to prevent recurrent emboli, depending on clinical response. The mother-infant relationship may be severely disrupted because of the mother's acute, life-threatening complication. Nursing measures to provide information and reduce knowledge deficits, to allay anxiety, and to minimize alterations in parenting are indicated.

Thrombophlebitis

PATHOPHYSIOLOGY

Thrombophlebitis is an infection of the vascular endothelium with clot formation attached to the vessel wall. The veins of the leg are most often involved, including the femoral, popliteal, and saphenous veins. Septic pelvic thrombophlebitis involving the ovarian and the uterine veins may accompany severe pelvic infections (Fig. 40-10).

Femoral thrombophlebitis usually appears about 10 days after delivery but can occur as late as the 20th day.

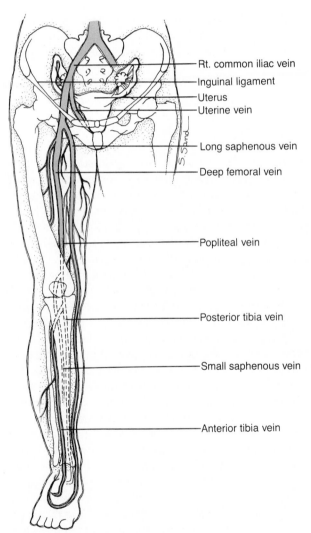

■ *Figure 40–10*
Sites of postpartum thrombophlebitis. Pelvic thrombophlebitis involves the uterine and ovarian veins. Femoral thrombophlebitis involves the femoral, popliteal, and long saphenous veins. When the small saphenous vein is involved, the term is phlebothrombosis, *because the thrombus is caused more by stasis than infection, although deep calf thrombi do become infected.*

It is characterized by pain, stiffness, pale skin, and swelling of the calf or thigh. These symptoms are caused by the formation of a clot in the veins which interferes with the return circulation of the blood. The woman often experiences malaise, chills, and fever. As in all acute febrile diseases occurring after labor, the secretion of milk may cease.

Pain may begin in the groin or the hip and extend downward, or it may begin in the calf of the leg and extend upward. In about 24 hours after the onset of pain, the leg begins to swell, and the pain may decrease. Often pain is severe enough to prevent sleep. The skin over the swollen area is shiny white. The acute symptoms last from a few days to a week, after which the pain gradually subsides and the patient slowly improves.

The course of the illness is 4 to 6 weeks. The affected leg is slow to return to its normal size and may remain enlarged and troublesome. In severe cases, abscesses may form, leading to serious infections, or clots may dislodge, causing pulmonary embolism. These complications can be life threatening.

NURSING PLANNING AND INTERVENTION

Treatment of femoral thrombophlebitis consists of rest, elevation of the affected leg, and analgesics as indicated for pain. Anticoagulants, such as heparin and dicumarol, may be prescribed to prevent further formation of thrombi. Antimicrobial drugs may be used to treat abscesses or generalized infection. The nurse administers medications and monitors their effects.

Nursing care includes using a bed cradle to keep the pressure of the bedclothes off the affected part. Heat or cold therapy may be used along the affected vessels. The affected part should not be rubbed or massaged. The leg is handled with care when changing dressings, applying bandages, making the bed, or giving a bath to avoid trauma and dislodgement of the clot.

Surgical treatment may be indicated in some severe or nonresponding cases and consists of incision of the affected vessel, removal of the clot, and repair of the vessel. Ligation of the major vessels may be necessary as a preventive measure for pulmonary embolism.

Pelvic thrombophlebitis is a serious complication and may accompany severe pelvic infections in the postpartum period. The onset usually occurs about the second week following delivery with severe, repeated chills and dramatic swings in temperature. The infection results from bacterial infection and is usually caused by anaerobic organisms. Antimicrobial therapy with broad-spectrum antibiotics and anticoagulant therapy are used.

Women with pelvic thrombophlebitis are often depressed and discouraged and feel physically unwell. Breast-feeding may be interrupted, and the significant emotional and physiological changes following childbirth may be compounded by the illness.

Nursing care includes accurate observation, recording, and reporting of signs and symptoms. The progress of the illness is monitored, and further complications should be detected early. Physical care focuses on comfort and prevention of further complications. Supportive care to help the mother and family work through the depression and discouragement is provided. The principles outlined in the discussion of grief are appropriate here (see Chap. 45).

Vulvar Hematomas

PATHOPHYSIOLOGY

Blood may escape into the connective tissue beneath the skin covering the external genitalia or beneath the vaginal mucosa to form vulvular and vaginal hematomas. Hematomas occur once in every 500 to 1000 deliveries and are usually caused by rupture or trauma to blood vessels without laceration of the superficial tissues. Delayed hematoma formation can result from sloughing of a necrotic blood vessel that was damaged by prolonged pressure during childbirth. Smaller hematomas may resorb spontaneously; larger hematomas often cause tissue necrosis, which can lead to rupture and profuse bleeding.

NURSING PLANNING AND INTERVENTION

Vulvar hematomas cause severe perineal pain with a tense, fluctuant, and sensitive tumorlike swelling of varying size covered by bluish-black skin. Vaginal hematomas may temporarily escape detection, but the client's pain and difficulty voiding alert the nurse to this complication. The client often reports perineal, vaginal, bladder, or rectal pressure that is not relieved by analgesia.

Small hematomas are usually treated supportively and allowed to resolve of their own accord. Heat and cold therapy can be used for pain relief.[12,13] If pain is severe or the hematoma enlarges, incision and evacuation of the blood, with ligation of bleeding points, is required. Large genital hematomas nearly always result in a blood loss that is more than the clinical estimate. Hypovolemia and anemia should be prevented by blood replacement as necessary.

Vulvar or vaginal hematomas may become infected, particularly those that are opened and drained. Aseptic technique and teaching the patient perineal and bowel hygiene reduce the risk of infection. Dressings or perineal pads must be changed frequently, and early signs of infection, such as foul-smelling discharge or tem-

perature elevation, must be reported at once. Broad-spectrum antibiotics may be administered.

■ POSTPARTUM DEPRESSION

Etiology and Psychopathology

During the postpartum period, women can exhibit a variety of emotional responses, ranging from "the blues" to deeper depression that may become incapacitating, or even psychotic reactions. Postpartum depression transcends culture, with no appreciable differences in incidence found between women in Western developed countries and various developing countries.[14,15] About 50% to 75% of postpartum women experience transitory "blues," with 10% to 20% undergoing significant depression. Postpartum psychosis develops in 1% to 2% of new mothers.[16] The frequency of depression increases with time after birth, with 8.5% of women depressed in the first several days and 14.2% depressed by 12 weeks. The overall rate of postpartum depression is 10.4%.[17]

Several types of postpartum depression have been described (Table 40-4). The most common type, postpartum blues, is an adjustment disorder to a life event (childbirth), with women experiencing a depressed mood. This type of depression usually occurs 3 to 5 days postpartum, with the mother feeling "down" and crying easily and frequently for no apparent reason. Many women have pronounced fatigue, feelings of loss and sadness, poor concentration, and feelings of hostility toward husbands or partners. These negative feelings are usually resolved by 4 to 5 days postpartum.[16]

Postpartum affective (neurotic) depression is a more severe depression that may occur within a few days of birth or may not be recognized for several months. The woman experiences a deep, persistent sense of loss and sadness accompanied by anxiety, irritability, sleep disturbances, lack of appetite, guilt, hypochondriasis, and, at times, phobias. Most women do not have suicide ideation or thoughts of harming the baby. This type of depression generally persists for about 1 year postpartum. Women with borderline personalities have many of the above symptoms, but additionally have feelings of helplessness, emptiness, nothingness, and aloneness following childbirth. These feelings may have been present before pregnancy but are accentuated by delivery. There may be transitory psychotic episodes with a sense of being out of control, fear of going crazy, and periods of depersonalization and disorientation.[16] Contact with reality usually is maintained. Infant abuse and neglect can occur, and suicide is a potential risk.

Postpartum psychosis (psychotic depression) usu-

TABLE 40-4. TYPES OF POSTPARTUM DEPRESSION

	Postpartum Blues	Neurotic Depression	Borderline Depression	Psychotic Depression
Onset	Transitory; usually strongest about 3–5 days after birth	May be up to 6 months after birth	Could be up to 12 months after birth	Usually within first month after birth. Most common onset after 2 weeks postpartum
Symptoms	Mild depression; tears; some feelings of loss and being overwhelmed with responsibility; fatigue; rapid mood changes; poor concentration	May include: anxiety states, phobias, fears of harming baby, hypochondriasis, loss of weight, insomnia, obsessive thoughts, irritability, feelings of guilt, apathy, lack of energy, feelings of loss of love and self-esteem	Could fluctuate from neurotic depression to periods of psychosis	Accompanied by delusions and hallucinations, disorientation, strong feelings of anger towards self and baby; may be paranoia, strong obsessive reaction. May be unipolar (only depression) or bipolar (swinging from mania to depression)
Contact with Reality	Maintained throughout	May be accompanied by feelings of depersonalization and disorientation with reality testing maintained	May have transitory loss of contact with reality. Depersonalization and acting out.	Loss of contact with reality
Risk Factors	Minimal	Suicide	Suicide	Suicide or infanticide or both
Incidence	75% of mothers	One in 10 (10–15%)	Not known	One in 500 to 700 births (2%)
Defenses	Usually get "primary maternal preoccupation" with infant, some sublimation, rationalization, intellectualization, and altruism	Mainly characterized by repression and restriction of ego functioning. May try and control through thinking, detachment, isolation, reaction formation, somatization, and introjection	Restriction of ego functioning, splitting, depersonalization and acting out	Severe regression, breakdown and splitting into primitive images. Primary process and magical thinking predominate, may get severe acting out including turning against self and infant
Organic Etiology	Minimal, although loss of sleep and endocrine change may contribute	May be some hormonal imbalance, depressive disposition associated with psychogenic factors	Possible vulnerability; no clear causality	May be strong organic predisposition to schizophrenia, etc.
Childhood History	No strong evidence of deprivation, loss, repression, or abuse in first 6 years of life	May be characterized by deprivation in early years and strong parental control during the years from 3 to 6	Typically experienced problems with separation–individualization	Often characterized by deprivation, loss or abuse in first year or two of life. Previous psychiatric illness common
Treatment	Opportunity to discuss feelings of loss and to ventilate feelings of anger, etc. Patience, support, and understanding	Insight-oriented psychotherapy; drug therapy and hospitalization may be necessary if anxiety and suicidal feelings persist.	Long-term intensive therapy required	Hospitalization. Supportive psychotherapy; drug therapy, ECT as a last resort

(continued)

TABLE 40–4. TYPES OF POSTPARTUM DEPRESSION *(continued)*

	Postpartum Blues	Neurotic Depression	Borderline Depression	Psychotic Depression
		Infant parent psychotherapy may be useful		
Prognosis	Excellent. Difficulties and feelings can usually be integrated into personality for growth	Good depending on previous history and willingness to remain in psychotherapy. Many women recover completely	Guarded without long-term intensive psychotherapy and help with parenting	Poor: may continue to need drug therapy
Effect on Infant	Minimal	May reduce orienting responses and cause delay of attachment and developmental milestones; may result in feeding or sleeping disorders	Abuse and neglect possible. Difficulties most likely in second year postpartum	If extreme and no substitute caregiver available could result in infant's withdrawal from animate and inanimate environment

ECT = electroconvulsive therapy.
Landy S, Montgomery J, Walsh S: Postpartum depression: A clinical view. Matern Child Nurs J 18(1):1–29, Spring 1989.

ally occurs within 2 to 4 weeks after birth. The woman loses contact with reality and experiences delusions, hallucinations, and disorientation. Common themes for delusions and hallucinations are associated with childbirth, the baby's health, and sexuality. There are often strong feelings of anger toward self and the baby, accompanied by delusions in which the woman believes she is being told to harm the baby. Paranoia and strong aggressive feelings may be present. Depression may be unipolar or bipolar (swinging between depression and mania). The risk of suicide or harming the baby is substantially increased.[18]

CAUSATIVE FACTORS IN POSTPARTUM DEPRESSION

Physiological factors have long been suspected of playing an important role in postpartum depression, although no evidence unequivocally makes this link. Given the massive physiological shifts of pregnancy and postpartum, the timing and transience of postpartum blues does suggest a hormonal etiology. These physiologic changes could trigger depressive reactions in women with predisposition or risk factors. Postpartum affective disorders and psychosis appear much less related to pregnancy and childbirth events.

Psychosocial stressors are more important than physiologic factors in causation of affective depression. A principal feature seen through several generations is the mother–daughter relationship that may lead to rejection of the reproductive role. Postpartum depression is associated with a lack of early support, attention, and

a dependable relationship with either parent; mothers who were not warm, nurturing, or dependable or who had negative attitudes toward their mothering roles; and fathers who were absent, preoccupied, or minimally available.[19]

Current life situation is important in postpartum depression. Any stressful life event, such as death of a loved one, loss of job, or change of residence, occurring around the vulnerable postpartum period will have an impact on the woman's mood. An unstable relationship with the husband or partner has a strong association with depression. Other factors that increase the risk of depression include inadequate financial resources, housing difficulties, and dissatisfaction with education. In this last area, the critical factor is not the level of education but the woman's satisfaction with that level and her disappointment in herself.

Coping with psychosocial stresses is more difficult when new adaptations are necessary, such as a new baby's caretaking and integrating into the family. Sleep deprivation, discomfort, and fatigue often contribute to overwhelming the mother's coping abilities. Lack of feelings of competence also appear significant in postpartum depression. Obtaining satisfactory information and feeling in control, both of self and over events during the childbirth experience, are positively related to postpartal psychological outcome.[20]

Nursing Assessment

Early identification of risk for postpartum depression will enable the nurse to take preventive steps so depressive disorders can be avoided or minimized. A history of previous postpartum depression, familial affective disorders, or depression not related to pregnancy alerts the nurse to a potential problem. Other risk factors include low socioeconomic status, marital instability, single parent with limited support systems, ambivalence or negativity about parenthood, history of abuse or neglect as a child, self-disappointment and criticism, feeling incompetent to care for infant, and recent stressful life events. In providing care during the postpartum period, the nurse also assesses for early predictive signs in the mother's behavior and interaction with the infant (see Assessment Tool: Early Predictive Signs of Postpartum Depression).

Nursing Diagnosis

Ineffective individual coping related to depression is a frequent nursing diagnosis for postpartum blues and affective depression. The identifiable stressor is childbirth; contributing factors may include negative self-concept, change in life pattern, loss, inadequate support system, and inadequate problem solving. More severe depressions lead to a diagnosis of impaired social interactions, in which the woman does not interact effectively with her environment. This is often related to chronic mental illness, substance abuse, social isolation, thought disturbances, and personality disorders.

Nursing Planning and Intervention

Nursing care for women with postpartum blues is mainly supportive, as the condition resolves spontaneously in a few days. The nurse assists the mother to understand the temporary nature of the condition, express her feelings in an accepting environment, and explore options for coping with her concerns. For milder affective depressions, emotional support in conjunction with some practical assistance, such as obtaining help with household tasks and infant care so the mother can sleep adequately, often is sufficient to enhance coping abilities and decrease depression. The nurse assists the woman to problem-solve constructively and teaches relaxation techniques. Strategies are encouraged that rely on her personal strengths and previous experiences and help establish a supportive network of understanding people. Self-help and support groups are excellent resources for supportive networks.

Women who experience more intense depression need mental health consultation and therapy. Counselling to deal with feelings and concerns may be behavioral, supportive, or insight oriented, depending on the mother's needs and capacity to integrate new perspectives into her functioning. Depending on resources available, the woman may obtain individual psychiatric therapy or group therapy or participate in self-help or support groups. Parenting groups, hot lines, and mental health drop-in centers provide additional sources of as-

Assessment Tool

Early Predictive Signs of Postpartum Depression

In providing care during the postpartum period, the nurse assesses the mother's behavior and interaction with the infant for these signs:

Lack of visitors, no sharing of news about birth with relatives or friends.

Spouse or partner not warm, supportive, or caring toward mother.

Mother expresses rejection or ambivalence toward pregnancy, childbirth, or the baby.

Mother views baby as rejecting her, behaving badly or aggressively, may call baby a "monster."

Mother experiences sleep disturbances or severe nightmares.

Mother demonstrates lack of warmth and interest in baby during feeding and caretaking; may not want to hold baby; does little verbalization; lacks eye-to-eye contact; exhibits little reciprocity.

Mother expresses intense feelings of loss involving body image, independence, personal routines, status, goals.

Mother shows extreme feelings of sadness, anxiety, guilt, and anger and cries frequently

Adapted from Landy S, Montgomery J, Walsh S: Postpartum depression: A clinical view. Matern Child Nurs J 18(1):1–29, 1989.

sistance. Psychotherapy for the mother (with the infant present), which focuses on confrontation and working through previously unresolved and unconscious conflicts related to her own experience of being parented, is often especially beneficial.[16]

For women with severe affective depressions, borderline personalities, or psychotic depression, tranquilizers or antidepressant medication are usually necessary. Psychiatric referral and management should be instituted as soon as possible. Hospitalization may be needed if the depression is not controlled with medication or the woman is acting out extremely, planning suicide, or posing a serious threat to the infant.

Evaluation

For postpartum blues and mild affective depression, nursing care is effective when the woman can express feelings, identify coping patterns and consequences, identify strengths and accept support from others, and make decisions and follow through with actions to accomplish goals or make desired changes. Depression either resolves or significantly decreases, and the mother assumes caretaking and family responsibilities with a more positive mood.

The longer-term prognosis for women with severe affective depression, borderline personalities, and psychotic depression varies; about 25% to 43% of women with postpartum depression still have some impairment a year after delivery. Services needed often are multifaceted, and not all communities have adequate mental health facilities. Effective nursing care guides the woman to appropriate treatment modalities that will aid her recovery, promote more adaptive individual coping behaviors, and reduce social isolation.

■ REFERENCES

1. Gall S: Therapeutic dilemmas in the treatment of pelvic infections. J Reprod Med 35(11)(Suppl):1091–1094, November 1990
2. Sweet RL: Role of cephamycins in obstetrics and gynecology. J Reprod Med 35(11)(Suppl):1064–1069, November 1990
3. Cox SM, Gilstrap LG: Postpartum endometritis. Obstet Gynecol Clin North Am 16(2):363–371, June 1989
4. Anderson GC: Risk in mother-infant separation postbirth. Image 21(4):196–199, Winter 1989
5. Soper DE, Kemmer CT, Conover WB: Abbreviated antibiotic therapy for the treatment of postpartum endometritis. Obstet Gynecol 69:127, 1987
6. Ledger WJ: Obstetrical and gynecological infections. In

Willson JR, Carrington ER (eds): Obstetrics and Gynecology, 8th ed. St. Louis, CV Mosby, 1989
7. Gibbs RS: Infection after cesarean section. Clin Obstet Gynecol 28:697–710, 1985
8. Watts DH, Krohn MA, Hillier SL, et al: Bacterial vaginosis as a risk factor for post-cesearean endometritis. Obstet Gynecol 75(1):52–58, January 1990
9. Galask RP: The challenge of prophylaxis in cesarean section in the 1990s. J Reprod Med 53(11)(Suppl): 1078–1081, November 1990
10. Stray-Pedersen G, Blakstad M, Bergan T: Bacteriuria in the puerperium. Am J Obstet Gynecol 162(2):792–797, March 1990
11. Robson SC, Boys RJ, Hunter S, et al: Maternal hemodynamics after normal delivery and delivery complicated by postpartum hemorrhage. Obstet Gynecol 74(2):234–238, August 1989
12. Hill PF: Effects of heat and cold on the perineum after episiotomy/laceration. JOGNN 18:124–129, 1989
13. LaFoy J, Geden EA: Postepisiotomy pain: Warm versus cold sitz bath. JOGNN 18:399–403, 1989
14. Cox JL: Postnatal depression: A comparison of African and Scottish women. Soc Psychiatry 18:25–28, 1983
15. Harris B: "Maternity blues" in East African clinic attenders. Arch Gen Psychiatr 38:1293–1295, 1981
16. Landy S, Montgomery J, Walsh S: Postpartum depression: A clinical view. Matern Child Nurse J 18(1):1–29, Spring 1989
17. Posner NA, Unterman RR, Williams KN: Postpartum depression: The obstetrician's concerns. In Inwood DG (ed): Recent Advances in Postpartum Psychiatric Disorders. Washington, DC, American Psychiatric Press, 1985
18. Zare-Parsi M, Hoffman BF: Postpartum mental disorders. Can Mental Health 37(1):13–16, 1989
19. Unterman RR, Posner NA, Williams KN: Postpartum depressive disorders: Changing trends. Birth 17(3):131–137, September 1990
20. Green JM, Coupland VA, Kitzinger JV: Expectations, experiences, and psychological outcomes of childbirth: A prospective study of 825 women. Birth 17(3):15–24, September 1990

■ SUGGESTED READING

Berman SM, Harrison HR, Boyce WT, et al: Low birth weight, prematurity, and postpartum endometritis. JAMA 257:1189–1194, 1987
Fowler JE: Urinary tract infections in women. Urol Clin North Am 13:673–683, 1986
Galask RP: Changing concepts in obstetric antibiotic prophylaxis. Am J Obstet Gynecol 157:491, 1987
Gilbert L, Porter W, Brown VA: Postpartum haemorrhage: A continuing problem. Br J Obstet Gynaecol 94:67–71, 1987
Gravett MG, Hummel D, Eschenbach DA, et al: Independent associations of bacterial vaginosis and *Chlamydia*

trachomatis infection with adverse pregnancy outcome. JAMA 256:1899–1903, 1986

Jones RN: Role of new cephamycins in the management of obstetric and gynecologic infections. J Reprod Med 35(11)(Suppl):1070–1077, November 1990

O'Hara MW: Social support, life events and depression during pregnancy and the puerperium. Arch Gen Psychiatr 43:569–573, 1986

O'Hara MW, Engeldinger J: Postpartum depression. Postgrad Obstet Gynecol 10(4):1–6, 1990

Robson SC, Hunter S, Moore M, et al: Haemodynamic changes during the puerperium: A Doppler and M-mode echocardiographic study. Br J Obstet Gynaecol 94:1028–1039, 1987

Sneddon J, Kerry RJ: The psychiatric mother and baby unit: A five-year study. In Ingwood DG (ed): Recent Advances in Postpartum Psychiatric Disorders. Washington, DC, American Psychiatric Press, 1985

Sweet RL, Gall SA, Gibbs RS, et al: Multicenter clinical trials comparing cefotetan with moxalactam or cefoxitin as therapy for obstetrics and gynecologic infections. Am J Surg 155:56, 1988

Watts DH, Eschenbach DA, Kenny GE: Early postpartum endometritis: The role of bacteria, genital mycoplasma, and *Chlamydia trachomatis*. Obstet Gynecol 73:52–60, 1989

41

Emergencies in Maternity Nursing

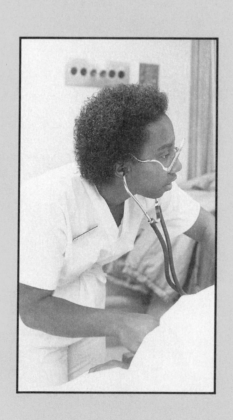

■ PRECIPITOUS LABOR AND DELIVERY

Precipitous labor progresses rapidly, lasting less than 3 hours from onset to spontaneous delivery. Precipitous delivery may occur with or without precipitous labor, and refers to an unexpected and sudden delivery, which often is unattended by professionals. Labor or delivery in a hospital setting occasionally progress so rapidly that the maternity nurse must deliver the infant.

Precipitous labor and delivery are most often related to unusually decreased resistance of birth canal tissues, which permits rapid passage of the fetus through the pelvis. Factors that predispose women to precipitous labor include multiparity, a history of rapid labors, premature or small fetus in vertex presentation, large bony pelvis, pliable pelvic tissues, and cocaine abuse. Abnormally strong and frequent uterine contractions can produce precipitous labor, as can unusually frequent contractions of normal amplitude. On rare occasions, unawareness of labor and lack of painful contractions are associated with rapid labor and delivery.

Maternal complications are infrequent in precipitous labor associated with pliable pelvic tissues. When maternal pelvic tissues are firm and resist stretching, or when the cervix is long and firm, there is substantial risk of injury. Strong uterine contractions forcing the fetal presenting part against firm, resistant maternal tissues increase the risk of uterine rupture, lacerations of the cervix and birth canal, and amniotic fluid embolism. Excessive uterine contractility during labor may predispose the woman to postpartum hemorrhage due to uterine atony.

Fetal and neonatal complications seldom occur when there are pliable maternal pelvic tissues and a large bony pelvis, providing minimal resistance to fetal descent and birth. There is the risk of decreased placental circulation associated with strong, frequent uterine contractions, which may result in fetal hypoxia. Adverse effects of hypoxia due to uterine hyperactivity are particularly likely if the fetus is chronically stressed. With bony and firm pelvic tissue providing resistance to descent and birth, trauma to the fetal head may occur.

Nursing Assessment

The maternity nurse assesses the frequency, strength, and duration of uterine contractions and notes when these are unusually close and vigorous. When assessment of the labor pattern indicates a rapidly progressing labor, the nurse ascertains the stage of cervical dilation and effacement more frequently. Fetal station and presentation are monitored frequently, and fetal heart rate is followed carefully for abnormalities.

When the labor pattern is indicative of precipitous labor, the nurse estimates the time delivery might be expected and determines whether physician attendance is likely. If delivery appears imminent without physician attendance, the nurse prepares to deliver the infant in a manner that ensures safety of both mother and infant.

Nursing Diagnosis

During the stage of active, precipitous labor, nursing diagnoses may include: Fear Related to Loss of Controllable Body Function and Unpredictable Outcomes, Alteration in Comfort: Pain Related to Intense Uterine Contractions, and High Risk for Trauma Related to Tissue Injury. After delivery especially if the woman felt a loss of control or was disappointed with the birth experience, nursing diagnoses may include: Situational Low Self-Esteem Related to Performance During Labor and Delivery, Body Image Disturbance Related to Unpredictable Body Functioning and Loss of Control, Impaired Tissue or Skin Integrity Related to Lacerations of the Birth Canal, Alterations in Comfort: Pain, and High Risk for Infection or Injury (hemorrhage, hematoma).

Nursing Planning and Intervention

The nurse takes action as feasible to notify the physician or midwife of the precipitous labor and impending delivery. Plans are made to obtain an emergency delivery pack and assistance from other personnel, if possible. Goals of nursing care are to ensure a safe birth and an emotionally satisfying experience for the mother, father, and others involved.

The nurse's composure and ability to convey calm are important for a successful delivery. Whenever possible, the mother should be told what to anticipate and what she can do to cooperate effectively. Teamwork with the mother is essential and can be accomplished if her confidence is supported through both physical and emotional aspects of care. If the father is present, he can help care for the mother and infant in whatever capacity seems most appropriate and in accord with his ability.

If the mother is on a delivery table, it is wise *not to break* the lower end. It takes practice to handle the infant over a dropped table while accomplishing the following three critical objectives:

Holding the baby close to the introitus to prevent tension and pulling on the cord
Holding the baby's head down to promote drainage of secretions
Holding the infant at or above the level of the introitus to prevent transfusion of the baby by gravity flow

Research Highlight

Pregnancy Outcomes After Trauma

Trauma during pregnancy is related to increased risk of spontaneous abortion, preterm labor, abruptio placentae, fetomaternal transfusion, and stillbirth. How frequently these complications occur and their time of onset are not well established. This controlled, prospective cohort study compared 85 women with varying degrees of trauma during pregnancy to a control group of 85 pregnant women matched for gestational age. The purpose of this study was to compare pregnancy outcomes between women experiencing trauma and uninjured pregnant women serving as controls.

Women beyond 12 weeks' gestation with trauma to the head and central body were included. Those beyond 20 weeks had at least 4 hours of cardiotocographic monitoring, ultrasound evaluation, and an acid elution assay to estimate volume of fetomaternal transfusion. History included type of injury, classified as motor vehicle accident with use of restraints noted, fall to horizontal or from height, or direct blow to the abdomen (kick, punch). There were no significant differences in demographic and obstetrical variables between the study and control groups.

Motor vehicle accidents were the most common type of injury (52%), followed by falls (26%) and direct blow to abdomen (14%). Of all the trauma victims, 88% had minor or no injuries on clinical examination (minor bruising, lacerations, contusions), 9% had moderate injuries (broken long bones, fractured ribs, extensive bruising), and 2.4% were critically ill. Immediate adverse outcomes occurred in 20% and included abruptio placentae, ruptured membranes, onset of labor, or fetal death. Abruptio placentae occurred more frequently among those less severely injured; neither the less severe injury nor the minimal physical findings ruled out immediate adverse effects.

The rate of fetomaternal transfusion was 31% in the trauma and 8% in the control group—a highly significant difference. The volume of transfusion was also greater in women with trauma. Anterior location of the placenta and uterine tenderness were the only physical signs associated with fetomaternal transfusion. Trauma subjects using restraints during motor vehicle accidents had a nonsignificant tendency to more frequent transfusions than those not wearing restraints.

Nearly two thirds of subjects had contractions every 2 to 5 minutes during the first hour of monitoring; only 6.7% had no uterine activity during 4 hours of monitoring. Contractions stopped in 90% of women without tocolysis. Ultrasonography accurately predicted abruptio placentae in 40% of the cases.

When immediate adverse effects were excluded, women with minor to moderate trauma had no differences in pregnancy outcomes from the control group in terms of birth weight, gestational age at delivery, or Apgar score. This finding is important for nurses to allay fears of pregnant families after trauma has been carefully evaluated, which includes at least 4 hours of cardiotocographic monitoring.

(Pearlman MD, Tintinalli JE, Lorenz RP: A prospective study of outcome after trauma during pregnancy. Am J Obstet Gynecol 162(6): 1502–1507, June 1990)

If the mother is on a flat labor bed or stretcher, there may not be sufficient space to deliver the shoulders. The perineum may not be readily visible, and it may be difficult to keep the infant's nose and mouth free from the blood and amniotic pool, making suctioning the infant difficult. The mother's hips should be elevated using an upside down padded bedpan (or similar object) that provides about 5 in of space between the perineum and the bed. If nothing is available, the mother is asked to raise her hips by placing her feet firmly on the bed, or another person can raise her buttocks a few inches off the bed until suctioning and delivery can be completed.

The mother's head needs to be elevated about 45 degrees by any means available. In the supine position during delivery, the mother's vena cava and aorta are compressed and the uteroplacental blood flow is compromised, which could result in a hypoxic infant. Elevating the head also helps the mother to maintain eye contact with her attendants, which can help allay fear and help her to see and hear instructions.

The lateral Sims' position often is recommended for emergency deliveries because it places the least strain on the perineum and affords the best possible visualization of the birth. It also allows for necessary space for delivering the shoulders.

Maintenance of clean technique is important, although sterility and asepsis are not priorities because vaginal intrusion and the use of instruments are not involved in these deliveries. The infant also does not need to be in a sterile environment after birth. The priorities for clean technique are as follows: (1) cleansing the nurse's hands, (2) cleansing the mother's skin, (3) putting on gloves if they are available, (4) placing clean or sterile drapes on the mother if they are available, and (5) preventing fecal contamination of the birth canal and baby.

The nurse protects the perineum by assisting a slow birth of the infant's head (Fig. 41-1A). Massaging and supporting the perineum may be helpful as described below. The inexperienced nurse should give priority to safe delivery of the infant over protecting the perineum.

DELIVERY OF THE HEAD

As the head distends the perineum at the acme of a contraction, gentle, even pressure is exerted against the head to control its progress and prevent perineal lacerations. This kind of *control applied* during each contraction prevents the head from suddenly pushing through the vulva and causing subsequent complications. *The head must never be held back.* The mother should be encouraged to pant through the contraction to prevent bearing down, particularly as the head, which

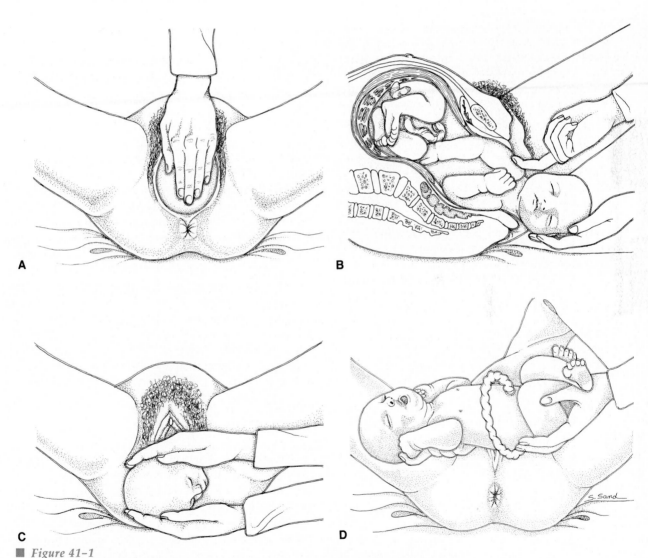

A   **B**

C   **D**

■ *Figure 41–1*

Assisting an emergency birth. (A) Apply gentle, even pressure with the flat of your hand, fingers and thumb close together, on the emerging head to slow the baby's progress and protect the mother's perineum. (B) While gently supporting the head, during restitution and external rotation, feel around the neck for the umbilical cord, pulling gently to slacken it if necessary. (C) Placing palms over baby's ears, apply gentle traction downward until the anterior shoulder appears fully at the introitus, then upward to lift out the other shoulder. (D) As the body emerges, slide your hand down the baby's back, cradling the buttocks in one hand, the head and the upper back in the other. Hold the head lower than the trunk.

is supported by the nurse, is being delivered. Preferably, the head is delivered between contractions.

The nurse can place the index finger inside the lower vagina and the thumb opposite on the perineum and gently massage the area to stretch perineal tissues and prevent lacerations. This is called "ironing the perineum." The nurse supports the perineum with one hand and controls the delivery of the head with the other hand. The head should be allowed to emerge slowly. Rapid delivery of the head can cause perineal tears, and the sudden change of pressure within the fetal skull may cause subdural or dural tears.

RUPTURE OF THE MEMBRANES

If the membranes have not ruptured previously, they may remain intact until they appear as a smooth, glistening object at the vulva. When they protrude, membranes may rupture with the subsequent contractions. If the membranes have not ruptured before the head is delivered, they must be broken immediately by the nurse to prevent aspiration of fluid when the infant takes its first breath.

MANAGEMENT OF THE UMBILICAL CORD

As soon as the head is delivered, the nurse should feel for a loop or loops of cord around the neck by inserting one or two fingers along the back of the fetal neck (see Fig. 41-1B). If the cord is found, it is gently slipped over the baby's head when this can be done easily, or pulled on gently to slacken it. If the cord is coiled too tightly to permit this, it must be double clamped and cut (between the clamps) before the rest of the body is delivered. One or more loops of cord around the fetal neck occur in about a quarter of all deliveries.

SUCTIONING

As the head extends upward, the infant's mouth and nose are wiped gently to remove mucus, blood, and fluid. The mouth, nasal passages, and throat are suctioned with a bulb syringe. Lacking these, the nurse can use a finger to wipe the throat and squeeze fluid from the nares.

DELIVERY OF THE INFANT'S BODY

After external rotation of the head, which is usually spontaneous, there is no occasion for haste in the delivery of the body. Gentle downward pressure with the hands on either side of the head, over the ears, may be exerted to direct the anterior shoulder under the symphysis pubis, then reversed upward to deliver the posterior shoulder over the perineum (see Fig. 41-1C). The *posterior* shoulder should be controlled by the nurse's

hand. When the axilla of *the anterior* shoulder is seen, the nurse slides a hand along the posterior shoulder to hold the arm close to the infant's body and prevent flapping with delivery, which can tear the mother's perineum. The infant's body follows easily and quickly and should be supported as it is born.

As the body emerges, the nurse can slide a hand down the baby's back, cradling the buttocks in one hand and the head and back in the other. The head is held lower than the trunk (see Fig. 41-1D). The newborn is kept close to the introitus to prevent tension on the cord and is held at the level of the uterus. The nose and mouth can be suctioned again, and the newborn is dried, including the head, to prevent heat loss.

IMMEDIATE CARE OF THE INFANT

Gently rubbing the back as the infant is dried is helpful to stimulate crying and respiration after the airway is clear. A clear airway is essential, because the newborn may aspirate material into the lungs if encouraged to cry with an occluded airway. The infant can be placed on the mother's abdomen and steadied until she can hold him. She should be helped to keep the head lower than the rest of the body.

The infant must be kept warm, which is most easily done by having the mother hold the baby skin-to-skin. The pair can be covered by warmed, dry blankets; or the baby can be wrapped in a separate blanket. The baby's head should be covered and dry because it is a major source of heat loss. If necessary, the airway can continue to be cleared and the Apgar can be done. After the airway is cleared, the mother is encouraged to put the baby to breast. Even if the infant only nuzzles or licks rather than sucks, oxytocin is released from the mother's pituitary, which stimulates uterine contractions and aids in the separation of the placenta and prevention of hemorrhage.

DELIVERY OF THE PLACENTA AND CUTTING THE CORD

Shortly after the Wharton's jelly in the cord is exposed to cool air, and the infant cries, the umbilical vessels stop pulsating and blood flow ceases. The baby on the mother's abdomen stimulates release of oxytocins that stimulate uterine contractions and aid placental separation. There is no rush to cut the cord; the nurse can wait until after delivery of the placenta. However, the cord should not be milked, because this can cause hypervolemia, leading to respiratory distress or hyperbilirubinemia and additional antibodies in cases of isoimmunization.

If the physician or midwife is still not present, the nurse proceeds with delivery of the placenta. It is important to *wait* for the placenta to separate before attempting to deliver it. The signs of placental separation are a slight gush of dark blood from the vagina, lengthening of the cord, and change in uterine contour from discoid to globular. The mother usually feels another urge to push, has a contraction, or feels pressure in her vagina. The nurse instructs the mother to push and can lift the placenta from the vagina by holding onto the umbilical cord. Uterine inversion can be guarded against by placing the flat of one hand gently but firmly on the lower abdomen just above the symphysis pubis. Force must not be used, and the placenta can be gently guided along the birth canal. If the umbilical cord is held near the introitus, it is less likely to break or tear than if held further back. The membranes may trail behind the placenta and can be teased out with a gentle up, down, and out motion. The nurse inspects the placenta to see if it is intact. The uterus can be massaged gently to maintain firmness and to help the uterine vessels constrict. Vigorous or continuous massage should be avoided to prevent muscle fatigue or prolapse or inversion of the uterus (see Chap. 22).

The umbilical cord is clamped by placing two sterile clamps about 2 to 4 in from the newborn's abdomen. The cord is cut between the clamps with sterile scissors. A sterile cord clamp or sterile cord ties are placed adjacent to the clamp on the newborn's umbilical cord. Only sterile equipment is used to clamp and cut the cord (Fig. 41-2). Double loops of tape must be placed around the cord and secured with at least two square knots. The cord should be observed frequently for any bleeding.

If the physician arrives soon after delivery, the nurse assists with examination of the mother, newborn, and placenta. An infant who is premature or who is having respiratory distress is transported to the nursery immediately. The newborn must be properly identified before leaving the delivery area.

EMOTIONAL CARE

The mother is assisted to express her feelings about the birth experience, to review the process, and to obtain information about what happened and why. Explanations and reassurance are provided for the mother and others involved, and they are complimented on their efforts in a difficult situation. The mother is helped to normalize the experience by understanding the processes involved and recognizing the frequency of such precipitous labors and deliveries.

Mother–infant bonding is supported by close contact, reassurance of normality as possible, and initial exploration of the infant. Being able to handle and put the baby to breast helps assure parents that the baby is normal and alleviates their fears about adverse effects from the precipitous birth.

RECORD KEEPING

The nurse records the following information on the delivery record: fetal presentation and position, presence of the cord around the neck, time of delivery, sex of infant, character of amniotic fluid, Apgar at 1 and 5 minutes, time of placental expulsion, intactness of placenta, condition of mother and infant, and any unusual occurrences.

Evaluation

Nursing intervention is effective when the mother experiences a safe delivery with prevention or minimization of complications. The infant is in good condition, and bonding between parents and infant occurs nor-

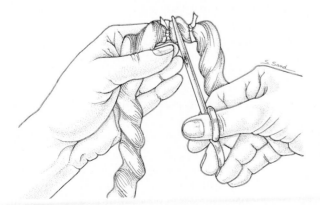

■ *Figure 41–2*
Placement of tapes and scissors for cutting the cord. To prevent the possibility of neonatal tetanus, it is important to use sterile materials.

Record Keeping for Emergency Delivery

Fetal presentation and position
Presence of cord around neck
Time of delivery
Apgar at 1 and 5 minutes
Sex of infant
Character of amniotic fluid
Time of placental expulsion
Intactness of placenta
Condition of mother after birth
Condition of infant after birth, anomalies
Medications given to mother or newborn
Unusual occurrences during the delivery

mally. The mother, father, and others present express understanding and acceptance of the precipitous labor and delivery, feel reassured that no significant adverse effects for mother or infant will result, and are able to accept and integrate their own behaviors and experiences.

Out of Hospital Delivery

Although labor may not be precipitous, the woman may be far from a hospital or birth center, or labor can be initiated unexpectedly. Emergency deliveries may occur in various locations outside of the hospital. Births at home are considered emergencies when they are unplanned and unexpected. Women in labor need to be transported to the nearest hospital or care facility whenever possible. When birth is imminent, however, transport should not be attempted and the delivery should be attended to by the most skilled person present. Important considerations for these deliveries include privacy, a clean place for the birth, and measures to protect the mother from infection and hemorrhage and the newborn from infection, chilling, and respiratory distress.

The nurse needs to provide a calm, competent image and to reassure the mother that all will be done to make the birth a safe and satisfying experience. The mother should not be separated from her partner or other support people, but does need to be screened from bystanders, both for privacy and asepsis. A clean surface for the birth should be provided using whatever clean material is available (newspapers, towels, blankets, garment bags turned inside out, coats or slacks turned inside out, and so forth).

A warm environment is important, if it can be provided. If clean water is available, the nurse or attendant should wash the hands using soap whenever possible.

The nurse gathers equipment and places it nearby. If delivery occurs in a shelter or other facility with an Emergency Delivery Pack, necessary equipment will be available. If not, substitutions must be made as needed. A clean, soft cloth can be used to wipe the newborn's face and mouth and dry the hair. New shoestrings can be used to tie the umbilical cord, and a new razor or scissors (clean or boiled) can be used to cut it. If these are not available, the cord may be left intact and the placenta may be wrapped in a blanket with the baby, making sure there is no traction on the cord.

The delivery is conducted as described for a hospital precipitous birth. Usually emergency deliveries proceed rapidly with few complications. The newborn must be protected from heat loss, infection, and overstimulation. Drying the newborn thoroughly and placing it skin-to-skin with the mother as they are both wrapped warmly

---

> **Emergency Delivery Pack**
>
> Drape for mother's buttocks to provide sterile field
>
> 4×4 gauze pads for wiping the newborn's face and removing secretions from mouth
>
> Bulb syringe to suction newborn's nose and mouth
>
> Two sterile clamps for umbilical cord (Kelly, Rochester)
>
> Sterile scissors to cut umbilical cord
>
> Sterile umbilical cord clamp (Hesseltine, Hollister)
>
> Package of sterile gloves
>
> Basin (round, emesis)
>
> Ophthalmic ointment or solution for baby's eyes
>
> Sterile water and eyedropper to rinse baby's eyes
>
> Blankets, sheets, towels, pillows
>
> Baby shirts, diapers, blankets
>
> Peripads, sanitary belt

---

prevents heat loss. Coats, garment bags turned inside out, blankets, towels, or even newspapers can be used to cover the mother and infant. Overstimulation is prevented by reducing the noise level and having dim lighting, when possible. People should be kept away (except the father and other close people) to reduce stimulation and the risk of infection.

If the newborn is having mild respiratory depression, the nurse must ascertain a clear airway, wipe mucus from the mouth and nares, facilitate mucus drainage by gravity, stimulate the newborn by rubbing the back and stroking the bottoms of the feet, and ensure the baby is dry and warm.

If the delivery occurs outside, in wilderness or parks, some form of shelter provides the warmest place, such as a tent, shower facility, or vehicle. When these are not available, building fires around the mother and infant can provide warmth. Insulation is provided by plastic or paper bags, newspapers, sleeping bags, coats, or tarps. Prevention of hypothermia is a major consideration in outdoor births.

Parent–infant bonding can be encouraged, even in the most unusual circumstances for birth. The parents are praised for coping with a difficult situation and reassured to the extent possible that mother and newborn are in good condition. The parents can be encouraged to hold, touch, and look at their newborn, and its normal behavior and appearance can be described. The mother can put the baby to breast when it nuzzles or sucks its fingers. Caring for the baby helps reassure parents about its condition and helps alleviate their fears about complications.

CONTINUING CARE FOR MOTHER AND INFANT

When the infant is breathing satisfactorily, he can remain skin-to-skin with the mother. The pair is covered with dry, clean covers as available. It is important that the infant's head is covered because it is the largest body area and heat dissipates readily with no covering. There is no need under emergency conditions to attempt to bathe the infant. The infant can also be allowed to nurse at will.

The mother is cleansed under the buttocks, and clean cloths are placed flat to absorb lochia. In general, cloths should not be placed against the perineum, to reduce the risk of infection. The perineum is inspected for lacerations. If there is active bleeding from lacerations, it is necessary to control this by pressing a clean cloth against the area and having the mother keep her thighs pressed together. Fundal firmness is checked, and the uterus is massaged gently as needed to stimulate contraction. To prevent or minimize hemorrhage, the uterus is kept contracted by gentle massage, expulsion of clots, avoiding bladder distention, and putting the infant to breast or manually stimulating the mother's breasts.

The nurse arranges to have someone call for emergency assistance, while remaining with the mother and newborn. If possible, the nurse should accompany them to the nearest health-care facility when transportation is available. The nurse clearly identifies the infant by keeping it with the mother at all times, or by securing a note to the infant's wrappings. The physician or provider at the health-care facility is provided a report by the nurse about the circumstances and details of the birth (see "Record Keeping for Emergency Delivery"). Whenever possible, the report should be written by the nurse.

■ TRAUMA IN THE PREGNANT WOMAN

Abdominal trauma during pregnancy is a common occurrence, and its consequences may be serious to the mother, infant, or both. The leading cause of death in women between the ages of 14 and 44 is accidents, principally related to automobiles. Because 23% of the U.S. population are women in this age group, including most pregnant women, it is estimated that 1 in 14 pregnant women will suffer some form of trauma. The rate of emergency department visits for trauma during pregnancy is about 24/1000 deliveries; major abdominal trauma occurs in 0.62/1000 pregnancies.[1]

Trauma during pregnancy is associated with an increased risk of spontaneous abortion, preterm labor, abruptio placentae, stillbirth, and fetomaternal transfusion.[2] The severity, frequency, and time of onset of these complications are related to the type and location of injury, gestational age, and severity of the injury. Abdominal trauma can be fatal to both the mother and fetus or may primarily affect the fetus. Direct blows to the maternal abdomen without overt maternal injury, as a result of motor vehicle accidents, falls, and assaults, may have little consequence to the mother but may have great significance for fetal well-being and survival.

Factors Determining Risk in Abdominal Trauma

GESTATIONAL AGE

When pregnancy is less than 16 weeks' gestation, the fetus is located deep in the pelvis and the risk of abruption from trauma is reduced. At later gestational ages, the fetus and placenta are higher in the abdomen and more susceptible to the effects of trauma. Even relatively minor deformation forces against the abdomen appear sufficient to shear the placental attachments away from the decidua basalis. Adverse effects are always possible from abdominal trauma, regardless of gestational age.

MINOR TRAUMA

Minor trauma involves limited bruising, lacerations, and contusions, usually from falls or blows to the abdomen, and occasionally from motor vehicle accidents. Most trauma (approximately 75%–85%) experienced by pregnant women is minor. The incidence of minor trauma increases with gestational age, with 80% of falls occurring after the 32nd week of pregnancy.[3] Pregnant women experience falls more frequently during the third trimester, related to the protuberant abdomen which affects balance, fatigue, hypotension and hyperventilation, and loosening of pelvic joints. Trauma from assaults (blows to the abdomen) is more frequent before 36 weeks, probably not occurring in late pregnancy due to social stigma associated with striking an obviously pregnant woman.[1]

After minor trauma, the incidence of abruptio placentae is about 4% to 5%.[2] Late placental abruptions, preterm labor, and ruptured membranes also occur infrequently.[4]

MAJOR TRAUMA

Moderate to major trauma involves broken long bones, fractured ribs, and extensive bruising, lacerations, and contusions. Women suffering major trauma often are critically ill on arrival at the hospital emergency room. About 9% to 10% of injuries to pregnant women involve moderate trauma, and 2% to 3% involve major trauma and critical condition.[2] Maternal death is usually caused by head and chest injuries rather than abdominal trauma. The leading cause of fetal death from trauma is maternal death. Most fetal deaths in which the mother survives trauma are due to abruptio placentae resulting from maternal shock or damage to the placenta or uterus.[3,4]

The incidence of abruptio placentae resulting from major trauma is between 6% and 35%, primarily associated with motor vehicle accidents and with the rate increasing with the severity of the injury.[2,5] Preterm labor is a common problem, occurring in about 20% of pregnant women suffering moderate to major trauma.[1] It is not unusual for contractions to occur after trauma, resulting from uterine contusion with extravasation of blood from myometrial capillaries and subsequent irritability. As the extravasated blood is resorbed, uterine irritability diminishes. In about 90% of women, contractions stop without tocolysis to interrupt labor.[2] Tocolysis may actually mask uterine activity resulting from abruptio placentae, presenting an increased threat to fetal survival.

Fetomaternal transfusion occurs in about 30% of major abdominal injuries during pregnancy, particularly when the placenta is located anteriorly. Uterine tenderness after injury has been associated with increased rates of fetomaternal transfusion, whereas contractions and fetal heart tracing abnormalities had no such association.[2] Ruptured membranes and abnormalities in fetal heart tracings may also occur, frequently in combination with preterm labor or abruptio placentae.

Gunshot Wounds in Pregnancy

The incidence of gunshot wounds in the U.S. population is increasing, and pregnant women are sustaining gunshot wounds to the abdomen more frequently. Although accidental deaths have decreased during the past decade, and motor vehicle accident deaths have decreased by 20%,[6] deaths caused by homicide and suicide have increased, especially those from handguns.[7]

As the uterus enlarges during pregnancy, it is more susceptible to gunshot injury. The musculature of the pregnant uterus is relatively dense, so most of the energy of a missile is transmitted to the muscle, and injury to other organs is relatively rare. Maternal morbidity and mortality from gunshots are low because of this; only 19% of women sustaining gunshot wounds to the pregnant uterus have associated visceral injuries. As pregnancy progresses, the ratio of fetus to amniotic fluid increases, and the fetus presents a larger target. Fetal injuries can range from minor to lethal. The incidence

of fetal injuries is between 60% and 90%, half of which are serious. In addition to direct injury to the fetus, the bullet may injure the cord, membranes, or placenta. Perinatal mortality resulting from gunshot wounds during pregnancy ranges between 47% and 70%.[7]

After gunshot injury to the pregnant uterus, abdominal tenderness often appears later than in the nonpregnant state. Guarding and rigidity are often diminished or absent. Changes of vital signs may not appear until a reduction of 35% of maternal blood volume has occurred, due to the hypervolemia of pregnancy. The risk to the fetus can be severe, because homeostasis is maintained in the mother at the expense of the fetus by reducing uteroplacental blood flow.

Self-inflicted gunshot wounds in an attempt to induce an abortion are rare, but seem to be increasing.[8] These tend to occur in women whose pregnancy had progressed too far to consider other ways of termination, and who are mentally disturbed or desperate.

Nursing Assessment

The maternity nurse often is involved in assessment and treatment of pregnant women with abdominal trauma, in conjunction with the emergency room team. The management of the injured pregnant woman usually occurs initially in the emergency room. The maternity nurse and obstetrician should be involved in treatment at an early point.

As for all types of serious trauma, initial assessments focus on adequacy of airway, presence of breathing, cardiovascular status, and extent of the injury. Fetal status is assessed, including heart rate and pattern and fetal movements, to evaluate for hypoxia. Uterine tenderness, tone and contractions, and vaginal bleeding or fluid leakage are assessed at an early point. The nurse carefully assesses for abruptio placentae. Presenting signs and symptoms of abruption may be minimal; when abruption results from trauma, bleeding is less common than in other causes. Vaginal bleeding was found as a presenting sign in only 20% of fetal deaths due to trauma-related abruption.[4]

Information about the circumstances of the injury is obtained to the extent possible. The mother's health and prenatal history are included in the assessment, to aid correct interpretation of vital signs and present symptoms.

Nursing Diagnosis

For all pregnant women experiencing abdominal trauma, *high risk for injury* is an important nursing diagnosis. Injury can be related to tissue hypoxia, hemorrhage, cardiovascular collapse, brain damage, and tissue damage. Other frequent nursing diagnoses include Alteration in Comfort: Acute Pain Related to Effects of Trauma; Fear Related to Danger to Self and Fetus; and Knowledge Deficit Related to Extent of Injuries and Required Treatment Procedures. There often is impaired skin or tissue integrity related to mechanical destruction, pressure, or shearing. Fluid volume deficit related to abnormal fluid loss may occur with hemorrhage.

Nursing Planning and Intervention

SEVERE TRAUMA

Immediate priorities are the same as those for the nonpregnant trauma victim. These include control of bleeding; ensuring airway patency; immobilization of fractured extremities, vertebrae, and pelvis in an effort to reduce blood loss in the surrounding tissues; and blood replacement.

The care of the pregnant woman experiencing trauma is different because of physiological changes of pregnancy and the need to care for a second patient, the fetus. Because blood volume is normally increased during pregnancy, blood replacement should be generous. If blood is not immediately available, fluid replacement should be substituted until it is. The pregnant woman maintains her vital signs for a longer period of time in the face of excessive hemorrhage than does the nonpregnant woman. Pulse and blood pressure may be sustained at virtually normal levels until almost immediately before vascular collapse. Failure to recognize and treat the difference in pregnancy can lead to sudden collapse and irreversible shock (see Chaps. 38 and 40).

When the woman is lying supine, in late pregnancy the weight of the uterus and its contents creates pressure on the vena cava. The resulting reduction in the return of venous blood to the heart reduces cardiac output and maternal blood pressure and reduces placental blood flow. It may also increase venous pressure in the lower half of the body, producing more bleeding in injured extremities. Pregnant women should be placed on their left side whenever feasible. This allows the uterus to fall forward and relieves vena cava pressure.

All women suffering major trauma to the uterus in mid to late pregnancy must be evaluated for signs of abruptio placentae and preterm labor. Evaluation consists of electronic fetal monitoring to obtain a reactive non-stress test (NST) and to rule out premature labor. Ultrasonography may be useful to evaluate the condition and placement of the placenta. The condition of the fetus must be monitored. The maternity nurse usually is responsible for appropriate monitoring to detect early signs of fetal distress and to initiate appropriate action. Assessment of fetal viability is an important part of the management of the pregnant trauma victim.

When the fetus is not viable, fetal monitoring is usually not required and the primary consideration is the mother's safety. In the event of premature labor with a viable fetus, preparation should be made to care for the premature infant on delivery. In some circumstances, a cesarean delivery may be necessary.

MODERATE TO MINOR TRAUMA

With a previable fetus, treatment is focused on the mother's safety and reduction of pain. In pregnancies greater than 20 weeks' gestation, a period of 4 to 24 hours of monitoring is recommended to assess for abruptio placentae.[2,3] Even if the women has no signs of fetal distress or injury, a period of monitoring is important, because abruption can be delayed by several hours to as late as 4 to 5 days.[2,9] With a reassuring fetal heart rate pattern and no evidence of abruptio placentae or preterm labor, women with minor trauma can be discharged within a few hours.

Women who are Rh negative with gestations of 12 or more weeks may be evaluated for fetomaternal transfusion; administration of Rh immune globulin prophylactically is recommended.[1,2]

Nursing care includes keeping mother and family informed about the condition of mother and fetus, the treatment plan, and the expected course and outcomes. Clear, simple explanations are necessary due to the high levels of anxiety and fear, which reduce the family's capacity to process information. Emotional support and reassurance to the extent possible are important. After the immediate crisis has passed, the nurse encourages the expression of feelings and reliving the events of the trauma to assist integration and acceptance. If fetal risk or loss occurs, the nurse supports the parent's grieving process (see Chap. 45).

GUNSHOT WOUNDS

Management of gunshot wounds is individualized according to the type and extent of injuries, and maternal and fetal condition. It is not necessary to explore the abdomen surgically in every case. Selective observation can often be used when the mother's condition is stable. If the entrance of the wound is below the fundus and the bullet can be seen on x-ray in the uterine muscle, less than 20% of patients require surgical management of a visceral wound. The bullet can be removed without an associated cesarean operation: the risk of precipitating labor is low if surgical procedures are carefully done. Cesarean delivery is necessary when the size of the uterus prohibits adequate exploration or repair of maternal injuries, or if the fetus is mature and is suspected of having sustained an injury. Delivery of a dead infant can await spontaneous labor or can be induced, depending on maternal condition and indications.[7]

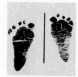

Nursing Care Plan

The Woman With Abdominal Trauma During Pregnancy

Patient Goals

1. Woman receives immediate life support and emergency care to control effects of trauma.
2. Adequate oxygenation is maintained and bleeding is controlled to ensure fetal well-being.
3. Woman obtains adequate pain relief.
4. Potential complications are identified early, and appropriate treatment is initiated.
5. Woman and family understand and accept the effects of trauma on her and the fetus.
6. Woman and family express feelings about effects of trauma and grieve losses.

Assessment	Potential Nursing Diagnosis	Planning and Intervention	Evaluation

Adequacy of airway, presence of breathing	Potential for injury related to tissue hypoxia, hemorrhage, cardiovascular collapse, brain damage, and tissue damage	Assist with emergency life support measures
		  Contol bleeding
		  Ensure patent airway
			Patent airway is maintained

Cardiovascular status (blood pressure, pulse, perfusion, hemorrhage)			Vital signs are stabilized
Extent of injury (minor, moderate, severe)	Alteration in comfort: acute pain related to effects of trauma	Immobilize fractured extremities, vertebra, pelvis	Bleeding, shock, or hemorrhage are controlled
Areas involved in injury	Fear related to danger to self and fetus	Institute intravenous fluids and blood replacement	Complications are detected early, and treatment controls problems
Potential fractures (extremiteis vertebra, pelvis, head)	Knowledge deficit related to extent of injuries and required treatment procedures	Cardiovascular resuscitation if necessary	Fetal condition remains good, heart rate and pattern are normal

Fetal status
  Fetal heart rate and pattern
		Monitor vital signs every 5–10 min
		  Blood pressure and pulse
		  Respiration
			Woman and family express understanding of events of trauma on her and fetus

Fetal movements	Impaired skin or tissue integrity related to mechanical destruction, pressure or shearing	Promote fetal well-being Monitor fetal heart rate and pattern frequently (external monitor, fetal head scope)	Parents express feelings and concerns, resolve fears about subsequent effects on mother or fetus
Uteroplacental status Tenderness, tone, contractions (frequency, intensity, duration)	Fluid volume related to abnormal fluid loss (hemorrhage)		
Vaginal bleeding or fluid leakage		Have mother lie on left side whenever feasible to reduce vena cava compression, promote fetoplacental oxygenation)	Parents accept the injury, understand factors connected with its occurrence, plan for reducing future risks
Circumstances of injury Type (motor vehicle, fall, blow to abdomen)			
Location (home, street, other buidling, outdoors, and so forth)		Evalutate maternal blood loss carefully, identify earliest signs of hypovolemic shock, assist immediate treatment	Pregnancy continues, and the mother successfully delivers a healthy, term infant
Persons present and immediate first aid			The woman fully recovers from all effects of trauma
Health and prenatal history		Administer oxygen to mother if BP drops, res-	When fetal death occurs parents grieve effectively

(continued)

Nursing Care Plan (continued)

Assessment	Potential Nursing Diagnosis	Planning and Intervention	Evaluation
Significant chronic illness or health problems		pirations labored, signs of shock	and move toward acceptance and integration of the loss
Prenatal problems and treatment		Detect preterm labor and abruptio placentae	
Current medications, activity restrictions		Electronic fetal monitoring, nonstress test (NST)	
Alcohol and street drug use		Ultrasonography for condition, placement of placenta	
Reactions of woman and family		Uterine tonus, contractions, tenderness	
Orientation, mentation		Assist with emergency procedures	
Emotional responses (fear, anger, anxiety, grief)		Intubation, resuscitation, ventilation	
Capacity for information and understanding		Preparation for surgery, cesarean delivery	
		Emotional support and reassurance	
		Keep woman and family informed about condition, test, procedures, expected results	
		Answer questions simply and directly	
		Remain calm, use reassuring manner, assure that all is being done to protect mother and fetus	
		After crisis, encourage expression of feelings, reliving events of trauma, understanding what happened and why	
		Support initial grieving if fetal loss occurs	

PREVENTION OF ABDOMINAL TRAUMA DURING PREGNANCY

The use of seatbelts during pregnancy should be reviewed with every pregnant woman by the maternity nurse. As term approaches, seatbelts are increasingly uncomfortable and the woman is disinclined to use them. Proper placement of seatbelts is critical during later pregnancy. Belts with shoulder harnesses are best, and the lower belt should be worn encircling the pelvis below the protruding abdomen (see Chap. 19). In a collision, the sudden deceleration that occurs on impact delivers substantially more force to the lower abdomen when a seatbelt is across it, with risk of contusion and

Client Education

Preventing Accidental Trauma

- Wear shoulder harness seatbelts 100% of the time; position lap belt across pelvis below abdomen.
- When driving an automobile, be sure you are seated comfortably, have good visibility, and can readily control the car.
- As pregnancy progresses, stay aware of changes in body posture and in your center of gravity.
- Avoid climbing ladders, fences, trees, and onto counters because this upsets your balance and can lead to falls.
- Avoid stretching to reach objects on high shelves, because this can upset your balance and lead to falls.
- Lift objects carefully, using good body mechanics (keep back straight, bend knees, and use thigh muscles); don't lift very heavy objects.
- Bathe and shower with care in late pregnancy; if your tub has a high edge, have assistance when you get in and out; use tub and shower mats to prevent slipping on wet surfaces.
- Remove obstacles in areas of routine traffic, throw rugs that might slip out from under you, sharp protruding corners.
- Wear comfortable, low-heeled shoes that provide good support and traction.
- Avoid dangerous situations for violence; do not provoke arguments, don't walk alone at night or frequent places where fights or arguments might occur.

compression. In pregnancies beyond 20 weeks, the sudden increase in intrauterine pressure directed upward through the amniotic fluid can result in abruptio placentae. When seatbelts are not worn, maternal deaths due to head trauma and internal injuries associated with motor vehicle accidents significantly increase. The nurse should emphasize that seatbelts must be worn during pregnancy and should teach proper placement.

Home safety and avoidance of falls are other important preventive measures. The nurse reviews sources of household hazards, and plans with the mother to reduce or eliminate these. The mother is taught how to move, sit, stoop and carry objects as pregnancy progresses toward term to avoid losing balance and falling. Factors that increase risk for family violence can be assessed and reviewed with the women (see Chap. 6).

Evaluation

Immediate intervention is effective when the pregnant trauma victim's vital signs stabilize, and immediate risks of hemorrhage, shock cardiac arrest, and further complications are controlled. Further success can be measured by early detection and management of complications such as preterm labor, abruptio placentae, and fetomaternal transfusion. The most optimal outcome is

full recovery and health of both mother and fetus; the fetal condition is good, and pregnancy continues without adverse effects.

Psychosocial interventions are effective when parents can express their feelings and concerns, resolve fears about subsequent effects on mother and infant, and express understanding of the events related to the trauma and its treatment. Parents who can accept the injury, understand factors connected with its occurrence, and plan for reducing risks of future injuries have benefited from nursing intervention. When fetal death occurs, parents are able to grieve effectively and move toward acceptance and integration of this loss.

■ REFERENCES

1. Williams JK, McClain L, Rosemurgy AS et al: Evaluation of blunt abdominal trauma in the third trimester of pregnancy: Maternal and fetal considerations. Obstet Gynecol 75(1):33–37, January 1990
2. Pearlman MD, Tintinalli JE, Lorenz RP: A prospective study of outcome after trauma during pregnancy. Am J Obstet Gynecol 162(6):1502–1507, June 1990
3. Rosenfeld JA: Abnormal trauma in pregnancy. Postgrad Med 88(6):89–94, November 1990

4. Kettel LM, Branch DW, Scott JR: Occult placental abruption after maternal trauma. Obstet Gynecol 71(3): 449–453, Pt 2, 1988

5. O'Keefe DF: When the accident victim is pregnant. Contemp Ob/Gyn 148–163, July 1985

6. 1980s saw record US progress in cutting accidental deaths. The Nation's Health 21(1):1, 12, January 1991

7. Franger AL, Buchsbaum HJ, Peaceman AM: Abdominal gunshot wounds in pregnancy. Am J Obstet Gynecol 160(5):1125–1127, Pt 1, May 1989

8. Buchsbaum HJ, Staples PP: Self-inflicted gunshot wound to the pregnant uterus: Report of two cases. Obstet Gynecol 65:32S–35S, 1985

9. Higgins SD, Garite TJ: Late abruptio placenta in trauma patients: Implications for monitoring. Obstet Gynecol 63:10S–12S, 1984

Study Aids

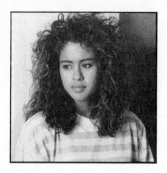

Unit VII
Assessment and Management of High Risk Maternal Conditions

CONFERENCE MATERIAL

1. A mother, para 2, is admitted to the hospital at 42 weeks' gestation for induction of labor. Her membranes have been artificially ruptured, and intravenous oxytocin has been started. Discuss the nursing care of this mother from this time until she is in active labor.

2. What specific nursing care would you give to a mother who sustained a third-degree perineal laceration as the result of a maximal breech delivery?

3. A 38-year-old gravida 5 had an uneventful pregnancy until the last trimester, when she developed preeclampsia. Now, at term, she is admitted to the hospital because of suspected abruptio placentae and after consultation is to have an emergency cesarean section. Identify three nursing diagnoses, and describe the related nursing care of this mother from time of admission until she is taken to the operating room for surgery.

4. A primigravida, who has 3-year-old adopted twins, is delivered by low cervical cesarean section because of pelvic injuries received in an auto accident 6 years earlier. Discuss the nursing care of this mother following cesarean section.

5. J.W. is a 25-year-old multipara whose labor was complicated by prolonged early rupture of the membranes. There were no complications of delivery. On her second postpartum day, her temperature spiked to 39°C with a pulse rate of 118. She also reported increased afterpains and headache. On examination, you note fundal tenderness and a foul odor to the lochia, which is decreased and red-brown in color. After the physician's examination, the diagnosis of endometritis is established, cultures are taken, and antibiotic therapy is begun. J.W. is breast-feeding her infant and planning to leave the hospital early tomorrow. How will you counsel her regarding (A) the infectious process and treatment, (B) breastfeeding, and (C) hospital discharge. What physical care activities will be added to the care plan as part of the management of her endometritis?

6. Three common infectious processes during the postpartum period are mastitis, urinary tract infection, and thrombophlebitis. For each of these conditions, discuss the following:

A. Measures that may be taken prenatally, intrapartally, and postpartally to prevent their development
B. The mechanisms by which these infections develop
C. Their clinical manifestations (signs and symptoms)
D. Their medical management and delegated nursing functions
E. The nursing care plan that you would institute, including the postpartal psychological processes, infant care and feeding, discharge planning, and follow-up care after hospitalization.

7. One of the responsibilities of the nurse in an antepartal clinic is to provide childbirth education classes to parents. In preparing material for these classes, you have decided to include a class on cesarean birth, even though the women are having normal pregnancies and are generally low-risk patients. Part of your reason for doing this is the knowledge of the rising cesarean rate, which in some medical centers is one of every four deliveries. Discuss in detail (a) how you decide which areas of content related to cesarean births you include in this 1-hour class, and (b) write a brief content outline of these topics and the specific points you plan to make in each area.

8. You are caring for a mother having her fourth child who is in very active labor. Suddenly, the membranes rupture, and she begins to bear down. As you observe the perineum, you see the infant's head crowning. Since you are alone with this mother at the time, what will you do?

9. You are taking an antepartal history and you suspect that the mother may have a drinking problem. She tells you that she smokes about a pack of cigarettes a day and "does a little grass" to keep her husband "company." Discuss in detail the specific points in the history taking that you would want to be sure to cover with this patient.

10. Develop a specific care plan for this patient which encompasses smoking cessation and cessation of alcohol and substance abuse.

MULTIPLE CHOICE

Read through the entire question and place your answer on the line to the right.

1. Which of the following signs and symptoms should the nurse anticipate when a pregnant client has a history of heart disease and is not receiving medication?
   A. Dyspnea
   B. Slow pulse rate
   C. Decrease in blood pressure
   D. Hemorrhage
   Select the number corresponding to the correct letter or letters.
   1. A only
   2. B only
   3. A, C, and D
   4. All of the above   ____

2. Which of the following factors influence the answer that you have given in Question 1?
   A. Increased need for oxygen intake
   B. Increased blood volume
   C. Toxic damage to the heart
   D. Failure of kidneys to excrete creatinine
   Select the number corresponding to the correct letters.
   1. A and B
   2. A and C
   3. B, C, and D
   4. All of the above   ____

3. Which of the following signs and symptoms would the client with a ruptured fallopian tube manifest?
   A. Hegar's sign
   B. Intense pain
   C. Profound shock
   D. Irregular fetal heart tones
   E. Vaginal bleeding
   Select the number corresponding to the correct letters.
   1. A, C, and D
   2. A, C, and E
   3. B, C, and E
   4. B, D, and E   ____

4. In the management of hypertensive disorders of pregnancy, which of the following symptoms during labor should be reported to the physician promptly?
   A. Regular uterine contractions
   B. Epigastric pain
   C. Dimness of vision
   D. Headache
   E. Decrease in urinary excretion
   Select the number corresponding to the correct letters.
   1. A, C, D and E
   2. B, D, and E
   3. A, C and E
   4. B, C, D and E   ____

5. Which of the following conditions are causes of bleeding in the first trimester of pregnancy?
   A. Threatened Abortion
   B. Abruptio placentae
   C. Hyperemesis Gravidarum
   D. Ectopic pregnancy
   Select the number corresponding to the correct letters.
   1. A and B
   2. A and D
   3. A, C, and D
   4. B, C, and D   ____

6. Which of the following are common causes of bleeding in the third trimester of pregnancy?
   A. Hyperemesis Gravidarum
   B. Habitual Abortion
   C. Abruptio placentae
   D. Placenta previa
   E. Ectopic pregnancy
   Select the number corresponding to the correct letters.
   1. A and B
   2. A, B, and C
   3. C and D
   4. A, C, and D   ____

7. By what criterion or criteria is an incomplete abortion distinguished from a threatened abortion?
   A. Dilatation of the cervix
   B. Bright red bleeding
   C. Passage of placental tissue
   D. Pain
   Select the number corresponding to the correct letter or letters.
   1. A and C
   2. A and B
   3. C only
   4. A, C, and D   ____

8. A client in the third trimester of pregnancy reports to the nurse by phone that she has experienced vaginal bleeding. This is unassociated with pain and she feels otherwise well. She should be advised
   A. To come to the hospital immediately for evaluation
   B. To go to bed and call again if bleeding persists
   C. To continue normal activities since this condition is commonly seen just prior to labor
   D. To report this to the physician at the time of the next prenatal visit   ____

9. The client described above continues to bleed vaginally. The most serious condition that must be ruled out is
   A. Placental abruption
   B. Ectopic pregnancy
   C. Uterine atony
   D. Hydatidiform mole   ____

10. All of the following are warning signals of preeclampsia that should be watched for during the course of routine prenatal care *except*
    A. Sudden excessive weight gain (greater than 5 lb/wk)
    B. Pedal edema
    C. An elevation of blood pressure greater than 15

mm Hg in diastolic pressure over previously
observed levels

D. An elevation of more than 30 mm Hg in systolic pressure above previously observed levels ____

11. Match the statements below with the number of the hemoglobinopathy they most accurately describe.
   A. No increased fetal morbidity or maternal morbidity, but an increased incidence of urinary tract infection in pregnancy ____
   B. Only slight increased perinatal mortality but greatly increased maternal morbidity and mortality ____
   C. Fifty percent of pregnancies end in spontaneous abortion, neonatal death, or stillbirth ____
      1. Sickle cell trait
      2. Sickle cell hemoglobin C disease
      3. Sickle cell anemia

12. Diabetes may have a deleterious effect in pregnancy in the following ways:
   A. Increased fetal size with a greater risk of difficult vaginal delivery
   B. A fourfold increase in the incidence of congenital anomalies
   C. An increased incidence of oligohydramnios
   D. Increased incidence of urinary tract infection
   Select the number corresponding to the correct letters.
   1. A, B and D
   2. A, C and D
   3. B and C
   4. All of the above ____

13. Match the following statements with the condition listed below.
   A. Potentially lethal infection of the newborn that may occur during delivery ____
   B. Eyes may be affected at birth and, unless promptly treated, blindness may result. ____
   C. Characterized by anorexia, nausea, vomiting, and elevated serum bilirubin levels ____
      1. Gonorrhea
      2. Herpes genitalis
      3. Viral hepatitis

14. Which is the most likely indication for a forceps delivery?
   1. The mother is too tired to push.
   2. The baby exhibits fetal distress in the second stage.
   3. The cervix fails to dilate.
   4. The umbilical cord has prolapsed. ____

15. The three most frequent causes of postpartum hemorrhage are
   A. Retained placental fragments
   B. Full bladder
   C. Uterine atony
   D. Lacerations of the perineum, cervix, and vagina
   E. Clotting defects
   F. Uterine infections

Select the number corresponding to the correct letters.
   1. A, B, and C
   2. A, C, and D
   3. B, C, and D
   4. C, E, and F
   5. B, C, and F ____

16. What is the effect of tetanic contractions on the pregnant uterus?
   A. Descent and rotation are hastened.
   B. Ruptured uterus is a great risk.
   C. Fetal head may be compressed and ruptured.
   D. Uterine inertia may follow.
   E. Perineal lacerations may occur.
   Select the number corresponding to the correct letter or letters.
   1. A only
   2. B only
   3. A, C, and D
   4. B, C, and E ____

17. A patient in the first stage of labor develops hypertonic dysfunction. Which of the following are important in the treatment of this condition?
   A. Pitocin
   B. Sedation
   C. Fluids
   D. Bed rest
   E. Ambulation
   Select the number corresponding to the correct letters.
   1. A, B, and D
   2. A, C, and E
   3. B, C, and D
   4. B, C, and E ____

18. Which of the following principles should be observed in the use of intravenous oxytocin to stimulate labor?
   A. The condition of the fetus must be satisfactory.
   B. It should be used only in cases of primary uterine inertia.
   C. It should not be given to a multipara who has had five or more full-term pregnancies.
   D. It should be used in cases of borderline pelvis.
   E. A responsible person should be in constant attendance while the mother is receiving intravenous oxytocin.
   Select the number corresponding to the correct letters.
   1. A and B
   2. A, C, and E
   3. B, D, and E
   4. All of the above ____

19. What specific treatment should be included in the care given a mother who has had a repair of a third-degree laceration of the perineum?
   A. Give daily routine perineal care.
   B. Begin stool softeners early.
   C. Omit enemas until the fifth postpartal day.
   D. Limit activities in regard to early ambulation.
   E. Encourage the mother not to sit erect until the wound has healed.

Select the number corresponding to the correct letter or letters.
1. A only
2. A and B
3. A, C, and D
4. All of the above _____

20. Which of the following structures are involved when an episiotomy is performed?
   A. The vaginal mucosa
   B. The levator ani muscle
   C. The glans clitoris
   D. The cardinal ligament
   E. The fourchette
Select the number corresponding to the correct letter or letters.
1. A only
2. A and B
3. A, B, and E
4. All of the above _____

21. Which of the following account for the increasing cesarean birth rate?
   a. Lack of medical education pertaining to forceps deliveries
   b. Increase in malpractice claims for birth related injuries
   c. Consumer demand for pain-free deliveries
   d. Changes in the definitions of dystocia and fetal distress
Select the number corresponding to the correct letters.
1. A, B, and C
2. B, C, and D
3. A, B, and D
4. A, C, and D _____

22. A. What type of fetal heart rate pattern would be most likely to appear if the cord prolapses?
   1. Combined acceleration waveform
   2. Isolated acceleration waveform
   3. Severe variable deceleration waveform
   4. Late deceleration waveform
   5. Early deceleration waveform _____
   B. If the nurse suspects a prolapsed cord, in what position should she place the mother with the hope of relieving pressure on the cord?
   1. Knee-chest or head-down position
   2. Fowler's position
   3. Sims's position
   4. A prone position _____
   C. In addition to changing the mother's position to relieve pressure on the cord, what other measures may the nurse employ if she observes the umbilical cord prolapsed out of the vagina?
   1. Immediately wash the cord with warm antiseptic solution and replace in vagina.
   2. Push the presenting part up with a sterile gloved hand in the vagina.
   3. Apply a clamp to the exposed cord and cover with a sterile towel.

4. Keep the cord warm and moist by continuous applications of sterile saline compresses. _____
   D. What is the main objective of emergency care when prolapsed cord occurs?
   1. To prevent cold air from prematurely stimulating respiration
   2. To prevent drying of the cord while it is still pulsating
   3. To stimulate and restore circulation in the cord by vasodilatation
   4. To prevent or relieve pressure on the cord _____

23. A major nursing goal in caring for the pregnant substance abuser is
   A. Immediate withdrawal from the drug(s)
   B. Initiation of childbirth instruction
   C. Provision for assuring return for prenatal care
   D. Psychiatric referral _____

24. An important approach in planning care with the pregnant smoker is
   A. Referral to a 12-step program
   B. Making a contract with the mother
   C. Making her aware of the complications that can arise for herself and fetus when she smokes
   D. Emphasizing the benefits from smoking cessation _____

25. Nurses providing antepartum counseling to women with cardiac disease should emphasize the importance of
   A. Avoiding all sexual activity during pregnancy
   B. Avoiding contact with individuals suffering from infectious disease
   C. Participating in a natural childbirth
   D. Restricting all physical activity _____

26. Mrs. Alvarez is diagnosed as having pregnancy-induced hypertension (PIH). The nurse would suspect this condition if she found which of the following data in her assessment?
   A. Ankle edema and glucosuria
   B. Glucosuria and proteinuria
   C. Proteinuria and hypertension
   D. Hypertension and hyporeflexia _____

27. All of the following physiologic changes may be present in Mrs. Alvarez except
   A. Increase in arterial blood pressure
   B. Decrease in peripheral vascular resistance
   C. Decrease of plasma renin activity
   D. Increase in pressor responsiveness to angiotensin 11 _____

28. Magnesium sulfate is ordered for Mrs. Alvarez. The nurse should withhold the medication if
   A. Respirations are 16 per minute
   B. Reflexes are 2+
   C. Irritability and nervousness are evident
   D. Urinary output is less than 20 ml/hr _____

29. The organisms that most often cause postpartal infections of the genital tract include
    A. Anaerobic nonhemolytic streptococci
    B. Beta-hemolytic streptococci
    C. Coliform bacteria and bacteroides
    D. Staphylococci
    E. Pseudomonas
    Select the number corresponding to the correct letters.
    1. A, B, and C
    2. B, C, and D
    3. A, C, and D
    4. B, C, and E
    5. All of the above   ____

30. By which routes do bacteria usually colonize genital tissues?
    A. Cervicovaginal organisms entering the uterine cavity during labor
    B. Amniotic fluid colonization prior to or during labor
    C. Colorectal organisms introduced vaginally by examinations
    D. Urinary colonization with vaginal contamination   ____

31. Risk factors that increase the probability of developing postpartal infection include
    A. Anemia
    B. Prolonged rupture of membranes
    C. Intrauterine fetal monitoring
    D. Manual removal of placenta
    E. Hemorrhage
    Select the number corresponding to the correct letters.
    1. A, B, and C
    2. B, C, and D
    3. C, D, and E
    4. All of the above   ____

32. Risk factors for developing wound infection after cesarean section include
    A. Obesity
    B. Diabetes
    C. Longer time in hospital prior to delivery
    D. Multiple vaginal examinations
    E. Longer duration of surgery
    Select the number corresponding to the correct letters.
    1. A, B, and C
    2. B, C, and D
    3. C, D, and E
    4. All of the above   ____

33. Signs and symptoms of pulmonary embolism include
    A. Sudden intense chest pain
    B. Severe dyspnea
    C. Flushing
    D. Irregular or feeble pulse
    E. Cyanosis
    Select the number corresponding to the correct letters.

1. A, B, and C
2. A, B, C, and D
3. A, B, D, and E
4. All of the above   ____

34. What is the treatment of puerperal mastitis before suppuration occurs?
    A. Antibiotics, breast support, ice application
    B. Antibiotics, breast support, heat application
    C. Antibiotics, aspiration, breast support
    D. Antibiotics, incision and drainage, breast support   ____

35. Measures to prevent puerperal mastitis include
    A. Keeping skin of nipples intact
    B. Careful asepsis in the nursery
    C. Conscientious handwashing by nursing personnel
    D. Regular nasopharyngeal cultures of nursery staff
    E. Prophylactic antibiotics to nursing mothers
    Select the number corresponding to the correct letters.
    1. A, B, and C
    2. A, B, C, and D
    3. A, B, C, and E
    4. All of the above   ____

36. Urinary tract infections during the postpartum period are common because of which of these contributing factors?
    A. Bladder trauma leading to decreased sensitivity to distention
    B. Distention leading to incomplete emptying of the bladder
    C. Urinary stasis due to residual urine
    D. Colonization of residual urine by rectogenital organisms
    E. Dehydration due to restriction of fluids during labor
    F. Diuresis due to rapid decrease in blood volume after delivery
    Select the number corresponding to the correct letters.
    1. A, B, C, and D
    2. A, B, C, D, and E
    3. A, B, C, E, and F
    4. All of the above   ____

DISCUSSION

37. List the four classic signs of endometritis.

38. How does peritonitis differ from parametritis?

39. List the signs and symptoms of femoral thrombophlebitis.

MULTIPLE CHOICE

40. The developmental tasks of adolescence include all of the following except
  A. Achievement of trust
  B. Achievement of a secure identity
  C. Achievement higher cognitive skills
  D. Achievement of physical maturation   ____

41. In counseling a sexually active adolescent girl about family planning, it is important for the nurse to understand that
  A. Knowledge about family planning methods is likely to increase the adolescent's effective use of contraceptives.
  B. Cognitive development in adolescence is a predictor of contraceptive choices.
  C. Adolescent girls depend on their partners' decision in selecting contraceptive methods.
  D. The diaphragm is the contraceptive method of choice for adolescent girls.
  Select the number corresponding to the correct letters.
  1. A and B
  2. A, C, and D
  3. B, C, and D
  4. A and C   ____

42. The population at greatest risk for medical complications during adolescent pregnancy is
  A. Nonwhite adolescents
  B. White adolescents
  C. Girls in early adolescence
  D. Girls in middle adolescence
  Select the number corresponding to the correct letters.
  1. A
  2. A and C
  3. B and C
  4. C   ____

43. The nurse assessing a pregnant adolescent should be particularly concerned about which of the following potential problems?
  A. Gestational diabetes and premature labor
  B. Increased weight gain and birth of a LGA infant
  C. Sexually transmitted diseases and nutritional deficiencies
  D. Bleeding disorders such as placenta previa and abruptio placentae   ____

44. In counseling the adolescent mother and father about parenting skills, it is *most* important for the nurse to emphasize the infant's need for
  A. Appropriate play materials
  B. Interaction with a variety of adults and infants
  C. Monthly well baby visits with the pediatrician or nurse practitioner
  D. Frequent and loving interaction with the parents   ____

UNIT VIII

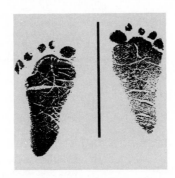

*Assessment
and
Management
of High Risk
Perinatal
Conditions*

42

Fetal Diagnosis and Treatment

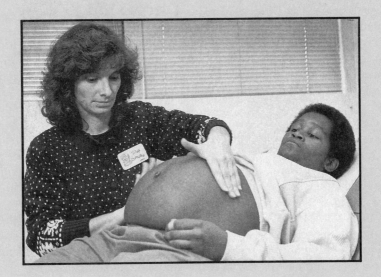

The concept of the fetus as an individual patient whose specific anatomic and physiologic problems are subject to diagnosis and treatment is relatively new to the practice of obstetrics. Prior to the 1960s, the diagnosis of fetal condition was limited to the assessment of fetal activity perceived by the mother, movement palpated by the physician, or simply auscultation of the fetal heartbeat. Plain x-rays offered a minimum of information, such as fetal position and major bony abnormalities, whereas amniograms (the introduction of radiopaque materials into the amniotic fluid) increased the risk of preterm labor or premature rupture of membranes without offering much more diagnostic data. In addition, x-rays were recognized as being potentially harmful to the developing fetus. In the last three decades, a series of rapidly evolving developments have opened the way to increasingly accurate approaches to fetal diagnosis. These developments include ultrasound techniques, safer use of amniocentesis (which has allowed greater access to amniotic fluid for cytogenetic and biochemical assessment of the fetus), and biochemical, behavioral, and electronic fetal monitoring.

Several circumstances exist in which the fetus might be in jeopardy that demand evaluation of fetal status. Such instances range from the first-trimester patient with a threatened abortion, with whom there is need to determine the viability of the pregnancy, to midtrimester pregnancy studies to determine congenital anatomical and chromosomal disorders. In the third trimester, serial evaluations are necessary in chronic maternal disorders such as diabetes and hypertension as well as in more acute problems such as preeclampsia and the postdate pregnancy. The application of sophisticated tests to determine fetal condition currently is limited to women with a determined fetal risk, whereas normal pregnancies are evaluated largely by clinical means. Some or all of these techniques may soon be routinely applied as a form of antenatal screening.

The action to be taken when the fetus at risk is definitely in jeopardy is determined by the period of gestation. If the pregnancy is determined to be nonviable in the first trimester, the uterus can be evacuated. This is basically an all-or-none evaluation. In the midtrimester, with a previable fetus, assessment of well-being is of variable moment. There are some instances in which in utero medical, surgical, and pharmacologic therapy can be directed toward the fetus, thereby allowing the pregnancy to continue. Many of these approaches, however, are investigative in nature. If in utero fetal therapy is not initiated, there may be no recourse if serious fetal problems are uncovered during the second trimester of pregnancy, given the fact that delivery is unacceptable. Fetal evaluations performed in the third trimester can present the perinatal health care team with a choice between delivery of a potentially viable premature infant or pro-

longation of intrauterine life with the risk of fetal death. When the indications of in utero jeopardy are severe, the decision to deliver often results in the birth of a seriously ill newborn and a potential neonatal death. More commonly, however, the studies are reassuring and permit prolongation of the pregnancy.

Advances in fetal assessment have led to advances in understanding that permit significant, albeit limited, treatment of the fetus beyond simply converting the fetus to a newborn. The proliferation of technology has been accompanied by a parallel rapid growth in the number and types of specialized professional and supportive personnel in the broad area of perinatology. Subspecialties have evolved for both maternal-fetal medical specialists and neonatologists. Obstetric anesthesia has emerged as a growing and well-defined area of study. Training programs have been developed for perinatal nurse clinicians, and the concept of the perinatal team has become well established. Such a team includes the obstetrician, neonatologist, anesthesiologist, nurse specialist, nutritionist, genetics counselor, social worker, and other supporting consultants. It is the combined efforts of this team that has resulted in a decrease in the incidence of perinatal morbidity and mortality.

■ NONINVASIVE METHODS OF FETAL DIAGNOSIS

Ultrasound

Only with the development of ultrasound was a noninvasive, direct visualization of the fetus in utero possible. Ultrasound has provided obstetric health caregivers a technique to delineate accurately normal and abnormal fetal anatomy with considerable detail. Fetal parts can be measured for growth and determination of gestational age. Heart motion can be seen and cardiac structure and function assessed. Fetal body and eye movements, breathing, sucking, swallowing, and urination are easily visualized with sonography. Under ultrasound guidance, a needle may be placed into the amniotic cavity, placenta, or the fetus itself in invasive diagnostic procedures such as amniocentesis, chorionic villus sampling, fetal blood sampling, and even tissue sampling, i.e., biopsies.

Ultrasound is the transmission of low-energy, high-frequency sound waves through a medium such as fluid or tissue and the recording of the intensity and the delay time for reflected echoes. A transducer containing piezoelectric crystals, i.e., crystals that vibrate in response to an electronic stimulus and conversely produce an electric signal if vibrated, generates sound waves. As

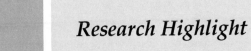

Research Highlight

Antepartum fetal surveillance in the high-risk pregnancy has been shown to reduce significantly both fetal and perinatal mortality. Nearly half of all stillbirths, however, are associated with no identifiable maternal or fetal risk factors. Moore and Piacquadio conducted a prospective study evaluating the effectiveness of a fetal movement screening program in reducing fetal mortality.

From 28 weeks' gestation, 256 low-risk women were asked to record the time interval to appreciate 10 fetal movements between 7:00 PM to 11:00 PM. Subjects who failed to perceive 10 movements in 2 hours were instructed to report for further evaluation.

The mean time interval of monitoring was 30 minutes. During the study period, the number of antepartum tests performed increased 13%. Fetal mortality among patients with decreased movement dropped from 44 per 1000 during the control period to 10 per 1000 births during the study period.

The authors conclude that the count-to-10 fetal movement screening program is a simple and effective method in reducing the rate of fetal demise. Nurses need to educate mothers on procedures of counting fetal movements and the importance of immediately reporting a decrease in fetal activity.

Moore TR, Piacquadio K: A prospective evaluation of fetal movement screening to reduce the incidence of antepartum fetal death. Am J Obstet Gynecol 160:1075–1080, 1989.

sound is generated, it passes through various tissues at different speeds based on the density and elasticity of the tissue structure. In general, the denser the tissue, the higher the velocity of sound transmission. Sound travels through tissue until it comes to another tissue of a different density, a tissue interface (boundary). The change in density results in a small proportion of sound energy being reflected back toward the transducer. The echoes are received by the transducer crystals, converted into electric signals, and displayed on a monitor as dots, the brightness of which reflects the strength of the signal. Traditionally, real-time B-scan can display black areas that are completely devoid of echoes. These regions are called *anechoic* and frequently relate to areas of fluid such as amniotic fluid. Bright white areas are generated by strong reflectors such as bone tissue. Gray areas are generated by small echoes arising from tissues of intermediate density such as cardiac, renal, or brain tissue. Currently, state-of-the-art equipment display signal strengths in 128 shades of gray, and prototype methods are available for color conversion of these images.

Ultrasonic information can be displayed in a variety of ways. Real-time B-scan is the mainstay of obstetric ultrasonic imaging. It displays motion picture–like, two-dimensional, sectional images of the fetal anatomic structure. Real-time scanning also provides a method of visualizing fetal heart activity, fetal behavior, and fetal bladder and stomach filling and emptying. Another display of information used in obstetric ultrasound is M-mode, which yields a group of lines that depict movement of anatomic structures versus time. M-mode provides valuable information about cardiac structure and dynamic changes occurring in the fetal heart. Finally, Doppler ultrasound analyzes data on the frequencies of returning echoes to determine the velocity of moving structures. The primary use of Doppler ultrasound in obstetrics has been to detect and measure blood flow in the uterine arteries and fetal umbilical, carotid, and intracranial vessels.

SAFETY OF ULTRASOUND

Obstetric ultrasound examinations are performed during the most sensitive periods of human growth and development. Diagnostic studies may be conducted during any or all three trimesters of pregnancy, including periods in which a disruption in normal embryonic process may have disastrous effects. Thus, the primary question that has been raised since the inception of obstetric ultrasonography more than 25 years ago is the safety of ultrasound to the fetus and mother. Extensive research has been done examining the possible deleterious effects of ultrasound.

The American Institute of Ultrasound in Medicine issued a report concerning the safety of ultrasound delivered at diagnostic intensities, stating that there has been no independently confirmed evidence of bioeffect of ultrasound delivered at diagnostic intensities.[1] Additionally, they state that "although the possibility exists that such biological effects may be identified in the future, current data indicate that the benefits to patients of the prudent use of diagnostic ultrasound outweigh the risks, if any, that may be present."

In 1984, the National Institutes of Health (NIH) and the US Food and Drug Administration (FDA) convened a Consensus Development Conference of Diagnostic Ultrasound Imaging in Pregnancy.[2] They determined that ultrasound should be performed only when there are firm clinical indications. Table 42-1 lists the indications for obstetric ultrasound as recommended by the NIH panel. These recommendations, however, have been questioned by many authors who advocate routine screening of obstetric patients.

THE ULTRASOUND EXAMINATION

Ultrasound examinations may take one of two forms: the basic examination and the targeted examination.[3] Every patient who undergoes ultrasound assessment should have a basic examination that includes the determination of fetal number, presentation, documentation of fetal life, placental localization, amniotic fluid volume, gestational dating, detection and evaluation of maternal pelvic masses, and a survey of fetal anatomy for gross malformations. This examination is adequate for most obstetric patients and takes an average of 20

TABLE 42-1. SUMMARY OF THE NIH GUIDELINES FOR THE USE OF DIAGNOSTIC ULTRASOUND IN OBSTETRICS

Ovarian follicle development surveillance

Suspected hydatidiform mole

Suspected ectopic pregnancy

Adjunct to cervical cerclage placement

Pelvic mass detected clinically

Suspected uterine abnormality

Intrauterine contraceptive device localization

Suspected fetal death

Suspected multiple gestation

Abnormal serum alpha-fetoprotein value

Suspected polyhydramnios or oligohydramnios

Follow-up observation of identified fetal anomaly

History of previous congenital anomaly

Adjunct to amniocentesis

Estimation of gestational age:
    1. In patients who are late registrants for prenatal care
    2. In patients who are to undergo elective termination of pregnancy

Evaluation of fetal growth
    1. In patients who have an identified etiology for uteroplacental insufficiency leading to intrauterine growth retardation
    2. In patients when macrosomia is suspected

Significant uterine size–clinical dates discrepancy

Serial evaluation of fetal growth in multiple gestation

Estimation of fetal weight and/or presentation in premature rupture of membranes and/ or premature labor

Vaginal bleeding of undetermined etiology

Suspected abruptio placentae

Biophysical profile for fetal well-being

Adjunct to special procedures

Adjunct to external version

Determination of fetal presentation in labor when the presenting part cannot be adequately assessed

Observation of intrapartum events

(Modified from Shearer MH: Revelations: A summary and analysis of the NIH Consensus Development Conference on ultrasound imaging in pregnancy. Birth 11:23, 1984)

minutes. However, a patient who has a fetus with a known or suspected defect should be sent for a targeted examination, i.e., an examination that is performed by a sonographer who has more expertise in sophisticated scanning techniques. An examination of this type may take up to 40 minutes to perform.

Obstetric ultrasound may be performed by two techniques: transabdominal scanning or transvaginal scanning. Transabdominal ultrasound is the more traditional method and can be used throughout all trimesters of pregnancy regardless of the size of the pregnant uterus.

In preparing the patient for a transabdominal ultrasound examination in the first trimester of pregnancy, it is important that she be instructed to drink four 8-oz glasses of water 2 hours prior to the examination and not to void. A filled bladder is required for the examination because most pelvic structures are located behind gas-filled loops of bowel. An ultrasound beam is unable to penetrate gas; water, however, is an excellent transmission medium. Bladder distension displaces the bowel out of the pelvis, lifts the uterus from behind the symphysis, and provides an "acoustic window" to the pelvic structures.[4] Bladder filling is not usually necessary for the second and third trimester scans because at this gestation there normally is sufficient amniotic fluid to serve as an acoustic window and the expanded uterus pushes the intestines out of the way. One of the exceptions to this is when a patient is undergoing sonographic examination for placental localization.

On arrival for a transabdominal scan, the patient does not have to change into a special gown. She should be instructed to lie supine on the examining table and either lift or lower her clothing to expose her abdomen from the costal margin to the symphysis. From approximately 20 weeks' gestation on, the patient should be observed for symptoms of supine hypotension that could result from compression of the vena cava by the enlarged uterus. These symptoms include sudden onset of faintness, dizziness, nausea, ringing in the ears, and numbing of the extremities. Immediate treatment of this phenomenon involves turning the patient on her left side to alleviate the compression.

After the patient is comfortably situated on the examining table, coupling gel is generously applied to the patient's abdomen to eliminate the air interface between the transducer and the patient's skin. Even though the gel is usually water soluble and does not stain, a towel or sheet should be provided to the patient to protect her clothing. Ultrasound gel is notoriously cold, and gel warmers can be used to ease patient discomfort.

Transvaginal ultrasound scanning consists of placing an elongated ultrasound transducer within the vagina to visualize the pelvic structures. One of the advantages of transvaginal ultrasound over abdominal scanning is that no acoustic window is required for transvaginal scanning. Patients, therefore, do not have to fill their bladders and may find this technique more comfortable. A second advantage is that the transvaginal probe is closer to the pelvic structures than the abdominal transducer, allowing these structures to be visualized more clearly.[5] This technique is especially useful in obese women, women with abdominal wall scarring, or patients who display interfering bowel gas. Obstetric indications for transvaginal scanning include documentation of early intrauterine pregnancy, identification of early ectopic pregnancy, assessment of embryonic development and detection of anomalies, and cervical incompetence.[6] Transvaginal ultrasound has limited use in fetal anatomic visualization and biometrics measurements after 16 weeks' postmenstrual age, being used primarily to evaluate the presenting fetal part in mid to late pregnancy.

No preexamination preparation is involved in transvaginal scanning. Upon arrival for the examination, the patient is asked to remove any clothing below the waist. She is placed in a lithotomy position, or a pillow may be placed under her buttocks to raise the pelvic area. A transducer sheath or a condom partially filled with coupling gel is placed over the vaginal transducer. A lubricant can be placed over the outside of the transducer sheath for ease of insertion. The transducer is then inserted through the introitus and into the midvagina. A female chaperon should be present when the transvaginal scan is performed. At the end of the examination, the condom is removed and the transducer is cleaned with Cidex or some other disinfectant.[6]

Important to any ultrasound examination is documentation of the study. A written report of the ultrasound findings should be included in the patient's medical record. The report should contain any measurements made as well as the anatomic findings observed during the examination. A permanent record of ultrasound images obtained during the examination should be added to the patient's record. There are various recording devices that can produce a record of an ultrasound examination. A multiformat camera uses x-ray film, which requires developing. Nine images can be recorded on a single sheet of film. Instant-film cameras, such as a Polaroid, are a common method of recording images. The major disadvantage of this method is the expense of the film; the cost per picture ranges from $0.75 to $0.95. A popular method of recording images is a video image recorder. This device records images on a sheet of thermal paper, resulting in a good-quality picture at a relatively inexpensive cost, i.e., approximately $0.06 per picture. Dynamic imaging as obtained by real-time ultrasound can be saved on a video recorder. The value of this device is that complete ultrasound examinations can be recorded and referred to another physician for a second opinion. Lastly, ultrasound images can be saved on computer discs, allowing approximately ten images per disc. The major disadvantage of this method is that it is time consuming. Whatever method is used for recording an ultrasound examination, the images should be labeled with the patient's name and the date of the examination.

CLINICAL APPLICATIONS OF ULTRASOUND

Detection of Early Intrauterine Pregnancy. Ultrasound in the first 11 postmenstrual weeks can have a significant role in the diagnosis of early intrauterine pregnancy and embryonic life. In a normal pregnancy, the gestational sac can routinely be detected with transvaginal ultrasound between 4 and 5 postmenstrual weeks.[7] The mean sac diameter should be measured; in a normally developing pregnancy, the sac should be 5 mm at 5 weeks.[8] The accuracy of the mean sac diameter for dating purposes is ±2 weeks.[9] During the middle of the fifth postmenstrual week, the embryo measures between 2 and 5 mm. After 6 postmenstrual weeks, heart pulsations can be detected with vaginal ultrasound, whereas abdominal ultrasound may detect heart motion between 7 and 8 weeks. By the end of the ninth week of development, the embryonic head, body, and extremities can clearly be identified with either abdominal or vaginal ultrasound, and fetal movements are clearly recognizable by this time. Deviation from normally identified sonographic signs could indicate complications of early pregnancy, such as blighted ovum, incomplete or complete abortion, or anembryonic pregnancy.[10]

Fetal Measurements. Sonographic measurement of the fetus throughout pregnancy is important in determining the gestational age of the fetus, evaluating fetal growth to identify of intrauterine growth retardation, and detecting congenital malformations. During the ultrasound examination, measurements are made with electronic calipers as the sonographer identifies the desired fetal part. Various tables and nomograms have been created to describe normal growth of various fetal parameters and can be located in any basic clinical ultrasound book.

CROWN-RUMP LENGTH. The crown-rump length (CRL) is the longest demonstrable length of the embryo or fetus, excluding the limbs and yolk sac.[11] The CRL is considered to be one of the most accurate indicators of fetal age due to the excellent correlation between length and age in early pregnancy when growth is rapid and minimally affected by pathologic disorders. The CRL can be used reliably until 12 weeks' gestation, after which a linear measurement of the fetus is difficult because of increasing flexion and extension of the fetal trunk. For purposes of dating, the accuracy of the CRL is ±3 days from 7 to 10 weeks' gestation and ±5 days betweens 10 and 14 weeks.[12]

MEASUREMENTS OF THE FETAL HEAD. The biparietal diameter (BPD) is the maximum distance between the two fetal parietal bones. It is one of the most widely used measurements in obstetric ultrasound because it is easy to obtain, has a distinctive appearance, and provides a relatively accurate measurement.[10] The BPD is used in determining gestational age and fetal weight and diagnosing anomalies such as microcephaly and hydrocephaly. The measurement is taken at the widest portion of the fetal skull with the thalamus positioned midline (Fig. 42-1).[13] The BPD can be measured as early as 9 to 10 weeks' gestation when the head can be differentiated from the rump; however, at this time, the internal anatomy of the head is not consistently visualized. This measurement can be used reliably by 12 weeks when internal structures of the head are routinely identified. Accuracy of the BPD decreases with increasing gestational age owing to shaping of the fetal head, growth disturbances, and individual variation. At 16 weeks' gestation, the BPD has an accuracy of ±5 to 7 days, whereas at more than 28 weeks' gestation, the accuracy is ±3 weeks.

Cephalic index (CI) is the ratio of the BPD to occipitofrontal diameter (OFD). The CI is used to determine if the shape of the fetal head is normal. During the course of pregnancy, pressure from the maternal parts, such as the ribs or pelvic bones, or tumors can result in an abnormal shaping of the fetal head. The fetal head can become dolichocephalic (flattened and elongated) or brachycephalic (short and widened). If these conditions occur, the BPD should not be used to determine gestational age. In normal conditions, the CI

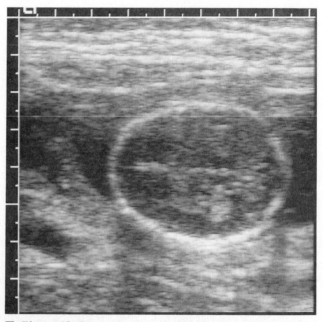

■ *Figure 42-1*
Normal fetal biparietal diameter (BPD).

ranges between 0.70 and 0.86 and should remain constant throughout pregnancy.[14]

Head circumference (HC) in the fetus can be computed from measurements of the BPD and the OFD (HC = [BPD + OFD] × 1.57) or directly measured with a digitizer, map reader, or the assistance of computer software installed in state-of-the-art ultrasound equipment. The HC is not affected by abnormal head shape as is the BPD; therefore, it can be used to determine gestational age. It is also used in the diagnosis of intrauterine growth retardation (IUGR) and various anomalies such as microcephaly.

MEASUREMENTS OF THE FETAL BODY. Abdominal circumference (AC) is used as a parameter in the diagnosis of IUGR. It is an estimation of the size of the fetus at the level of the liver. The measurement of the abdomen is taken at this location because the fetal liver is the organ that will be most severely affected in growth-retarded fetuses.[4] The AC also reflects subcutaneous fat, which has an influence on fetal weight. AC is also used in the determination of gestational age. As in HC, the AC can be measured mechanically, electronically, or computationally (AC = [transverse diameter of the abdomen + anteroposterior diameter] × 1.57). The AC should be measured at the level of the left portal vein.

MEASUREMENT OF THE FETAL EXTREMITIES. Fetal long bones are good indicators of fetal growth because the bones are not subject to changes in shape due to pressure or position. Although all long bones of the fetus can be identified and measured with real-time ultrasound, the femur length (FL) is the most widely used parameter. The fetal femur is the largest, easiest to identify, and least movable of the long bones of the fetal body. It is also one of the most reproducibly measured structures obtained in obstetric ultrasound. FL is used as a parameter in determining gestational age and is considered to be as accurate as the BPD by some investigators.[15,16] It is also used in the diagnosis of skeletal dysplasias. The femur is measured from the origin to the distal end of the shaft (Fig. 42-2) and can be obtained as early as 10 weeks' gestation.

Determination of Fetal Age. Although it is customary to use Nägele's rule to determine the period of gestation and estimated date of confinement (EDC) from the first day of the last menstrual period, this method is fraught with error for various reasons. In at least 20% of women, menstrual age is not a reliable factor in determining gestational age because of oligomenorrhea, bleeding in the first trimester, becoming pregnant after the use of oral contraceptive, or during the postpartum period. In addition, there are a significant number of women who fail to remember exact dates. In these women, only 70% delivered within ±2 weeks of their EDC.[17] Physical measurements, such as fundal height, have an increasing inaccuracy as the woman approaches term. In the first trimester, a physical examination may predict fetal age to ±2 weeks; by the third trimester, the fundal height may vary by as much as ±4 to 6 weeks.[18] In the case of an uncomplicated pregnancy, not knowing the exact length of gestation may not represent a serious problem. In the high-risk mother for whom timing of the delivery is critical, however, the information is vital.

Real-time ultrasound has become the gold standard for the determination of gestational age. There are, however, some constraints on the use of ultrasound as a dating tool. As a rule, the most accurate sonographic measurements of gestational age are those made early in pregnancy before individual growth patterns have

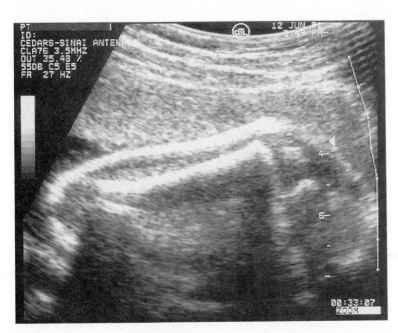

■ *Figure 42–2*
Normal fetal femur.

much effect on the fetus. These individual patterns emerge in the third trimester of pregnancy and account for the lack of precision in sonographic dating after 28 weeks' gestation. Second, although any of the published fetal size–age nomograms can be used for dating purposes, some differences in normal growth patterns may exist owing to environmental and genetic factors such as altitude and race. Even though in most instances these differences are small, ideally, nomograms should be developed for each specific population being served. This, however, is not always practical or possible. It would behoove the examiner, therefore, to select nomograms that were generated from a population that most closely mirrors the population being examined.

Other than crown-rump length, a single morphometric measurement is not accurate for dating purposes, especially during the third trimester of pregnancy. An average of sonographically determined ages of multiple fetal parameters (BPD, HC, AC, and FL) have been found to yield a more accurate estimation of fetal age throughout gestation than any single parameter used alone.[19] Using multiple parameters tends to minimize operator errors and limitations in instrumentation and average out normal individual variations in fetal anatomy.[20]

Determination of Fetal Growth

INTRAUTERINE GROWTH RETARDATION. One of the most commonly recognized abnormalities of the fetus is *intrauterine growth retardation* (IUGR), a term applied to the clinical syndrome in which the fetus fails to prosper in utero. It is known to be a compounding factor in one out of four stillbirths.[21] It occurs in 5% to 10% of fetuses and carries up to a sevenfold increased risk of perinatal mortality and significant morbidity.[22] Additionally, 25% of IUGR fetuses have been noted to have long-term neurologic deficits.[23]

IUGR has been defined in a variety of ways. Fetuses with an estimated weight below the 10th percentile are commonly classified as growth retarded; however, an estimated fetal weight below the 3rd percentile has also been used to define IUGR. Streeter and Manning[24] demonstrated a progressive increase in the incidence of serious morbidity as birthweight percentile decreased. Their results ranged from a morbidity of less than 10% in the 5th to 10th percentile to as high as 36% below the 5th percentile. Thus, if 3rd percentile is accepted as the cutoff for normal growth, a higher percentage of abnormal fetuses will be missed than if cutoff is set at the 10th percentile. Conversely, if the 10th percentile cutoff is accepted, more normal fetuses will be followed with high-risk management than necessary. Most institutions follow the conservative definition of IUGR as estimated fetal weight below the 10th percentile.

There are two types of abnormal growth patterns commonly recognized. Asymmetrical IUGR occurs when the fetus grows normally until the third trimester.

After 28 weeks' gestation, growth of the fetal trunk slows relative to head growth, a result of "brain sparing." Brain sparing results from a hypoxemic reflex redistribution of cardiac output. Preferential channeling of oxygen and nutrient rich blood from the placenta to the brain results in an increased cerebral blood flow and a reduction in perfusion of the kidney and lung, which results in diminished amniotic fluid production.[22] The etiology of asymmetrical IUGR is uteroplacental insufficiency due a variety of maternal disorders, including chronic hypertension, collagen vascular disease, chronic renal disease, preeclampsia, and class F/R diabetes. Symmetrical IUGR is a growth lag of both the fetal head and body, i.e., the entire fetus is proportionately small for gestational age. The insult in this disorder occurs within the first trimester and is so severe that the brain is not spared as in asymmetrical IUGR. TORCH infections, congenital malformations, drugs, and chromosomal abnormalities are causative factors of symmetrical IUGR.

Clinical diagnosis of IUGR includes measurement of fundal height, maternal weight gain assessment, and estimation of fetal weight by palpation. These methods have been shown to be insufficiently accurate in identifying the growth-retarded fetus.[25,26] IUGR is clinically undiagnosed in 50% of the cases prior to birth. Accurate diagnosis of IUGR depends on ultrasonic morphometric assessment. Sonographic parameters that are employed in the evaluation of IUGR include BPD, HC, AC, and FL. Additionally, body proportionality indices (e.g., the ratio of the HC to AC) are used in the determination of asymmetrical IUGR. Serial measurements of growth parameters are recommended for all fetuses with proven or suspected IUGR. The interval between examinations varies with gestational age, severity of growth retardation, fetal well-being, and maternal condition at the time of diagnosis. The usual interval between examinations, however, is 2 weeks to minimize biologic variation and measurement error. Estimation of fetal weight (EFW) can be computed by a number of formulas utilizing various sonographic measurements, but it has a ±15% estimate of error[27,28] and therefore is not a reliable independent indicator of IUGR.

LARGE-FOR-GESTATIONAL-AGE FETUS. The fetus at risk for macrosomia, the large-for-gestational-age (LGA) fetus, presents a number of problems for the obstetric team. Fetuses who are suspected of being LGA are at risk for intrapartum complications, including cephalopelvic disproportion, shoulder dystocia and asphyxia. The detection of the LGA fetus provides the obstetric team with information for selecting the timing and route of delivery.[29] Etiologic factors of macrosomia include diabetes, postdatism, maternal obesity, and previous delivery of a macrosomic infant. Macrosomia, defined as birthweight in excess of 4000 to 45000 g, is present in 1% of all deliveries. Sonographic growth parameters used to diagnosis LGA include BPD, AC, and EFW.

EFW, however, is biased toward underestimation of true weight in LGA fetuses. As in evaluation of growth retardation, fetuses with suspected LGA should have serial scans to assist in the obstetric management of these patients.

Detection of Congenital Anomalies. A congenital anomaly consists of a departure from the normal anatomical structure of an organ or system. Major structural anomalies are identified in 7% of newborns and account for 20% of perinatal deaths.[30,31] Infants with nonlethal malformations may require major surgery and have neurologic abnormalities and psychiatric deficits that impose an economic burden on society and significant financial and emotional stresses on their families. For these reasons, the detection of congenital anomalies is considered an important goal of prenatal care.

Antenatal detection of fetal malformations is not performed for the purpose of termination of undesirable pregnancies. Although the recognition of fetal anomalies can provide parents with an opportunity to interrupt pregnancy if they desire, prenatal diagnosis enhances the obstetric management of the dysmorphic pregnancy in several ways. It allows a predelivery consideration of referral for a prepared delivery at a perinatal center that can provide immediate care for neonatal medical and surgical problems. Prenatal diagnosis can result in further testing, such as chromosome analysis or magnetic resonance imaging, which can better define the anomaly. Parents can be afforded prebirth counseling to prepare them for the appearance and postnatal care of their affected infant. Heroic intrapartum interventions can be avoided if the anomaly is demonstrated to be lethal, as in the case of anencephaly and acardia. Lastly, early antenatal detection can result in the initiation of in utero fetal therapy if appropriate.

Ultrasound plays a key role in the management of developmental anomalies. All ultrasound examinations should include a detailed review of fetal anatomy. The sonographer focuses on the recognition of a departure from normal fetal anatomy (Fig. 42-3) such as the absence of a normal structure (Fig. 42-4); the presence of an abnormal structure; a disruption of the shape, size, or location of a normal structure; abnormal measurements; or abnormal fetal motion.[32] Accuracy of diagnosis is based on the gestational age at the time of the examination. Many malformations are not apparent until 16 to 18 weeks' gestation, and others may not be expressed until much later. A scan in early pregnancy, therefore, does not exclude the presence of anomalies. Accuracy of the examination is also affected by the index of the sonographer's suspicion at the time of the examination. An examination of the fetal spine will be more detailed in a patient with an elevated maternal serum alpha-fetoprotein than a routine scan for gestational age determination. Finally, the accuracy of detection varies with the expertise of the sonographer.

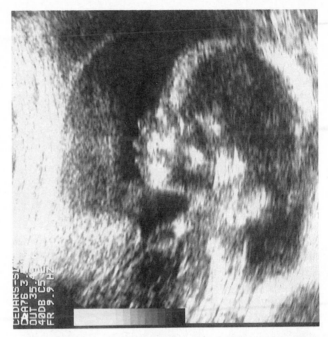

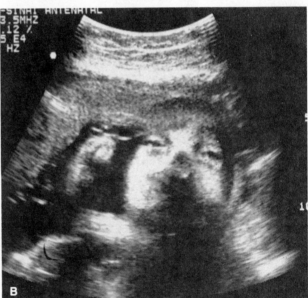

■ *Figure 42–3*

(A) *Fetal facial profile showing normal contour. An abnormal profile could be indicative of a number of abnormalities such as micrognathia. (B) Ultrasound image of the face used to visualize the retinas of the fetus. Fetal eye movements can be detected as early as 16 weeks' gestation.*

Sonographer experience, as well as recent advances in ultrasound technology, has permitted the detailed prenatal diagnosis of multiple congenital anomalies. If the anomalies fit a pattern, chromosomal studies are warranted. Obstetric management and patient counseling on the prognosis of morbidity and mortality may alter with a diagnosis of a lethal aneuploidy such as trisomy 18. Suggestive markers of the aneuploidic fetus include abnormalities of the hands, feet, and limbs (Fig. 42-5),[33–37] abnormalities of the face and head,[35] diaphrag-

■ *Figure 42-4*
Ultrasound can be used to detect a number of congenital anomalies. (A) Severe hydrocephalus. Lack of visualization of the normal internal structures of the fetal brain in conjunction with ventricular dilatation and macrocephaly are indicative of this congenital disorder. (B) Anomalies also can be detected by the presence of an abnormal structure. Transverse scan of the fetal abdomen at the insertion of the umbilical cord illustrates an omphalocele. Fetal intestines can be seen within the umbilical cord. The umbilical vein, viewed with color flow Doppler imaging, surrounds the abnormally placed bowel.

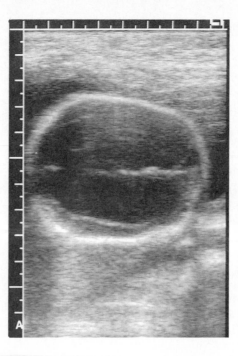
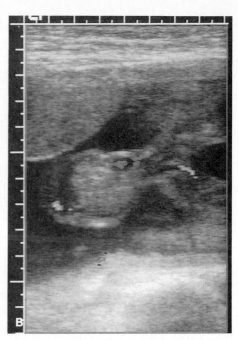

matic hernia,[35] thickened nuchal skin folds,[38] congenital heart defects,[39,40] and fetal choroid plexus cysts.[41]

Assessment of the Fetal Environment

AMNIOTIC FLUID ASSESSMENT. Ultrasound assessment of amniotic fluid plays a crucial role in pregnancy assessment. In the last decade, there have been several reports documenting the methodology of measurement of amniotic fluid. One of the most common methods is

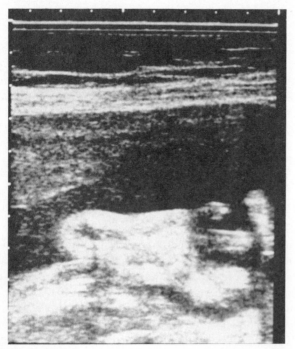

■ *Figure 42-5*
Wide spacing of the second toe on the foot of a fetus diagnosed with Trisomy 18.

the single measurement of the vertical axis of the largest pocket of amniotic fluid.[42,43] In this method, decreased fluid (oligohydramnios) is defined as an amniotic fluid pocket measurement < 2 cm (<3 cm in some institutions), whereas increased fluid (hydramnios) is described as a single vertical amniotic fluid pocket ≥ 8 cm. A technique that has recently gained popularity is a four-quadrant approach called the *amniotic fluid index* (AFI).[44] The AFI involves dividing the maternal abdomen into four quadrants using the umbilicus and linea nigra as the horizontal and vertical reference points of division. Holding the ultrasound transducer perpendicular to the floor, the vertical diameter of the largest pocket of amniotic fluid is identified and measured. The numbers from each quadrant are summed, the result of which is the AFI (Fig. 42-6). For clinical purposes, decreased amniotic fluid is defined by an AFI ≤ 5 cm, whereas increased amniotic fluid is an AFI ≥ 24 cm.[45]

Oligohydramnios is associated with postterm gestation, IUGR, renal dysfunction, obstructive uropathy, and rupture of membranes. Oligohydramnios predisposes the fetus to cord compression, which can lead to fetal distress in labor or fetal demise. If prolonged, decreased fluid can result in fetal pulmonary hypoplasia. Hydramnios is associated with maternal illness such as diabetes and anemia. It is also related to congenital anomalies of the central nervous system (anencephaly) and the gastrointestinal system (tracheoesophageal fistula, upper gastrointestinal tract obstruction); idiopathic macrosomia; hydrops fetalis; and aneuploidy. An increased volume of amniotic fluid can result in preterm labor, premature rupture of membranes, cord prolapse, and perinatal death.

PLACENTA. The placenta is easily assessed by ultrasound and is used in the diagnosis of placenta previa and abruptio placentae as discussed in Chapter 33.

AMNIOTIC FLUID INDEX
AFI = 15.0 cm

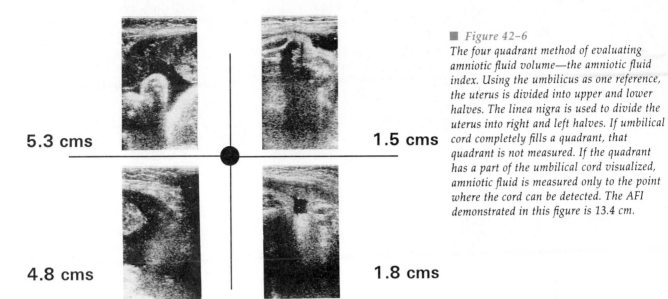

5.3 cms

1.5 cms

4.8 cms

1.8 cms

■ *Figure 42–6*
The four quadrant method of evaluating amniotic fluid volume—the amniotic fluid index. Using the umbilicus as one reference, the uterus is divided into upper and lower halves. The linea nigra is used to divide the uterus into right and left halves. If umbilical cord completely fills a quadrant, that quadrant is not measured. If the quadrant has a part of the umbilical cord visualized, amniotic fluid is measured only to the point where the cord can be detected. The AFI demonstrated in this figure is 13.4 cm.

The most common abnormality of the placenta assessed with ultrasound is variation in size in certain high-risk pregnancies. The placenta may be markedly enlarged in cases of hemolytic disease of the newborn, diabetes, and anemia due to edema of the chorionic villi.[46] Placentas from preeclamptic mothers tend to be smaller than the norm. The observations of the size of placentas may assist in diagnosing the presence and severity of these diseases.

Placental maturational changes can be evaluated during the sonographic examination. Placental calcium deposition is a normal physiologic process that occurs throughout pregnancy. The incidence of placental calcification increases exponentially with increasing gestational age, beginning around 29 weeks' gestation. Calcium is deposited in the basal and chorionic plate, as well as in the perivillous and subchorionic spaces. A sonographic grading system (grade 0 to grade III) has been developed to describe the presence of echogenic areas within the placenta: grade 0 is the least calcified placenta, and grade III demonstrates significant calcification.[47] Placental grading in conjunction with BPD and FL has been used as a noninvasive method to evaluate fetal lung maturity and determine the timing of elective deliveries.

MULTIPLE GESTATION. Assessment of the uterine environment includes the determination of the number of fetuses in utero. Ultrasound is used to diagnosis multiple pregnancies and conjoined twins. It is also used to assess characteristics of the placenta and membrane, providing information about zygosity and relative risks. Monoamniotic twins have an increased incidence of fetal wastage.[48] Twin-to-twin transfusions resulting from placental arteriovenous anastomoses may occur in monochorionic twins. The donor twin is usually growth retarded and has a marked reduction of amniotic fluid. The recipient twin may suffer from complications of overperfusion such as cardiomegaly, fetal hydrops, and polyhydramnios.

M-MODE ECHOCARDIOGRAPHY

Real-time directed M-mode echocardiography is a useful supplement to cross-sectional (real-time B-scan) imaging for evaluating myocardial wall thickness, chamber dimension, and valve and wall motion (Fig. 42-7).[49–51] M-mode is used in the detection of fetal arrhythmias, congenital heart block, and congenital heart defects, such as tetralogy of Fallot.[52] The most common fetal arrhythmias are premature atrial contractions and premature ventricular contractions. They are usually benign in healthy fetuses.[53] Supraventricular tachyarrhythmias (paroxysmal atrial tachycardia, atrial flutter), however, can be lethal. Unless maternally treated with digoxin and/or other antiarrhythmic drugs, in utero heart failure can occur resulting in pericardial effusion, fetal hydrops, and death.[54]

DOPPLER ULTRASOUND

Doppler ultrasound technology is based on the Doppler effect; i.e., when a sound wave of a defined frequency is reflected from moving matter, the shift in reflected frequency provides a measure of the speed of move-

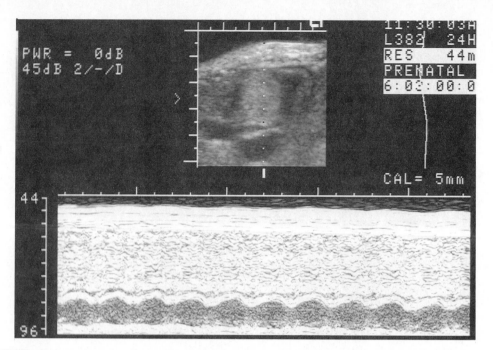

■ *Figure 42–7*
Movement of the cardiac valves and walls can be studied using M-mode ultrasound of the fetal heart. This case demonstrates a fetal cardiac tumor (rhabdomyoma).

ment. The Doppler effect has applications in everyday life ranging from police radar detectors to home burglar alarms. In obstetrics, Doppler detects the movement of red blood cells in vessels and is used to measure blood velocity and flow.

Currently, the implementation of Doppler ultrasound is achieved in three modes: (1) continuous wave Doppler, (2) pulsed wave Doppler, and (3) two-dimensional Doppler color-flow imaging. In continuous wave Doppler, the transducer contains two piezoelectric crystals, one for the transmission of sound, the other for reception of the echo. The frequency of the received echo is compared to the frequency of the transmitted echo to derive the Doppler shift. Any motion within the region of the overlapping beams is capable of producing the shift. Continuous wave Doppler is, therefore, unable to measure the depth or range, i.e., the source, of the shift.[55]

In pulsed wave Doppler, the transducer contains a single crystal that both emits short bursts of sound and receives the reflected signals after a variable time delay during the interpulse interval. In general, pulsed wave Doppler transmits a signal 0.1% of the time while receiving returning signals 99.9% of the time. The location, range, or depth of the sound, can be determined by adjusting the gate, i.e., the sending and receiving times for the crystal.[55] A duplex ultrasound system combines pulsed wave Doppler with real-time imaging to directly visualize and sample vessels at specific anatomical locations.

Whereas pulsed wave Doppler is based on a range-gated signal at a single location at a time, color-flow Doppler image uses multiple gates, measuring mean frequency shifts at multiple points and at multiple ranges. The resulting information is represented as color-coded flow patterns superimposed on real-time images of fetal anatomy (Fig. 42-8).[55] The choice of color assignment for the received echo is determined by the direction of motion with respect to the transducer. Conventionally, a red color is assigned to designate flow toward the transducer and a blue color to flow away from the transducer. Because color assignment depends only on flow direction, tortuous vessels will vary in color assignment as their orientation with respect to the transducer changes.

A Doppler waveform of a vessel represents the velocity waveform, which in turn reflects the upstream and downstream circulatory condition, i.e., systole and diastole. These waveforms have been described in several ways, the most common of which use qualitative ratios to eliminate inaccuracies of Doppler measurements. Doppler measurements relate maximum frequencies observed during end diastole (D) to those noted during peak systole (S). These include the simple S/D ratio, the Pourcelot's resistance index (RI = $[S - D]/S$), and the pulsatility index (PI = $[S - D]$/mean value of the maximum frequencies).

Doppler has been used to measure the velocity in several vessels in the maternal-fetal unit, including the intracerebral, renal, internal iliac, femoral and umbilical arteries. The widest application of Doppler in obstetrics is umbilical artery Doppler studies, which measure the velocity of blood returning from the fetus to the placenta. During pregnancy, flow in the umbilical artery is determined primarily by cardiac contractility upstream and by placental impedance downstream. Increasing volume flow in the umbilical circulation is related to a decrease in vascular resistance. Thus, as gestation ad-

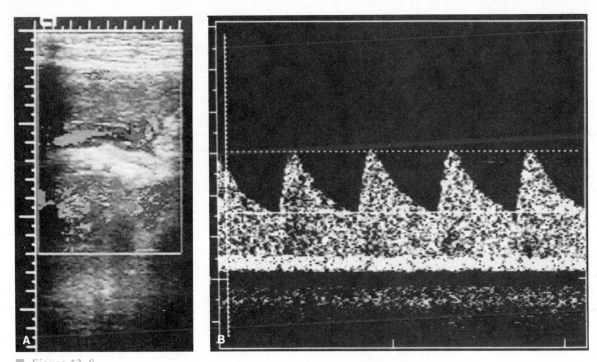

■ *Figure 42–8*

Doppler velocity waveforms. (A) Color flow Doppler imaging is used to detect a location for amniocentesis. When only real-time B-scan was utilized, the top colored area appeared black, seeming to contain only amniotic fluid. Color flow imaging demonstrates that this pocket is packed with umbilical cord. (B) Normal Doppler waveform of the umbilical artery.

vances, relative flow in diastole increases.[56,57] Approximate values of normal S/D ratios are 4.0 at 20 weeks', 3.0 at 30 weeks', and 2.0 at 40 weeks' gestation.

Studies that compare values of normal fetuses with values from fetuses suspected of being growth retarded have found that if the values are elevated for gestational age, the fetus is more likely to have IUGR.[58] Fetuses with absent end-diastolic velocities in the umbilical artery appear to be at higher risk than the average. These fetuses have an increase in congenital anomalies, perinatal mortality, delivery by cesarean section, and fetal distress.[59,60] Although these reports are promising, the sensitivity of Doppler in the prediction of diagnosis of growth retardation ultrasound ranges from 55%[61] to 78.3%.[58] In an effort to improve the sensitivity of Doppler as a test, other vessels in the fetal circulatory system have been investigated. Internal carotid artery velocities were chosen for study because fetuses with growth retardation are thought to have an increase of blood flow to the brain in asymmetrical growth retardation.[62,63] These studies demonstrated that the proportion of blood flowing during diastole in the cerebral vasculature increased with advancing gestation, whereas there was a decline in diastolic flow in the umbilical circulation in growth retarded fetuses. Although Doppler ultrasound apparently has potential as a quick, noninvasive, and relatively easy diagnostic tool in predicting perinatal outcome, additional prospective studies are needed prior to the widespread clinical use.

Color-flow imaging is the most recent of Doppler techniques to be used in obstetrics. A number of established uses of this diagnostic modality have been identified. Color Doppler can be used in the evaluation of placenta previa by better determining what portion of the placenta is in continuity with the cervix. Imaging of the placenta with color can also be used to trace out the fetal circulation in multiple gestations in which a twin-to-twin transfusion is suspected. Color is valuable in umbilical cord identification as an adjunct to percutaneous umbilical blood sampling and amniocentesis. In the former procedure, it is essential that the proper sampling site on the cord is penetrated, whereas in the latter, it is equally important that the umbilical cord should be devoid of puncture. Several congenital anomalies can be detected with color-flow imaging. These include intracranial anomalies such as hydrocephalus, renal anomalies, and anomalies of the umbilical cord or vein. Doppler color-flow imaging is also used in fetal echocardiography to detect intracardiac and great vessel flow disturbances and diagnose structural malformations of the heart.

Magnetic Resonance Imaging

Obstetric magnetic resonance imaging (MRI) is a new noninvasive diagnostic tool that provides high-resolution cross-sectional images of soft tissues in the reproductive system, including the fetus, placenta, and uterus. MRI is dependent on the physical property of nuclear magnetism, which is possessed by some but not all atomic nuclei. The presence of a nuclear magnetic moment is dependent on the structure of the nucleus of an atom. Nuclei without magnetic moments will not be visible by MRI. This is why structures like bone are not seen on MRI. MRI uses information from nuclear magnetic moments to characterize the structure of the tissue being studied.[64] Images are produced using an interaction between hydrogen nuclei, static magnetic fields, and radio waves.[65] The images that are produced are often as precise as can be seen by direct visual examination.

MRI is specifically suited for the detection of soft-tissue abnormalities that cannot be identified by ultrasound. Obstetric applications for MRI include known or suspected hydatidiform mole[66]; placenta previa[67]; fetal anomalies, including hydrocephaly, cystic hygroma, urethral obstruction, hydronephrosis, and anencephaly[68,69]; and IUGR.[70]

The advantages of MRI over ultrasound is that MRI can be used in adverse scanning conditions. These include maternal obesity, overlying bony structures, and gas-filled intestines, which may interfere with optimal sonographic imaging. MRI has a particular advantage over ultrasound in patients with oligohydramnios because ultrasound diagnosis is often difficult in patients with decreased amniotic fluid. Oligohydramnios is not a limiting factor in MRI diagnosis because amniotic fluid is not required for fetal visualization in this technique. On the contrary, decreased amniotic fluid may be a benefit because it can restrict fetal movement, which in itself is a disadvantage in MRI. Other disadvantages of MRI are the expense and the length of the examination, which may be 1 to 2 hours.[65]

A second exciting developing technology of magnetic resonance technology is nuclear magnetic resonance spectroscopy (NMRS). The concentrations of various metabolites (adenosine diphosphate, adenosine triphosphate, and creatinine phosphate) within select target tissue are possible with NMRS and are now being measured in the newborn.[71] It is hoped that the future application of this technique will allow the determination of an in utero asphyxial insult on brain metabolism to assist in the obstetric management of high-risk pregnancies.

■ INVASIVE METHODS OF FETAL DIAGNOSIS

Amniocentesis

Amniocentesis, the oldest prenatal invasive procedure, has been in use for over 100 years. Initial use of am-

niocentesis in the nineteenth century was the treatment of polyhydramnios.[72] Since that time it has been employed in amniography, elective termination of pregnancy, management of isoimmunized pregnancies, diagnosis of chromosomal and metabolic disorders, detection of neural tube defects, evaluation of fetal lung maturity, and detection of intraamniotic infections.

The most common indication for amniocentesis is prenatal diagnosis, followed by the evaluation of lung maturity in the third trimester of pregnancy.

The technical aspects of amniocentesis and related nursing care are discussed in Chapter 14.

Percutaneous Umbilical Blood Sampling

In utero blood sampling has been possible since 1972 when Valenti obtained samples under endoscopic visualization.[73] Prior to 1982, blood sampling was performed by fetoscopy, which is a difficult and invasive technique that has a significant associated fetal risk. In 1983, Daffos and associates were the first to report percutaneous umbilical blood sampling (PUBS), also known as cordocentesis, under direct ultrasound guidance.[74]

Indications for PUBS are risk of fetal hemolytic disease, rapid karyotype, the diagnosis of congenital infection, hemoglobinopathies, coagulopathies, immunodeficiency syndromes, and fetal well-being.[75] Additionally, PUBS is performed to study the development of various fetal biologic parameters. Prior to PUBS, these factors could only be studied in products of abortion. Fetal blood can now be studied for hematologic, biochemical, hemostasis, endocrinologic, immunologic, and acid-base parameters.[76]

PUBS can be performed as either an inpatient or outpatient procedure. Immediately before the procedure, a complete ultrasound examination is performed. The insertion site of the umbilical cord in the placenta is then identified. This site is preferred for sampling because the cord is in its most fixed position and can be punctured more easily at this point. Free-floating cord is more difficult to penetrate because it slips away from the needle. Color-flow Doppler is useful in locating the proper location. The site may be obstructed by the fetus, and, on occasion, it may be necessary to empty or fill the bladder or manipulate the fetus manually to gain access to the umbilical cord.

The maternal abdomen is draped and cleaned with an antiseptic solution. Local anesthesia is used at the puncture site. A 20 or 22 gauge spinal needle is inserted under ultrasonic guidance (Fig. 42-9). Recently, needles designed to optimize sonographic visualization have been used. After the needle enters the cord, the stylet is removed and fetal blood is drawn into a syringe containing a small amount of anticoagulant or normal saline at-

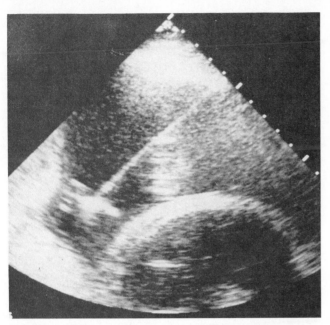

■ *Figure 42–9*
A needle penetrating the umbilical cord in percutaneous
umbilical blood sampling.

tached to the hub of the needle. As soon as blood flows into the syringe and dilutes the solution, this syringe is replaced with a second syringe, which is used for collection purposes. Heparin may be placed in the second syringe if the blood is to be used for blood gas analysis. The amount of blood aspirated depends on the indication for PUBS; it is rarely more than 5 ml. Transfer of the blood to the appropriate tubes should occur immediately after collection. On completion of sampling, the needle is withdrawn and ultrasound is used to determine fetal status. The fetal heart rate is then monitored for 1 to 2 hours following the procedure.[75]

The sampling procedure is relatively short, taking approximately 10 minutes to perform.[76] Complications of PUBS include a spontaneous abortion rate of 0.8%, whereas fetal demise occurs in 1.1% of the procedures. Additional complications associated with the procedure are bleeding from the puncture site, fetal bradycardia, infection, thrombosis of the umbilical vein, and formation of umbilical cord hematoma.[77–80]

Chorionic Villus Sampling

Chorionic villus sampling is an effective method for obtaining living trophoblastic tissue for genetic diagnosis in the first trimester of pregnancy. The tissue can be tested for a rapidly increasing number of biochemical and chromosomal disorders of the fetus. A detailed discussion of chorionic villus sampling is presented in Chapter 14.

Fetal Tissue Sampling

There are several genetic disorders that are not amenable to diagnosis by chromosomal analysis. In these cases, direct sampling of fetal tissue can be performed. Fetal skin sampling is performed if there is a suspicion of genodermatoses, severe skin disorders associated with high rates of morbidity and mortality. In this procedure, biopsy forceps are inserted through an Angiocath. Under continuous ultrasound guidance, the biopsy forceps are used to take fetal skin samples.[81]

Fetal liver biopsy is performed to diagnose inborn errors of metabolism limited to liver enzyme abnormalities. The biopsy is performed under continuous ultrasound guidance. A biopsy needle is inserted directly into the fetal liver, and fetal liver tissue is aspirated.[81]

Tissue sampling techniques are investigational in nature and are not widely used.

■ BIOCHEMICAL ASSESSMENT OF THE FETUS

Maternal Serum Studies

ALPHA-FETOPROTEIN

Since it was first introduced as a method to identify the fetus at risk for a neural tube defect, maternal serum alpha-fetoprotein (MSAFP) screening has now incorporated a whole new area of high-risk patients. This includes those at risk for fetal growth disturbances, preterm labor, and chromosomal disorders.[82,83] A detailed discussion of alpha-fetoprotein can be found in Chapter 14.

HUMAN CHORIONIC GONADOTROPIN

Human chorionic gonadotropin (hCG), a glycoprotein hormone, is exclusively produced during pregnancy. Produced principally in syncytiotrophoblasts, hCG is detectable in maternal plasma soon after implantation. Plasma levels rise rapidly and double in concentration every 1.4 to 2.5 days, peaking at about 10 weeks' gestation, and fall off to relatively low levels in the second and third trimesters. The function of this hormone is to maintain corpus luteum function during early pregnancy.[84] It is the basis for most pregnancy tests.

Values of hCG that deviate from the norm are suggestive of an abnormally developing pregnancy. Abnormally slow production of hCG in early pregnancy is associated with threatened abortion or ectopic pregnancy.[85,86] Fifteen percent of normal intrauterine pregnancies, however, demonstrate a slow production. Ultrasound in conjunction with hCG determinations can be used to differentiate normal from abortive or ectopic pregnancies.[87]

Elevated hCG levels are associated with hydatidiform mole. Values that remain elevated after 100 days of pregnancy are strongly suggestive of a molar pregnancy. Values that are increased prior to this period are not necessarily due to a mole but may be due to multiple pregnancy. Evaluation with ultrasound is used to make a differential diagnosis.[87]

Recently it has been demonstrated that hCG levels in midtrimester pregnancies may be predictive of Down syndrome in conjunction with maternal age, maternal serum alpha-fetoprotein levels, and maternal serum estriol levels (see Chapter 14).

ESTROGEN-ESTRIOL

Prior to maternal serum alpha-fetoprotein testing for gestational screening, serial plasma or urinary estriol (E3) determinations were the most widely used markers of fetoplacental well-being. Estrogen levels in maternal serum and urine rise progressively during the course of normal pregnancy. Although estrone and estradiol also increase during pregnancy, it is estriol that is the predominant estrogen, increasing 1000-fold and accounting for 90% of the total estrogen. At least 90% of the estrogen precursors are produced by the fetal adrenal cortex. The conversion of these precursors to estriol is a function of the placenta. The basis of monitoring the fetus with estriol determinations is that if either the fetus or the placenta becomes compromised, decreased production of E3 is expected to occur.[84,88] Abnormal estriol levels have been thought to be a predictor of poor perinatal outcome.

Serum and urine estriol levels have been used extensively in the past to determine fetal condition in a number of high-risk pregnancies, including diabetes, postterm pregnancies, hypertension, preeclampsia, and intrauterine growth retardation. Currently, however, estriol determinations are not used clinically in the obstetric management of these complicated pregnancies.

Maternal serum estriol levels in midtrimester pregnancies may be predictive of Down syndrome in conjunction with maternal age, maternal serum alpha-fetoprotein levels, and hCG levels (see Chapter 14).

PROGESTERONE

Progesterone, a steroid hormone, is produced by the placenta in progressively increasing quantities during pregnancy. It can be measured as serum progesterone or urinary pregnanediol but has little value in evaluating fetal well-being, because progesterone does not require fetal precursors and can, in fact, persist in significant

quantities even after an intrauterine fetal death has occurred.

HUMAN PLACENTAL LACTOGEN

Also known as human chorionic somatomammotropin, human placental lactogen (hPL) is synthesized by the syncytiotrophoblast of the placenta in progressively increasing quantities throughout pregnancy. This hormone presently is not used in clinical management of high-risk pregnancies.

MATERNAL BLOOD ENZYME MEASUREMENT

A number of enzymes increase in concentration in maternal serum during pregnancy, including heat-stable alkaline phosphatase (HSAP), diamine oxidase (DAO), and oxytocinase. The measurement of these enzymes is not currently used in the assessment of fetal well-being.

Amniotic Fluid Studies

PHOSPHOLIPIDS: ASSESSMENT OF FETAL LUNG MATURITY

Assessment of fetal lung maturity has evolved through extensive investigation of fetal pulmonary fluids. Because there are respiratory movements in utero, the composition of amniotic fluid reflects the content of pulmonary fluids. Analysis of amniotic fluid phospholipids is the most accurate method of determining the degree of fetal lung maturity. This analysis is recommended when elective preterm delivery is anticipated or required and when elective term delivery is planned but gestational age is uncertain.

The stability of lung airway spaces is dependent on the presence of adequate amounts of surfactant. Synthesized by the type II pneumocytes in the lung, surfactant promotes lung airway space stability by reducing alveolar surface tension. Although it is present in small quantities from midpregnancy and increases slowly with advancing gestation, the mature pathway for surfactant synthesis is activated at 35 weeks in the normal pregnancy. In certain stressful circumstances, such as preeclampsia, class D and F diabetes, and IUGR, the process is accelerated. In others, such as class A, B, and C diabetes, it may be delayed.

There are several techniques for measuring this activity, including the "Shake" test, lecithin/sphingomyelin (L/S) ratio, latex agglutination of phosphatidylglycerol, and optical density at 650 nm (OD650). The Shake test determines the stability of foam on the surface of mixtures of ethyl alcohol and various dilutions of amniotic fluid (Fig. 42-10). Maturity is indicated when

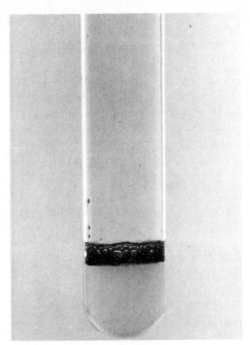

Shake test. Note bubbles on the surface maintained by surfactant in the amniotic fluid.

the foam is stable in the presence of a 2:1 dilution. A kit (Lumadex-FSI Test) that uses these principles but varies the concentrations of ethanol and amniotic fluid has the advantage of being commercially available and prepackaged. Used carefully under controlled conditions, the Shake test has been shown to be quite accurate in predicting lung maturity.

The most widely used technique is the L/S ratio. Lecithin is a major constituent of surfactant. Because the concentration of sphingomyelin remains relatively constant, a rising L/S ratio indicates increasing surfactant production. The separation of lecithin and sphingomyelin is achieved by thin-layer chromatography. The ratio is determined either by visual inspection or by densitometry. Pulmonary maturity is established when the L/S ratio exceeds 2:1. The chances of encountering severe neonatal respiratory distress syndrome with an L/S ratio greater than 2:1 is extremely low.

A specific phospholipid in amniotic fluid, phosphatidylglycerol, has proven to be valuable in borderline instances of the L/S ratio and in women with class A, B, and C diabetes in whom fetal pulmonary maturity is often delayed to 37 weeks or later. The presence of phosphatidylglycerol in more than trace amounts, associated with an L/S ratio of more than 2:1, virtually ensures fetal pulmonary maturity.

Slide agglutination tests for the presence of phosphatidylglycerol are available. They appear to predict reliably the absence of respiratory distress syndrome when positive. When the slide test is negative, perfor-

mance of more definitive test (such as chromatography) is recommended.

Recently, optical density measurement of amniotic fluid has been used as a rapid screening test of lung maturity. The determination of the absorbance of light by amniotic fluid of 650 nm wavelength has been adopted by some institutions.

BILIRUBIN: ASSESSMENT OF THE ISOIMMUNIZED PREGNANCY

Hemolytic disease is one of the complications of pregnancy in which there may be devastating fetal effects with virtually no maternal risk. Although the fetal pathology of severe hemolytic disease had been described before the turn of the century, the exact nature of the problem was not known until after the discovery of the Rh factor in 1940. Most of the attention has been focused on the Rh factor (D antigen) as a cause, but the ABO blood groups may also cause a form of hemolytic disease, as do other lesser blood factors such as Kell, c, E, and C.

There is an overall decline in this disease in the United States. In 1970, the incidence of hemolytic disease in newborns was approximately 45 in 10,000 births. By 1980, it had dropped to 13 in 10,000 births. The majority of new cases result from failure to prevent maternal sensitization by not administering or administering an inadequate dose of Rh immunoglobulin when indicated during the antenatal and postpartum periods.

All pregnant women should be tested for ABO and Rh types and screened for antibodies to these and other red blood cell antigens. Any red blood cell antibody present must be specifically identified and appropriate titers must be obtained to determine whether there is a risk to the fetus. If an antibody is present that is known to cause fetal or newborn hemolytic disease, the father's blood type and zygosity for that antigen should be determined whenever possible.

Anti-D Globulin. The ability to prevent Rh sensitization has been an established fact since Rh (anti-D) globulin became commercially available in 1969. It prevents sensitization by clearing the fetal cells from the maternal circulation and perhaps also by depressing the patient's immune response. A single dose (300 μg) is capable of clearing up to 15 ml of fetal erythrocytes. Microdoses (50 μg) have been made available for use in situations in which only small fetomaternal hemorrhages are likely.

Candidates for Rh immunoglobulin are unsensitized Rh-negative patients who (1) have delivered Rh-positive babies, (2) have had untypeable pregnancies such as stillborns, ectopic pregnancies, or spontaneous or induced abortions, (3) have received ABO-compatible Rh-positive blood, or (4) have had an invasive diagnostic procedure such as amniocentesis. It is of no value in the patient who is already sensitized. It should be administered within 3 days of delivery.

Pathophysiology. Even though the maternal and fetal circulation are normally completely separated, breaks in this barrier permit the entry of fetal red blood cells into the maternal circulation during the second and third trimesters and at delivery in up to 50% of pregnancies. Such breaks also occur with abortions beyond 6 to 8 weeks of pregnancy. Isoimmune hemolytic disease of the fetus and newborn is caused by a fetal-maternal blood group incompatibility, with maternal immunization against a fetal blood group antigen. Maternal antibodies bind fetal circulation and trigger fetal reticuloendothelial system digestion of fetal red blood cells. Deformed cells are removed from circulation and disposed of by hemolysis and phagocytosis. With worsening anemia, the fetus compensates by maximizing red blood cell production. Hemolysis continues, so the anemia remains uncorrected and worsens. In the worse possible case, hydrops fetalis occurs, resulting in ascites, pericardial effusion, cardiac failure, impaired placental circulation, and finally, fetal death.[89]

Management. It has been well established that the severity of the hemolytic anemia in the fetus can be determined by the quantity of bilirubin in the amniotic fluid, i.e., the higher the bilirubin level, the lower the fetal hemoglobin. Thus, amniocentesis with analysis of bilirubin in the fluid is used for making therapeutic decisions in sensitized women. Using spectrophotometry, bilirubin produces an optical density peak at 450 nm, and it is the height of this peak (or OD450) that is used to evaluate fetal involvement (Fig. 42-11). In most laboratories, a significant antibody titer below which fetal morbidity is unlikely can be determined. Although this varies from institution to institution, titers above 1:8 to 1:16 are generally considered significant. Amniocentesis can be instituted as early as 20 weeks' gestation. The frequency of repeated amniocentesis is determined by the level of the OD450, weekly taps being indicated if values are high.

The common method for evaluating OD450 is the Liley chart, which is illustrated in Figure 42-11. Values in the lower zone for the particular gestation indicate a mildly affected or even unaffected fetus, whereas those in the middle zone indicate an affected fetus but one not in the immediate danger of death. Values in the

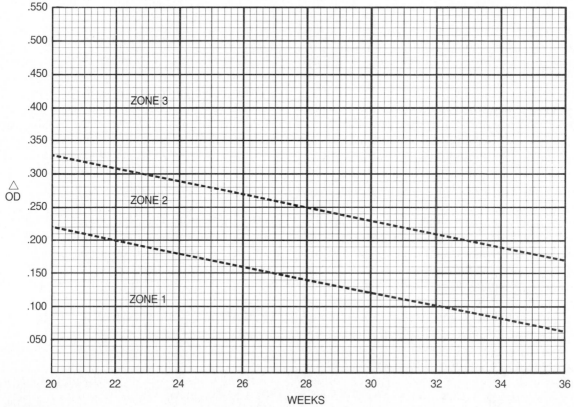

■ *Figure 42-11*
Modified Liley graph for relating OD450 to weeks of gestation in determining the severity of hemolytic disease. (Management of Erythroblastosis [Technical Bulletin, No. 17]. ACOG, Chicago, July, 1972.)

upper zone suggest the fetus will not survive 10 to 14 days without intervention. Management decisions are not based on single values but rather on the trend. If the OD450 remains in the lower zone, no interference is indicated and the pregnancy can be allowed to proceed to term. If the values remain in the middle zone, the fetus is best delivered as soon as there is evidence of maturity. Upper-zone values indicate immediate intervention by delivery if beyond 33 to 34 weeks' gestation or by intrauterine transfusion if before that age.

Ultrasound is a vital element in the management of the isoimmunized fetus. The fetus is examined for signs of congenital abnormalities as well as signs of edema or ascites (Fig. 42-12). Routine measurements are obtained to verify gestational age to assure proper usage of the Liley chart. When measurements are made, any changes in the abdominal circumference that may be due to hepatosplenomegaly are specifically noted. M-mode ultrasound has been found to be effective in identifying pericardial effusions.[90] Doppler ultrasound has several uses in the assessment of the isoimmunized fetus; e.g., affected fetuses have been found to have higher than usual velocities in umbilical arteries when the fetus is anemic,[91] whereas color-flow imaging can be used to visualize the umbilical cord for purposes of fetal blood sampling to diagnose fetal anemia directly.

■ BIOPHYSICAL ASSESSMENT OF THE FETUS

Fetal Behavior

Within the past decade, obstetric medicine has shifted away from the use of maternal clinical and biochemical markers such as fundal height measurements and estriol determinations toward more specific and direct examination of the fetus made possible with the development of high-resolution real-time ultrasound. The ability to visualize directly the fetus and monitor fetal activities and responses to stimuli has provided insight into the functional maturation of the fetal central nervous system. Behavioral patterns (states) and fetal reactions to stimuli indicate that several stages of neurologic organization can be defined in relation to other parameters of intrauterine development. Associated with the direct observation of fetal behavior comes an increasing recognition of fetal disease and the opportunity to effect treatment.

FETAL MOVEMENT

There is a successive development of simple movement involving the entire fetal body to more complex move-

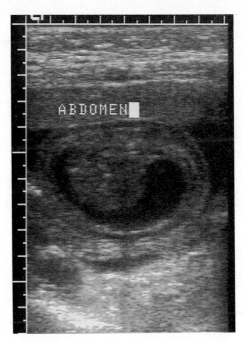

■ *Figure 42–12*
Fetal ascites in a fetus with severe hemolytic disease as detected with ultrasound.

ments of individual fetal parts. Movements can be discerned with ultrasound as early as 7 weeks' gestation. By 8 weeks, general movements of the limbs trunk and head can be appreciated. Hiccoughs are observed as early as 9 weeks, and fetal breathing is initiated at 10 weeks. By 12 weeks of pregnancy, sucking and swallowing are incorporated into the repertoire of fetal movement.[92] All movements that can be identified in the term fetus are present by 15 weeks' gestational age.

What occurs in the second and third trimesters of pregnancy is the development of periodicity of individual movements, fixed combinations of individual movements, and the association of fetal heart rate patterns and fetal motility. In general, there is a normal decrease of movement with increasing gestational age. The maximum incidence of motor activity in the 20 to 22-week fetus is 21%, whereas it is only 10% in the 30 to 40-week fetus. The quality of movement patterns is also age dependent in that the frequency of rest-activity cycles decreases with gestational age. The younger fetus moves an average of 10 minutes, then rests for 9 minutes, thus having three rest-activity periods within a 1-hour interval. The average term fetus, however, will move for 23 minutes, then rest for 40 minutes having only one rest-activity pattern within an hour. Individual variations do occur. Up to 90 minutes may elapse before movement can be detected in a normal fetus. A diurnal rhythmicity of movement develops during the second trimester of pregnancy, with the 24 to 28-week fetus moving more often in the late night–early morning hours (11:00 PM to 8:00 AM). The third trimester fetus, however, has a burst of activity between 9:00 PM to 1:00 AM. Correlations of fetal movements with fetal heart rate have been found as early as 20 to 22 weeks, with this interaction increasing with gestational age. The number and amplitude of fetal heart rate accelerations associated with movements increase as the fetus approaches 32 weeks.[93–96]

FETAL BREATHING MOVEMENTS

Although fetal breathing movements are considered as a preparatory exercise for extrauterine breathing, they are essential for fetal lung growth. Fetal respiratory activity enhances both neuromuscular and skeletal development of the respiratory system and makes the appropriate respiratory epithelial development of the gas-exchanging surfaces of the fetal lung possible.[97] Fetal breathing is detected at 10 weeks' gestation and increases with gestational age. The frequency of breathing decreases, however, as early as 3 days prior to the initiation of labor and persists until delivery. A circadian pattern of fetal breathing appears at 24 weeks' gestation in which breathing occurs more frequently between 11:00 PM and 2:00 AM. The 30 to 39-week fetus has a higher incidence of breathing between 4:00 and 7:00 AM.[98–100]

EFFECTS OF ASPHYXIA ON FETAL BIOPHYSICAL ACTIVITIES

As in the extrauterine patient, asphyxia (insufficient intake of oxygen) produces effects on multiple organ systems in the fetus including the lungs, kidneys, and central nervous system. Signs of fetal asphyxia are dependent on the extent, duration, and chronicity of the asphyxial insult. Acute episodes of asphyxia result in a shunting of blood from the fetal lung and kidney to the brain. If the insult is prolonged, diminished amniotic fluid production occurs owing to decreased urine production and lung fluid flow. If an acute episode of total asphyxia (no oxygen is delivered to the fetus) or a prolonged partial asphyxia occurs, the fetal central nervous system can become affected, resulting in alterations in the frequency and patterning of fetal behavior. In extreme cases, hypotonia, absent fetal breathing, absent fetal movements, and absent heart rate reactivity can progressively be observed. In the human fetus, asphyxia commonly occurs as a result of a chronic reduction in uteroplacental perfusion.

FETAL BEHAVIORAL STATES

Behavioral states are stable periods of specific, fixed combinations of several physiologic variables that recur over time. Well-developed behavioral states are exhibited by the human neonate born at or near term.[101] The assessment of neonatal behavioral states is important because these states influence the responsiveness of the infant during a neurologic examination. Behavioral states are considered to be indicators of the functional condition of the central nervous system.[102]

Behavioral states have been studied in the 32 weeks to term fetus, based on the criteria of body movements, breathing movements, eye movements, and heart rate patterns (Table 42-2). In general, the term fetus spends approximately 98% of the time in either quiet or active sleep (state 1 or state 2), which is similar to the normal newborn. The fetus alternates between these two states over a 20 to 40-minute period. States 3 and 4 (quiet and active awake states) are recognized only 2% of the time.[103,104]

TABLE 42-2. FETAL BEHAVIORAL STATE CRITERIA

State Criteria	State 1F	State 2F	State 3F	State 4F
Body movements	Incidental	Periodic	Absent	Continuous
Eye movements	Absent	Present	Present	Present
Heart rate pattern	Stable, little variability, isolated accelerations	Greater variability than 1F, frequent accelerations	Greater variability than 1F, no accelerations	Unstable, large, and long-lasting accelerations, often fused into sustained tachycardia
Breathing movements	Regular	Irregular	Irregular	Irregular

(Adapted from Nijhuis JG, Prechtl HFR, Martin CB Jr., et al: Are there behavioral states in the human fetus? Early Human Dev 6:177–195, 1982; Nijhuis JG, Martin CB Jr., Gommers S, et al: The rhythmicity of fetal breathing varies with behavioral state in the human fetus. Early Human Dev 9:1–7, 1983.)

The influence of behavioral states on fetal biophysical activities is of major importance in the interpretation of fetal behavior. The observation of normal biophysical activities indicates a functional and therefore nonasphyxiated fetal central nervous system. Consideration of fetal behavioral state is, therefore, unnecessary. In contrast, failure to recognize the presence of normal biophysical activities requires consideration of fetal behavioral state. Differentiating between a normal sleep state and asphyxiation can be determined by extending the observation of the fetus for a period beyond the time for pattern shift or repeating the observation at some later point. In either instance, subsequent observation of normal activities confirms normality, whereas persistent absence of activities suggests asphyxia.

FETAL BIOPHYSICAL PROFILE

Fetal biophysical profile (FBP) scoring is a method of fetal surveillance based on a composite assessment of several markers of fetal disease.[105–107] The basic premise of the FBP is that the observation of a number of biophysical variables is superior in predictive accuracy to that achieved by the observation of any one variable. Thus, the compromised fetus can be better identified by consideration of variables that reflect immediate fetal condition (heart rate reactivity [the nonstress test], fetal movement, fetal breathing, and fetal tone) and a variable that reflects fetal condition over a long period (amniotic fluid volume). Except for fetal heart rate activity, all variables are measured by real-time ultrasound. For scoring purposes, each variable is assigned a score of 2 when normal and a score of 0 when abnormal. The variable is coded as normal whenever fixed criteria (Table 42-3) are reached regardless of the duration of observation, up to a maximum of 30 minutes. The highest possible combined score obtainable is 10. The lowest score that can be observed when all the parameters are abnormal is 0. A combined score of 10 or 8 is regarded as normal. A combined score of 6 is equivocal and indicates that the profile should be repeated within 24 hours. A combined score of 4, 2, or 0 is indicative of fetal compromise and delivery of the fetus should be considered. A deviation in this system is in the case of oligohydramnios. In any fetus with decreased amniotic fluid and intact membranes, and all other FBP variables are normal, delivery is considered at many institutions.[43,108]

Clinical experience with the FBP as a measure of fetal compromise has yielded encouraging results. Manning and associates[107] have reported on FBP results of more than 26,000 high-risk patients and demonstrated that a significant exponential rise in perinatal morbidity as well as mortality occurs with decreasing profile scores. Other prospective studies have shown similar results.[106,109]

MATERNAL PERCEPTION OF FETAL MOVEMENT

Although maternal perception of fetal movement is the oldest and least expensive means of monitoring fetal

TABLE 42–3. CHARACTERISTICS OF THE FETAL BIOPHYSICAL PROFILE

Parameter	Score 2 (Normal)	Score 0 (Abnormal)
Nonstress test	Reactive: 2 or more fetal heart rate accelerations of at least 15 beats per minute in amplitude and at least 15-sec duration in 10 min within a 40-min testing period	Nonreactive: 1 or less fetal heart rate acceleration of at least 15 beats per min and 15-sec duration in 10 min within a 40-min testing period
Fetal breathing movements	At least 1 episode of fetal breathing of at least 30-sec duration in 30-min observational period	Absence of fetal breathing or less than 30 sec of breathing within a 30-min observation period
Fetal body movements	At least 3 discrete episodes of fetal movements in a 30-min period; episodes of active continuous movement counted as a single movement	2 or less discrete fetal movements in a 30-min observation period
Fetal tone	At least 1 episode of extension of extremities, hand, or trunk with return to position of flexion	Extremities in position of extension or partial flexion; spine in position in full extension; fetal movement not followed by return to flexion
Amniotic fluid volume	Amniotic fluid index > 5 cm	Amniotic fluid index ≤ 5 cm

(Modified from Walla CA, Platt LD: Observing fetal maturation through fetal movement and fetal behavior. In Berman M (ed): Diagnostic Medical Sonography, vol I. Obstetrics and Gynecology. Philadelphia, JB Lippincott, 1991)

condition, only recently has it re-emerged as an effective screening tool in both high- and low-risk pregnancies. Several studies have reported that a reduced or total absence of fetal activity is associated with fetal compromise.[110–112]

Numerous protocols have been proposed to record maternal perception of fetal movement. They all involve either (1) counting for a fixed time period and recording the number of movements, or (2) recording the time taken to count a fixed number of movements. One frequently used method is the Cardiff "count-to-ten" chart,[113] which involves having the mother note fetal movements up to a maximum of ten. When ten movements are felt, she discontinues counting. Less than ten movements within a 12-hour period are to be reported to her care provider. Variations on this technique involve a reduction in time defining the counting period to eliminate having abnormal results reported in the evening when further fetal evaluation is difficult to arrange (see Research Highlight).

The effectiveness of this assessment technique is based on several factors. An adequate explanation must be given to the patient on how to keep a movement chart. She must also be instructed on the importance of reporting a reduction in fetal movements.[114] Additionally, maternal compliance is more favorable when counting is for 1 hour or less each day and when her risk factors are specifically defined.[115]

Antepartum Fetal Heart Rate Monitoring

Periodic electronic fetal monitoring during the third trimester has become a common method for evaluating the fetus in a high-risk pregnancy (Table 42-4). As with many other forms of fetal assessment, a normal result is highly accurate in indicating fetal well-being. On the other hand, false-positive results occur with a relatively high frequency. This has required that two or more different tests of fetal well-being be carried out before premature delivery or other remedial measures are instituted.

The observation of changes in fetal heart rate associated with spontaneous or evoked fetal movement has become known as the *nonstress test* (NST). Evaluation of fetal heart rate in the presence of spontaneous or oxytocin-induced contractions is termed the *contraction stress test* (CST) or *oxytocin challenge test* (OCT). The CST was widely applied clinically prior to the more recent development of the NST. The ease of performing the NST (Fig. 42-13) and its apparent reliability as a screening tool have greatly reduced the number of CSTs performed. An example of a clinical protocol for per-

forming these tests is given in the nursing guidelines for these tests.

CONTRACTION STRESS TEST

The CST requires administration of oxytocin by intravenous infusion. Continuous external fetal monitoring is applied, and oxytocin is administered in increasing dosages until uterine contractions occur. The occurrence of repeated late decelerations with contractions is classified as a positive or abnormal test. The lack of late decelerations with each of three contractions during a 10-minute interval is classified as a negative result or a passed test (Fig. 42-14).

Other terms used for classification of tests include *unsatisfactory, suspicious,* and *equivocal.* Unsatisfactory tests occur when interpretable tracings cannot be obtained or the criterion of three contractions in a 10-minute interval is not met. Unsatisfactory tests are repeated within a short time (usually 24 hours). It has been suggested that the interpretation of the test should be based on a 10-minute testing segment known as a "testing window." The classification of *equivocal* and elimination of the term *suspicious tests* (occasional decelerations) have been proposed in conjunction with the concept of a 10-minute testing window. Equivocal tests are those in which nonrepetitive late decelerations are observed (i.e., no positive or negative testing window) or in which decelerations are associated with maternal hypotension or uterine hyperstimulation. Because external methods of pressure monitoring are used, uterine hyperstimulation cannot be defined on the basis of true intrauterine pressure (mm Hg) but rather is defined on the basis of the frequency of contractions (more than three contractions in 10 minutes) or a tetanic contraction. It is suggested that equivocal tests be repeated in 24 hours. In some areas of the country, the CST is interpreted without the use of the testing window. If the test shows any late decelerations, it is considered equivocal and is repeated within 24 hours.

Early investigators found that positive CSTs were associated with a relatively high frequency of poor outcome, such as intrauterine fetal death, fetal distress, or poor condition of the infant at birth. A normal CST gave a high degree of confidence for continued fetal survival in utero during an arbitrarily set limit of 1 week. Further experience has confirmed this observation. Instances of fetal death within 1 week of a negative CST are infrequent. When this has occurred, the fetal deaths have often been attributed to factors other than the primary indication for testing (e.g., abruptio placentae or fetal malformation). Some have suggested performing CSTs more frequently when there is deterioration of the maternal condition (e.g., increasing severity of

Nursing Guidelines for Performing the Contraction Stress Test

A. Procedure for the CST

1. Take client to a labor room or antepartal testing unit.
2. Explain to client the testing procedure and the time involved. (The test itself requires an average of about 90 minutes, but it is not uncommon for the procedure to take 3 hours.)
3. Have client change into a gown.
4. Place client in a semi-Fowler's position at a 30 to 45-degree angle with a slight left tilt.
5. Place client on an external monitor. A phonotransducer or ultrasound transducer is used to record the fetal heart rate (FHR) and a tocodynamometer to measure uterine contractions (UC).
6. Record client's blood pressure initially and at 5- to 10-minute intervals.
7. Obtain at least a 10-minute baseline recording of FHR and observe for spontaneous UC.
   If spontaneous UCs without late decelerations are noted at a frequency of <3 in 10 minutes or no spontaneous uterine activity is observed, proceed with oxytocin infusion.
8. Prepare and begin an oxytocin infusion according to the institutional protocol or as indicated by the physician.

(Courtesy of Patricia M. Graef, BSNEd)

a. Start the oxytocin infusion (secondary line) by inserting the needle into the connector of the primary line at the connector most proximal to the primary line. Be sure to keep primary line running at a slow rate.
b. Client is evaluated by the physician when the dosage of oxytocin reaches 10 mU/min. If the oxytocin infusion is to be continued, the physician must write an order to increase the dosage.

B. Interpretation of the CST

1. Test is read as:
   a. Negative—no late deceleration of the FHR when an adequate frequency of 3 contractions in 10 minutes has been established, a "negative window"
   b. Positive—late decelerations occurring with 3 contractions in 10 minutes, a "positive window"
   c. Equivocal—no positive or negative window
   d. Hyperstimulation—excessive uterine activity is present in association with a deceleration of the FHR
   e. Unsatisfactory—inadequate UC or FHR record

---

pregnancy-induced hypertension) or in certain very high-risk disorders (e.g., diabetes with vascular disease).

Clinical studies in which clients were induced to labor and electronically monitored following a positive CST have demonstrated a high false-positive rate (25%–40%), that is, late decelerations did not recur in labor. Because of this experience, it has been suggested that more than one test of fetal well-being should be carried out before a preterm delivery for fetal compromise is indicated. Clearly, the greatest benefit of the CST lies in the reassurance that allows continuation of a high-risk pregnancy when the test result is normal.

NIPPLE STIMULATION TEST

Another noninvasive technique has been developed in antepartal testing for the achievement of a CST. It is called the *nipple stimulation test*. This technique is based on the principle that nipple stimulation causes oxytocin to be released from the neurohypophysis, and, if successful, the need for intravenous infusion of Pitocin is eliminated. Several methods have been suggested to achieve an adequate test without effecting uterine hyperstimulation. The following protocol has been used successfully in a number of institutions. In this method, the patient is instructed to roll both nipples between her fingers for a total of 2 minutes. The patient then rests for 3 minutes, then the procedure is repeated. Stimulation is continued for 20 minutes. If inadequate uterine contractions occur, the patient increases stimulation to 3 minutes and resting to 2 minutes. Stimulation is discontinued if 3 contractions occur in 10 minutes, if a positive CST is observed, if a prolonged fetal heart rate deceleration occurs, or if hyperstimulation is observed. If, after 60 minutes, adequate contraction frequency is not achieved, an oxytocin challenge test is initiated.

The CST is an invasive and lengthy test. An average CST takes up to 90 minutes or more to achieve adequate contraction frequency. Because of the simplicity of nipple stimulation, the disadvantages of the CST can be avoided. Several reports have demonstrated that nipple stimulation is efficacious and has a predictive value similar to that of the CST.[116-118]

TABLE 42-4. INDICATIONS FOR ANTEPARTUM FETAL SURVEILLANCE*

Medical Problems

Diabetics:
  DMA1: 40 weeks (280 days)
  DMA1 with previous stillborn
  DMA1 with added medical problems
  DMA2—R

Cardiac disease

Chronic hypertension

Collagen-vascular diseases

Renal disease

Thyroid disease

Sickle cell disease

Obstetric Problems

Abnormal fetal heart tones, arrhythmias

Amniotic fluid: increased, decreased, meconium stained

Fetal anomalies

Decreased fetal movement: one test only at the time of the complaint

IUGR: when diagnosed—According to ultrasound assessment and evaluation in IUGR
  clinic. Testing will be terminated if IUGR is ruled out.

Placenta previa

Postdates: testing initiated at 41 weeks (≥287 days)

Pregnancy-induced hypertension

Previous stillborn: started 1 week before previous loss or 34 weeks

SPROM (spontaneous premature rupture of membranes): daily testing—if the patient
  reaccumulates her fluid and her nonstress test remains normal, twice weekly testing
  should be considered

Multiple gestation
  Concordant growth: Stated at 38 weeks' gestation
  Discordant growth (≥20% difference in EFWs): started when IUGR diagnosed

Rh disease

  * The earliest that antepartum fetal surveillance will be initiated is an estimated fetal weight of >750 g or 26-
week gestational age. Testing is performed twice a week unless otherwise noted.
  (Courtesy of Paula M. Broussard, RN, BS)

NONSTRESS TEST

Observation of accelerated fetal heart rate associated with fetal movements led to the development of the NST. This form of testing does not require intravenous administration of drugs and thus can be safely and more quickly performed in an outpatient area. These features, coupled with the apparent reliability of the NST as a screening test, have resulted in a marked reduction in the number of CSTs performed.

Various criteria have been applied for interpreting the NST. The occurrence of five accelerations of greater than 15 beats per minute for more than 15 seconds in 20 minutes was initially required as a normal or reactive test (Fig. 42-15). More recent studies have suggested that fewer accelerations of the same magnitude may be adequate. Many institutions define a reactive NST as the occurrence of two qualifying accelerations within a 10-minute period. Because the fetus has cyclic periods of rest, external stimulation has been used to elicit movement for the testing. Failure to demonstrate a reactive pattern owing either to lack of accelerations with movement or to lack of fetal movement is taken as an indication for further evaluation of the fetus by a CST or FBP (Fig. 42-16).

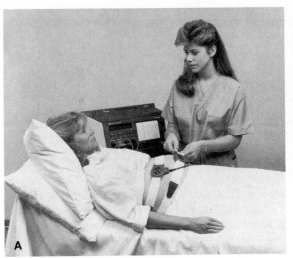

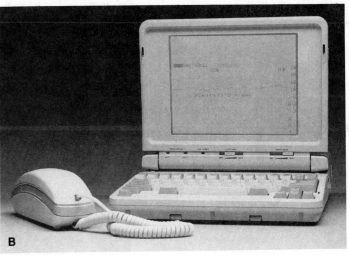

■ *Figure 42–13*

(A) *Patient undergoing a nonstress test in a hospital setting. (Courtesy: Corometrics Medical Systems, Inc. Wallingford, Connecticut.) (B) Antepartum fetal heart rate monitoring also can be performed in the patient's home utilizing a portable monitoring system. Several manufacturers have produced machines to achieve this function. One example is a lap-top computer that allows for transmission of on-going monitoring to a physician by using a modem. (Courtesy: Peritronics Medical Inc., Brea, California.)*

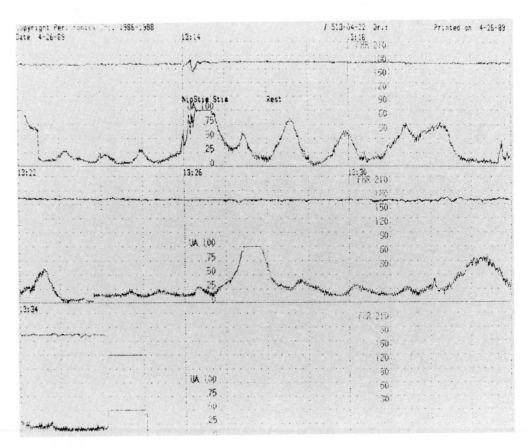

■ *Figure 42–14*
Computer print out of a negative CST performed with nipple stimulation.

Nursing Guidelines for Performing the Nonstress Test (NST)

A. Procedure for the NST

1. Take client to the antepartial testing unit.
2. Explain the procedure to the client, including the time involved. The test requires an average of 30 minutes.
3. Have client change into a gown.
4. Place client in a semi-Fowler's position at a 30 to 45-degree angle with a slight left tilt.
5. Place client on an external monitor using ultrasound transducer or phonotransducer to record the fetal heart rate (FHR). A tocodynamometer is used to document fetal activity and spontaneous uterine activity.
6. Record client's blood pressure initially and at 5- to 10-minute intervals.

(Courtesy of Patricia M. Graef, BSNEd)

7. The strip is run for a maximum of 40 minutes.

B. Interpretation of the NST

1. Test is read as:
   a. Reactive—2 FHR accelerations greater than 15 beats per minute above the baseline and lasting 15 seconds or more with fetal movement in 10-minute period
   b. Nonreactive—no or one FHR acceleration greater than 15 beats per minute and lasting 15 seconds or more with fetal movement in a 10-minute period or accelerations less than 15 beats per minute or lasting less than 15 seconds

VIBROACOUSTIC STIMULATION

The reactive NST has been found to be a safe and reliable indicator of fetal well-being. Although a nonreactive NST may be a useful test of fetal compromise, episodes of nonreactivity are often related to fetal behavioral state. One of the problems with antepartum fetal heart rate testing is the difficulty in separating healthy fetuses at rest from sick fetuses who are not moving because of asphyxia. Various attempts to stimulate the fetus have proven ineffective. These include

the administration of orange juice prior to testing and manual manipulation of the maternal abdomen.[119,120] Vibroacoustic stimulation is performed as an adjunct to improve the efficacy of antepartum fetal heart rate testing. It is used to reduce the incidence of falsely nonreactive tests presumably secondary to fetal sleep states and overall testing time. The stimulus is generated by an artificial larynx that provides both acoustic and vibratory stimuli (Figs. 42-17 and 42-18). This device emits fundamental tones of approximately 85 to 100 dB with a fundamental frequency of 850 Hz. When applied to

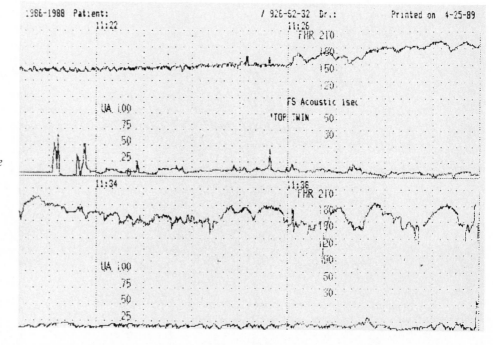

■ *Figure 42–15*
Computer print out of a reactive NST performed with vibroacoustic stimulation.

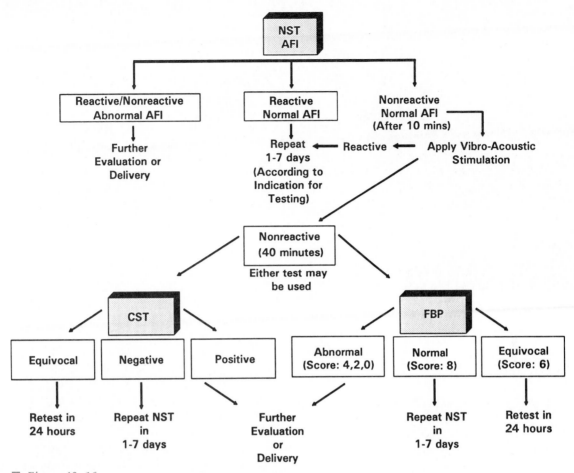

■ *Figure 42–16*
An example of a management scheme of antepartum fetal surveillance.

the maternal abdomen, the fetus changes state and reacts with a startle response. The vibroacoustic stimulator has received FDA approval for antepartum use between 28 and 42 weeks' gestation.

Vibroacoustic stimulation is initiated in nonstress testing after 10 minutes of nonreactivity. The stimulator

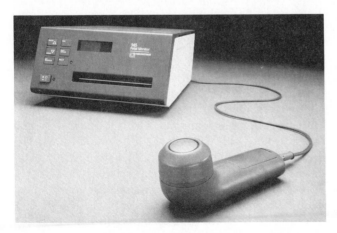

■ *Figure 42–17*
Vibroacoustic stimulator. (Courtesy: Corometrics Medical Systems, Inc. Wallingford, Connecticut.)

is applied to the maternal abdomen for 1 second and fetal heart rate response is observed for 1 minute. If the criteria for adequate accelerations are not met, the fetus is stimulated for 2 seconds. If accelerations are not achieved after an additional 1-minute observation, a third application of stimulation is performed for 3 seconds. The fetal heart rate is then observed until it becomes reactive or 40 minutes have elapsed. Several studies have reported that the use of vibroacoustic stimulation results in a significant reduction in the number of nonreactive nonstress tests and a decrease in the time required for a reactive test to occur.[121,122] Reactivity achieved with stimulation was found to have equal predictive value to that of a spontaneously reactive NST.

MODIFIED BIOPHYSICAL PROFILE

Many institutions advocate the use of a modified biophysical profile (the NST and amniotic fluid index) as the primary testing mode of fetal surveillance. If nonreactivity is observed, the remaining three variables of the FBP can be performed to assure fetal well-being.

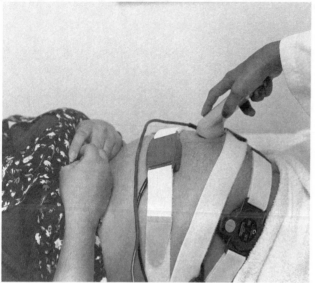

■ *Figure 42–18*

Application of vibroacoustic stimulation. Initial studies were performed with the stimulator placed over the fetal head. Effective stimulation can, however, be achieved by placing the stimulator on any location on the maternal abdomen.

This method of testing has been found to be equal in predictive value of the CST and FBP.[122]

■ FETAL TREATMENT

The art of fetal treatment is far less developed than that of fetal diagnosis. The most common approach to the fetus by the obstetrician is to select an appropriate time for delivery, convert the fetus to a newborn, and thus allow active treatment by the neonatologist. Perhaps the most important approach to the fetus is to provide appropriate support throughout the pregnancy. This includes adequate prenatal diet, as well as glucose and oxygen during labor, especially if there is fetal distress.

Treatment in the case of a positive prenatal diagnosis of severe congenital disease is generally limited to therapeutic abortion. In some instances, however, in utero treatment may correct an increasing number of fetal defects and diseases.

Pharmacologic and Nutritional Therapy

Many drugs administered to the mother cross the placenta into the fetal circulation. Transplacental passage is generally a function of the molecular size of the drug. Substances with molecular weights less than 500 cross

readily by simple diffusion. Although there should always be concern over the possible deleterious effects of drugs, one can sometimes achieve a desirable therapeutic effect in the fetus by treating the mother. An example of this is the administration of digitalis to the mother when the fetus is found to suffer from supraventricular tachycardia. This cardiac arrhythmia is suspected when there is an elevated fetal heart rate and is confirmed by fetal echocardiography. Administering digitalis through the mother to the fetus is the treatment of choice.

Another example of fetal drug therapy is the administration of glucocorticoids to the mother to induce the production of surfactant by the type II cells of the fetal lung and thereby reduce the risk of respiratory distress syndrome. The evidence is that if this is done between 26 to 28 and 32 to 34 weeks of gestation, and if delivery can be delayed for 24 to 48 hours, there will be a significant reduction in respiratory distress. The effect appears to be transient; the frequency of respiratory distress increases when delivery is delayed for more than 7 days following treatment. The effectiveness of this approach is still under investigation. Those who do not favor its use point out that the long-term effects on the child of exposure to glucocorticoids in utero are not known and that glucocorticoids may increase the risk of in utero infection.

Nutritional supplementation has been proposed as a method for treating IUGR. Supplemental nutrients can be provided to the growth-retarded fetus by three main routes: maternal administration, amniotic fluid, and direct administration to the fetus. These methods are experimental, and research is ongoing.[123]

Transfusion

Intrauterine fetal transfusion in Rh disease is the most publicized form of fetal treatment. When the hematocrit determined by fetal blood sampling is low, or hydrops is present, intrauterine transfusion is indicated. Prior to PUBS, intraperitoneal transfusion was the treatment of choice of the isoimmunized fetus. The direct intravascular route for fetal transfusions, however, is now favored over the intraperitoneal route because it yields direct information with regard to the severity of the disease, corrects fetal anemia more physiologically, and is associated with a lesser risk of complications. The survival rate reaches 80% to 90% even in hydropic fetuses. Transfusions can be performed from 18 to 34 weeks' gestation by a technique similar to that for fetal blood sampling. Type O Rh-negative blood that is packed to a hematocrit of 65% to 85% is infused at a rate of 5 to 10 ml/min. The amount of transfused blood is calculated according to the estimated fetoplacental blood volume for gestational age and fetal pretransfusion hematocrit.[124] Intravascular transfusion has transformed the prognosis for immune hydrops, particularly if it is already present before 25 weeks.

Intrauterine intravascular transfusions have also been used to infuse platelets into the fetus diagnosed with severe thrombocytopenia. The fetus is transfused at 37 weeks to allow vaginal delivery. Cesarean section does not eliminate the risk of hemorrhage in the fetus and is unnecessary in most cases.[125]

Surgery and Needle Aspiration

Refinements in sonography have resulted in earlier and more accurate diagnosis of fetal abnormalities. Efforts to treat these have received substantial press coverage, captured public attention, and engendered substantial public and professional debate. Successful intrauterine treatment of obstruction of the lower urinary tract that would otherwise result in extensive kidney damage has been reported. Particularly noteworthy is the intrauterine treatment of hydrocephalus. Efforts have been made to relieve the hydrocephalus by intermittent sonographically directed needle aspiration through the mother's abdomen or even by the surgical insertion of a shunt to provide continuous drainage into the amniotic sac. The risk/benefit ratio of these procedures is not established, and they must still be considered experimental. Clearly, there are substantial ethical issues, as such treatment could allow the survival of a severely retarded child who might otherwise have died in utero.

Future Therapy

The future undoubtedly holds many advances—from the prenatal correction of congenital defects to the unscrambling of genetic mishaps. There may well be treatments of maladies that are presently unknown in this rapidly developing area of fetal medicine.

■ NURSING CARE OF THE FETUS AND FAMILY AT RISK

Nursing Process

The nursing process is designed to accomplish the major patient goals of care of the fetus and family at risk, as follows:

1. The fetus maintains optimal health.
2. The compromised fetus is detected and treated to permit appropriate delivery and neonatal care.

3. The patient and family indicates knowledge of fetal diagnostic and treatment procedures.
4. The patient and family psychologically adjusts to the defective or compromised fetus.

Nursing care is planned in conjunction with the desires of the mother and the family involved as well as with various members of the perinatal team, including the perinatologist, sonographer, laboratory personnel, and neonatologist. Fetal diagnostic techniques are most often performed as outpatient procedures, allowing the nurse minimal time and patient contact to achieve effective and therapeutic care as proposed by the perinatal team. A wide base of knowledge of diagnostic methodologies and fetal disease processes, communications skills, and an organized plan of care are essential in assisting the fetus and its family accomplish desired goals in a timely manner.

Nursing Assessment

Assessment of the fetus is initiated by obtaining a complete medical and obstetric history on the patient's arrival for testing. Factors that may alter fetal diagnosis and treatment can be identified at this time. Psychosocial factors are appraised to determine the level of anxiety and stress the mother and family are experiencing in relation to the possibility of having an abnormal fetus. The family may be grieving and experiencing a sense of loss of their anticipated "perfect" child. Capacity of learning should be assessed to ascertain the level of knowledge the family can absorb. When the family is faced with the possibility of having a defective child, they are often unable to assimilate information relating to either the diagnostic procedure or the prognosis of their child.

Potential Nursing Diagnoses

Nursing assessment can result in identifying several potential diagnoses relating to the fetus in jeopardy as well as its family. In terms of the fetus, included are the high risks for fetal injury and alteration in nutritional status. The family may be diagnosed as having ineffective coping mechanisms as well as a knowledge deficit of fetal diagnosis, treatment, and prognosis.

Nursing Intervention

Several clinical evaluations of the fetus can be accomplished by the nurse. These include fundal height, determination of estimated date of delivery, and maternal weight. Education of fetal activity counting is also a

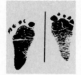

Nursing Care Plan

The Fetus and Family at Risk

Patient Goals
1. Fetus maintains optimal health.
2. Compromised fetus is detected and treated to allow for appropriate delivery and neonatal care.
3. Patient indicates knowledge of fetal diagnostic and treatment procedures.
4. Patient and family psychologically adjust to the defective or compromised fetus.

Assessment	Potential Nursing Diagnosis	Planning and Intervention	Evaluation
Care of the Fetus			

Gestational age
  Nägele's rule
  Fundal height
  Ultrasound
	Potential for injury (asphyxia, meconium aspiration, hypoglycemia, polycythemia, specific health problems) related to early delivery or complications	Review prenatal record
		
		Obtain history from mother
		
		Calculate gestational age
		
		Perform fundal height measurement
		
		Prepare mother for ultrasound
			The fetus' age is determined and documented
			
			The fetus is delivered as close to term as possible
			
			The fetus survives birth with no or few complications

Nutrition Growth and development of the fetus	Potential alteration in nutritional status: less than body requirements related to disease process (i.e., chronic hypertension, prolonged pregnancy)	Do serial fundal heights with prenatal care Provide nutritional counseling for the mother Take maternal weight at each prenatal visit Ultrasound examination Fetal activity determination Results reported to physician Initiate antepartal testing if appropriate	Fetal well-being is determined and maintained Fetus is delivered at appropriate time if it is in jeopardy
Need for delivery of the high-risk infant Level of care the hospital provides		Monitor fetal heart rate and report findings to physician Facilitate transfer if needed Prepare for high-risk delivery Have appropriate neonatal resuscitation equipment available and in working condition Have qualified personnel present to care for the infant at the delivery	High-risk infant is born in a hospital that can provide appropriate care

(continued)

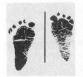

Nursing Care Plan *(continued)*

Assessment	Potential Nursing Diagnosis	Planning and Intervention	Evaluation
Care of Mother and Her Support System			
Communication Coping behaviors	Fear of injury to, or death of, infant related to high-risk factors	Allow communication by using open-ended questions	Client/family communicates freely with each other and staff
	Ineffective individual coping (depression, guilt) related to perceived parental role failure	Allow time for the parents to ask questions and voice fears	Client/family voices fears
		Assist and promote effective coping behavior	Client/family indicate understanding of procedures by repeating and discussing information
		Explain procedures	Client/family develop coping behaviors indicated by their words and actions
		Facilitate the parents' meeting with the neonatal staff prior to the birth	
Learning capabilities Determine factors or situations causing learning deficit Assess readiness to learn	Knowledge deficit of etiologic factors and care related to the high-risk condition	Develop a teaching plan Provide teaching that is client/family specific	Client/family achieves learning goals Client/family participate actively in health management plan

vital nursing function. The majority of diagnostic techniques, however, are usually performed by sonographic and laboratory specialists, as well as the perinatologist. It is often the responsibility of the nurse to explain the indications, risks, accuracy, and methodology of the procedures as well as the rationale for their use. The family must be allowed to ask questions about the tests as well express their fears and concerns about their fetus.

Many nurses across the country are now performing expanded roles as nurse specialists in the field of antepartum fetal surveillance. With specialized training, these nurses have the ability to perform not only antepartum fetal heart rate monitoring but also various sonographic procedures including, but not limited to, the FBP, gestational age determinations, growth evaluations, and Doppler ultrasound.

Evaluation

The fetus and the family must be re-evaluated in light of the results of the diagnostic procedures. It is anticipated that the fetus will maintain optimal health as a result of assessment and intervention. It is also desirable that the family understands the reasons for testing and the treatment that may ensue as a result of the diagnostic outcome. Finally, it is expected that the family members will have the ability to communicate freely among themselves and staff members about their fears and concerns.

■ REFERENCES

1. AIUM Bioeffects Reports Subcommittee: Bioeffects considerations for the study of diagnostic ultrasound. J Ultrasound Med 7:S4, 1988
2. NICHD consensus report: Diagnostic ultrasound imaging in pregnancy. Washington, DC, US Department of Health and Human Services, PHS, NIH Publication No. 84-667, 1984
3. Ultrasound in Pregnancy. Washington, DC, American College of Obstetrics and Gynecology Technical Bulletin No. 116, 1988
4. Jeanty P, Romero R: Obstetrical Ultrasound. New York, McGraw-Hill, 1984
5. Rebar RW: Transvaginal sonography. J Reproductive Med 33:931–938, 1988

6. Berman MC: Principles of scanning technique in obstetric and gynecologic ultrasound. In Berman MC (ed): Diagnostic Medical Sonography, vol I. Obstetric and Gynecology, pp 3–18. Philadelphia, JB Lippincott, 1991

7. deCrespigny L, Cooper D, McKenna M: Early detection of intrauterine pregnancy with ultrasound. J Ultrasound Med 7:7–10, 1988

8. Nyberg DA, Filly RA, Mahony BS, et al: Early gestation: Correlation of hCG levels and sonographic identification. Am J Radiol 144:451–454, 1985

9. DuBose TJ: Assessment of fetal age and size: Techniques and criteria. In Berman MC (ed): Diagnostic Medical Sonography, vol I. Obstetrics and Gynecology, pp 273–300. Philadelphia, JB Lippincott, 1991

10. Fleischer AC, Pennell RG, Sacks GA, et al: Sonography in early intrauterine pregnancy emphasizing transvaginal scanning. In Fleischer AC, Romero R, Manning FA, et al (eds): The Principles and Practice of Ultrasonography in Obstetrics and Gynecology, pp 39–56. Norwalk, CT, Appleton & Lange, 1991

11. Robinson HP, Fleming JEE: A critical evaluation of sonar crown-rump length measurements. Br J Obstet Gynaecol 82:702–710, 1975

12. Jeanty P: Fetal biometry. In Fleischer AC, Romero R, Manning FA, et al (eds): The Principles and Practice of Ultrasonography in Obstetrics and Gynecology, pp 93–108. Norwalk, CT, Appleton & Lange, 1991

13. Hadlock FP, Deter RL, Harrist RB, et al: Fetal biparietal diameter: Rational choice of plane of section for sonographic measurement. Am J Radiol 138:871–874, 1982

14. Hadlock FP, Deter RL, Carpenter RJ, et al: Estimating fetal age: Effect of head shape on BPD. Am J Radiol 137:83–85, 1981

15. Jeanty P, Rodesch R, Delbekd D, et al: Estimation of gestational age from measurement of fetal long bones. J Ultrasound Med 3:75–79, 1984

16. Wolfson RN, Peisner DB, Chik LL, et al: Comparison of biparietal diameter and femur length in the third trimester: Effects of gestational age and variation in fetal growth. J Ultrasound Med 5:145, 1986

17. Campbell S, Warsof SL, Little D, et al: Routine ultrasound screening for the prediction of gestational age. Obstet Gynecol 65:613, 1985

18. Kurtz AB, Needleman L: Ultrasound assessment of fetal age. In Callen PW (ed): Ultrasonography in Obstetrics and Gynecology. Philadelphia, WB Saunders, 1988

19. Hadlock FP, Harrist RB, Shah YP, et al: Estimating fetal age using multiple parameters: A prospective evaluation in a racially mixed population. Am J Obstet Gynecol 156:955, 1987

20. DuBose TJ: Fetal biometry: Vertical calvarial diameter and calvarial volume. J Diagn Med Ultrason 1:205–217, 1985

21. Morrison I, Olson J: Weight specific stillbirths and associated causes of death: An analysis of 765 consecutive stillbirths. Am J Obstet Gynecol 152:975, 1985

22. Manning FA, Hohler C: Intrauterine growth retardation: Diagnosis, prognostication, and management based on ultrasound methods. In Fleischer AC, Romero R, Manning FA, et al (eds): The Principles and Practice of Ultrasonography in Obstetrics and Gynecology, pp 331–348. Norwalk, CT, Appleton & Lange, 1991

23. Fitzhardinge PM, Steven EM: The small-for-dates infant: II. Neurological and intellectual sequelae. Pediatrics 50:50, 1972

24. Streeter H, Manning FA: Classification of neonatal morbidity and mortality by birth weight percentile in IUGR neonates (abstract). Proc Soc Obstet Gynecol Can 1980

25. Andersen HF, Johnson TRB, Barclay ML, et al: Gestational age assessment: I. Analysis of individual clinical observations. Am J Obstet Gynecol 139:173, 1981

26. Beazley JM, Underhill RA: Fallacy of the fundal height. Br Med J 4:404, 1970

27. Hadlock FP, Deter R, Harrist R, et al: A date-independent predictor of intrauterine growth retardation: Femur length/abdominal circumference ratio. Am J Radiol 141:979, 1983

28. Campbell S, Wilkin P: Ultrasonic measurement of fetal abdominal circumference in the estimation of fetal weight. Br J Obstet Gynaecol 82:689–697, 1975

29. Acker DB, Sachs BP, Friedman EA: Risk factors for shoulder dystocia. Obstet Gynecol 66:762, 1985

30. Chung CS, Myrianthopoulos NC: Congenital anomalies: Mortality and morbidity, burden and classification. Am J Med Genet 27:508, 1987

31. Myrianthopoulos NC, Chung CS: Congenital malformation in singleton: Epidemiologic survey. In Bergsma D (ed): Birth Defects. New York, Stratton Inter-cont Medical Book, 1974

32. Romero R, Oyarzun E, Sirtori M, et al: Prenatal detection of anatomic congenital anomalies. In Fleischer AC, Romero R, Manning FA, et al (eds): The Principles and Practice of Ultrasonography in Obstetrics and Gynecology, pp 193–210. Norwalk, CT, Appleton & Lange, 1991

33. Chervenak FA, Tortora M, Hobbins JC: Antenatal sonographic diagnosis of clubfoot. J Ultrasound Med 4:49–50, 1985

34. Jeanty P, Romero R, d'Alton M, et al: In utero sonographic detection of hand and foot deformities. J Ultrasound Med 4:595–601, 1985

35. Benacerraf BR, Miller WA, Frigoletto FD: Sonographic detection of fetuses with trisomies 13 and 18: Accuracy and limitations. Am J Obstet Gynecol 158:404–409, 1988

36. Benacerraf BR, Osathanondh R, Frigoletto FD: Sonographic demonstration of hypoplasia of the middle phalanx of the fifth digit: A finding associated with Down syndrome. Am J Obstet Gynecol 159:181–183, 1988

37. Jeanty P: Prenatal detection of simian crease. J Ultrasound Med 9:131–136, 1990

38. Benacerraf B, Gelman R, Frigoletto FD: Sonographic identification of second trimester fetuses with Down's syndrome. N Engl J Med 317:1371–1376, 1987

39. Copel JA, Cullen M, Green JJ, et al: The frequency of aneuploidy in prenatally diagnosed congenital heart disease: An indication for fetal karyotyping. Am J Obstet Gynecol 158:409–413, 1988

40. Bundy AL, Saltzman DH, Pober B, et al: Antenatal sonographic findings in Trisomy 18. J Ultrasound Med 5:361–364, 1986

41. Platt LD, Carlson DE, Medearis AL, et al: Fetal choroid plexus cysts in the second trimester of pregnancy: A cause for concern. Am J Obstet Gynecol 164:1652–1656, 1991

42. Manning FA, Hill LM, Platt LD: Qualitative amniotic fluid volume determination by ultrasound: Antepartum detection of intrauterine growth retardation. Am J Obstet Gynecol 139:254–258, 1981

43. Chamberlain PF, Manning FA, Morrison I, et al: Ultrasound evaluation of amniotic fluid volume: I. The relationship of marginal and decreased amniotic fluid volumes to perinatal outcome. Am J Obstet Gynecol 150:245–249, 1984

44. Phelan JP, Smith CV, Broussard P, et al: Amniotic fluid volume assessment with the four-quadrant technique at 36–42 weeks gestation. J Reprod Med 32:540–542, 1987

45. Carlson DE, Platt LD, Medearis AL, et al: Quantifiable polyhydramnios: Diagnosis and management. Obstet Gynecol 75:989–992, 1990

46. Perrin EVDK, Sander CH: How to examine the placenta and why. In Perrin EVDK (ed): Pathology of the Placenta. New York, Churchill Livingstone, 1984

47. Grannum PAT, Berkowitz RL, Hobbins JC: The ultrasonic changes in the maturing placenta and their relation to fetal pulmonic maturity. Am J Obstet Gynecol 133:915–922, 1979

48. Mahony BS, Filly RA, Callen PW: Amnioticity and chorionicity in twin pregnancies: Prediction using ultrasound. Radiology 167:383–385, 1985

49. DeVore GR: The prenatal diagnosis of congenital heart disease: A practical approach for the fetal sonographer. J Clin Ultrasound 13:229–245, 1985

50. DeVore GR, Siassi B, Platt LD: Fetal echocardiography: IV. M-mode assessment of ventricular size and contractility during the second and third trimesters of pregnancy in the normal fetus. Am J Obstet Gynecol 150:981–988, 1984

51. DeVore GR, Siassi B, Platt LD: M-mode echocardiography of the aortic root and aortic valve in second and third trimester normal human fetuses. Am J Obstet Gynecol 152:543–550, 1985

52. DeVore GR, Siassi B, Platt LD: Fetal echocardiography: VIII. Aortic root dilatation: A marker for tetralogy of Fallot. Am J Obstet Gynecol 159:129–136, 1988

53. DeVore, Siassi B, Platt LD: Fetal echocardiography: III. The diagnosis of cardiac arrhythmias using real-time-directed M-mode ultrasound. Am J Obstet Gynecol 146:792, 1983

54. Kleinman CS, Copel JA, Weinstein EM, et al: Treatment of fetal supraventricular tachyarrhythmias. J Clin Ultrasound 13:265–273, 1985

55. Maulik D, Yarlagadda P, Downing G: Doppler velocimetry in obstetrics. Obstet Gynecol Clin North Am 17:163–186, 1990

56. Stuart B, Drumm J, FitzGerald DE, et al: Fetal blood velocity waveforms in normal pregnancy. Br J Obstet Gynaecol 87:708–785, 1980

57. Trudinger BJ, Giles WB, Cook CM, et al: Fetal umbilical artery flow velocity waveforms and placental resistance: Clinical significance. Br J Obstet Gynaecol 92:23–30, 1985

58. Fleischer A, Schulman H, Farmakides G, et al: Umbilical artery velocity waveforms and intrauterine growth retardation. Am J Obstet Gynecol 151:502–505, 1985

59. Rochelson B, Schulman H, Farmakides G, et al: The significance of absent end-diastolic velocity in umbilical artery velocity waveforms. Am J Obstet Gynecol 156:1213–1218, 1987

60. Woo JSK, Liang ST, Lo RLS: Significance of an absent or reversed end-diastolic flow in Doppler umbilical artery waveforms. J Ultrasound Med 6:291, 1987

61. Berkowitz GS, Chitkara U, Rosenberg J, et al: Sonographic estimation of fetal weight and Doppler analysis of umbilical artery velocimetry in the prediction of intrauterine growth retardation: A prospective study. Am J Obstet Gynecol 158:1149–1153, 1988

62. Wladimiroff JW, vd Wijngaard JA, Degani S, et al: Cerebral and umbilical arterial blood flow velocity waveforms in normal and growth retarded pregnancies. Obstet Gynecol 69:705–709, 1987

63. Arduini D, Rizzo G, Romanni C, et al: Fetal blood flow velocity waveforms as predictors of growth retardation. Obstet Gynecol 70:7, 1987

64. Mattison DR, Angtuaco T, Miller FC, et al: Magnetic resonance imaging in maternal and fetal medicine. J Perinatol 9:411–419, 1989

65. Lowe TW, Weinreb J, Santos-Ramos R, et al: Magnetic resonance imaging in human pregnancy. Obstet Gynecol 66:629–633, 1985

66. Powell MC, Buckley J, Worthington BS, et al: Magnetic resonance imaging and hydatidiform mole. Br J Radiol 59:561, 1986

67. Powell MC, Buckley J, Price H, et al: Magnetic resonance imaging and placenta previa. Am J Obstet Gynecol 154:565–569, 1986

68. McCarthy S, Filly R, Stark D, et al: Magnetic resonance imaging of fetal anomalies in utero: Early experience. Am J Radiol 145:677–682, 1985

69. Thickman D, Mintz M, Mennuti M, et al: MR imaging of cerebral abnormalities in utero. J Comput Assist Tomogr 8:1058, 1984

70. Stark D, McCarthy S, Filly R, et al: Intrauterine growth retardation: Evaluation by magnetic resonance. Radiology 155:425–427, 1985

71. Manning FA: Reflections on future directions of perinatal medicine. Semin Perinatol 13:342–351, 1989

72. Romero R, Pupkin M, Oyarzun E, et al: Amniocentesis. In Fleischer AC, Romero R, Manning FA, et al (eds): The Principles and Practice of Ultrasonography in Obstetrics and Gynecology, pp 439–454. Norwalk, CT, Appleton & Lange, 1991

73. Valenti C: Endoamnioscopy and fetal biopsy: A new technique. Am J Obstet Gynecol 114:561–564, 1972

74. Daffos F, Capella-Pavlovsky M, Forestier F: A new procedure for fetal blood sampling in utero: Preliminary results of fifty-three cases. Am J Obstet Gynecol 146:985–987, 1983

75. Romero R, Athanassiadis AP, Inati M: Fetal blood sam-

pling. In Fleischer AC, Romero R, Manning FA, et al (eds): The Principles and Practice of Ultrasonography in Obstetrics and Gynecology, pp 455–474. Norwalk, CT, Appleton & Lange, 1991

76. Daffos F: Fetal blood sampling. In Harrison MR, Golbus MS, Filly RA (eds): The Unborn Patient, pp 75–81. Philadelphia, WB Saunders, 1990

77. Daffos F, Capella-Pavlovsky M, Forestier F: Fetal blood sampling during pregnancy with use of a needle guided by ultrasound: A study of 606 consecutive cases. Am J Obstet Gynecol 153:655, 1985

78. Muller J, Giovangrandi Y, Parnet-Mathieu F, et al: Acute fetal distress after blood sampling (case report). Eur J Obstet Gynecol 28:269, 1988

79. Jauniaux E, Donner C, Simon P, et al: Pathologic aspects of the umbilical cord after percutaneous umbilical blood sampling. Obstet Gynecol 73:215, 1989

80. Pielet BW, Socol ML, MacGregor SN, et al: Cordocentesis: An appraisal of risks. Am J Obstet Gynecol 159:1497, 1988

81. Shulman LP, Elias S: Percutaneous umbilical blood sampling, fetal skin sampling, and fetal liver biopsy. Semin Perinatol 14:456–464, 1990

82. Wald N, Cuckle H, Densem J, et al: Maternal serum screening for Down's syndrome in early pregnancy. Br Med J 297:883–887, 1988

83. Burton BK: Elevated maternal serum alpha-fetoprotein (MSAFP): Interpretation and follow-up. Clin Obstet Gynecol 31:293–305, 1988

84. Martin JN, Cowan BD: Biochemical assessment and prediction of gestational well-being. Obstet Gynecol Clin North Am 17:81–93, 1990

85. Kadar N, Caldwell B, Romero R: A method of screening for ectopic pregnancy and its indications. Obstet Gynecol 58:162–166, 1981

86. Pittaway DE, Reish RL, Wentz AC: Doubling times of human chorionic gonadotropin increase in early viable intrauterine pregnancies. Am J Obstet Gynecol 152:299, 1985

87. Coleman BG, Arger PH: Ultrasound in early pregnancy complications. Clin Obstet Gynecol 31:3–18, 1988

88. Ray DA: Biochemical fetal assessment. Clin Obstet Gynecol 30:887–898, 1987

89. Harman CR: Ultrasound in the management of the alloimmunized pregnancy. In Fleischer AC, Romero R, Manning FA, et al (eds): The Principles and Practice of Ultrasonography in Obstetrics and Gynecology, pp 393–416. Norwalk, CT, Appleton & Lange, 1991

90. DeVore GR, Donnerstein RI, Kleinman CS, et al: Fetal echocardiography: II. The diagnosis and significance of a pericardial effusion in the fetus using realtime-directed M-mode ultrasound. Am J Obstet Gynecol 144:693–701, 1982

91. Copel JA, Grannum PA, Belanger K, et al: Pulsed Doppler flow-velocity waveforms before and after intrauterine intravascular transfusion for severe erythroblastosis fetalis. Am J Obstet Gynecol 158:768–774, 1988

92. deVries JIP, Visser GH, Prechtl HFR: Fetal motility in the first half of pregnancy. Clin Develop Med 94:46–64, 1984

93. deVries JIP, Visser GHA, Mulder EJH, et al: Diurnal and other variations in fetal movement and heart rate patterns at 20–22 weeks. Early Human Develop 15:333–348, 1987

94. Patrick J, Campbell K, Carmichael L, et al: Patterns of gross fetal body movements over 24-hours observation during the last 10 weeks of pregnancy. Am J Obstet Gynecol 142:363–371, 1982

95. deVries JIP, Visser GHA, Prechtl HFR: The emergence of fetal behaviour: I. Qualitative aspects. Early Human Develop 7:301–322, 1982

96. Dierker LJ, Rosen MG, Pillay S, et al: The correlation between gestational age and fetal activity periods. Biol Neonate 42:66–72, 1982

97. Maloney JE, Alcorn D, Bowes G, et al: Development of the future respiratory system before birth. Semin Perinatol 4:251–260, 1980

98. Patrick J, Campbell K, Carmichael L, et al: Patterns of human fetal breathing during the last 10 weeks of pregnancy. Obstet Gynecol 56:24–30, 1980

99. Natale R, Nasell-Paterson C, Connors G, et al: Patterns of fetal breathing activity in the human fetus at 24–28 weeks of gestation. Am J Obstet Gynecol 158:317–321, 1988

100. Carmichael L, Campbell K, Patrick J: Fetal breathing, gross fetal body movements, and maternal fetal heart rates before spontaneous labor at term. Am J Obstet Gynecol 148:675–679, 1984

101. Nijhuis JG, Martin CB Jr, Prechtl HFR: Behavioral states of the human fetus. Clin Develop Med 94:65–78, 1984

102. Junge HD: Behavioral states and state related fetal heart rate and motor activity patterns in the newborn infant and the fetus antepartum: A comparative study. J Perinatol Med 7:85, 1979

103. Arduini D, Rizzo G, Giorlandino C, et al: The development of fetal behavioral states: A longitudinal study. Prenat Diagn 6:117–124, 1986

104. Arduini D, Rizzo G, Giorlandino C, et al: The fetal behavioral states: An ultrasonic study. Prenat Diagn 5:269–276, 1985

105. Manning FA, Platt LD, Sipos L: Antepartum fetal evaluation: Development of a fetal biophysical profile score. Am J Obstet Gynecol 136:787–795, 1980

106. Platt LD, Walla CA, Paul RH, et al: A prospective trial of the fetal biophysical profile versus the nonstress test in the management of high-risk pregnancies. Am J Obstet Gynecol 153:624–633, 1985

107. Manning FA, Harman CR, Morrison I, et al: Fetal assessment based on fetal biophysical profile scoring: IV. An analysis of perinatal morbidity and mortality. Am J Obstet Gynecol 162:703–709, 1990

108. Bastide A, Manning FA, Harman CR, et al: Ultrasound evaluation of amniotic fluid: Outcome of pregnancies with severe oligohydramnios. Am J Obstet Gynecol 154:895, 1986

109. Baskett TF, Allen AC, Gray JH, et al: Fetal biophysical profile and perinatal death. Obstet Gynecol 70:357–360, 1987

110. Sadovsky E, Polishuk WZ: Fetal movements in utero:

Nature, assessment, prognostic value, timing of delivery. Obstet Gynecol 50:49–55, 1977

111. Liston RM, Cohen AW, Mennuti MT, et al: Antepartum fetal evaluation by maternal perception of fetal movement. Obstet Gynecol 60:424–426, 1982

112. Rayburn WF: Clinical implications from monitoring fetal activity. Am J Obstet Gynecol 144:967–980, 1982

113. Pearson JF, Weaver JB: Fetal activity and fetal well-being: An evaluation. Br Med J 1:1305–1307, 1976

114. Draper J, Field S, Thomas H, et al: Womens' views on keeping fetal movement charts. Br J Obstet Gynaecol 93:334–338, 1986

115. Eggertsen SC, Benedetti TJ: Maternal response to daily fetal movement counting in primary care settings. Am J Perinatol 4:327–330, 1987

116. Oki EY, Keegan KA, Freeman RK, et al: The breast stimulated contraction stress test. J Reprod Med 32:919, 1987

117. Huddleston JF, Sutliff G, Robinson D: Contraction stress test by intermittent nipple stimulation. Obstet Gynecol 63:669, 1984

118. Rosenzweig BA, Levy JS, Schipious P, et al: Comparison of the nipple stimulation and exogenous oxytocin contraction stress tests. J Reprod Med 34:950–954, 1989

119. Eglinton GS, Paul RH, Broussard PM, et al: Antepartum fetal heart rate testing: XI. Stimulation with orange juice. Am J Obstet Gynecol 150:97–99, 1984

120. Druzin ML, Gratacos J, Paul RH, et al: Antepartum fetal heart rate testing: XII. The effect of manual manipulation of the fetus on the nonstress test. Am J Obstet Gynecol 151:61, 1985

121. Smith CV, Phelan JP, Platt LD, et al: Fetal acoustic stimulation test: II. A randomized clinical comparison with the nonstress test. Am J Obstet Gynecol 155:131–134, 1986

122. Clark SL, Sabey P, Jolley K: Nonstress testing with acoustic stimulation and amniotic fluid volume assessment: 5973 tests without unexpected fetal death. Am J Obstet Gynecol 160:694–697, 1989

123. Harding JE, Charlton V: Experimental nutritional supplementation for intrauterine growth retardation. In Harrison MR, Golbus MS, Filly RA (eds): The Unborn Patient, pp 598–610. Philadelphia, WB Saunders, 1990

124. Nicolaides KH, Soothill PW, Rodeck CH, et al: Rh disease: Intravascular fetal blood transfusion by cordocentesis. Fetal Ther 1:185, 1986

125. Daffos F, Forestier F, Muller JY, et al: In utero platelet transfusion in alloimmune thrombocytopenia. Lancet 2:1103, 1984

43

Intrapartum Fetal Monitoring and Care

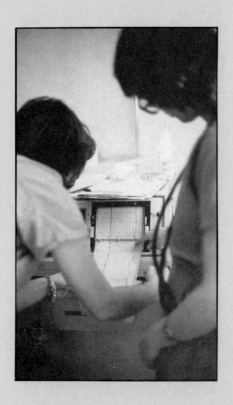

The primary goal of intrapartum fetal monitoring is to detect fetal stress and distress at a time when appropriate actions can be undertaken by the perinatal team. Timely actions are vital during the labor process for the delivery of a physically and neurologically intact infant. For many years, the forces of labor and the well-being of the fetus were evaluated by palpation of the maternal abdomen and by periodic sampling of the fetal heart rate (FHR) through auscultation. These methods were the mainstay of fetal intrapartum surveillance until the advent of continuous electronic monitoring of the fetal heart and uterine activity (UA) 30 years ago.

Fetal monitoring, whether by auscultation or electronic means, has expanded the role of the nurse in caring for the family during labor and delivery (Fig. 43-1). With this expanded role have come additional responsibilities in parent education, counseling, patient care, and surveillance.

■ FETAL HEART RATE AUSCULTATION

Pros and Cons

Lack of enthusiasm for the use of auscultation as a method of evaluating fetal condition was sparked by a number of nonrandomized studies comparing fetal and neonatal outcome in patients having continuous electronic fetal monitoring as opposed to patients undergoing intermittent auscultation.[1-4] These investigations suggested that most intrapartum fetal deaths are avoidable and neonatal morbidity is decreased when the FHR is monitored continuously. Most obstetricians believe that continuous as opposed to intermittent sampling of fetal monitoring offers substantial benefit in this regard. Prospective, randomized clinical trials of its value, however, have produced conflicting results, especially concerning its use in low-risk clients during normal labor.[5-10] Two of the recent clinical studies demonstrated that fetal and neonatal death rates were similar in women monitored with auscultation and those monitored with electronic fetal monitoring.[8,10] A significant advantage of continuous electronic monitoring over intermittent auscultation was found in evaluating newborn status in two investigations,[7,10] whereas no difference was found between these groups in other studies. Additionally, most of the studies reported a significant increase in the rate of both vaginal and abdominal operative deliveries in women who received continuous monitoring. Thus, although the observation of normal fetal monitoring data is predictive of a good fetal outcome, the interpretation of abnormal patterns has been fraught with difficulty and with considerable false-positive diagnosis (i.e., an apparently abnormal finding when the fetus is well) leading to operative deliveries. All of this conflicting information has led the medical community, governmental agencies, and the consumer to question the value of routine continuous electronic fetal monitoring.

In 1988, the American Academy of Pediatrics (AAP) and the American College of Obstetricians and Gynecologists (ACOG) published new guidelines for FHR assessment during labor[11] (Table 43-1). These guidelines state that both continuous FHR monitoring and intermittent auscultation are acceptable methods of monitoring the fetus in both low- and high-risk pregnancies. The guidelines are based on protocols delineated in randomized clinical trials. In these investigations, however, there was usually one nurse dedicated to one patient in the intermittent auscultation group, a situation that may not be available on many labor and delivery services. Because of economic implications, many institutions can meet the AAP–ACOG guidelines only by providing their laboring patients with continuous electronic fetal monitoring.

Techniques of Auscultation

Auscultation of the fetal heart rate can be performed with a DeLee stethoscope or a Doppler ultrasound device (Fig. 43-2). The DeLee stethoscope (fetoscope) was

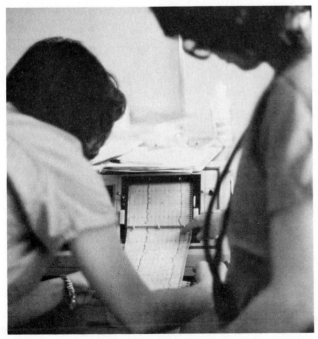

■ *Figure 43–1*
Professional labor nurses are trained to apply and read monitor equipment. (Photo by Kathy Sloane.)

Research Highlight

Acoustic stimulation has been used as an adjunct to antepartum testing and to clarify fetal acid-base status in the presence of abnormal intrapartum (FHR) patterns. The purpose of this study is to evaluate the usefulness of fetal acoustic stimulation in the early intrapartum period as a predictor of subsequent fetal distress.

The study group consisted of 201 women with uncomplicated, singleton, vertex-presenting pregnancies in the latent phase of labor. Fetal acoustic stimulation was performed after a 40-minute baseline FHR monitor tracing was obtained on admission for labor. Fetuses who showed a nonreactive response to stimulation were found to be at significantly greater risk of initial and subsequent abnormal FHR patterns, meconium staining, cesarean delivery because of fetal distress, and Apgar scores <7 at both 1 and 5 minutes.

Fetal acoustic stimulation could be valuable in the early intrapartum period as an admission test in early labor to triage fetuses to a low- or high-risk category for intrapartum fetal distress. Low-risk patient with a reactive response to stimulation may be managed by intermittent auscultation or intermittent electronic fetal monitoring in the active phase of labor, or ambulation in the latent phase of labor without telemetry.

Sarno AP, Ahn MO, Phelan JP, et al. Fetal acoustic stimulation in the early intrapartum period as a predictor of subsequent fetal condition. Am J Obstet Gynecol 162:762–767, 1990.

first used in 1917 and has changed little in appearance since that time. The fetoscope has a stethoscope attached to a curved piece of metal that is placed on the examiner's head. Conduction of sound through the frontal bone of the head is used to assist in amplifying the heart beat. The Doppler device is a continuous-wave ultrasound that uses sound to detect cardiac wall or valve motion.

Leopold's maneuvers (described in Chapter 20) may be performed to assist in determining fetal presentation and position. In the cephalic presentation and LOA or LOP position (fetal head down and back to the mother's left side), fetal heart tones are best heard in the lower left quadrant of the maternal abdomen. In the breech presentation, the fetal heart sounds are heard at or above the level of the umbilicus.

After locating the fetal heart, the baseline FHR, rhythm, and presence or absence of nonperiodic changes (accelerations and decelerations not associated with uterine contractions [UC]) can be detected by auscultating between contractions.[12] The fetal heart beat can be counted for 15 seconds and multiplied by 4, 30 seconds and multiplied by 2, or a full 60 seconds to determine the baseline rate. If a fetal heart beat less than 100 beats per minute is auscultated, the mother's pulse should be taken to differentiate between the maternal and fetal rate. The minimal standard practice is to evaluate and record the FHR during a contraction

TABLE 43–1. GUIDELINES FOR INTRAPARTUM FETAL HEART RATE MONITORING

	Rate of Assessment	
	High-Risk Pregnancy	*Low-Risk Pregnancy*
Intermittent Auscultation		
1st stage of labor		
Latent phase	Every 30 min	Every 60 min
Active phase	Every 15 min	Every 30 min
2nd stage of labor	Every 5 min	Every 15 min
Continuous Electronic Fetal Monitoring		
1st stage of labor	Every 15 min	Every 30 min
2nd stage of labor	Every 5 min	Every 15 min

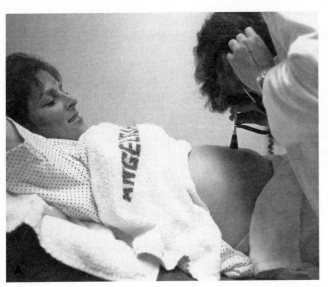
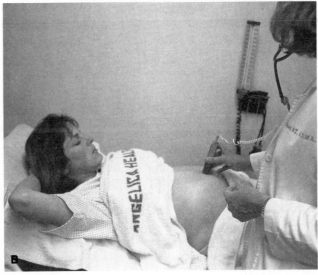

■ *Figure 43–2*
Auscultation of the fetal heart rate. (A) DeLee stethoscope, also known as a fetoscope.
(B) Doppler ultrasound.

and for 30 seconds thereafter[13] to determine the presence or absence of periodic changes (accelerations or decelerations associated with UC) in the FHR.

Nonreassuring FHR patterns observed during auscultation include a fetal baseline heart rate less than 100 beats per minute between UC, a rate less than 100 beats per minute 30 seconds after a UC, or an unexplained baseline tachycardia greater than 160 beats per minute.[13] Continuous electronic monitoring can be initiated in patients exhibiting nonreassuring patterns.

Documentation of auscultated FHR monitoring should include assessment of FHR and UA data, nursing interventions, and patient responses to the interventions. Statements concerning the FHR, rhythm, and the nature of identified FHR changes should be recorded in the patient's chart.[12] Documentation of FHR monitoring is further discussed later in this chapter.

■ ELECTRONIC FETAL HEART RATE MONITORING

Methods of Monitoring

UTERINE ACTIVITY

UA may be monitored by either external or internal methods. External monitoring provides a recording of the frequency and duration of UC, whereas internal monitoring provides an accurate measurement of intra-uterine pressure for assessing both baseline tone and the intensity of contractions.

The use of an internal-pressure catheter permits the most accurate assessment of UA, both quantitatively and temporally. Thus, the internal method is particularly useful in evaluating clients receiving oxytocic drugs or in instances when the temporal relationship of changes in FHR to UC is unclear. Internal uterine monitoring is also helpful in documenting the adequacy of labor in clients who experience an arrest of cervical dilatation. Often a labor pattern of frequent contractions of low intensity will appear impressively strong when using the external technique. The clinical impression of weak contractions perceived by an experienced nurse may be confirmed with internal-pressure monitoring. In such cases, oxytocin augmentation may be necessary. Nevertheless, most labors that are monitored can be adequately assessed by the external method. The method used and any change of method should be noted directly on the fetal monitoring record as well as in the nursing note or nursing flow sheet.

External-Pressure Monitor. UA is monitored by a pressure transducer called a *tocodynamometer* (Figs. 43-3 and 43-4). A transducer converts one form of energy to another; this transducer converts pressure to electrical signals. The tocodynamometer is a flat disk with a flush plunger. It is secured to the mother's abdomen with an elastic belt. As the uterus contracts, the abdominal wall rises and presses against the transducer. The subsequent movement of the plunger is converted into an electrical signal and is recorded on the paper, giving a continuous record of the frequency and duration of contractions.

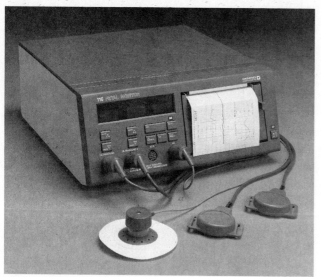

■ *Figure 43–3*

A typical fetal heart rate monitor with a beltless tocodynamometer and Doppler transducer. Note that there are two Doppler transducers present for the simultaneous monitoring of twins. (Courtesy: Corometrics Medical Systems, Inc. Wallingford, Connecticut.)

Correct placement of the tocodynamometer is necessary if interpretable data are to be gathered (see the Nursing Guidelines for Application of the External Fetal Monitor). The transducer is placed over the area where the greatest displacement of the uterus occurs during a contraction (i.e., the uterine fundus). Displacement of the abdominal wall by the uterus may not be adequate to record UC in a client with a small uterus (i.e., less than 20 weeks' gestation) or in one who is extremely overweight. Movement of the maternal abdominal wall caused by respirations, coughing, or position changes may be reflected on the fetal monitoring record. Any

such interfering factors should be noted as such on the monitor tracing. It may not be possible to obtain consistent data with this method from clients who are extremely restless. Occasionally, clients who are experiencing pain find that the firm elastic straps become uncomfortable or interfere with breathing techniques and effleurage. When this occurs, repositioning the tocodynamometer and straps may be useful.

Internal-Pressure Method. A soft plastic catheter filled with sterile water is passed, usually by a physician, into the uterus beyond the presenting fetal part by means of a firmer plastic introducer (Fig. 43-5). This, of course, requires that the cervix be partially dilated. Although a catheter or balloon may be placed extra-amniotically, for clinical use, the placement is intra-amniotic and requires that the membranes be previously ruptured. The catheter is connected to a pressure transducer (strain gauge). The intrauterine pressure is transmitted from the amniotic fluid through the sterile water in the catheter to the pressure transducer. The transducer produces an electrical signal that is amplified by the recorder. Changes in the intrauterine pressure that occur with contractions or increased intra-abdominal pressure from, for example, the Valsalva maneuver or coughing are recorded on the monitor (see Nursing Guidelines for Application of the Intrauterine Pressure Catheter).

The internal-pressure catheter provides a means of sampling amniotic fluid for meconium or bacteria during labor if this becomes clinically useful. If the catheter becomes plugged by vernix, meconium, or blood, intrauterine pressure will not be transmitted to the transducer. Flushing with small amounts of sterile water usually corrects the problem. When this fails, the catheter should be withdrawn slightly and repositioned. This may relieve kinking of the catheter or entrapment between the lower uterine segment and fetus. The portion

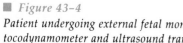

■ *Figure 43–4*

Patient undergoing external fetal monitoring. Both the tocodynamometer and ultrasound transducer are secured to the mother's abdomen with an elastic belt.

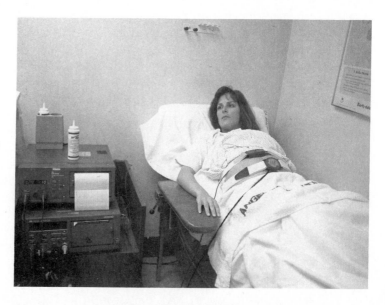

Nursing Guidelines for Application of the External Fetal Monitor

Equipment Needed

Fetal monitor

Monitor paper

Ultrasound transducer

Tocodynamometer

2 straps and buttons

Conductive jelly

Preparation of Equipment

Plug ultrasound transducer into outlet on front of monitor.

Plyg tocodynamometer into outlet on front of monitor

Turn monitor on.

Test monitor by pushing FHR button.

Procedure

Nursing Intervention	Rationale
1. Explain procedure to mother and support person.	• Allays fears and gains cooperation; promotes compliance
2. Elevate head of bed 15–30 degrees	• Decreases aorta and vena caval compression
3. Powder 2 straps and place under client.	• Promotes comfort
4. Apply conductive jelly to ultrasound	• Aids in transmission of ultrasound wave
5. Place ultrasound on client's abdomen and move around until strong FHR is heard and consistent waveform appears on oscilloscope.	• Locates the point of maximum FHR; verifies clarity of input
6. Attach straps to ultrasound using buttons to fasten.	• Should be firmly attached but not tight
7. Push recorder button if haven't done so already.	• Will not record otherwise
8. Place tocodynamometer on the fundal portion of uterus.	• Location of greatest uterine displacement
9. Attach straps to tocodynamometer using buttons to fasten.	• Should be firmly attached but not tight
10. Adjust sound and equipment as needed, particularly when a procedure is performed or client's position is changed.	• Monitor sensitive to change or disturbance to equipment

of the catheter in the vagina or outside the client should not be advanced into the uterus. Not only may this result in bacterial contamination, but it is generally ineffective because the flexibility of the catheter will cause it to coil alongside the presenting fetal part. Perforation of the uterus and injury to the placenta should be considered when excessive vaginal bleeding occurs after placement of the catheter and when UC fail to be recorded. Perforation into the broad ligament has been reported, in which case hemorrhage was concealed. The presence of maternal hypotension and tachycardia following catheter insertion might suggest this rare complication.

Several modifications of the traditional internal-pressure catheters have been manufactured. A model that has gained popularity is a catheter that has a pressure sensor in its tip and transmits measured uterine pressure directly to the fetal monitor through the transducer port. This type of catheter is disposable, easily calibrated, and does not require any water column or irrigation to transmit intrauterine pressure data accurately.[14] Disadvantages of the sensor-tipped catheter are the increased diameter of the tip as well as the increased stiffness of the catheter, which could promote greater patient discomfort and increased risk of uterine perforation.[14]

A second modification made on the pressure catheter is the addition of a second lumen. This device can be used to measure intrauterine pressure through one lumen and infuse fluids into the uterus through the second lumen for purposes such as amnioinfusion.

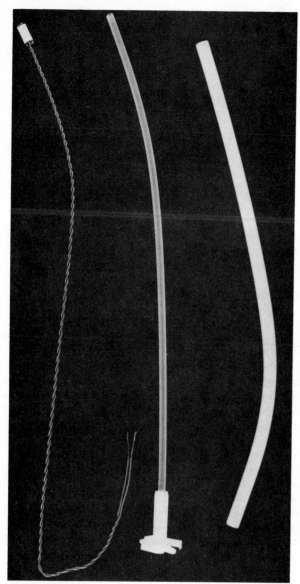

■ *Figure 43-6*
Scalp electrode and introducer for fetal heart monitoring.

Nursing Guidelines for Application of a Fetal Scalp Electrode

Equipment Needed

Fetal monitor

Monitor paper

Leg plate

Leg strap

Fetal scalp electrode

Procedure

1. Explain purpose, indications, and procedure for internal FHR monitoring to the client and the support person.
2. Test leg plate before beginning the procedure by plugging into monitor where indicated. It should read out a test rate of 120 beats per minute.
3. Position client for a vaginal examination.
4. Open spiral electrode pack with sterile technique.
5. Remove applicator and attach color-coded wires to appropriate push post on the leg plate following application of spiral electrode to baby's scalp by physician or certified nurse.
6. Apply electrode paste to leg plate and secure firmly with leg strap to mid-inner or anterior thigh.
7. Observe oscilloscope for FECG waveform, making sure it correlates simultaneously with an audible signal and a clear, interpretable tracing.

or after delivery by gentle counterclockwise rotation of the attached wires.

CENTRALIZED FETAL HEART RATE MONITORING

Recent advances in technology have permitted centralized fetal monitoring, that is, a monitoring system that allows a simultaneous display of every monitored bed in a labor and delivery unit (Fig. 43-7). Real-time tracings of the FHR can be displayed as well as status screens that provide an overview of patient data. These displays can be placed at the nurses' station, allowing constant surveillance of the patient even when a nurse is not physically present in the patient's room. An additional

advantage of such a system is that FHR tracings and related nursing notes can be saved on an optical computer disk (Fig. 43-8) and, therefore, permanently archived.

DETERMINATION OF FETAL BLOOD pH

Scalp Sampling. Determination of pH of fetal scalp blood is clinically useful for the diagnosis of fetal distress. For this measurement, a small volume of fetal blood may be obtained by puncturing the fetal scalp and collecting the blood samples in fine glass capillary tubes. To perform this procedure, the membranes must be ruptured, the cervix must be dilated 3 to 4 cm, and the fetal presenting part must be fixed in the pelvis. The procedure requires the client to be in the lithotomy position. It may be performed in bed or in the delivery room. Serial determinations are often obtained 20 to 30 minutes apart. Regardless of where the procedure is carried out, the obstetric team must be prepared to act immediately should the pH determination reveal severe fetal acidosis (pH $\leq$ 7.20).

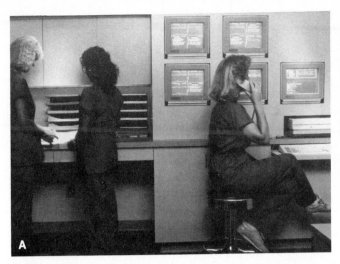

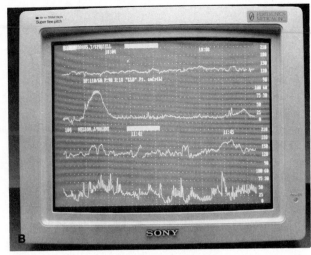

■ *Figure 43–7*
(A) Example of a centralized fetal heart rate monitoring system, and (B) a status screen
revealing patient status and fetal heart rate tracings. (Courtesy: Peritronics Medical Inc., Brea,
California.)

A conical vaginal endoscope is used to visualize the vertex of the fetus during fetal blood sampling (Fig. 43-9). Because of the invasive nature of the procedure, sterile technique is used throughout. The perineum is covered with sterile drapes and prepared with a povidone-iodine solution. The amnioscope is inserted into the vagina and the dilated cervix. A light source is then attached to the amnioscope. A light film of silicone jelly is applied to the scalp. This causes droplets of fetal blood to bead and aggregate, making it easier to collect the blood samples in the capillary tubes. A small metal blade attached to a long handle is used to puncture the scalp. The narrow 2 × 2-mm detachable blades are

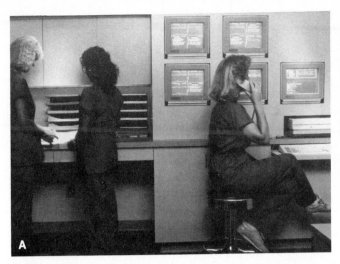

■ *Figure 43–8*
Optical disk used to archive fetal monitoring tracings and
relevant patient data. (Courtesy: Peritronics Medical Inc., Brea,
California.)

mounted in plastic to control the depth of the puncture. A single brisk motion is used to penetrate the skin in a manner similar to that used to obtain a "finger stick." The scalp sampling should not be performed overlying a suture line or fontanelle. The beaded drops of fetal blood are allowed to aggregate and are collected in the long, heparinized capillary tubes. Heparinized capillary tubes hold 250 μl of fetal blood when full. Modern instruments require only 25 to 40 μl of fetal blood to obtain a determination of blood gases. The tube is then passed to the waiting nurse, who inserts a fine metal bead or short wire into the capillary tube prior to sealing it with wax. A magnet passed along the outside of the tube moves the metal wire and stirs the sample to prevent clotting. Exposing the sample to atmospheric air can cause an exchange of oxygen and carbon dioxide, which will alter the hydrogen ion concentration. Placing the capillary tube on ice will retard cellular respiration and thus retards a change in *p*H.

After an adequate sample of scalp blood is obtained, the physician applies firm pressure to the puncture site through the next two contractions to guarantee adequate hemostasis. The site should be observed through a third contraction, and if there is no bleeding, the endoscope may be removed. Repeated scalp blood sampling may be safely performed if necessary. The risks of the procedure include continued bleeding from the puncture site, ecchymosis, hematoma, and infection.

Following scalp blood sampling, the nurse should observe the client for excessive vaginal bleeding that may be fetal in origin. In addition, sustained fetal tachycardia may be observed on the monitor tracing when fetal blood loss occurs externally or a massive hematoma forms.

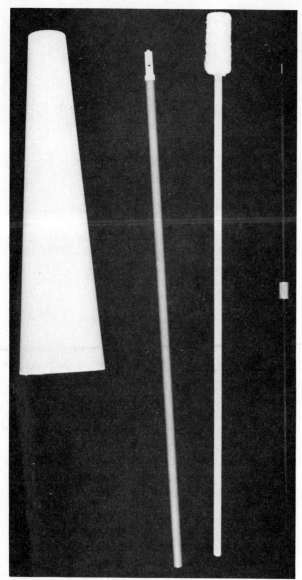

■ *Figure 43–9*
Scalp sampling equipment includes plastic amnioscope, scalpel, cotton sponge, and heparinized capillary tube.

CARE OF THE NEWBORN. When assessing the newborn, the nurse should closely inspect the scalp of the infant to identify the puncture site(s). In many institutions, cleansing with an antiseptic solution and applying an antibiotic ointment are routine. Personnel in the nursery should be alerted to the number and the status of scalp puncture sites at the time the infant is transferred to the nursery. In this way, any complications resulting from the procedure can be detected immediately and treated.

CLINICAL INTERPRETATION OF FETAL SCALP pH. The partial pressure of oxygen and carbon dioxide, as well as bicarbonate ion concentration, can be measured on fetal scalp blood values. The pH, however, has proven to be the simplest, most rapid, and most clinically useful measurement that can be performed on a small sample of blood. The pH of the fetal scalp blood normally ranges between 7.25 and 7.35 during labor. This correlates well with the acid-base status of the blood in the umbilical vessels. A mild progressive decline of pH within the normal range has been noted with contractions and as labor progresses. When the fetus becomes hypoxic, anaerobic glycolysis occurs, resulting in an excess production of lactic acid and an increase in hydrogen ion concentration. The increased hydrogen ion concentration is measured as a decrease in pH (acidosis). Thus, the development of acidosis reflects the effects of hypoxia on respiration or cellular metabolism.

Generally, cord compression with resultant variable decelerations results in a rapid increase in fetal PCO_2, resulting in a mild respiratory acidosis that quickly subsides. Persistent variable decelerations and late decelerations are strongly suggestive of fetal metabolic acidosis.

Clinical studies have demonstrated a correlation between the pH of fetal scalp blood and abnormalities in FHR, Apgar scores, and umbilical cord pH. As a result of these observations, the measurement of the pH of fetal scalp blood has become an increasingly important method for diagnosing and confirming fetal distress. This measurement helps when the interpretation of fetal monitoring data is unclear and reduces the chances of false-positive diagnoses of fetal distress using fetal monitoring. Traditionally, a scalp blood pH of 7.20 or less is considered to be indicative of fetal acidosis or fetal distress; pH values between 7.20 and 7.25 are borderline and warrant repeat sampling. Generally, one does not act on a single pH determination. Equivocal and low values should be repeated while the physician is preparing for a possible rapid delivery.

As is true of other antepartal and intrapartum methods of fetal evaluation, measurement of scalp blood pH may produce false-negative results (normal values when the fetus is hypoxic). Events that occur following fetal blood sampling, but before delivery (e.g., continued cord compression), may account for many of the false-negative results observed. Abnormal maternal acid-base status may be transmitted passively to the fetus through the placenta and account for a portion of the false-positive cases (abnormal values when the fetus is well). This is possible in the diabetic client who is prone to develop ketoacidosis. For this reason, obtaining a simultaneous blood sample from the mother to determine the pH of her blood is occasionally of value in interpreting the fetal pH and will reduce the frequency of false-positive results. Because these problems occur in only a small proportion of cases, they do not detract substantially from the clinical value of fetal pH measurement. In fact, it has been suggested by some physicians that the diagnosis of fetal distress should always be based on the finding of fetal acidosis; however, rapid fetal deterioration, inability to obtain samples, or suspicion of false-negative results makes this test impractical as an absolute criterion in all cases.

Although fetal scalp sampling is a valuable tool in certain clinical situations, many institutions seldom use this technique.[15,16] Newer techniques of fetal scalp and vibroacoustic stimulation in conjunction with careful FHR monitoring have been found to be reasonable alternatives to fetal scalp sampling.[14] With these techniques, it has been estimated that less than 0.5% of patients would need a fetal scalp blood pH.[16]

Scalp Stimulation. Observations have been made that acceleration of the fetal heart rate is associated with the puncturing of the fetal scalp during blood sampling in fetuses with a scalp pH greater than 7.20.[15] Subsequent to these observations, Clark and Paul[16] have described a correlation between heart rate accelerations in response to a tactile stimulation of the fetal scalp and normal scalp pH. During the first stage of labor, 15 seconds of digital pressure on the fetal scalp followed (if needed) by a gentle pinch with an atraumatic (Allis) clamp has been found to stimulate a FHR acceleration of 15 beats per minute lasting at least 15 seconds in the normal fetus. A response to scalp stimulation is an excellent predictor of fetal well-being. If accelerations occur, a normal fetal pH (pH greater than 7.19) can be assumed. If no accelerations are present, however, an abnormal pH is not necessarily present. As with most forms of fetal assessment, scalp stimulation is less accurate in predicting poor outcome or fetal compromise. The use of scalp stimulation, however, can reduce the necessity of scalp blood sampling by approximately 50% in the presence of a FHR pattern suggesting acidosis.

Acoustic Stimulation. Fetal vibroacoustic stimulation has proven effective in the reduction of nonreactive nonstress tests during antepartum fetal surveillance (see Chapter 42). A similar technique has been used in the intrapartum period. Vibroacoustically stimulated fetal accelerations in labor can be elicited in a fetus with a scalp pH above 7.25.[19] Intrapartum sound stimulation is applied to the maternal abdomen for ≤3 seconds. The response is termed *reactive* if an immediate acceleration of 15 beats per minute in 15 seconds is evident. If a qualifying acceleration is not present, the stimulus is repeated for a maximum of three times. As in scalp stimulation, vibroacoustic stimulation has been found to be an excellent predictor of fetal well-being; however, it is less accurate in predicting poor outcome or fetal compromise. The need for scalp sampling can also be reduced by at least 50% when this technique is used.

Percutaneous Umbilical Blood Sampling. Percutaneous umbilical blood sampling (PUBS) is under investigation as a technique for intrapartum fetal evaluation.

(Refer to Chapter 42 for a description of this procedure.) PUBS allows for a direct in utero sampling of umbilical cord blood that can be analyzed for respiratory gases, acid-base status, and lactate concentration.[20,21] Although the diagnosis of fetal acidosis can be made with scalp sampling, an accurate differentiation between acute (respiratory acidosis) or chronic (metabolic acidosis) fetal distress can be made with PUBS.

Umbilical Cord Blood Sampling at Delivery. Following delivery of an infant in whom fetal distress has been suspected, umbilical venous and arterial blood samples should be obtained from a doubly clamped segment of the cord. Measurement of blood gases and pH on these samples makes it easier to correlate the fetal monitor tracing, the scalp blood pH measurements, and the neonatal condition. Cord blood sampling can also provide direction in the management of the newborn.

The technique involves clamping a 10 to 20-cm (4–8 in) length of cord immediately at birth. A 1 ml heparinized syringe with a small-gauge needle, bevel side up, is inserted into the umbilical artery and a sample is withdrawn. After residual air is removed from the syringe, the sample is capped. The syringe can be placed on ice; however, recent investigations have indicated that there is little change in either pH or blood gases when left at room temperature for 30 minutes.[22] Although blood samples from the umbilical vein can also be removed, fetal status is better reflected by arterial cord blood samples. Normal values for umbilical cord blood are listed in Table 43-2.

Application of the Fetal Monitor

The decision to apply the fetal monitor should be based on institutional policy. In many institutions, continuous electronic fetal monitoring is employed in all laboring clients. In other institutions, the responsibility for selection of clients to be monitored rests with the physician and with the nurse. The nurse's role in selection is particularly important when the number of clients who are

TABLE 43–2. NORMAL VALUES FOR UMBILICAL CORD BOOD

Cord Blood	pH	P_{CO_2} (mm Hg)	P_{O_2} (mm Hg)	Bicarbonate (mEq/L)
Arterial	7.28	49.2	18.0	22.3
Venous	7.35	38.2	29.2	20.4

(Adapted from Yeomans ER, Hauth JC, Gilstrap LC, et al: Umbilical cord pH, pCO_2 and bicarbonate following uncomplicated term vaginal deliveries. Am J Obstet Gynecol 151:798–800, 1985)

in labor exceeds the number of available monitors and priorities for monitoring must be established. The decision to monitor generally is made on the basis of one of the following primary indications:

1. Antepartum risk factors, including maternal complications such as diabetes, hypertension, and cardiac, renal, and hematologic diseases. Fetal problems such as suspected intrauterine growth retardation or postdate pregnancy are included.
2. Intrapartum risk factors, such as third-trimester bleeding, passage of meconium, or abnormalities of FHR determined by auscultation.
3. Other obstetric factors (e.g., to evaluate abnormal progress of labor or the effects of drugs such as oxytocics and some anesthetic agents)

After the decision has been made to monitor a client, the method of monitoring is selected. This is contingent on four factors: (1) status of the cervix and membranes, (2) indication for monitoring, (3) client acceptance, and (4) availability. When the membranes are intact or the cervix is not dilated, external methods of monitoring must be used. If adequate data cannot be obtained with the available external systems, internal monitoring should be considered. In cases in which the most accurate data are required (e.g., true beat-to-beat variation, temporal relationship of decelerations to contractions, or true intrauterine pressures), internal monitoring must be used.

See the Nursing Guidelines for Care During FHR Monitoring.

Fetal Monitor Tracing

Fetal monitors are equipped to provide a continuous recording of FHR and UA. This information is recorded on perforated paper that folds "accordion style" (Fig. 43-10). The UA is generally recorded on the lower channel. The recording paper provides a vertical scale for measuring the intrauterine pressure, usually in millimeters of mercury (mm Hg). Most monitors are

---

Nursing Guidelines for Care During FHR Monitoring

1. Continue to perform nursing care that is given to all laboring mothers.
2. Explain to mother and support person what fetal monitoring consists of.
   - Allow mother to express herself and to participate in decision making.
   - Obtain a signed consent form if institution requires it.
   - If FHR monitoring is routine for all clients and this mother refuses, follow institution guidelines for releasing institution and personnel from liability.
3. Explain steps involved for FHR monitoring before or while applying either external or internal monitoring.
4. Recognize mother's fears, concerns, and needs for reinforcement and support. Common fears include the following:
   - Harm to baby from ultrasound
   - Harm to baby from scalp clip to head
   - Something wrong with baby
5. The following procedures can be done to maximaze client comfort:
   - Noisy machine volume can be adjusted so that mother can relax and be comfortable.
   - The mother will have to stay in bed but may change her position frequently to feel less confined.
   - If available, monitoring by telemetry would further allow client mobility.
   - Powdering and reapplying the monitor straps every 2 hours may minimize discomfort from tight straps.
6. Remember always to greet and speak to the client before evaluating the monitor tracing. The laboring mother and fetus are our main focus. The monitor assists with their care.

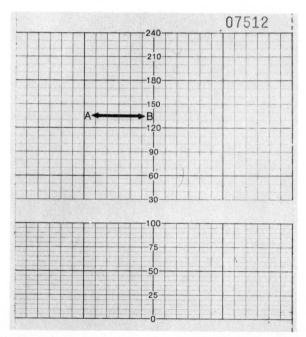

■ *Figure 43–10*

Recording paper for fetal monitor. Note fetal heart rate (beats per minute) recorded on upper channel, UA (mm Hg) recorded on lower channel, and panel number at top of sheet. Distance from A to B equals 1 minute when paper speed is 3 cm/min.

equipped with a zeroing and calibration device to ensure that the record accurately reflects the true intrauterine pressure. The FHR in beats per minute is displayed on the upper channel. Some monitors are also equipped with a digital display of the FHR and a small oscilloscope screen for viewing the FECG.

The paper speed is usually set at 3 cm/min. Divisions on the horizontal scale provide a measurement of the time elapsed and are useful as markers to correlate events on both channels. Numbering on the individual sheets of the record provides a reference for rapid calculation of elapsed time for longer intervals.

Documentation of Fetal Heart Rate Data

Because the data obtained become a part of the client's permanent record, it is important that a systematic method of identification be used at the beginning of each new fetal monitor tracing paper and subsequent delivery. A sample format for identification is shown in Figure 43-11. In addition, the clock-time and important clinical data should be identified on the strip as well as in the patient's record. These include vital signs, vaginal examinations, rupture of membranes, physician review of the tracing, medications (dose and route of administration), and client activity. This information is important for interpreting the record, retrospectively reviewing the tracing for teaching purposes, and defending against litigation.[23]

Nursing documentation of the FHR data must also be recorded either on a flow sheet or in a nurse's note. A joint statement[24] prepared by ACOG and the Nurses Association of the American College of Obstetricians and Gynecologists has stipulated that nurses must use descriptive names, such as *early, late,* and *variable decelerations* in documentation. The patient's record should include nursing assessments of the FHR and UA. Identification of nonreassuring FHR patterns demand initiation of appropriate nursing interventions and physician notification. The attending physician is expected to respond. If the physician does not respond or is unfamiliar with monitoring, the nurse should follow hospital protocol for dealing with the situation.[24] These actions must be documented in the patient chart. If they are not documented, in a logical, retrospective review of the chart, one can only assume that these nursing interventions were not performed.

In charting, the nurse's note should include appropriate terminology, as follows:

2/8/91

0930 Continuous fetal internal monitoring. FHR ranges between 130 and 142 bpm with variability ranging between 6 and 8 bpm since 0800. Refer to flow sheet.

1000 Uterine contractions occurring every 3 minutes with intensity to 75 mm Hg. Repetitive late decelerations. Decreased FHR variability. Dr. Smith notified at

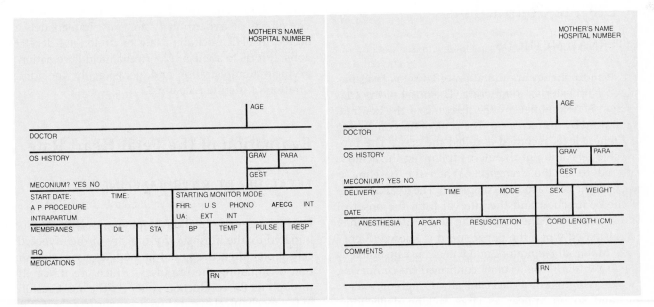

■ *Figure 43–11*
(Left) Label provides identification and clinical information for interpretation of tracing and is applied when monitoring is initiated and at the start of each new monitor strip. (Right) Label provides identification and clinical information for correlation of monitor data with neonatal condition and is applied following delivery.

Nursing Guidelines for Intervention for Fetal Heart Rate Patterns (continued)

Nursing Intervention	*Rationale*
1. Recognize the pattern and assess the frequency, depth, and duration of the deceleration.	There is correlation between the severity of the variable deceleration and fetal condition.
2. Follow institution policy: do you assess before notifying the physician and carrying out the interventions of #3?	Some institutions have 24-hour physician coverage on the unit; in other institutions the nurse must inform the physician by phone, because they have standing orders. Changing position may help to remove the pressure on the cord. If this is not effective, physician may attempt upward displacement of presenting part.
3. Turn client to her left side or to knee–chest position and give oxygen 10 L/min by mask.	

III. *Baseline Changes*
A. Tachycardia

Description

A baseline FHR of more than 160 beats per minute persisting 10 to 15 minutes
Mild: 160–179 beats per minute
Marked: 180 or more beats per minute

Pathophysiology:

Fetal hypoxia, maternal fever, idiopathic maternal anxiety, prematurity, drug related, fetal arrhythmia

Nursing Intervention	*Rationale*
1. Confirm by auscultating FHR.	Confirm that monitor is operating properly and FHR has increased. Tachycardia may be in response to fetal movement.
2. Monitor maternal vital signs.	Tachycardia may be due to maternal fever.
3. Monitor contractions.	FHR may increase in response to excessive contractions.
4. Change maternal position.	Aortoiliac compression is alleviated.
5. Continue to watch closely by reviewing tracings for changing patterns.	Etiologic factors might be identified. Tachycardia may be a sign of fetal distress; arrhythmias may be identified by FECG.
6. Chart descriptive note or chart on flow sheet.	Nursing management is dictated by institution policies.

B. Bradycardia

Description:

An FHR of less than 120 beats per minute persisting 10 to 15 minutes
Mild: 100–119 beats per minute
Marked: Less than 100 beats per minute

Nursing Intervention	*Rationale*
1. Change maternal position	Changing position alleviates uterine pressure on the aorta and vena cava.
2. Give oxygen by mask @ 10 L/min.	Fetus may have congenital heart abnormality.
3. Continue to watch closely for:	Ominous signs indicate fetal distress, even impending death.
Marked bradycardia with loss of variability and late decelerations.	This is a sign of fetal distress.

(continued)

Nursing Guidelines for Intervention for Fetal Heart Rate Patterns (continued)

Nursing Intervention	Rationale
Mild bradycardia with good FHR variability and absence of late decelerations.	This is generally not a sign of fetal distress.
Bradycardia due to heart block.	This is not a sign of acute fetal distress.
4. Chart descriptive note or chart on flow sheet.	Nursing management is dictated by institution policies.

C. Variability

Description

A variation of the resting FHR
Average: 6–10 beats per minute
Minimal: 3–5 beats per minute
None: 0–2 beats per minute

Pathophysiology:

Maternal medication, fetal acidosis, fetal neurologic immaturity

Nursing Intervention	Rationale
1. Observe variability of the FHR.	Variability is an indication of normal neurologic control of heart rate and a measure of fetal reserve.
2. Increased variability requires no nursing intervention.	This may be due to external uterine palpitation, UC, fetal activity, or maternal activity
3. Decreased variability: follow physician's order based on cause.	Possible causes include prematurity, drugs, hypoxia and acidosis, fetal sleep, fetal cardiac arrhythmias.
4. Chart descriptive note or chart on flow sheet.	Nursing management is dictated by institution policies.

TACHYCARDIA AND BRADYCARDIA

The FHR decreases slightly as pregnancy advances and normally ranges between 120 and 160 beats per minute. Elevation of the FHR baseline above 160 for periods greater than 10 minutes is referred to as *baseline tachycardia*. Rates between 161 and 180 are classified as *mild tachycardia* and those greater than 180 as *marked tachycardia*. Rates below 120 are referred to as *bradycardia*. Those between 100 and 119 are classified as *mild bradycardia* and those less than 100 as *marked bradycardia*. Either fetal tachycardia or bradycardia may be related to fetal hypoxia (low oxygen content of the fetal blood or inadequate delivery of oxygen to the fetal tissues). Fetal tachycardia may be an early warning sign of fetal hypoxia, whereas fetal bradycardia occurs somewhat later in the sequence of events. Abnormalities in baseline FHR may also be due to arrhythmias (abnormal discharge or transmission of impulses through the conduction system of the heart). These are usually benign and transient but may, at times, be associated with congenital heart defects or heart failure. Fetal tachycardia may also be associated with maternal fever, fetal infec-

tion, maternal thyrotoxicosis, fetal anemia, and fetal tachyarrhythmias. Because core temperature (internal body temperature) rises earlier and is higher than that measured either orally or rectally, fetal tachycardia may precede maternal fever by a short time. Likewise, fetal bradycardia may be associated with maternal hypothermia, but this is an unusual event clinically. Fetal bradycardia may also be caused by drugs administered to the mother, such as beta-blockers. Fetal congenital heart block may produce a baseline bradycardia. This phenomenon has been observed in infants of mothers with systemic lupus erythematosus, who produce an antibody that crosses the placenta and destroys the fetal conducting system.

VARIABILITY

As fetal development advances, the autonomic nervous system assumes an increasingly important role in modulating FHR. Discharge of sympathetic nerves causes an increase in rate, whereas discharge of parasympathetic nerves causes a slowing of the heart rate. The normal continuous opposition of these two stimuli results in the beat-to-beat variability noted in the heart rate of the normal fetus. It is reflected by the fine irregularity seen on the normal FHR tracing (Fig. 43-12). A fetus of at least 28 weeks' gestational age should demonstrate normal beat-to-beat variability that usually ranges from 2 to 10 beats per minute around the average heart rate.

It is important to note that true beat-to-beat variability can be assessed only by direct fetal electrography (i.e., internal monitoring using the spiral electrode). In the past, variability of the FHR baseline was often overlooked as an indicator of fetal status; however, it is now apparent that normal beat-to-beat variability is probably the most reliable indication of fetal well-being. When beat-to-beat variability is normal (i.e., ≥6 beats per minute), it is thought to indicate an intact nervous system with normal regulatory influence over the FHR. Whereas several factors may be responsible for the loss of heart rate variability, a flat FHR baseline in the absence of explainable causes is considered ominous and potentially indicative of hypoxia (Fig. 43-13).

Nowhere in FHR monitoring is the influence of drugs more obvious than in the assessment of FHR variability. It has become increasingly apparent that a large proportion of drugs administered to the mother will cause diminished or absent FHR variability. Specific drugs that decrease variability include narcotics, barbiturates, phenothiazines, atropine, and tranquilizers. For this reason, it is often useful to evaluate FHR variability by internal monitoring before these drugs are administered.

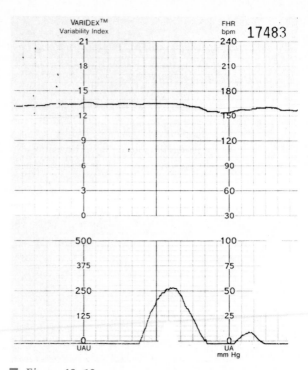

■ *Figure 43–13*

Fetal heart rate tracing with absent beat-to-beat variability. Note subtle late deceleration.

PERIODIC CHANGES

When changes in the FHR occur in association with uterine contractions, they are described as being *periodic.* The fetus is equipped with cardiovascular reflexes that may cause periodic or transient changes in the FHR from its normal baseline. Some of these responses (e.g., accelerations with fetal movement) are indicative of normal fetal status, whereas others (e.g., variable deceleration with cord compression) are designed to compensate for alterations in cardiovascular dynamics. Both periodic and nonperiodic changes require careful evaluation for the diagnosis of fetal stress and distress.

Accelerations. Transient increases of the FHR (>15 beats per minute for >15 sec) have been noted during labor since fetal monitoring was first used (Fig. 43-14). They are, at times, associated with contractions but often are unrelated to UA. The outcome of fetuses demonstrating accelerations in labor has been uniformly good. It is believed that the increased FHR is due to transient discharges of the sympathetic nervous system. It has also been suggested that accelerations associated with contractions might be caused by partial compression of the cord, which results in selective occlusion of the umbilical vein and causes fetal hypotension and a transient increase in the FHR. The observation that accelerations are associated with fetal movement in the healthy fetus

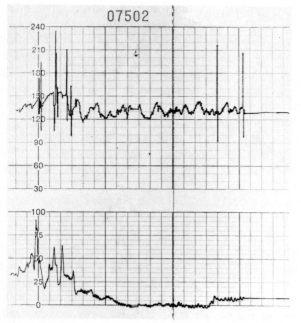

■ *Figure 43–12*

Fetal heart rate tracing. Note fine irregularity or beat-to-beat variability.

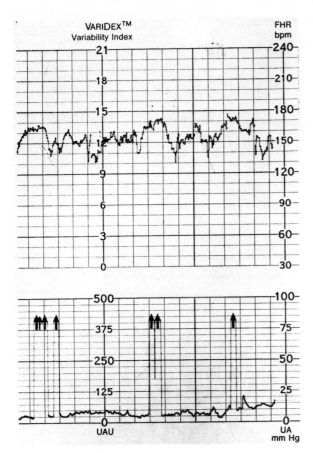

■ *Figure 43–14*

Transient accelerations of fetal heart rate noted during NST. Arrows were made by the client to indicate when fetal movements were perceived.

is the basis of the nonstress test for antepartal evaluation of the high-risk fetus.

Early Decelerations. Transient slowing of the FHR in a pattern that is almost a mirror image of the contractions is known as an *early deceleration*. These decelerations are believed to be related to the fetal head compression associated with the contraction, resulting in a parasympathetic discharge mediated by the vagus nerve. Parasympathetic stimulation results in slowing of the FHR. This pattern represents a normal response of the fetus to this stimulus and, in the absence of other periodic FHR changes, is associated with a uniformly good outcome.

Characteristically, these decelerations have a waveform that coincides with and resembles an inverted UC (Fig. 43-15). They are uniform in shape, of short duration, and of low amplitude. The FHR at the *nadir* (lowest point) of the deceleration is usually 100 beats per minute or greater. When slower FHRs are observed with contractions, the decelerations are usually of the variable type (see below). Early decelerations do not respond to oxygen administered to the mother or to

position change. They may be abolished when atropine (a vagolytic agent) is administered. Because of the benign nature of this pattern, however, remedial action is not necessary.

Late Decelerations. Like the term *early decelerations*, the designation *late decelerations* indicates a uniform shape and a consistent relationship of the deceleration to contractions. In contrast to early decelerations, the onset of the late deceleration, its nadir, and its recovery do not coincide with the onset, amplitude, and recovery of the UC but rather are delayed (Fig. 43-16). Unlike variable decelerations, late decelerations may be quite subtle, entirely within the normal FHR range and yet ominous. This is particularly true if FHR variability is absent or diminished. Several studies have demonstrated that subtle late decelerations accompanied by reduced heart rate variability are more likely to be associated with fetal acidosis than are more obvious late decelerations in which variability is preserved. A classification of late decelerations is given in Table 43-3.

Late decelerations are thought to reflect the effects of intermittent hypoxia on the fetal autonomic nervous system, causing transient fetal hypertension and triggering a vagally mediated bradycardia. Prolonged tissue hypoxia will lead to the accumulation of lactate and result in fetal acidosis. Such effects on acid base balance may have a direct effect on the fetal myocardium and conducting system, causing slowing of the heart rate.

The hypoxia reflected in late decelerations results from the reduced oxygen delivered by the placenta as a result of the diminished intervillous blood flow that occurs with the UC. A direct and specific relationship between hypoxia and late decelerations has been demonstrated experimentally in monkeys. Hypoxia causing late decelerations may be elicited when less oxygen is delivered to the uterus (e.g., with maternal hypoxia or hypotension), when abnormally strong UC occur (hypertonus), or when relative placental insufficiency exists (e.g., intrauterine growth retardation or hypertensive disorders of pregnancy).

Transient late decelerations associated with maternal hypotension or uterine hypertonus that responds to remedial action are thought to signal fetal stress. Removing or correcting the stress often results in fetal recovery. On the other hand, a pattern of consistent and persistent late decelerations that do not respond to remedial measures suggests fetal distress and is often associated with hypoxia, acidosis, and low Apgar scores at birth. This latter group of findings, of course, indicates prompt delivery.

Variable Decelerations. Variable deceleration is the most commonly observed FHR change during labor. The nomenclature of this pattern is based on the fact that the relationships of these decelerations to the con-

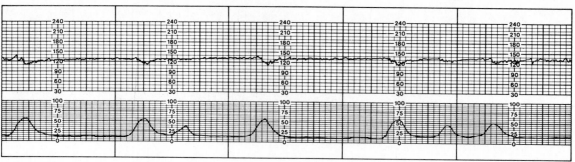

■ *Figure 43–15*

Early deceleration. The fetal heart rate baseline is in the normal range with diminished variability. Uterine activity is normal with oxytocin augmentation. Early deceleration patterns are evident, approximating a mirror image of the uterine pressure curve. The nadir of the early deceleration occurs at the same time as the peak of the uterine contraction. (Puttler OL Jr: Continuous electronic monitoring during labor: Pattern recognition. Freeman RK: In Freeman RK (ed): A Clinical Approach to Fetal Monitoring. San Leandro, CA, Berkeley Bio-Engineering, 1974.)

tractions and the waveform are both variable (Fig. 43-17). These decelerations represent a reflex response to umbilical cord compression. They are often observed in association with UC, a situation in which cord compression is more likely to occur; the cord can be wrapped around the fetal trunk, the neck, or an extremity. They may also represent compression of the cord against the uterine wall during a contraction. Variable decelerations are often seen when oligohydramnios is present. This is a circumstance during which the cord is particularly vulnerable. When the umbilical cord is compressed, fetal peripheral resistance rises. The fetal PO_2 falls and PCO_2 rises. This triggers baroreceptors, which stimulate the vagus nerve and cause a fall in the FHR. The firing of the vagus nerve is erratic, resulting in the variable onset, shape, severity, and dura-

tion of the contraction. The sudden hypoxia from cord compression may trigger aortic arch chemoreceptors also playing a role in the pathogenesis of these decelerations.

Variable decelerations may be classified as mild, moderate, or severe (see Table 43-3). Because there is a correlation between the severity of variable decelerations and fetal condition, it is important that the nurse evaluate the frequency, depth, and duration of these decelerations.

The variable decelerations must be judged in context with the entire fetal tracing. What is the baseline FHR? Has it shifted upward or downward during the course of labor? Is the baseline variability acceptable? The answers to these questions will help the nurse and physician decide whether these variable decelerations are the harbinger of poor fetal outcome or whether they

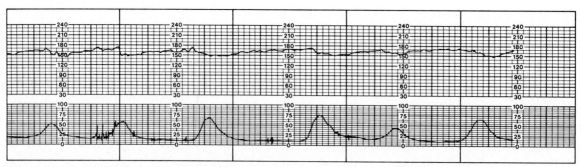

■ *Figure 43–16*

Moderate late deceleration. There is a mild fetal tachycardia, ranging between 160 and 170 beats per minute, with decreased variability. Uterine activity is normal. The nadir of late deceleration occurs when the uterine contraction is nearly over. A scalp capillary blood sample had been taken just prior to the first portion of this pane, and mild fetal acidosis was demonstrated with scalp blood pH 7.21. (Putter OL Jr.: Continuous electronic monitoring during labor: Pattern recognition. In Freeman RK (ed): A Clinical Approach to Fetal Monitoring. San Leandro, CA, Berkeley Bio-Engineering, 1974.)

TABLE 43-3. PRINCIPLES OF GRADING VARIABLE AND LATE DECELERATIONS

	Criteria of Grading		
	Mild	*Moderate*	*Severe*
Variable Deceleration			
Level to which FHR drops and duration of deceleration	<30-sec duration irrespective of level >80 bpm irrespective of duration 70–80bpm <60 sec	<70 bpm <30 <60 sec 70–80 bpm >60 sec	<70 bpm >60 sec
Late Deceleration			
Amplitude of drop in FHR	<15 bpm	15–45 bpm	>45 bpm

bpm = beats per minute.

represent a period of transient cord compression. Anytime a fetus experiences repetitive variable decelerations, the nurse should take initiative and institute maternal position change in an attempt to relieve the cord compression. The usual first move is to roll the client in the left lateral recumbent position. If this is ineffective, other position changes should be attempted to relieve the decelerations. If the client is receiving oxytocin and persistent, severe variable decelerations are present, oxytocin infusion should be stopped until the physician has the opportunity to evaluate the tracing.

Mild variable decelerations are usually of little clinical significance. Moderate and severe variable decelerations can cause a significant reduction in umbilical blood flow, resulting in an increase in fetal P_{CO_2} and a transient respiratory acidosis. Repetitive severe variable decelerations can result in fetal metabolic acidosis. This requires early intervention by the physician. Therefore, with repetitive moderate and severe variable de-

celerations, fetal scalp sampling or delivery should be performed.

AMINOINFUSION. A factor related to the occurrence of variable decelerations is oligohydramnios, i.e., an inverse relationship exists between the amount of amniotic fluid and the frequency of variable decelerations.[25] This relationship appears strongest with an amniotic fluid index (AFI) of less than 8 cm. Maintenance of an adequate amniotic fluid volume during labor provides protective cushioning of the umbilical cord, thereby minimizing cord compression. Amnioinfusion, the infusion of normal saline into the amniotic cavity through an intrauterine pressure catheter, can be used to decrease the frequency and severity of variable decelerations during labor.[26-28]

Indications for amnioinfusion include patients with premature rupture of membranes or intrauterine growth retarded fetuses experiencing mild variable decelerations; decreased AFI less than or equal to 5 cm; or any

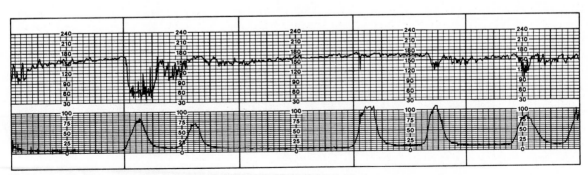

■ *Figure 43–17*

Severe variable deceleration. There is a mild fetal tachycardia with normal baseline variability. Uterine activity is normal. The deceleration is corrected by changing the client's position. Subsequent deceleration patterns are much less severe. (Puttler OL Jr.: Continuous electronic monitoring during labor: Pattern recognition. In Freeman RK (ed): A Clinical Approach to Fetal Monitoring. San Leandro, CA, Berkeley Bio-Engineering, 1974.)

patient in labor with ruptured membranes who is experiencing frequent, prolonged, or severe variable decelerations. Contraindications to the procedure include late decelerations; moderate or severe variable decelerations; diminished baseline variability; chorioamnionitis; meconium-stained amniotic fluid; vaginal bleeding; and fetal or uterine anomalies.

Amnioinfusion can be performed through either a single- or double-lumen pressure catheter. The procedure is initiated by providing the patient with a thorough explanation of amnioinfusion and obtaining a informed consent. The AFI is determined with an ultrasound examination. (The procedure for measuring the AFI is described in Chapter 42.) A vaginal examination is performed to rule out cord prolapse and to determine fetal presentation and cervical dilatation. If direct continuous electronic fetal monitoring has not already been initiated, a scalp electrode and intrauterine pressure catheter are established. The patient should be placed in a left lateral recumbent position to prevent supine hypotension. Normal saline that has been warmed to body temperature is infused by gravity at a rate of 10 to 20 ml/min. A common method of heating the amnioinfusate is to place the bag or bottle of saline in a blood warmer. The amount of saline infused is variable. Some institutions infuse saline at a rate of 10 ml/min for 1 hour, after which it is reduced to 3 ml/min until delivery.[29] However, amnioinfusion has been found to increase uterine tone significantly during and after the infusion.[30] To decrease the risk of increased intrauterine pressure resulting in decreased uteroplacental perfusion,[31] some institutions prefer to limit the total volume of infusion. In women with oligohydramnios, an infusion of 250 ml saline has been found to increase the AFI by approximately 4 cm.[32] A total of 500 ml amnioinfusate will achieve an AFI greater than or equal to 8 cm.[28,30] Infused patients undergo hourly AFI determinations, and repeat

amnioinfusion is performed whenever the AFI drops below 8 cm. Studies are ongoing to determine the optimal method of infusion and the amount of saline used during the procedure.

SINUSOIDAL PATTERN

An unusual abnormality in FHR in which there is a repetitive undulation of the baseline resembling a "sine wave" has been called a *sinusoidal pattern* (Fig. 43-18). Occasionally, tracings of a normal fetus appear to have a transient sinusoidal pattern. This has not been correlated with any particular fetal abnormality. A persistent sinusoidal pattern sometimes is indicative of fetal hypoxia or severe fetal anemia. The latter is most frequently observed in fetuses suffering from hydrops fetalis due to Rh isoimmunization.

Severe fetal anemia can also be seen in cases of fetal maternal hemorrhage. This can occur spontaneously from a chronic placental abruption or following transplacental amniocentesis.

The pathophysiology of the development of a sinusoidal pattern is not understood. It has been hypothesized that this pattern may reflect an absence of autonomic nervous control over the FHR due to severe hypoxia. This pattern has been observed and is considered ominous in the hydropic fetus.

■ PSYCHOLOGICAL ASPECTS OF FETAL MONITORING

Fetal monitoring can occasionally have an important psychological impact on the clients. It is hoped that the

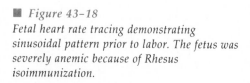

■ *Figure 43–18*
Fetal heart rate tracing demonstrating sinusoidal pattern prior to labor. The fetus was severely anemic because of Rhesus isoimmunization.

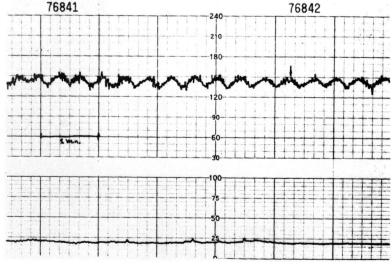

need for fetal monitoring has been discussed with the client before the onset of labor. If it has not, this task may fall on the labor room nurse. It is important to stress to the parents that the purpose of monitoring is to detect any evidence of fetal distress before the fetus is damaged, *not* because the physician believes that the fetus is already in danger. This will usually alleviate much of the client's fear. The nurse must make the client aware that the FHR is consistently changing and that there is a wide range of normal variation. The nurse must also assure the client that with external FHR tracing, movement by the mother or fetus can cause a temporary loss of the FHR on the monitor. The client must know that this is a mechanical phenomenon and does not reflect a real loss of the FHR. Often the nurse is also called on to explain to the client that internal monitoring is safe for the fetus.

Because most clients desire to observe the monitor tracing, the equipment should be placed in view of the mother, father, and nurse (Fig. 43-19). Couples often find that observing the onset and decrement (down-slope) of the contractions is useful in applying breathing techniques. This is particularly true for the father. The reassurance obtained from observing or listening to the fetal heartbeat during labor is often a secondary benefit to the couple.

Fetal monitoring requires a nurse who is professional, composed, and diplomatic. The nurse must be ready to take initiative. If an abnormal FHR pattern is noted, the nurse must take immediate action and, at the same time, allay the client's anxiety and notify the physician. Also, should scalp *p*H sampling or cesarean delivery become necessary, the nurse must exert a calming influence on the client while helping prepare her and the equipment for the appropriate procedure.

Indeed, the responsibility of helping the mother cope with the psychological aspects of fetal monitoring usually rests with the labor nurse. This nurse must be a competent, compassionate, secure person who can help the client understand the purpose of and procedures involved in fetal monitoring. This person should also be able to act swiftly in the event of an emergency and still maintain the client's confidence and allay her fears.

■ NURSING CARE OF THE WOMAN PARTICIPATING IN INTRAPARTUM FETAL MONITORING

Nursing Process

The nursing process is designed to accomplish the major patient goals of care of the woman participating in intrapartum fetal monitoring, as follows:

1. Mother and fetus maintain optimal health.
2. Mother indicates knowledge of the purpose of fetal monitoring.
3. Mother psychologically adjusts to continuous electronic fetal monitoring and uses it for breathing and relaxation techniques.

The role of the nurse during labor has expanded to caring for the fetus as well as for the mother. As with other diagnostic procedures, it is the nurses's responsibility to inform the client about the purpose and the procedure of the monitoring and to screen and interpret the data initially.

With consumerism becoming an increasingly important factor in the delivery of obstetric care, the need

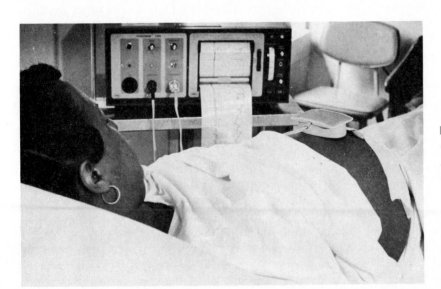

■ *Figure 43–19*
Client with external fetal monitor applied. Note that the monitor function can be observed by the client.

for fetal monitoring by those women intent on natural, nonintervention childbirth has been questioned. The principles of fetal monitoring and the scientific basis for interpreting the data have become well understood. Although it seems logical to presume that the detection and alleviation of fetal stress or the detection of fetal distress should be of benefit to all, the long-term benefits of clinically applied fetal monitoring are not as yet well substantiated. In counseling parents, the nurse should state the intended benefits of fetal monitoring without ignoring the infrequent complications. The nurse should never tell the family that intrapartum monitoring guarantees a healthy neonate.

Continuing interpretation of data and the use of new equipment or tests are imperative. In many institutions, nursing guidelines have been established concerning the application of fetal monitors, the interpretation of data, and the institution of remedial change when abnormalities are detected. Thus, to use the fetal monitor, the nurse must be familiar with the equipment, have an understanding of the fundamental principles involved, and have access to updated information concerning interpretation and management of the data.

When fetal monitoring first became widely used, concerns were raised that there would be a tendency to nurse the monitor rather than the client. On the contrary, fetal monitoring has had the beneficial result of freeing the nurse from repetitious tasks and providing an opportunity for more and better quality care for the mother and the fetus. In applying monitoring, the nurse makes independent assessments of maternal and fetal pathophysiology and initiates action to correct abnormalities as they develop. These tasks have led to the concept of the nurse caring for a high-risk mother and fetus as an "intensivist." As a result, greater appreciation of the need for primary personal continuous nursing care during labor and delivery has developed. Thus, monitoring is an important factor in enhancing the quality of nursing care during labor and delivery.

Nursing Assessment

Assessment of the intrapartum monitored patient is initiated with an evaluation of the clinical status of both the mother and fetus. This includes maternal vital signs, assessment of the amount of amniotic fluid, and baseline data of the FHR and UA. As labor progresses, ongoing data are compared to the data obtained at admission. FHR and UC pattern recognition and interpretation should be related to maternal condition. An elevation of the maternal temperature, hyperactivity of the uterus related to the use of oxytocin, or a supine position of the mother can precipitate ominous FHR patterns. Heart rate abnormalities can often be corrected with an alteration of the mother's physical status. If membranes

rupture after admission to the labor unit, the quality and quantity of fluid should be evaluated.

Other factors that should be assessed during this phase of nursing process should include an evaluation of the mother's support system and level of coping. Additionally, both the mother and her accompanying partner's level of knowledge of fetal monitoring should be assessed. They should be evaluated for their understanding of the purposes, procedures, and interpretations of monitoring data and how they relate to fetal condition.

Potential Nursing Diagnoses

A variety of nursing diagnoses may be made through the various stages of intrapartum fetal monitoring. Examples are anxiety related to the perceived loss of the fetus; alterations in comfort: pain, related to the position or equipment used in monitoring; ineffective individual coping related to an unsatisfactory support system; knowledge deficit of monitoring procedures related to inability to concentrate or understand nurses' instructions; and powerlessness related to being confined to bed by monitoring equipment.

Nursing Planning and Intervention: Remedial Measures for Fetal Distress

ABNORMALITIES IN FETAL HEART RATE

The keys to excellent nursing care in the client with abnormalities in the FHR tracing are careful attention to detail and fast, calm action. Early decelerations do not usually require intervention.

In the event of repetitive late decelerations, oxytocin should be discontinued if it is being used. Oxygen should be delivered by face mask at 5 to 6 L/min. Maternal blood pressure should be ascertained. If the client is hypotensive, an attempt should be made physiologically to raise the blood pressure. This can be accomplished by maternal position change and increase in the rate of intravenous crystalloid infusion. If the client has received regional anesthesia and this has caused hypotension, an anesthesiologist should be summoned so that an appropriate vasopressor agent can be administered.

In the event of repetitive late decelerations that do not correct with the above measures, fetal scalp sampling should be performed quickly or delivery should be effected.

If severe variable decelerations occur, the same steps should be taken as in the case of late decelerations. Also, an immediate vaginal examination should be done

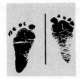

Nursing Care Plan

The Woman Participating in Intrapartum Fetal Monitoring

Patient Goals
1. Mother and fetus maintain optimal health.
2. Mother indicates knowledge of the purpose of fetal monitoring.
3. Mother psychologically adjusts to continuous electronic fetal monitoring and uses it for breathing and relaxation techniques.

Assessment	Potential Nursing Diagnosis	Planning and Intervention	Evaluation
Determination of Need for Electronic Fetal Monitoring (EFM)			
Assess current maternal physical status	Potential for injury (fetal distress) related to unexpected factors	Review maternal records and fetal data if available	Mother's data are within normal limits; EFM may not be needed
		Check maternal vital signs and question regarding maternal subjective impressions and observations regarding physical status	Mother's data show prenatal factors associated with possible fetal distress; monitor is indicated
Assess labor progress		Review chart and question mother regarding onset and quality of contraction, condition of the membranes, and other pertinent data	Mother's assessment indicates abnormal labor pattern; monitor is indicated
		Observe for behavioral manifestation of normal or abnormal labor progress	
		Report and record as necessary (to be done as indicated throughout)	
Assess FHR		Auscultate FHR	FHR abnormalities; apply monitor
Assess amniotic fluid at time of rupture of membranes		Observe or review records as to quality and quantity	Scant, excessive, or meconium-stained fluid may indicate fetal disease, abnormality, or distress; monitor indicated
Assess Couple's Knowledge of EFM	Knowledge deficit of fetal monitoring related to purpose	Review records for evidence of prenatal preparation classes	Couple exhibits satisfactory knowledge
		Question couple, allowing time for feedback	
Assessment Indicates Application of EFM	Knowledge deficit of fetal monitoring procedures re-	Apply EFM—external or internal as indicated	Parents understand rationale for use, procedure for

(continued)

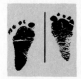

Nursing Care Plan (continued)

Assessment	Potential Nursing Diagnosis	Planning and Intervention	Evaluation
	lated to lack of interest or opportunity to discuss earlier	Explain (or reexplain) rationale for use	monitoring, and interpretation of EFM data
		Explain methods to be used	Parents participate in decision making
		Apply monitor so that mother is comfortable; explain about position changes	Mother is comfortable and understands need for position changes
		Place monitor in mother's view; review initial tracings	Mother understands timing for breathing and relaxation techniques
		Review tracings with parents periodically; answer *all* questions	Parents understand labor course
			Parents observe labor progress with data
Problem Assessment			
Determine baseline bradycardia by strip review and observations of mother's verbal and behavioral input	Fear of possible loss of fetus related to unknown outcome	Evaluate FECG; identify arrhythmia	Client appreciates support of nurse
	Powerlessness related to outcome	Review tracing for periodic deceleration and baseline variability	Client discusses fears
	Alteration in comfort: pain, related to immobility	Review record for drugs	Client understands and asks for comfort measures
		Institute remedial measures for fetal distress	Client understands possible outcomes and verbalizes
		Turn to left lateral recumbent position	Client asks questions concerning procedures
		Discontinue oxytocin if applicable	Support person is a comfort to the woman
		Adminster O₂ by mask	
		Report and record verbally and in writing	
		Remain with client; institute primary nursing (one-to-one); answer questions	
		Comfort measures as necessary	
		Be alert for possible deterioration	
		Review strips frequently and regularly	
		Confirm by auscultation	
		Evaluate FECG; identify arrhythmais	
		Take maternal temperature	

(continued)

Nursing Care Plan   (continued)

Assessment	Potential Nursing Diagnosis	Planning and Intervention	Evaluation
		Review drugs adminstered to mother Review tracings for periodic decelerations and baseline variability Institute remedial measures for fetal distress as outlined above	

to rule out an occult prolapse of the umbilical cord. If cord prolapse is found, the fetal head should be elevated vaginally and the client placed in the Trendelenburg or knee–chest position and taken to the delivery room immediately.

IMPAIRED MATERNAL OXYGEN DELIVERY

Impaired delivery of maternal oxygen may result from a number of maternal disorders. Maternal pulmonary dysfunction, associated with an acute severe asthmatic attack, amniotic fluid embolism, thromboembolism, tonic–clonic seizure, or general anesthesia, may result in maternal hypoxia delivering less oxygen to the placenta and fetus. Heart failure and hypotension can keep normally oxygenated blood from reaching the uterus. Hypotension may be caused by maternal blood loss, compression of the vena cava by the gravid uterus, or autonomic blockade associated with conduction anesthesia.

When maternal oxygen uptake or delivery of oxygen to the uterus is impaired, oxygen should be administered by mask and the mother turned to the left lateral recumbent position. This position displaces the gravid uterus off the inferior vena cava, thus promoting venous return to the heart and improved cardiovascular function. Then, if necessary, pharmacologic correction of the respiratory, cardiac, or autonomic disorder can be initiated.

IMPAIRED PLACENTAL EXCHANGE OF OXYGEN

The cause of impaired placental oxygen exchange may be placental insufficiency. This may be caused by ex-

cessively strong contractions that either occur spontaneously or are caused by hyperstimulation with oxytocin. Such contractions result in transient interruption of blood flow in the intervillous space and thus diminish oxygen exchange. When this occurs, administration of oxytocin should be discontinued if it is being used. Improving maternal oxygenation and oxygen delivery by administration of oxygen and use of the left lateral position are also helpful. Uteroplacental insufficiency may also be seen in intrauterine growth retardation, placental abruption, and postdate pregnancy.

IMPAIRED FETAL CIRCULATION OR OXYGEN TRANSPORT

Cord compression is the most common cause of compromised fetal circulation. In this situation, prolapse of the cord should be determined rapidly by perineal inspection and vaginal examination. This complication requires prompt delivery, usually by cesarean section. When there is evidence of cord compression, the previously mentioned measures should be initiated (i.e., maternal oxygen administration, left lateral position, and discontinuation of oxytocics). Positions other than left lateral (e.g., right lateral or knee–chest) may also be useful in alleviating variable decelerations and should be tried when the pattern does not respond to the initial remedial measures. Fetal oxygen transport to the tissues may also be impaired when there is severe fetal anemia, as is seen in Rh isoimmunization and fetal maternal hemorrhage. When the fetal tracing does not respond to appropriate nursing measures, the physician may elect to obtain a fetal scalp pH determination or proceed with immediate delivery.

Evaluation

Evaluation of the mother and fetus undergoing intrapartum monitoring is a continuous process until the delivery of the infant. FHR and UA pattern recognition in light of maternal and fetal condition must be constantly reassessed. The continuation of the nursing process is based on the maternal and fetal responses to the nursing and medical interventions provided. It is anticipated that both the mother and fetus will maintain optimal health as a result of intrapartum monitoring.

■ REFERENCES

1. Benson R, Shubeck R, Deutschberger J, et al: Fetal heart rate as a predictor of fetal distress: A report from the collaborative project. Obstet Gynecol 32:259–266, 1968
2. Shenker L, Post RC, Seiler JS: Routine electronic monitoring of fetal heart rate and uterine activity during labor. Obstet Gynecol 46:185, 1975
3. Lee WK, Baggish MS: The effect of unselected intrapartum fetal monitoring. Obstet Gynecol 47:516, 1976
4. Paul RH, Huey JR, Yaeger CF: Clinical fetal monitoring—Its effect on cesarean section rate and perinatal mortality: Five year trends. Postgrad Med 61:160–166, 1977
5. Haverkamp AD, Orleans M, Langendoerfer S, et al: A controlled trial of the differential effects of intrapartum fetal monitoring. Am J Obstet Gynecol 134:399–412, 1979
6. Wood C, Renou P, Oates J, et al: A controlled trial of fetal heart rate monitoring in a low-risk population. Am J Obstet Gynecol 141:527–534, 1981
7. Renou P, Chang A, Anderson I, et al: Controlled trial of fetal intensive care. Am J Obstet Gynecol 126:470–476, 1976
8. Leveno KJ, Cunningham FG, Nelson S, et al: A prospective comparison of selective and universal electronic fetal monitoring in 34,995 pregnancies. N Engl J Med 315:615–619, 1986
9. Shy KK, Luthy DA, Bennett FC, et al: Effects of electronic fetal-heart rate monitoring, as compared with periodic auscultation, on the neurologic development of premature infants. N Engl J Med 322:588–593, 1990
10. McDonald D, Grant A, Sheridan-Pereira M, et al: The Dublin randomized controlled trial of intrapartum fetal heart rate monitoring. Am J Obstet Gynecol 152:524–539, 1985
11. American Academy of Pediatrics, American College of Obstetricians and Gynecologists: Guidelines for Perinatal Care, 2nd ed, p 67. Washington DC, AAP, ACOG, 1988
12. Nurses Association of American College of Obstetricians and Gynecologists: OGN Nursing Practice Resource: Fetal Heart Rate Auscultation. Washington DC, NAACOG, 1990
13. American College of Obstetricians and Gynecologists: ACOG Technical Bulletin No. 132: Intrapartum Fetal Heart Rate Monitoring. Washington DC, ACOG, 1989
14. Freeman RK, Garite TJ, Nageotte MP: Fetal Heart Rate Monitoring, 2nd ed. Baltimore, William & Wilkins, 1991
15. Perkins R: Perinatal observations in a high-risk population managed without intrapartum fetal pH studies. Am J Obstet Gynecol 149:327, 1984
16. Clark SL, Paul RH: Intrapartum fetal surveillance: The role of fetal scalp blood sampling. Am J Obstet Gynecol 153:717–720, 1985
17. Clark SL, Gimovsky ML, Miller FC: Fetal heart rate response to scalp blood sampling. Am J Obstet Gynecol 144:706–709, 1982
18. Clark SL, Gimovsky ML, Miller FC: The scalp stimulation test: A clinical alternative to fetal scalp blood sampling. Am J Obstet Gynecol 148:274–277, 1984
19. Smith CV, Nguyen HN, Phelan JP, et al: Intrapartum assessment of fetal well-being: A comparison of fetal acoustic stimulation with acid-base determinations. Am J Obstet Gynecol 155:726–728, 1986
20. Pardi G, Buscaglia M, Ferrazzi E, et al: Cord sampling for the evaluation of oxygenation and acid-base balance in growth-retarded fetuses. Am J Obstet Gynecol 157:1221–1228, 1987
21. Shah DM, Boehm FH: Fetal blood gas analysis from cordocentesis for abnormal fetal heart rate patterns. Am J Obstet Gynecol 161:374–376, 1989
22. Strickland DM, Gilstrap LC, Hauth JC, et al: Umbilical cord pH and pCO_2: Effect of interval from delivery to determination. Am J Obstet Gynecol 148:191–193, 1984
23. Eganhouse DJ: Electronic fetal monitoring: Education and quality assurance. JOGNN 20:16–22, 1991
24. Nurses Association of American College of Obstetricians and Gynecologists: Electronic Fetal Monitoring: Nursing Practice Competencies and Educational Guidelines. Washington, DC, NAACOG, 1986
25. Rutherford SE, Phelan JP, Smith CV, et al: The four quadrant assessment of amniotic fluid volume: An adjunct to antepartum fetal heart rate testing. Obstet Gynecol 70:353–356, 1987
26. Miyazaki FS, Nevarez F: Saline amnioinfusion for relief of repetitive variable decelerations: A prospective randomized study. Am J Obstet Gynecol 153:301–306, 1985
27. Nageotte MP, Freeman RK, Garite TJ, et al: Prophylactic intrapartum amnioinfusion in patients with preterm premature rupture of membranes. Am J Obstet Gynecol 153:557–562, 1985
28. Strong TH, Hetzler G, Sarno AP, et al: Prophylactic intrapartum amnioinfusion: A randomized clinical trial. Am J Obstet Gynecol 162:746–748, 1990
29. Nageotte MP, Bertucci L, Towers CV, et al: Prophylactic amnioinfusion in pregnancies complicated by oligohydramnios: A prospective study. Obstet Gynecol 77:677–680, 1991

30. Posner MD, Ballagh SA, Paul RH: The effect of amnioinfusion on uterine pressure and activity: A preliminary report. Am J Obstet Gynecol 163:813–818, 1990

31. Tabor BL, Maier JA: Polyhydramnios and elevated intrauterine pressure during amnioinfusion. Am J Obstet Gynecol 156:130–131, 1987

32. Strong TH, Hetzler G, Paul RH: Amniotic fluid volume increase after amnioinfusion of a fixed volume. Am J Obstet Gynecol 162:746–748, 1990

■ SUGGESTED READING

Afriat CI: The nurse's role in fetal heart rate monitoring. Perinatol Neonatol 7:29–32, 1983

Afriat CI: Electronic Fetal Monitoring. Rockville, MD, Aspen Publishers, 1989

Applegate J, Haverkamp AD, Orleans M, et al: Electronic fetal monitoring: Implications for obstetrical nursing. Nurs Res 28:369–371, 1979

Blank J: Electronic fetal monitoring nursing management defined. JOGNN 14:463–467, 1985

Freeman RK, Garite TJ, Nageotte MP: Fetal Heart Rate Monitoring. Baltimore: Williams & Wilkins, 1991

Gilstrap LC, Hauth JC, Hankins GDV, et al: Second-stage fetal heart rate abnormalities and type of neonatal acidemia. Obstet Gynecol 70:191–195, 1987

Goodlin RC: History of fetal monitoring. Am J Obstet Gynecol 133:323, 1979

Komaromy B, Gaal J, Lampe L: Fetal arrhythmia during pregnancy and labor. Br J Obstet Gynaecol 84:492, 1977

Kubli FW, Hon EH, Khazin AF, et al: Observations on heart rate and pH in the human fetus during labor. Am J Obstet Gynecol 104:1190–1206, 1969

Niswander KR: Asphyxia in the fetus and cerebral palsy. In Pitkin RM, Zlatnik FJ (eds): Yearbook of Obstetrics and Gynecology. 1983. Chicago, Yearbook Medical Publishers, 1983

Schneiderman CI, Waxman B, Goodman CJ Jr: Maternal-fetal electrocardiogram conduction with intrapartum death. Am J Obstet Gynecol 113:1130, 1972

Shiono PH, McNellis D, Rhoads GG: Reasons for the rising cesarean delivery rates, 1978–1984. Obstet Gynecol 69:696–700, 1987

Snydal SH: Methods of fetal heart rate monitoring during labor: A selective review of the literature. J Nurse Midwif 33:4–14, 1988

Thacker SD: The efficacy of intrapartum electronic fetal monitoring. Am J Obstet Gynecol 156:24–30, 1987

44

Disorders of Gestational Age and Birth Weight

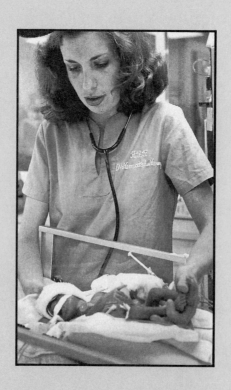

The particular, precise, and highly specialized practice of neonatal nursing could cover an entire text. The neonate and the family's complete dependence on the skill of the primary caretaker, the neonatal nurse, makes the nurse's task that much more demanding, challenging, rewarding, stressful, and draining.

From the time of birth, resuscitation, stabilization, possible transport, and continued care in the neonatal intensive care unit (NICU), the neonate is cared for by an ever-vigilant specialized team.

■ OVERVIEW

Disorders of Gestational Age and Birth Weight

The size of an infant at birth is influenced by many factors that affect the maternal and fetal environments. The relationship between low birth weight and perinatal morbidity and mortality has long been recognized. Only recently, however, have the different implications of birth weight relative to gestational age been established. Infants of low birth weight may be of appropriate size for their gestational age but immature because they are born before pregnancy has progressed to full term. These infants are classically "premature"—born before their organ systems have matured to the point of physiological functioning. Other low-birth-weight infants may be undersized for the length of their gestation, whether delivered before or at term. These infants are called *small for gestational age*. Often they are physiologically mature but have not attained the size and weight appropriate for gestational age for numerous reasons.

Infants experiencing disorders of gestational age and birth weight also include those who are large for gestational age and who are postmature—born after pregnancy has progressed beyond full term. The associated problems and potential causes are different among these various types of altered fetal growth, requiring individualized assessment and approaches to management. The particular causes of alterations in fetal growth also determine the newborn's immediate and long-term prognosis. The challenge to effective assessment and management of fetal growth disorders begins with an understanding of the intricate and complex mechanisms that control normal fetal growth.

Classification of Infants by Birth Weight and Gestational Age

In the past, all newborns weighing 2500 g or less were termed *premature* and those weighing more than 2500 g were designated *full term*. This approach assumed that intrauterine growth rates were essentially the same for all fetuses and that birth weight corresponded to gestational age. A considerable amount of data has now accumulated to demonstrate the inaccuracy of this assumption, and the two dimensions of *birth weight* and *gestational age* are now considered separately.

The World Health Organization (WHO) has designated a *term birth* as one occurring between 38 and 42 weeks' gestation, with age calculated from the date of the onset of the mother's last menstrual period. WHO advises that newborns not be classified as *premature* on the basis of weight alone. Gestational age must be used to assign categories of preterm, term, and postterm births. Also, it must be recognized that an infant weighing less than 2500 g is not necessarily premature.

Intrauterine growth standards are used to compare an infant's weight and gestational age with population averages. Although these have shortcomings in application to particular situations (e.g., differences in weight due to race, parity, sex, altitude), they are useful as guides in the assessment of high-risk infants. The most widely used growth chart was developed in Colorado and gives percentiles of intrauterine growth for weight, length, and head circumference. However, the altitude effects made this estimate low for the rest of the country. A more recent fetal growth chart includes correction factors for parity, race, and sex and presents average fetal weights for the 10th, 25th, 50th, 75th, and 90th percentiles (Fig. 44-1). Infants may be classified in any one of nine groups (Fig. 44-2).

Weight serves in the assessment of growth, and gestational age in the assessment of maturity. An infant born at 40 week's gestation and weighing less than 2500 g (below the 10th percentile for weight of length) would be mature but undergrown. This disorder is called *intrauterine growth retardation*, with the infant classified as *small for gestational age* (SGA). An infant born at 36 weeks' gestation and weighing 3500 g (above the 90th percentile for weight) would be immature but overgrown. Such *large-for-gestational-age* (LGA) infants are typical for diabetic mothers. Although this infant has attained average term weight, it is actually premature, with incomplete maturation of organ systems.

The term *premature* seems appropriate for the *preterm*, immature infant, regardless of birth weight. Preterm infants are those infants born before 37 weeks' gestation. Preterm infants may also be SGA, implying that at least two factors are involved, that one causing the early delivery and that one retarding the growth rate *in utero*.

The term *low-birth-weight infant* defines any liveborn infant weighing 2500 g or less. A *very-low-birth-weight infant* weighs 1500 g or less (Figs. 44-3 and 44-4).

Infants are at risk for various medical problems, depending on their gestational age. See Table 44-1,

(Text continues on page 1116)

Research Highlight

Variations exist in the techniques used to perform manual ventilation in neonates and in the proficiency levels of nurses in NICUs who perform the procedure. Howard-Glenn and Koniak-Griffin investigated (1) whether significant differences exist in nurses' ability accurately to control prescribed peak inspiratory pressure (PIP) when using manometers as compared to when they are not used, during manual ventilation in NICU infants; and (2) whether the number of years of NICU work experience is related to manometer use and success in controlling prescribed PIP.

A convenience sample of 60 professional nurses whose work experience ranged from 1 to 26 years participated in the study. Each nurse was observed performing one manual ventilation procedure. Pneumogards provided recordings of peak airway pressures during manual ventilation. Observation was made of the number of times the nurse looked at the manometer for insufflations during the ventilation procedure. Scores were given for successful PIP achievement while using the manometer and compared with successful PIP achievement without using the manometer.

Results revealed that 78% of the nurses using the manometers achieved successful PIP, whereas 41% of the nurses not using the manometers achieved successful PIP. This difference was statistically significant and supports nurses' need to use manometers to control PIP successfully. Analysis also showed that the greater the nurses' NICU work experience, the less likely they were to use the manometer during manual ventilation; however, the correlation between the number of years' experience and success controlling PIP was insignificant.

Supplementary findings included the following: (1) 49% of the time, nurses used the manometer with 60% accuracy; (2) nurses used the manometer more during initiation of ventilation, with use declining in the middle and rising at the end of the procedure; (3) the successful control of PIP increased correspondingly to use of the manometer; and (4) as manometer use declined, accuracy was maintained for several insufflations, then declined until the manometer was used again.

Howard-Glenn L, Koniak-Griffin D: Evaluation of manometer use in manual ventilation of infants in neonatal intensive care units. Heart Lung 19(6): 620–627, 1990.

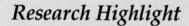

Research Highlight

Although early, frequent parent-infant contact is supported in the literature, little data are available regarding patterns of parental visiting and telephoning to the nursery throughout the hospitalization. In addition, data were lacking regarding factors associated with family visiting and telephoning. The purposes of this study were to examine (1) parental and family visiting and telephoning patterns to very-low-birth-weight infants over a 6-week period; and (2) factors associated with the frequency of visiting and telephoning.

Data concerning visiting and telephoning and demographic data were collected by a chart review of a sample of 65 infants with birth weights less than 1500 g born at an urban tertiary-care center. Data indicated that a typical mother visited a mean 2.2 times a week, and a typical father 1.5 times a week. A typical mother telephoned a mean 3.1 times a weeks, and a typical father never telephoned the nursery. Factors significantly related to visiting were: married parents, higher level of family income, private medical insurance, and ownership of a car.

Nurses need to consider all family members and encourage them to be more involved, relieving a mother who may already be overwhelmed by her own physical and emotional problems. Nurses need to use interventions that would promote more sustained contact. More research needs to be done regarding reasons for limited contact so that assistance can be provided to these families.

Brown L, et al: Very low birth infants: Parental visiting and telephoning during initial infant hospitalization. Nurs Res 38(4):233–235, July/August 1989.

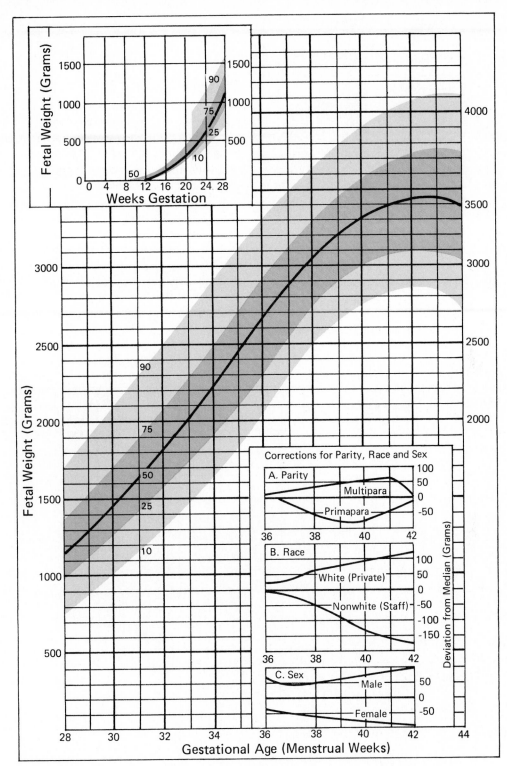

■ *Figure 44–1*

Fetal weight. The 10th, 25th, 50th, 75th, and 90th percentiles of fetal weight in g throughout pregnancy and correction factors for parity, race (socioeconomic status), and sex are graphed. Data were obtained from 31,202 prostaglandin-induced abortions and spontaneous deliveries. (Brenner WE, Edelman DA, Hendricks CH: A standard of fetal growth for the United States of America. Am J Obstet Gynecol 126:555–564, 1976)

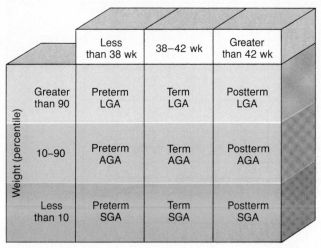

■ *Figure 44–2*
Birth weight–gestational age groups as defined by Lubchenko and coworkers. (Clewell WH: Prematurity. J Reprod Med 23(5): 237–244, 1979)

"Problems Associated With Specific Gestational Age Groups."

Factors That Affect Fetal Growth

Fetal growth is influenced by a variety of factors of maternal, placental, and fetal origin. Genetic predispositions, the mother's nutritional and health status, fetal nutrition, fetal and maternal endocrine functions, developmental insults, environmental stressors, and placental function are variably involved in this process. Maturation is affected by biochemical determinants, enzymes, genes, and hormones, particularly adrenal and thyroid. Development of the various organs follows a different time sequence, with hormonal action triggering a certain organ to grow and mature at a particular time during gestation. As different organs mature at different times, there are critical periods when stressors can alter

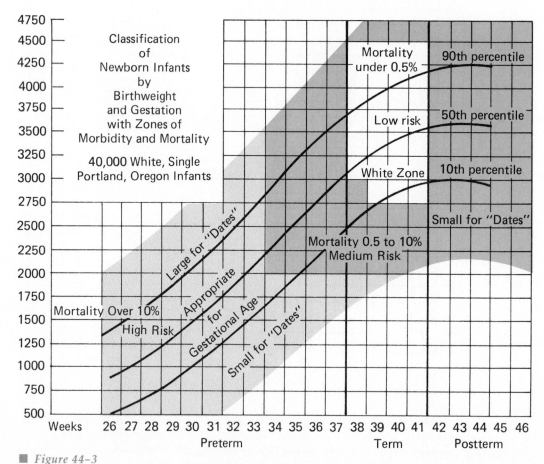

■ *Figure 44–3*
Classification of newborn by birth weight and gestation with areas of morbidity and mortality. (Babson SG, Benson RC, Pernoll ML, et al: Management of High-Risk Pregnancy and Intensive Care of the Neonate. St Louis, CV Mosby, 1975)

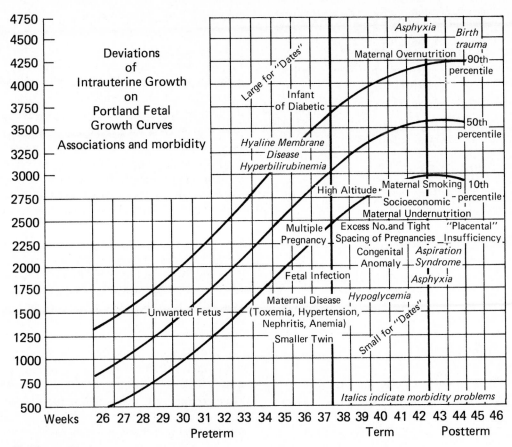

■ *Figure 44–4*

Intrauterine growth curves and associations with perinatal mortality and morbidity. (Babson SG, Benson RC, Pernoll ML, et al: Management of High-Risk Pregnancy and Intensive Care of the Neonate. St Louis, CV Mosby, 1975)

normal development significantly. After these critical periods, the organ is less susceptible to damage and more capable of functioning in the extrauterine environment.

MATERNAL FACTORS

Although genetic factors certainly play an important role in determining fetal measurements and weight, other environmental influences also have been associated with fetal growth. Maternal nutritional status, as measured by prepregnancy weight and the slow, steady weight gain experienced during pregnancy, is a definitive influencing factor. (See Chap. 18 for further discussion on adequate maternal nutrition to promote fetal growth.) Adjunct risk factors in this area include those women who are experiencing malnutrition for various reasons, pregnant adolescents, women of low socioeconomic status, women with low pregnancy weight or inadequate weight gain during pregnancy, women of short stature, women having frequent pregnancies, and

women who have delivered other infants of low birth weight.[1]

Pregnancy-induced hypertension poses a threat to fetal growth because it promotes a decrease in uterine blood flow. (See Chap. 33 for more discussion of this maternal syndrome.) Advanced maternal diabetes mellitus and its accompanying vascular insufficiency promote intrauterine growth retardation.

Substance abuse of alcohol and heroin has been correlated with decreased fetal growth. The use of prescribed drugs, such as propranolol, warfarin, and steroids, has also been correlated with SGA infants. Cigarette smoking is directly related to SGA births, with the number of cigarettes smoked and the duration of smoking implicated in the fetal weight result. Birth weight is decreased on the average of 170 g as a result of 10 cigarettes smoked a day and 300 g as a result of 15 cigarettes smoked a day.[1]

It has been demonstrated that infants born at higher altitudes experience decreased birth weight as a result of the decrease in oxygen tension.

TABLE 44-1. PROBLEMS ASSOCIATED WITH SPECIFIC GESTATIONAL AGE GROUPS

SGA Term (<2500 g; >37 weeks)

Perinatal asphyxia

Meconium aspiration

Persistent fetal circulation syndrome (PFC)

Hypoglycemia

Thermal instability

Polycythemia-hyperviscosity

Major congenital malformations

Nonbacterial intrauterine infection

Multiple birth (e.g., twins, triplets)

Intrauterine parabiotic syndrome

AGA Premature (<2500 g; ≤37 weeks)

Hyaline membrane disease and immature lung syndrome

Patent ductus arteriosus

Intraventricular-periventricular hemorrhage

Hydrocephaly

Retinopathy of prematurity (retrolental fibroplasia)

Necrotizing enterocolitis

Undernutrition

Thermal instability

Hyperbilirubinemia

Anemia of prematurity

Anemia caused by vitamin E deficiency

Inguinal hernia

LGA Term (<4000 g; >37 weeks)

Perinatal asphyxia

Spontaneous pneumothorax, pneumomediastinum

Birth trauma

  Fractured humerus
  Brachial plexus palsy
  Facial palsy
  Depressed skull fracture

Transposition of great vessels

Postmature (any weight; ≥42 weeks)

AGA or SGA

Perinatal asphyxia

Meconium aspiration

Malnutrition; wasting

Thermal instability

Polycythemia-hyperviscosity syndrome

(Sheldon B, Korones SB: High-Risk Newborn Infants, p 145. St. Louis, CV Mosby, 1986.)

PLACENTAL INFLUENCES

Under normal conditions, the size of the placenta is a major determinant of fetal size. When there is severe maternal nutritional deprivation, the maintenance needs of the placenta apparently are met first, leading to reduction of fetal growth. In a fetus with growth retardation, however, the placenta is relatively smaller than with a normally growing fetus of the same gestational age. This is associated with higher levels of asphyxia at birth and perinatal morbidity seen among SGA infants. Placental mechanisms for maintaining optimal transfer of nutrients and gases between maternal and fetal blood are necessary for an adequate supply of growth-promoting substances to the fetus. The diffusion capacity of the placenta increases proportionately with fetal weight during pregnancy. Any impairment of oxygen transfer has a deleterious effect on fetal growth. Transfers of minerals, electrolytes, and trace metals, which are necessary in an adequate supply for proper fetal growth, are also related to placental function.[2]

There appears to be no single placental abnormality common to infants who are SGA, and placental and cord defects are present in only a small number of cases. When lesions are present, the most common are infarction, circumvallate placenta, velamentous cord insertion, and marginal cord insertion.

FETAL ENDOCRINE INFLUENCES

The hypothalamic-pituitary axis acts through the pancreas to modify fetal growth. This is an interactional situation between mother and fetus. In the normal-birth-weight fetus of a normal mother, the pancreas has 2% endocrine tissue with 40% beta cells. In infants of gestational diabetic mothers, endocrine tissue is 10% with 60% beta cells, leading to significantly higher fetal insulin levels. The percentages of endocrine tissue and insulin levels are directly proportional to the excess fetal weight observed in infants of diabetic mothers. There appears to be a competitive effect between adrenal cortical hormones and insulin. This relates to lung maturation and the formation of surfactant. Cortisol slows cell growth but enhances an antagonist to glucocorticoids. This effect seems related to the higher incidence of respiratory distress syndrome (RDS) in infants of diabetic mothers. A similar relationship between insulin levels and glucocorticoids occurs with enzyme and glucose metabolism in the liver. Insulin, acting unopposed in the fetus, directly influences cytoplasmic growth and increases triglyceride concentrations in the brain, liver, and lung.[2]

Thyroid and adrenal hormones are important to fetal maturation. Inadequate levels of thyroid hormone are associated with decreased fetal size, delayed skeletal ossification, delayed maturation, and mental retardation. Infants of hyperthyroid mothers may have advanced neurologic development for gestational age, greater body weight, greater placental weight, and advanced skeletal development. They appear several weeks older than their gestational age. Corticosteroids are used to induce organ maturation, for instance, to promote lung maturation. They also affect maturation of the foregut (absorption of antibodies), pancreas, liver, and small bowel. Liver glycogen depends on the presence of corticosteroids. It is possible that growth hormone may play a role in brain growth. Somatomedins (growth hormone ancillary factors) may be important in cell multiplication in the fetus, as high levels are found in large infants at birth and low levels are found in SGA infants. Through an endocrine chain, hormonal regulation of fetal growth may be finely regulated by the central nervous system.[2]

OTHER FETAL FACTORS

Infants of multiple gestation have a more pronounced decrease in growth late in the third trimester. Certain congenital malformations, chromosomal disorders, and congenital infections promote intrauterine growth retardation. Examples of such disorders are trisomies 8, 13, 18, and 21, congenital heart disease, and rubella. Prolonged pregnancy and family history of small neonates are additional related factors.[3]

Assessment (Identification) of the High-Risk Neonate

Although the causes of prematurity and altered fetal growth are not completely understood, several associated factors have been identified that alert nurses and physicians to the possibility of these problems. Early recognition of mothers with high-risk pregnancies and careful prenatal care can often contribute to a better outcome for the infant and the mother.

Many of the factors contributing to the birth of a high-risk infant are not specific for a particular problem or condition but are generally related to increased morbidity and mortality. Others have specific associations with neonatal disorders or fetal abnormalities. Those related to prematurity include diabetes, placental insufficiency, multiple pregnancy, preeclampsia and hypertensive disorders, and infection. Several overlap with increased incidence of SGA infants, including preeclampsia and hypertensive disorders, placental insufficiency, infections, discordant twin, and altitude. Con-

genital anomalies are more highly correlated to term SGA infants.

Chapter 29 covers assessment of gestational age. Assessment considerations related to SGA and LGA neonates may be found in those sections of this chapter. Factors associated with high-risk infants are listed in Table 44-2.

■ SMALL-FOR-GESTATIONAL-AGE INFANTS (INTRAUTERINE GROWTH RETARDATION)

SIGNIFICANCE OF GESTATIONAL AGE

Infants whose weights fall below the 10th percentile for their gestational age have experienced impairment of the normal growth process during the prenatal period. Some physicians use the limiting criterion of birth weight of two standard deviations below the mean of gestational age. This condition may occur at any gestational age, but most SGA infants are born at, or close to, term and weigh less than 2500 g. Under the old classification, these infants would have been called *premature*, although their period of intrauterine life was not significantly shortened. Although small, these infants are mature in comparison with infants of similar weight but lower gestational age.

Growth-retarded infants have an increased risk of perinatal morbidity and mortality. The infant's condition is a product of a process of intrauterine deprivation that begins many weeks before birth. It is often related to abnormalities of the pregnancy or of the fetus.

There are two types of intrauterine growth retardation, and these types may occur separately or simultaneously. Fetal growth involves both an increase in the number of cells (hyperplasia) and an increase in the size of cells (hypertrophy). Embryonic growth involves a rapid increase in the number of cells as the organs and body structures are formed. These cells increase in size later in pregnancy. If an insult to the fetus occurs early in gestation, mitosis is impaired and fewer new cells are formed. This results in small organs of subnormal weight. The cells, however, are of normal size. This type of growth disruption is not reversible despite a change in maternal nutrition.[4] If interference with growth occurs later, the cells are normal in number but smaller in size, again resulting in smaller organs, but in this instance as a result of reduced amounts of cytoplasm. This type of impairment may be reversible with optimum maternal nutrition.[4] An intrauterine insult

TABLE 44–2. IDENTIFICATION OF HIGH-RISK INFANT: ASSOCIATED FACTORS

Antepartal Factors

Maternal Characteristics

Age <15 or >35

Low socioeconomic status

Unmarried

Family or marital conflicts

Emotional illness or family history of mental illness

Persistent ambivalence or conflicts about the pregnancy

Stature under 5 ft

20% underweight or overweight

Malnutrition

Reproductive History

Parity ≥ 3 or more previous abortions

Previous stillborn or neonatal death

Previous premature labor or low-birth-weight infant (<2500 g)

Previous excessively large infant (>4000 g)

Infant with isoimmunization or ABO incompatibility

Infant with congential anomaly, genetic disorder, or birth trauma

Prior preeclampsia or eclampsia

Uterine fibroids >5 cm or submucous

Abnormal Pap smear

Infertility

Prior Cesarean section

Prior fetal malpresentations

Contracted pelvis

Ovarian masses

Genital tract abnormalities (incompetent cervix, subseptate or bicornate uterus)

Pregnancy occurring 3 months or less after last delivery

Previous prolonged labor or significant dystocia

Prior multiple birth

Substance Abuse

Drugs

Alcohol

Smoking

Environmental hazards

Exposure to known tertogens

Anemias with hemoglobin <9 g and hematocrit <32%

Pulmonary disease

Endocrine disorders

Gastrointestinal or liver disease

Epilepsy

Malignancy

Complications of Present Pregnancy

Low or excessive weight gain

Hypertension (mean arterial pressure >90, blood pressure 140/90, increase >30 mmHg systolic or >20 mm Hg diastolic)

Recurrent glycosuria and abnormal fasting blood sugar or glucose tolerance test

Uterine size inappropriate for gestation age (either too large or too small)

Recurrent urinary tract infections

Severe varicosities or thrombophlebitis

Recurrent vaginal bleeding

Premature rupture of membranes

Multiple pregnancy

Hydramnios with a single fetus

Rh negative with a rising titer

Late or no prenatal care

Viral infections (rubella, cytomegalovirus, herpes, mumps, rubeola, chickenpox, shingles, smallpox, vaccinia, influenza, poliomyelitis, hepatitis, Western equine encephalitis, coxsackie virus B)

Syphilis, especially late pregnancy

Bacterial infections (gonorrhea, tuberculosis, listeriosis, severe acute infection)

Protozoan infections (toxoplasmosis, malaria)

Postmaturity

Anemia with hemoglobin of 9 g or less

Severe pregnancy-induced hypertension

Abnormal fetal assessment tests

Intrapartum Factors

Complications of Labor and Delivery

Labor longer than 24 hours in primigravida

Labor longer than 12 h in multigravida

Second stage longer than 1 h

Ruptured membranes more than 24 h

Abnormal presentation or position

Heavy sedation or injudicious anesthesia

Maternal fever or infection

Placenta previa or abruptio placentae

Cesarean section

Meconium-stained amniotic fluid

Fetal distress demonstrated by monitoring or scalp blood sampling

Prolapsed cord

High forceps or midforceps delivery: difficult or operative delivery

Premature labor

Severe pregnancy-induced hypertension

Precipitous labor less than 3 h

Elective induction

Oxytocin (Pitocin) augmentation

Immediate Problems of Infant

Malformation or other significant abnormality

Birth injury

Asphyxia (Apgar <6 at 5 min)

Neonatal Factors

Charcteristics of Infant

Preterm

SGA or LGA

Birth weight <5½ lb or > 9 lb

Low-set ears

Enlargement of one or both kidneys

Single palmar crease

Single umbilical artery

Small head size

(continued)

TABLE 44–2. IDENTIFICATION OF HIGH-RISK INFANT: ASSOCIATED FACTORS *(continued)*

Medical Problems	*Clinical Problems*
Chronic hypertension	Feeding problems
Renal disease	Anemia
Diabetes mellitus	Hyperbilirubinemia
Heart disease	Temperature instability
Sickle cell trait or disease	Respiratory distress
	Hypoglycemia
	Polycythemia
	Sepsis
	Rh or ABO incompatibilities
	Hypocalcemia
	Persistent cyanosis
	Shock
	Seizures
	Heart murmur

throughout both phases of growth results in cells that are fewer in number and smaller in size. The classic example of the latter condition is the infant with the rubella syndrome.

Maternal preeclampsia, which tends to be more prominent during later pregnancy, creates the second type of growth retardation in which cell numbers are normal but cell size is reduced.[4]

Nursing Assessment

Most growth-retarded infants resemble appropriate-for-gestational-age, preterm infants. Common physical characteristics of the SGA infant with extreme growth retardation are listed below.

Common Physical Characteristics of SGA Infant

- Decrease in subcutaneous tissue
- Loose, dry skin
- Decrease in normal chest and abdominal circumference
- Sunken abdomen
- Thin, slightly yellow, dull, dry umbilical cord
- Sparse scalp hair
- Wide-eyed look[4]

However, assessment of gestational age according to physical characteristics may be altered or misleading for several reasons. Vernix is often decreased or absent. Consequently, the skin is more exposed to amniotic fluid. As a result, sole creases appear more mature than is actually true. Breast tissue formation is reduced in SGA infants. In females, the adipose tissue covering the labia is decreased; thus, external genitalia appear less mature. In the SGA infant, neurologic criteria tend to be more accurate than physical criteria.[1]

Physiological Problems

In adaptation to extrauterine life, the problems encountered by the SGA infant are different from those of the appropriate-for-gestational age, preterm infant. If the problem of poor growth in utero has been detected during pregnancy, nurses and physicians skilled in resuscitation should be present at delivery.

Certain disorders tend to occur more frequently in the SGA infant, as discussed in the following sections, and therefore should be anticipated by the caregiver.

ASPHYXIA

Any neonate may be a victim of asphyxia during the labor and delivery process or immediately after birth. Moreover, SGA infants appear to be particularly vulnerable to this immediate neonatal complication.

The process of asphyxia may be a result of one of the following three mechanisms:

1. Fetal asphyxia from lack of umbilical circulation
2. Fetal asphyxia due to lack of placental exchange, as in abruptio placentae, or the SGA infant's chronic hypoxia in utero
3. Fetal asphyxia from inadequate perfusion of the maternal side of the placenta

Furthermore, neonatal asphyxia may be the result of excess fluid in the lungs, airway obstruction, or ineffective respiratory effort.[5]

The failure to initiate or maintain normal respirations at birth is a severe, life-threatening emergency requiring immediate intervention to prevent anoxic cellular damage and to save the infant's life.

Nursing personnel need to be able to predict when an asphyxiated infant may be born and require a resuscitative effort. Fetal monitoring during labor and delivery plays a significant role in that process. Indications of fetal distress on the monitor assist the staff and prepare them for a depressed infant. (See Chap. 43 for more details on monitoring and indications of fetal distress). Other maternal indices are prolapsed cord, uterine rupture, abruptio placentae, placenta previa, chorioamnionitis, premature labor, malpresentation, maternal diabetes, polyhydramnios, and oligohydramnios. These occurrences compromise fetal oxygenation status and thus promote fetal asphyxia.

The Apgar score is the most universally known indicator of neonatal well-being at 1 and 5 minutes of life. Usually, normal respiratory patterns are established almost immediately, and by 1 minute the infant is pink, crying, and active, with a heart rate of 120 to 160 beats per minute, normal reflexes and muscle tone, and an Apgar score of 8 to 10. If asphyxia has occurred, the infant is apneic.

Primary apnea occurs when asphyxia has been prolonged over 1 to 2 minutes, with mild bradycardia and hypotension. The newborn is cyanotic, with diminished reflexes, bradycardia of 60 to 100 beats per minute, and an Apgar score of 3 to 5. Following gentle suctioning and the administration of oxygen, gasping respirations usually begin after about 2 minutes. Rapid improvement often follows, with the 5-minute Apgar score reaching 8 to 10. Without other complicating conditions, these infants have an excellent immediate and long-term prognosis.

Secondary apnea occurs when there is severe bradycardia and hypotension, and death follows shortly if there is not immediate resuscitation. The newborn is ashen; heart sounds are distant, with weak pulses and bradycardia between 20 and 60 beats per minute; reflexes are absent; and the Apgar score is 1 to 3. No gasping movements are initiated with stimulation, and the infant must be resuscitated (see further discussion in this chapter). Spontaneous respiration may not begin for 5 to 15 minutes after resuscitation is started. There

is danger of irreversible effects of anoxia, with long-term disabilities.[6]

The three causes of intrauterine injury of the central nervous system, narcosis, hypoxia, and brain hemorrhage, all produce a similar clinical syndrome of asphyxia, characterized by apnea. The course and prognosis of this syndrome vary with the degree of hypoxia, the location and extent of the hemorrhage, and the degree of hypercapnia and acidosis. This acidotic asphyxial state is more injurious and difficult to correct than hypoxia alone.

The normal oxygen saturation of the arterial blood of the fetus at birth is approximately 60%, but in severe cases it may drop to as low as 12%. In addition, the blood of these infants has a high concentration of lactic acid and a very low *p*H.

Management is aimed at correcting metabolic acidosis as well as maintaining tissue oxygenation. Any underlying disorder (hypoglycemia, anemia) must also be identified and corrected.

MECONIUM ASPIRATION SYNDROME

Infants at risk for developing meconium aspiration syndrome are term, postterm, or SGA infants. Aspiration of meconium into the alveoli, occurring in utero or at birth, may result from fetal hypoxia. The etiology may be multifactorial because fetal distress and asphyxia do not always result in meconium aspiration syndrome. The fetal response to hypoxia includes reflex relaxation of the anal sphincter and accelerated intestinal peristalsis, in addition to reflex gasping, which draws the meconium into the tracheobronchial system.[4,7]

Meconium in the respiratory tract acts like a foreign body and blocks the flow of air into the alveoli. Increasing inflation of the alveoli distal to the obstruction can lead to their rupture and the leakage of air into the interstitial tissue (Fig. 44-5). This initiates a series of complications, such as pulmonary interstitial emphysema, pneumomediastinum, pneumothorax, and persistent pulmonary hypertension. The asphyxia that results from these meconium effects on the lungs may lead to various metabolic abnormalities, central nervous system dysfunction, renal failure, and other complications.

The syndrome may be prevented or minimized through appropriate obstetric management of the mother in whom there is evidence of meconium-stained amniotic fluid and prompt removal of meconium from the infant's upper respiratory tract immediately after birth.[4] Direct visualization and suctioning are essential preventive measures. Despite preventive efforts, the infant may require neonatal intensive care for stabilization and prevention of further complications. Management required may include conventional assisted ventilation, extracorporeal membrane oxygenation, or jet ventilation.

Nursing care primarily focuses on continuing ob-

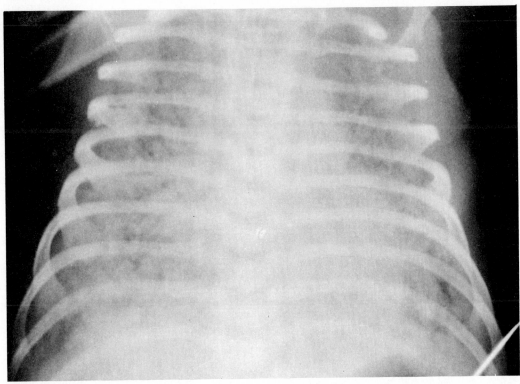

■ *Figure 44–5*
Severe meconium aspiration syndrome, showing shaggy heart border and irregular densities throughout both lungs, and having a wooly quality in this patient. (Avery GB: Neonatology: Pathophysiology and Management of the Newborn, 3rd ed. Philadelphia, JB Lippincott, 1987)

servations, assessments, and interventions involving the neonate's respiratory system. In addition to ventilator care, assessment of respiratory status includes frequent documentation of transcutaneous oxygen monitor or pulse oximeter readings. The nurse's knowledge of potential complications requires diligent observation for seizures, gastrointestinal bleeding, and renal failure.[8]

HYPOGLYCEMIA

Neonatal hypoglycemia is a frequent occurrence in SGA infants as well as infants of diabetic mothers, erythroblastotic infants, preterm infants, and others.[4]

Hypoglycemia is defined as a blood glucose level of 20 to 25 mg/dl in the low-birth-weight infant and 30 to 35 mg/dl in the infant weighing more than 2500 g during the first 3 days of life. After 72 hours of life, glucose should be at least 40 mg/dl.[4] However, because the effects of minimal blood sugars are unknown and screening for blood sugars are not as accurate as the laboratory chemical values, in practice it is recommended that the blood sugar be maintained at 40 mg/dl in infants of all gestational ages.

The blood glucose concentration may be monitored by the screening tests of Dextrostix (Ames Laboratories, Elkhart, IN), Chemstrip Glucoscan Test Strips (Lifescan,

Inc, Mountain View, CA), or other screening device. It is essential to follow the directions carefully to achieve the most accurate reading. Any low or questionable reading should be checked by laboratory determination. Blood sugars must be carefully monitored and early feedings with D_5W or formula given if necessary. Boluses of intravenous $D_{10}W$ glucose mixtures may be required in symptomatic infants or those who do not tolerate feedings.[9]

Symptoms such as tremors, cyanosis, convulsions, apnea, abnormal cry, cardiac arrest, hypotonia, hypothermia, and tachypnea are often nonspecific. Continuous low blood sugar may result in increased risk of cerebral damage.

Finally, infants with hypoglycemia as a result of a specific medical problem, such as sepsis, must be treated for that problem specifically as well as the alleviation of hypoglycemia.[10]

THERMAL REGULATION

Lacking subcutaneous tissue and fat, SGA infants have difficulty maintaining body temperature. In addition to body composition, basal metabolic rates differ from normal. Effects of asphyxia are aggravated by cold stress.

POLYCYTHEMIA

On the average, SGA infants have a higher plasma volume than appropriate-for-gestational-age infants. This polycythemia–hyperviscosity state may be due to intrauterine hypoxia, which stimulates erythropoiesis. Furthermore, a placental-fetal blood shift may occur during labor or as a result of fetal asphyxia. The alteration in blood viscosity leads to hypoxia and hypoglycemia. With a hematocrit greater than 65 and symptoms of hypoxia and hypoglycemia present, treatment is required. A partial exchange transfusion may be necessary.[1]

Nursing Diagnoses

Potential nursing diagnoses in the care of the SGA infant include the following: impaired gas exchange, alteration in nutrition less than body requirements, alteration in tissue perfusion, high risk for injury, and parental knowledge deficit.

Nursing Interventions

The nurse is prepared to intervene, based on maternal risk factors, gestational age, weight, length, head circumference, and other characteristic observations. The nurse is knowledgeable about various complications that may occur (see Nursing Care Plan: Small-for-Gestational-Age Infant).

The nurse is prepared for resuscitation of an asphyxiated infant by reviewing any pertinent risk factors and labor record. The nurse is aware of any meconium-stained amniotic fluid, which necessitates visualization and suctioning at the time of delivery, as well as subsequent respiratory assessment. Nutritional requirements need to be met from the time of delivery, whether parenterally or orally. It is imperative that the nurse screen the neonate's blood glucose according to the unit protocol, acting to provide a glucose source if necessary. Because the SGA neonate is at risk for temperature instability, the nurse assesses the temperature frequently while preventing cold stress and providing a neutral thermal environment. The nurse monitors the neonate's hematocrit for abnormal increases and reports any deviations from the normal range.

Evaluation

On successful completion of the nursing process with the SGA infant, the following will have been accomplished:

1. The infant maintains spontaneous, unassisted, and regular respirations.
2. Arterial blood gases are within normal limits.
3. Transcutaneous oxygen monitor demonstrates adequate oxygenation.
4. The infant has minimal or absent lung disease.
5. The infant receives adequate nutritional intake for maintenance of homeostasis.
6. The infant's Dextrostix determinations are normal.
7. The infant exhibits the absence of cold stress.
8. The infant exhibits the absence of any complications associated with this gestational age.
9. Parents demonstrate an understanding of the neonate's potential and actual needs.

■ POSTTERM INFANTS

Considering an accurate gestational age of greater than 42 weeks, the postterm infant may experience the effects of the placental insufficiency due to aging. Because this infant is usually larger than the term infant, cephalopelvic disproportion may be a problem during the birth process. Resultant birth trauma may also present significant problems as a result of vaginal deliveries. With placental insufficiency occurring in the latter part of the gestation, physical characteristics resemble those of the SGA infant.

Nursing Process

The nurse is knowledgeable about the potential complications that may affect the postterm infant and prepares accordingly. The nurse uses a plan of care geared toward accurate assessment of gestational age, prevention of further complications, and education and support of the parents.

Nursing Assessment

The nurse ascertains that the pregnancy is at 42 weeks or longer with the use of a gestational assessment tool to verify the postterm infant status. The nurse assesses the infant for characteristic physiological abnormalities and potential physiological complications.

Physical characteristics of postmature infants include decreased or absent vernix caseosa/lanugo, abundant scalp hair; dry, cracked, thin skin; little subcutaneous fat; yellow staining of skin, nails, and cord; and an alert, wide-eyed look.

Clinical problems of postterm infants include hypoxia, perinatal asphyxia, meconium aspiration, hy-

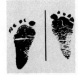

Nursing Care Plan

Small-for-Gestational-Age Infant

Patient Goals

1. The infant maintains spontaneous, unassisted and regular respirations.
2. Arterial blood gases are within normal limits.
3. Transcutaneous oxygen monitor demonstrates adequate oxygenation.
4. The infant has minimal or absent lung disease.
5. The infant receives adequate nutritional intake for maintenance of homeostasis.
6. The infant's Dextrostix are normal.
7. The infant exhibits the absence of cold stress.
8. The infant exhibits the absence of any complications associated with this gestational age.
9. Parents demonstrate an understanding of the neonate's potential and actual needs

Assessment	Potential Nursing Diagnosis	Planning and Intervention	Evaluation

Observation of infant for SGA characteristics
  Decrease in subcutaneous tissue
  Loose, dry skin
  Decrease in normal chest and abdominal circumference
  Sunken abdomen
  Thin, slightly yellow, dull, dry umbilical cord
  Sparse scalp hair
  Wide-eyed look
 	
Gestational-age assessment and weight
 	
Risks: maternal nutrition problems, pregnancy-induced hypertension, advanced maternal diabetes, maternal smoker, maternal abuse of drugs/alcohol, multiple gestation, congenital infections, chromosomal disorders, congenital malformations, meconium-stained amniotic fluid
	Impaired gas exchange
	
	Alteration in body requirements, less than body requirements
	
	Alteration in tissue perfusion
	
	High risk for injury
	
	Parental knowledge of injury
		Prepare for possible resuscitation of asphyxiated infant at delivery
		
		Perform direct visualization and suctioning when meconium is present in amniotic fluid
		
		Assess respiratory status of the infant on an ongoing basis
		
		Monitor arterial blood gases, if needed
		
		Monitor transcutaneous oxygen readings
		
		Provide nutritional source, whether parenteral or oral
		
		Monitor Dextrostix until stable
		
		Provide neutral thermal environment and monitor temperature continuously
		
		Monitor hematocrit and report abnormalities
		
		Monitor infant for any other potential complications
		
		Inform parents of infant's condition, support, and provide resources as necessary
			The infant maintains spontaneous, unassisted, and regular respirations
			
			Arterial blood gases are within normal limits
			
			Transcutaneous oxygen monitor demonstrates adequate oxygenation.
			
			The infant has minimal or absent lung disease
			
			The infant receives adequate nutritional intake for maintenance of homeostasis
			
			The infant's Dextrostix are normal
			
			The infant exhibits the absence of cold stress
			
			The infant exhibits the absence of any complications associated with this gestational age
			
			Parents demonstrate an understanding of the neonate's potential and actual needs

poglycemia, polycythemia, and thermal regulation problems.

Potential Nursing Diagnoses

Nursing diagnoses that may apply to the postterm infant include the following: impaired gas exchange; alteration in nutrition, less than body requirements; alteration in tissue perfusion; high risk for injury (birth trauma) related to vaginal delivery of a large infant; and parental knowledge deficit.

Planning and Intervention

The nurse is prepared for the birth of an infant with injuries resulting from birth trauma or asphyxia. Using the Apgar score and immediate observations, the nurse in the delivery area may need to provide resuscitation and other immediate support to the neonate. The nurse provides parenteral and other forms of nutrition to the infant as needed as soon as possible after birth. Heelstick Dextrostix must be monitored frequently to detect hypoglycemia. The nurse monitors the hematocrit and reports any deviations from normal; assesses temperature frequently and provides the appropriate environmental temperature; and informs parents about the infant's condition and provides support and resources as needed (see Nursing Care Plan: Postterm Infant).

Evaluation

On successful completion of nursing interventions, the following patient goals should be accomplished:

1. The infant maintains spontaneous, unassisted, and regular respirations.
2. Arterial blood gases are within normal limits.
3. Transcutaneous oxygen monitor demonstrates adequate oxygenation.
4. The infant receives adequate nutritional intake for the maintenance of homeostasis.
5. The infant's Dextrostix determinations are within normal limits.
6. The infant exhibits the absence of cold stress.
7. The infant exhibits the absence of any complications associated with this gestational age.
8. Parents demonstrate an understanding of the neonate's potential and actual needs.
9. Birth trauma is absent or minimal.

■ LARGE-FOR-GESTATIONAL-AGE INFANTS

The LGA infant is the infant who fits into the 90th percentile or above on the growth chart. Excessive birth weight often is the result of genetic influence. LGA infants are susceptible to hypoglycemia and potential birth trauma as a result of their size. For further discussion of an example of an LGA infant, see the section on the infant of diabetic mother in Chapter 46.

■ PRETERM OR PREMATURE INFANTS

Factors That Affect Prematurity

Premature or preterm infants are born before the 37th week of gestation, regardless of birth weight. Most babies who weigh less than 2500 g at birth are premature, as are almost all those weighing less than 1500 g. As previously stated, however, not all infants weighing less than 2500 g are necessarily premature. The main criterion is gestational age. Most of these preterm infants are appropriate for gestational age but some are SGA.

A number of factors have been identified that are associated with preterm labor (Table 44-3). For a further discussion on preterm labor, see Chapter 38.

OVERVIEW

As neonatal technology advances, the survival of infants of very low birth weight has improved year by year. One study has demonstrated an improvement over time in the survival rate of neonates weighing less than 800 g, although the severity of central nervous defects increased for those survivors.[11] Controversy exists concerning the level of management of very-low-birth-weight infants versus financial costs and risks of handicaps.

Physiological Problems

CARDIOVASCULAR SYSTEM

Changes in fetal circulation that occur at birth are covered in Chapter 10. The most common cardiovascular defect occurring in the preterm infant is the patent ductus arteriosus. The ductus, being the fetal structure act-

(Text continues on page 1131)

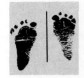

Nursing Care Plan

Postterm Infant

Patient Goals

1. The infant maintains spontaneous, unassisted, and regular respirations.
2. Arterial blood gases are within normal limits.
3. Transcutaneous oxygen monitor demonstrates adequate oxygenation.
4. The infant receives adequate nutritional intake for the maintenance of homeostasis.
5. The infant's Dextrostix are within normal limits.
6. The infant exhibits the absence of cold stress.
7. The infant exhibits the absence of any complications associated with this gestational age.
8. Parents demonstrate an understanding of the neonate's potential and actual needs.
9. Birth trauma is absent or minimal.

Assessment	Potential Nursing Diagnosis	Planning and Intervention	Evaluation
Gestational-age assessment	Impaired gas exchange	Prepare for possible resuscitation of asphyxiated infant at delivery	The infant maintains spontaneous, unassisted, and regular respirations
Birth weight	Alteration in nutrition, less than body requirements	Perform direct visualization and suctioning when meconium is present in amniotic fluid	Arterial blood gases are within normal limits
Maternal diabetes	Alteration in tissue perfusion		Transcutaneous oxygen monitor demonstrates adequate oxygenation
Genetic influences	High risk for injury (birth trauma)	Monitor oxygenation by invasive or noninvasive means	
Gestation of 42 weeks or more	Parental knowledge deficit related to care of postterm infant	Ongoing assessment of respiratory status	The infant receives adequate nutritional intake for the maintenance of homeostasis
Decreased or absent vernix caseosa/lungs		Monitor Dextrostix frequently	
Abundant scalp hair		Monitor hematocrit and report any abnormalities	The infant's Dextrostix are within normal limits
Dry, cracked, thin skin		Provide nutritional support as needed	The infant exhibits the absence of cold stress
Yellow staining of skin, nails, cord		Observe, document and report any signs of birth injuries: limpness, abnormal movement of extremities	The infant exhibits the absence of any complications associated with this gestational age
Alert, wide-eyed look		Provide neutral thermal environment	Parents demonstrate an understanding of the neonate's potential and actual needs
		Provide information, support, and resources for parents	Any injury as a result of traumatic birth is absent or minimal

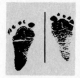

Nursing Care Plan

Preterm Infant and Family

Patient Goals

1. Infant breathes normally or at ease with ventilator assistance, without evidence of respiratory distress.
2. Noninvasive monitoring indicates adequate oxygenation.
3. Infant maintains normal fluid/electrolyte balance.
4. Infant loses minimal birth weight and gains steadily.
5. Infant adjusts to method of feeding.
6. Infant maintains normal bowel movements.
7. Infant maintains healthy, intact skin.
8. Infant does not experience cold stress.
9. Infant maintains stable temperature.
10. Infant remains or becomes infection free.
11. Infant demonstrates level of comfort.
12. Parents indicate knowledge and skill by performing caretaking tasks.
13. Parents voice confidence in caring for the infant.
14. Parents follow through on referrals.

Assessment	Potential Nursing Diagnosis	Planning and Intervention	Evaluation
Maternal Factors			
Placenta previa	Impaired gas exchange related to lack of surfactant	Observe, record, and report signs and symptoms of respiratory distress	Infant breathes normally or at ease with ventilator without evidence of respiratory distress
Abruptio placentae		Tachypnea	
Hypertensive disease of pregnancy		Cyanosis	
Cervical incompetence		Retractions	
Premature rupture of membranes		Grunting	
Uterine anomalies		Nasal flaring	
Infections		Diminished breath sounds	
Previous preterm delivery		Keep airway open by suctioning as needed	
		Administer oxygen along with appropriate monitoring of blood gases	
		Monitor ventilator function and settings	
		Change position frequently; use chest physical therapy	
		Maintain intravenous lines and monitor closely for any infiltration	Infant maintains normal fluid and electolyte balance
Fetal Factors			
Multiple gestation	Fluid-volume deficit related to insensible water loss and inadequate fluid intake	Administer correct fluid and correct amount per hour	Infant loses minimal birth weight and gains steadily
Infections			

(continued)

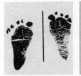

Nursing Care Plan (continued)

Assessment	Potential Nursing Diagnosis	Planning and Intervention	Evaluation
		Total intake per shift and daily	
		Observe for signs of dehydration	

		Check skin turgor
		  Check urine output
		  Check mucous
		    membranes
		  Check character of
		    fontanel	

		Monitor color, odor, specific gravity, Clinitest, and amount of urine	
		Weigh daily at approximately the same time	
		Use heat shields or plastic sheeting with radiant warmers	
	Alteration in nutrition: less than body requirements related to actual intake less than caloric requirements	Provide adequate calorie intake with most efficient method according to individual needs	Infant adjusts to method of feeding

		Nipple
		  Breast
		  Gavage
		  Nasojejunal
		  Gastrostomy
			Infant maintains normal bowel movements

		Measure abdominal girth as needed	
		Measure residuals and replace	
		Allow parents to participate in feeding plan	
		Observe stool patterns closely and report any abnormalities	
	Impairment in skin integrity related to tapes and other abrasive materials used with monitoring devices	Place as little tape as possible on skin	Infant maintains healthy, intact skin
		Use OpSite for other skin devices	
		Keep any lotions having direct skin contact to a minimun	

(continued)

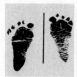

Nursing Care Plan (continued)

Assessment	Potential Nursing Diagnosis	Planning and Intervention	Evaluation
		Place infant on water bed or sheepskin	
		Turn and reposition frequently	
	High risk for injury (cold stress) related to immature temperature-regulating mechanism	Maintain neutral thermal environment	Infant does not experience cold stress
		Monitor skin temperature by probe method	Infant maintains stable temperature
		Frequently check temperature of heating unit	
		Avoid subjecting infant to heat losses by evaporation, convection, conduction, and radiation	
	High risk of infection related to immature immune system	See Care Plan for infection, Chap. 46	Infant remains or becomes infection free
	Anticipatory grief of parents related to loss of perfect infant	See Care Plan for grieving family, Chap. 45	
	Parental knowledge deficit related to care of the preterm infant	Give parents adequate and realistic information regarding infant's condition	Parents indicate knowledge and skill by performing caretaking tasks
		Encourage parents to perform many caretaking tasks	Parents voice confidence in caring for the infant
		Refer to home health care, social services, parental support group	Parents follow through on referrals
Numerous invasive painful procedures	Alteration in comfort related to invasive, painful procedures	Administration of pain medications	Infant exhibits absence of painful behaviors and demonstrates comfort level
Crying		Swaddle	
Grimace		Use of pacifier	
Rigid posture		Tactile stimulation	
Heart rate and blood pressure increase		Rocking	
Oxygen saturation decrease			

TABLE 44–3. FACTORS ASSOCIATED WITH PRETERM LABOR AND DELIVERY

Maternal history	Chronic disease
	Diabetes
	Renal disease
	Cardiovascular disease
	Respiratory disease
	In utero exposure to diethylstilbestrol (DES)
	Reproductive tract anomalies
	Underweight (prior to pregnancy)
	Smoking
	Age extremes (<18, >40)
	Previous preterm labor
This pregnancy	Inadequate weight gain
	Acute maternal illness
	Pregnancy-induced hypertension
	Urinary tract infection
	Chorioamnionitis, vaginal infection
	Antepartum hemorrhage
	Isoimmunization
	Premature rupture of membranes (PROM)
	Multiple gestation
	Polyhydramnios
	Retained IUD
Fetal factors	Fetal anomalies
	Intrauterine fetal demise
	Infection

(Bartram J, Clewell WH: Prenatal environment: Impact on neonatal outcome. In Merenstein GB, Gardner SL. [eds]: Handbook of Neonatal Intensive Care, 2nd ed, p 42. St. Louis, CV Mosby, 1989.)

ing as a pathway for blood between the pulmonary artery and aorta, remains open owing to the preterm birth. The preterm infant has a lower pulmonary vascular resistance as a consequence of decrease in the muscular development of the pulmonary arterioles. Vasoconstrictive efforts are not as responsive to increases in oxygen levels. While the ductus remains open, there is an increase in the amount of blood shunted to the pulmonary circuit, leading ultimately to pulmonary edema and increases in respiratory effort and oxygen consumption. About 15% of infants with patent ductus arteriosus have additional cardiac defects.

RESPIRATORY SYSTEM

The preterm infant is at risk for respiratory problems. The lungs are not fully mature until after 35 weeks' gestation. Surfactant, acting as an agent to decrease surface tension in the lung, is deficient in the preterm infant. In addition, it is not until 34 to 36 weeks that mature alveoli are present in the fetal lung. (For further discussion of the problem of respiratory distress syndrome and other respiratory disorders, see the section, Special Health Problems of the Preterm Infant.)

Apnea. Generally speaking, the preterm infant's respiratory patterns may be regular or may exhibit increasing and frequent periods of apnea. Apnea is a common clinical problem experienced in neonatal intensive care. Preterm infants' immature respiratory centers do not respond readily to elevated levels of $Paco_2$ as do term infants. As a result, hypoventilation and hypercapnia occur.

Patterns of periodic breathing in the preterm (pauses of 5–10 seconds) have been reported quite commonly. True apneic episodes, however, last for 10 to 15 seconds, accompanied by pallor, cyanosis, hypotonia, and bradycardia. Repeated apneic episodes occur most often in preterm infants weighing less than 1000 g. This disorder represents immaturity of the respiratory control systems in the brain. Apneic episodes in the neonate, which must be treated promptly, if possible, may be precipitated by the following disorders:

1. Temperature instability
2. Central nervous system problems
3. Drugs (maternal-fetal)
4. Infection
5. Metabolic disorders
6. Neonatal asphyxia
7. Abdominal distention

All infants at risk should be placed on an apnea monitor for the first 2 weeks of life. The use of tactile stimulation and repositioning to avoid pharyngeal obstruction by hyperflexion of the neck has been helpful in managing and preventing apneic episodes. Other management techniques include low nasal continuous positive airway pressure (CPAP) at 3 to 5 cm H_2O, xanthine drugs, and doxapram.[12]

GASTROINTESTINAL SYSTEM

Maturity of the gastrointestinal tract is established by 36 to 38 weeks' gestation. Therefore, the preterm infant's gastrointestinal tract is not as functional as its mature potential. The preterm infant is subject to the following factors, which may interfere with mature gastrointestinal functioning:

1. Uncoordinated sucking and swallowing until 34 to 35 weeks
2. Incompetent cardiac sphincter
3. Delayed gastric emptying time
4. Decreased absorption of fat
5. Incomplete digestion of protein
6. Decreased or uncoordinated motility[13]

CENTRAL NERVOUS SYSTEM

Sleep–wake cycles are difficult to evaluate in the preterm infant. Preterm infants experience more quiet sleep, less active sleep, and higher pO_2 levels in the prone position. More quiet sleep is experienced in a neutral thermal environment.

Little facial expression is noted before 30 to 32 weeks' gestation. Little spontaneous crying occurs before 30 to 32 weeks. From this time on, hunger is expressed by crying. Rhythmic, nonnutritive sucking is noted only after 33 weeks' gestation. The auditory system functions from 26 weeks' gestation. Consistent auditory responses are noted at 32 to 34 weeks.

A gradual increase in muscle tone is noted with increasing gestational age. As muscle tone increases, the extremities gradually assume a flexed position. This posturing and flexible nature of the extremities represent a part of the gestational age assessment scoring. By 36 weeks, muscle movements become more coordinated.

The stage of development of the nervous system at birth is dependent on the degree of maturity. The fetus has a majority of neurons by 18 to 20 weeks' gestational age. The basement membrane of brain capillaries is of minimum thickness compared with the adult brain. This phenomenon may be one factor predisposing the preterm infant to subependymal and intraventricular hemorrhage (IVH). Reflexes, such as Moro and tonic neck, are present in the preterm infant.[14]

RENAL SYSTEM

In the preterm infant, the kidneys and related urinary structures have immature properties. The kidneys do not concentrate urine well or excrete large amounts of fluid. Further, drug excretion takes longer. Glomerular filtration rate efficiency parallels gestational age. The buffering capacity of the kidneys is low, predisposing the neonate to acidosis with decreased excretion of bicarbonate and acid.[15]

HEPATIC SYSTEM

The preterm infant's immature liver presents serious problems during the immediate neonatal period. Bilirubin levels rise more rapidly than in the term infant, owing to inability of the liver to process bilirubin. Infants weighing less than 1500 g may be placed on prophylactic phototherapy.[16]

Hypoglycemia of the neonate may be due to low liver glycogen stores. Lower serum protein levels, deficiency of blood-clotting factors, and deficient conjugation and detoxification of certain drugs are all attributed to liver immaturity.

IMMUNOLOGIC PROBLEMS

The preterm infant has lower levels of IgG, which largely is acquired during the last trimester. IgA and IgM, present in colostrum, may not be received by the neonate who is given nothing by mouth (NPO) due to illness.

Elevated levels of IgM or IgA in cord blood may reflect an exposure of the fetus to an antigen in utero. If maternal to fetal transplacental bleeding has occurred, elevated levels of IgM or IgA may also be found.[17] Preterm infants' white blood cells do not function as well in the disposition of bacteria.

INTEGUMENTARY PROBLEMS

The skin of the preterm is thin, transparent, and covered with abundant vernix. There is a high rate of insensible water loss, especially with infants of less than 30 weeks' gestational age. Further, the preterm infant's skin absorbs chemicals readily, so precautions must be taken with topical ointments and solutions covering the skin. Finally, the skin is extremely vulnerable to damage from adhesive materials, so care must be taken with the amount and kind of adhesive used with monitors and other items placed on the skin.[18]

THERMAL REGULATION

The following factors foster temperature regulation problems in the preterm infant:

1. High surface:mass ratio
2. Reduced brown fat stores
3. Increase in insensible water loss
4. Respiratory distress, fostering insensible water loss with work of breathing
5. Extended posture of extremities
6. Immature vasomotor control[4]

Special Health Problems of the Preterm Infant

RESPIRATORY DISTRESS SYNDROME

Previously known as hyaline membrane disease (HMD), RDS type I is a developmental disease of preterm infants appropriate for gestational age.[19] By estimate, 50,000 infants develop RDS each year in the United States. RDS is the most common single cause of respiratory distress in neonates, almost exclusively occurring in the preterm. Although advances in neonatal care have improved the prognosis of these infants, RDS is still a leading cause of neonatal mortality.

Pathophysiology. RDS is a partial persistence of the fetal cardiopulmonary state. The disease is primarily a developmental disorder because the synthesis of surfactant in utero must have taken place for lung maturation to be complete at about 35 weeks' gestation. Surfactant is a complex biochemical substance composed of phospholipids and proteins. Surfactant exerts a detergent-like action over the inner surface of the alveoli, decreasing their tendency to collapse. During low surfactant production by the type II alveolar cells, alveolar collapse, atelectasis, and decreased lung compliance occur. The combination of atelectasis and pulmonary hypoperfusion from vasospasm leads to hypoxia and hypercapnia. Prolonged hypoxia and hypercapnia result in metabolic and respiratory acidotic states. Hypoxic and acidotic states aggravate vasospasm, which increases pulmonary hypoperfusion. Hypoxia and acidosis also cause destruction of capillaries and alveoli. Capillary damage and destruction of alveoli lead to an increase in surfactant deficiency. Right-to-left shunting of blood may persist at the foramen ovale and ductus arteriosus as a result of increased blood pressure in the pulmonary circuit. Blood is thus diverted from the lungs, enhancing their hypoperfusion.[4]

Perinatal complications that may increase the incidence or severity of RDS are asphyxia, maternal diabetes, and possibly cesarean birth. RDS occurs more often in males than females and in the second of twins. Factors enhancing the production of surfactant and lung maturation include the stress of intrauterine infections, premature rupture of membranes, maternal hypertensive disorders, and maternal administration of glucocorticoids.

Clinical Manifestations. Assessment of the neonate reveals respiratory distress, usually within 4 hours after birth (Fig. 44-6). Distress is a result of the diminished lung compliance and atelectasis that significantly increase the work of breathing. The Silverman score (Fig. 44-7) is an index of measuring observations indicating respiratory distress. The index reflects other diseases as well as that are the result of respiratory compromise in the neonate. The major signs exhibited are cyanosis, tachypnea, retractions, grunting, nasal flaring, and seesaw respirations. Breath sounds are diminished. Hypotension may be present (Fig. 44-8).

Laboratory Data. Arterial blood gas analysis shows hypoxia, hypercapnia, and respiratory or metabolic acidosis. The typical x-ray appearance shows a diffuse reticulogranular pattern over both lungs, peripheral air bronchograms, and loss of lung volume (Fig. 44-9).

Management. Management is geared toward correcting hypoxia and acidosis, alleviating the work of breathing, and maintaining homeostasis. Measures include the

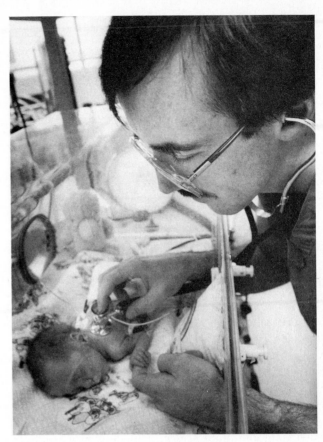

■ *Figure 44–6*
The nurse performs a respiration assessment. (Courtesy of The Children's Hospital of Philadelphia)

administration of oxygen, assisted ventilation with continuous distending pressure, conventional mechanical ventilation, or high-frequency ventilation.[20] Final approval has come from the Food and Drug Administration for use of synthetic surfactant, which has proven to decrease the morbidity and mortality in infants with RDS.

Prognosis. Usually, symptoms begin to lessen as surfactant production is established at about 48 to 72 hours of life. The following complications may occur as a result of RDS[21]:

- Respiratory—pneumothorax, pneumomediastinum, bronchopulmonary dysplasia
- Cardiovascular—hypotension, hypovolemia, hypoxemia, myocardial failure, patent ductus arteriosus
- Central nervous system—cerebral edema, intracranial hemorrhage
- Sepsis
- Renal failure

Nursing Process. The nurse uses the nursing process with the neonate diagnosed with respiratory distress

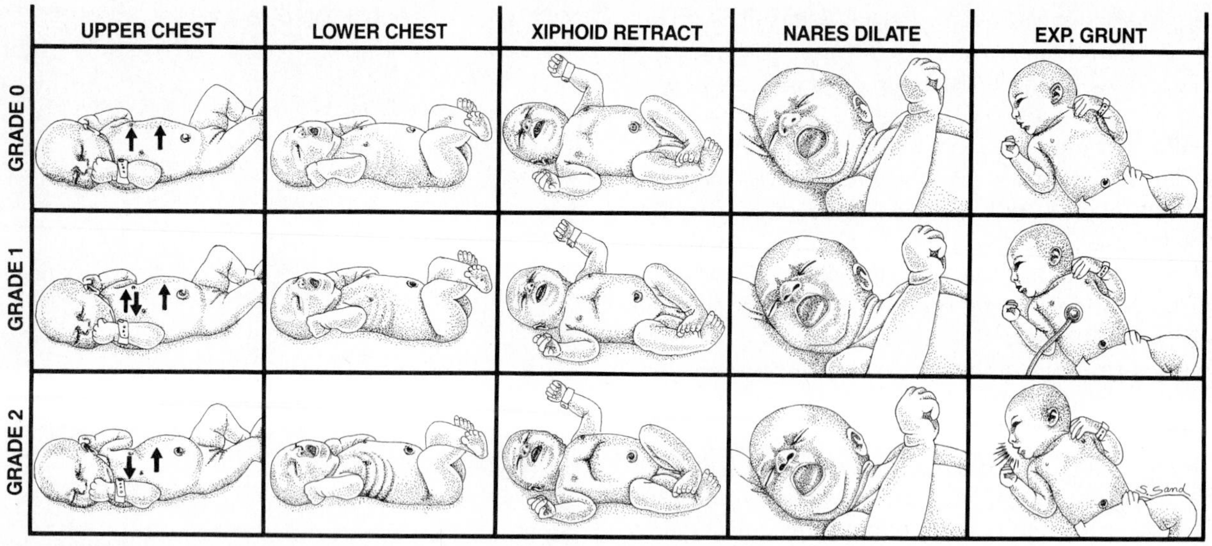

	UPPER CHEST	LOWER CHEST	XIPHOID RETRACT	NARES DILATE	EXP. GRUNT
GRADE 0					
GRADE 1					
GRADE 2					

■ *Figure 44–7*

Observation of retractions using the Silverman score. An index of respiratory distress is determined by grading each of five arbitrary criteria. Grade 0 indicates no difficulty; grade 1 indicates moderate difficulty; and grade 2 indicates maximum respiratory difficulty. The retraction score is the sum of these values; a total score of 0 indicates no dyspnea, whereas a total score of ten denotes maximal respiratory distress.

syndrome to achieve the objectives of recognizing and assessing the infant at risk, stabilizing the critically ill infant, preventing further complications, and providing support for the family in crisis.

Nursing Assessment. By performing a gestational age assessment correctly, the nurse can ascertain quickly that the infant is preterm and therefore at risk for RDS. Consequently, the nurse is alert for the characteristic signs of respiratory distress, as previously described. The nurse also provides continuous respiratory assessment as well as observes for potential complications associated with RDS.

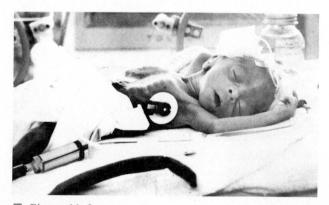

■ *Figure 44–8*

Respiratory distress syndrome. This infant exhibits marked substernal and intercostal retractions, "seesaw" respirations, and nasal flaring.

Potential Nursing Diagnosis. Nursing diagnoses that may apply to the neonate with RDS include the following: impaired gas exchange related to lack of lung surfactant; ineffective airway clearance related to an increase in secretion production; ineffective breathing pattern; alteration in nutrition, less than body requirements, related to larger caloric expenditure than intake, potential complications related to RDS and preterm status; and parental knowledge deficit related to disease process.

Nursing Planning and Intervention. Nursing priorities in care should focus primarily on the respiratory system and alleviation of the work of breathing. The nurse monitors the respiratory status of the infant by physical assessment and the use of invasive and noninvasive measurements of oxygenation. The nurse administers oxygen and other respiratory medications as ordered, monitoring for therapeutic and adverse effects. Provision of ventilator care is an important component of the plan. Nutritional status, fluids, and acid-base balance must be frequently assessed and corrected as needed. The nurse is knowledgeable about potential complications associated with respiratory distress syndrome and is alert to those clinical manifestations. Parents and other family members are kept informed, encouraged to visit and provide caretaking of the infant, and supported psychosocially.

Further details regarding nursing interventions are provided in the nursing care plan and in the section, Planning and Intervention in High-Risk Neonatal Care.

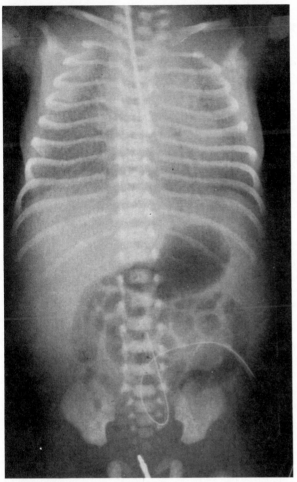

■ *Figure 44–9*
Severe hyaline membrane disease. Note diffuse density of the lung fields compared with intestinal gas, with well-defined air bronchograms. Both lungs are uniformly involved. An umbilical artery catheter lies at the aortic bifurcation (third lumbar vertebra). (Avery GB: Neonatology: Pathophysiology and Management of the Newborn, 3rd ed. Philadelphia, JB Lippincott, 1987)

BRONCHOPULMONARY DYSPLASIA

Bronchopulmonary dysplasia is a significant chronic lung disorder in neonates. The definition includes neonates who, following mechanical ventilation during the first week of life, remain dependent on oxygen for more than 28 days and have persistent increased densities on chest radiographs. Incidence and severity vary widely, ranging from 15% to 50% of infants weighing less than 1500 g who required assisted ventilation. Diagnosis is made when an infant demonstrates prolonged requirement for ventilator and oxygen therapy. Characteristic radiologic changes are seen weeks later.[22]

Bronchopulmonary dysplasia appears to be the result of numerous risk factors, such as pulmonary immaturity, endotracheal intubation, oxygen admin-

istration, mechanical ventilation, and patent ductus arteriosus.[4]

Pathophysiology. There are destructive inflammatory changes in the lung tissue described as thickening and eventual destruction of alveolar walls, basement membrane, and bronchiolar epithelial lining layers. Fibrosis and atelectasis are present.

Clinical Manifestations. Clinical characteristics include respiratory distress, oxygen dependence, retractions, rales, CO_2 retention, respiratory acidosis, and potential congestive heart failure.

Prognosis. In those infants who recover, repeated pulmonary infections and wheezing are common.

Nursing Process. Goals of the nurse's efforts are maintaining oxygenation, maintaining fluid balance and optimal nutrition, and preventing infection.

Nursing Assessment. The nurse performs a thorough respiratory assessment to determine the severity of respiratory distress present. Ongoing invasive and noninvasive oxygenation determinations are a priority because the infant's status can change dramatically with the smallest change in oxygen therapy.

The nurse assesses nutritional and fluid balance status on a regular basis. Provision of adequate nutrition is of primary concern, because malnutrition will delay development of new alveoli and predispose to infection. Signs of sepsis and respiratory infection must be recognized as early as possible to initiate treatment.

Potential Nursing Diagnosis. Potential nursing diagnoses for the infant with bronchopulmonary dysplasia are: impaired gas exchange; alteration in nutrition, less than body requirements; and high risk for infection.

Nursing Planning and Intervention. The nurse must maintain diligent monitoring of respiratory status. Respiratory assessment, oxygen administration, ventilator care, and chest physiotherapy are integral components of this care. Weaning the infant from oxygen with extreme caution is an ongoing intervention. The provision of adequate nutrition via parenteral and oral caloric intake is crucial to maintain optimal status. Signs of fluid overload, such as increase in weight, rales, edema, and hepatomegaly, are noted and reported because these infants are subject to congestive heart failure.

Accurate and safe administration of diuretics, bronchodilators, and antibiotics is an ongoing part of the nurse's plan of care as needed.

Evaluation. The nursing process has been effective when the patient goals have been met. The infant dem-
(Text continues on page 1139)

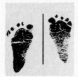

Nursing Care Plan

The Family and Neonate With Respiratory Distress Syndrome

Patient Goals

1. Infant receives ventilatory assistance as needed.
2. Infant demonstrates normal acid-base balance.
3. Infant demonstrates adequate oxygenation.
4. Infant maintains patent airway.
5. Infant demonstrates steady weight gain.
6. Infant receives adequate caloric intake for weight.
7. Infant demonstrates absence of feeding intolerance.
8. Infant maintains stable temperature.
9. Typical complications are absent or minimal.
10. Infant demonstrates evidence of hydration.
11. Parents visit the infant regularly.
12. Parents provide caretaking.
13. Parents demonstrate understanding of prognoses by discussing problems freely.

Assessment	Potential Nursing Diagnosis	Planning and Intervention	Evaluation
Preterm delivery	Impaired gas exchange related to lack of lung surfactant	Deliver oxygen according to needs displayed by transcutaneous readings or arterial blood gas samples	Infant receives ventilatory assistance
Evidence of fetal hypoxic episode			Infant returns to normal acid-base balance
Previous family history		Use appropriate delivery method	Oxygenation is within acceptable limits
Evidence of respiratory distress		Oxygen hood Flooding of isolette	
		Check oxygen concentration every hour	
		Calibrate oxygen sensors as per protocol	
	Ineffective breathing pattern related to disease process	Manage ventilatory assistance	
		CPAP	
		Monitor pressure readings	
		Check nasal prongs for patency	
		Lubricate nasal prongs	
		Check nares for pressure areas	
		Ventilator	
		Maintain ordered settings	
		Keep bag and mask nearby in case of ventilator failure or extubation	

(continued)

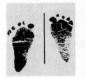

Nursing Care Plan (continued)

Assessment	Potential Nursing Diagnosis	Planning and Intervention	Evaluation
		Monitor blood gases soon after ventilator or oxygen changes made	
		Observe color	
		Observe respiratory effort	
		Auscultate and assess breath sounds, heart rate	
		Observe general activity	
		Recognize and promptly correct alterations in acid–base balances by	

		Changes in ventilator settings
		  Bagging
		  Administration of drugs
		  Volume replacement	

	Ineffective airway clearance related to an increase in secretion production and inability to clear airway by coughing	Use suction for brief periods using intermittent pressures	Infant maintains patent airway
		Use sterile procedure with saline instillation with endotracheal tube Bag before and after suctioning with 100% oxygen to prevent atelectasis	
		Suction only as needed	
		Observe and describe infant's tolerance to the procedure as well as the amount, color, and character of secretions	
		Turn frequently and use chest postural draininge to mobilize secretions	
		Keep well hydrated to promote secretion liquefaction	
	Fluid volume and electrolyte imbalances related to disease, sensible and insensible water losses, and use of parenteral fluids	Record daily weights	Infant establishes balanced intake and output
		Monitor laboratory values as ordered	Infant reaches and maintains fluid and electrolyte balance
		Observe for signs and symptoms of electrolyte imbalances, fluid overload, and dehydration	Infant steadily gains weight

(continued)

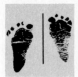

Nursing Care Plan (continued)

Assessment	Potential Nursing Diagnosis	Planning and Intervention	Evaluation
		Deliver correct type and amount of intravenous fluid	Infant maintains skin integrity
		Monitor output; check specific gravity, Clinitest, color, odor	
		Maintain positioning of peripheral IV site	
		Observe site for infiltration	
		Restrain infant as needed	
		Secure umbilical catheter as needed to prevent any dislodgment from tubing	
		Observe extremities for blanching or discoloration of hands and feet	
		If discoloration or blanching occurs, contralateral foot may be wrapped briefly—if adverse reaction of vasospasm not relieved, removal of catheter is required	
		For subclavian catheter, change dressing as per protocol using sterile technique	
		For all intravenous lines, change tubing every 24 hours	
	Alteration in nutrition, less than body requirements, related to larger caloric expenditure than intake	Provide adequate calories per kilogram of body weight	Infant demonstrates absence of feeding intolerance
		Minimize volume by using special higher caloric preterm formulas	Infant maintains stable temperature
			Infant demonstrates steady weight gain
	Ineffective thermoregulation, related to preterm status	Minimize caloric expenditure with heat loss by maintaining thermoneutral environment	Infant receives adequate caloric intake for weight
		Use hats when out of isolette	

(continued)

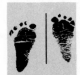

Nursing Care Plan   (continued)

Assessment	Potential Nursing Diagnosis	Planning and Intervention	Evaluation
		Conserve energy by minimizing bottle feedings	
		Gavage feed as necessary	
		Place head of bed up after feedings	
		Measure residuals and abdominal girth	
	Parental knowledge deficit related to disease process	Provide informative, realistic explanations to parents regarding short-term and long-term prognosis	Parents visit NICU regularly
			Parents provide caretaking
		Encourage parents to visit and provide caretaking tasks for infant	Parents demonstrate understanding of prognoses by discussing problems freely.
	Potential injury related to complications	Observe for and record signs and symptoms of	
		Bronchopulmonary dysplasia	
		Pneumothorax	Complications are absent or minimal
		Retrolental fibroplasia	
		Necrotizing enterocolitis	
		Intraventricular hemorrhage	
		Patent ductus arteriosus	

onstrates adequate or stable oxygenation, with minimal assistance of oxygen or ventilator. Infants may continue to require this assistance at home, necessitating parental involvement, education, and support. The infant is free of any clinical signs of sepsis. The infant demonstrates signs of adequate hydration and nutritional status.

PNEUMOTHORAX

Pneumothorax is a potential complication of assisted ventilation and positive end-expiratory pressure (PEEP).

Clinical signs indicate a sudden, rapid deterioration in condition, especially in an infant with respiratory disease. Tachypnea, grunting, pallor, or cyanosis may occur. Breath sounds may be decreased. Cardiac apex may shift away from the affected side. Bradycardia and hypotension may occur.

Diagnosis may be ascertained by transillumination of the chest followed by definitive chest films.

High oxygen administration alone or further intervention may be necessary to reinflate the affected lung. The air leak can be decompressed by needle aspiration and subsequent placement of a chest tube with water-seal drainage and suction of 10 to 20 cm H_2O. When air movement in the tube and bubbling cease, the tube is clamped and removed in 24 hours if the infant's condition remains stable.

RETINOPATHY OF PREMATURITY

Retinopathy of prematurity is an acquired disease in the low-birth-weight infant. Although oxygen administration has been implicated in the past, evidence exists that other factors contribute to its development. The very-low-birth-weight infants weighing 500 to 750 g have an incidence of 42% compared with 7% in infants weighing between 1001 and 1500 g. According to current literature, retinopathy of prematurity is not a preventable disease because the causes are unknown.[4]

The progression of the disease ranges from dilation and tortuosity of retinal vessels to retinal detachment.

Management. Infants at risk because they meet the following criteria receive routine ophthalmologic examinations in the NICU:

1. Birth weight less than 1500 g
2. Mechanical ventilation administered more than 24 hours
3. Oxygen required more than 40% for more than 12 hours

Infants with advanced disease may benefit from transscleral cryotherapy, which freezes scarred retinal vessels. Cryotherapy has been shown to decrease the risk of blinding complications of retinopathy of prematurity by 50%. Routine follow-up is essential to detect and treat vision problems as the infants grow.[23]

INTRAVENTRICULAR HEMORRHAGE

IVH occurs in the preterm infant and is recognized as a major disorder with increasing frequency. Incidence increases with decreasing gestational age. IVH is a leading cause of death. Survivors may experience no impairment to severe impairment.

Risk Factors. Obstetric and neonatal factors that may serve as stimuli for bleeding include birth asphyxia, hypotension, assisted ventilation, RDS, pneumothorax, hypercarbia, thrombocytopenia, fluid and electrolyte imbalances, and volume expanders.

Pathophysiology. A highly vascular area, the subependymal germinal matrix, is very evident between 28 and 32 weeks. Little of this structure is present at term. The subependymal germinal matrix is located at the level of the foramen of Monro and the head of the caudate nucleus. Bleeding is thought to originate from the capillaries of the germinal matrix.

As a stimulus to increased cerebral blood flow and resultant venous congestion, hypoxia and hypercarbia dilate cerebral vessels. Further, hypoxia and acidosis injure the endothelium of the vessels, making them rupture easily.

In preterm infants, the mechanism for keeping cerebral blood flow constant may be impaired. Arterioles dilate as stimulated by hypoxia or hypercarbia. A rise in blood pressure at this point may result in capillary rupture and hemorrhage. Bleeding may be isolated in the subependymal germinal matrix or extended into the neighboring ventricles.[25] The classification system shown in the box can be used to isolate the severity of the hemorrhage.

Classification of Severity of Intraventricular Hemorrhage

Grade I: Isolated subependymal hemorrhage

Grade II: Intraventricular hemorrhage without ventricular dilation

Grade III: Intraventricular hemorrhage with ventricular dilation

Grade IV: Intraventricular hemorrhage with ventricular hemorrhage and hemorrhage into the parenchyma of the brain[24]

Clinical Manifestations. Clinical signs may range from none to a dramatic change in condition. Observations of a deterioration may come about very quickly. The nurse may notice apnea, bradycardia, hypotension, seizures, or decerebrate posturing. The anterior fontanel bulges, and the temperature becomes unstable, indicating increasing intracranial pressure.

Diagnosis. Spinal fluid shows an increased number of red blood cells, elevated protein, and low glucose. Computed tomography (CT) and ultrasound techniques can pinpoint the location and size of the hemorrhage.

Prevention. Studies are ongoing to determine the usefulness of drugs in preventing hemorrhage (i.e., phenobarbital and ethamsylate).[25] Nurses can prevent intracranial insult by identifying the infant who is at risk for IVH and providing as safe an environment as possible, given the many factors involved.

Careful monitoring of intake and output and its subsequent effects on blood pressure is advised. Avoidance of the head-down position as used frequently in chest physiotherapy is essential. Administration of sodium bicarbonate, slowly and well diluted, is recommended. Avoidance of stress for the infant, which can raise the blood pressure, may be accomplished by grouping nursing activities and providing rest periods. Activities that lead to hypoxia, such as suctioning and intubation, should be time limited. Administration of preoxygenation and postoxygenation by bag and mask is essential.

Treatment. The activity of hemorrhage can be monitored by CT scan and ultrasound. Small hemorrhages will not require any treatment and resolve spontaneously. Others will require removal of the blood by spinal tap, direct ventricular puncture, or ventricular reservoir. Daily lumbar punctures may be required.

If posthemorrhagic hydrocephalus occurs, surgery is required to place a ventriculoperitoneal shunt. This shunt drains the accumulated cerebrospinal fluid into the peritoneal cavity, where it is reabsorbed.

Nursing Assessment and Interventions. Continuing observation of the neonate at risk can alert the nurse to those subtle cues indicative of a change in status. Status of the fontanels (i.e., flat, full, tense, or bulging) should be noted regularly. Seizure activity may be extremely subtle (i.e., brief apnea) and may be difficult to pick up.

In an infant diagnosed with IVH, the nurse must continue to be alert for signs of increasing intracranial pressure, such as apnea, bradycardia, hypotension, and temperature instability. Repeat measurements of head circumferences and observation of fontanels are required. Assistance with treatment procedures and care of drains may be essential.

PATENT DUCTUS ARTERIOSUS

The process of the patent ductus arteriosus is more likely in the preterm infant than in the term infant.

Physiology. The ductus arteriosus in the fetus serves as a connection between the pulmonary artery and the aorta. It functions as a bypass for the lungs and, possibly, as a volume recipient from the left ventricle.

In the term infant, the ductus arteriosus closes in stages. Early or functional closure occurs in the first 24 hours. Later or anatomical closure of the tissue occurs in a few days. In the preterm infant, these events occur also, but at a later time, when age and weight approach that of a term infant.

The appearance of clinical signs of patent ductus arteriosus depends on the balance between the pulmonary and systemic vascular beds. If the pulmonary vascular resistance is low, there may be a left-to-right shunt, increasing the work of breathing for the neonate. If there is severe RDS, pulmonary vascular resistance is high, resulting in a right-to-left shunt.

Clinical Manifestations. Signs are more evident on the third or fourth day, when RDS would be resolving. Murmurs can be auscultated. Wide pulse pressures, tachycardia, and bounding pulses are noted. Signs and symptoms of pulmonary edema occur, such as tachypnea, grunting, retractions, and rales.[26]

Elevation of $paCO_2$, recurrent apnea, and increasing need for oxygen are noted.

Diagnosis. In addition to clinical manifestations, chest x-ray, contrast echocardiography, and Doppler evaluation are used to make the diagnosis.

Treatment. Fluid restriction is necessary to decrease the work load of the heart. Adjustments are necessary in the case of the use of overhead warmers to combat insensible water loss. Diuretics such as furosemide (Lasix) may be used to control volume on board. Controversy exists as to whether the use of digoxin in the preterm infants is really therapeutic. Preterm infants exhibit a high incidence of arrhythmias. Because anemia can increase the heart's work load, the hematocrit needs to be kept as close to 45 as possible.[26]

The role of prostaglandins and indomethacin's inhibitory effect are fairly recent medical advances in the treatment of patent ductus arteriosus. Overall, indomethacin has been successful, although in some neonates the ductus has reopened. Because it affects the kidney, indomethacin should not be administered if the blood urea nitrogen is above 25 or the creatinine is above 1.8.[26] Renal function will be affected, with a decrease in urine output, decrease in serum sodium, and increase in potassium. These effects last only 72 hours. A total of three doses is given every 12 hours intravenously, orally, or rectally. If there is not subsequent improvement in status, surgical intervention may be necessary. The timing of medical or surgical intervention and the choice of candidates remain open to debate and the individual situation.

Nursing Process. Care of an infant with a congenital heart defect is described in detail in Chapter 45.

NECROTIZING ENTEROCOLITIS

Necrotizing enterocolitis (NEC), a disease of the neonate characterized by necrosis of the bowel, occurs in 3% to 5% of neonates admitted to the NICU.[27] Mortality figures range widely from 10% to 55%. NEC is the most frequent preoperative diagnosis for infants going to surgery. The average age of onset of the disease is 4 days. Most infants with NEC are low-birth-weight, preterm infants.[28] The majority are 33 weeks' gestation and weigh less than 1500 g. Predisposing factors are numerous.

Etiology and Pathophysiology. Factors that have been cited in the literature that lead to an episode of NEC are feeding, mucosal injury in the bowel, and bacterial colonization.[27]

Most infants developing NEC were fed a cow's milk formula; few were fed only breast milk. Intestinal ischemia may be a result of vasospasm in response to asphyxia as blood is shunted to vital organs of the heart and brain. Bacterial colonization of the gut normally begins at delivery and progresses to 10 days in a healthy neonate. Infants in the NICU experience a more sterile environment, however, and colonization is delayed. Bacteria most commonly tied to NEC are normal flora: *Escherichia coli, Aerobacter, Klebsiella,* and *Pseudomonas.*[29]

Clinical Manifestations. Signs indicative of NEC are abdominal distention along with gastric retention and vomiting. Others mentioned are lethargy, irritability, apnea, diarrhea, unstable temperature, respiratory distress, metabolic acidosis, and gastrointestinal bleeding. X-ray films of the abdomen indicate multiple dilated loops of bowel and pneumatosis.

Diagnostic laboratory work includes complete blood count, platelets, electrolytes, arterial blood gases, and blood cultures.

Treatment.

MEDICAL. The neonate is place on NPO status to rest the bowel. Intravenous fluids are given, a nasogastric tube is placed to low suction, and intravenous or gastric antibiotics are given. Serial abdominal films are obtained to monitor any changes in the gut. Other management is supportive.

SURGICAL. Resection of necrotic segments of bowel and enterostomy are performed if the disease progresses to intestinal perforation and peritonitis.

Nursing Process. The plan of care begins when the nurse is aware of infants at risk for NEC. The nurse's observations are crucial in establishing the correct diagnosis and subsequent management.

Assessment. Infants at risk are identified. The preterm infant is observed for tolerance to feedings.

Potential Nursing Diagnosis. Nursing diagnoses that may be applicable to the infant with NEC are high risk for infection; alteration in nutrition, less than body requirements; thermoregulation, ineffective; and alteration in comfort.

Planning and Interventions. Nurses must be aware of the risk factors that may contribute to gut ischemia. Once an at-risk infant has been identified, the nurse should promote NPO status and initiate IV maintenance, permitting the intestinal wall to heal. Once feedings are initiated, the administration of fresh breast milk via nasogastric tube is optimal to check gastric residuals. Nasojejunal tubes should be avoided because the introduction of formula into the bowel may cause mucosal damage and subsequent bowel perforation. A neutral thermal environment must be maintained because hypothermia contributes to NEC by promoting bowel ischemia. Umbilical catheters should be discontinued as soon as possible because they have been noted as a risk factor for NEC.[29] Infants with NEC usually are placed on long-term total parenteral nutrition (TPN) therapy until the bowel is rested or reanastomosed. Promotion of comfort may be achieved by careful positioning, stroking and tactile stimulation, and administration of pain medications.

Evaluation. The infant with NEC, on receiving optimal nursing care, will (1) demonstrate absence of further signs of infection; (2) demonstrate adequate signs of hydration and optimum nutrition; (3) demonstrate absence of discomfort; and (4) maintain normal temperature.

■ NURSING PROCESS IN HIGH-RISK NEONATAL CARE

In the formulation of the plan of care, the nurse takes into consideration the risk factors and the probable gestational age of the infant about to be born. The remainder of this chapter focuses on planning and intervention in high-risk neonatal care. Although the examples given are usually discussing the preterm infant, the term infant could also receive similar interventions.

■ NURSING DIAGNOSIS IN HIGH-RISK NEONATAL CARE

To intervene most successfully, the nurse needs to formulate appropriate nursing diagnoses. The following are examples of nursing diagnoses pertaining to the preterm neonate: potential fluid volume deficit related to insensible water loss and inadequate fluid intake; high risk for impairment of gas exchange related to lack of surfactant; high risk for cold stress related to immature temperature-regulating mechanism; and high risk of infection related to immature immune system.

■ PLANNING AND INTERVENTION IN HIGH-RISK NEONATAL CARE

Resuscitation

Elements of successful resuscitation include anticipation, adequate preparation, and appropriate management. An NICU nurse, neonatologist, and respiratory therapist should attend all high-risk deliveries. These personnel should also be on rotating call in the event that unanticipated problems occur with the neonate. Obstetric and neonatal nurses should all be trained in resuscitation and delivery areas or labor rooms appropriately equipped. Equipment needs to be replaced as it is used, and the cart should be checked for inventory, expiration

Neonatal Resuscitation Equipment

1. Oxygen and air tanks with oxygen diluter, corrugated tubing
2. Infant warmer with suction machine, thermometer, 2 bottles of sterile water for suctioning, and stethoscope
3. Cardiac monitor with leads, strain gauge (to be brought to room when delivery expected)

Shelf Supplies

IV instrument tray

Catheter-assist tray (see next section)

Blood-culture tube, culturettes

Blood-collecting tubes

Dextrostix with heelstick equipment

Hematocrit tubes with sealing material

Extra syringes—8 each of tuberculin, 3 ml, 5 ml, and 10 ml

Safety pins

Feeding tubes—2 No. 8

Suction supplies—1 connecting tube; 2 each of numbers 5, 8, and 10 DeLee

Endotracheal suction tubes (2) and adapter

Sterile gloves—4 of each size

Sterile drapes (2 packs)

Sterile towels (4)

Ice basins for blood gases

Infant hood

2 continuous positive airway pressure (CPAP) setups— 1 always set up and 1 extra

Face masks—1 each of 3 different infant sizes

Chart and pens on clipboard

Oxygen analyzer—brought in before delivery

Lab slips and white tape for identification labels

Stop watch

Stockinette and safety pins for restraints

1 hemoset

1 metriset

1 250-ml $D_{10}W$

1 150-ml $D_5/2$ NS

Betadine

Needle electrodes

Catheter-assist Tray

1 20-ml syringe

2 10-ml syringes

2 5-ml syringes

5 3-ml syringes

5 tuberculin syringes

4 packages 4-0 silk suture

4 No. 20 knife blades

4 disposable No. 16 blunt needles (Luer stub adapters)

4 disposable Tomac stopcocks

4 No. 5 arterial catheters

4 No. 3½ arterial catheters

1 roll of 1-in pink tape

Cord clamp and cord tie

Disposable scalpels

Alcohol sponges

Corks

Extra 2 × 2 gauzes

4 steri-drapes

2 intraflo

Medicine Tray

4 heparin, 100 U/ml

1 20-ml vial of 1% lidocaine and 1% lidocaine for IV use

2 calcium gluceptate, 200 mg/ml

2 sodium bicarbonate

2 each normal saline and sterile water vials

1 KCl vial; 1 NaCl vial

1 salt-poor 25% albumin

2 adrenalin 1:1000 (dilute 0.1 ml to total volume of 1 ml)

Neosporin ointment

Narcan 0.4 mg/ml, 1 vial

50% dextrose, 50-ml bottle

Intubation Tray

Laryngoscope with regular and premature size blades and batteries

Forregger tubes—1 each of sizes 2.5, 3.0, 3.5, 4.0, 8, 10, 12, 14, 16

Portex tubes—2 each of sizes 2.5, 3.0, 3.5, and 4.0

Benzoin and cotton swabs

Elastoplast, pink tape, precut tapes (preemie and regular)

Pneumothorax equipment

Needle holder, tweezers, and scissors

4-0 sutures and stylette

(Waechter EH, Phillips J, Holaday B: Nursing Care of Children, 10th ed. Philadelphia, JB Lippincott, 1985; adopted from the *Nursing Manual*, Nursery, Mt. Zion Hospital and Medical Center, San Francisco, CA)

dates, and drugs every shift (see Neonatal Resuscitation Equipment). As part of preparation, personnel should be comfortable working with the equipment.[30]

Chapter 25 discusses the universally known Apgar scoring system, which provides an assessment and guide for resuscitation required. Although this score is a guideline, the caregiver should evaluate the neonate immediately and proceed with intervention (not wait for 1 minute).

Resuscitation technique encompasses the skills of maintaining an open airway, assistance with breathing, and maintaining circulation, the ABCs of cardiopulmonary resuscitation (Fig. 44-10). All procedures should be carried out under the open radiant warmer to allow easy access along with continuous temperature moni-

toring of the neonate. The neonate should be dried thoroughly to avoid evaporative heat loss.

AIRWAY

As the head emerges at the time of birth, the nose and mouth are cleared of mucus with a bulb syringe or Delee trap.

If further suctioning is required, the infant should be placed in the radiant warmer. The mouth is again suctioned first, followed by the nose, to avoid reflex aspiration if the nose is stimulated first. Intermittent suction with a suction catheter for brief periods (10–15 seconds) is recommended. Continuous heart rate monitoring should be maintained, because suctioning can

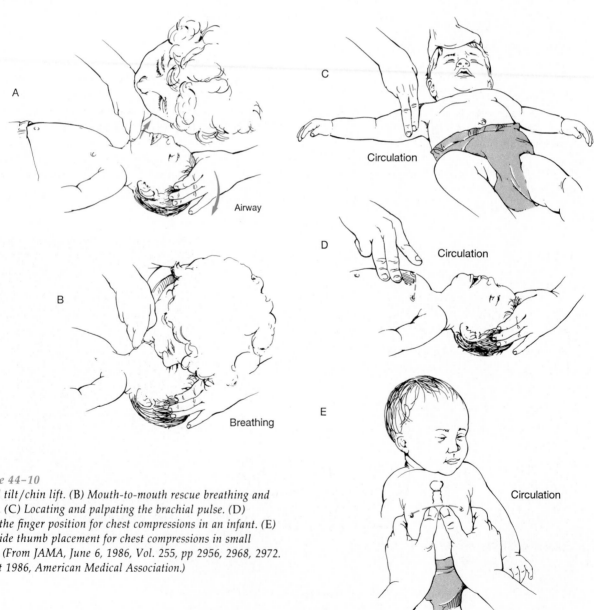

■ *Figure 44–10*
(A) *Head tilt/chin lift.* (B) *Mouth-to-mouth rescue breathing and nose seal.* (C) *Locating and palpating the brachial pulse.* (D) *Locating the finger position for chest compressions in an infant.* (E) *Side-by-side thumb placement for chest compressions in small neonates. (From JAMA, June 6, 1986, Vol. 255, pp 2956, 2968, 2972. Copyright 1986, American Medical Association.)*

stimulate the vagus, resulting in bradycardia. Oxygen should be administered under intermittent positive-pressure ventilation at 3 to 4 L/min. The neonate should be mechanically ventilated between suctioning if he or she is apneic.[31]

BREATHING

Bag and Mask. The infant is placed in the so-called sniffing position, without hyperextension of the neck; some neonates may require a towel roll under the shoulders to maintain this position. The mask is placed over the nose and mouth to create a seal. Various mask sizes should be available, because mask size must be appropriate for each particular infant. The bag should have a one-way valve on the neck piece to allow for expiration. The bag should also have a collar and reservoir to permit 100% oxygen to be administered. Some bags have a pop-off valve to control maximum peak pressures, although others have attached gauges to give this information.[32] One type of bag is shown in Figure 44-11.

OXYGEN CONCENTRATION. Most infants require 100% oxygen during a resuscitation effort. Some infants already receiving oxygen therapy may require only the percentage they are receiving.

RATE. The usual rate for hand bagging is from 40 to 60 breaths per minute to stimulate the usual respiratory rate (Table 44-4).

AMOUNTS OF PRESSURE. Peak pressure is the highest pressure in the lungs during normal inspiration. It is recommended to use 40 to 60 cm H_2O pressure from the first breath of assisted hand ventilation and 16 to 20 cm H_2O pressure for subsequent ventilation in neonates with normal lungs. In neonates with diagnosed lung disease, 20 to 25 cm H_2O pressure may be necessary. Excess pressure could cause pneumothorax.

PEEP is the lowest positive pressure measured during expiration. If the pressure is not allowed to drop to zero, then PEEP is given. Infants with diseased lungs may require some small PEEP pressures, whereas infants with normal lungs do not require any PEEP.[32]

Chest movement should be observed with each mechanical breath. Some respiratory effort and improvement of color should ensue. If spontaneous respirations do not occur quickly, endotracheal intubation should be quickly accomplished by an experienced resuscitator.

Endotracheal Intubation. The infant is again placed in the proper position to straighten the airway. Once positioning is accomplished, the laryngoscope is inserted and the endotracheal tube of correct size is inserted on the right side of the mouth and advanced into the trachea. If is helpful to measure the distance from mouth to suprasternal notch before placing the tube (Fig. 44-12). The pressure of bilateral breath sounds when bagged with 100% oxygen means that placement is ac-

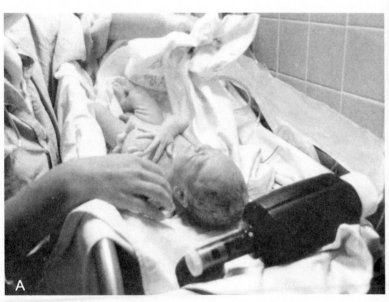
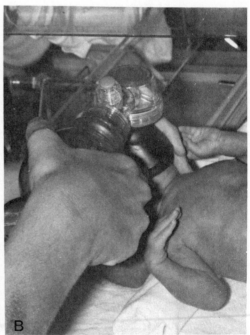

■ *Figure 44-11*

Bagging in resuscitation. (A) An Ambu resuscitation bag stands ready in case it is needed. (B) Appropriate technique for bagging. A towel is placed under the newborn's shoulders to maintain the sniffing position. (A, courtesy of Booth Maternity Center, Philadelphia)

TABLE 44-4. SUGGESTED METHODS OF EMERGENCY HAND VENTILATION

Condition of Neonate	Rate in Breaths per Minute (BPM)	Concentration of Inspired Oxygen (F_{IO}^2)	Peak Pressure (cm H_2O pressure)	Positive End Expiratory Pressure-PEEP (cm H_2O pressure)
Depressed neonate in delivery room (state of lungs unknown)	40–60	100%	Very first breath: 40–60 Other breaths: 16–25	0
Neonate with normal lungs (acute distress)	40–60	If witnessed deterioration, may try less than 100% If unwitnessed, 100%	16–20	0
Neonate with known diseased lungs (as initial stabilization before transport)	40–60	100%	16–25	Up to +5

* If efforts do not result in improvement of neonate's condition, other appropriate measures to be taken include (1) reassessment of airway (i.e., need for suctioning and intubation); (2) emergency medicines, including correction of hypovolemia; and (3) use of other bagging techniques such as increasing the F_{IO_2}, increasing the rate, using a PEEP or increasing the PEEP, and carefully increasing peak pressure (these techniques create increased risk of complications).

(Mason TN: A hand ventilation technique for infants. MCN 7(6):367, November/December 1982. Copyright © 1982, American Journal of Nursing Company.)

curate. If one side has diminished breath sounds, the tube is probably placed too far. An x-ray film will confirm placement, which really cannot be done during a delivery area resuscitation. After insertion is accomplished, the infant is mechanically ventilated by rapid bagging with 100% oxygen. It is important to secure the tube somewhat before transporting the infant from the delivery area. Application of tincture of benzoin to the upper lip and cheeks followed by adhesive strips helps stabilize the tube until it can be more permanently secured for long-term care (Fig. 44-13).[31]

CIRCULATION

While other resuscitative measures are being accomplished, the pulse should be monitored and cardiac compression performed in the event of cardiac arrest. Two fingers should be placed in the middle of the sternum and compressed ½ to 1 in at a rate of 100 to 120 per minute. The hand-encircling method can also be used.

It is imperative to maintain the cardiac massage and the ventilation. This can be accomplished by alternating the two maneuvers. A 5:1 ratio of cardiac massage to assisted ventilation of 100% oxygen should be used. The two procedures must not be performed simultaneously because the pressure applied during cardiac massage may rupture a lung that has just been inflated by the ventilation. If the procedure is effective, the femoral or brachial artery pulses are palpable in synchrony with depression of the sternum. The procedure is to be discontinued periodically to determine the presence of spontaneous cardiac activity. When this occurs, cardiac compression may be discontinued.

MEDICATIONS

Medications may be required in a resuscitative effort (Table 44-5). Medications are not the primary emphasis in a resuscitative effort, but their indications and usual dosages should be reviewed.

ENVIRONMENT

Infants who are at risk for cold stress are low birth weight, SGA, preterm, or asphyxiated. These infants are at risk owing to the lack of fat deposits and less brown fat available for generation of heat. Less subcutaneous fat is available for heat conservation. Brown fat thermogenesis is decreased in the asphyxiated infant who has been hypoxic. Precautions must be taken to observe these infants closely to prevent any further environmental insult. Once other resuscitative measures have been accomplished—airway, breathing, circulation, and drugs—the infant's axillary temperature should be taken. Controlled heat and slow rewarming are recommended, with continuous temperature monitoring by temperature probe taped to the abdomen. The infant with cold stress may exhibit RDS symptoms of tachypnea, flaring, grunting, and retractions. These symptoms disappear as the temperature returns to normal.[31]

Once the infant is supported and stabilized, immediate transport to the NICU is recommended, whether in-house or to a regional center. Parents should be informed of all events and permitted to see their infant as soon as possible.

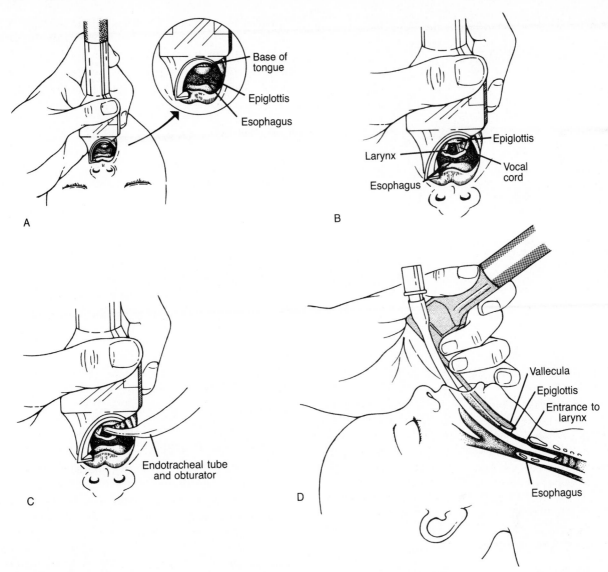

■ *Figure 44–12*

Technique of endotracheal intubation. (A and B) The Miller blade should be inserted near the midline and moved to the left side of the mouth, gently deflecting the tongue. As it is advanced, the base of the tongue and epiglottis are visualized. (C and D) The blade should be advanced in the same plane of movement into the vallecula (see D); as the blade is gently raised, the epiglottis swings anteriorly, revealing the opening of the larynx. If secretions or meconium is noted, gentle suctioning should be done before insertion of the endotracheal tube. On certain occasions when the epiglottis is not adequately raised, the blade tip may be placed posterior to the epiglottis, which can then be gently raised to expose the vocal cords. The endotracheal tube is advanced from the right corner of the mouth and inserted while maintaining direct visualization. The laryngoscope blade is then carefully withdrawn while the position of the tube is maintained by the right hand on the infant's face. Note the tip of the blade in the vallecula.

Transport of the Infant at Risk

Recent advances and specialization in the care of the neonate have resulted in the regionalization of services for the high-risk neonate.

Transport is accomplished when sick infants are identified and admitted to a tertiary-care center. In some cases, in utero transport can be carried out when the birth of a critically ill neonate is anticipated. Unfortu-nately, it is not always possible to transport the mother, so most centers have a transport team available to ac-company the neonate from the referral hospital to the center. Transportation is accomplished by ground or air ambulance. The transport team usually consists of a registered nurse or physician and a registered respiratory therapist. General indications for neonatal transport and the equipment required are listed in the box.

It is essential that the parents have the opportunity

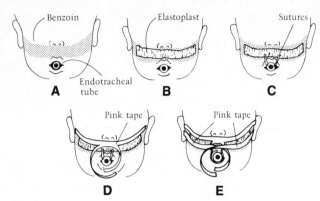

■ *Figure 44–13*
Technique for securing an orotracheal tube. (Redrawn from Gregory GA: Respiratory care of newborn infants. Pediatr Clin North Am 19:317, 1972)

to see the infant before the transport team departs. It is helpful for the parents to have a picture of the infant to keep with them.

Neonatal Intensive Care Unit

NICUs, developed to provide highly skilled nursing and medical care to the high-risk neonate, require extensive sophisticated equipment (Fig. 44-14). The first of such types of nurseries emerged in the mid-1960s in the United States. Nurses provide 24-hour care, with one

---

Neonatal Transport

General neonatal indications for transport:
• Low birth weight or preterm
• Respiratory assistance needed
• High acuity level
• Life-threatening surgery
• Seizures
• Persistent fetal circulation

Equipment required:

Battery-operated monitors for vital signs, blood pressure

Transcutaneous oxygen monitor

Suction equipment

Intravenous pump, equipment

Respirator

Blood-drawing equipment

Resuscitation equipment

Transport equipment should be checked every shift*

* For details, see OGN Nursing Practice Resource, Maternal-Neonatal Transport, No. 8, June 1983.

---

nurse for every one or two critically ill neonates. With the emphasis now on the development of the whole infant and family, sole physical care is obsolete. Nurseries are designed with infant stimulation in mind as well as a comfortable setting for the families involved.

Continuing Management

PROVIDING A NEUTRAL THERMAL ENVIRONMENT

A neutral thermal environment keeps the infant's metabolic rate and oxygen consumption at a minimum and temperature within normal range. Skin temperature should be maintained between 36.1 and 36.7°C (96.8–97.8°F). Axillary temperature should be kept at or about 36.7°C (97.8°F). Infants of low birth weight have more difficulty maintaining a normal temperature owing to a decrease in subcutaneous fat; a small body mass in relation to a larger surface area; thin, fragile skin; and an extended-limbs posture.[33]

Temperature of the neonate may be assessed by one or several of the following means:

• Probe taped to skin
• Axillary temperature
• Anal (core) temperature

Environmental temperature should be assessed frequently in conjunction with the infant's temperature.

Several types of equipment may be used for the provision of heat in the neonate. The standard isolette does not provide as much accessibility as the overhead warmer. Isolettes can provide humidity and isolation (Fig. 44-15). The isolette can be flooded with oxygen but only to a maximum of about 40%. The temperature of the isolette can be adapted by a servocontrol mechanism and Thermistor probe taped to the skin.

Infants in isolettes gain heat by convection but lose heat by evaporation, conduction, and radiation. When portholes are opened, cooler nursery air is sucked in and warm air escapes, increasing convective loss. Cuffs around the portholes can help with this problem. Dressing the infant without interfering with assessment and apparatus helps to protect the infant against heat loss.[34]

The radiant overhead warmer provides improved visibility and accessibility to the neonate (Fig. 44-16). A temperature probe unit adjusts the heat flow in accordance with the infant's skin temperature. One significant disadvantage of the radiant warmer is insensible water loss. Insensible water loss represents the water that is lost from the lungs and skin through the mechanisms of convection and evaporation. The use of plastic sheeting has been found most effective in reducing insensible water loss. The use of heat shields may interfere

TABLE 44-5. DRUGS USED IN THE RESUSCITATION OF INFANTS AND CHILDREN

Agent*	How Supplied	Recommended Dose†	Uses
Atropine sulfate	0.4 mg/ml ampule	IV 0.01–0.05 mg/kg/dose	To reverse or prevent the effects of the vagus nerve on the heart, tracheobronchial tree, and mucous membranes
Calcium	Calcium gluconate, a 10% solution containing 100 mg Ca gluconate/ml (9.7 mg elemental calcium/ml)	100 mg/kg day (1–2 ml/kg/day) or 0.1–0.2 ml/kg 1 dose IV slowly, with heart rate monitored for bradycardia	Calcium is a potent stimulant of cardiac contractile force, used to increase cardiac output
	Calcium chloride, a 10% solution containing 100 mg Ca chloride/ml (27.2 mg elemental calcium/ml)	10 mg/kg (0.1 ml/kg) IV slowly, with the same precautions as for gluconate. May repeat every 3–5 min to maximum dose of 2 ml/kg	
Dextrose (50%)	50-ml ampules, vials	1 ml/kg initially. May be repeated	Used to correct hypoglycemia; stimulates cardiac contractile force
Dopamine	200 mg in 5 ml	Dilute 100 mg in 100 ml normal saline to produce solution of 1 mg/ml. Give 5–10 μg/kg/min initially, titrate up to 50 μg/kg/min	Used as a support for failing circulation
Epinephrine (Adrenalin)	1:1000 solution	Dilute to 1 mg/10 ml by adding 1 ml of 1:1000 epinephrine to 9 ml of normal saline. Give 0.1 ml of this solution/kg body weight (0.01 mg/kg)	A potent stimulant of cardiac contractile force and excitation; valuable for initiating contraction in the arrested heart
Isoproterenol	0.2 mg/ml 1.0 mg/5 ml	Dilute 1 mg in 100 ml normal saline to produce solution of 10 μg/ml, or 1 mg in 250 ml normal saline to produce solution of 4 μg/ml. Give 0.05–0.5 μg/kg/min, IV	Cardiac stimulant that increases cardiac output; used to maintain blood pressure in shock; smooth muscle relaxant used for severe bronchospasm
Lidocaine	1% solution (10 mg/ml)	0.5–1 mg/kg slowly IV every 20 min‡	Used to decrease ventricular irritability, maintain a normal rhythm following defibrillation, and increase the chances of successful defibrillation
Sodium bicarbonate	Ampules of 50 mEq/50 ml or 10 mEq/10 ml	2–5 mEq/kg slowly IV. May repeat at 5–10 min intervals, if needed	Used to correct acidosis, which is always associated with inadequate circulation and reduced peripheral perfusion occurring during an arrest

Defibrillation: 2–5 watt-sec/kg initially

* Most emergency drugs are toxic. Review the package insert for complete information about dosage and side effects, toxicities, containdications, and need for special monitoring.
  † Consult package insert for information about administration and maximum doses.
  ‡ Doses not definitely established for infants and children.
  (Waechter EH, Phillips J, Holaday B: Nursing Care of Children, 16th ed. Philadelphia, JB Lippincott, 1985.)

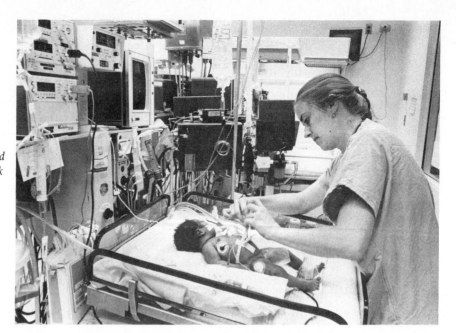

■ *Figure 44-14*
Sophisticated equipment and highly skilled nursing and medical care are the hallmark of the NICU. (Courtesy of The Children's Hospital of Philadelphia)

with radiant heat transfer and impede the servocontrol function.[33]

It is impossible to combat all drafts that might occur. The use of stockinette caps may not be as effective in preventing heat loss in radiant warmers. One study demonstrated that infants wearing a stockinette head covering did not maintain heat as well as infants wearing insulated bonnets or no head covering at all.[35]

All equipment used must be checked thoroughly and frequently for correct functioning. Temperature probes used must be kept taped on the skin. Units housing infants should be kept away from drafts.

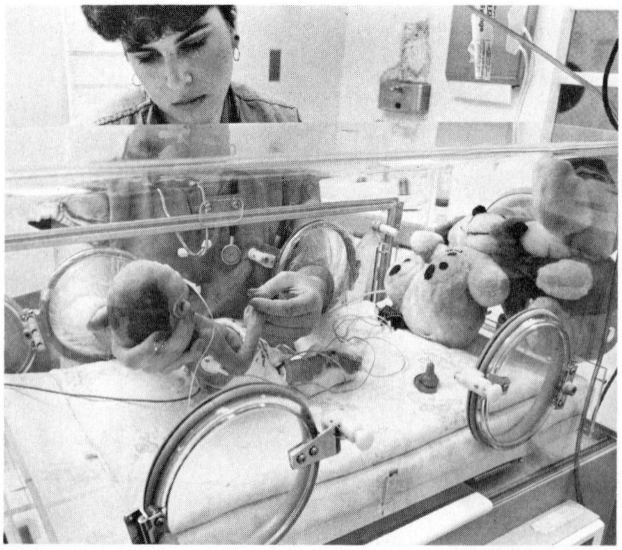

All those caring for infants should always apply warm hands, warm surfaces, warmed oxygen. All procedures should be carried out in a warm area or under a radiant heat source.

Nurses should observe infants for signs of cold stress, such as tachypnea, apneic spells, color changes, hypoglycemia, and metabolic acidosis.

If infants do become chilled, they should be warmed slowly over a period of hours to avoid apnea. The heating unit's desired temperature should be increased very gradually until the infant's temperature is stable. The infant may require a calorie source to correct hypoglycemia and/or to stabilize blood gases.

As the infants' condition stabilizes, they can be weaned slowly from an isolette. Initially, they are dressed in a shirt and diaper as the isolette's temperature is gradually lowered. If this is successful, the portholes are opened, the heat is turned off, and the infants eventually are transferred to an open crib.

MAINTAINING SKIN INTEGRITY

The skin functions as a barrier against infection, helps regulate body temperature, stores fats, discharges electrolytes and water, and protects organs.

The preterm's skin is particularly fragile and susceptible to trauma and irritation. The outside layer of the epidermis, the stratum corneum, becomes thicker as maturation occurs. Skin permeability decreases with increasing gestational age. Finally, bonds between the layers of epidermis and dermis strengthen with increasing gestational age.[36]

■ *Figure 44-15*
Isolette. Access to the neonate is provided through hand holes so that the carefully controlled environment will not be disturbed. (Courtesy of The Children's Hospital of Philadelphia)

their application. Bathing frequency should be decreased to one to two times a week to maintain the acid mantle of the skin as a barrier to infection.

PREVENTING INFECTION

The nurse is responsible for minimizing the neonate's exposure to invasive microorganisms. The high-risk infant is at risk for infection. The preterm infant is vulnerable as a consequence of its immature immunologic state, as described previously. Many neonates require invasive procedures and diagnostic tests that can serve as routes for organisms.

Handwashing and Dress Code. All caregivers, parents, and visitors who come into contact with the high-risk neonate must be instructed in and follow the handwashing procedure required by the NICU. In addition, the nursery dress codes, as described in detail in Chapter 30, must be adhered to. Refer to Chapter 30 for guidelines for staff members' health status.

Universal precautions are required in the care of the high-risk neonate.

Equipment. Isolettes and radiant warmers should be changed weekly. Intravenous tubing and solutions should be changed using aseptic technique according to agency policy. Other equipment used must be cleaned according to policy.

RESPIRATORY CARE

Assessment. Observation of the preterm infant provides numerous clues as to respiratory status.

Respirations should be counted for a full minute, because irregularity is common (Fig. 44–17). Instances of periodic breathing are to be expected; however, apnea may be of a more pathologic nature. The usual respiratory rate ranges from 40 to 60 breaths per minute.

The infant's color should be generally pink. In the first few hours after birth, acrocyanosis may occur owing to vasomotor instability.

Respiratory movements should be symmetrical. The abdomen can be seen rising and falling as breaths are inspired and expired. Respiratory distress is indicated by tachypnea, retractions, grunting, nasal flaring, cyanosis, pallor, hypotonia, and bradycardia.

Additional data regarding respiratory status are provided by auscultation to ascertain abnormal breath sounds and indications of airway obstructions. Accurate identification of abnormal breath sounds requires considerable practice and skill on the part of the nurse. The infant's chest size requires the use of a stethoscope with a small diaphragm so that it picks up more local sounds than those transmitted across the small chest. Breath sounds should be auscultated bilaterally, moving the

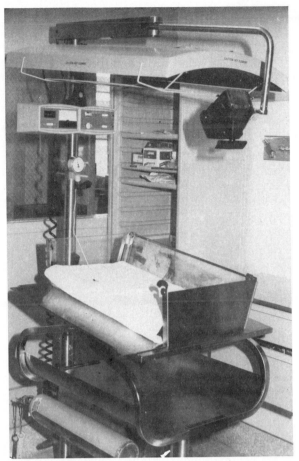

■ *Figure 44–16*
The radiant overhead warmer. Although visibility and accessibility are provided with the radiant warmer, a problem is insensible water loss.

The use of tape is necessary to secure monitor leads and other pieces of equipment used in the NICU. The choice of tape deserves due consideration, as well as the amount and placement. Skin blankets with porous adhesive backing, such a HolliHesive and Stomahesive, have been used with success in some neonatal units. This material is pliable and easy to remove, and it can be cut into various shapes. Tape can then be placed on top of the "skin blanket" without directly touching the skin.[36] One study demonstrated that this type of pectin-based barrier proved invaluable because it produced less skin irritation and was effective in securing devices.[37]

Problems are encountered with electrodes, which must be in direct skin contact. Electrodes can be wrapped on with Kling bandage. The use of limb electrodes is a possibility.

OpSite, when used for a dressing for burns and other skin problems, is very useful owing to its transparent and waterproof nature.

The preterm infant's skin is extremely permeable to topical ointments, so great care should be taken with

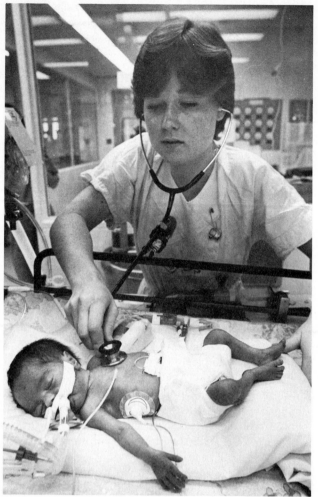

■ *Figure 44–17*
Respirations are assessed by the nurse for a full minute. The usual rate ranges from 40 to 60 breaths per minute. (Courtesy of The Children's Hospital of Philadephia)

samples analyzed to titrate oxygen requirements and ventilatory settings.

Arterial blood is sampled intermittently by arterial puncture or from an indwelling arterial catheter. Intermittent arterial sticks are painful, and test results are altered by crying and breath holding. The use of an umbilical arterial line provides ready access for withdrawing frequent and accurate blood gas samples (Fig. 44-18). Placement of the umbilical line is a sterile procedure; confirmation is made by radiograph. Complications of arterial lines include hemorrhage, ischemic damage to organs, and thrombus formation. The nurse must be alert to blanching or cyanosis of one or both extremities, necessitating removal of the catheter.

Percutaneous arterial placement is an alternative to the umbilical line. Sites of placement are the radial, dorsalis pedis, temporal, or posttibial arteries. Extremities must be assessed for adequate circulation.[38]

Capillary blood samples have been found to correlate closely with arterial blood, especially in infants older than 24 hours (Table 44-6). The extremity must be warmed prior to collection of sample for adequate capillary arterial flow. The site should be cleaned with alcohol and dried. Any alcohol residue can cause hemolysis. The first drop obtained after puncture should be discarded because it contains more interstitial fluid than subsequent blood flow.

NONINVASIVE MONITORING. Transcutaneous oxygen tension (TcPo$_2$) monitoring is noninvasive and pro-

stethoscope down the chest along the midaxillary line both laterally and anteriorly.[19] Abnormal or diminished breath sounds should be noted. Infants may present with rales, rhonchi, or decreased breath sounds in various disease states. Breath sounds should be equal bilaterally.

On auscultation of the chest, the heart sounds are assessed by counting the rate and describing the quality and location of the point of maximal impulse (PMI). Murmurs may be noted as well as displacement of the PMI. The PMI is usually located in the fourth intercostal space to the left of the sternum in the midclavicular line. A displacement of the PMI may be indicative of pneumothorax.

Monitoring of Blood Gas Status.

INVASIVE MONITORING. Those infants experiencing respiratory distress and thus requiring additional oxygen or ventilatory support must have frequent blood gas

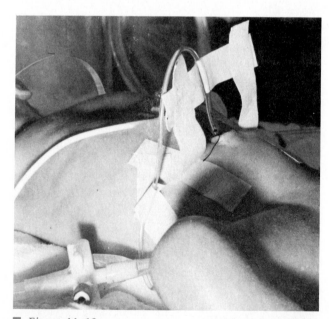

■ *Figure 44–18*
An umbilical artery catheter is used to monitor blood pressure. This is a sterile procedure. A bridge is taped over the catheter to secure it. (Symansky MR, Fox HA: Umbilical vessel catheterization: Indications, management, and evaluation of the technique. J Pediatr 80:820, 1972)

TABLE 44-6. NORMAL VALUES FOR BLOOD GAS PARAMETERS

Parameter	Arterial	Capillary
pH	7.35–7.45	7.35–7.44
PCO_2	35–45 mm Hg	35–45 mm Hg
PO_2	50–80 mm Hg	40–50 mm Hg
HCO_3	20–26 mEq/L	20–26 mEq/L
Base excess	+4 to −4 mEq/L	+4 to −4 mEq/L

(Clancy GT: Blood gas monitoring and management of neonates with respiratory distress. J Perinat Neonat Nurs 1(1):77, 1987.)

vides continuous monitoring of PO_2 readings. The monitoring of continuous status is helpful to observe the neonate's response to nursing interventions such as weighing, nasogastric feedings, suctioning, and postural drainage. One nursing research study demonstrated significant decrease in $TcPO_2$ during suctioning and repositioning but not during heelstick procedures.[39] Another study showed a modest increase in $TcPO_2$ and heart rate during nonnutritive sucking in preterm infants of less than 33 weeks' gestation and weighing less than 1500 g.[40] Placement of the electrode requires a space with good capillary blood flow and little fat. The electrode should not be placed on a bony prominence. Commonly used sites are the upper chest, abdomen, and inner thigh. The site should be changed and the electrode recalibrated minimally every 4 hours.[19] Some reports of skin erosion beneath the electrode make diligent assessment of skin a vital task.

Pulse oximetry is the newest noninvasive method of oxygen monitoring, using an infrared light source to determine the amount of saturated oxygen in tissues and read out the patient's pulse rate. The probe can be left in place indefinitely, as the sensor is wrapped around an extremity, that is, a finger or toe. Significant complications have not been reported; however, oximeters are very sensitive to patient movement and work optimally when the patient is resting quietly or sleeping. Because pulse oximetry indicates hemoglobin saturation and not arterial oxygen tension, once the hemoglobin saturation reaches 90% to 95%, the arterial oxygen tension must be checked. Pulse oximetry enables the nurse to position the neonate and perform procedures with optimal oxygenation results.[41]

Administration of Oxygen and Ventilatory Support.

Flooding of the isolette with oxygen presents problems because the maximum concentration able to be maintained is probably no more than 30% to 40%. Frequent opening of the portholes makes maintaining a constant flow impossible.

When other ventilator support is not necessary, administration of oxygen by hood is an option (Fig. 44-19). An oxygen analyzer must be kept in the hood to measure the percent of oxygen administered. Oxygen should be warm and kept at a stable temperature. The neonate should be suctioned periodically to maintain the open airway. Blood gases should be monitored every 4 hours and 10 to 20 minutes following each change in fraction of inspired oxygen (fIO_2).

Continuous positive airway pressure results from a machine applying pressure throughout the lungs of the neonate. This type of pressure helps to keep the alveoli open, thus decreasing the work of breathing and oxygen requirements. Infants with RDS benefit the most from CPAP, because atelectasis is a common complication. The use of CPAP is indicated for a paO_2 of less than 50 mm Hg in the presence of 60% oxygen.[19]

CPAP pressure is measured in centimeters of H_2O. The initial amount delivered is usually 4 to 6 cm H_2O, and this pressure is slowly increased until oxygenation is sufficient as measured by blood gas readings. CPAP is usually delivered by nasal prongs or endotracheal intubation (Fig. 44-20).

The neonate on nasal CPAP must have frequent nares care. Nasal prongs need to be removed periodically and cleaned with sterile water and cotton-tipped applicators. The nasopharynx and oropharynx should be suctioned with a bulb syringe. Nasal prongs must be anchored securely at all times. If the prongs are too loose, effective therapy will not be achieved; if they are too tight, erosion of the nasal membranes may occur. The infant may require an orogastric tube to prevent abdominal distension. Sucking on a pacifier may promote ventilation through the nose.[42]

Conventional Mechanical Ventilation. In the event of apnea or inability to maintain adequate oxygenation with CPAP, endotracheal intubation and positive-pressure ventilation may be essential for respiratory assistance. paO_2 of less than 50 mm Hg, $paCO_2$ of greater than 60, and pH of less than 7.25 in 100% oxygen with CPAP indicate that respiratory assistance is required. Other indicators are apnea, severe retractions, respiratory rate over 80, and cyanosis.[43]

In the preterm infant with RDS, the ideal paO_2 should be maintained between 50 and 75 mm Hg to avoid complications of retinopathy of prematurity and bronchopulmonary dysplasia.

Several kinds of positive-pressure ventilators are available (Table 44-7). The nurse must become intimately familiar with the particular machine used in the unit as well as the implications of the various settings. Various parameters that may be altered to provide maximal assistance for each individual patient are peak inspiratory pressure, respiratory rate, inspiratory:expiratory ratio, PEEP, and oxygen flow rate delivered (FIO_2).

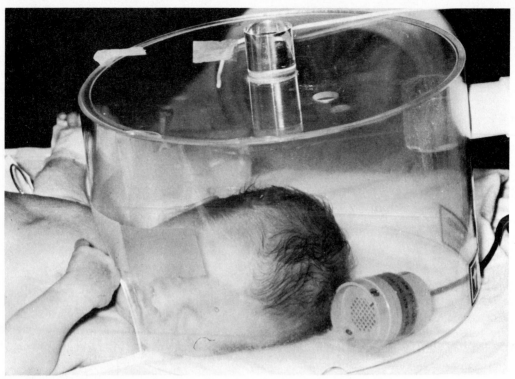

■ *Figure 44–19*
Oxygen hood for administration of controlled oxygen concentration. Note the temperature probe passing through the lid and the sensor of oxygen analyzer next to infant's face. (Avery GB: Neonatology: Pathophysiology and Management of the Newborn, 3rd ed. Philadelphia, JB Lippincott, 1987)

It is important once the endotracheal tube is placed for the infant to be bagged to estimate ventilator settings before placing the infant on the ventilator itself.

Endotracheal Tube. Selection of the tube size is based on the infant's weight, gestational age, and unit protocol. The nurse is responsible for assessment of placement. Auscultation of the lungs should reveal equality of breath sounds. Radiography will confirm placement.[34]

Securing of the tube is essential for anticipated long-term therapy.

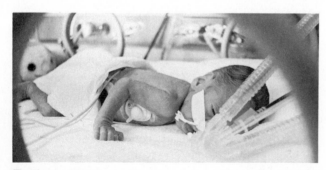

■ *Figure 44–20*
Nasal continuous positive airway pressure (CPAP). (Courtesy of The Children's Hospital of Philadelphia)

Once the infant is placed on the respirator, ventilator settings and alarms must be checked frequently. Blood gases must be checked at least every 4 hours and 10 to 20 minutes past a change in ventilator settings.

Suctioning is essential to keep the airway open. The suction catheter size can be estimated by multiplying the endotracheal tube size by two. The next size suction catheter above this size should pass into the tube. Negative effects of suctioning include hypoxemia; changes in heart rate, blood pressure, and intracranial pressure; and pneumothoraces. Other possible long-term effects include mucosal trauma and sepsis. Negative effects can be minimized by preoxygenation with hyperventilation or continuous oxygen administration, limiting the depth of catheter insertion to just beyond the distance of the tube, use of sedation, and minimal infant handling.[44]

Chest physical therapy may be necessary to assist in the mobilization of secretions (Fig. 44-21). Various devices, such as padded nipples and electric toothbrushes, may be used for percussion and vibration techniques.[45]

High-Frequency Ventilation. To attempt to reduce the effects of barotrauma or the progression of injury in infants with advanced lung disease, a new method of high-frequency ventilation has been developed. High-

TABLE 44-7. COMMONLY USED POSITIVE-PRESSURE VENTILATORS

Volume Type

Bournes LS 104–150 (Bournes Medical Systems, Riverside, CA)

Servo 900B (Siemens Corporation, Union, NJ)

Pressure Type

Time Cycled

Bournes BP 200 (Bournes Medical Systems, Riverside, CA)

Bear BP 2001 (Bear Intermed, Riverside, CA)

Healthdyne 100 (Healthdyne, Inc., Marietta, GA)

Sechrist IV-100 (Sechrist Industries, Inc., Anaheim, CA)

Pressure Cycled

Baby Bird II (Bird Corporation, Palm Springs, CA)

Cavitron PV-10 (Healthdyne, Inc., Marietta, GA)

(Spitzer AR, Fox WW: Use and abuse of mechanical ventilators. In Stern L (ed): Hyaline Membrane Disease: Pathogenesis and Pathophysiology. Orlando, Grune & Stratton, 1984.)

frequency ventilation may be a future alternative to conventional ventilation methods for infants with severe RDS and bronchopulmonary dysplasia.

Extracorporeal Membrane Oxygenator (ECMO). ECMO is a method of establishing a pulmonary bypass circuit, permitting the exchange of gases to occur outside of the lung in the machine. This therapy allows the lung to rest and has been used in infants with severe RDS, meconium aspiration syndrome, and persistent pulmonary hypertension.

Muscle Paralysis. Skeletal muscle paralysis may be required to achieve normal muscle tone in the ventilated infant. Pancuronium (Pavulon) may be administered to block transmission of acetylcholine across the neuromuscular synapse. Because painful stimuli are still perceived, morphine sulfate may be required to promote comfort.

NUTRITIONAL SUPPORT

Fluid Therapy. Because preterm infants are particularly susceptible to water losses due to the high surface:body mass ratio, permeable skin, radiant warmers, phototherapy, increase in urine volume, and abnormal fluid losses due to diarrhea, they require adequate fluid intake at all times. Further, most preterm infants initially are too critically ill to tolerate enteral feedings. Several routes of parenteral fluid administration may be used.

Peripheral or central catheters may be used for the administration of fluids. When administration of fluids is supplemented or considered temporary, peripheral lines may be the optimum route. Peripheral lines may be used in scalp veins or extremities. Teflon angiocaths are preferred to steel scalp vein needles because the line can be maintained longer with less risk of infiltration. The nurse inserts the device, using aseptic technique, and carefully secures it, allowing for the opportunity to observe the site for signs of infiltration. Intravenous fluids should be administered at the prescribed rate using infusion pumps, minidrip, and a fluid reservoir such as a drip controlled chamber or burette. The extremity may need to be restrained to maintain the line. The site and extremity need to be assessed frequently for signs of infiltration and circulatory adequacy.

If long-term therapy is anticipated, especially with TPN, placement of a central line into the internal and external jugular is warranted. The catheter is threaded into the superior vena cava. This placement facilitates the use of hyperosmolar solutions and high-dextrose solutions such as TPN.

Determination of fluid requirements can be estimated by taking into account daily weights, fluid intake and output, and urine specific gravity. Smaller infants may require 180 to 200 ml/kg/day, with initial restrictions of 60 to 75 ml/kg/day. High fluid intake has been associated with patent ductus arteriosus, bronchopulmonary dysplasia, and NEC.[46] Certain criteria may be assessed by the nurse to ensure fluid balance (Table 44-8).

Accurate assessment of intake and output is essential. All gains and losses must be accounted for, such as catheter flushes. The prescribed amount of intravenous fluid must be administered per hour.

Infants should be observed for electrolyte imbal-

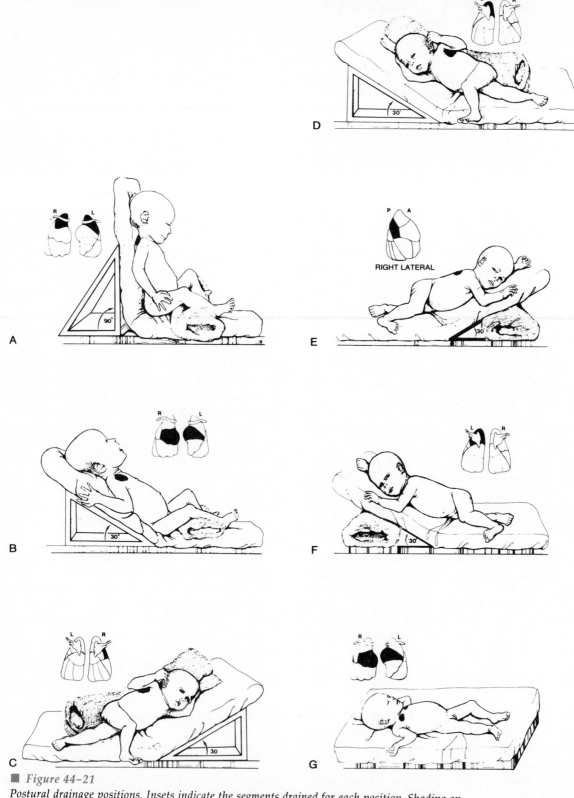

■ *Figure 44–21*

Postural drainage positions. Insets indicate the segments drained for each position. Shading on the infant indicates the area for chest percussion and vibrations. The dependent-head position should be used with caution. (Fletcher MA, MacDonald M, Avery G: Atlas of Procedures in Neonatology. Philadelphia, JB Lippincott, 1983)

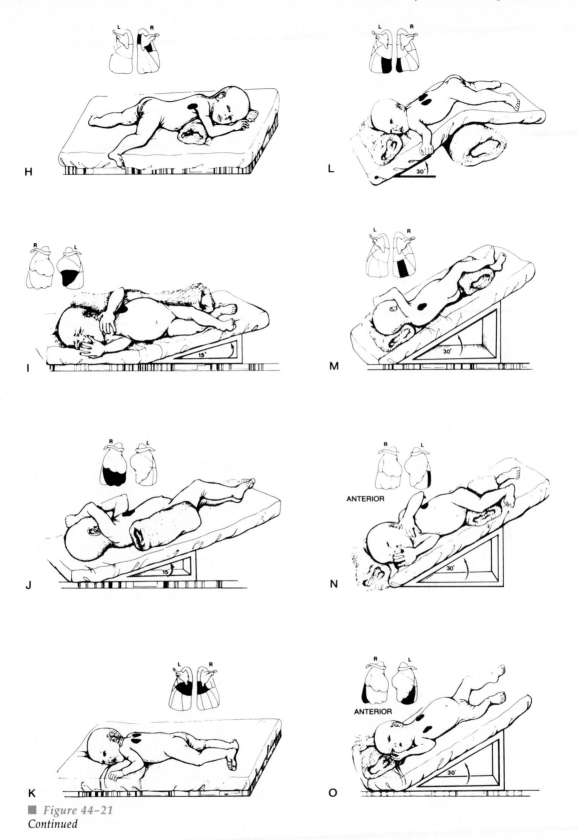

■ *Figure 44–21*
Continued

ances. Frequent monitoring of serum and urine electrolytes is an ongoing concern.

Types of Feeding. Formulas especially composed for the preterm infant are available; such formulas use the type of proteins similar to that of human milk. There is controversy regarding the adequacy of breast milk for promotion of growth in the preterm versus cow's milk formulas. The advantages of breast milk are well known, especially the immunologic ones. Disadvantages remain

TABLE 44-8. OBSERVATIONS FOR HYDRATION STATUS

Parameter	Fluid Overload	Dehydration
Urine volume	Often increased (>3–5 cc/kg/h)	<0.5 cc/kg/h
Urine specific gravity	<1.005	>1.015
Skin	Edema; dependent or pitting	Dry mucous membranes; poor turgor
Eyes	Orbital edema	Sunken eyes
Fontanelles	May be bulging	Depressed
Liver size	Increased (a sign of heart failure)	—
Respiratory tract	Thin secretions, rales, increased P_{CO_2}, increased F_{IO_2}*	Thick endotracheal secretions
Weight	2–3% above expected weight *or* gain 2% of previous day's weight	>3–4% below expected weight or loss 3–4% of previous day's weight

Fluid imbalance is a syndrome that affects all body tissues. If fluid imbalance is present, more than one sign will be present on exam.

* P_{CO_2}, carbon dioxide pressure; F_{IO_2}, fractional inspired oxygen.

(Harkavy KL: Fluids, electrolytes, and nutrition for neonates. In Daze AM, Scanlon JW: Neonatal Nursing, p 49. Baltimore, University Park Press, 1985.)

regarding the storage of breast milk. Freezing of breast milk destroys the antibodies. Although antibodies are preserved for human milk stored at 4°C, dangers also remain of contamination by bacteria. A new approach to adapt breast milk for use by the preterm is commercial breast milk additives.

Feeding Schedule. Very-low-birth-weight infants may require hourly or every 2- to 3-hour feedings. Volumes are begun with small amounts, and increases are gradually introduced.

Feeding Techniques.

GAVAGE FEEDING. Feeding by gavage, whether intermittent or continuous, is a common means of feeding infants who cannot tolerate oral feedings for a period of time and whose gastrointestinal tract is intact. Infants who may require this feeding assistance include those of less than 32 weeks' gestation and those with central nervous system depression and poor sucking reflexes. Appropriate-for-gestational-age infants who become very tired may require gavage to avoid needless energy expenditure and loss of calories.

For intermittent gavage feeding, a 5 Fr or 8 Fr feeding tube is chosen according to the infant's size and tolerance. Vagal stimulation with subsequent bradycardia may be a problem as the tube is introduced. The tube is measured from the tip of the nose or mouth to the tip of the earlobe, ending at the tip of the xiphoid process (Fig. 44-22).

Another method is to measure from nose or mouth to earlobe and then to a point midway between the termination of the xiphoid process and the umbilicus. One study showed a high error rate in measurement and correct tube placement in the preterm infant.[47] The tube is then marked at the point of measurement, ensuring that it will be inserted only to that point.

Infants are positioned either on their back or on their side with their head elevated. They may need to be restrained in a mummy restraint or held during the procedure.

After the tube is lubricated with sterile water, the infant's head is held still with one hand and the tube is inserted up to the mark with the other hand. Tubes may be inserted through the mouth or the nares. Nose insertion may obstruct the passage of a nose breather and irritate the nasal mucosa (Fig. 44-23).

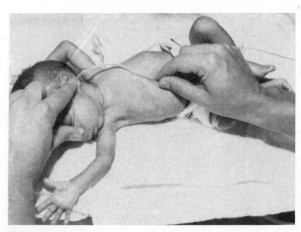

■ *Figure 44–22*

Measurement for gavage feeding.

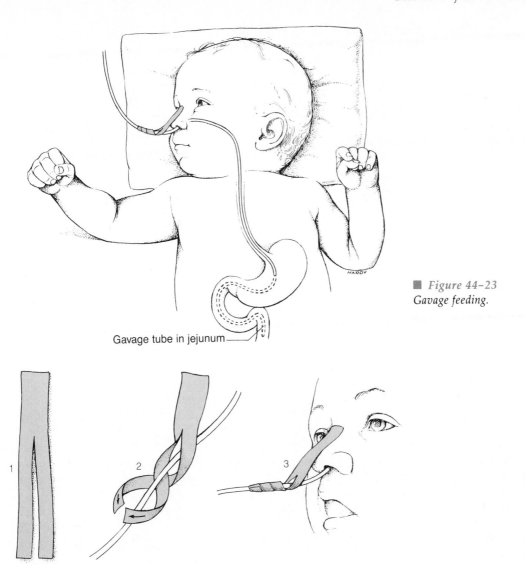

■ *Figure 44–23*
Gavage feeding.

Gavage tube in jejunum

Correct placement of the feeding tube may be checked by aspiration of the gastric residuum and injection of air while listening with the stethoscope. Gastric residual should be measured and returned to the stomach unless otherwise ordered. The amount of residual may be subtracted from the ordered amount of feeding. Increasing amounts of residual, abdominal distension, or absent bowel sounds should be documented and reported. If cyanosis, severe gagging, or coughing ensues, the tube may be misplaced and should be removed and reinserted properly.

On ascertaining correct placement, the syringe is separated from the tube. The plunger is then removed from the barrel, and the barrel is reconnected to the tube. The desired amount of formula is poured into the syringe. The syringe is elevated 6 to 8 in over the infant's head, and the feeding is allowed to flow in by gravity.

When the formula is absorbed, the tube is rinsed with 2 to 3 ml of sterile water. The tube is folded over onto itself and removed with one smooth motion.

If infants could not be held during the feeding, this is an appropriate time to hold them. Some infants enjoy sucking on a pacifier during the feeding. Sucking helps them practice the reflex and associate it with a full stomach.

After feeding, infants should be positioned on their right side or their abdomen with the head slightly elevated to facilitate digestion.

Continuous gavage feedings by nasogastric tube may minimize problems of distension and aspiration. While a nasogastric tube is left securely taped in place, formula is pumped in by continuous drip. The tube may be clamped or removed when each feeding is complete. Residual as well as abdominal circumferences are checked frequently.

TRANSPYLORIC FEEDINGS. Continuous infusions by the transpyloric route represent alternative methods of nutritional support. The tube is passed into the stomach, and placement is checked by x-ray film when a gastric residual pH of 7 is obtained. Continuous infusion, advancing from glucose water to the infant's full fluid and caloric requirement, may be given. Hypertonic formulas should not be introduced directly into the small intestine. Perforations have been reported, because polyvinyl or polyethylene catheters become stiff after a week or so of continuous use. Oral feedings should be begun as soon as the infant's condition permits.[48]

The nurse needs to assess the infant for signs of abdominal distention by inspection and measurement of abdominal girth. Tubing is changed routinely to prevent bacterial growth. Residual is also checked and reported as per agency policy. A stool guaiac test needs to be performed to see that the infant is tolerating the feedings. Infants may need some form of restraint so that the tube will not be pulled out. Nonnutritive sucking may be enjoyed by the infant.[49]

ORAL FEEDING. Behaviors indicating that the infant may be ready to advance to oral feeding include a strong, vigorous suck, coordination of sucking and swallowing, sucking in response to the gavage tube, and wakefulness before feedings. The infant may be challenged with feedings slowly. Oral feedings could begin with once a day, then once every 8 hours, then every other feeding, and so on, as tolerated. If the infant requires more than 30 minutes to finish the feeding, the next feeding should be a gavage feeding.

If the infant is expending too much energy on the work of feeding, the result could be a weight loss instead of steady gain. Special "preemie" soft nipples are available to facilitate the sucking process. The nurse performs a thorough abdominal assessment to assess the infant's tolerance to the feeding challenge. See Chapter 30 for further details regarding oral nutrition for the neonate. See Chapter 30 for further technical details.

BREASTFEEDING. Chapter 30 discusses breastfeeding of the normal newborn at length.

Traditional methods of establishing breastfeeding in the preterm infant have begun with the mother expressing milk until the infant is at least 34 to 35 weeks' gestation. Bottle feedings are then introduced. When the infant has been taking the desired amount without distress, breastfeeding is permitted. Often not enough time has elapsed from the onset of breastfeeding to discharge for the mother to feel comfortable with breastfeeding the small neonate.

Some data suggest that stable preterm infants can breast feed prior to 34 weeks and weighing less than 1500 g. Infants can be monitored in a noninvasive manner for fatigue and weighed before and after feeding to estimate intake. Breastfeeding the low-birth-weight infant is an area worthy of ongoing nursing research.[50]

TOTAL PARENTERAL NUTRITION. TPN, also known as *hyperalimentation*, is an aseptically prepared hypertonic solution composed of protein, carbohydrates, electrolytes, vitamins, and minerals (Table 44-9).

In cases in which oral feedings must be delayed for a long time, TPN has been able to provide adequate

TABLE 44-9. DAILY REQUIREMENTS OF TOTAL PARENTERAL NUTRITION

Protein	2.5–3.5 g/kg
Fat emulsion	2–4 g/kg
Calories	90–110 kcal/kg
H_2O	125–150 ml/kg or as needed
Na	3–4 mEq/kg
K	2–3 mEq/kg
Ca	50–100 mg/kg depending on size of infant
P	1–1.5 mmol/kg
Mg	1 mEq/kg
Multivitamins* (MVI Pediatric)	10 ml (65% of dosage to infants <3 kg; 30% to infants <1 kg)

* Multivitamin preparations are undergoing scrutiny because of the preservatives in them. Practitioners must keep abreast of current recommendations.
(From Avery GB, Fletcher AB: Nutrition. In Avery GB (ed): Neonatology, 3rd ed. Philadelphia, JB Lippincott, 1987.)

nutrition to the neonate. Indications for the use of TPN include low-birth-weight infants, surgical infants in whom the gut needs to be rested, NEC, and prolonged diarrhea.[48]

Central catheters for TPN infusion may be inserted in various sites: external or internal jugular, or internal jugular into superior vena cava (Fig. 44-24). Peripheral lines may also be used. TPN is infused at a carefully calculated rate by way of an infusion pump. A filter is placed close to the insertion site to help prevent infection. A sterile dressing is placed securely over the insertion site. Neither medications nor blood should be given through the line.

Nursing care for the infant receiving TPN involves monitoring the equipment, the infusion, and the infant.

The solution is prepared aseptically in the pharmacy and refrigerated until used. The solution container, tubing, and filter must be changed minimally every 24 hours and labeled. The container label is carefully checked against the physician's order for correct ingredients and amounts.

Peripheral lines must be watched carefully for any signs of infiltration. Severe tissue necrosis and sloughing can occur owing to the hyperosmolar solution. The insertion site dressing is changed at least three times a week using strict aseptic technique and following agency procedure. The infusion itself is maintained at the desired rate.

Various parameters are measured, such as Dextrostix, urine specific gravity, sugar and acetone, intake and output, and daily weights. Blood studies are done frequently to check electrolyte requirements (i.e., hemoglobin, hematocrit, electrolytes, and serum osmolarity). The infant's sucking needs may be satisfied by a pacifier.

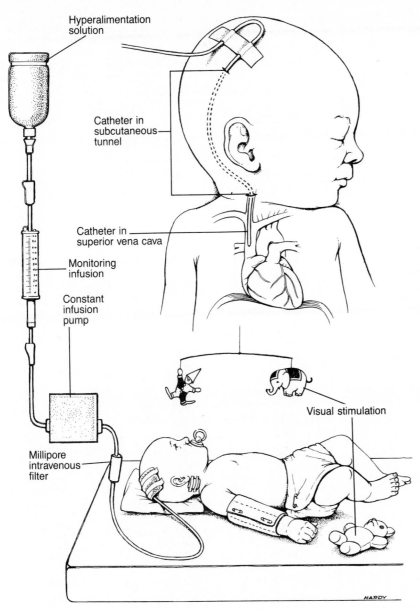

Hyperalimentation solution

Catheter in subcutaneous tunnel

Catheter in superior vena cava

Monitoring infusion

Constant infusion pump

Millipore intravenous filter

Visual stimulation

HARDY

■ *Figure 44–24*
Hyperalimentation (total parenteral nutrition) aseptically feeds the infant through, in this case, the superior vena cava. The solution is infused at a carefully calculated rate by way of an infusion pump.

INTRALIPID. Intralipid is a Swedish soybean oil–egg emulsion designed to deliver extra calories and lower glucose concentration in addition to TPN. Infants on TPN alone develop fatty acid deficiencies quite rapidly.

Intralipid should be infused slowly (preferably for 24 hours) in a line separate from other intravenous solutions, but may be run in the same line through a Y connector or close to the insertion site. Serum is checked for turbidity daily to ensure fat clearance. Serum fatty acids and triglyceride levels should be monitored weekly. The American Association of Pediatrics recommends that amount of lipids not exceed 3 g/kg/day, or 33 calories.[51]

ALTERATION IN COMFORT

In today's technologically advanced NICU environment, preterm infants undergo numerous invasive and painful procedures.

To intervene effectively, it is essential for the nurse to make an accurate assessment of behaviors indicating pain versus irritability (Table 44-10). Both pharmacologic and nonpharmacologic interventions may be effective in promoting comfort in the neonate (Tables 44-11 and 44-12).[52]

Care of the Parents

The parents of high-risk newborns often have adaptational needs or problems that necessitate sensitive and thoughtful nursing care. Not only are they making the transition to new parenthood, with all its requirements, but they must cope with the unusual situation of a small, different, and often sick baby. The importance of the early postpartum period for the establishment of bonds between the parents and the newborn and the laying

TABLE 44-10. PAIN AND AGITATION BEHAVIORS OF PREMATURE NEONATES

Mode of Expression	Pain Behaviors	Irritable Behaviors
Verbal	Crying, often sudden and loud	Whining cry
Nonverbal	Decreased activity	Frown
	Grimace	Flailing of extremities
	Flexing extremities	Random movements of head and body
	Tensing muscles	Rigid posture
	Rigid posture	Altered feeding patterns
	Flushed face	
	Decreased period of alertness (withdrawal)	
Physiologic	Sudden heart rate increase, up to 40% (may follow temporary initial decrease)	Heart rate and blood pressure increase only with activity
	Blood pressure increase	No diaphoresis
	Duskiness	No color changes unless prolonged
	Oxygen saturation decrease	No oxygen saturation decrease unless prolonged

(Broome ME, Tanzillo H: Differentiating between pain and agitation in premature neonates. J Perinat Neonat Nurs 4(1):55, 1990.)

TABLE 44-11. PHARMACOLOGIC MANAGEMENT OF NEONATAL PAIN AND RESTLESSNESS

Drug	Dose	Route	Frequency	Comments	Side Effects
Analgesic					
Morphine	15 μg/kg/h	IV	Continuous infusion without loading dose	Inexpensive, well studied, very effective	Dose-related respiratory depression and sedation; decreased intestinal motility
Fentanyl	2–4 μg/kg	IV	Every 1–2 h, given over minimum of 2 min	Monitor plasma levels if given frequently; particularly useful for short procedures	
Anesthetic					
Lidocaine (for use during painful procedures	0.2–0.8 ml	Intradermal	2–3 min prior to procedure		Hypotension, restlessness uncommon
Sedation					
Chloral hydrate	6–8 mg/kg	po			Nausea, increased peristalsis, paradoxic excitement

IV = intravenous; po = per os (by mouth).
(Broome ME, Tanzillo H: Differentiating between pain and agitation in premature neonates. J Perinat Neonat Nurs 4(1):57, 1990.)

TABLE 44-12. NONPHARMACOLOGIC MANAGEMENT OF NEONATAL PAIN AND IRRITABILITY

Pain

Swaddling or containment during procedure

Alternative distraction: music, light, conversation

Pacifier during and after procedure

Calming before and after procedure

Tactile stimulation

Rocking

Irritability

Swaddling

Decreased light and noise

Decreased handling; increased rest periods between procedures

Rhythmic activities; stroking, patting

Vestibular stimulation: upright positioning

(Broome ME, Tanzillo H: Differentiating between pain and agitation in premature neonates. J Perinat Neonat Nurs 4(1):59, 1990.)

of the groundwork for healthy attitudes toward future relationships with the child must not be underestimated.

INTERACTIONAL DEPRIVATION

Prolonged mother-infant separation has been studied for its effects on attachment. As soon as possible after the infant's birth, the mothers in the early-contact group were admitted into the nursery and encouraged to touch their babies and to perform such caretaking duties as the infant's condition allowed. Mothers in the late-contact group were not permitted into the nursery until after their infants reach almost 1 month of age. Results revealed detectable differences in mothering perfor-

---

Psychological Processes Parents Go Through After Birth of a High-Risk Infant

Shock, disbelief, and denial

Anger and searching self and others for causes

Grieving over loss of fantasized perfect infant

Grieving over own inability to produce perfect infant

Anticipatory worrying over loss of infant

Initiation of contact with infant

Belief and desire that infant will live

Readiness to establish caretaking relationship

---

mance between these two groups. In one study, high-contact mothers had higher scores on an attachment interview, on maternal performance, on *en face* feeding, and on the amount of fondling of infants when tested 1 month after delivery (Fig. 44-25).[53] In another study comparing late- and early-contact mothers 1 month after discharge of the infants, and after 200 feedings at home, the late-contact mothers held their babies differently and changed their positions less, bubbled their infants less frequently, and were not as skillful in feeding.[54] Some mothers who were barred from interaction with their babies in the nursery resumed prior interests when they returned home. The babies then had to compete with these interests when they were discharged.

Such studies suggest that prolonged separation may adversely affect commitment or attachment between mother and infant, may reduce confidence in mothering abilities, and may interfere with the mother's ability to develop an efficient routine of care. When mothers were allowed into the high-risk nursery for early and frequent contact and caretaking of their infants, there was no increase in nursery infections or disruption of nursery routine.[55]

Modifying hospital routine to allow mothers early contact with their high-risk infants appears to have a positive effect on later maternal behavior. This lends support to the concept of a sensitive time for bonding to occur between the mother and her infant. This time is probably within the first several hours of delivery.

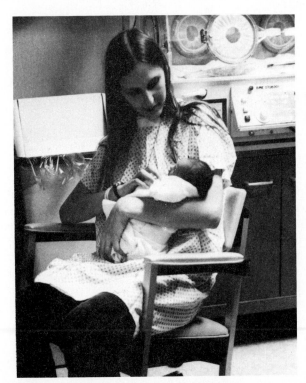

■ *Figure 44-25*
En face *contact between mother and infant should be encouraged when the infant is removed from the Isolette.*

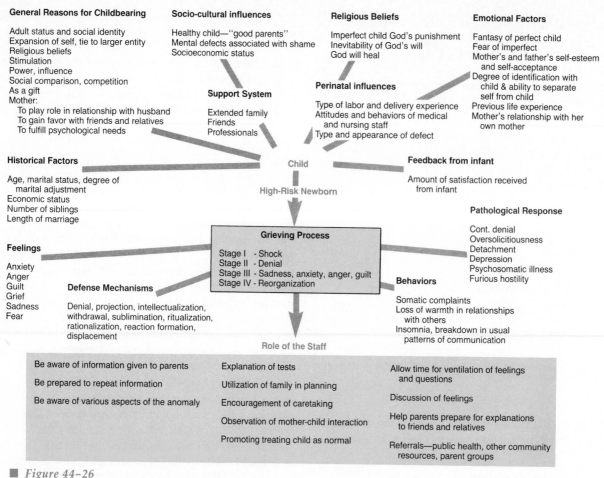

General Reasons for Childbearing

Adult status and social identity
Expansion of self, tie to larger entity
Religious beliefs
Stimulation
Power, influence
Social comparison, competition
As a gift
Mother:
   To play role in relationship with husband
   To gain favor with friends and relatives
   To fulfill psychological needs

Socio-cultural influences

Healthy child—"good parents"
Mental defects associated with shame
Socioeconomic status

Support System

Extended family
Friends
Professionals

Religious Beliefs

Imperfect child God's punishment
Inevitability of God's will
God will heal

Perinatal influences

Type of labor and delivery experience
Attitudes and behaviors of medical
   and nursing staff
Type and appearance of defect

Emotional Factors

Fantasy of perfect child
Fear of imperfect
Mother's and father's self-esteem
   and self-acceptance
Degree of identification with
   child & ability to separate
   self from child
Previous life experience
Mother's relationship with her
   own mother

Historical Factors

Age, marital status, degree of
   marital adjustment
Economic status
Number of siblings
Length of marriage

Child

High-Risk Newborn

Feedback from infant

Amount of satisfaction received
   from infant

Pathological Response

Cont. denial
Oversolicitiousness
Detachment
Depression
Psychosomatic illness
Furious hostility

Feelings

Anxiety
Anger
Guilt
Grief
Sadness
Fear

Defense Mechanisms

Denial, projection, intellectualization,
   withdrawal, sublimation, ritualization,
   rationalization, reaction formation,
   displacement

Grieving Process

Stage I - Shock
Stage II - Denial
Stage III - Sadness, anxiety, anger, guilt
Stage IV - Reorganization

Behaviors

Somatic complaints
Loss of warmth in relationships
   with others
Insomnia, breakdown in usual
   patterns of communication

Role of the Staff

Be aware of information given to parents

Be prepared to repeat information

Be aware of various aspects of the anomaly

Explanation of tests

Utilization of family in planning

Encouragement of caretaking

Observation of mother-child interaction

Promoting treating child as normal

Allow time for ventilation of feelings
   and questions

Discussion of feelings

Help parents prepare for explanations
   to friends and relatives

Referrals—public health, other community
   resources, parent groups

■ *Figure 44–26*
Parental response to the high-risk newborn.

Greater maternal attentiveness and better caretaking seem related to later exploratory behavior in infants; thus, removing barriers to maternal attachment during the sensitive period may have a potent influence on the later development of these babies.

PARENTAL REACTIONS AND PSYCHOLOGICAL TASKS

The birth of a premature or high-risk infant is often experienced as an acute emotional crisis by the family. This causes a certain amount of disorganization in the parents before they are able to master their feelings and come to accept the event (Fig. 44-26). Because the baby may be born before term, parents are often deprived of the last 6 to 8 weeks in which the final psychological (and sometimes material) preparation for the birth is made.

PLANNING AND INTERVENTIONS

The nurse's first action is to assess the parents' reactions to the high-risk birth, based on the knowledge that cer-

tain behaviors may be anticipated. The nurse assists the parents to work through the grieving process by allowing expression of feelings, facilitating communication with health-care team members, providing support, information, and referrals as needed. Parents are encouraged to visit and telephone at any time, whether the infant is cared at the birth medical center or transported to a tertiary-care facility.

In the event that the infant is transported to a tertiary-care center, the parents need to be informed of the circumstances and encouraged to see and touch the infant before transport occurs. It is helpful for the parents to be given a snapshot of the infant. Some nurseries have developed a pamphlet describing the unit.

Visiting the NICU. The father may often be the first parent to visit the neonatal unit and assume the role of communicator to the mother. Either the mother is not housed at the transport hospital or her physical condition may not permit her to visit immediately.

The father's first visit may be overwhelming at first, although the nurse may have tried to prepare him in advance. It is best to simply explain the equipment and its functions and then allow the father to ask questions. The nurse may encourage him to touch the baby and begin the attachment process at a tolerable pace.

The mother's first visit can be handled in a similar fashion. If she plans to breastfeed, she should be taught how to express and save her milk. This is a positive act that can definitely enhance the mother-child relationship.

As visits continue, parents may be encouraged to bring small objects from homes, such as toys and clothes. Siblings and other relatives may be allowed to visit, depending on the unit policy.

As time goes by, specific caretaking tasks may be assumed by the parents under the nurse's supervision. This will prepare the parents gradually for the time of discharge, greatly enhance their self-confidence, and promote attachment. Any pamphlets that will help stress important information are always appreciated.

In the event that the tertiary-care center is far from the parents' home, a return transport may be offered and be acceptable to the parents.[56]

Evaluation

The nursing process in high-risk neonatal care is challenging, stressful, yet also rewarding. This highly specialized area seeks to intervene successfully for the critically ill neonate. The many technical aspects are beyond the scope of this text, and the reader is referred to one of the many texts on the subject of neonatal intensive care.

■ REFERENCES

1. Kliegman RM, Hulman SE: Intrauterine growth retardation: Determinants of aberrant fetal growth. In Fanaroff AA, Martin RJ (eds): Neonatal-Perinatal Medicine, pp 69–100. St. Louis, CV Mosby, 1987
2. Cheek DB, Graystone JE, Niall M: Factors controlling fetal growth. Clin Obstet Gynecol 20(4):925–942, December 1977
3. Pernoll M, Benda GI, Babson SG: Diagnosis and Management of the Fetus and Neonate at Risk: A Guide for Team Care, 5th ed, p 178. St. Louis, CV Mosby, 1986
4. Korones SB: High Risk Newborn Infants, 4th ed, pp 126–138, 178, 263–268, 277, 338. St. Louis, CV Mosby, 1986
5. Phibbs RH: Delivery room management of the newborn. In Avery GB (ed): Neonatology: Pathophysiology and Management of the Newborn, pp 182–201. Philadelphia, JB Lippincott, 1981
6. Pilkin RM, Scott JR: The Yearbook of Obstetrics and Gynecology, pp 1973, 1978. Chicago, Year Book Medical Publishers, 1978
7. Olds SB, London ML, Ladewig PA: Maternal-Newborn Nursing, p 1013. Menlo Park, CA, Addison-Wesley, 1988
8. Turnage CS: Meconium aspiration syndrome. J Perinat Neonat Nurs 3(2):69–80, 1989
9. Schreiner RL, Bradburn NC: Care of the Newborn, 2nd ed, pp 56. New York, Raven Press, 1988
10. DiGiacomo JE, Hagedorn MI, Hay WW: Glucose homeostasis. In Merenstein GB, Gardner SL: Handbook of Neonatal Care, p 223. St. Louis, CV Mosby, 1989
11. Hoffman EL, Bennett FC: Birth Weight Less than 800 Grams: Changing Outcomes and Influences of Gender and Gestation Number. Pediatrics 86(1):27–33, 1990
12. Marchal FM, Bairam A, Vert P: Neonatal apnea and apneic syndromes. Clin Perinatol 14(3):509–523, 1987
13. Bucuvalas JC, Balistreri WF: The neonatal gastrointestinal tract: development. In Fanaroff AA, Martin RJ (eds): Neonatal-Perinatal Medicine, p 899. St. Louis, CV Mosby, 1987
14. Hack M: Sensorimotor development of the preterm infant. In Fanaroff AA, Martin RJ (eds): Neonatal-Perinatal Medicine, pp 473–491. St. Louis, CV Mosby, 1987
15. Spitzer A, Bernstein J, Edelmann CM, et al: The kidney and urinary tract. In Fanaroff AA, Martin RJ (eds): Neonatal-Perinatal Medicine, pp 981–1009. St. Louis, CV Mosby, 1987
16. Morechi R, Gartner, LM, Lee KS: Jaundice and liver disease. In Fanaroff AA, Martin RJ (eds): Behrman's Neonatal-Perinatal Medicine, p 768. St. Louis, CV Mosby, 1983
17. Polmar SH, Manthei V: Immunology. In Fanaroff AA, Martin RJ (eds): Neonatal-Perinatal Medicine, p 752. St. Louis, CV Mosby, 1987
18. NAACOG OGN Nursing Practice Resource: Neonatal Skin Care. No. 12, pp 1–6, March 1985
19. Nugent J: Acute respiratory care of the newborn. JOGN Nurs 12(3)(suppl):31s–44s, 1983
20. Walsh MC, Carlo WA, Miller MJ: Respiratory disease of the newborn. In Carlo WA, Chatburn RL (eds): Neonatal Respiratory Care, pp 260–288. Chicago, Year Book Medical Publisher, 1988
21. Vidysagar D: Clinical features of RDS. In Stern LB (ed): Hyaline Membrane Disease, pp 97–117. Orlando, Grune and Stratton, 1984
22. Martin RJ, Fanaroff AA: Complications of neonatal respiratory care. In Carlo WA, Chatburn RL (eds): Neonatal Respiratory Care, p 355. Chicago, Year Book Medical Publishers, 1988
23. Long C: Cryotherapy: A new treatment for retinopathy of prematurity. Pediatr Nurs 15(3):269–272, 1989
24. Donlen JM, Budd RA: The low birth weight infant: A nursing perspective. In Stahler-Miller K (ed): Neonatal and Pediatric Critical Care Nursing, p 13. New York, Churchill Livingstone, 1983
25. Carey B: Intraventricular hemorrhage in the preterm infant. JOGN Nurs 12(3)(suppl):61s–65s, 1983
26. Dooley KJ: Management of the premature infant with a patent ductus arteriosus. Pediatr Clin North Am 31(6): 1160–1171, 1984

27. Harrison E: Necrotizing enterocolitis. J Enterostomal Ther 11:233, 1984

28. Brown EG, Sweet AY: Neonatal necrotizing enterocolitis. Pediatr Clin North Am 29(6):1149–1153, 1982

29. Amspacher KA: Necrotizing enterocolitis: The never-ending challenge. J Perinat Neonat Nurs 3(2):58–67, 1989

30. Perehudoff B: Newborn resuscitation in the delivery room. J Perinat Neonat Nurs 3(2):81–90, 1989

31. Daze AM, Scanlon JW: Code Pink: A Practical System for Neonatal/Perinatal Resuscitation, pp 89–124. Baltimore, University Park Press, 1981

32. Mason TN: A hand ventilation technique for neonates. MCN 7(6):367–368, 1982

33. McCormick A: Special considerations in the nursing care of the very low birth weight infant. JOGN Nurs 13(6):358–361, 1984

34. Williams J: Assessment and stabilization of the newborn. In Daze AM, Scanlon JW (eds): Neonatal Nursing, pp 18–32. Baltimore, University Park Press, 1985

35. Greer PS: Head coverings for newborns under radiant warmers. JOGNN 17(4):265–271, 1988

36. Kuller JM, Lund C, Tobin C: Improved skin care for premature infants. MCN 8(3):200–201, 1983

37. Lund C, Kuller JM, Tobin C, et al: Evaluation of a pectin-based barrier under tape to protect neonatal skin. JOGNN 15(1):39–43, 1986

38. Clancy G: Blood gas monitoring and management of neonates with respiratory distress. J Perinat Neonat Nurs 1(1):72–83, 1987

39. Norris S, Campbell L, Brenkert S: Nursing procedures and alterations in transcutaneous oxygen tension in premature infants. Nurs Res 31(6):330–335, 1982

40. Paludetto R, Robertson SS, Hack M, et al: Transcutaneous oxygen tension during nonnutritive sucking in preterm infants. Pediatrics 74(4):539–542, October 1984

41. Riedel K: Pulse oximetry: A new technology to assess patient oxygen needs in the neonatal intensive care unit. J Perinat Neonat Nurs 1(1):49–57, 1987

42. Hazinski MF, Pacetti AS: Nursing care of the infant with respiratory disease. In Carlo WA, Chatburn RL (eds): Neonatal Respiratory Care, p 198. Chicago, Year Book Medical Publishers, 1988

43. Spitzer AR, Fox WW: Use and abuse of mechanical ventilators. In Stern LB (ed): Hyaline Membrane Disease, pp 149–159. Orlando, Grune and Stratton, 1984

44. Shorten DR: Effects of tracheal suctioning on neonates: A review of the literature. Intensive Care Nurs 5:167–170, 1989

45. Curran CL, Kachoyeanos MK: The effects on neonates of two methods of chest physical therapy. MCN 4(5):309–313, 1979

46. Kilbride HW, Forlaw L: Total parenteral nutrition. In Merenstein GB, Gardner SL: Handbook of Neonatal Care, p 264. St. Louis, CV Mosby, 1989

47. Weibley T, Adamson M, Clinkscales N, et al: Gavage tube insertion in the premature infant. MCN 12(1):24–27, 1987

48. Avery GB: The newborn. In Jelliffe DB, Jelliffe EF (eds): Nutrition and Growth, pp 129–152. New York, Plenum Press, 1979

49. Price E, Gyotoku S: Using the nasojejunal feeding technique in a neonatal intensive care unit. MCN 3(6):364–365, 1978

50. McCoy R, Kadowaki C, Wilks S, et al: Nursing management of breast feeding preterm infants. J Perinat Neonat Nurs 2(1):42–55, 1988

51. Sterk MB: Understanding parenteral nutrition. JOGN Nurs 12(3)(suppl):47s, 1983

52. Broome ME, Tanzillo H: Differentiating between pain and agitation in premature neonates. J Perinat Neonat Nurs 4(1):53–62, 1990

53. Klaus MH, Jerauld R, Kreger N, et al: Maternal attachment: Importance of the first postpartum days. N Engl J Med 286:460, 1972

54. Klaus MH, Kennell JH: Mothers separated from their newborn infants. Pediatr Clin North Am 17:1015–1037, 1970

55. Barnett C, Leidermann P, Grobstein R, et al: Neonatal separation: The maternal side of interactional deprivation. Pediatrics 45:197, 1970

56. Thornton J, Berry J, Dal Santo J: Neonatal intensive care: The nurse's role in supporting the family. Nurs Clin North Am 19(1):125–137, March 1984

■ SUGGESTED READING

Avery GB (ed): Neonatology. Philadelphia, JB Lippincott, 1987

Beckholt AP: Breast milk for infants who cannot breastfeed. JOGNN 19(3):216–220, 1990

Beckmann CA: Postterm pregnancy: Effects on temperature and glucose regulation. Nurs Res 39(1):21–24, 1990

Bull MJ, Weber K, Stroup KB, et al: Automotive restraint systems for premature infants. J Pediatr 112(3):385–388, March 1988

Cerase P: Ethical dilemmas in the resuscitation of the very low birth weight infant. J Perinat Neonat Nurs 1(3):69–76, 1988

Cohen SP: Bacterial sepsis in the very low birth weight infant. Neonat Network 2(1):56–65, July 1988

Franck LS: Pain in the nonverbal patient: Advocating for the critically ill neonate. Pediatr Nurs 15(1):65–68, 1989

George DS, Stephen S, Fellows RR, et al: The latest on the retinopathy of prematurity. MCN 13(4):254–258, 1988

Glass SM, Giacoia GP: Intravenous drug therapy in premature infants: Practical aspects. JOGNN 16(5):310–318, 1989

Harrison LL, Twardosz S: Teaching mothers about their preterm infants. JOGNN 15(2):165–171, 1986

Jacono J, Hicks G, Antonioni C, et al: Comparison of perceived needs of family members between registered nurses and family members of critically ill patients in intensive care and neonatal intensive care units. Heart Lung 19(1):72–78, 1990

Klaus MH, Fanaroff AA: Care of the High Risk Neonate. Philadelphia, WB Saunders, 1987

Korones SB: High-Risk Newborn Infants. St. Louis, CV Mosby, 1986

Lemons P, Stuart M, Lemons JA, et al: Breast feeding the premature infant. Clin Perinatol 13(1):111, 1986

Lynch TM: Invasive and noninvasive pressure monitoring in neonates. J Perinat Neonat Nurs 1(1):58–71, 1987

Meier P, Anderson GC: Responses of small preterm infants to bottle and breast-feeding. MCN 12(2):97–105, 1987

Merenstein GB, Gardner SL: Handbook of Neonatal Intensive Care, 2nd ed. St. Louis, CV Mosby, 1989

Penticuff JH: Infant suffering and nurse advocacy in neonatal intensive care. Nurs Clin North Am 24(4):987–997, 1989

Pinch WJ, Spielman ML: Ethical decision making for high-risk infants: The parents' perspective. Nurs Clin North Am 24(4):1017–1021, 1989

Richardson C: Hyaline membrane disease: Future treatment modalities. J Perinat Neonat Nurs 2(1):78–88, 1988

Short BL, Miller MK, Anderson KD: Extracorporeal membrane oxygenation in the management of respiratory failure in the newborn. Clin Perinatol 14(3):737–745, 1987

Streeter NS (ed): High-Risk Neonatal Care. Rockville, MD, Aspen, 1986

Thomas KA: How the NICU environment sounds to a preterm infant. MCN 14(4):249–251, 1989

Vidyasagar D, Shimada S: Pulmonary surfactant replacement in respiratory distress syndrome. Clin Perinatol 14(4):991–1011, 1987

Wilks S, Meier P: Helping mothers express milk suitable for preterm and high risk infant feeding. MCN 13(2):121–123, 1988

45

The High-Risk Infant: Developmental Disorders

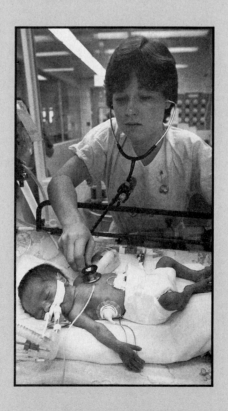

During labor, delivery, and the first several hours of neonatal life, many changes occur in the fetus and neonate that allow physiological adaptation to extrauterine life. Developmental characteristics of the infant may have significant influence on this process of moving from intrauterine to extrauterine life, such as genetic or congenital abnormalities and size and gestational age (see Chap. 44). Perinatal teams must be constantly alert to signs of complications in the neonate, with the objectives of identifying problems early, correcting disorders quickly (or minimizing subsequent effects), preventing permanent disabilities, and promoting the parental bonding process.

■ PARENTAL AND STAFF REACTIONS TO DEFECTS AND DISORDERS

The birth of an infant with congenital anomalies or development defects presents significant psychosocial stresses for the family and precipitates an adaptive crisis. A variety of emotional difficulties may interfere with the parents' relationship with the infant and disrupt functioning of the family. Parents often express feelings of anxiety, guilt, fear, inadequacy, helplessness, failure, and anger. The way in which parents cope with crisis and work through their feelings will influence how realistically they perceive their infant's medical condition and needs, how they are able to adapt to the infant's hospital environment, their ability to assume the primary caretaking role, their ability to assume responsibility for the infant's care after discharge, and, for some, how they will cope with the death of their infant (Fig. 45-1).

Grief

Grief is the characteristic response to the loss of a valued object. A grief reaction may be precipitated by certain perinatal situations, such as abortion, stillbirth, preterm birth, infant deformity or illness, neonatal death, and relinquishment of a neonate.[1]

STAGES OF THE GRIEVING PROCESS

The grieving process has been studied at length and in various settings. The various common behaviors noted during grief have been grouped into stages. Stages may be labeled differently but basically contain the same behaviors. Grieving parents may not exhibit all of the behaviors, and they may repeat behaviors during the process.

Shock. Shock, denial, disbelief, and withdrawal behaviors characterize the first phase. Parents may experience a feeling of numbness. Physiological reactions are loss of appetite, palpitations, fatigue, shortness of breath, and so on. A tendency to withdraw from the situation may be observed in the case of a defective or critically ill neonate. This coping mechanism allows the potential loss to be less painful if attachment has not occurred.

Searching. The second stage involves seeking an answer or reason for the event by the parents. Behaviors of anger, guilt, hostility, and emptiness are commonly seen. Parents may feel that their actions are to blame for the loss. Health-care professionals may be the target of their anger.

Disorientation. Disorientation is a bridge stage to reorganization. During this time, gradual change to normal activities will occur. Parents may still be experiencing depression and may have little emotional energy to deal with setbacks (e.g., a complication in the health course of the preterm infant).

Reorganization. Over a considerable period of time, parents accommodate to the loss. Minimal energy is devoted to the grief process, and most energy is directed toward normal living.[2]

NURSING PROCESS

An outline of the nursing process is found in the Nursing Care Plan: The Grieving Family.

Assessment. Nursing assessment begins with the establishment that an actual or potential perinatal loss has occurred. Variables that the nurse considers in planning care are the family's past experiences and usual coping strategies in dealing with loss or crisis, support systems available, cultural and religious factors, and age and maturity level of the parents.

Nursing Diagnosis. Potential nursing diagnoses are anticipatory or dysfunctional grieving related to a perinatal loss, self-concept, disturbance in self-esteem, and knowledge deficit related to a perinatal loss.

Planning and Intervention. The nurse plans to facilitate and support the family's grieving process. In addition, the nurse provides the family with information regarding the loss, including any implications for future childbearing.

Research Highlight

Few studies have investigated perinatal bereavement or aspects of it.

The authors wished to answer three questions in their exploratory–descriptive study: (1) How much contact do parents have with their baby at the time of the child's death? (2) What factors are significantly associated with the reasons why parents do or do not hold their baby? (3) What are the positive and negative aspects of contact or lack of contact? Contact was separated into actual physical contact or visual contact.

A nonrandom sample of 39 individuals responded to a questionnaire. Nineteen parents held their babies; 20 did not hold them. Of the 20 who did not hold their babies, nine saw their babies and 11 did not. Of the "no hold" group, 80% did not hold because of a health professional's decision. Of parents who held their babies, 100% made positive comments on the experience, although some negative comments also were made. Of the nine parents who saw but did not hold their baby, four (40%) reported positive experiences, including relief that the baby looked normal. Five (55%) reported regrets that they had not held their baby. Of the 11 "no contact" parents, only three (27%) had any positive comments about the absence of contact. Most comments made by parents in the "no contact" group were negative. Ten of the parents (91%) in the "no contact" group reported problems with resolution of the grief process.

Nurses and other health professionals need to look closely at their interventions with the bereaved parents. Clearly their influence is crucial concerning parents' decisions to see and hold their infants at the time of a perinatal death.

Ransohoff-Adler M, Berger CS: When newborns die: Do we practice what we preach? *J Perinatol* 9(3):311–316, 1989

Evaluation. Adaptive responses to a crisis such as a perinatal loss are described in the nursing care plan and Figure 45-1.

■ CONGENITAL AND GENETIC ABNORMALITIES

A congenital disorder is one that is present at birth and can be transmitted by genetic or environmental factors or both. A genetic disorder is one that is transmitted from generation to generation. See Chapter 14 for a detailed discussion of genetic disorders. Approximately 250,000 infants are born each year with abnormalities significantly altering the structure and function of their bodies. As a result of the varied and complex nature of congenital and genetic disorders, an organized multidisciplinary approach is required, including medical, surgical, rehabilitation, financial, and community health resources. Enormous psychological and financial burdens can be overwhelming to the parents without competent resources at their disposal. As time goes on, prevention, detection, and various treatment modalities are improving.

The reader needs to keep in mind that the disorders discussed represent those more commonly dealt with in the perinatal setting.

Congenital Heart Disease

Changes in the fetal circulation after birth are discussed in Chapter 10.

Congenital heart disease has an incidence of about 7 per 1000 at birth. Cardiovascular malformations account for approximately 1.2 in 1000 deaths during infancy. Most congenital heart disease is thought to be multifactorial in origin—implying both genetic and environmental factors. Some congenital heart diseases are associated with syndromes, such as trisomy 21 and Turner's syndrome. Some defects are associated with maternal rubella, maternal anticonvulsant medications, or maternal alcohol consumption.

TYPES OF CONGENITAL CARDIAC ANOMALIES

Major types of congenital cardiac anomalies are illustrated and described in Figure 45-2.

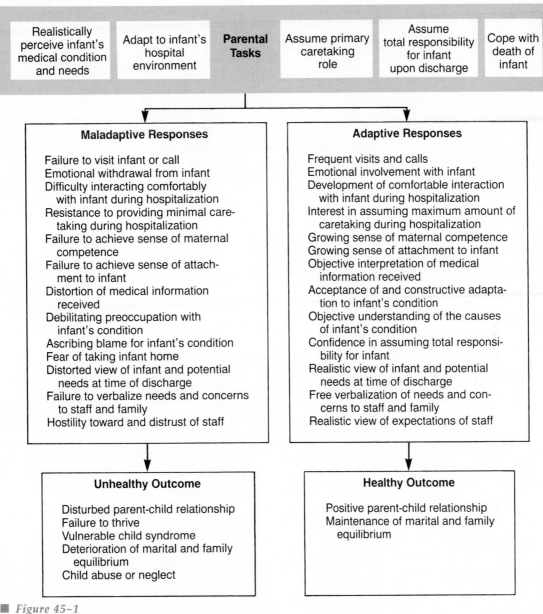

Parental Tasks
Realistically perceive infant's medical condition and needs · Adapt to infant's hospital environment · Assume primary caretaking role · Assume total responsibility for infant upon discharge · Cope with death of infant

Maladaptive Responses

Failure to visit infant or call
Emotional withdrawal from infant
Difficulty interacting comfortably with infant during hospitalization
Resistance to providing minimal care-taking during hospitalization
Failure to achieve sense of maternal competence
Failure to achieve sense of attach-ment to infant
Distortion of medical information received
Debilitating preoccupation with infant's condition
Ascribing blame for infant's condition
Fear of taking infant home
Distorted view of infant and potential needs at time of discharge
Failure to verbalize needs and concerns to staff and family
Hostility toward and distrust of staff

Adaptive Responses

Frequent visits and calls
Emotional involvement with infant
Development of comfortable interaction with infant during hospitalization
Interest in assuming maximum amount of caretaking during hospitalization
Growing sense of maternal competence
Growing sense of attachment to infant
Objective interpretation of medical information received
Acceptance of and constructive adapta-tion to infant's condition
Objective understanding of the causes of infant's condition
Confidence in assuming total responsi-bility for infant
Realistic view of infant and potential needs at time of discharge
Free verbalization of needs and con-cerns to staff and family
Realistic view of expectations of staff

Unhealthy Outcome

Disturbed parent-child relationship
Failure to thrive
Vulnerable child syndrome
Deterioration of marital and family equilibrium
Child abuse or neglect

Healthy Outcome

Positive parent-child relationship
Maintenance of marital and family equilibrium

■ *Figure 45–1*
Parental response during crisis period. (Grant P: Psychosocial needs of families of high-risk infants. Fam Community Health 1(3):93, November 1978)

ASSESSMENT

The nurse reads the history for evidence of familial congenital heart defects. The nurse assesses the new-born for one of the following: cyanosis, respiratory dis-tress, congestive heart failure and decreased cardiac output, abnormal cardiac rhythm, and cardiac murmurs.

Congestive heart failure implies that the heart is unable to pump effectively enough to meet the body's circulatory requirements. The nurse assesses the neonate for evidence of diminished cardiac output and decreased tissue perfusion. The infant with congestive heart failure may exhibit the following: tachycardia, cardiac enlarge-ment, tachypnea, gallop rhythm, decreased peripheral pulses, decreased urine output, edema, diaphoresis, hepatomegaly, decreased exercise tolerance, failure to thrive and feeding problems, and decreased cardiac output.

Medical Diagnosis. Diagnostic tools used include ar-terial blood gases, chest x-ray, electrocardiogram, echo-cardiogram, and cardiac catheterization. Whether car-diac catheterization is used in the neonatal period

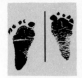

Nursing Care Plan

The Grieving Family

Patient Goals

1. The family members are supportive of one another.
2. The family applies its energy to working through grief.
3. The family uses healthy coping mechanisms.
4. The family adapts to crisis.
5. The parents verbally repeat understanding of prognosis and resources.
6. Parents of ill infants visit the nursery.
7. Family is able to verbalize positive self-esteem.
8. Family verbalizes information related to loss.

Assessment	Potential Nursing Diagnosis	Planning and Intervention	Evaluation

Perinatal loss
  Abortion
  Stillbirth
  Neonatal death
	Anticipatory or dysfunctional grieving related to a perinatal loss	Anticipate various stages of the grief process	Family is supportive of one another

Intrauterine fetal death		Allow family time to ventilate feelings	Family applies its energy to working through grief
Infant of low birth weight or preterm		Provide facts sought by family	Family applies healthy coping mechanisms
Infant with a congenital anomaly		Allow family time to see and hold baby—describe how baby will look, and wrap as a normal newborn	Family adapts to crisis
Infant with a life-threatening illness		Ask if parents wish to name baby	Parents verbally repeat understanding of prognosis and resources
Family support systems available		Provide photographs or other remembrances of baby if family wishes	Parents of ill infants visit nursery
Past grief experiences		Seek parents' permission for an autopsy	
Religious beliefs		Ask if parents wish baby baptized	
Age and maturity level of parents		Notify clergy if family wishes	
Cultural considerations		Provide information on hospital policy regarding funeral options	
Usual coping methods for crises		Refer to a community support group, social worker, counselor as needed	
		Provide follow-up care as needed	
		In case of ill baby, encourage parents to visit nursery as much as possible	

(continued)

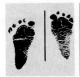

Nursing Care Plan (continued)

Assessment	Potential Nursing Diagnosis	Planning and Intervention	Evaluation
		Assist in mobilization of resources	
		Be realistic regarding prognosis and any long-term ramifications	
		Discuss talking to siblings about death	
Repeat abortions, fetal, or neonatal deaths	Self-concept, disturbance in self-esteem	Observe and assess family responses to loss, especially any expression of guilt	Family is able to verbalize positive self-esteem
Verbalizing of guilt feelings			Family identifies positive coping behaviors
Perinatal loss as a result of trauma, teratogenic exposure, or genetic problem		Be available and listen to expression of feelings	
		Assist with referrals as needed	
		Discuss parents' strengths in parenting other siblings, as appropriate	
Verbalization of concerns and questions	Knowledge deficit related to perinatal loss	Assess family's ability to process information	Family verbalizes information related to loss
		Provide information and review events as appropriate	
		Provide information regarding grief, what to expect with siblings	
		Clarify any misunderstandings	

depends on the accuracy of other diagnostic tools and the type of lesion suspected.

In the cardiac catheterization procedure, a radiopaque catheter is inserted through a peripheral blood vessel, usually the femoral vein, into the heart. Angiography is carried out by the injection of dye through the circulation. The data obtained indicate anatomical defects; pressure changes and oxygen saturation of blood in the chambers of the heart and great vessels; and changes in cardiac output or stroke volume. Complications of this procedure are hemorrhage, arrhythmias, infection, reactions to dye, and obstruction in the vessels.[3] The data obtained from this procedure greatly assist the surgical team if surgery is warranted. Once the lesion is definitely identified, the decision of whether medical or surgical intervention is the best approach can be made.

Nursing Diagnosis. Potential nursing diagnoses include: ineffective breathing patterns related to congestive heart failure; impaired gas exchange related to congenital cardiac defect; alteration in nutrition, less than body requirements, related to difficulty breathing, sucking, and swallowing; fluid-volume excess related to congestive heart failure; and decreased cardiac output related to congestive heart failure and congenital heart defect.

Planning and Nursing Interventions When the neonate is suspected of having congenital heart disease, the

Transposition of the great arteries

This anomaly is an embryologic defect caused by a straight division of the bulbar trunk without normal spiraling. As a result, the aorta originates from the right ventricle, and the pulmonary artery from the left ventricle. An abnormal communication between the two circulations must be present to sustain life.

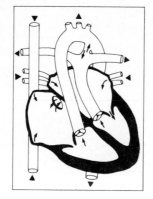

Atrial septal defect

An atrial septal defect is an abnormal opening between the right and left atria. Basically, three types of abnormalities result from incorrect development of the atrial septum. An incompetent foramen ovale is the most common defect. The high ostium secundum defect results from abnormal development of the septum secundum. Improper development of the septum primum produces a basal opening known as an ostium primum defect, frequently involving the atrioventricular valves. In general, left to right shunting of blood occurs in all atrial septal defects.

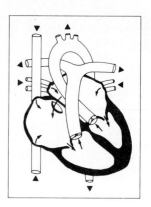

Patent ductus arteriosus

The patent ductus arteriosus is a vascular connection that, during fetal life, short circuits the pulmonary vascular bed and directs blood from the pulmonary artery to the aorta. Functional closure of the ductus normally occurs soon after birth. If the ductus remains patent after birth, the direction of blood flow in the ductus is reversed by the higher pressure in the aorta.

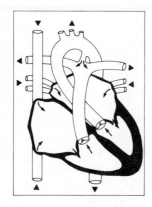

Ventricular septal defect

A ventricular septal defect is an abnormal opening between the right and left ventricle. Ventricular septal defects vary in size and may occur in either the membranous or muscular portion of the ventricular septum. Due to higher pressure in the left ventricle, a shunting of blood from the left to right ventricle occurs during systole. If pulmonary vascular resistance produces pulmonary hypertension, the shunt of blood is then reversed from the right to the left ventricle resulting in cyanosis.

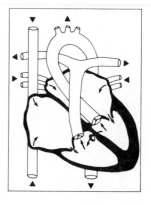

Coarctation of the aorta

Coarctation of the aorta is characterized by a narrowed aortic lumen. It exists as a preductal or postductal obstruction, depending on the position of the obstruction in relation to the ductus arteriosus. Coarctations exist with great variation in anatomical features. The lesion produces an obstruction to the flow of blood through the aorta causing an increased left ventricular pressure and work load.

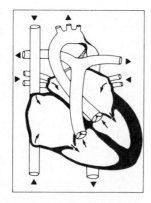

Tetralogy of Fallot

Tetralogy of Fallot is characterized by the combination of four defects—(1) pulmonary stenosis, (2) ventricular septal defect, (3) overriding aorta, and (4) hypertrophy of right ventricle. It is the most common defect causing cyanosis in patients surviving beyond two years of age. The severity of symptoms depends on the degree of pulmonary stenosis, the size of the ventricular septal defect, and the degree to which the aorta overrides the septal defect.

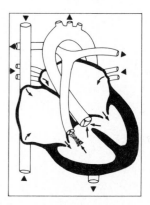

■ *Figure 45–2*

Six types of congenital anomalies. (Courtesy of Ross Laboratories)

nurse is involved in gathering observational data, assisting, and preparing the infant for various diagnostic procedures. Small, frequent oral feedings should be tried to avoid overtiring the infant. Strict intake and output records are kept, as well as daily weights. Parenteral nutrition may be necessary if oral feedings are not tolerated.

When oral feedings are tolerated, a low-sodium formula may be used, such as Lonalac or Similac PM 60/40. Oxygen is administered safely as needed while blood gas status is monitored. Digoxin is administered safely by checking the dosage and route with another nurse. The apical pulse is counted prior to administration, and the drug is held if the pulse is less than 90 to 100 beats per minute. If diuretics are being given, potassium levels are monitored frequently and adjusted with supplements in intravenous fluid or given orally. Cardiovascular drugs and nursing considerations are listed in Table 45-1.

Parents need experience and teaching for planned home interventions.

POSTOPERATIVE AND POSTCATHETERIZATION NURSING CARE. Areas of particular importance to note following cardiac catheterization are the equality of peripheral pulses and the temperature and color of the affected extremity.

Postoperatively, the neonate requires close observation in the intensive care unit. Monitors are attached for constant recording of vital signs, including blood pressure. All readings should be compared with the baseline. Environmental and anesthetic influences may decrease the temperature initially. In addition, some temperature elevation due to the inflammatory process

may be noted in the first 24 to 48 hours postoperatively. Any temperature elevation after this time may be indicative of infection.

All intravenous lines and dressings are observed and changed as needed. An intraarterial line with heparinized saline is suggested. Central venous pressure readings are taken frequently.

Respiratory status is monitored carefully by turning, postural drainage, and assessment of breath sounds. Suctioning accompanied by prebagging and postbagging with oxygen may be necessary to remove secretions. Chest tubes are in place postoperatively. The Pleurevac system is checked for adequate functioning and color and amount of drainage.

Fluid and electrolyte requirements are calculated according to the infant's weight and electrolyte reports. Initial fluids are parenteral, because feedings are gradually resumed. Blood replacement may be necessary; frequent monitoring of hematocrit, hemoglobin, and blood levels is essential.

All nursing activities are designed to allow maximum rest periods for the neonate.[3] Other steps in the nursing process are in the Nursing Care Plan: The Infant With a Congenital Heart Defect.

Cleft Lip and Cleft Palate

The cleft lip and the cleft palate, which may occur separately or in combination, result from the failure of the soft or bony tissues of the palate and the upper jaw to unite during the fifth to twelfth weeks of gestation. The defect may be unilateral or bilateral or, rarely, midline and incomplete or complete (Fig. 45-3). Only the lip may be involved, or the disunion may extend into the upper jaw or the nasal cavity.

Each year about 1 in 700 infants are born with a cleft lip or cleft palate, making this condition one of the most common birth defects. More males than females appear to be affected by the combination cleft lip and cleft palate disorder. Cleft palate alone has an increased incidence in females. These disorders may be associated with various other syndromes.

A clear-cut etiologic pattern for these deformities remains obscure. Variables found to be associated with them include genetic factors, drugs (particularly corticosteroids), radiation, hypoxia in utero, maternal viral illness during pregnancy, and dietary influences. The hypothesis has been put forward that palatolabial defects may be due to sex-modified multifactorial inheritance.[5]

TREATMENT

Surgical repair for the lip is occasionally performed immediately after birth, but more often, the surgery is

TABLE 45-1. CARDIOVASCULAR DRUGS AND DIURETICS

Drug	Dosage and Route	Nursing Considerations
Digoxin	Premature: 0.02–0.04 mg/kg IV (total digitalizing dose) 0.01 mg/kg/day divided every 12 h (maintenance) Full term: 0.04 mg/kg IV (total digitalizing dose) 0.01 mg/kg/day divided every 12 h PO (maintenance)	**Cardiotonic** Monitor apical pulse for bradycardia Monitor serum potassium Watch for nausea, vomiting Check dosage carefully Observe for ECG changes
Hydralazine	0.2 mg/kg/dose or 1.7–3.5 mg/kg/day divided every 4–6 h IV, IM 1 mg/kg/day divided every 6 h to increase as needed up to 7.5 mg/kg/day	**Antihypertensive** Monitor blood pressure and apical pulse Watch for nausea, vomiting, diarrhea
Lidocaine	0.5–1.5 mg/kg/dose by slow IV push; may be repeated every 5–10 min as needed 20–50 μ/kg/min continuous IV infusion	**Antiarrhythmic** Use infusion pump for accurate IV administration Use cardiac monitor
Procainamide	2 mg/kg/dose given over 5 min IV 40–60 mg/kg/day divided every 6 h PO	**Antiarrhythmic** Use with caution in congestive heart failure Monitor blood pressure, ECG
Propranolol	0.01–0.15 mg/kg/dose by slow IV push; then 0.5–1.0 mg/kg/day divided every 6 h PO Starting dose: 1 mg/kg/day divided every 6 h PO 0.15–0.25 mg/kg/dose IV	**Antiarrhythmic** Check apical pulse rate Monitor blood pressure, ECG, pulse
Chlorothiazide	20–30 mg/kg/day divided every 12 h PO	Monitor intake/output, serum electrolytes Monitor serum creatinine and blood urea nitrogen levels
Ethacrynic acid	2–3 mg/kg/day divided every 12 h PO 0.5–2.0 mg/kg/dose IV	Very potent diuretic Monitor potassium levels Oral solutions should be stored in refrigerator
Furosemide	1–2 mg/kg/dose every 6–8 h PO 0.5–2.0 mg/kg/dose every 12 h IM or IV	Potent loop diuretic Monitor serum potassium
Spironolactone	1.7–3.3 mg/kg/dose divided every 6–8 h	When used alone diuretic effect may take 2–3 days; may be used in addition to another diuretic Potassium-sparing diuretic Monitor potassium, electrolytes, intake/output, weight

postponed until the infant demonstrates steady weight gain and is past the neonatal period. Surgery is more often accomplished when the infant is 1 or 2 months of age or weighs at least 10 lb. The timing for cleft palate repair depends on the severity of the defect. Most often, this surgery is scheduled when the child is between 6 and 18 months of age. For severe defects, the surgical repair may require stages until the child is 4 or 5 years old.

When surgery is performed later, a prosthetic speech device usually is fitted so that speech development may not be hindered. Cleft palates usually involve other difficulties, such as frequent respiratory tract infections and orthodontia and speech problems.

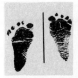

Nursing Care Plan

The Infant With a Congenital Heart Defect

Patient Goals

1. Infant exhibits the absence of respiratory distress.
2. Infant tolerates regular feeding pattern.
3. Infant's respiratory and heart rates stabilize.
4. Infant maintains fluid balance status.

Assessment	Potential Nursing Diagnosis	Planning and Intervention	Evaluation

Familial history of congenital heart defects	Ineffective breathing patterns related to congestive heart failure	Observe infant for
		  Cyanosis
		  Murmurs, arrhythmias
		  Absent or unequal pulses
		  Tachypnea
		  Retractions
		  Grunting
		  Nasal flaring
		  Edema
		  Decrease in urine output
		  Difficulty in coordination of breathing, sucking, swallowing
			Infant exhibits lack of respiratory distress

Presence of
  Cyanosis
  Murmur
  Congestive heart failure
  Respiratory distress
	Impaired gas exchange related to congenital cardiac defect		Infant returns to normal feedings

Other congenital anomaly present	Alteration in nutrition, less than body requirements, related to difficulty breathing, sucking, and swallowing		Infant's respiratory and heart rates stabilize
	Fluid-volume excess related to congestive heart failure		Infant maintains fluid balance
	Decreased cardiac output related to congestive heart failure, congenital heart defect	Provide continuous monitoring	
		Monitor vital signs frequently	

		Provide assistance with diagnostic procedures
		  Chest film
		  Echocardiogram
		  Cardiac catheterization	

		Give small, frequent feedings with rest periods	
		Put up head of bed after feeding	
		Record strict intake and output	
		Monitor daily weights	
		Administer drugs as ordered	
		Administer oxygen	

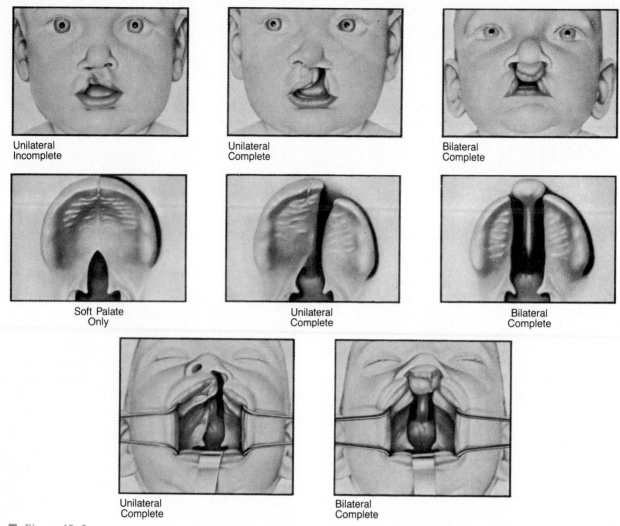

Unilateral
Incomplete

Unilateral
Complete

Bilateral
Complete

Soft Palate
Only

Unilateral
Complete

Bilateral
Complete

Unilateral
Complete

Bilateral
Complete

■ *Figure 45–3*
Illustrations of cleft lip and cleft palate. (Redrawn from drawing provided by Ross Laboratories)

Therefore, the care of these children requires a coordinated, multidisciplinary effort. Professionals from a craniofacial team may include a pediatrician, audiologist, otolaryngologist, speech pathologist, geneticist, dental specialists, surgeons, nurses, and social workers.

NURSING ASSESSMENT

The family is assessed for grief and loss behaviors, coping methods, and strengths. Parents are encouraged to hold and provide caretaking activities for the infants. The infant is assessed for the severity of the defect. The infant also is assessed thoroughly for any respiratory distress, airway obstruction, and feeding ability and tolerance. Early assessment should be made by the craniofacial team.

NURSING DIAGNOSIS

Potential nursing diagnoses include potential parental knowledge deficit related to infant care; high risk for

dysfunctional grieving; potential alteration in parenting; high risk for alteration in nutrition, less than body requirements; and high risk for airway obstruction.

PLANNING AND INTERVENTION

The nurse provides the family with clear explanations and addresses questions as needed. The family must see the infant immediately after birth. Positive aspects of the infant's appearance should be emphasized, and the infant should be accepted by the nurses as all the other infants in the nursery are. Nurses can expect that parents will display grief behaviors and have a need to ventilate. Providing assistance with feeding will help to decrease any parental anxieties. The nurse should encourage parental caretaking because bonding may be initially delayed.

Feeding. Potential feeding problems include ineffective suck and difficulty swallowing properly, thereby allowing secretions to pool in the nasopharynx and predisposing to aspiration. Because the infant can have difficulty creating an effective seal, nutritional intake could be compromised. Considering the variables affecting the situation, such as the severity of the defect, the nurse promotes the most natural feeding method possible. Infants with less severe defects may be able to breast-feed successfully. The let-down reflex can be stimulated with the use of a breast pump. The nurse may refer the mother to a lactation specialist or home health agency for further assistance after discharge. For bottle-fed infants, various special types of long nipples and soft bottles are available for use (Fig. 45-4). The parents are

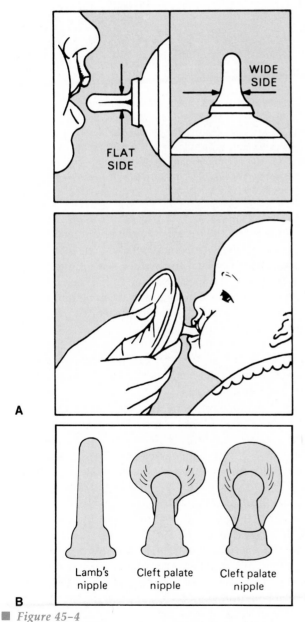

■ *Figure 45–4*
Nipples used for feeding babies with cleft lip and palate. (A) Beniflex Nurser. (B) Other types of nipples. (Beniflex Nurser courtesy of Mead Johnson)

instructed to hold the infant as upright as possible during the feeding and aim the nipple toward the intact part of the palate. The caregiver may need to use squeezes of the bottle to assist the infant. The use of an acrylic prosthetic device may be used to create a seal over the defect. Occasionally, other feeding methods such as gavage or rubber-tipped asepto syringe feeder may be necessary.

Preoperative and Postoperative Nursing Interventions. Parents require information concerning the surgery, such as the type of anesthesia, extent of parental involvement and participation permitted, and special types of restraints and other apparatus to be expected postoperatively.

Postoperatively, elbow restraints to prevent flexion may be required. Lip care as prescribed is carried out. The use of a Logan's bow is optional to prevent tension on the suture line. Most centers resume feedings 24 hours after lip surgery and 48 hours after palate surgery.[6] Children with palatal repairs may have a suture through the tip of the tongue secured to the cheek during the first 24 hours to maximize airway management. A mist tent may be used to treat upper airway congestion.

EVALUATION

As a result of appropriate nursing interventions, the family should experience an adequate knowledge base, be given the opportunity to grieve, as well as to provide caretaking to the infant. The infant will not experience respiratory distress and will receive adequate nutritional intake for body requirements.

Hypospadias

Hypospadias is a disorder in which the urethral meatus lies somewhere proximal to the tip of the glans penis, either on the ventral surface of the glans or penile shaft, or, in severe cases, on the perineum. In contrast, epispadius is a congenital anomaly in which the urethral meatus is located on the dorsal surface of the penis (Fig. 45-5). Hypospadias is the second most common genital abnormality (after cryptorchidism) in the male newborn. Infants with hypospadias have familial histories and sometimes have associated urinary tract anomalies. Severe hypospadias may be associated with other genital abnormalities such as endocrine, intersex, or chromosomal abnormalities. Hypospadias may also occur in some rare syndromes that have poor prognoses.

MANAGEMENT

Management includes maternal history taking for evidence of possible maternal progestin or estrogen ex-

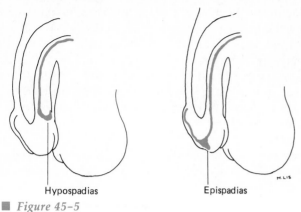

■ *Figure 45–5*
Illustration of hypospadias and epispadias.

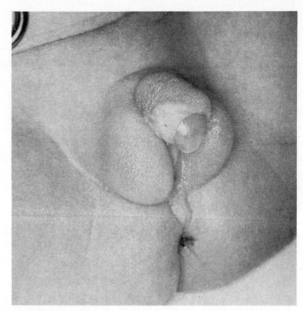

■ *Figure 45–6*
Infant born with ambiguous genitalia. From this photograph it is difficult to tell whether this patient has an atypical penis with penoscrotal hypospadias or whether there is extreme masculinization of the clitoris and scrotal changes of the labia majora. (Avery GB: Neonatology: Pathophysiology and Management of the Newborn, 3rd ed. Philadelphia, JB Lippincott, 1987)

posure and family history of hypospadias, endocrine, or other intersex problems.

Maternal progestin exposure may have occurred at 8 to 14 weeks' gestation. The infant is assessed for any urinary tract abnormalities and the extent of the hypospadias. Sexual organs are assessed to rule out any potential intersex problems. Circumcision is withheld, selection of sex is accomplished, and the infant is evaluated for any rare associated syndromes.

Surgical repair ideally is carried out during the first year of life. A severe form of hypospadias may require staged surgeries.[7]

Intersex Problems

Any discrepancy in the genetic, gonadal, or genital makeup of a person is defined as an intersex problem (Fig. 45-6). The reader may wish to review Chapter 10 for normal fetal differentiation and Chapter 14 for genetic defects in sex chromosomes. It is essential for the identification and diagnosis of intersex problems to be carried out in an expedient manner to be able to provide sex assignment, identify any associated anomalies requiring treatment, provide genetic counselling, and correct problems early so that the patient will have a strong sense of gender identity. The complexity and number of intersex problems are beyond the scope of this text; the reader is referred to the Suggested Reading list. In terms of management, if an intersex problem is suspected, the parents should be told that sexual assignment is delayed until definitive diagnostic evaluation is made, which should require only 2 to 3 days.

Diagnostic evaluation begins with a history and physical examination and chromosomal analysis. Various biochemical studies and hormonal assays are completed. Internal genital structures are assessed by way of endoscopy.

Based on complex selection criteria, selection of sex is made. Subsequent management of the patient may involve hormonal treatment and various reconstructive surgery. Surgery for the patient to be reared as a female should be completed in the first year. Surgery for the male should be done in infancy so that he can stand to urinate and have a normal genital appearance.[7]

The family is provided with genetic counseling once the specific diagnosis is known.

Spina Bifida

Spina bifida is a rather common malformation (1 in 500 live births) and is the result of the congenital lack of one or more vertebral arches, usually at the lumbar site (Fig. 45-7A). When the membranes covering the spinal cord bulge through the opening, the condition is known as *meningocele* (Fig. 45-7A). It forms a soft, fluctuating tumor filled with cerebrospinal fluid. The extrusion of the cord along with the meninges is known as *meningomyelocele* (Fig. 45-7A and B).

The degree of neurologic deficit is determined by the level of lesion. Surgical closure should take place within 24 hours to prevent further deterioration of the spinal cord and roots.[8]

The decision to intervene surgically is made by physician and family, bearing in mind the associated complications and long-term follow-up required.

Hydrocephalus may develop, depending on the site

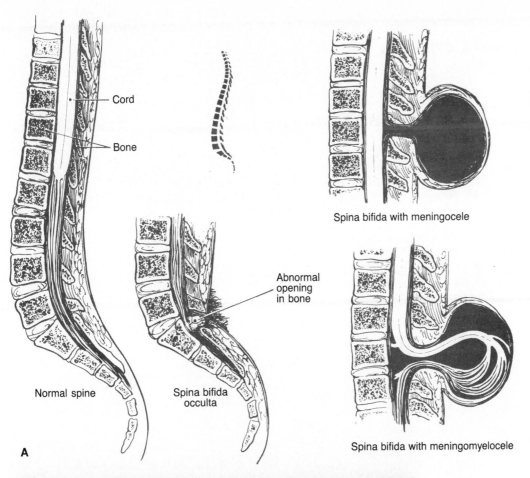

Cord

Bone

Normal spine

Spina bifida occulta

Abnormal opening in bone

Spina bifida with meningocele

Spina bifida with meningomyelocele

A

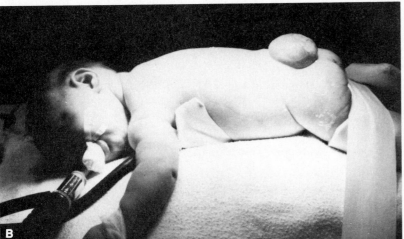

B

■ *Figure 45–7*
(A) *Spina bifida. (Spina Bifida: Hope Through Research. PHS Publication No. 1023, Health Information Series No. 103, 1970) (B) Meningomyelocele in the lumbosacral area. The patient is in a prone position with supporting blanket rolls beneath a heating blanket. (The heating blanket is not shown.) (Mayer BW: Pediatric Anesthesia: A Guide to Its Administration. Philadelphia, JB Lippincott, 1981)*

of the lesion, requiring serial shunts. Bowel and bladder involvement frequently is present. Orthopedic devices and surgery may be required, depending again on the site of the lesion.

ASSESSMENT

The family's level of understanding is evaluated as well as strengths, coping strategies, and grief. The infant is assessed for associated bowel and bladder complications as well as motor and sensory functions of the lower extremities. Assessment for potential of hydrocephalus is made because a strong association is prevalent.

NURSING DIAGNOSIS

Nursing diagnoses are delineated in the Nursing Care Plan: Family of Neonate With Meningomyelocele as

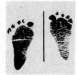

Nursing Care Plan

The Family of the Neonate With Meningomyelocele

Patient Goals

1. The neonate's lesion site is identified early, and related involvement is established.
2. The lesion site is infection free.
3. The neonate does not experience trauma to the lower extremities.
4. Any developing hydrocephalus or increased intracranial pressure is identified.
5. The neonate's bowel and bladder functions are maintained.
6. The parents are informed regarding long-term care and prognosis.
7. The parents follow through with demonstration of infant caretaking and any referrals as necessary.

Assessment	Potential Nursing Diagnosis	Planning and Intervention	Evaluation
Neural tube dysfunction ascertained during pregnancy testing	Infection related to neural tube defect and occasional leakage of fluid	*Preoperatively*	Neonate's vital signs are stable
Herniated sac noted at delivery		Protect sac by carefully positioning neonate on abdomen or side	
Complications of disease process		Cover defect with dressing as ordered	
Decrease in sensation and movement below lesion		Use doughnut-shaped device for support	
Bowel and bladder dysfunction		Observe sac for fluid drainage	
High risk for hydrocephalus		*Postoperatively*	
		Protect incisional site from contamination by urine or feces	
		Position on side or abdomen	
		Take temperature frequently	
		Inspect incisional site for redness or swelling	
	High risk for injury: trauma to lower extremities related to level of defect and lack of motion and sensation	Provide passive exercises to lower extremities frequently	Neonate responds to passive exercise
		Change position frequently	Neonate demonstrates absence of discomfort
		Refer to physical therapy	
	Alteration in bowel and bladder function related to level of nerve involvement	Note urine function—if stream or frequent dribbling	Neonate empties bladder
		Use Credé's method of emptying bladder	

(continued)

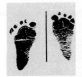

Nursing Care Plan (continued)

Assessment	Potential Nursing Diagnosis	Planning and Intervention	Evaluation
		Observe anal sphincter functioning by stimulation	Neonate responds to stimulation of anal sphincter
	High risk for injury: hydrocephalus related to meningomyelocele	Measure head circumference daily	Neonate's head grows at acceptable rate
		Observe for signs of increasing intracranial pressure	Neonate demonstrates absence of intracranial pressure
		Note bulging or tenseness of fontanel	
		Observe for irritability, change in behavior	Neonate behaves normally
	Impaired physical mobility related to loss of nerve innervation below lesion	Provide frequent range of motion exercises	Neonate responds to exercises
		Change position	Neonate is comfortable
		Support extremities	
		Consider long-term referral	
	Parental anxiety related to uncertainty of long-term diagnosis	Allow parents to discuss situation at length	Parents freely discuss the situation and prognosis
		Provide realistic information regarding long-term care and prognosis	Parents acknowledge understanding of long-term care
		Teach parents signs of increasing intracranial pressure, how to Credé bladder, how to provide range of motion exercises	Parents identify signs of increasing intracranial pressure
			Parents perform return demonstration on teaching
			Parents care for infant under supervision in the nursery setting
		Refer to multidisciplinary agencies, parental support group, spina bifida clinic	Parents follow through on support groups

well as the nursing care plan of the family experiencing grief found earlier in this chapter.

PLANNING AND INTERVENTION

Preoperatively, the nurse provides parental support and referral to the appropriate health-care professionals, especially physicians and spina bifida clinical specialist; social service; home health care; and parental support groups. The nurse provides information to the parents and promotes caretaking and bonding activities. The nurse positions the infant comfortably and protects the sac from trauma and infection.

Postoperatively, the nurse positions the infant, usually in the prone or the lateral positions so that the incisional site is kept infection free. Passive range of motion exercises are given to the lower extremities. Physical therapists may be able to assist in providing appropriate exercises. The nurse assists with bowel and bladder function, noting patterns. The bladder may need to be emptied by Credé's method.

EVALUATION

As a result of interventions, the neonate exhibits stable vital signs, responds to passive range of motion, has no discomfort, maintains bowel and bladder function, and demonstrates no evidence of hydrocephalus. Parents are able to discuss their feelings, ask pertinent questions, demonstrate appropriate caretaking, and use support groups as needed.

Hydrocephalus

Hydrocephalus results from an excess accumulation of cerebrospinal fluid in the ventricles of the brain. Normal cerebrospinal fluid circulation is impaired. The neonate demonstrates enlargement of the head as a result of increased intraventricular cerebrospinal fluid pressure. Additional signs are "setting sun" appearance of the eyes, separated sutures, tense fontanels, and prominence of the forehead (Fig. 45-8). Neurologic deficits may result, despite surgical shunting. The abnormal accumulation of fluid may occur between the brain and dura mater (external) or in the ventricular system of the brain (internal). As a result of the enlarged head, the fetus is often breech, necessitating cesarean delivery as a result of cephalopelvic disproportion.

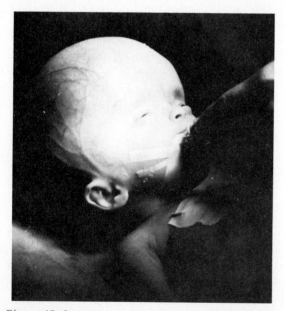

■ *Figure 45–8*

Hydrocephalus. Note the enlargement of the head, the prominent veins in the skin, and the "setting sun" appearance of the eyes. (Mayer BW: Pediatric Anesthesia: A Guide to Its Administration. Philadelphia, JB Lippincott, 1981)

NURSING INTERVENTIONS

The nurse provides skin care to prevent pressure areas and infection of the skin. The head must be supported with care when handling and feeding are done. Documentation of any possible sign of increased intracranial pressure is essential. The head circumference is serially assessed, as are enlarging fontanels and sutures, lethargy, vomiting, or irritability.

If a shunt procedure is performed, the neonate's shunt site is assessed for signs and symptoms of infection, and the neonate is positioned off the site initially, and in a flat plane to avoid sudden decompression and evacuation of the shunt. Parents are taught to assess the neonate for signs of increasing intracranial pressure and infection.

Anencephaly

In anencephaly, there is complete or partial absence of the infant's brain and of the skull overlying the brain. The cause is not known. Although there is a familial tendency in occurrences, multiple environmental factors seem to be involved. About 70% of anencephalic infants are female. Fifty percent of pregnancies involve polyhydramnios. If infants survive labor and delivery, their life expectancy is quite short. Supportive care is provided the infants; they seldom live more than a few days. The parents also need much support in grieving and integrating this traumatic situation.

Microcephaly

The microcephalic infant has an occipital frontal head circumference that is greater than three standard deviations below the mean or less than the 3rd percentile.[8] Microcephaly may be congenital or acquired. A maternal virus may be implicated, or microcephaly may be the result of a chromosomal abnormality. Acquired microcephaly may occur as a result of maternal herpes, ischemic insults, hypothyroidism, or aminoacidurias. Diagnostic evaluation includes a torch titer, skull x-rays, and amino acid screenings. No treatment is carried out.

Congenital Diaphragmatic Hernia

Congenital diaphragmatic hernia is a defect that is surgically correctable by removing the herniated viscera from the thorax and repairing the diaphragm. This defect is caused by the failure of the pleuroperitoneal cavity to fuse at 7 to 8 weeks' gestation (Fig. 45-9). Despite advances in care, the mortality rate remains at 50% to 80%. The left side is affected in 85% to 90% of the cases

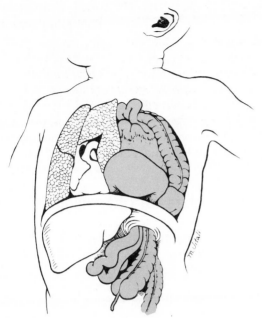

■ *Figure 45–9*
Diaphragmatic hernia showing abdominal contents within the
thoracic cavity. This is considered a true pediatric emergency.
(Mayer BW: Pediatric Anesthesia: A Guide to Its
Administration. Philadelphia, JB Lippincott, 1981)

as a result of later closure of the left posterolateral pleuroperitoneal membrane and the protection given to the
right posterolateral pleuroperitoneal membrane by the
liver. Herniation of the small intestine occurs in most
cases, and about half involve herniation of the liver. In
most cases, intestinal malrotation occurs. As a result of
pressure of the herniated bowel against the developing
lung, lung maturity is arrested, resulting in varying
degrees of pulmonary hypoplasia. Other related lung
disorders are abnormalities of pulmonary arteries, decreased number of pulmonary vessels, and predisposition for persistent pulmonary hypertension.[9]

ASSESSMENT

The neonate is noted to be in varying degrees of respiratory distress, depending on the extent of lung hypoplasia. Because of the mediastinal shift, venous return
is decreased, compromising cardiac output. The neonate
may be cyanotic and in a shocky state. The most common defect is in the left diaphragm. Breath sounds may
be decreased on the left side; a barrel or asymmetrical
chest results. The abdomen is scaphoid and empty. In
severe cases, the Apgar score is low and does not
improve.

POTENTIAL NURSING DIAGNOSES

Nursing diagnoses may include impaired gas exchange
related to hypoplastic lung syndrome; altered cardio-

pulmonary tissue perfusion; ineffective breathing pattern as a result of hypoplastic lungs; and alteration in
comfort related to the congenital defect.

PLANNING AND INTERVENTION

Major resuscitation efforts are attempted to reverse cardiopulmonary shock. A nasogastric tube is inserted to
prevent further bowel distension. Oxygen and ventilatory support are indicated. Intubation may be necessary with the lowest pulmonary pressures possible
and low positive end-expiratory pressure. High-
frequency, low-pressure ventilatory systems may be required. High-frequency jet ventilators have been used
with variable results.[9] Intubation and ventilation could
promote rupture in the hypoplastic lung so the neonate
needs to be monitored closely in the event that emergency surgery (such as a thoracotomy) is required. An
intravenous line is inserted to administer vasopressors
and volume expanders as ordered. Dopamine or tolazo-
line drips may be administered. Blood transfusions may
be necessary. Pulse oximetry and arterial blood gases
are required for monitoring respiratory status. Medications such as sodium bicarbonate may be administered
to promote acid-base balance.

MANAGEMENT

On medical stabilization of the neonate, surgical repair
is accomplished. The transabdominal approach remains
the method of choice, with the transthoracic another
alternative.

Postoperative Management. Priorities in the care of
the neonate postoperatively are the promotion of effective breathing patterns. Administration of oxygen
and maintenance of assisted ventilation are essential.
Other modes of ventilatory therapy such as extracorporeal membrane oxygenation have been used with
some success.[10,11]

Prevention of respiratory complications, such as
pneumothorax and acid-base imbalances, is a crucial
element in care. Vasodilators and vasopressors may be
necessary to promote adequate circulation.

EVALUATION

The prognosis of the neonate with this severe respiratory
involvement depends on the speed and efficiency of the
management effort.

Esophageal Atresia and
Tracheoesophageal Fistula

Esophageal atresia and tracheoesophageal fistula are
common anomalies. Pure esophageal atresia with no

connection to the trachea accounts for a small portion of these defects. Of the four types of tracheoesophageal fistulas, the most common is the esophageal atresia with a distal fistula to the trachea (occurrence rate of 80–90%). See Figure 45-10 for an illustration of the types of atresia.

DIAGNOSIS AND MEDICAL MANAGEMENT

The neonate has difficulty swallowing secretions, feeding, and maintaining an open airway. A history of maternal polyhydramnios is common. Diagnosis is made by passage of a radiopaque tube without contrast. Once diagnosis is established, a double-lumen tube is placed to low suction to prevent aspiration. The mouth and nose may need to be suctioned periodically. The infant may be placed in the prone or head-up position, depending on the type of defect. An intravenous line is inserted. Broad-spectrum prophylactic antibiotics may be administered to prevent infection.

Postoperatively, whether the neonate has a gastrostomy tube depends on the surgeon's preference and the type of defect. With a blind esophageal pouch, the prone position is preferred to promote drainage. Postoperative ventilatory assistance may be necessary. For suctioning purposes, the catheter is marked to prevent any damage to the suture line. Eight centimeters is the permitted distance for suctioning. For neonates with endotracheal tubes, suctioning should be permitted only to the length of the endotracheal tube.[1] Before feedings are resumed, a contrast study may be performed to determine if any leaks will occur. A retropleural tube is placed to gravity flow. Antibiotics are continued. Major postoperative complications are stricture, abnormal esophageal motility, and a leak at the anastomotic site.

Bowel Atresia and Stenosis

Any portion of the bowel may be narrow, but certain areas have a higher risk for abnormalities. The duodenum at the entrance of the common duct is the most common site for atresia or stenosis.[1]

ASSESSMENT

A maternal history of polyhydramnios is common. Gestational age assessment often reveals a small-for-gestational-age infant. Infants have difficulty feeding, and abdominal distension occurs. If the defect is beyond

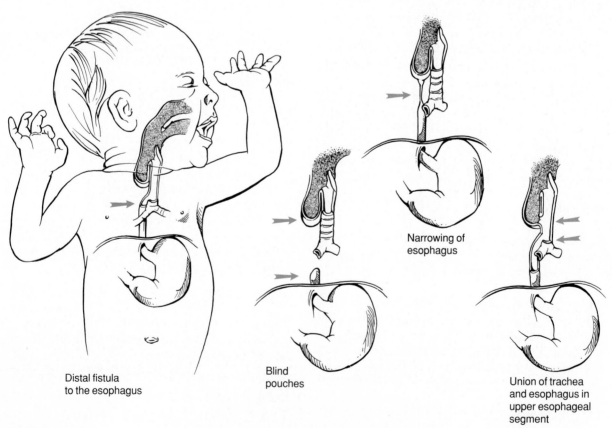

Narrowing of esophagus

Distal fistula to the esophagus

Blind pouches

Union of trachea and esophagus in upper esophageal segment

■ *Figure 45–10*
Esophageal atresia. (A) The most common form of esophageal atresia. (B) Both segments of the esophagus are blind pouches. (C) The esophagus is continuous, but with a narrowed segment. (D) The upper segment of the esophagus opens into the trachea.

the entrance of the common duct, bile-stained vomiting occurs. If the stenosis is above the common bile duct, the vomiting will not be bile stained but will be saliva or undigested milk.

MANAGEMENT

On diagnosis by x-ray, surgery is indicated. A classic "double bubble" is demonstrated on an abdominal upright film in duodenal atresia. Surgical repair may be accomplished by end-to-end anastomosis or various types of ostomies if end-to-end anastomosis is not possible.

PLANNING AND INTERVENTION

Preoperatively, an orogastric tube is inserted and maintained postoperatively to prevent abdominal distension. Fluids are administered intravenously; a Broviac catheter may be inserted in surgery for the purposes of admin-

istering total parenteral nutrition. The ostomy site is covered with a saline sponge until the stoma begins to function and an appliance can be placed. Accurate gastric output is kept, because fluid and electrolyte balance depends on intravenous replacement of fluid losses (see Nursing Care Plan: Infant With a Tracheoesophageal Fistula).

Imperforate Anus

Imperforate anus consists of atresia of the anus, with the rectum ending in a blind pouch (Fig. 45-11). There are approximately 34 major categories. The imperforate anus may be a high or low defect, with or without fistula to the bladder, vagina, or urethra[1] (Fig. 45-12). The male usually has a high lesion and the female a low lesion. The defect is obvious on physical examination. Ultrasound assists in establishing the exact level of obstruc-

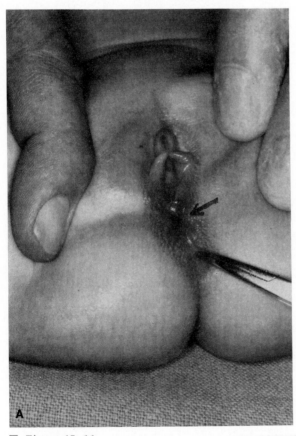
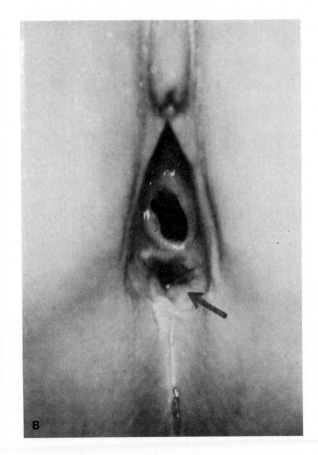

■ *Figure 45–11*

(A) Female with imperforate anus. The arrow demonstrates perineal fistula opening. The clamp is at the point where a normal anus would open. (B) Closeup of female with imperforate anus and an introital fistula just inside the labia minora and immediately beneath the hymenal ring. This is the most common form of fistulous opening in female imperforate anus. (Avery GB: Neonatology: Pathophysiology and Management of the Newborn, 3rd ed. Philadelphia, JB Lippincott, 1987)

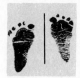

Nursing Care Plan

The Infant With a Tracheoesophageal Fistula

Patient Goals

1. The neonate remains infection free.
2. The neonate maintains adequate nutritional and fluid status.
3. The neonate demonstrates absence of complications.

Assessment	Potential Nursing Diagnosis	Planning and Intervention	Evaluation
Maternal history of hydramnios	Ineffective airway clearance related to structural defect	*Preoperatively*	Neonate remains free of aspiration pneumonia
Neonatal regurgitation and cyanosis with first feeding	Impaired gas exchange related to aspiration	If suspected anomaly due to large amounts of secretions and respiratory distress, do not feed	
Inability to pass nasogastric tube		Use sterile water for first feedings, if necessary	
Respiratory distress		Assist with diagnostic tests	
		Manage double-lumen indwelling suction tubing	
		Raise head of bed slightly	
		Postoperatively	Neonate's nutrition is adequate to prevent dehydration and promote weight gain
		Chest tube maintenance Keep tube secure Keep clamp nearby in case of dislodgement; clamp close to chest wall Record and describe drainage from chest tube Position with head of bed raised	Neonate remains free of postoperative complications
	Alteration in nutrition: less than body requirements, related to surgical procedure (inability to feed immediately postoperatively)	Administer oxygen as ordered	
		Monitor intake/output	
		Administer gastrostomy feedings as tolerated and as ordered	
		Suction gently—mark suction catheter to minimize vigorous suctioning and any damage to suture lines	

tion and ruling out a fistula. Types of surgical interventions range from a primary perineal repair to a colostomy procedure.

A corrective pull-through for the colostomy patient can be done at 1 year of age. The neonate with a high lesion with urinary fistula must be also assessed for renal and vertebral anomalies. Infants have chronic constipation following the pull-through procedure, thus requiring a high residue diet with occasional enemas or suppositories.

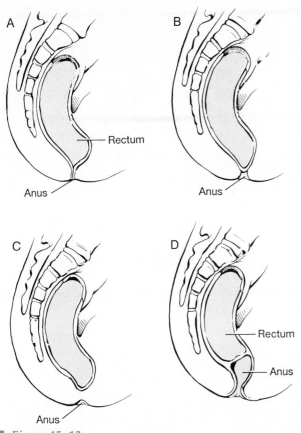

■ *Figure 45–12*

(A) Anal stenosis—Anal opening is present but constricted. (B) Membranous atresia—Anal and rectal structures appear normal except for a shiny, translucent membrane. (C) Anal agenesis—Rectum terminates in a blind pouch (80% of all anorectal abnormalities). (D) Rectal atresia—Anal canal is developed but does not communicate with the rectum.

Abdominal Wall Defects

OMPHALOCELE

Omphalocele is a congenital abdominal wall defect, occurring in 1 in 5000 births, in which an amount of the abdominal contents protrudes at the base of the umbilicus (Fig. 45-13). Omphaloceles develop between the tenth and twelfth week of fetal life. The mass is covered with a layer of peritoneum and amnion and may rupture at delivery. Omphaloceles are often seen in conjunction with other cardiac, genitourinary, neurologic, or chromosomal anomalies.

Before surgery, the bowel should be cleansed gently, covered with a plastic sac, layer of plastic food wrap, or saline-soaked sponge covered with a dressing. This covering assists in thermoregulation by decreasing evaporative loss and prevents contamination and trauma.[1] An orogastric tube is placed. The neonate should be positioned in the lateral position and the

bowel supported to prevent injury to the mesenteric blood supply. Antibiotics are administered. Maintenance and replacement intravenous fluids are administered. Volume expanders such as normal saline, albumin, or plasma protein fraction (Plasmanate) assist in maintaining intravascular integrity. Postoperatively, the neonate may require a Broviac catheter placement for long-term total parenteral nutrition. Several postoperative complications could occur. Respiratory distress could occur as a result of the increase in abdominal pressure. Ventilatory assistance may be needed. The abdominal vessels may be compressed by the surgical replacement of abdominal contents. The result can be a decrease in cardiac return. Edema of the lower extremities results from third spacing of fluid into tissue and an increase in extravascular volume. Elevation of the extremities may alleviate swelling. Finally, infection is a major postoperative problem.

GASTROSCHISIS

Gastroschisis, "ruptured omphalocele," is currently occurring more frequently than omphalocele, reversing previous trends.[1] Neonates with gastroschisis are often small for gestational age and preterm. Unlike omphalocele, gastroschisis has few associated anomalies.

The lesion is not covered with membrane, and the umbilical cord protrudes lateral to the defect in the abdominal wall (Fig. 45-14). Treatment is similar to that for omphalocele.

■ CHROMOSOMAL ANOMALIES

Chapter 17 discusses genetic disorders in depth. This section describes typical neonates with trisomy 13, 18, and 21.

Trisomy 13, or D

Trisomy 13 is characterized by an extra chromosome in the D group, which includes pairs 13 through 15 (see Chap. 14). Infants with this abnormality frequently have difficulty establishing and maintaining respiration. One of the most striking features is the abnormal cranial development. The cranium is usually small, with a sloping forehead. The ears may be malformed and low set, and the eyes usually have some defect (cataracts, iris defects, unusual smallness), often bilaterally. Cleft palate and lip are commonly present. In addition, the hands and feet are often grossly deformed. Extra digits are common on both hands and feet. The thumbs may be retroflexible (double jointed). The foot frequently has

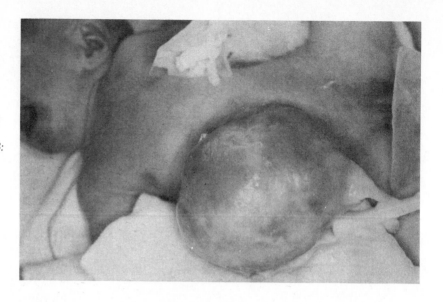

■ *Figure 45–13*
Large omphalocele. Note covering of the sac and its relationship to the umbilicus, which protrudes from the lower portion. (Avery GB: Neonatology: Pathophysiology and Management of the Newborn, 3rd ed. Philadelphia, JB Lippincott, 1987)

a posterior prominence of the heel sometimes accompanied by a convex sole, known as ''rocker-bottom'' foot. Other defects may include a bulbous nose, umbilical and diaphragmatic hernias, abnormal genitalia, scalp defects, and extensive capillary hemangiomatas far in excess of what is usually found in the normal newborn.

Neurologic examination reveals these infants to have a weak or absent Moro reflex and little or no response to loud noises; hence, they appear to be deaf. They are prone to develop myoclonic seizures. All suffer from apneic spells of unknown origin. Autopsy often reveals the complete lack of olfactory nerves and tracts. All of these infants are mentally retarded, and most have severe cardiac defects (dextroposition of the heart, ventricular septal defect), which are the major contributors to death. The average life span is less than a year, although several have lived to the age of 5 years.[12]

Trisomy 18, or E

Trisomy 18 is characterized by an extra chromosome in the E group, which includes pairs 17 and 18 (see Chap. 14). These babies are usually born at term, but are small, averaging about 2 kg (5 lb). Their placentas are often very small. The head is small with an occiput that is prominent but proportionate to the body size. The eyes are usually normal, but the ears are generally malformed and low set. The mouth appears small because of the short upper lip, and the mandible is small, giving a receding chin.

The hands of these babies are always malformed, but in a different way from those in trisomy 13 infants, and they give the best diagnostic clue to the condition. These babies keep their fists clenched most of the time, with the index finger overlying the third finger.

Profuse lanugo covers the forehead, back, and ex-

■ *Figure 45–14*
Patient with gastroschisis. Note edematous, matted bowel, the result of the intestines floating freely in the amniotic fluid. Remarkably, these distorted viscera will ultimately fit back into the abdominal cavity and will finally assume a normal appearance and function. (Avery GB: Neonatology: Pathophysiology and Management of the Newborn, 3rd ed. Philadelphia, JB Lippincott, 1987)

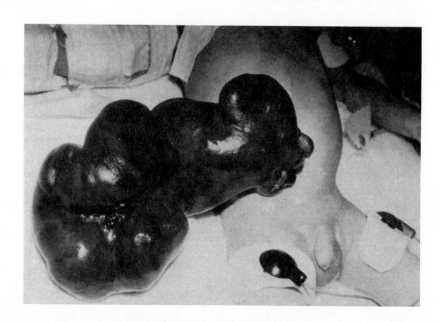

tremities, and the skin usually has a mottled appearance. The sternum is very short; thus, the abdomen appears long. The pelvis is small, with limited abduction of the hips. There also may be abnormal genitalia. Inguinal and umbilical hernias are frequent; diaphragmatic eventration (elevation of a thinned portion of the diaphragm) occurs more often than frank hernia in these patients.

Neurologic examination reveals abnormal muscle tone. These babies progress from a hypertonic state to frank opisthotonos. Opisthotonos is a dorsal arched position of the body in which the feet and head touch the floor or bed. Because the sucking reflex is poor, gavage feeding is often instituted. Unlike trisomy 13, trisomy 18 babies demonstrate no gross brain abnormalities. Cardiac abnormalities are common, and either these or aspiration accounts for the death of these babies.

The life span of these infants is less than 6 months on the average. During this time, they become progressively undernourished and present a failure-to-thrive syndrome. As with trisomy 13, some infants have survived to childhood, so that death in infancy cannot be predicted.[12]

Trisomy 21, or Down's Syndrome

In Down's syndrome, an extra chromosome belonging to pair 21 or pair 22 or a translocation of 15/21 is found (see Chap. 14). Although these babies are apt to have congenital defects and are more susceptible to infection, they can be expected to live much longer and have less severe mental retardation (although it can be very severe) than the other trisomy infants.

The eyes are set close together and are slanting, have narrow palpebral fissures, and contain Brushfield's spots. The nose is flat. The tongue is large and fissured and usually is very obvious because it protrudes from the open mouth. The head is small, and posteriorly the occiput appears flat above the broad, pudgy neck (Fig. 45-15). The hands are short and thick, especially the fingers (the little finger is curved), with simian creases apparent on the palmar surfaces. In addition to having defective mentality and the deformities mentioned above, these infants have underdeveloped muscles, loose joints, and heart and alimentary tract abnormalities.[12]

Incidence and Etiology. The incidence of Down's syndrome has been estimated at 1 in 500 births. This ratio, however, has dropped with the lowering of maternal age. For statistics on incidence with increasing maternal age, see Chapter 14.

Types. The most common chromosomal defect of the ovum in Down's syndrome is trisomy of chromosome 21 or 22. This results in a total chromosomal count of

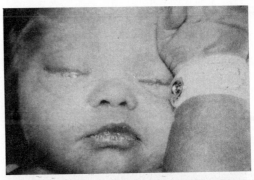
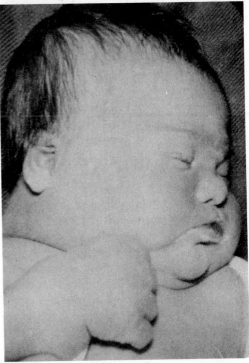

■ *Figure 45–15*
Patient with Down syndrome. (Avery GB: Neonatology: Pathophysiology and Management of the Newborn, 3rd ed. Philadelphia, JB Lippincott, 1987)

47 instead of the normal number of 46. This type, commonly referred to as *standard trisomy*, usually occurs in infants born to older women and is rarely familial. The incidence of standard trisomy is 1 in 600 births.

The second type of abnormality results from a 15/21 translocation; in this type the actual chromosomal count is 46. The translocation type of Down's syndrome usually occurs in infants born to younger parents, is of the familial type, and is rare.

The third type of the disorder, *mosaicism*, is very rare. A unique factor in mosaicism is that one person may have cells with different chromosomal counts. Laboratory tests may demonstrate that the affected person's blood cells, for example, have 47 chromosomes, whereas the skin cells may show 46 chromosomes. This is not a familial type of Down's syndrome, and, moreover, the abnormalities may be less severe.

Prognosis. The usual causes of death in these babies are heart defects and infectious illnesses. The survival rate is variable.

Planning and Intervention

Immediate care is supportive for the infant. Warmth, prevention of infection, maintenance of fluid and electrolyte balance, and, often, oxygen therapy are provided. Nursing interventions are aimed primarily at supporting the parents in helping them to work through their grief. The supportive aspect is particularly important because of the grave prognosis for these babies. It is often helpful to institute home health care for long-term referrals.

■ INBORN ERRORS OF METABOLISM

Numerous metabolic disorders, so-called inborn errors of metabolism, are now known to originate from mutations in the genes that alter the genetic constitution of a person to the extent that normal function is disrupted. These biochemical disorders arise because of the disturbance (mutation) in a molecule of the gene itself. They do not stem from some mishap or alteration during the embryonic development of tissue or organs. The mode of transmission of these inborn errors usually is recessive (i.e., to be affected, an infant must receive a pair of defective genes, one from the mother and one from the father). The mother and father in these cases would be carriers of the defective genes but would not be affected by the resulting disorder *per se.* Fortunately, defective genes are found rather infrequently in the general population, and the chance of their joining is rare; hence, the diseases they produce are rare.

It is important to remember that these inborn errors of metabolism do not usually produce symptoms that are apparent at birth. Therefore, maternity nurses will rarely see evidence of these disorders although they are involved in neonatal screening tests.

Neonatal Screening Tests

Screening for inborn errors of metabolism varies among states and countries. Testing for phenylketonuria is universal. Other tests available on a statewide basis are (in order of incidence) congenital hypothyroidism, galactosemia, maple syrup urine disease, homocystinuria,

biotinidase deficiency, sickle cell disease, congenital adrenal hyperplasia, and cystic fibrosis. Treatment is available for 66% of inborn errors of metabolism.[13]

Phenylketonuria

Phenylketonuria, the result of an inborn error of metabolism, reflects the absence of the liver enzyme phenylalanine hydroxylase. Without this enzyme, phenylalanine cannot be converted to tyrosine. As a result, toxic levels of phenylalanine and its metabolites, phenylpyruvic acid and phenylacetic acid, accumulate in blood, urine, and the central nervous system. The affected child has a musty odor, decreased pigmentation of skin and hair, and progressive mental retardation. The incidence is about 1 in 1500 live births. Minimal central nervous system damage will be done if early diagnosis is made and treatment is begun before 3 months of age.

Even with diet, children demonstrate lower school achievement and mean intelligence quotient than their siblings.

The most commonly used screening method is the Guthrie method, which uses small amounts of blood placed on filter paper. Accuracy of the test depends on adequate ingestion of protein for 24 to 48 hours. With current short hospital stays, a repeat test may be necessary in a few weeks. Phenylalanine levels of about 4 to 8 mg/dl are considered a presumptive positive. Parents can also check the infant's urine against a test strip at about 6 weeks of age. A green color reaction is positive. Treatment must begin before 3 months of age to prevent mental retardation.

The only treatment is dietary restriction to keep phenylalanine levels between 8 and 10 mg/dl.[13]

Diet needs to be low in phenylalanine, yet with sufficient blood phenylalanine levels to allow for growth. The infant may receive Lofenalac (low phenylalanine) in combination with a routine formula. Another diet is a formula containing no phenylalanine (Analog XP) in combination with breast milk. Frequent monitoring of phenylalanine levels is essential. Parents require multidisciplinary support.

Galactosemia

Galactosemia is an autosomal recessive disease and an inborn error of carbohydrate metabolism. The body is unable to metabolize galactose and lactose owing to lack of complex enzyme structures. Levels of galactose in the blood lead to cataract formation, renal disease, liver dysfunction, and some degree of mental retardation. Formulas such as Nutramigen or ProSobee may be used as treatment because they are lactose free. Other treatment may be necessary for concomitant clinical problems.

Congenital Hypothyroidism

Thyroid deficiency is believed to have been present at or before birth. Factors that may be responsible are inborn error of metabolism, maternal iodine deficiency, or maternal ingestion of antithyroid drugs.

Early signs include hypotonia, lethargy, large fontanels, respiratory distress, feeding problems, hypothermia, constipation, pallor, and poor cry.

Classic features that appear at about 6 weeks of age include depressed nasal bridge; relatively narrow forehead; puffy eyelids; coarse hair; large tongue; thick, dry, cold skin; abdominal distention; bradycardia; hypotension; and hyporeflexia.

Treatment consisting of thyroid replacement should be initiated immediately. Although physical recovery is usually good, the outlook for mental recovery is less favorable.[14] Authorities differ on the merits of treatment in the prevention of mental retardation.

Maple Syrup Urine Disorder

In maple syrup urine disease, three branched-chain amino acids are unable to be metabolized. The result is a rapidly progressing disease characterized by severe depression of the central nervous system and ultimately death from respiratory failure. Some degree of success is reported in a diet low in leucine, isoleucine, and valine. Frequent monitoring of these amino acids is essential to provide for adequate growth but not excess amino acids.[15]

Homocystinuria

Homocystinuria is an autosomal recessive disease with progressive clinical symptoms. There is a reduction in the activity of cystathionine synthetase, which leads to the building of homocystine in the blood and urine and methionine in the blood. A gradual buildup of metabolites does not clinically present until 2½ to 3⅓ years.

Signs are dislocation of lenses, skeletal deformities, thrombotic episodes, and mental retardation. Treatment is the administration of pyridoxine or a diet low in methionine and high cystine.[15]

■ MUSCULOSKELETAL DISORDERS

Talipes Equinovarus (Clubfoot)

Clubfoot occurs twice as often in males as in females, with an overall incidence of 1 in 1000 births.[16] The three elements of this deformity are equinus or plantar flexion of the foot at the ankle, varus or inversion deformity of the heel, and forefoot adduction (Fig. 45-16). All three are present in classic talipes equinovarus. Infants with this deformity should be examined for associated anomalies, especially those of the spine. There is a hereditary pattern in some families. Clubfoot may also be part of a generalized neuromuscular syndrome. Therapy begins early. If the foot can be manipulated to the other direction, simple exercise may correct the abnormality. Plaster casts may be applied after the affected foot structures have been stretched and manipulated. Casts are applied sequentially, correcting first the forefoot adduction, then inversion of the heel, and, lastly, the equinus flexion at the ankle. Serial casting is needed as the infant grows. After correction is obtained, braces are usually needed for months to years to prevent recurrences of the deformities. Surgery is rarely required.[16]

Congenital Hip Dysplasia

Congenital hip dysplasia refers to malformations of the hip involving various degrees of deformity that are present at birth. Congenital hip dysplasia occurs in 1 in 4 to 7 per 1000 births. It occurs more frequently in females than in males. One fourth of the cases are bilat-

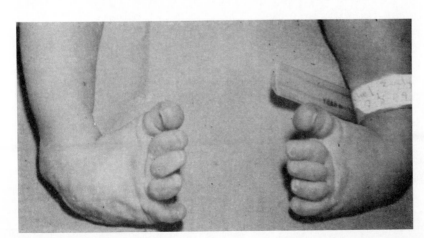

■ *Figure 45–16*
Talipes equinovarus (clubfoot). (Avery GB: Neonatology: Pathophysiology and Management of the Newborn, 3rd ed. Philadelphia, JB Lippincott, 1987)

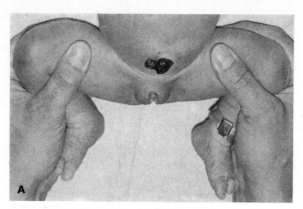
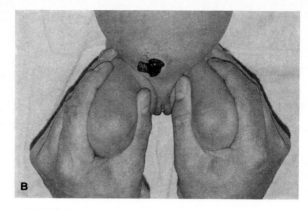

■ *Figure 45–17*

(A) Ortolani's sign. The fingers are on the trochanter and the thumb grips the femur as shown. The femur is lifted forward as the thighs are abducted. If the head was dislocated, it can be felt to reduce. (B) The thighs are adducted, and if the head dislocates, it will be both felt and seen as it suddenly jerks over the acetabulum. (Avery GB: Neonatology: Pathophysiology and Management of the Newborn, 3rd ed. Philadelphia, JB Lippincott, 1987)

eral; if unilateral, the left hip is involved more often than the right.

There is a significantly higher incidence of congenital hip disorders and breech presentation. Dislocation (luxation) refers to the femoral head lying outside the acetabulum but still within the stretched and elongated capsule. Subluxation of the femoral head refers to the head riding on the edge of the acetabulum.

When either dislocation or subluxation occurs, acetabular dysplasia results.

ASSESSMENT

Ortolani's maneuver is carried out when the infant is supine with the knees bent and hips flexed to 90 degrees and fully abducted (Fig. 45-17). When the hip is reduced by abduction, a click is felt as the femoral head slides across the posterior aspect of the acetabulum and enters the socket. With hip adduction, the femoral head redislocates out of the acetabulum with a click.

Barlow's maneuver, a modification of Ortolani's,

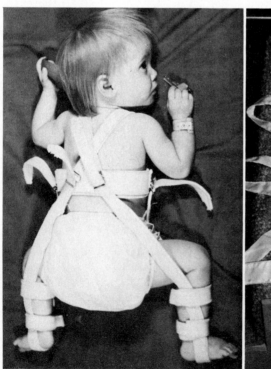
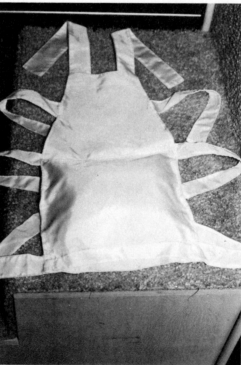

■ *Figure 45–18*

Nonrigid Frejka apron, an abduction device used to correct a dislocated hip. (Coleman S: Congenital Dysplasia and Dislocation of the Hip. St Louis, CV Mosby, 1978)

will detect almost all congenital hip dislocations; Ortolani's misses some cases in the neonatal period. In Barlow's test, the infant is supine with hips flexed to 90 degrees and the knees are fully flexed. The index finger of each hand is placed over the greater trochanter and the thumbs opposite the lesser trochanter, in the femoral triangle. The hips are placed in midabduction and thumb pressure applied posteriorly over the lesser trochanter; a congenital hip will dislocate across the acetabular posterior rim. When the thumbs are released, the femoral head will be reduced back into the hip socket.

Ultrasound assists with physical assessment and diagnosis.

PLANNING AND INTERVENTION

Early diagnosis and intervention are essential for the prevention of chronic deformity. No matter the type of deformity, the hip needs to be maintained in a position of flexion and abduction. Methods used vary from triple diapers to orthopedic splints, or Frejka pillow splint (Fig. 45-18). If these methods are ineffective, a hip spica cast may be applied, to be followed by a brace. Successful treatment is usually accomplished in 3 to 4 months.[16]

Parents need education and support in applying corrective measures or appliances, using adaptive feeding and holding techniques, and understanding the course of treatment and expected results. If the patient is identified and treated early, the long-term prognosis for correction is good.

Polydactyly

Polydactyly, a hereditary condition, consists of extra digits on the hands and feet. If the digits do not include bones, ligation with a silk suture during the neonatal period is often adequate to cause sloughing of the tissue, leaving only a small scar after a few days. Surgery is required if bones are present in the extra digits. Surgery should wait until the function of each of the duplicated digits is certain.

■ REFERENCES

1. Merenstein G, Gardner SL: Handbook of Neonatal Intensive Care, pp 539–547, 593–595. St. Louis, CV Mosby, 1989
2. NAACOG OGN Nursing Practice Resource: Grief Related to Perinatal Death. 13:2–3, June 1985
3. Whaley LF, Wong DL: Nursing Care of Infants and Children, pp 383, 1283–1286. St Louis, CV Mosby, 1983
4. Lees MH, King DH: The cardiovascular system. In Fanaroff AA, Martin RJ (eds): Neonatal-Perinatal Medicine, pp 639–743. St. Louis, CV Mosby, 1987
5. Kurczynski TW: Congenital malformations. In Fanaroff AA, Martin RJ (eds): Neonatal-Perinatal Medicine, pp 253–277. St. Louis, CV Mosby, 1987
6. Curtin G: The infant with cleft lip or palate: More than a surgical problem. J Perinat Neonat Nurs 3(3):80–89, 1990
7. Danish RK: Metabolic and endocrine disorders: Part V. Abnormalities of sexual differentiation. In Fanaroff AA, Martin RJ (eds): Neonatal-Perinatal Medicine, pp 1155–1166. St. Louis, CV Mosby, 1987
8. Brann AW, Schwartz JF: Central nervous system disturbances: Developmental anomalies and neuro-muscular disorders. In Fanaroff AA, Martin RJ (eds): Neonatal-Perinatal Medicine, pp 534–552. St. Louis, CV Mosby, 1987
9. Theorell CJ: Congenital diaphragmatic hernia: A physiologic approach to management. J Perinat Neonat Nurs 3(3):66–79, 1990
10. Gerraughty AB, Younie LJ: ECMO: The artificial lung for gravely ill newborns. Am J Nurs 87:655–658, 1987
11. Roberts PM, Jones MB: Extracorporeal membrane oxygenation and indications for cardiopulmonary bypass in the neonate. JOGNN 19(5):391–400, 1990
12. Polin RA, Mennuti MT: Genetic disease and chromosomal anomalies. In Fanaroff AA, Martin RJ (eds): Neonatal-Perinatal Medicine, pp 231–252. St. Louis, CV Mosby, 1987
13. Schmidt K: A primer to inborn errors of metabolism for perinatal and neonatal nurses. J Perinat Neonat Nurs 2(4):60–71, 1989
14. Morishima A: Metabolic and endocrine disorders: Thyroid disorders. In Fanaroff AA, Martin RJ (eds): Neonatal-Perinatal Medicine, pp 1102–1105. St. Louis, CV Mosby, 1987
15. Nicholson JF: Inborn errors of metabolism. In Fanaroff AA, Martin RJ (eds): Neonatal-Perinatal Medicine, pp 1016–1048. St. Louis, CV Mosby, 1987
16. Dick HM: Orthopedic problems. In Fanaroff AA, Martin RJ (eds): Neonatal-Perinatal Medicine, pp 1235–1243. St. Louis, CV Mosby, 1987

■ SUGGESTED READING

Baker K, Kuhlmann T, Magliaro B, et al: Homeward bound: Discharge teaching for parents of newborns with special needs. Nurs Clin North Am 24(3):655–664.
Lynch ME: Congenital defects: Parental issues and nursing supports. J Perinat Neonat Nurs 2(4):53–56, 1989
Fink B: Congenital Heart Disease. Chicago, Year Book Medical Publishers, 1985
Paxton JM: Transport of the surgical neonate. J Perinat Neonat Nurs 3(3):43–49, 1990
Shaw N: Common surgical problems in the newborn. J Perinat Neonat Nurs 3(3):50–65, 1990
Walden BJ: The newborn infant with Down Syndrome: Realities and possibilities. J Perinat Neonat Nurs 2(4):72–82, 1989

46

The High-Risk Infant: Acquired Disorders

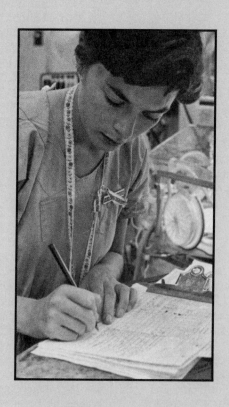

Certain factors have an impact on the neonate's transition to extrauterine life. These include maternal disorders, birth trauma, and postnatal infections and physiological processes as affected by the newborn's environmental systems. Most neonates make the transition to extrauterine life smoothly. For those neonates that do not, the professional's skills in the delivery room and the nursery are important to their future development.

Infants with acquired disorders may be only mildly affected, or they may be confined to an intensive care unit for months. Parents of these infants need teaching from nurses to be able to cope with any unexpected illness of the infant. Parents also need assistance in dealing with guilt associated with this traumatic experience.

■ BIRTH TRAUMA

Assessment

Immediate observation of the newborn in the delivery room usually permits the nurse to identify injuries or anoxia resulting from the birth process. A thorough neonatal assessment (discussed in Chap. 29), alertness to subtle changes in the newborn's behavior and condition, and careful recording of observations are important in the ongoing care.

Nursing Diagnosis

Nursing diagnoses will help to determine intervention in physical problems of the neonate and psychosocial problems concerning the family. Diagnoses of the newborn may include such items as alternation in comfort, pain related to the specific injury; impairment of skin integrity related to immobility (in casting of fractures); and high risk for injury, shock related to intracranial hemorrhage.

Knowledge deficit related to the type of disorder, its prognosis, and home care may be an important diagnosis concerning the family.

Planning and Intervention

Some kinds of birth trauma require emergency intervention to save the infant's life; others can be treated later or resolve spontaneously in several days. Facility with emergency techniques enables the nurse to promote the well-being of the high-risk infant with an acquired disorder.

After managing the emergency situation, the major responsibility of the nurse is to minimize the pain. The nurse must use judgment in using procedures that will alleviate pain or lessen it as much as possible. Gentle handling of the infant is important. Positioning will also aid in pain relief. The newborn's vital functions must be supported.

In some cases, immobilization of a fracture will be necessary, and the nurse must take steps to avoid skin breakdown. Observations and management used in general cast care are adapted to the newborn.

Communicating with parents by providing information and support is a major nursing responsibility (see Chap. 45). The nurse should share with the parents the description of the condition and possible outcomes. They should be shown how to handle the baby and be given time for touching and stroking if the newborn's movements must be kept to a minimum. Training in home care will give the family confidence in its ability to care for newborns when they are released. Follow-up appointments should be made and a telephone number provided that the parents may call for additional help.

Specific interventions are included in the discussion of each condition.

Evaluation

As mentioned earlier, some injuries will resolve spontaneously. Other newborns may be moved to a neonatal intensive care unit, and still others will go home with their parents. Evaluations will differ in each case. Major concerns will be that the newborn has little pain or is pain free; that the newborn has stable vital signs; and that the parents are knowledgeable about their newborn's condition and confident about their ability to care for the infant at home.

Head Trauma

CAPUT SUCCEDANEUM

Soft, edematous swelling of the scalp frequently occurs over a portion of the presenting part. Pressure from the uterus or birth canal can precipitate the accumulation of serum or blood above the periosteum. Swelling may cross suture lines. No treatment is indicated. A caput succedaneum usually resolves spontaneously in a few days (Fig. 46-1).[1]

CEPHALHEMATOMA

Cephalhematoma is not as common as caput succedaneum. The incidence is 0.4% to 2.5% of all live births.

Research Highlight

The technical aspects of the operation of the transcutaneous bilirubinometer, potential problems that may be encountered by the user, and research concerning the instrument's validity and reliability have been written about. The transcutaneous bilirubinometer can be a useful tool for nursing research as well as a tool to evaluate neonatal jaundice in the home setting. The instrument can identify those infants requiring serum bilirubin determinations as well as prevent other infants from being subjected to unnecessary blood sampling. Responses to treatment such as home phototherapy can be evaluated by the nurse using the instrument as a guide.

Brown L, et al: Transcutaneous bilirubinometer: An instrument for clinical research. Nurs Res 39(4):241–243, 1990)

Cephalhematoma is caused by a collection of blood between the bone and periosteum. The suture lines are not crossed by this hematoma. Usually it is unilateral, but it may be bilateral. Cephalhematoma occurs during labor and delivery owing to the rupture of blood vessels crossing the skull to the periosteum. It may be precipitated by prolonged labor or the use of forceps. Because the bleeding is a slow process, it may take hours or days for the swelling to be noticeable. It may be obvious by the second or third day. Most cephalhematomas resolve in 2 weeks to 3 months, with the majority resolving by 6 weeks of life (Figs. 46-2 and 46-3.)[2]

A skull fracture is present in 10% to 25% of affected infants.[2]

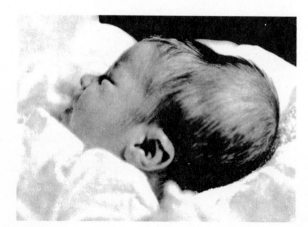

■ *Figure 46–1*
Caput succedaneum. (Courtesy of MacDonald House, University Hospitals of Cleveland)

The nurse's role in caring for infants with caput succedaneum and cephalhematoma is the reassurance of parents that both conditions will resolve without treatment.

INTRACRANIAL HEMORRHAGE

The following categories of intracranial hemorrhage in the newborn can be associated with birth trauma.

Subarachnoid Hemorrhage. Subarachnoid hemorrhage is the most common type of neonatal intracranial hemorrhage. Trauma is the most common cause in term infants; hypoxia is the most common in preterm infants. Subdural hemorrhage is more common in term infants than in preterm infants as a result of trauma tearing veins and venous sinuses.

ASSESSMENT. Irritability, decreased level of consciousness, seizures, and apnea may occur in subarachnoid hemorrhage. Lumbar punctures and computed tomography scans assist in and confirm the diagnosis. Subdural hemorrhage causes definitive neurologic abnormalities such as apnea, coma, unequal pupils, nuchal rigidity, and opisthotonos.

INTERVENTIONS. Parent teaching and referral to support groups are essential, gearing information to particular infant prognosis. Complications of subdural hemorrhage may range from none to permanent neurologic deficits. The major potential complication of subarachnoid hemorrhage is hydrocephalus.[2]

Perinatal Hemorrhage and Shock

Blood loss from hemorrhage can occur at any time in the perinatal period: prenatal, intranatal, or neonatal. If there are significant amounts of blood loss, the end result may be shock. Anemia occurring early in neonatal life may also be due to some form of perinatal hemorrhage.

PERINATAL INFLUENCES

Fetal–maternal transfusion is common but not usually severe enough to cause anemia in the newborn. Fetal-to-fetal transfusion occurs only in identical twins. Significant anemia occurs in only 15% of the cases. Major blood loss can occur from various obstetric problems[3] (Table 46-1).

ASSESSMENT

A neonate in hypovolemic shock has cool, clammy skin, mottled or gray extremities, diminished pulses, and decreased capillary refill. Low blood pressure and central venous pressure (CVP) will be evident along with com-

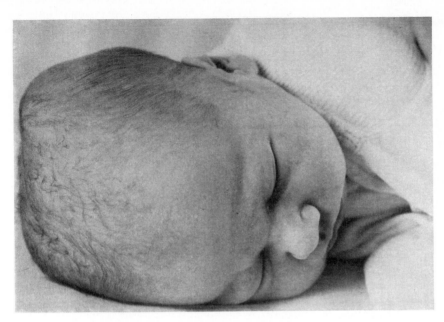

■ *Figure 46–2*
Cephalhematoma. (Courtesy of Mead Johnson Laboratories)

pensatory tachycardia. Dehydration is evident by dry mucous membranes, poor skin turgor, and sunken fontanels.

Laboratory values may indicate electrolyte imbalances, metabolic acidosis, hypoglycemia, and abnormal coagulation patterns (Table 46-2). Because renal blood flow is dependent on cardiac output, any decrease leads to decrease in urine output.

TREATMENT

Immediate treatment is resuscitative in nature. Central and peripheral intravenous lines are inserted. Critical care monitoring is employed, including electrocardiogram, CVP, pulmonary artery catheter, pulse oximetry, or transcutaneous oxygen monitor. Fluid replacement is administered by the use of various kinds of volume expanders. Blood and blood products are administered as needed (Table 46-3).[4] Pharmacologic interventions may be necessary (Table 46-4).

Nervous System Problems

FACIAL PARALYSIS

Facial paralysis due to pressure on cranial nerve VII may occur as a result of a difficult vaginal delivery or pressure of forceps on the facial nerve, which may cause temporary paralysis of the muscles of one side of the face so that the mouth is drawn to the other side. This will be particularly noticeable when the infant cries. Other signs noted are inability to close the eye on the affected side and absence of wrinkling of the forehead. The condition is usually transitory and disappears in a few days, often in a few hours. No medical treatment is necessary. Because the infant can look grotesque, the parents will need an explanation concerning the temporary nature of this affliction (Fig. 46-4).

If the mother is allowed to feed the baby, the nurse should be with her consistently during the first feedings

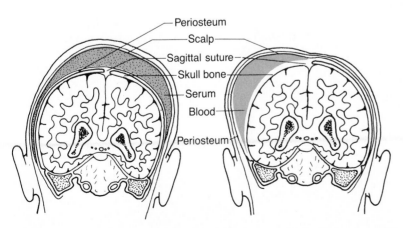

■ *Figure 46-3*
Comparative diagram of the underlying pathophysiology in caput succedaneum (left) and cephalhematoma (right).

TABLE 46-1. TYPES OF BLOOD LOSS EXPERIENCED BY THE NEONATE

Perinatal	Neonatal
Fetal-maternal transfusion	Intracranial hemorrhage
Fetal-to-fetal transfusion	Intraventricular hemorrhage
Rupture of umbilical cord	Organ hemorrhages
Rupture of placental vessels	Cephalhematomas
Placenta previa	Iatrogenic loss due to blood
Abruptio placentae	sampling[3]

(Adapted from Braune KW, Lacey L: Common hematologic problems of the immediate newborn period. JOGN Nurs 12(3) (Suppl): 19s–26s.)

to help her as necessary. Sucking may be difficult for the infant, and the mother needs to develop patience and skill in the feeding of her baby.

If one eye remains open because of the affected muscles, the physician prescribes such treatment as is appropriate. Artificial tears may need to be instilled daily to prevent drying, or a protective eye patch may be used. Any necessary instruction regarding continuing care after discharge should be given to the mother before she leaves the hospital.

Often, when disorders occur, parents are afraid to handle their infant for fear of hurting him or her. This may happen even if the condition is short term and fairly innocuous. Thus, parents should be encouraged to hold and cuddle their infants whenever their condition permits.

ARM PARALYSIS

Brachial plexus injury is the most common nerve injury of the newborn. Damage to the upper plexus (Erb's palsy) is more common than damage to the lower plexus (Klumpke's palsy).

Erb's palsy usually occurs as a result of pulling or stretching the shoulder away from the head, a result of vertex or breech delivery. Symptoms are a limp arm with elbow extended, wrist pronated, and arms internally rotated. The grasp reflex is present, but the deep tendon reflex is absent. The Moro reflex is lessened or absent on the affected side (Fig. 46-5).

Treatment includes maintaining the correct alignment by proper positioning, intermittent immobilization, and frequent full range of motion exercises to prevent contractures. Immobilization may be completed by a splint or pinning the shirt sleeve to the mattress.

Symptoms of lower plexus injury are limited to the forearm and hand. There may be edema and cyanosis of the part. The wrist and hand are limp and the deep tendon reflex is present, but the grasp is absent. Treatment is similar to that for Erb's palsy.[1]

PHRENIC NERVE INJURY

Phrenic nerve injuries occur most often in conjunction with brachial palsy, which is usually the result of a difficult breech delivery. Because the phrenic nerve is the only nerve innervating the diaphragm, paralysis of the diaphragm occurs, usually unilaterally. Symptoms are those of respiratory distress. The infant should be positioned on the affected side and given intravenous

TABLE 46-2. NORMAL HEMATOLOGIC VALUES DURING THE FIRST WEEK OF POSTNATAL LIFE IN THE PRETERM AND TERM INFANT

Value	Cord Blood	1 Week (postnatal age)
Preterm (≤1500 g)		
Hemoglobin (g/dl)	13.0–18.5	14.8
Hematocrit (vol %)	49.0	45.0
Reticulocytes (% of erythrocytes)	10	3
Platelets		150,000–350,000
Term		
Hemoglobin (g/dl)	14–20	17.0
Hematocrit (vol %)	53.0	54.0
Reticulocytes (% of erythrocytes)	3–7	0–1
Platelets		200,000–400,000

(Braune KW, Lacey L: Common hematologic problems of the immediate newborn period. JOGN Nurs 12(3)(Suppl): 19S–26S, 1983; Adapted from Oski F, Naiman J: Hematologic Problems in the Newborn, 2nd ed. Philadelphia, WB Saunders, 1972)

TABLE 46-3. GUIDELINES FOR SAFE TRANSFUSIONS

Risk	Nursing Interventions
Volume overload	Adjust fluid intake as prescribed, report excessive weight gains and symptoms of congestive heart failure. Monitor fluid intake and output. Except in emergencies, give routine transfusions slowly over 3–4 h
Thromboemboli	Avoid using regional arterial lines; use venous lines when possible. Use saline flushes before and after transfusion. (Glucose flushes will cause clotting when in contact with blood for transfusion.)

Infection
  Cytomegalovirus (CMV)
  Hepatitis
  Acquired immune deficiency Syndrome (AIDS)
	Use CMV negative blood. Use blood screened for hepatitis and AIDS.

Hemolytic transfusion reactions	Type and crossmatch blood, then identify correct recipient of the blood product by double-checking patient's ID number and name with another qualified staff member.
Graft-versus-host disease (GVHD)	Use irradiated blood components for patients susceptible to GVHD.

Metabolic derangements
  Hypothermia
  Acidosis/alkalosis*
  Hyperkalemia*
 	
  Hypocalcemia*
 	
  Hypoglycemia
	
	Warm blood before giving.
	Monitor blood pH values as indicated, especially with exchange transfusion.
	Usually only with exchange transfusion: monitor serum potassium levels and report abnormal values.
	Usually only with exchange transfusion: monitor calcium levels; watch for cardiac arrhythmias.
	Monitor blood sugar levels according to established unit policy. Maintain levels at 45 mg/percent or above.

* These problems can be minimized if fresh blood (stored no longer than 5–6 days) is used for exchange transfusions.
(Kelting S, Johnson C: Erythropoiesis and neonatal blood transfusions. MCN 12(3):176, 1987)

fluids and oxygen if necessary. More severe respiratory distress may require mechanical ventilation. Surgical intervention to move the diaphragm down may be necessary if spontaneous recovery does not occur over time. Most infants recover spontaneously in weeks or months with supportive treatment. A potential complication is the occurrence of pneumonia in the atelectatic lung.[1]

Fractures

CLAVICLE

The clavicle is the bone most commonly fractured during delivery, usually as a result of dystocia (i.e., shoulder delivery in vertex or extended arms in breech). The infant may be asymptomatic. Symptoms that might be observed are decreased or absent mobility of the affected arm, discoloration of the site, crepitus along the clavicle, and absence of the Moro reflex on the affected side. No treatment or interventions are necessary other than gentle handling to minimize pain and proper alignment.[1]

LONG BONES

The humerus is the bone most often fractured following the clavicle. Fracture of the femur is the most common fracture of the lower extremities.

Fracture of the humerus occurs with difficult delivery of the arms or shoulders in a vertex delivery. The sign noted is immobility of the affected arm. The Moro reflex is absent on the affected side. The affected arm must be immobilized in the adducted position for 2 to 4 weeks to allow healing to occur. Immobilization may be carried out by splints or a cast.

Fracture of the femur may occur during a breech delivery. Deformity of the thigh, swelling, or immobility may be noted. Treatment is traction, suspension, and casting for about 3 to 4 weeks.[1]

SKULL

Because of the flexibility and molding of the infant's head, skull fractures are uncommon. They occur as a result of prolonged, difficult labor or forceps delivery. Fractures may be linear or depressed; most are linear.

TABLE 46–4. CARDIOVASCULAR DRUGS USED IN THE TREATMENT OF PEDIATRIC SHOCK

Drug	Usual Intravenous Dose	Comments
Isoproterenol	0.05–1.5 mcg/kg per min	Increases strength and rate of cardiac contraction. Dilates peripheral vessels. May increase myocardial work and oxygen consumption. May include arrhythmias.
Epinephrine	0.05–0.5 mcg/kg per min	At low doses, increases strength and rate of cardiac contraction to moderate degree and causes systemic vascular resistance (SVR) to decrease slightly at low doses. At high doses, causes marked increase in strength and rate of cardiac contraction and severe vasoconstriction of peripheral vasculature (increased SVR). As epinephrine may decrease renal blood flow significantly, monitor urine output.
Dopamine	1–20 mcg/kg per min (higher doses may be used)	Effects vary with dose: low dose response primarily dopaminergic; mid-range cause moderate increase in heart rate and contractility; high doses (10–20 mcg/kg/min) vasoconstriction predominates. May cause arrhythmias.
Dobutamine	2–15 mcg/kg per min (higher doses may be used)	Increases strength of cardiac contraction but causes minimal change in heart rate. On occasion, causes tachycardia and hypertension.
Amrinone	0.75 mg/kg initially; 5–10 mcg/kg per min (adult dose recommendation)	Increases strength of cardiac contraction and relaxes vascular smooth muscle, causing decreased afterload and preload. Clinical studies regarding use in children are ongoing.
Nitroprusside	0.5–10 mcg/kg per min	Dilates peripheral arteries and veins. May produce severe hypotension. Do not use in boluses. Immediate onset and short duration (2–4 sec) of action. Protect from light.
Phentolamine	1–20 mcg/kg per min	Dilates peripheral arteries and, to a lesser extent, veins. Also causes cardiac stimulation. May cause marked hypotension, tachycardia, and arrhythmias.
Hydralazine	0.1–0.5 mg/kg per dose every 3–6 h	Primarily vasodilates peripheral arteries. Also maintains or increases renal and cerebral blood flow. May cause tachycardia.
Tolazoline	1–2 mg/kg initially; 1–2 mg/kg per h	Decreases peripheral resistance and increases venous capacitance. Causes cardiac stimulation. Reduces pulmonary arterial pressure and resistance.

(Rimar JM: Shock in infants and children: Assessment and treatment. MCN 13(2):100, March/April 1988)

The infant will be asymptomatic with a linear fracture unless blood vessels become involved, leading to a subdural hematoma. Depressed fractures may require surgery if brain tissue is involved.[2]

■ NEONATAL INFECTIONS

Infectious diseases during pregnancy are discussed in Chapter 34. The following is a continuation of the discussion of those diseases as found in the neonate. The neonate is particularly vulnerable to infection for two reasons: the protective environment of the uterus is no longer available, and the neonate has not acquired defenses against disease. The fetus may have become infected in utero, or the neonate may become infected during passage through the birth canal or when exposed to the environment of the hospital and caregivers.

Assessment

Nurses are the chief observers of the neonate. They are in the presence of the neonate for longer periods of time than other caregivers, are experienced in recognizing signs and symptoms of sepsis, and can be aware of even slight changes in the newborn's condition. The behaviors, signs, and symptoms of sepsis in the neonate are often subtle and are noticed only by experienced caregivers. Neonatal nurses have the responsibility to note such behaviors so that diagnosis and treatment may be begun early. Their observations also may prevent an epidemic of infection within the newborn nursery (see Box).

NEONATES AT RISK

Maternal factors influencing neonatal sepsis include symptomatic bacteriuria during pregnancy, smoking

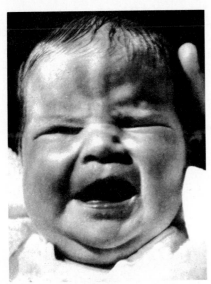

■ *Figure 46–4*
Facial nerve paralysis. Note the asymmetry of the mouth during crying.

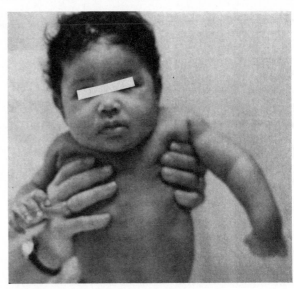

■ *Figure 46–5*
A 2-month-old baby girl with a left Erb's palsy. (Avery GB: Neonatology: Pathophysiology and Management of the Newborn, 3rd ed. Philadelphia, JB Lippincott, 1987)

Clinical Signs of Sepsis in the Neonate

Central Nervous System

Full fontanel
Lethargy
Jitteriness
Temperature instability
Irritability
Hypotonia
Tremors and seizures

Gastrointestinal

Feeding problems
Vomiting
Diarrhea

Skin

Rashes
Jaundice

Respiratory

Apnea
Cyanosis
Grunting

Laboratory

Positive blood cultures
White blood count > 35,000, < 25,000
Sedimentation rate > 5 mm/h

(indirectly promotes low birth weight), low socioeconomic status, and minority race.

At delivery, mothers with bacterial or viral infections of the urinary tract, vagina, or cervix may infect their infant during the birth process. Rupture of the membranes for longer than a 24-hour period has been associated with increased incidence of neonatal infection. Other factors associated with neonatal infection are bleeding secondary to placenta previa or abruptio placentae, fetal distress, and prolonged second stage of labor.[5] Scalp abscesses have been observed following internal fetal monitoring. Cephalhematomas occasionally lead to complications of osteomyelitis of the skull.

Male infants are more often infected than females. The neonate is more vulnerable to infection than even older children. Antibody levels are low, particularly IgA and IgM, because IgG is the only immunoglobulin acquired transplacentally. Decrease in the bacterial capacity, deficient leukocyte response, and deficient phagocytosis have been documented in the neonate. Serum complement components of Cl_Q, C3, and C5 and low levels of serum properdin have been demonstrated. Colostrum has been demonstrated to be effective protection against infection.[5]

Nursing Diagnosis

Nursing diagnosis involving the newborn may include the following: alteration in bowel elimination, diarrhea related to the infection; fluid-volume deficit related to vomiting, diarrhea, or feeding problems; alteration in respiratory functions, ineffective airway clearance related to specific infection; and alteration in comfort, pain related to the infection.

The family may be diagnosed for the following: knowledge deficit of care related to specific infection; and alteration in family processes related to stress of involvement and care.

Planning and Intervention

An important aspect of infection control is prevention (see Chap. 30). Once an infection is found in a neonate, steps must be taken to prevent further spread. Antibiotics used in infection management are listed in Table 46-5. Further interventions are discussed with each condition and in the nursing care plan at the end of this section.

Bacterial Infections

GASTROENTERITIS

Agents most commonly associated with gastroenteritis are enteropathogenic *Escherichia coli* (EPEC), *Salmonella,*

TABLE 46-5. DOSAGE SCHEDULES FOR ANTIBIOTICS FREQUENTLY USED IN NEWBORN INFANTS

		Daily Dosage per kg (No. of Doses)	
Drug	Route*	Infants < 1 wk Old†	Infants 1–4 wk Old
Amikacin	IV, IM	15–20 mg (2)**	20–30 mg (3)**
Ampicillin	IV, IM	50–75 mg (2 or 3)	75–100 mg (3 or 4)
For meningitis		100–150 mg (2 or 3)	150–200 mg (3 or 4)
Carbenicillin	IV, IM	200 mg (2)	300–400 mg (3 or 4)**
Cefazolin	IV, IM	40 mg (2)	40–60 mg (2 or 3)
Cefotaxime	IV, IM	100 mg (2)	150 mg (3)
Ceftazidime	IV, IM	100 mg (2 or 3)	150 mg (3)
Ceftriaxone	IV, IM	50 mg (1)	50–75 mg (1)
Cephalothin	IV	40–60 mg (2 or 3)	60–80 mg (3 or 4)
Chloramphenicol	IV, PO	25 mg (1)	25–50 mg (1 or 2)‡
Clindamycin	IV, IM, PO	10–15 mg (2 or 3)	15–20 mg (3 or 4)
Colistin sulfate	PO	15–20 mg (4)	15–20 mg (4)
Erythromycin	PO	20 mg (2)	30–40 mg (3)
Gentamicin	IV, IM	5 mg (2)	7.5 mg (3)
Kanamycin	IV, IM	15–20 mg (2)**	20–30 mg (3)**
Methicillin	IV, IM	50–75 mg (2 or 3)	75–100 mg (3 or 4)
For meningitis		100–150 mg (2 or 3)	150–200 mg (3 or 4)
Mezlocillin	IV, IM	150 mg (2)	225 mg (3)
Moxalactam	IV	100 mg (2)	150 mg (3)
Nafcillin	IV, IM	50 mg (2 or 3)	75 mg (3 or 4)
Neomycin	PO	100 mg (4)	100 mg (4)
Netilmicin	IV, IM	5 mg (2)	7.5 mg (3)
Oxacillin	IV, IM	50–75 mg (2 or 3)	100–150 mg (3 or 4)
Penicillin G	IV	50,000 units (2 or 3)	75,000–100,000 units (3 or 4)
For meningitis		100,000–150,000 units (2 or 3)	150,000–200,000 units (3 or 4)
Procaine penicillin G	IM	50,000 units (1)	50,000 units (1)
Ticarcillin	IV, IM	150–225 mg (2 or 3)	225–300 mg (3 or 4)**
Tobramycin	IV, IM	4 mg (2)	6 mg (3)
Vancomycin	IV	30 mg (2)	45 mg (3)

(Remington JS, Klein, JO: Infectious Diseases of the Fetus and Newborn Infant, 3rd ed, p 1067. Philadelphia, WB Saunders, 1990)
* Abbreviations: PO, oral: IM, intramuscular: IV, intravenous
† Lower dosages and less frequent administration may be needed in low birth-weight infants (see text).
** See text for more specific recommendations or explanation.
‡ Dosage should be based on serum concentrations achieved.

Shigella, Yersinia, Campylobacter, and, rarely, *Pseudomonas, Klebsiella, Enterobacter,* and *Candida albicans.* Classic symptoms are fever, vomiting, abdominal distention, and severe diarrhea.[5]

Management and Prevention. Any infant suspected of harboring an infection should be isolated as defined by agency procedure. In the case of diarrhea, stool culture should be taken from the suspect infant, as well as from others in the nursery. Prior to receiving culture reports, therapy for the primary infant and prophylactic therapy for other infants may be instituted. Medications of choice for EPEC are *neomycin* or *colistin sulfate.* Other therapy includes fluid and electrolyte maintenance through parenteral or oral routes.

An outbreak of diarrhea in the nursery may necessitate closure of the nursery to new admissions and a thorough cleaning of the physical environment. All personnel who come in contact with newborns should review infection control techniques as a preventive measure against future outbreaks.

INFECTIONS OF THE SKIN

Various lesions of the skin and subcutaneous tissue that result from bacterial infection include maculopapular rashes, vesicles, pustules, bullae, abscesses, cellulitis, impetigo, erythema multiforme, and petechiae or purpura. Most skin infections are the result of *Staphylococcus aureus.* Skin infection may occur as a primary event or may be part of a systemic infection. Diagnosis is accomplished by smear and culture of aspirated material from the lesion. The treatment of skin lesions (with the exception of those associated with systemic infection) consists of local antiseptic, systemic antimicrobial agents, and incision and drainage.[6]

SYPHILIS

Congenital syphilis occurs most often by transplacental passage of *Treponema pallidum* from an infected mother, although infection can also occur from contact with an infected lesion at birth.

The extent of the disease in the newborn depends on the time during gestation that the diagnosis was made, the extent of the disease in the mother, and the success of maternal treatment. If the mother is treated before the 18th gestational week, disease in the fetus is almost always prevented. Langhans' layer of the chorion, which provides a protective barrier, deteriorates between 16 and 18 weeks. Treatment after the 18th week may cure fetal spirochetemia in organ systems, but late changes of congenital syphilis may still occur.

A neonate with early congenital syphilis may be born prematurely. Other clinical indicators are hepatosplenomegaly; generalized lymphadenopathy; he-matologic abnormalities; mucocutaneous manifestations, such as a maculopapular coppery brown rash; bony lesions; nephrotic syndrome; neurologic manifestations; chorioretinitis; and intrauterine growth retardation. Definitive diagnosis is made by the observation of one or more of the signs and symptoms and positive laboratory findings of serologic tests.

Symptomatic congenital syphilis should be treated with penicillin in two intramuscular or daily intravenous doses for 10 days.

Late congenital syphilis may still appear with more complications of interstitial keratitis, deafness, bone, joint, and skin involvement.[5]

CONJUNCTIVITIS

Conjunctivitis in the newborn is most likely due to infection with *Neisseria gonorrhoeae,* inclusion conjunctivitis caused by *Chlamydia trachomatis,* or chemical conjunctivitis induced by silver nitrate solution. Infection with *N. gonorrhoeae* is characterized by edema, chemosis, and a profuse, purulent conjunctival exudate, occurring 2 to 5 days after birth. Infants with documented gonococcal infections should be treated with parenteral ceftriaxone or cefotaxime. Eyes are irrigated with saline until the discharge has cleared. Topical antibiotics are not effective alone. Prompt treatment protects against corneal involvement.

Inclusion conjunctivitis occurs from 5 to 14 days after delivery, presenting with watery eye discharge, changing to purulent with edema. Treatment is ophthalmic ointment or drops of tetracycline, erythromycin, or sulfonamides. Pneumonia may occur in these infants. Chemical conjunctivitis occurs anywhere from 6 to 24 hours after birth.[6] Chapter 25 discusses neonatal eye prophylaxis.

THRUSH

Thrush is an infection of the mouth caused by the organism *C. albicans,* the organism that causes maternal monilial vaginitis.

The condition appears as small, white patches (due to the fungus growth) on the tongue and in the mouth. Nystatin (Mycostatin) is the drug of choice in treating oral monilial infections.

PNEUMONIA

Pneumonia is a significant factor in 10% of neonatal deaths. Three types of pneumonia exist, depending on the time of presentation and the route of acquisition.

Transplacental pneumonitis is a congenital infection acquired in utero. Symptoms are manifested early and may be connected with infections such as cytomegalovirus, herpes, rubella, toxoplasmosis, and *Listeria monocytogenes.*

Aspiration pneumonia, acquired as part of the birth process, is manifested in the first few days of life. Organisms most often involved are group B β-hemolytic streptococci, group D streptococci, pneumococci, and coliform organisms.

Acquired pneumonia at delivery or in the postpartum period is the third type. *S. aureus* and coliform organisms are commonly implicated in postnatally acquired pneumonia. Symptoms of respiratory distress may vary but include nasal flaring, tachypnea, retractions, diminished breath sounds, and rales.

Diagnosis is based on blood cultures and chest roentgenogram.

Treatment consists of appropriate antibiotic therapy, oxygen, and supportive measures.

GROUP B STREPTOCOCCI

Group B streptococci are now the leading cause of early neonatal sepsis. Previously, coliform organisms retained this distinction. Five types of group B streptococci have been isolated. Sites of culture of the organisms are the throat, stools, and genital tract. The maternal carrier rate is about 30%, remaining relatively the same regardless of trimester. Incidence is about 1 to 3 in 1000 live births, with a mortality rate of 40% to 75%.

Two separate clinical syndromes have been identified. The early-onset type has a higher mortality rate than the late-onset type. Early-onset disease usually is manifested within 3 to 5 days of life and most often within 12 to 24 hours. Early-onset symptoms closely resemble those of respiratory distress syndrome.[7] It produces a fulminant pneumonia with an extremely high mortality rate (greater than 40%). The organism is sexually transmitted and is carried asymptomatically in the cervix and vagina in a significant number (over 20%) of pregnant women. The infection is thought to be contracted by contact during the birth process and is especially likely to occur when predisposing factors, such as prematurity, prolonged labor, and premature rupture of the membranes, exist. The rate of newborn colonization is high; however, the attack (infection) rate is low (1%–2% of colonized babies become infected). Screening of all gravidas and treatment of carriers has been recommended, but the practicality of the approach is open to serious question.

The late-onset syndrome, occurring between 10 and 50 days of age, presents as nonspecific signs of irritability, lethargy, apnea, failure to nurse, and fever. Meningitis often is the consequence of late-onset disease. The source is not necessarily the cervix, vagina, or even the mother. Mortality in late-onset infection is considerably less than the early-onset syndrome.

Diagnosis is presumed based on isolation of the organism from the neonate's gastric contents and confirmed by positive blood or cerebrospinal fluid cultures.

Treatment is supportive in addition to appropriate therapy following laboratory studies. Medications of choice include penicillin, ampicillin, vancomycin, semisynthetic penicillins, and first-, second-, or third-generation cephalosporins.[7]

TORCH Viruses

There are more than a dozen viral infections that the newborn may contract during the prenatal, intrapartum, and postpartum periods. They are categorized in the acronym TORCH, which represents *t*oxoplasmosis, *o*ther, *r*ubella, *c*ytomegalovirus, and *h*erpes simplex virus.

Maternal aspects of viral infections are discussed in Chapter 34.

TOXOPLASMOSIS

Congenital toxoplasmosis results from transplacental transfer of the parasite *Toxoplasma gondii* to the fetus. The neonatal incidence is 0.3 to 6 per 1000 live births. Not all infants born to a mother infected with toxoplasmosis during the pregnancy are affected by this disease. Most infants are without symptoms at birth (60%–75%).

Classic congenital defects are chorioretinitis, microcephaly, hydrocephalus, and cerebral calcifications.[8] Other indications of the disease include prematurity, intrauterine growth retardation, seizure disorders, and hepatosplenomegaly.[9]

Laboratory diagnosis isolates anti-Toxoplasma IgM fluorescent antibodies in cord or neonatal blood. Drugs of choice are pyrimethamine (1 mg/kg/day orally) and sulfadiazine (50–100 mg/kg/day).[10] Both drugs should be administered over a 21- to 30-day period. Folinic acid, 2 to 6 mg, should also be given three times a week to prevent anemia. These drugs may not reverse neurologic damage already incurred but may prevent further adverse effects.[9]

OTHER VIRAL INFECTIONS

Hepatitis B Virus. The incidence of hepatitis B virus (HBV) infecting the newborn is 0 to 7 per 1000 live births. Routes of transmission are varied. Most infants are affected primarily during the last trimester of gestation or at the time of delivery from contaminated secretions in the birth canal.[9] Other potential routes in the postpartum period are contact with infected maternal saliva, urine, feces, serum, or breast milk.

Acquisition of the virus in utero may lead to low birth weight of the newborn. A small number of infants infected with HBV around the time of delivery may present with acute hepatitis accompanied by liver changes. Most remain asymptomatic. HBV may be cultured from amniotic fluid as a diagnostic measure. The presence of IgM may be noted in cord blood or neonatal serum. It is recommended that hepatitis B immune globulin be given to infants of infected mothers.[11]

RUBELLA

The incidence of congenital rubella has been noted as 0.5 to 0.7 per 1000 or 3 to 5 per 1000 during epidemics. Although rubella is generally considered to be a relatively mild illness, for the fetus whose mother has been exposed with subsequent transplacental transmission, the consequences may be disastrous. Damage to the fetus may occur without obvious illness in the mother. Consequences in the fetus depend on the virulence of the virus and the gestational age of the fetus. The fetus is at a critical development stage during the first 4 weeks of pregnancy, when there is a 50% chance of a resulting anomaly. From the fifth to the eight week, chances decrease to 25%. From the ninth to the twelfth week, an 8% to 17% chance exists. There is a low percentage of 10% resulting in defects when maternal rubella occurs between 13 and 24 weeks.[12]

Major defects identified with infection occurring up to 4 weeks prior to pregnancy or during the first trimester are cardiac defects, cataracts, and deafness. There is a higher rate of spontaneous abortions and stillbirths. Some additional problems of infants infected in the first trimester are intrauterine growth retardation, glaucoma, hepatosplenomegaly, hepatitis, lesions in long bones, meningitis, and pneumonia.[12] Psychomotor retardation, microcephaly, and deafness result from second-trimester infection. Infection during the last trimester of pregnancy may also result in problems.[9] Approximately two thirds of neonates are asymptomatic.

In addition, the effects of the disease may be evident later, usually by age 5. Some may even exhibit neurologic deficits after age 10.

Diagnosis is established by hemagglutination inhibition or complement fixation antibodies in blood or rubella-specific IgM from cord or neonatal serum. Finally, rubella virus can be cultured from amniotic fluid, the placenta, and the neonate's throat, urine, or spinal fluid.

Treatment of the neonate consists in supportive management, surgical correction of defects as feasible, and multidisciplinary referral.

CYTOMEGALOVIRUS

Cytomegalovirus (CMV) is the most common of perinatal infections. In addition to transplacental transmission, contact with contaminated vaginal or nasopharyngeal secretions, urine, or feces can transmit the virus. Finally, less frequently, viral transmission occurs from blood transfusion or breast milk. CMV has been noted in preterm infants receiving multiple transfusions.[9] The incidence of congenital occurrence in the neonate is 0.5% to 1% of infants born each year in the United States. As with other congenital viruses, many neonates are asymptomatic. Congenital defects include bone lesions, anemia, low birth weight, hepatomegaly, splenomegaly, jaundice, petechiae, heart disease, pneumonia, cataracts, chorioretinitis, microcephaly, obstructive hydrocephaly, intracranial calcifications, and encephalitis. The most common findings are hepatosplenomegaly and jaundice.[9]

Diagnostic tools are positive viral cultures of amniotic fluid or neonatal serum, anti-CMV IgM antibodies in cord or neonatal serum, or the presence of CMV inclusion cells in urine or cerebrospinal fluid.

Treatment is supportive. Long-term follow-up is essential to monitor growth and development. Immunization to prevent infection is in the experimental stages. Drug therapy with antimetabolites and antiviral agents is also experimental.

HERPES SIMPLEX VIRUS (HSV)

Most neonates with herpesvirus infection are infected by herpes simplex, type 2, the genital version. Other neonates are infected by type 1, the oral virus. Herpes is the most common virus in pregnant women following CMV.

Most of these neonates come in contact with the virus at delivery when the infant passes through the infected maternal birth canal. The virus, however, also can ascend during pregnancy or following rupture of the membranes. Some cases of transplacental infection have been reported.[9] Finally, sites other than the genital area in the mother and other nonmaternal sources have been demonstrated.

The incidence in the neonate is 0.03 to 0.05 per 1000 live births. The greatest risk to the neonate at delivery occurs when the mother has had a primary herpetic lesion during at last 3 weeks of pregnancy. Thirty to 50% of neonates delivered through the infected birth canal are affected. Cesarean delivery should be performed when active lesions or positive herpes cultures are noted during the previous 2 weeks and when the membranes have been ruptured less than 6 hours or are intact.[9] A significant decrease in neonatal infection has been demonstrated if cesarean delivery is performed within 4 hours of membrane rupture.[8]

The incubation period for neonatal herpes is usually 6 to 11 days from birth to onset of disease. Some infants may be asymptomatic. Lesions may be seen in the eyes, throat, mouth, and skin. Disseminated disease is indicated by jaundice, purpura, respiratory distress, shock, and central nervous system involvement. Diagnosis is established by viral cultures of eyes, nose, throat, blood, urine, or cerebrospinal fluid. In addition, identification of herpes-specific IgM antibodies in cord or neonatal serum can be made. Vidarabine and acyclovir are drugs of choice.

Acquired Immunodeficiency Syndrome (AIDS)

Statistics place the number of pediatric AIDS cases at 1346 in the United States.[13]

By 1991, the number is expected to increase to 3200 to 10,000 cases.[14] Numbers of pediatric AIDS cases represent about 1% to 2% of the general AIDS population. HIV-infected children exhibit high morbidity and mortality rates.

Etiology. AIDS is an infectious disease caused by the human immunodeficiency virus, a virus that invades the T4 "helper" lymphocytes. As a result, the neonate's immune system is compromised as evidenced by lower resistance to infections.

Mode of Transmission. Wide variation in data exists concerning rates of transmission from seropositive mothers to neonates. It is unknown why some infants of HIV-positive mothers are not affected. Transmission of the virus occurs during prepartum, intrapartum, or postpartum periods by cross-placental transmission or exposure to vaginal secretions at birth. Breast milk is thought to be a possible source of transmission. The average age of onset of clinical signs is approximately 4 to 6 months of age. Most infants are diagnosed between 6 and 12 months of age. Diagnostic tests used to detect the HIV antibody are the ELISA test followed by the Western blot to confirm diagnoses and rule out false-positive results. Infants tested before 6 months of age may demonstrate false-positive results as a consequence of maternally transmitted antibodies. These infants' tests must be repeated at 6 months of age. Centers for Disease Control guidelines for positive diagnosis include the following:

Seropositive test for HIV antibody
Evidence of immunosuppression
Wasting syndrome
Encephalopathy
Presence of opportunistic disease[15]

Assessment. Common clinical findings are persistent oral candidiasis with failure to thrive, generalized lymphadenopathy, hepatosplenomegaly, and parotitis. Other bacterial infections to which they are susceptible are meningitis, pneumonia, septic arthritis, osteomyelitis, urinary tract infections, otitis media, and skin infections. Common opportunistic infections to which these children are vulnerable are *Pneumocystis carinii* pneumonia; oral candidiasis and esophagitis; recurrent diarrhea or severe diarrhea with malabsorption; and lymphoid interstitial pneumonitis.[13] Other clinical findings are central nervous dysfunction with developmental delay, nephropathy, hepatic abnormalities, anemia, leukopenia, and thrombocytopenia. Some dysmorphic features that have been documented are microcephaly, ocular hypertelorism, prominent boxlike appearance of the forehead, flat nasal bridge, mild upward or downward obliquity of the eyes, long palpebral fissures with blue sclerae, short nose with flattened columella, well-formed triangular philtrum, and patulous lips.[16]

Clinical Management. Medications used in the treatment plan are antimicrobials, AZT (azidothymidine), and intravenous gamma globulin. Other supportive care is given as indicated by any specific opportunistic disease present.

Potential Nursing Diagnoses. Potential nursing diagnoses include: high risk for infection; alteration in nutrition; high risk for spontaneous bleeding; alteration in respiratory function; alteration in elimination; alteration in comfort; social isolation; and knowledge deficit.

Nursing Interventions. The nurse assesses the neonate for signs and symptoms of infection. Vital signs are monitored, including temperature. The skin and oral mucous membranes are inspected; thorough, gentle mouth and skin care is provided. Aseptic technique is used for all invasive procedures. Visitors and staff are monitored for signs of infection.

The nurse monitors intake and daily weights. Supplemental nasogastric feedings or total parenteral nutrition may be indicated. Breastfeeding is contraindicated because the virus is thought to be transmitted via breast milk.

Trauma to skin is minimized or avoided. The nurse monitors for signs of bleeding.

Baseline respiratory status is documented and changes noted. Hydration status is maintained. Chest physiotherapy and suctioning are used as needed. Oxygen therapy may be indicated. The neonate is positioned to maintain an open airway. Resuscitation masks are available at the bedside for use in the event of a respiratory arrest.

Stool elimination patterns are monitored along with any signs or symptoms of dehydration.

Comfort measures, such as repositioning, pacifier use, touch, and administration of pain medications are used.

Parents are provided with information regarding the disease as well as the opportunity to verbalize feelings. Parents' emotional distress may necessitate referrals to support groups and mental health professionals.

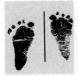

Nursing Care Plan

Neonates With Infections (Prevention and Management)

Patient Goals

1. Infected infants are identified and managed immediately.
2. Infants at risk for infection are assessed.
3. The infant is isolated, and spread of infection is curtailed.
4. Bowel patterns are adequate.
5. Fluid balance is present.
6. Infant demonstrates adequate weight gain.
7. Infant's respiratory status is stable.
8. Infant's vital signs remain stable.
9. Infant exhibits comfort behaviors.
10. Other infants in the nursery remain symptom free.

Assessment	Potential Nursing Diagnosis	Planning and Intervention	Evaluation
Maternal Factors			
Smoking	High risk for infection related to immature immune system, environmental factors, maternal exposure or actual infectious disease process, sharing of nursery	Continue to observe newborn for signs and symptoms	Infected infants are identified and managed immediately
Low socioeconomic status		Skin: rashes, lesions, jaundice	Infants at risk for infection are assessed
Bacterial or viral infections of the urinary tract, vagina, or cervix		Central nervous system: hypotonia, temperature instability, irritability, lethargy, full or bulging fontanel	The infant is isolated, and the spread of infection is curtailed
Rupture of membranes more than 24 h	Alteration in bowel elimination, diarrhea related to infection		Bowel patterns are adequate
Amnionitis			
Maternal bleeding			Fluid balance is present
Neonatal Factors			
Male sex	Fluid-volume deficit related to vomiting, diarrhea, or feeding problems	Respiratory: tachypnea, apnea, cyanosis, grunting, retractions, nasal flaring	Infant demonstrates adequate weight gain
Preterm			Infant's respiratory status is stable
Invasive procedures (surgery, diagnostic)	Alteration in respiratory functions, inefficient airway clearance related to specific infection	Gastrointestinal: vomiting and diarrhea, feeding problems	Infant's vital signs remain stable
Certain congenital malformations (i.e., meningomyelocele, gastroschisis)		Circulatory: hypotension; cool skin, mottling	Infant exhibits comfort behaviors
		Provide assistance in performing diagnostic tests	Other infants in the nursery remain symptom free
		Obtain various laboratory specimens as ordered	
		Frequently monitor vital signs and intake and output	

(continued)

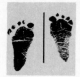

Nursing Care Plan (continued)

Assessment	Potential Nursing Diagnosis	Planning and Intervention	Evaluation
		Pay careful attention to environmental temperature	
		Administer antibiotics as ordered	
		Use infection protocol as per agency procedure– strict handwashing and any required isolation	

Family members have identified the need for a support person, especially for home-care situations.

Family members need to be taught precautionary measures regarding HIV transmission.

Evaluation. Nursing care has been effective when infection is recognized and minimized, no spontaneous bleeding occurs, nutritional status is adequate for growth and development, oxygenation needs are met, eliminatory patterns are adequate, comfort behaviors are exhibited, and parents are knowledgeable about the disease and have access to functional support systems.

Precautions for Nurses, Health Care Workers, and Family Members. Once an infectious process is diagnosed, the neonate is isolated as indicated by the specific disease process. The neonate may even be isolated if an infection is suspected, pending the results of diagnostic tests.

Disposable items are used in the provision of care. Soiled linens, diapers, and other contaminated items are disposed of in the appropriate plastic bags, according to agency policy. Handwashing is carried out before and after providing care. Gloves are worn when contact with mucous membranes, nonintact skin, blood, and other body fluids is anticipated, particularly when dressings and diapers are changed. Protective covers such as gloves, gowns, aprons, masks, and eye or face shields are worn during invasive procedures that may contaminate the eyes or face. Bulb syringes or wall suction units are used for suctioning. When performing heelsticks and venipunctures and inserting and discontinuing intravenous catheters, gloves are worn. Needles should not be recapped. Any needle sticks must be reported, according to agency procedure.

■ INFANT OF A DIABETIC MOTHER

The successful control of diabetes with insulin has led to survival and fertility of an increasing number of women. Better control of the diabetic state during pregnancy has increased the infant's chances for a healthy state of birth. The infant of a diabetic mother (IDM), however, still presents with a number of clinical problems that are best dealt with in the intensive care nursery setting.

IDMs may be large for gestational age, but most are appropriate for gestational age. Typically, the infant has a round face, soft skin, an abundance of subcutaneous fat tissue (Fig. 46-6), and a plethoric appearance.

Clinical Problems and Related Management

HYPOGLYCEMIA

Infants of class A to C or type I diabetic mothers are at risk for hypoglycemia. Maternal hyperglycemia is accompanied by fetal hyperglycemia. The fetal pancreas is thus stimulated, leading to hypertrophy of islet cells and hyperplasia of beta cells with subsequent increase

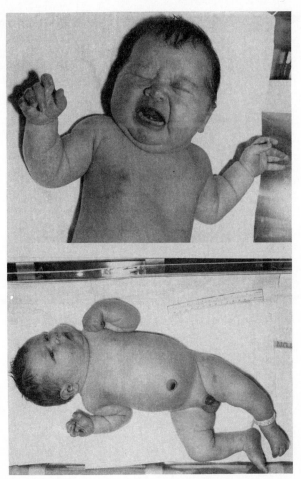

■ *Figure 46–6*
The infant of a diabetic mother showing typical features. (Avery GB: Neonatology: Pathophysiology and Management of the Newborn, 3rd ed. Philadelphia, JB Lippincott, 1987)

in insulin content. On delivery, the neonate is no longer dependent on maternal glucose; thus, a hypoglycemic state ensues. Because insulin acts to stimulate fetal organ growth, a hyperinsulin state produces an increase in organ size and macrosomia (large for gestational age). There is an impetus for increased deposition of fat in the third trimester. Potential birth injuries may occur with attempted vaginal delivery of very large neonates. These potential birth injuries include cephalhematoma, subdural hemorrhage, facial palsy, ocular hemorrhage, clavicular fracture, and brachial plexus injury.[17] Hypoglycemia is defined as a plasma concentration of less than 40 mg/dl in the term infant and 30 mg/dl in the preterm infant. It may also be defined as a glucose strip determination (Dextrostix, Chemstrip) of less than 45 mg/dl. Glucose test strips should be confirmed by a blood glucose determination. Blood glucose levels usually drop within the first 30 to 60 minutes of life. Most IDMs are asymptomatic. Signs or symptoms that do occur are lethargy, irritability, coarse tremors, apnea, and convulsions.[17] Treatment is the administration of intravenous glucose, by constant infusion, calculated according to the weight of the neonate. In lieu of intravenous administration, early feedings may be begun within the first 30 minutes after delivery.

HYPOCALCEMIA

Hypocalcemia is defined as a calcium level below 7 mg/dl and is one of the most common clinical problems for the IDM. About 50% of infants born to insulin-dependent women experience hypocalcemia during the first 3 days of life. During pregnancy, a maternal hyperparathyroid state exists that seeks to increase maternal calcium that has been diverted to the fetus. After delivery, serum calcium falls owing to the levels of parathyroid hormone, vitamin D, and calcitonin. Subsequently, parathyroid hormone and vitamin D levels rise to correct this deficiency. Symptoms of hypocalcemia are jitteriness, convulsions, and twitching. Calcium in oral form may be administered with feedings when calcium levels are stabilized.

HYPERBILIRUBINEMIA

The etiology of hyperbilirubinemia in IDMs is not clear, although several theories have been postulated. Of these, polycythemia commonly seen in IDMs emerges as a significant factor associated with hyperbilirubinemia. Treatment is the same as for jaundice due to other factors.

RESPIRATORY DISEASE

The IDM appears to develop hyaline membrane disease later than other neonates.[17] Some clinicians also note problems due to transient tachypnea of the newborn. The fetus's hyperinsulin state may interfere with the ability of the lungs to use phospholipids. There appears to be an increased number of "false-positive" lecithin/sphingomyelin (L/S) ratios among all diabetic classes. Respiratory distress syndrome has been noted with an L/S ratio of greater than 2.0 in the IDM.[18] See Chapter 44 for management.

BIRTH DEFECTS

An increase in congenital defects has been noted in infants of diabetic mothers. For further discussion of the fetus of a diabetic mother, see Chapter 42 and the Nursing Care Plan: Infant of a Diabetic Mother.

■ JAUNDICE IN THE NEONATE

Hyperbilirubinemia in the neonate may occur due to numerous causes. Physiologic jaundice, evident after

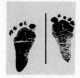

Nursing Care Plan

Infant of a Diabetic Mother

Patient Goals

1. Infants at risk are identified.
2. Birth injuries are identified and managed promptly.
3. Metabolic problems are identified and managed promptly.
4. Infant maintains fluid and electrolyte balance.

Assessment	Potential Nursing Diagnosis	Planning and Intervention	Evaluation
History			
Maternal diabetic classification and method of control during pregnancy	High risk for birth injury (cephalhematoma, subdural hemorrhage, facial palsy, ocular hemorrhage, clavicular fracture, brachial plexus injury) related to macrosomia	Identify the infant of a diabetic mother from history and neonatal physical characteristics	Infants at risk are identified
			Birth injuries are identified and managed promptly
Neonatal			
Weight	Fluid-volume deficit related to maternal diabetes	Document characteristics	Metabolic problems are identified and managed promptly
Apgar score		Plethora	
Gestational age		Round face	Infant maintains fluid and electrolyte balance
		Soft skin	
		Abundance of subcutaneous tissue	
		Observe for metabolic problems	
		Hypoglycemia	
		Jitteriness	
		Irritability	
		Apnea	
		Dextrostix < 45	
		Continue to monitor frequent Dextrostix	
		Check with blood glucose as needed. Must be above 30 mg/dl in term infant and 20 mg/dl in the preterm	
		Carry out treatment orders if required	
		Frequent, early feedings	
		Intravenous fluids	
		Hypocalcemia	
		Tremors, convulsions, twitching	
		Prolonged QT interval	

(continued)

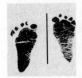

Nursing Care Plan (continued)

Assessment	Potential Nursing Diagnosis	Planning and Intervention	Evaluation
		Calcium levels < 7 mg/ dl	
		Carry out orders for calcium replacement (either intravenous or oral)	
		Hyperbilirubinemia, respiratory distress syndrome	
		See related care plans	

24 hours of age, is a common phenomenon (see Chap. 29).

Pathologic forms of jaundice may be the result of a variety of factors. Hemolytic disease of the newborn (e.g., Rh or ABO incompatibility) is significant but decreasing in severity owing to preventive measures. The administration of anti-D globulin (RhoGAM) to eligible women has been an important intervention combating Rh incompatibility and erythroblastosis fetalis. ABO incompatibility has always been less of a threat to the newborn than the Rh problem. For extensive discussion of the pathophysiology of these entities, see Chapter 42.

In addition to hemolytic disease of the newborn, pathologic hyperbilirubinemia can result from increased production or decreased excretion of bilirubin or, infrequently, a combination of these two processes.

Examples of overproduction of bilirubin are hemolytic disease of the newborn, hereditary hemolytic anemias, glucose-6-phosphate dehydrogenase deficiency, polycythemia, enclosed hemorrhage (e.g., cephalhematoma, extensive bruising), swallowed maternal blood, increased enterohepatic circulation, and oxytocin-induced labor.

Decreased hepatic uptake of bilirubin and decreased bilirubin conjugation result from undersecretion of bilirubin. Hepatitis, biliary duct obstruction, and galactosemia can lead to impaired excretion of bilirubin. Bacterial infections or intrauterine viral infections can result in increased bilirubin production along with decreased hepatic clearance.[19]

Obstetric factors related to the incidence of jaundice are labor induction, epidural anesthesia, the use of intravenous fluids during labor, and delayed or limited feeding during the infant's first 24 hours of life.[20]

Pathologic forms of jaundice pose a serious threat to the neonate owing to the possibility of the complication of kernicterus. Kernicterus results from the accumulation of unconjugated and unbound bilirubin in brain cells. Neurologic signs occur, and ultimately intellectual function is impaired. The exact bilirubin level at which kernicterus occurs varies with each individual infant, occurring sooner in the preterm infant.

Assessment

Chapter 29 discusses the physical assessment of an infant suspected of being jaundiced.

Pathologic disease may be suspected if jaundice is evident within the first 24 hours of life and lasts more than 7 days in the term infant or 10 days in the preterm infant or if serum bilirubin increases by greater than 5 mg/dl every 24 hours. Further investigation is also needed if bilirubin levels are greater than 12.9 mg/dl in the term infant and 15 mg/dl in the preterm infant during the first 48 hours.[19] Finally, infants with erythroblastosis fetalis (severe isoimmunization) present with generalized edema, pallor, hepatosplenomegaly, hydrothorax, and severe anemia.

Diagnostic tests that may be used are direct and total serum bilirubin, blood typing of mother and baby, complete blood count, total serum protein, and direct Coombs' test. The direct Coombs' test is performed on neonatal cord blood, measuring whether neonatal red blood cells are coated with maternal antibodies.

A noninvasive screening tool that may be used to correlate skin color with a total serum bilirubin value is transcutaneous bilirubinometry. A hand-held fiberoptic instrument illuminates the skin and measures the intensity of the yellow color. This method should be accompanied by a total serum bilirubin test and should not be relied upon solely to institute treatment.

Nursing Diagnosis

Potential for injury is high on the list of possible nursing diagnoses. These potential injuries might include kernicterus related to elevated bilirubin levels; dehydration or hyperthermia related to phototherapy; and hyperbilirubinemia, electrolyte imbalances, hypoglycemia, and hypothermia related to exchange transfusion rebound. There may also be an alteration in bowel elimination (diarrhea) related to phototherapy. Alteration in family processes is another potential problem related to the infant's eyes being covered during phototherapy and even the confinement during phototherapy.

Planning and Intervention

In the event of a positive Coombs' test or a very-low-birth-weight infant, phototherapy may often be initiated without waiting for bilirubin results. Treatment could involve immediate exchange transfusion, as in the event of a hydropic infant. More often than not, however, the more conservative treatment of phototherapy is used.

The decision to initiate phototherapy is somewhat individualized, with criteria varying from center to center. Some physicians may elect to adopt a "wait and see" attitude in the absence of acute pathology. Phototherapy can be viewed as a preventive measure more than a treatment, and, as such, is not usually used for healthy infants with physiologic jaundice.

PHOTOTHERAPY

The use of intense fluorescent light to reduce serum bilirubin has gained acceptance in the treatment of hyperbilirubinemia (Fig 46-7).

Phototherapy, by the processes of photoisomerization and photooxidation, results in more water-soluble bilirubin end products, which are rapidly excreted in urine and bile. Phototherapy generally consists of a single quartz halogen lamp or a bank of four to eight cool-white, daybright, or special blue fluorescent bulbs covered by a Plexiglas shield and positioned 12 to 30 inches from the patient. The energy output from the lights must be checked periodically to confirm the desired output. The success of phototherapy depends on the energy output in the blue spectrum of the lights and on the surface area of the neonate exposed to the treatment. Once phototherapy has been initiated, serum bilirubin levels must be frequently monitored, because visual assessment of any jaundice is no longer valid.

Ongoing studies continue to investigate the possibility of any long-term or permanent side effects of phototherapy. So far, none are known. The nurse focuses on the care of the infant receiving phototherapy and any subsequent short-term side effects.

Although no long-term effects have been demonstrated in humans, to prevent any potential retinal side effects, the infant's eyes are shielded from the light by means of patches (Fig. 46-8). The nurse should make sure that the lids are closed when the patches are applied. The nurse must check frequently for correct positioning of the eye patches, that the eyes are indeed covered, and that the nares are not occluded. The eye patches are to be removed at least once each shift to inspect the eyes for conjunctivitis and to allow eye contact with parents and visual stimulation.

Because diapers may cover a large amount of surface area in small infants, the nurses may choose to use a tie on surgeon's mask as a small "bikini diaper" to collect stool and urine. By changing the infant's position frequently, maximal exposure to the lights' benefits is achieved.

Monitoring of temperature is important because additional heat from the light necessitates adjustments in environmental temperature. Infants in open cribs may exhibit heat loss. Fluids need to be increased to compensate for insensible water loss. Daily weights are monitored. Expected changes in elimination patterns are loose green stools and green urine. Meticulous skin care is required to maintain intact skin. Lotions and ointments should not be used on the infant's skin because their use may lead to increased risk of burns. Bronze-baby syndrome may occur in some infants, as exhibited by a dark-grayish–brown discoloration of the skin, serum, and urine. This effect disappears when treatment is discontinued. Finally, the neonate needs to have tactile stimulation as often as possible, whether with parents or the nursing staff. Parental contact will provide reassurance to the family of the infant's progress.

Once phototherapy is discontinued, bilirubin levels must be followed for at least 24 hours to assess any possible rebound effect.

Home Phototherapy. Home phototherapy may be an optimal alternative when used carefully with families meeting the program's criteria. Benefits include financial savings, uninterrupted maternal-infant bonding, and parental satisfaction. With the trend toward early discharge, home phototherapy can prevent readmission should hyperbilirubinemia occur. Parental education regarding infant care and home visits by a home health

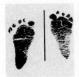

Nursing Care Plan

Neonate With Pathologic Jaundice

Patient Goals

1. Infants at risk for hemolytic disease are identified.
2. Infants are free of kernicterus.
3. Infant's vital signs are stable.
4. Infant maintains fluid and electrolyte balance.
5. Infant maintains intact skin.
6. Infant receives appropriate stimulation.
7. Infant interacts with parents.

Assessment	Potential Nursing Diagnosis	Planning and Intervention	Evaluation
Jaundice noted within first 24 h	High risk for injury, kernicterus related to elevated bilirubin levels	Observe for levels of jaundice, note any progression	A risk infant is identified
Positive direct Coombs' test	High risk for injury, dehydration, hyperthermia related to phototherapy treatment	Use transcutaneous bilirubinometry as a screening tool	Infants are free of kernicterus
Maternal-neonatal blood typing indicative of Rh or ABO incompatibility	Alteration in bowel elimination, diarrhea related to phototherapy	Obtain bilirubin specimens, monitor laboratory results	Infant's vital signs are stable
Presence of other risk factors	High risk for injury, (hyperbilirubinemia, electrolyte imbalances, hypoglycemia, hypothermia) related to exchange transfusion rebound	Give frequent feedings and monitor intake and output, skin turgor, weight	Infant maintains fluid and electrolyte balance
		Initiate phototherapy as ordered	Infant maintains intact skin
		Remove infant's clothing	Infant receives appropriate stimulation
		Place eye shield securely on infant. Remove at least every 4 h to observe for conjunctivitis and allow for visual stimulation	Infant interacts with parents
		Monitor temperature of infant and of isolette or warmer frequently	
		Observe diaper area for loose stools	
		Keep skin as clean as possible	
		Change position frequently	
		Remove from phototherapy for interaction and feeding with parents PRN	
		Prepare infant for exchange transfusion—restraints, monitors	

(continued)

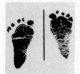

Nursing Care Plan (continued)

Assessment	Potential Nursing Diagnosis	Planning and Intervention	Evaluation
		Assist with insertion of catheter	
		Assist with collection of all blood samples	
		Check blood for correct typing	
		Use blood-warming equipment for procedure	

care nurse are essential components of a home phototherapy program. Risks of home therapy programs are reported to be minimal.

EXCHANGE TRANSFUSION

Exchange transfusions are performed in those infants subjected to hemolytic disease (e.g., Rh incompatibility or ABO incompatibility; Table 46-6). The exchange transfusion will decrease levels of bilirubin and correct any anemia. The donor blood used must be compatible with both infant's and mother's serum.[20]

Procedure. An exchange transfusion alternately removes a small amount of blood from the infant and replaces it with the same amount of donor blood. An umbilical catheter is used to perform the exchange, usually a double-volume type. In a double-volume exchange, the amount of donor blood is twice that of the newborn volume. Small amounts up to 20 ml are exchanged at a time. An infusion of albumin can be given several hours prior to the procedure to increase the number of bilirubin binding sites. This would make the exchange more efficient.

■ *Figure 46–7*
Phototherapy, using fluorescent lights, is considered conservative treatment for jaundice.

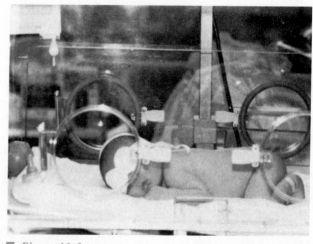

■ *Figure 46-8*
A full-term newborn receiving phototherapy in a closed isolette for hyperbilirubinemia. (Photo: BABES, Inc.)

TABLE 46–6. INDICATIONS AND BLOOD PRODUCTS FOR EXCHANGE TRANSFUSIONS IN HEMOLYTIC DISEASE OF THE NEWBORN

Indications for Exchange Transfusions	Type of Donor Blood Used for Exchange Transfusions

Rh incompatibility
   Anemia (hematocrit < 45%)
   Positive Coombs' test and rate of rise in serum bilirubin
     > 0.5 mg/h
	Rh incompatibility
	1. Rh-negative blood of infant's type that crossmatches with mother's serum
	2. Type O, Rh-negative red blood cells, Rh-negative plasma
	3. Type O, Rh-negative "low titer" whole blood

ABO incompatibility Rate of rise in serum bilirubin > 1.0 mg/h	ABO incompatibility 1. Type O, Rh-specific with low titers of anti-A antibody and anti-B antibody 2. Type O, Rh-negative red blood cells resuspended in type AB, Rh-negative plasma

(Braune KW, Lacey L: Common hematologic problems of the immediate newborn period. JOGN Nurs 12(3)(Suppl):19S–26S, May/June 1983; Adapted from Klaus M, Fanaroff A: Care of the High-Risk Neonate. Philadelphia, WB Saunders, 1979, and Katlwinkel J, Cook LJ, Ivey HH, et al: Book II, Newborn Care: Concepts and Procedures. Charlottesville, University of Virginia Medical Center, Unit 16, 1979)

Preexchange. The nurse is the primary caregiver who assesses the infant's color as becoming more jaundiced and behavior as increasingly lethargic, necessitating more diagnostic work-up. The nurse checks to see that all preexchange blood samples have been collected. An informed consent must be signed by the parents. Donor blood ordered must be checked for the type, unit number, and expiration date. Usually a hematocrit of donor blood is obtained. The desirable donor hematocrit is between 45 and 55. Blood must be warmed slowly. Blood-warming units keep blood at an even temperature during the procedure. The infant must be placed on monitors and restrained. The nurse prepares the infant for umbilical artery catheterization, if needed, by restraining the infant and setting up the sterile tray, solutions, and surgical gloves.

Procedural Tasks. The infant's temperature and other vital signs are taken and recorded at frequent intervals during the procedure. Vital signs are recorded on the infant's flow sheet as well as the exchange record itself. An exchange record is provided in the standard exchange transfusion tray. The amount of blood placed in and out is recorded on the exchange transfer sheet as well as any drugs given. For example, a dose of calcium may be given for every 100 ml exchanged. Total amounts of blood infused and withdrawn are recorded. Postexchange blood samples are withdrawn at the end of the procedure.

Posttransfusion. Frequent vital signs continue following the procedure. Some complications to anticipate and keep in mind are rebound hyperbilirubinemia, electrolyte imbalances, hypoglycemia, and hypothermia.

Evaluation

Evaluation and reassessment indicate that the newborn retains healthy eyes during phototherapy. Time is allowed for eye contact with the parents and visual stimulation. Tactile stimulation is given as often as possible. Despite the use of monitors and restraints during exchange transfusions, the neonate receives as much tactile stimulation and care as possible.

Fluid and electrolyte balance and temperature must be maintained, and the infant's temperature and vital signs are stabilized.

Breast Milk Jaundice

The incidence of increased bilirubin at about the fourth to seventh day, with a peak at 2 weeks, has been reported in 1% to 2% of breastfed babies.[20]

The exact etiology of breast milk jaundice is unknown. Theories have focused on the roles of pregnanediol, increased enzyme activity, and increased free fatty acids in breast milk.

A most recent hypothesis proposes that breast milk jaundice occurs as a result of increased amounts of β-glucuronidase in breast milk, which leads to increased intestinal absorption of bilirubin. Breastfeeding-associated jaundice, a different phenomenon, appears to correlate with infants' success at breastfeeding. Research indicates that infants who do not nurse well tend to have higher average bilirubin levels than those infants who nurse often and well.[20]

Treatment for elevated bilirubin levels due to breast milk jaundice may vary. Whether or not the temporary

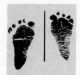

Nursing Care Plan

Infants Born to Drug Abusers

Patient Goals

1. Infant receives adequate nutritioin.
2. Infant maintains fluid-volume balance.
3. Irritability and muscle rigidity are lessened.
4. Maternal-infant interactions are ongoing and positive.
5. Maternal caretaking is competent and ongoing.
6. A safe home environment is established prior to discharge.
7. Follow-up care is planned.

Assessment	Potential Nursing Diagnosis	Planning and Intervention	Evaluation
Known history of maternal drug abuse	Alteration in nutrition, less than body requirements, related to uncoordinated and ineffective sucking and swallowing reflexes	Provide small, frequent feedings	Infant receives adequate nutrition
Amount, type of drug, and type of last dosage		Gavage feed if necessary	Infant maintains fluid-volume balance
Positive maternal and neonatal drug screens		Feed in upright position	Irritability and muscle rigidity are lessened
Noted associated congenital anomalies	High risk for fluid-volume deficit related to inadequate fluid intake, vomiting, diarrhea	Provide support to chin with hand to promote effective sucking	Maternal-infant interactions are ongoing and positive
Characteristic behaviors observed and documented		Begin intravenous fluid administration	Maternal caretaking is competent and ongoing
Lack of quiet sleep	Altered growth and development related to exposure to toxic substances prenatally	Monitor intake and output	A safe home environment is established prior to discharge
Nonnutritive sucking patterns		Assess mucous membranes, skin turgor for hydration status	Follow-up care is planned
Tremors	High risk for alteration in parenting	Reduce stimuli in environment	
Irritability		Hold infant firmly, close	
Vomiting		Provide background noise, music	
Diarrhea		Position to avoid arms in "W" posture	
Constipation		Promote maternal-infant interaction and caretaking	
		Provide information as needed	
		Multidisciplinary referral	

termination of breastfeeding is appropriate is debatable. Some physicians may simply monitor bilirubin levels closely and use phototherapy as deemed appropriate. Others may have the mother discontinue breastfeeding and substitute formula during the few days of peak bilirubin level.

Nurses need to give information to the parents, assuring them that this condition is only temporary. The mother may need help in learning to pump her breasts, if cessation of breastfeeding is recommended.

■ INFANTS OF DRUG-ADDICTED MOTHERS

The life-style of addicted women during the childbearing years promotes other health problems affecting the fetus and subsequently the neonate.

Chapter 36, Addictive Disorders in Pregnancy, discusses the typical effects on the fetus and neonate of smoking, drugs, and alcohol. This section will focus on the nursing process used in the care of neonates born to addicted mothers.

Nursing Assessment

Infants exposed prenatally to toxic substances exhibit characteristic appearances and behaviors described in detail in Chapter 36. If there is a known positive maternal history for drug or alcohol abuse, assessment priority focuses on any obvious congenital anomalies.

Prominent behavior alterations are demonstrated in the gastrointestinal and central nervous systems. Infants may display vomiting, intermittent constipation and diarrhea, and ineffective feeding patterns as a result of uncoordinated sucking and swallowing.

Numerous central nervous system abnormalities can be noted with varying developmental implications. Infant's behaviors range from highly irritable to passive, with most displaying irritability and difficulty sleeping. Tremors of hands, arms, legs, chin, and tongue are common, increasing as the infant fatigues. Increased muscle tone interferes with normal motor development; pull to sit is delayed and arms are typically widespread in "W" position. Resistance is exhibited in bringing arms to the midline. This increased muscle tone inhibits development of fine motor skills. Life-long developmental disabilities such as short- and long-term learning problems, slower intellectual development, emotional and behavioral differences, and delayed language development become increasingly evident as the infant grows and matures.[21]

Potential Nursing Diagnoses

Various physiological and psychosocial nursing diagnoses are possible for infants exposed prenatally to drugs and alcohol. Potential nursing diagnoses are: alteration in nutrition, less than body requirements related to uncoordinated and ineffective sucking and swallowing reflexes; high risk for fluid-volume deficit related to vomiting and/or diarrhea; altered growth and development related to exposure of toxic substances prenatally; and high risk for alteration in parenting related to infant's altered response patterns and potential continuation of maternal drug abuse patterns.

Interventions

The nurse assists with nutritional deficits by providing small, frequent feedings, rest periods, gavage feedings if necessary, feeding in an upright position, and supporting infant's chin with a hand to facilitate sucking.

To help diminish the infant's irritability and tremors, the nurse adjusts the environment by decreasing noise and dimming lights. Soft music or background noise may have a calming effect. Swaddling the infant, holding the infant close, rocking the infant, carrying the infant in a front-pouch carrier, and offering the infant a pacifier may assist in soothing the infant. Sedatives may be administered as ordered to assist in promoting less irritability and tremors.[21]

Infants may be swaddled, carried, or held in positions that facilitate arm placement at midline rather than in "W" position. Separation between mother and infant should be minimized, and the mother's active participation in caregiving should be encouraged. Multidisciplinary referrals are essential to attempt to establish a safe home environment for the infant. Follow-up care and ongoing assessment of the home are vital in light of the evidence that these infants are at high risk for abuse and neglect.

Evaluation

As a result of effective nursing interventions, the infant receives adequate nutrition, maintains adequate fluid volume, and demonstrates less irritability and muscle rigidity. Maternal-infant interactions are ongoing and positive; maternal caretaking is facilitated. A multidisciplinary approach, set in motion by referral, establishes that the infant is returning to a safe environment and that ongoing follow-up is carried out (see Nursing Care Plan: Infants Born to Drug Abusers).

■ REFERENCES

1. Mangurten HC: Birth injuries. In Fanaroff AB, Martin RJ (eds): Behrman's Neonatal-Perinatal Medicine. St Louis, CV Mosby, 1983

2. Minarcik, Chester J Jr, Beachy P: Neurologic disorders. In Merenstein GB, Gardner SL (eds): Handbook of Neonatal Intensive Care. St. Louis, CV Mosby, 1989

3. Braune KW, Lacey L: Common hematologic problems of the immediate newborn period. JOGN Nurs 12(3)(suppl):19s–26s, 1983

4. Rimar JM: Shock in infants and children: Assessment and treatment. MCN 13:2:98–105, 1988

5. Feigin RD, Callanan DL: Postnatally acquired infections. In Fanaroff AB, Martin RJ (eds): Behrman's Neonatal-Perinatal Medicine. St Louis, CV Mosby, 1983

6. Marcy M, Klein JO: Focal bacterial infections. In Remington JS, Klein JO (eds): Infectious Diseases of the Fe-

tus and Newborn Infant. Philadelphia, WB Saunders, 1990

7. Baker CJ, Edwards MS: Group B Streptococcal Infections. In Remington JS, Klein JO (eds): Infectious Diseases of the Fetus and Newborn Infant. Philadelphia, WB Saunders, 1990

8. Devore N, Jackson V, Piening SL: Torch infections. Am J Nurs 83(12):1660–1665, December 1983

9. Samson L: Perinatal viral infections and neonates. Journal of Perinatal and Neonatal Nursing 1(4):56–65, 1988

10. Remington JS, Desmonts G: Toxoplasmosis. In Remington JS, Klein JO (eds): Infectious Diseases of the Fetus and Newborn Infant. Philadelphia, WB Saunders, 1990

11. Zeldis JB, Crumpacker CS: Hepatitis. In Remington JS, Klein JO (eds): Infectious Diseases of the Fetus and Newborn Infant. Philadelphia, WB Saunders, 1990

12. Haggerty L: TORCH: A literature review and implications for practice. JOGN Nurs 14(2):124–129, 1985

13. Thurber F, Berry B: Children with AIDS: Issues and future directions. J Pediatr Nurs 5(3):168–177, 1990

14. Williams AD: Nursing management of the child with AIDS. Pediatr Nurs 15(3):259–261, 1989

15. Boland M: Care of HIV-infected children. AJN Continuing Education, pp 1–5, 1989

16. Ippolito C, Gibes RM: AIDS and the newborn. J Perinat Neonat Nurs 1(4):78–86, 1988

17. Epstein MF: Medical parental expectations in the care of the infant of a diabetic mother. Diabetes Educat 9(2):44s–46s, Summer 1983

18. Cowett RM, Schwartz R: The infant of the diabetic mother. Pediatr Clin North Am 29(5):1213–1231, October 1982

19. Frank CG, Turner BS, Merenstein GB: Jaundice. In Merenstein GB, Gardner SL: Handbook of Neonatal Intensive Care. St. Louis, CV Mosby, 1989

20. Wilkerson NN: A comprehensive look at hyperbilirubinemia. MCN 13(5):360–364, 1988

21. Lewis KD, Bennett B, Schmeder NH: The care of infants menaced by cocaine abuse. MCN 14(5):324–329, 1989

■ SUGGESTED READING

Boland M, Klug RM: AIDS: The implications for home care. MCN 11(6):404–411, 1986

Cerase PA: Neonatal sepsis. J Perinat Neonat Nurs 3(2):48–54, 1989

Dunn PA, Bhutani V, Weiner S, et al: Care of the neonate with erythroblastosis fetalis. JOGNN 17(6):395–386, 1988

Eliason MJ, Williams JK: Fetal alcohol syndrome and the neonate. J Perinat Neonat Nurs 3(4):64–72, 1990

Hill AS, Cochran CK, Dickerson C, et al: Nursing care of an infant with erythroblastosis fetalis. J Pediatr Nurs 4(6):395–402, 1989

Husson RN, Comeau AM, Hoff R, et al: Diagnosis of human immunodeficiency virus infection in infants and children. Pediatrics 86(1):1–8, 1990

Jones MB: A physiologic approach to identifying neonates at risk for kernicterus. JOGNN 19(4):313–318, 1989

Kelting S, Johnson C: Erythropoiesis and neonatal blood transfusion. MCN 12(3):172–177, 1987

Kennard MJ: Cocaine use during pregnancy: Fetal and neonatal effects. J Perinat Neonat Nurs 3(4):53–63, 1990

Klisch ML: Caring with persons with AIDS: Student reactions. Nurse Educat 15(4):16–19, 1990

Kuller JM: Effects on the fetus and newborn of medications commonly used during pregnancy. J Perinat Neonat Nurs 3(4):73–87, 1990

Lynch M, McKeon VA: Cocaine use during pregnancy-research findings and clinical implications. JOGNN 19(4):285–292, 1989

Smith J: The dangers of prenatal cocaine use. MCN 13(3):174–179, 1988

Wiley K, Grohar J: Human immunodeficiency virus and precautions for obstetric, gynecologic and neonatal nurses. JOGNN 17(3):165–168, 1988

Wilkerson NN: Treating hyperbilirubinemia. MCN 13(5):360–364, 1988

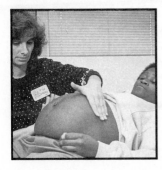

Unit VIII
Assessment and Management of High Risk Perinatal Conditions

CONFERENCE MATERIAL

1. In your own hospital setting, evaluate the facilities for and the care of the newborn infants in relation to the prevention of infection.

2. A mother's firstborn infant has a cleft lip and cleft palate. The infant is apparently normal otherwise. The distraught mother can see only "my poor deformed baby girl" and blames herself for this "tragedy," because she did not follow her physician's instructions during pregnancy, particularly in relation to good nutrition. How might the nurse handle the nursing problems in this situation?

3. How do you account for the high infant mortality during the neonatal period?

4. What community agencies in your city render services for developmentally disabled children? What is the procedure for making the referral to such agencies? How can the community health nurse intervene most effectively in such cases?

5. What services are available for parents of newborns with AIDS?

6. What methods are used by your hospital, well-baby clinics, or other community agencies for the detection of phenylketonuria?

MULTIPLE CHOICE

Read through the entire question and place your answer on the line to the right.

1. Which of the following factors may predispose to the production of an erythroblastotic infant?
   A. Rh-negative mother
   B. Rh-positive father
   C. Rh-positive fetus
   D. Rh-positive substance from the fetus finds its way into the mother's bloodstream to build up antibodies
   E. Mother has had a previous Rh-positive pregnancy or transfusion.
   Select the number corresponding to the correct letters.

1. A and D
2. A, C, and D
3. B, C, and E
4. All of the above   ____

2. Which of the following statements concerning diabetes complicated by pregnancy are correct?
   A. The size of the placenta tends to be in direct relation to the size of the infant.
   B. Toxemia occurs more frequently than in nondiabetic pregnancies.
   C. Deliveries are always performed by cesarean section, usually 2 weeks prior to term.
   D. The fetus tends to be large.
   E. Hypoglycemia occurs in the infant following delivery.
   Select the number corresponding to the correct letters.
   1. A and B
   2. B, D, and E
   3. B, C, D, and E
   4. All of the above   ____

3. The most effective treatment of erythroblastosis is accomplished by blood transfusion. Which of the following is the best method to use?
   A. Exchange transfusion with Rh-negative blood
   B. Exchange transfusion with Rh-positive blood
   C. Exchange transfusion with blood plasma
   D. Repeated small transfusions with Rh-negative blood
   E. Repeated small transfusions with Rh-positive blood
   F. Repeated small transfusions with blood plasma   ____

4. Hemolytic disease of the newborn may be produced by the union of parents with which of the following blood types?
   A. Rh-positive mother with Rh-negative father
   B. Rh-negative mother with Rh-negative father
   C. Rh-negative mother with Rh-positive father
   D. Type O mother with type A father
   E. Type A mother with type B father
   Select the number corresponding to the correct letters.
   1. A and C
   2. B and D
   3. C and D
   4. All of the above   ____

5. Which one of the following infectious diseases, when contracted by the mother during the first trimester of pregnancy, will most often produce congenital anomalies in the infant?
   A. Scarlet fever
   B. Rubella
   C. Diphtheria
   D. Rubeola
   E. Typhoid fever ____

6. Some disorders that affect the infant in the neonatal period are manifestations of inborn errors of metabolism. Which of the following conditions would this include?
   A. Phenylketonuria
   B. Icterus neonatorum
   C. Galactosemia
   D. Down's syndrome
   E. Erythroblastosis fetalis
   Select the number corresponding to the correct letter or letters.
   1. A only
   2. A and C
   3. B, C, and D
   4. B, D, and E ____

7. What has recently become the best method to prevent erythroblastosis fetalis?
   A. Injection of the mother soon after delivery with Rh-immune globulin to prevent maternal sensitization
   B. Transfusing the mother during pregnancy
   C. Transfusing all Rh-negative fathers
   D. Transfusing all Rh-negative babies
   E. Repeated small transfusions of Rh-positive blood to the mother
   Select the number corresponding to the correct letter or letters.
   1. A only
   2. A and B
   3. B, C, and D
   4. C, D, and E ____

8. Sampling of amniotic fluid can be useful in determining fetal lung maturity. The determination that is carried out for this purpose is
   A. Bilirubin
   B. Cytology
   C. Creatinine
   D. Lecithin–sphingomyelin (L/S) ratio ____

9. Certain behaviors indicate that a preterm infant may be ready to advance from gavage feedings to nipple feedings. Which of the following are these behaviors?
   A. Strong, vigorous suck
   B. Sucking and swallowing coordinated
   C. Competent gag reflex
   D. Sucking on gavage tube
   E. Wakefulness before feeding time
   Select the number corresponding to the correct letters.
   1. B, C, and E
   2. C and D

3. A and C
4. All of the above ____

10. Nursing care of an infant receiving TPN includes which of the following interventions?
   A. Changing tubing every 48 hours
   B. Changing the insertion site dressing once a week
   C. Frequent checking of Dextrostix
   D. Measuring head circumference
   E. Offering pacifier to infant
   Select the number corresponding to the correct letters.
   1. A, B, and E
   2. B and C
   3. A and D
   4. All of the above ____

11. Small-for-gestational age infants exhibit which of the following clinical problems?
   A. Hyperglycemia
   B. Anemia
   C. Congenital disorders
   D. Hypercalcemia
   E. Temperature instability
   Select the number corresponding to the correct letter or letters.
   1. A and B
   2. B, C, and E
   3. C and E
   4. All of the above ____

12. When the mother learned that her preterm infant was receiving gavage feedings, she asked the nurse why this was being done. Which of the following reasons may be correct for the nurse to reply?
   A. "This method of feeding your baby was indicated because he became exhausted when he tried to swallow."
   B. "Feeding your baby this way prevents him from vomiting and thus eliminates the danger of his aspirating formula into his lungs."
   C. "Feeding your baby this way conserves his strength and permits him to receive food into his stomach when sucking or swallowing may be difficult."
   D. "Your baby can be given his formula quickly this way and thus he does not have to be handled as much."
   E. "A tiny baby's resistance to infection is poor, so gavage feeding is really a protective measure against such infections as thrush, which he might acquire if he were bottle-fed."
   Select the number corresponding to the correct letter or letters.
   1. A only
   2. C only
   3. B, C, and D
   4. B, D, and E ____

13. Signs of neonatal congestive heart failure include
   A. Tachypnea
   B. Bradycardia

C. Hepatomegaly
D. Edema
E. Sternal retractions
Select the number corresponding to the correct letters.
1. A, C, D, and E
2. B, C, and E
3. A and D
4. B and E

14. Which of the following conditions are congenital disorders?
A. Patent ductus arteriosus
B. Brachial palsy
C. Hydrocephalus
D. Retrolental fibroplasia
E. Caput succedaneum
Select the number corresponding to the correct letter or letters.
1. A and C
2. B, C, and D
3. B, D, and E
4. All of the above   ____

15. Factors that may produce hyperbilirubinemia by the overproduction of unconjugated bilirubin are
A. Rh incompatibility
B. Asphyxia
C. Ecchymosis from bruising
D. Liver cell damage due to sepsis
E. Hepatitis

Select the number corresponding to the correct letters.
1. B, C, and D
2. A, D, and E
3. A and C
4. All of the above   ____

16. The following are examples of viral infections in the neonate:
A. Herpes simplex type II
B. Rubella
C. Syphilis
D. Toxoplasmosis
E. Cytomegalovirus
Select the number corresponding to the correct letters.
1. A, B, C, and E
2. B, C, D, and E
3. A and C
4. All of the above   ____

17. Which of the following clinical problems are possible in the infant of a diabetic mother?
A. Small-for-gestational age
B. Respiratory distress syndrome
C. Hyperglycemia
D. Hyperbilirubinemia
E. Hypercalcemia
Select the number corresponding to the correct letters.
1. A, C, and E
2. B and D
3. B, C, and E
4. All of the above   ____

UNIT IX

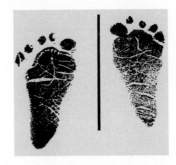

*Assessment
and
Management
of Women's
Health
Promotion*

47

Promoting Gynecologic Health

NURSING ASSESSMENT
Women's Health History
Gynecologic Physical Examination
Periodic Screening
NURSING DIAGNOSIS
NURSING PLANNING AND INTERVENTION

Breast Conditions
   Benign Breast Conditions
   Carcinoma of the Breast
Cervical Conditions
Pelvic Masses
Uterine Masses
WOMEN AND STRESS

FAMILY VIOLENCE AGAINST WOMEN
Factors Contributing to Spouse Abuse
Characteristics of Battered Women and Battering Men
Cycles of Family Violence

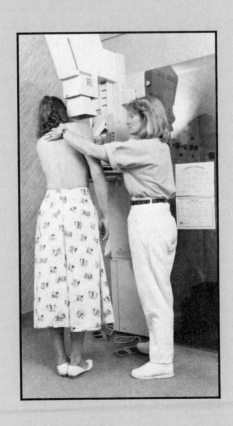

Nurses who provide care to women have many opportunities to promote individual and family health and to help reduce the risk of illness in their clients. The roles of nurses in maternity care have blended into various areas of women's health care, depending on the setting and client needs. The nurse working on the maternity unit, in the obstetrics-gynecology clinic, or in the physician's office may respond to health-care needs that encompass reproductive as well as gynecologic care. Health promotion and the prevention or early detection of illness are important responsibilities.

Common areas of gynecologic health care include health promotion; growth and development (including such life stages as adolescence and menopause); and common gynecologic disorders such as menstrual problems, breast problems, and genital infections. Many nurses are particularly sensitive to women's problems because of mutual perceptions and common experiences. Nursing care provided by women is often highly acceptable to the female client, because nurse and client often share perspectives, and the nurse represents a care provider who is understanding, is attuned to women's concerns, and keeps communications open. Male nurses may also have a particular sensitivity to women's health needs.

■ NURSING ASSESSMENT

Women's Health History

The assessment process may include a general health history, or it may be focused on particular systems or areas of concern. The nurse must decide how broad or focused the assessment will be, depending on the clinical setting, the major purpose of the client encounter, and the health needs or problems of the client. A postpartum nurse may need to assess the new mother's concern about possible exposure to diethylstilbestrol (DES) with a focused health history. The clinic nurse may do a thorough health history at an intake visit for a gynecologic problem.

A more thorough history usually includes identifying data, occupation, family structure, menstrual history, obstetric history, significant illnesses (with emphasis on gynecologic problems), immunizations, life-style and behaviors history, sexual history, and family health history. A review of systems often is included to assess their current status.

An important component of the history is a review of periodic screening procedures that are recommended for early detection of gynecologic problems, such as breast and cervical cancer. The woman is asked about her performance of breast self-examination (BSE) and about her most recent Papanicolaou (Pap) smear and the results. Particular risks that are suggested by the history are further explored. For example, women with multiple sexual partners are at higher risk for sexually transmitted disease, and those with rectal bleeding are at greater risk for polyps or cancer of the colon. Occupational hazards and high stress levels that place women at risk can also be identified and further explored.

The health history includes personal data; menstrual history; pregnancy history; contraceptive use; family health history; major illness; and questions about current health practices, life-style, occupational and environmental conditions, and health concepts (see Gynecologic Health History). Specific points in the health history relevant to developmental needs and gynecologic health promotion and problems are covered in the sections that follow.

Gynecologic Physical Examination

The nurse assists with an appropriate physical examination, depending on the systems involved or the purpose of the visit. Examinations may be focused on specific systems or may be general, as with the health history. The format closely follows that described in Chapter 19. Age and risk status of clients direct the examination to emphasize certain systems or parts.

For the adolescent, particular attention is paid to the progress of sexual development by noting stage of the secondary sex characteristics (see Sex Maturity Ratings in Girls, Chap. 8). Examination for scoliosis also is important for adolescents. The pelvic examination is often critical, as the most common health problems of adolescent girls include dysmenorrhea, irregular menses, vaginitis, and contraception. The first pelvic examination must be conducted gently and with great sensitivity. Special techniques for the first pelvic examination have been described.[1] The nurse's attitudes and actions at this time may affect the adolescent's emerging sexual identify either positively or negatively, an influence that could remain for many years.

Women in young and middle adulthood generally have health needs or problems centering around contraception, pregnancy, menstrual problems, vaginal and urinary infections, and neoplasms of the breasts or reproductive organs. Examinations focus on these areas, especially the breast and reproductive systems. In older adulthood, menopausal concerns become important, and the physical examination can focus on physiological changes expected with declining hormonal function. Cancers of the breast, reproductive organs, and colon

Research Highlight

Passive Smoke Increases Nicotine Levels in Cervical Secretions

Women exposed to cigarette smoke in the environment have biochemical evidence of nicotine in saliva, serum, and urine. Reports have suggested that the cerival mucus of passive smokers might contain nicotine and its metabolites. To confirm this report, the study was designed to measure concentrations of nicotine in cervical lavages taken from cytologically normal, nonsmoking women and compare concentrations in women with passive exposure to smoke and those not exposed.

Subjects were part of a larger study of cervical neoplasia. A sample of 145 nonsmokers with normal cervical cytology on routine Pap smears were interviewed about environmental exposure to tobacco smoke. The interview included questions about exposure inside and outside the home in the prior 24 hours, time since last exposure, number of active smokers in the home and smokers' relationships, usual intensity of smoking and products smoked. A 3 ml saline lavage of the cervix was collected and kept frozen until tested. Laboratory analyses were performed without knowledge of the smoke exposure history. Nicotine was extracted from savage samples and measured by gas chromatography-mass spectroscopy.

Women were divided into three groups: those exposed to smoke only inside their homes, those exposed only outside their homes, and those not exposed. The study population was 6.3% black with a median age of 30 years; neither race nor age was associated with environmental tobacco smoke exposure. Nicotine levels were highest among women exposed in the home (0.8 ng/ml), intermediate in those exposed outside the home (0.4 ng/ml), and lowest in those not exposed (0.2 ng/ml). Nicotine values ranges from below the limit of detection (<0.2) to 8.2 ng/ml. No associations were found between nicotine levels and the woman's exposure to number of smokers, smoking intensity, or time of last exposure.

The level of nicotine obtained in these nonsmoking women exposed to passive smoke was lower than that found in cervical lavages taken from active smokers (median values 11.8 ng/ml). The clear although small elevation of nicotine levels in cervical fluid of passive smokers supports the concept that even low-level exposure to tobacco smoke in the environment might result in systemic effects. Passive smoking should be further evaluated as a risk factor for cervical disease.

Nurses need to inform clients of the potential risks associated with passive exposure to environmental cigarette smoke. Women with relatively high levels of passive smoking are encouraged to have regular, at least annual Pap smears.

Jones CJ, Schiffman MH, Kurman R, et al: Elevated nicotine levels in cervical lavages from passive smokers. Am J Public Health 81(3):378–379, March 1991.

become a greater risk, which must be carefully assessed during examination.

Periodic Screening

Women at different ages are particularly susceptible to certain diseases. Periodic screening tests or examinations have been recommended according to an age-related schedule. The most critical screening procedures for women include breast examination, mammography, pelvic examination, Pap smear, hematocrit or hemoglobin, rectal examination, stool guaiac, and height, weight, and blood pressure. The nurse can perform many of these procedures both in the hospital and in the clinic or office. A schedule for screening tests and examinations is suggested in Table 47-1.

■ NURSING DIAGNOSIS

Data from the assessment process provide the foundation for making the nursing diagnosis. A common diagnosis might be alterations in health maintenance, in which the woman experiences or is at risk of experiencing a disruption in her state of wellness. These disruptions are often caused by inadequate preventive measures or an unhealthy life-style. Many factors may contribute to alterations in health maintenance, including lack of knowledge, poor learning skills, crisis or changing support systems, health or religious beliefs, financial changes, and poor self-esteem.

Health-seeking behaviors is an appropriate nursing diagnosis related to promoting gynecologic health, when

Assessment Tool

Women's Health History

Personal Data

Age, marital or relationship status

Education and occupation

Cultural or ethnic group

Children or persons living in home

Religion

Support systems

Menstrual History

Menarche or menopause

Menstrual cycle characteristics
  Length of cycle
  Days of flow
  Character of flow
  Premenstrual symptoms
  Degree of discomfort
  Medications or remedies used

Date and results of last Pap smear

If menopausal, any vaginal bleeding or other symptoms

If menstruating, any irregular bleeding

Pregnancy History

Age at first pregnancy

Total number of pregnancies and outcomes

Pregnancy complications

Contraceptive History

Current contraceptive (if any)

Other contraceptives used

Satisfaction and problems with contraceptive methods

Future fertility plans

Major Illnesses or Health Problem

Date and type of illness or health problem

Date and type of operations or hospitalizations

Current medical treatment and medications

Family Health History

Type of illness or health problems of relatives
  Heart attack   High blood pressure
  Stroke   Blood clots (lungs, legs)
  Cancer   Mental illness
  Diabetes   Obesity

Current Health Status

Client's definition of state of health

Concerns about symptoms or possible problems

Self-care activities

Last physical, gynecologic, and dental examination

Life-Style and Habits

Nutrition and eating patterns

Sleep and rest

Exercise and recreation

Elimination (bladder, bowel, skin)

Sexual patterns

Stress and stress management

Leisure activities

Environment at home and work (hazards, satisfactions, concerns)

Smoking

Alcohol use

Drug use (prescription, over-the-counter, recreational)

---

a woman in stable health is actively seeking ways to move toward a higher level of wellness. The woman desires information for health promotion, wants to increase control of her health practices, may be concerned about current environmental conditions that could affect health, or may be undergoing changes that affect her personal life situation (marriage, parenthood, retirement, menopause).

Depending on assessment data, the nursing diagnosis might also be noncompliance; high risk for injury; alterations in nutrition; diversional activity deficit; ineffective coping; or powerlessness. Women who do not follow health-related advice given by the nurse may have a nonsupportive family, may lack autonomy in health-seeking behavior, or may not have an effective therapeutic relationship with the nurse. When nutrition

TABLE 47–1. SCHEDULE FOR PERIODIC SCREENING FOR WOMEN

Screening Test or Examination	Age of Woman (years)			
	12 to 20	*20 to 40*	*40 to 60*	*60 to 80*
Breast examination	Annual	Annual	Annual	Annual
Mammogram	*	Baseline	Every 1 to 2 years depending on risk	Every 1 to 2 years depending on risk
Pelvic examination/Pap smear	Annual if sexually active	Annual	Annual	Annual or every 2 years
Hematocrit/hemoglobin	Every 2 years	Every 2 years	Every 5 years	Every 5 years
Rectal examination	*	*	Annual	Annual
Stool guaiac	*	*	Annual	Annual
Height and weight	Annual	Annual	Annual	Annual
Blood pressure	Every 2 years	Every 2 years	Annual	Annual
Urinalysis	*	Every 5 years	Every 5 years	Annual

* Not indicated unless increased risks or symptoms are present.

is in excess of body requirements, the weight gain may be associated with anxiety or depression, stress, sedentary life-style, or lack of nutritional knowledge. Powerlessness can be a problem in carrying out health-promoting behaviors when the woman experiences social displacement, insufficient finances, adolescent dependence on peer groups, or (in the elderly) sensorimotor deficits.

■ NURSING PLANNING AND INTERVENTION

The nursing care plan and nursing actions follow directly from the assessment and diagnosis. Key points in assessment, diagnosis, and nursing care are discussed for several common gynecologic health conditions.

Breast Conditions

Every nurse should be well versed in teaching BSE. This is a professional service nurses are in unique positions to offer clients in a variety of settings. BSE is important in early detection of minimal breast lesions.[2] BSE is usually taught initially at an adolescent health examination and should be reviewed and reinforced by the nurse every 2 to 3 years. It is recommended that women perform BSE every month about 1 week after their menses. The American Cancer Society's approach to teaching BSE is shown in the box on client teaching.

Clients with problems involving the breasts may present with various symptoms and signs, such as pain, lumps, nipple discharge, skin rashes or discolorations, and changes in size or shape. Any of these signs could be benign, or they could signal a malignant neoplasm. Differentiating breast problems is often complex and difficult. Any sign or symptom that cannot be identified readily as a benign problem should be referred to the physician for further evaluation. The nurse can obtain additional data by asking questions about the following:

How long the lump, thickening, or other symptom
    has been present and whether it has changed
Character of breast pain, if present
Presence and characteristics of nipple discharge
Presence of rash or eczema on the nipple
History of breast trauma, family history of cancer risk

In the physical examination, the nurse particularly assesses any skin changes (dimpling, erythema, rash), nipple discharge, and thickenings or lumps felt. It is important to perform the examination with the client in both sitting and supine positions. Characteristics of lumps help differentiate among various types of lesions. When examination data are combined with information from the history and data on incidence, conclusions can be drawn about the probable nature of the breast lesion (Table 47-2).

Mammography is an important screening and diagnostic procedure for breast conditions. More than 90%

Client Teaching

Breast Self-Examination Technique

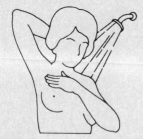

1. In the shower.

Examine your breasts during bath or shower; hands glide easily over wet skin. With fingers flat, move then gently over every part of each breast. Check for any lump, hard knot, or thickening.

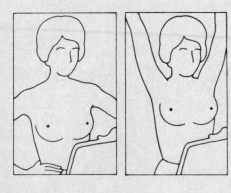

2. Before a mirror.

Inspect your breasts with arms at your sides. Next, raise your arms high overhead. Look for any changes in contour of each breast—a swelling, dimpling of skin, or changes in the nipple. Then rest palms on hips and press down firmly to flex your chest muscles. Left and right breast will not match exactly—few women's breasts do. Regular inspection shows what is normal for you and will give you confidence in your evaluation.

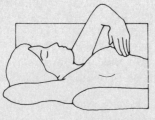

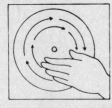

3. Lying down.

To examine your right breast put a pillow or folded towel under your right shoulder. Place your right hand behind your head—this distributes breast tissue more evenly on the chest. With left hand, press gently in small circular motions around an imaginary clock face. Begin at outermost top of your right breast for 12 o'clock, then move to 1 o'clock, and so on around the circle back to 12. A ridge of firm tissue in the lower curve of each breast is normal. Then move in an inch, toward the nipple, keep circling to examine every part of your breast, including the nipple. This requires at least three more circles. Now slowly repeat the procedure on your left breast with a pillow under your left shoulder and your left hand behind your head. Notice how your breast structure feels. Finally, squeeze the nipple of each breast gently between your thumb and index finger. Any discharge, clear or blody, should be reported to your physician immediately.

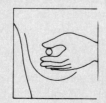

TABLE 47–2. DIFFERENTIATING AMONG BREAST MASSES

	Fibrocystic Disease	Fibroadenoma	Cancer
Usual age	30 to 55, regresses after menopause	15 to 20+, occurs up to 55	30 to 80, peak incidence 42–48
Number	Usually multiple, may be single	Usually single, may be multiple	Usually single, but may coexist with other lesions
Shape	Round	Round, discoid, or lobular	Irregular or stellate
Consistency	Soft to firm, bumpy nodular breasts	Usually firm, may be soft	Firm or hard
Delimitation	Usually well delineated	Well-delineated, clear margins	Not clearly delineated from surrounding tissue
Mobility	Mobile	Very mobile, slippery	May be fixed to skin or underlying tissue
Tenderness	Often tender	Usually nontender	Usually nontender, but not always
Retraction signs	Absent	Absent	Often present

of breast cancers can be detected by mammography; of these lesions, between 20% and 50% can be found only by mammography. Breast examination can detect about one third of minimal cancers; mammography finds smaller cancers earlier with less metastases to lymph nodes.[3] The American Cancer Society recommends a baseline mammogram between the ages of 35 and 40 years, mammogram every 1 to 2 years from ages 40 to 50, and annual mammogram after age 50. Radiation risks are minimal, as dedicated mammographic machines deliver 0.07 to 0.22 rad (0.0007–0.0022 Gy) per exposure, well below the limit of 0.5 rad (0.0005 Gy) established by the American Cancer Society.

BENIGN BREAST CONDITIONS

Fibrocystic change is the most common benign breast problem among women aged 25 to mid-40s; it usually subsides with menopause. This condition is also called *chronic cystic mastitis* and *cystic hyperplasia* and is thought to be estrogen related because its symptoms follow menstrual cycles and decrease after menopause. Fibrocystic change is characterized by multiple, usually bilateral breast lumps that become more tender prior to menses. The lumps are usually firm, mobile, well defined, and tender to palpation. They increase in size premenstrually, can fluctuate rapidly in size, and regress after menses. The most common location is the upper outer breast quadrants, although the lumps may occur in any area of breast tissue. Nipple discharge is rare.

Diagnosis is often based on history and physical examination that reveal the above patterns. Any lumps that are unusual in size, shape, consistency, or behavior should be referred for aspiration or biopsy. A baseline mammogram is strongly recommended, because it is difficult to distinguish cystic lumps from early breast cancer. Alteration in comfort: pain is a common nursing diagnosis, because many women experience quite severe discomfort of a cyclic nature. Knowledge deficit related to the medical condition, diagnostic procedures, and treatments is usually present. The woman also may have little knowledge of breast physiology and cyclic changes. Disturbance in self-concept related to pain or potential loss of body part or function also can occur. Women often fear cancer when they experience breast lumps and pain, so a nursing diagnosis of fear related to possible surgery, life-threatening disease, loss of body part or function, and other factors may be indicated.

Nursing care focuses on pain relief, education, and emotional support. The woman is advised to wear a good supportive brassiere both day and night and to avoid trauma to the breasts. Dietary factors may affect the extent of breast pain, and the nurse can recommend avoiding chocolate, coffee, and black tea and restricting sodium intake. When pain is acute, ice packs to the tender areas may help, and pain relievers such as salicylates or antiinflammatory medications may be used. The hormone inhibitor danazol (Danocrine) may be ordered when these therapies are not effective. As many as 70% to 80% of women using danazol report relief of pain and nodularity; however, the side effects include menstrual pattern changes and weight gain.[4]

Health teaching is an important intervention. Women must learn BSE thoroughly and feel confident in identifying unusual lumps or changes in their breasts. By explaining the relationship of fibrocystic disease to the monthly cycle, the nurse can help alleviate fears of cancer while reinforcing the need for further evaluation of suspected abnormalities. Providing support for discussion of the client's emotional responses to the threat of cancer can dissipate fears and develop effective coping strategies. Women with fibrocystic changes are encouraged to have regular breast examinations by a physician or nurse practitioner and periodic mammography, as indicated.

Fibroadenoma is the third most common breast tumor (following fibrocystic changes and carcinoma) and occurs primarily in women in their teens and early 20s. In adolescents, the cause is associated with breast hypertrophy during the pubertal growth spurt. The lump is typically well defined, firm and rubbery, freely movable, rounded, and nontender. A solitary nodule ranging from 1 to 5 cm is common, but multiple tumors occur in about 15% of cases. These tumors are responsive to hormones and can increase rapidly in size. There is no significant association with malignancy.

Diagnosis is based on tumor characteristics identified during examination. If there are unusual characteristics, a biopsy or mammogram may be necessary. Watchful observation with eventual surgical excision is the usual course of treatment. Although cancer is unlikely, it cannot be completely ruled out in any discrete lump. Nursing diagnoses could include knowledge deficit, disturbance in self-concept, and fear. Nursing care includes education and support similar to that described for fibrocystic changes, with explanations appropriate for fibroadenoma.

Intraductal papillomas are tiny tumors (2–3 mm) most commonly located in a major subareolar collection duct. They have a central fibrovascular stalk with delicate papillae and are often too small to palpate. Tumors are usually single but may be multiple. No particular age group is typical for occurrence. The most common presenting symptom is serosanguineous nipple discharge. During examination, the location of the affected duct may be found by gently pressing with the fingertip at successive points around the circumference of the areola. A point may be found where pressure produces the discharge. A small lump or thickening also may be felt. If no lump is palpable and the lesion cannot be localized, mammography is used to locate the papilloma.

Although papillomas are usually benign, low-grade malignancy may exist. The lesion must be excised and examined histologically. Excision is the definitive treatment for papillomas, with follow-up because they may recur. Multiple lesions are more difficult to manage, requiring several excisions. Nursing diagnoses can include knowledge deficit, disturbance in self-concept, and fear, with nursing care as described above.

CARCINOMA OF THE BREAST

Breast cancer is among the three most common causes of breast lumps in women and is the leading cause of

cancer deaths in women. One woman in 11 will develop breast cancer during her lifetime. Each year, more than 140,000 new cases are diagnosed, and 38,000 deaths from breast cancer are reported.[5] Women are most likely to develop breast cancer after the age of 35, with the peak incidence between the ages of 40 and 60. Individual risk increases steadily with age. Theories of causality include hormonal mechanisms involving endogenous steroids, viral agents, genetic transmission, and immunologic deficiencies.

Risk factors have been identified that place women at increased risk for breast cancer. Risk increases with age, and 75% of breast cancers occur after age 40. Race is a factor, with white women at higher risk than nonwhite. Reproductive factors increasing risk include nulliparity, early menarche (before age 12), late menopause (more than 30 years after menarche), first pregnancy after age 35, and oophorectomy before age 40.

Nutritional patterns associated with increased risk include diets high in fat and protein and low in selenium. Other possible factors include exposure to radiation, having other malignancies, experiencing chronic psychological stress, and being of higher socioeconomic status (see Assessment Tool: Risk Factors for Gynecologic Cancer).

Genetic risk factors have been identified for women in families with a history of breast cancer. When two or more first- or second-degree relatives have breast cancer, a woman's risk is increased threefold over that of women without this family history. This familial breast cancer is common and accounts for about 25% of all breast cancers. A more specific genetic linkage has been found for *hereditary breast cancer (HBC)* by epidemiological studies of family histories. HBC results from an autosomal dominant gene and is characterized by early age of onset (average 44 years), high degree of bilateral breast cancer, multiple sites of primary cancer with integral tumor patterns consonant with specific HBC syndrome, and improved survival rates.[5] About 9% of all breast cancer is due to HBC; the risk of transmission by an affected woman is 50%.[6] Biomolecular studies of cancer support the concept of suppressor genes (antioncogenes) that protect against the development of cancer. Inactivation or loss (deletion from a chromosome) of these genes is part of a cumulative series of steps leading to malignant transformation. The investigation of families that are prone to breast cancer has focused attention on chromosomes 11, 13, and 17 as a genetic locus for allele loss associated with HBC.[5,7]

Nursing Assessment. A breast mass is the most common sign of breast cancer. It is usually discovered by the woman or her sexual partner. In early stages, the lump is usually single, firm, and dense, may be movable or fixed to skin or underlying tissue, and may be circumscribed or irregular. The most frequent location is the upper outer quadrant of the breast. Other signs that

Assessment Tool

Risk Factors for Gynecologic Cancer

Breast Cancer

Over 40 years of age

White

Living in cold climate, Western hemisphere

Unmarried

Higher socioeconomic status

Nulliparous or first pregnancy after age 35

Family history of breast cancer (grandmother, mother, sister, daughter)

Previous breast cancer or fibrocystic breast disease

Early menarche (before age 12)

Late menopause (more than 30 years after menarche or after age 50)

Diet high in fat and protein, low in selenium

Other malignancies, lowered immunocompetency

Cervical Cancer

Multiple sexual partners

Beginning sexual contact before age 20

First pregnancy at an early age

High parity

Intercourse with men who have had venereal disease or prostatic cancer

History of sexually transmitted disease (herpes, trichomoniasis, chlamydia, genital warts, syphilis)

Ovarian Cancer

Delayed onset of childbearing

Low parity

Infertility

Nulliparity

Several spontaneous abortions

Family history of ovarian cancer

White of European or North American origin

Endometrial Cancer

White, middle class

Irregular menses

Infertility

Late menopause

Obesity, hypertension, and diabetes mellitus

Personal or family history of other cancers

History of atypical endometrial hyperplasia

Postmenopausal bleeding

---

usually appear later may include nipple discharge or retraction, skin edema or dimpling, and enlarged axillary lymph nodes. Breast cancer is usually nontender, but tenderness may occur and the woman may report pain or tingling sensations.

There are several types of breast cancer with differing rates of growth and severity. The two most common types are adenocarcinomas and ductal carcinomas (comprising about 65% of all breast cancers). Breast cancers tend to be spatially and temporally multicentric. Over half of the carcinomas have been found with multiple sites of apparently primary lesion, often microscopic in size and only identifiable by pathologic examination. Metastasis occurs early, and by the time a breast cancer is palpable (about 1 cm), micrometastases are almost certainly present. The length of time required for cancers to grow to 1 cm in size has been estimated

at between 3 months and 2½ years. It may take as long as 30 years for malignancies to progress from a single cell to a palpable mass. Metastasis first occurs in surrounding tissue, then through the ductal system, lymph channels, and circulatory system to distant metastatic sites such as bones, liver, and lungs.

DIAGNOSIS. Diagnostic tests most often used for evaluation of suspected breast cancer are mammography and biopsy.

Both film screen mammography and xeromammography are highly accurate and detect more than 90% of breast cancers. Malignant masses classically appear as stellate forms with radiating fibrils, or they may be irregular and poorly defined. Malignant calcifications may appear as tiny rods (0.25–1.5 mm) or may be punctate. Isolated, clustered microcalcifications are the most common mammographic sign of occult malignancy and are associated with 40% to 60% of positive biopsies.[8] Mammography often detects small breast cancers that cannot be palpated on breast examination.

With a suspicious breast mass, biopsy must be performed. Needle or aspiration biopsy withdraws a core of tumor cells or cystic fluid for microscopic examination. Incisional biopsy, which can be done under local anesthesia, removes a portion of tumor for cytologic examination.

If biopsy confirms malignancy, staging is done to determine if the disease is local (confined to the breast) or if metastasis has occurred. Chest x-ray films, lung scans, blood tests (primarily for alkaline phosphatase), and liver and bone scans are usually done. Node biopsies may also be indicated. This information permits staging or classification of the tumor to decide on the most appropriate treatment (see Staging [Classification] of Breast Cancer).

Nursing Diagnoses. Several nursing diagnoses may be appropriate for clients with breast cancer. Knowledge deficit related to medical condition, tests, and surgical procedures is likely to be present. Ineffective coping patterns related to anxiety may affect cognitive abilities.

Disturbance in self-concept related to potential loss of body part or function is probable, because therapy often involves some degree of breast removal. Fear related to anticipated pain, surgery, life-threatening disease, loss of body part or function, or change in the relationship with a partner may be present. During hospitalization and recovery, numerous other nursing diagnoses could be relevant, such as alterations in bowel elimination; alterations in comfort; ineffective individual coping; alterations in family processes; and powerlessness.

Staging (Classification) of Breast Cancer

The TNM* System of the American Joint Committee for Cancer Staging

Stage I

(T) Tumor less than 2 cm diameter

(N) Nodes in axilla, if present, not felt to contain metastasis

(M) No distant metastases

Stage II

(T) Tumor less than 5 cm diameter

(N) Nodes in axilla, if present, not fixed

(M) No distant metastases

Stage III

(T) Tumor greater than 5 cm or tumor of any size with skin invasion or attachment

(N) Nodes in supraclavicular area

(M) No distant metastases

Stage IV

(T) Tumor of any size with extension to chest wall and skin

(N) Any amount of nodal involvement

(M) Distant metastases are present

* (T, tumor; N, nodes; M, metastases)

Types of Surgery for Breast Lesions

Radical mastectomy (Classical, Halsted). Through a vertical incision the entire breast is removed with a significant margin of skin around nipple and areola and tumor. The pectoralis major and minor muscles are removed, the axillary vein is dissected, and the axillary lymph nodes are dissected. A skin-thin surgical flap is left, but depending on the amount of skin removed, skin grafting may be necessary.

Extended radical mastectomy. Includes the above procedure plus excision of the internal mammary lymph nodes. Some sections of the ribs must be removed to reach the internal mammary nodes. The supraclavicular nodes may also be removed. This operation is rarely done today.

Modified radical mastectomy. The entire breast and most of the axillary lymph nodes are removed, but the pectoralis muscles are preserved. Some surgeons dissect the entire axillary chain, whereas others leave the upper third intact. The axillary vein is stripped.

Simple (or total) mastectomy. The entire breast is removed, but the axillary nodes and pectoralis muscles are not. Some surgeons biopsy the last lymph node in the tail of the breast. If it has been invaded, either the axilla is irradiated or a radical mastectomy is done.

Partial mastectomy (segmental resection, wedge resection). The tumor and a wide segment of surrounding breast tissue, underlying fascia, and overlying skin are removed, usually about one third of the breast. Some surgeons also dissect the axillary nodes.

Lumpectomy, tylectomy, or local excision. The tumor and 3 to 5 cm of tissue on either side are removed, retaining other breast tissue and skin.

Subcutaneous mastectomy. Breast tissue, including the axillary tail, is removed through an incision beneath the breast. All breast skin, including the nipple and areola and a small button of tissue under the nipple, remains. A silicone implant is inserted, either during the initial surgery or several months later.

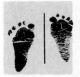

Nursing Care Plan

The Woman with Breast Problems

Nursing Goals

1. The woman will identify her risk factors for breast problems.
2. The woman will be aware of her risks for breast cancer.
3. The woman will understand risks and characteristics of breast problems.
4. The woman will prevent breast problems by reducing risk whenever possible.
5. The woman will perform regular BSE and follow recommended screening.
6. The woman will seek timely treatment for breast problems.

Assessment	Potential Nursing Diagnosis	Planning and Intervention	Evaluation

Risk factors
  Age, race
  Family history
  Menstrual patterns
  Pregnancy history
  Dietary patterns
  Life-style patterns
	Knowledge deficit related to risk factors for various breast problems	Teach BSE
		
		Teach risk factors for cancer
		
		Teach characteristics of women with benign breast diseases
			Client performs BSE correctly and verbalizes confidence in evaluating breast tissue
			
			Client can describe risk factors
			
			Client can describe characteristics of women with benign breast disease

History of problem, physical examination, and laboratory tests	Anxiety or fear related to potentially serious breast mass	Explain procedures and possible outcomes; provide support	Client less anxious, able to cope with waiting for results, understands rationales

Benign breast disease
  Fibrocystic disease
  Fibroadenoma
  Intraductal papilloma
	Knowledge deficit related to medical condition
	
	Alterations in comfort: pain
		Teach client about type of breast disease
		
		Provide pain relief measures (medications); teach client self-care methods of pain relief
			Client relates understanding of her type of breast problem
			
			Client obtains relief of pain through self-care methods of medications

	Disturbance in self-concept related to pain or potential loss of body part or function	Encourage client to express her concerns; clarify misconceptions	Client verbalizes concerns, understands risk, and accepts self-concept
	Fear related to potential life-threatening disease, surgery, or loss of body part or function	Encourage client to express fears and clarify her misconceptions	Client verbalizes fears, has realistic view of risk, carries out prevention and early detection measures
Breast cancer	Anxiety or fear related to effects of cancer, such as surgery, pain, death, loss of body part or function, change in relationships	Encourage client to express fears and clarify her misconceptions	Client verbalizes fears, finds ways of coping, is able to accept loss of breast
	Knowledge deficit related to medical condition, tests,	Teach client about procedures and routines related to treatment	Client describes procedures and routine, under-

(continued)

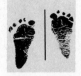

Nursing Care Plan (continued)

Assessment	Potential Nursing Diagnosis	Planning and Intervention	Evaluation
	hospitalization and surgical procedures, recovery		stands treatment and recovery process
	Disturbance in self-concept, related to loss of body part or function	Encourage client to express her concerns and feelings	Client verbalizes feelings and concerns, is able to accept altered self-concept
	Ineffective individual coping, related to anxiety, interpersonal conflicts, disfigurement, altered appearance, inadequate resources	Assist client to identify ineffective coping and find more effective approaches	Client voices problems affecting coping, can describe other approaches, is able to carry out normal daily activities and interests
	Sexual dysfunction related to loss of body part, disrupted relationship with partner	Encourage expression of feelings and involve sexual partner, promote comfort with body changes, refer to sexual counseling	Client and partner express feelings about body changes and sexuality, accept breast loss, resume satisfying sexual relationship, or seek sexual counseling
	During hospitalization: numerous physiological disruptions (circulatory, respiratory, infection, elimination, fluids) as well as above	Monitor vital signs, dressings, wound; promote respiratory and eliminative functions; promote hydration and nutrition; provide pain relief, minimize side effects of surgery or other therapy	Stable physiological function, wound heals, client recovers strength, discomfort is managed, side effects of therapy do not interfere significantly with daily activities and interests

Treatment. Surgical treatment for breast cancer ranges from local excision of the tumor to total resection of the breast, chest wall muscles, and axilla. The extent of surgery depends on the clinical staging of the disease, the histologic characteristics of the tumor, and other considerations, such as age and health status. Conservative breast surgery combined with radiotherapy or chemotherapy yields survival rates similar to those with more extensive mastectomy. Radiation therapy is often used as an adjunct to local excision or simple mastectomy, to shrink large tumors to operable dimensions, and as primary treatment for inflammatory breast cancer or inoperable tumors (see Types of Surgery for Breast Lesions).

Medical oncology uses antineoplastic drugs and endocrine therapy to affect tumor growth. Chemotherapy is often used as preferred adjuvant therapy to surgery when there is axillary node involvement. The systemic effects of drugs halt microscopic metastatic disease and can lengthen the period before relapse. For advanced breast cancer, chemotherapy is primarily palliative. When breast tumors are hormone sensitive, their growth can be retarded by using estrogen, androgen, or progestin, depending on tumor receptors.

Planning and Intervention. Significant side effects are caused by chemotherapy radiation and hormone therapy, making alterations in comfort a common nursing diagnosis.

Nursing care is related to the stage of the disease, the point in medical or surgical therapy, and the nursing diagnoses identified. Interventions commonly used include client teaching, support during procedures, emotional support and counseling, physiological monitoring and technical procedures, comfort measures, family counseling, and coordination of resources for family support and recovery (see Nursing Care Plan).

A specific screening and surveillance protocol is recommended for women from families with HBC. This begins with education about inherited risks and the natural history of HBC in the midteens. These young women are taught BSE and encouraged to examine their breasts at monthly intervals. By age 18, they should receive periodic physician examinations, which become semiannual by age 20. Baseline mammography is obtained by age 25, or 5 years earlier than the earliest age of breast cancer diagnosis in the family. Mammography is done annually thereafter. Surveillance is also provided for other forms of cancer, including ovarian, lung, and brain cancer and leukemia.[5]

Cervical Conditions

Maternity nurses need to be conversant with Pap smears and the management of cervical intraepithelial neoplasia. Women of all ages are concerned about cervical cancer, and the widespread use of Pap smears for screening has increased awareness over the past several decades.

Cancer of the cervix is the second most frequent cancer in women (after breast cancer), and about 2% of women will develop it before the age of 80. The death rate from cervical cancer has fallen steadily over the past 40 years, with most cases diagnosed as carcinoma in situ because of Pap smear screening. The average age at diagnosis of carcinoma in situ is 35 years and at diagnosis of invasive disease, 45 years. Increasing numbers of women in their teens and early 20s are being diagnosed in both stages of disease. Cervical cancer is progressive, with most untreated clients developing invasive disease in 5 to 9 years after carcinoma in situ.

Women are at increased risk for cervical cancer when they have multiple sexual partners, begin sexual contact before age 20, have their first pregnancy at an early age, have high parity, have intercourse with men who have had venereal disease or prostatic cancer, and have had sexually transmitted diseases themselves (such as herpes, trichomoniasis, chlamydial disease, genital warts, or syphilis).

All types of cervical dysplasia, from moderate through actual carcinoma in situ, may be considered part of the same process called cervical intraepithelial neoplasia (CIN). Histologically, the changes in tissue involve the same processes but are a matter of degree. When normal squamous metaplasia proceeds to atypical changes, these cells over many years can result in a cervical epithelium having varying degrees of dysplasia.[9]

Pap Smear Screening. Pap smear screening intervals ranging from 1 to 3 years are recommended by the American College of Obstetricians and Gynecologists and the American Cancer Society.[10,11] Investigations have found a significantly elevated risk for invasive cervical cancer associated with Pap smear screening intervals of 3 to 4 years or greater. Greater benefits from an annual Pap smear over a 2-year screening interval were not observed.[12,13] Women with 3-year screening intervals had greater than three times the risk of squamous cell cervical cancer as did women with annual screening intervals. The risk of cervical cancer was not increased for women screened every 2 years. Women with four or more lifetime sexual partners and Pap smear screening intervals of 3 years or more had more than three times the risk of cervical cancer as did women with fewer sexual partners and the same screening intervals. Pap smears appear to offer less protection against adenocarcinoma and other nonsquamous cell cervical cancers.[12]

Screening intervals that occur in actual practice often do not meet the 1- to 3-year recommendation. About half of the women screened received an annual Pap smear, and 30% had smears at 3-year intervals or greater. Women also may overreport their last screening interval, as obtaining Pap smears is socially acceptable and expected behavior. Recommending a 3-year interval for Pap screening appears to increase the woman's risk for more advanced cervical cancer. Pap smear screening should occur every 1 to 2 years.

Nursing Assessment. Nurses must be able to identify women at increased risk for cervical cancer, and many nurses have the skills to perform vaginal examinations and Pap smears. Women often have no symptoms associated with CIN, and the condition usually is detected on routine Pap smear. Associated conditions, such as vaginal infections or cervicitis, may cause symptoms and signs of increased or odorous vaginal discharge, itching or burning of the perineum, urinary frequency or burning, dyspareunia, or lower abdominal discomfort. A history of sexual, menstrual, and pregnancy patterns is critical in evaluating cervical conditions.

A complete pelvic examination is done, including speculum examination, bimanual examination, and collection of specimens. Before taking the Pap smear, the cervix is inspected and its condition noted. Findings may include nabothian cysts, ectropion, erosion, cervicitis, polyps, or other lesions, such as leukoplakia, herpes, or frank carcinoma (Fig. 47-1).

Nurses have increasing responsibility for Pap smear screening, particularly those in extended roles such as nurse practitioners and clinical specialists. The Pap smear is taken using a cotton-tipped applicator or cytobrush and a spatula (wooden or plastic). The cervix

Normal nulliparous cervix

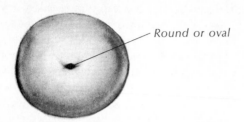

Round or oval

The nulliparous cervical os is small and either round or oval. The cervix is covered by smooth pink epithelium.

Normal parous cervix

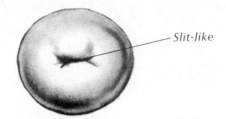

Slit-like

After childbirth, the cervical os presents a slit-like appearance.

Cervical polyp

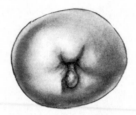

Cervical polyps usually arise from the endocervical canal, becoming visible when they protrude through the cervical os. They are bright red, soft and rather fragile. When only the tips are seen they cannot be clinically differentiated from polyps originating in the endometrium.

Nabothian or retention cysts

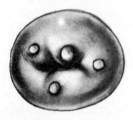

Retention or Nabothian cysts are another accompaniment of chronic cervicitis. Variable in size, single or multiple, they appear as translucent nodules on the cervical surface.

Ectropion & erosion

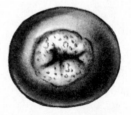

Ectropion is extension of endocervical columnar epithelium (reddish, bumpy) onto the ectocervix. This physiologic condition often occurs with increased estrogen activity (eg, pregnancy). If inflammation or infection occurs, the tissue becomes friable and bleeds easily. This is referred to as erosion.

■ *Figure 47–1*
Common cervical conditions.

is wiped gently only if there is excessive mucus. Lubricating jelly should not be used because it distorts the cell sample; water is permissible to aid speculum insertion. Samples are taken from the endocervical canal with the cotton-tipped applicator, which may be wetted with saline, or the cytobrush. The applicator is placed high in the cervix, rotated a few times, then withdrawn and applied to a slide by gentle rolling. The spatula, with the long tip placed into the cervical os, is used to scrape the ectocervix. The material is spread thinly on a slide.

Slides are sprayed or immersed immediately in a fixative; air drying can distort cells. The presence of inflammation or infection should be noted on the Pap request form.

Vaginal pool specimens are recommended for women over the age of 50, when they can be helpful in detecting endometrial cancer.[14] Depending on symptoms and vaginal or cervical signs, other specimens may be taken for microscopic examination, such as wet mounts prepared with saline or potassium hydroxide, or chlamydia or gonorrhea cultures. With a history of exposure to DES, samples are obtained with a spatula by scraping the vaginal walls, placing on a slide, and fixing as above.

DIAGNOSIS. Pap smears generally are reported descriptively and identify the degree of cervical epithelial change that has occurred (see Papanicolaou Smear Cytology Reports). If the report is abnormal, further evaluation is necessary. Women with an atypical Pap smear that also identifies the presence of a microorganism (with or without inflammation) are treated with the appropriate medication, such as antifungal, antitrichomonal, or antibiotic drugs. The Pap smear is then repeated in 3 to 6 months. If significant atypia still is present, the woman is referred for colposcopy or biopsy.

Women with Pap smears showing dysplasia require prompt management because this can be a precursor to cancer. Initial treatment consists in colposcopy and biopsy. Colposcopy uses a binocular stereoscopic microscope of low magnification to view the cervix through a vaginal speculum. The cervix is swabbed to remove mucus, and 2% acetic acid is applied to enhance cellular patterns. A green filter and Schiller's iodine solution may also be used to accentuate vascular patterns and identify suspicious cells. The transformation zone of the cervix (area of change from squamous to columnar epithelium) is carefully examined for vascular patterns, intercapillary distance, surface patterns, color tone and opacity, clarity, and demarcation. Typical findings include white epithelium, mosaic structure, punctation, and leukoplakia.

Biopsy specimens are taken from suspicious areas of the cervix. This is usually adequate if the upper margin of the transformation zone can be seen on the ectocervix. If the upper margin is not visible, endocervical curettage is necessary to sample the transformation zone adequately. Based on cytologic examination of these specimens, medical treatment can be planned.

Nursing Diagnoses. Nursing diagnoses related to CIN are similar to those for breast tumors. Both conditions potentially involve cancer, which is life-threatening and may require loss of body parts. Common nursing diagnoses might be knowledge deficit; ineffective coping patterns; disturbance in self-concept; anxiety; fear; sexual dysfunction; and powerlessness.

Treatment. Medical treatment depends on the extensiveness of the CIN. If cells from the endocervical canal have been found free of disease, and the abnormal cells from the cervix range from mild to moderate dysplasia to carcinoma in situ, techniques are used that completely destroy the surface of the transformation zone and penetrate at least 4 to 5 mm to destroy any dysplastic extensions into the gland crypts. Cryosurgery, carbon dioxide laser therapy, and radical electrocautery are all effective techniques that can be performed on an outpatient basis or in surgical centers. Local or general anesthesia can be used, and pain during the healing process is usually minimal.[9]

When CIN has progressed to the microinvasive stage, surgical conization is the initial treatment. It is used when colposcopy and biopsy fail to reveal the source of abnormal cells and when the upper margin of the transformation zone cannot be visualized. Surgical conization removes a cone-shaped wedge from the cervical canal with a knife. Depending on the extent of invasion, hysterectomy may follow conization.

Invasive cervical cancer is staged according to extent of stromal involvement and whether vaginal or pelvic wall extension, rectal or bladder extension, kidney involvement, and distant metastases have occurred (see Staging of Cervical Cancer). Treatment consists in hysterectomy (simple or radical), irradiation, or chemotherapy, depending on the extensiveness of disease, the woman's age and general health, and the presence of other abnormalities.

Papanicolaou Smear Cytology Reports

Pap smear reports usually provide a description of the cervical cells and other characteristics of the smear, such as hormonal status and whether the smear was satisfactory and contained endocervical cells. The following is a typical organization of a Pap smear report:

Cellular characteristics
- ☐ Within normal limits (class I)
- ☐ Inflammatory atypica (class II)
  - ☐ Reactive atypia
  - ☐ Squamous metaplasia
  - ☐ Trichomonas
  - ☐ Candida
  - ☐ Gardnerella
  - ☐ Radiation effect
- ☐ Squamous cell abnormality (class III)
  - ☐ Atypical squamous metaplasia
  - ☐ Reactive
  - ☐ Intraepithelial lesion (dysplasia) ☐ Low grade
  - ☐ High grade
- ☐ Squamous carcinoma (class IV)
- ☐ Glandular abnormalities
  - ☐ Endometrial cells present
  - ☐ Atypical glandular cells
  - ☐ Adenocarcinoma

Hormonal evaluation

	Estrogen Effect
_____ % Basal	☐ High
_____ % Intermediate	☐ Moderate
_____ % Superficial	☐ Low

Staging of Cervical Cancer

Stage 0		Carcinoma in situ, intraepithelial carcinoma
Stage I		Carcinoma strictly confined to the cervix
	IA	Microinvasive carcinoma (early stromal invasion)
	IB	All other cases of stage I (occult cancer = occ)
Stage II		Carcinoma extends beyond the cervix but has not extended to the pelvic wall. The carcinoma involves the vagina, but not as far as the lower third.
	IIA	No obvious parametrial involvement
	IIB	Obvious parametrial involvement
Stage III		Carcinoma has extended to the pelvic wall. On rectal examination, there is no cancer-free space between the tumor and the pelvic wall. The tumor involves the lower third of the vagina.
	IIA	No extension to the pelvic wall
	IIB	Extension to the pelvic wall or hydronephrosis or nonfunctioning kidney
Stage IV		Carcinoma has extended beyond the true pelvis or has clinically involved the mucosa of the bladder or rectum.
	IVA	Spread of carcinoma to adjacent organs
	IVB	Spread to distant organs

Nomenclature of the International Federation of Gynecology and Obstetrics.

Stage IA cancer of the cervix is treated with either hysterectomy or radiotherapy, as the cancer is confined to the cervix. Stages IB and IIA are treated with total hysterectomy and bilateral lymphadenectomy. Stages IIB through IVB involve spread of cancer beyond the cervix to other organs, and the treatment of choice usually is radiotherapy.[15]

Planning and Intervention. Nursing care is similar to that for breast problems and breast cancer (see Nursing Care Plan in earlier section). Of particular consideration is the meaning of reproductive ability to the woman and her partner. Some women suffer severe alterations in self-concept when they can no longer have babies, and their spouses often hold similar attitudes that devalue nonprocreative women. Interventions in these cases focus on the process of accepting physical and psychological changes and finding other qualities for which the woman can be valued. In other instances, loss of the uterus and reproductive capacity does not significantly diminish self-concept. The woman may have other valued roles or may be at a time in life when childbearing is no longer desired. For some women who have been experiencing considerable pain with menses and disruption in routines, hysterectomy may be viewed with relief. If cancer is diagnosed, many women find the threat to life vastly more important than the loss of reproductive capacity. Nursing interventions then focus on the client's expressing fear, placing realistic parameters on expectations, clarifying values and spiritual supports, enhancing family and community resources, and finding personal strengths for coping.

Prevention. Nursing care for women includes education about the risk factors for cervical cancer and ways that risk can be reduced. Young women need to be informed that early sexual activity and multiple sexual partners place them at increased risk for cervical cancer. The avoidance of sexually transmitted disease exposure can reduce risk. The importance of regular, frequent Pap smears is emphasized, with a screening interval of 1 to 2 years. Women are informed that longer screening intervals increase their risk of more advanced cervical cancer.

Diet may act as a factor in development of cervical cancer. Low intake of vitamin A, beta carotene, vitamin C, or folic acid is consistently correlated with an increased prevalence of cervical neoplasia. Vitamin A and its precursors exert effects by inhibiting steps in the chain of carcinogenesis, controlling cellular differentiation, or blocking the effects of transforming growth factors. Retinoids may stimulate immunologic defense mechanisms, thus interfering with carcinogenesis. Vitamin C helps to maintain normal epithelium and to provide protection against the effects of potential carcinogens. It acts by altering the structure of carcinogens and preventing access of carcinogens to the target tissue by competitive inhibition. Folate may inhibit or stimulate specific enzymes that are particularly important for cells undergoing mitosis.[16–18]

Vitamin A has been found to revert the metaplastic process. Cervical cancer is believed to begin in the metaplastic process in the transformation zone of the cervix. Studies have shown a marked deficiency or absence of Vitamin A binding proteins in cervical neoplastic tissues and that beta carotene has a protective effect against cervical cancer.[16]

Although specific causality has not been proven, most studies show a consistent inverse association between vitamin consumption and risk of cervical neoplasia. Nursing care includes advising women of the importance of adequate vitamin intake, especially vitamins A and C. Dietary counseling can ensure adequate food sources, or vitamin supplementation can be advised.

Pelvic Masses

Conditions involving pelvic organs and producing varying degrees of pain are common among women of reproductive age. Maternity nurses may be consulted about pelvic symptoms and need a working knowledge of the kinds of conditions that might be involved. Menstrual and bleeding problems are covered in Chapter 48. Common pelvic masses are discussed here, particularly ovarian tumors and uterine masses. Among younger women, these conditions tend to be benign; the risk of cancer increases with age. Cancer, however, must be considered in every type of pelvic mass until diagnosed otherwise.

Ovarian masses common among women between 20 and 40 years of age include functional ovarian cysts, cystadenomas, cystic teratomas, fibromas, endometriomas (chocolate cysts), and tuboovarian pregnancies (Table 47-3). Unless quite large, these masses usually cause no symptoms and are discovered incidentally during an examination. When symptoms are present, they are usually vague and may include lower abdominal discomfort or aching; feelings of fullness, pressure, dyspareunia; or discomfort with menstruation or defecation. Tuboovarian pregnancies cause acute abdominal pain prior to and during rupture and are discussed in Chapter 33.

The relative frequency of malignant ovarian neoplasms increases with each decade of life, ranging from 4% in the age range of 20 to 29 years to 49% in the age range of 60 to 69 years. In premenopausal women, the overall risk that an ovarian neoplasm is malignant is 13%; this risk increases to 45% in postmenopausal women.[19] Factors that increase the risk of ovarian cancer include delayed onset of childbearing, low parity, infertility, nulliparity, several spontaneous abortions, and family history of ovarian cancer. White women of European and North American origin are more likely to contract ovarian cancer than African-American women of African origin or Oriental women of Asian origin. There is some evidence that women with irregular menses and premenstrual tension may be at increased risk.[20]

Ovarian cancer is generally silent, making its diagnosis in early stages difficult. The most common types are cystadenocarcinomas and adenocarcinomas, which may be either solid or cystic. Ovarian metastasis from other primary cancers may occur. In early stages, ovarian cancer may feel no different from benign cystic or solid ovarian masses. Later, cancers may become fixed, heavy, and hard and have ill-defined margins. Malignant tumors frequently are nontender and cause few symptoms except vague pelvic fullness or aching. Infectious ovarian or pelvic masses are usually readily identifiable because of associated findings of fever, leukocytosis, tenderness, nausea, and vomiting.

Nursing Assessment. The health history focuses on age, menstrual history, present menstrual status, parturition history, family history—especially of cancers—and race. Symptoms involving the lower abdomen and reproductive organs are explored. Weight gain must be carefully evaluated; it may be related to ascites or ovarian enlargement. Some women may notice increased abdominal girth but may interpret this as midriff bulge or middle age. As the tumor enlarges, it progressively compresses surrounding pelvic structures and blood vessels, leading to urinary frequency, edema of lower extremities, constipation, and pelvic discomfort. Gastrointestinal symptoms may include heartburn, bloating, anorexia, and food intolerance. Unusual vaginal bleeding is a common symptom during reproductive years, including amenorrhea and irregular or excessive menses. Many types of ovarian tumors can affect menstrual patterns. Late signs of cancer are pelvic pain, cachexia, and anemia; unfortunately, much ovarian cancer is not discovered until an advanced stage with such signs, and prognosis is poor.

Physical examination usually reveals an ovarian enlargement; specific characteristics depend on the type of tumor (see Table 47-3). An experienced examiner often can make a reliable assessment based on tumor characteristics and associated history of symptoms, taking risk characteristics into consideration. Functional ovarian cysts that fail to resolve with conservative management must be further evaluated, as are solid masses, using such techniques as ultrasonography, laparoscopic examination, and biopsy.

DIAGNOSIS. Medical diagnosis is based on tumor characteristics and results of diagnostic tests. In some instances, surgical removal of the tumor with pathologic examination establishes the diagnosis. When ovarian cancer is diagnosed, it must be staged so appropriate therapy can be planned. An international system for staging ovarian cancer has been developed. Pap tests of vaginal, pleural, or peritoneal fluids; lung and bone scans; blood tests; and radiographic studies of chest, kidneys, and gastrointestinal system complete the diagnostic work-up.

Nursing Diagnosis. Nursing diagnoses may include knowledge deficit; disturbance in self-concept; ineffective coping; fear; anxiety; powerlessness; alterations in comfort; sexual dysfunction; and spiritual distress.

Treatment. Functional ovarian cysts may be managed conservatively, because these usually resolve sponta-

TABLE 47–3. CHARACTERISTICS OF PELVIC TUMORS

Condition	Location	Size	Consistency	Mobility
Ovary				
Functional cyst (follicular, corpus luteum)	Adnexa, usually unilateral	5 to 6 cm	Cystic	Mobile
Benign neoplastic (cystadenoma, cystic teratoma)	Adnexa, usually unilateral	6 to 12 cm	Cystic	Mobile unless large
Malignant (cystadenocarcinoma, adenocarcinoma)	Adnexa, usually unilateral	5 to 25 cm	Cystic or solid	Mobile early, fixed or frozen late
Endometrioma (chocolate cyst)	Adnexa, usually unilateral; cul-de-sac	>10 cm	Cystic	Usually fixed
Fallopian tubes				
Tuboovarian abscess	Adnexa, bilateral; cul-de-sac	Varies	Solid	Fixed
Parovarian cyst	Adnexa, usually unilateral	5 to 8 cm	Cystic	Mobile
Ectopia pregnancy	Adnexa, unilateral; cul-de-sac	5 to 6 cm	Solid	Mobile
Uterus				
Fibroid pedunculated	Midline; adnexa or cul-de-sac	Varies	Firm and rubbery	Mobile
Adenomyosis	Midline	8 to 12 cm	Firm to hard	Mobile uterus
Endometrial carcinoma	Midline	Often normal	Firm	Mobile uterus
Endometritis	Midline	Often normal	Firm	Mobile uterus

neously within several weeks. The client is reexamined during different phases of the menstrual cycle after an interval of 1 to 3 months. Failure of the mass to resolve by 12 weeks requires further diagnostic procedures. Solid benign tumors generally are removed surgically, with ovarian resection or removal depending on extent of tumor involvement. Ovarian cancer is treated according to stage of the disease. Surgical removal of as much of the tumor as possible is usually done first and

can range from simple removal of one ovary to radical hysterectomy and bilateral salpingo-oophorectomy. Chemotherapy or radiotherapy often follows, the combinations and extent dependent on the stage of cancer and aggressiveness of the malignancy.

Planning and Intervention. Nursing care is related to the type of ovarian tumor, medical treatment, and client and family responses. For simple benign problems, in-

Shape	Tenderness	Pain	Fever	Nausea, Vomitting, and Diarrhea	Other Associated Factors
Round to ovoid	None to slight	None to dull, aching	No	No	Delayed menses; spontaneous resorption in 6 to 12 weeks
Round to ovoid	None	None or vague fullness, aching	No	No	Disturbed menses ±
Varies	None	None or vague fullness, aching	No	No	Disturbed menses ±
Irregular	±	±	No	No	Nodules on uterosacral ligaments; fixed retroflexed uterus; cul-de-sac nodules
Poorly defined	++++	Severe constant	Yes	Nausea/vomiting	Elevated white blood cells, erythrocyte sedimentation rate; history of venereal disease or pelvic inflammatory disease ±; movement of cervix painful
Round to ovoid	None	None or vague, aching	No	No	Ovary separately palpable
Ovoid	++ to ++++	Mild to severe	No	Nausea/vomitting	Menstrual irregularities; signs, symptoms of pregnancy; peritonitis if ruptured
Irregular	No	None or vague aching	No	No	Uterus enlarged, nodular, irregular contour; pressure; irregular menses
Uterus globular	+++	Cramps	No	No	Abnormal bleeding, dysmenorrhea; multipara age 40 to 50
Usual	None	None usually	No	No	Abnormal bleeding
Usual	+++	Cramps, aching	±	±	History of venereal disease, vaginal discharge; menstrual changes

terventions emphasize client teaching, support during procedures, and emotional support to cope with fear and anxiety. When ovarian cancer is present, interventions include the above as well as physiological monitoring and technical procedures, comfort measures, support for family coping and adjustment, expressing and dealing with fear, coordinating resources for family support and recovery, clarifying values and spiritual supports, and finding personal strengths for coping.

Uterine Masses

Uterine masses often present as an enlarged or irregularly shaped uterus, although a pedunculated fibroid can be felt as an apparently separate pelvic mass. Evaluation of an enlarged uterus is to some extent related to age; certainly among women in the childbearing age pregnancy must always be considered. Infections, adenomyosis, polyps, fibroids, hyperplasia, and malignancy are among the more common causes of uterine enlargement. Endometrial carcinoma is the third most frequent malignancy in women; 90% of these are adenocarcinomas. The peak incidence is between ages 50 and 70, and it is more common in postmenopausal women. The etiology of endometrial cancer is unclear; it is possibly triggered by metabolic abnormalities involving pituitary hyperactivity and impaired glucose metabolism. Prolonged exogenous estrogen use, especially in postmenopausal women, has been associated with increased incidence of endometrial cancer.

Nursing Assessment. Risk for endometrial cancer is greater in white, middle-class women who experience irregular menses, infertility, or late menopause. An association has long been observed between obesity, hypertension, and diabetes mellitus and endometrial cancer, but the causal connections are not well understood. Other risk factors include personal or family history of cancers, atypical endometrial hyperplasia, and postmenopausal bleeding.

The history includes exploration of the above risk factors and questions about related symptoms. Fever, abdominal pain, nausea, and anorexia are indicative of an infection. Urinary frequency, nausea and vomiting, breast tenderness, and amenorrhea suggest possible pregnancy. Bleeding patterns are extremely important; irregular menses and abnormal bleeding are the most common symptoms of endometrial cancer. Postmenopausal bleeding requires immediate investigation because cancer is more frequent in this age group and bleeding is a hallmark symptom. Hormone use must be carefully assessed.

Pelvic examination is done to determine size, shape, and consistency of the uterus and to evaluate the ovaries and adnexa. Depending on symptoms and risk factors, endometrial biopsy or fractional curettage of the endocervix and endometrium often is done. Over 80% of endometrial cancers will be diagnosed with these methods. The Gravlee Jet Washer is another diagnostic aid used in women over the age of 35. This method obtains endometrial cells by washing the uterine cavity with normal saline in a collecting system.

DIAGNOSIS. Clinical findings may be used for initial diagnosis of uterine masses thought to be benign, such as fibroids or adenomyosis. Diagnostic tests help establish other causes, such as pregnancy test for pregnancy and biopsy or curettage for hyperplasia or cancer. Blood tests such as white blood cell count with differential and erythrocyte sedimentation rate aid the diagnosis of infections.

Nursing Diagnosis. Nursing diagnoses are related to the type of medical problem, the stage of disease if cancer is diagnosed, and the responses of the client and her family. Refer to discussion under ovarian tumors.

Treatment. Benign conditions such as uterine fibroids are often managed conservatively if the tumors are not increasing in size significantly. Management includes regular evaluation by pelvic examination and diagnostic tests. If the fibroids enlarge or other signs or symptoms cause concern, abdominal surgery may be required, with possible tumor resection or hysterectomy. The management of adenomyosis and hyperplasia is discussed in Chapter 48. Endometrial cancer is treated according to its stage and the age and health status of the client (see Staging for Endometrial Cancer). For early stages of adenocarcinoma (stage I), total abdominal hysterectomy with bilateral salpingo-oophorectomy (TAH-BSO) is the usual treatment. Stage II cancers, which extend beyond the corpus to the cervix, are treated with TAH-BSO accompanied by lymph node dissection, which is followed by radiation therapy. Stages III and IV are usually treated with intrauterine radiation or external radiotherapy. Chemotherapy and hormone therapy in various combinations may also be used.

Planning and Intervention. Nursing care for uterine masses follows the general approaches previously described for benign and malignant ovarian and breast conditions. Care for clients who are pregnant has been presented earlier; care for infectious conditions and

---

Staging for Endometrial Cancer

Stage I — The carcinoma is confined to the uterine corpus.

   IA — The length of the uterine cavity is 8 cm or less.

   IB — The length of the uterine cavity is more than 8 cm.

Stage II — The carcinoma involves the corpus and the cervix.

Stage III — The carcinoma has extended outside the uterus but not outside the true pelvis.

Stage IV — The carcinoma has extended outside the true pelvis or has involved the mucosa of the bladder or rectum.

The Stage I cases are subgrouped by histologic type of adenocarcinoma as follows:

   G1 — Highly differentiated adenomatous carcinomas

   G2 — Differentiated adenomatous carcinomas with partly solid areas

   G3 — Predominantly solid or undifferentiated carcinomas

Classification system developed by the International Federation of Gynecology and Obstetrics.

bleeding-related problems is discussed in Chapters 35 and 48, respectively.

Evaluation. Nursing intervention is evaluated by observing for changes in the client's behavior, level of knowledge, and attitudes. The client is able to express a clear understanding of the health problem and its cause, treatment, and outcomes. She understands measures that can be taken to prevent illness or complications and expresses a willingness to undertake these. Behavioral changes might be observed that indicate therapeutic progress, such as weight loss, normal physiological tests, medication compliance, general appearance, and affect. A positive attitude and seeking family support indicate effective emotional responses to health problems. Following through on referrals for psychological counseling or social support agencies indicates effective intervention. Regular BSE and having regular Pap smears are evidence that preventive measures are being carried out. Rapport with the nurse is shown when the client openly discusses concerns and asks questions.

■ WOMEN AND STRESS

Stress is an unavoidable part of life. Nurses providing care to gynecologic and maternity clients will have numerous opportunities to intervene in stress-related problems. Stress is conceptualized as a person-environment relationship that taxes or exceeds the resources of the person to deal with the resulting demands.[21] The body's response to stress includes physical, mental, emotional, and chemical reactions. Factors that contribute to stress are those that frighten, excite, confuse, endanger, or irritate the person. A certain amount of stress is natural and probably necessary for life, but continuous stress at a sufficiently high level can have adverse effects on health.

Various factors contribute to the stressors women encounter as well as to women's reactions to stress. There are biologic differences between women and men that lead to characteristic patterns and rates of illness, longevity, and causes of death. Although women are more resistant to infectious and degenerative disease and to major illness (e.g., cancer, heart disease), they do have more acute, limited conditions than men. Women seek care earlier, more often, and for less serious problems than do men.

Research indicates that higher levels of symptoms are experienced by those people with oppressive life conditions, such as financial insecurity, abusive families, unemployment, and social isolation. Women, minorities, and the poor with such oppressive conditions have more physical and emotional health problems.[22]

Such factors as changing family patterns, divorce, employment and unemployment, inequities in earnings and promotions, sexual discrimination, discounting the female experience, and learned helplessness influence women's experiences of and responses to stress.

Stress and Work. The number of women in the work force has increased dramatically. Forty-five percent of all workers are women; this proportion has increased from 35% in 1954 and 41% in 1980. More than 90% of all women work for at least some period during their lives. Although about half of women workers are responsible for financially maintaining their families, they continue to earn less than men with the same education.

Women have established an impressive presence in occupations previously reserved mostly for men. Nearly 18% of physicians, 22% of lawyers, 32% of computer systems analysts, and 50% of accountants and auditors are women. Few women have progressed from middle management to the top executive positions in business, however. A 1990 survey of Fortune 1000 companies showed only 3% of the top five chief-executive-officer positions were held by women, up from 1% a decade ago.[23]

The composition of the labor force is changing dramatically. Although only about half as many new workers will enter the labor force in the coming decade, two thirds of these will be women starting or returning to work. Minority men and immigrants will account for most of the rest. The needs, work styles, and career goals of this labor force will be very different. Young women now beginning careers want recognition of family and parenting needs, flexible work patterns, the ability to advance without workaholism, and successful blending of home and work responsibilities with cooperative, adaptable spouses. Although only 25% of young women plan to be housewives, 66% would like to stay home for a time to raise children. Surprisingly, 48% of young men also want the opportunity to be home with children.[23]

Women face multiple demands both at home and at work that can create role conflicts. The International Labor Office calculates that the average woman worldwide works 80 hours each week at home and at work, while the average man works 50 hours each week at home and at work.[24] Women, in effect, have two full-time jobs. This dual employment of women leads to considerable stress as they continue with primary responsibility for home activities, such as cooking, cleaning, and child care. Women with multiple roles of wife, mother, and career woman report coping with more stressful life events than single working women or married women at home but appear to be least vulnerable to both illness and depression. Women in multiple roles seem to have more resources for coping from a blend of family emotional support and work success.[25]

WORKPLACE HAZARDS. Workplace hazards may have different impacts on women than men. Unless tools, equipment, and work environments are designed to accommodate women's smaller muscle mass and strength, women have increased risk of musculoskeletal trauma. Women have less heat tolerance and reduced sweating, because of a greater proportion of body fat. Most protective equipment for chemical toxins is designed to fit men, and threshold safety limits have been established through research done on the male population.

The number of women moving into male-dominated jobs has decreased. Women are being employed in traditionally female jobs. These jobs have characteristics that are associated with high stress levels. Jobs in food service, health care, manufacturing, and clerical work are characterized by lack of control over work and environment, powerlessness, less recognition, excessive hours of work, low pay, underutilization of skills, and demanding requirements. This often leads to job dissatisfaction, which is a significant risk factor for coronary artery disease, hypertension, and ulcers.

Clerical workers using video display terminals full-time for information processing were found to have high levels of stress. Although the electromagnetic fields and radiation near computer terminals fall below government-established limits, it is not known whether these low-level fields are biologic hazards. Glare filters can reduce eye strain but do not affect electromagnetic fields.

Nurses face significant work-related stress because of work characteristics and chemical and physical hazards. Most nurses are women (94%) and have a dual role as wage earner and homemaker. They perceive their pay as inequitable (male nurses earn 10% more than female nurses), have limited opportunities for advancement within the hospital structure, and often find their work task oriented and repetitious. Hospitals are based on authoritarian power models, and many nurses experience a lack of independent decision-making opportunities or subtle discrimination within this masculine-value–dominated environment. Nurses, however, do not seem to have greater stress than other working women. When nurses and other female hospital employees were compared on a stress scale with other employed women, their mean scores were in the average or below-average ranges.[26]

HAZARDS OF MEDICAL TREATMENT. Many types of medical treatment recommended for both men and women have been tested only on men. Little evidence exists about the safety and efficacy for women of such therapies as cholesterol-lowering drugs, acquired immunodeficiency syndrome treatments, and antidepressants. Drugs are developed with incomplete data on metabolic differences between the sexes, particularly the effects of hormonal changes during the menstrual cycle. Women often are excluded as research subjects because they increase the cost and complexity of the study

through such factors as risk of pregnancy and menstrual hormone changes. Breast cancer, contraception, and menopause receive relatively little federal research support. Overall, the National Institutes of Health (NIH) spend about 13% of its budget directly on women's health issues.[27]

To strengthen and enhance the efforts of NIH research related to diseases and conditions affecting women, the Office of Research on Women's Health was established in 1990. Researchers with NIH grants and contracts will need to include women in clinical studies proportional to the degree the condition affects women. Through conferences, a focused research agenda, and communication of study findings, the Office will attempt to make changes in the health care system to improve women's health.

SUBSTANCE ABUSE. Substance abuse among women in the workplace is a significant stressor of increasing dimensions. Current estimates are that 50% of all alcoholics are women, but a lower proportion of clients in workplace alcoholism programs are females. Data on drug use show more younger people use illicit drugs and indicate that women use more prescription and over-the-counter drugs than men. Multiple drug use and abuse are increasing, including combining drugs and alcohol. Women are not being reached effectively by traditional identification and referral mechanisms, and research has focused on male behavioral models rather than female.

Stress levels have been tied generally to substance abuse. Being both a woman and a parent increases stress symptoms, and working exacerbates these problems. The origins, context, and control of employed women's substance abuse differ from those of men and seem related to issues of familial responsibilities, low self-esteem, job and pay discrimination, sex-role conflicts, and stress and conflict management.[28]

Women's drinking behavior often changes over time, related to shifting roles, contexts, and circumstances. Younger women show more onset and remission of problem drinking, whereas middle-aged women have more chronic problem drinking. The strongest predictors of alcohol dependence are sexual dysfunction and depression. Other predictors of chronic drinking problems include never being married, part-time employment or unemployment, and cohabitating. Divorce, separation, or children's departure from home are more likely to follow than to precede problem drinking. The onset of problem drinking may be facilitated by long-term use of psychoactive drugs (see Chap. 36).[29]

CIGARETTE SMOKING. Tobacco is a substance with great health risks that is used by many women. Although smoking rates have dropped substantially for men, the decline among women has been much smaller. Smoking prevalence rates in adolescent and young adult women are beginning to exceed those among men.

Smoking by women poses hazards to their own long-term health and has important impacts on reproductive function and the health of children.

The health consequences of smoking can be severe, including such diseases as emphysema, hypertension, coronary artery disease, and lung cancer. The incidence of lung cancer among women is increasing. Women smokers using oral contraceptives are at greatly increased risk for heart attack, especially after the ages of 35 to 40. Smoking during pregnancy retards fetal growth and increases the rates of spontaneous abortion and perinatal mortality. Women who smoke have 50% to 150% higher risk for invasive cervical neoplasia, CIN, and other severe cervical abnormalities.[30,31]

Women who smoke are relatively estrogen deficient, through the effects of nicotine and hydrocarbons on the ovaries, pituitary and adrenal glands, and hypothalamus. The metabolism of estrogen is changed in smokers, who have serum levels of estrone and estradiol reduced to 50% of nonsmokers' levels. Menopause occurs about 1½ years earlier in smokers, who also have a two to threefold increased risk for osteoporotic fractures of the spine and hip. Smoking's antiestrogenic effects are beneficial in diseases caused by estrogen excess. Smokers have decreased incidence of endometrial cancer, uterine fibroids, endometrial hyperplasia, and endometriosis. Menstrual irregularities and menopausal symptoms appear to be aggravated by smoking. The risks of breast cancer do not appear much affected by cigarette smoking.[30,32,33]

Nonsmokers also are harmed by "sidestream smoke," because this smoke coming directly from the burning tip of the cigarette contains higher concentrations of toxic chemicals than smoke inhaled into the lungs through a filter. Cigarette smoke is a mixture of particles and gases that contain 3800 to 4000 chemicals, of which more than 50 are known carcinogens. Nonsmoking women with normal Pap smears were tested for the presence of nicotine in cervical secretions. Those exposed to tobacco smoke in the home had the highest nicotine levels, with intermediate levels in women exposed only outside the home. Women with no reported exposure had very low nicotine levels.[34] Even low levels of exposure to tobacco smoke can have systemic effects and may be a risk factor for cervical disease.

Nurses continue to smoke at higher rates than other professional women and physicians. In the 1980s, 25% of nurses were still smokers. Psychiatric and mental-health nurses tend to smoke more than those in other specialties, reported at 48% to 52%.[35] Smoking among women has been related to work characteristics, stress, and concerns about weight. Young adult women are twice as likely as young adult men to report weight gain with smoking cessation and were much more worried about gaining weight when considering quitting. Women feel more social pressure to quit, 70% having been urged by people close to them and 30% by health providers.[36]

Nursing Assessment. Stress in women may be assessed by observation and by history taking. A person under severe stress usually manifests it by appearance and behavior: looking drawn, haggard, or poorly groomed and exhibiting a number of behavioral symptoms such as irritation, fatigue, anxiety, nervousness, confusion, distraction, or depression. Many people express stress through physical symptoms such as headaches, back pain, constipation or diarrhea, gastric distress, anorexia or overeating, palpitations, hyperventilation, insomnia, and increased susceptibility to infections. When the nurse suspects that stress is related to the client's symptoms or problems, further assessment can be done using a stress assessment tool. Involving the client in self-assessment is integral to using such tools for assessing stress levels. Coping strategies are usually included in the assessment process.

Substance abuse may require a somewhat different focus in assessment, because indicators are often subtle. Early indicators may include depression, dependency, low self-esteem, and learning problems. These are often followed by insomnia, anxiety, worry, inadequacy either felt or expressed through poor role performance, few leisure activities, missing appointments, and evasiveness. Late indicators include disrupted social relations, severe depression, inability to work, gastritis, fractures and injuries from falls, suicidal tendencies, and isolation. Other clues the nurse might observe are changes in appearance, heavy perfume or mouthwash, emphasis on somatic complaints (especially menstrually related), and concealing parts of the body (arms, legs). On physical examination, alcoholics may have spider angiomas, tender or enlarged liver, tachycardia, hypertension, and gastric tenderness. Depending on route of administration, drug users may have tracks on arms or legs.

Smokers usually do no attempt to conceal their cigarette use. Signs that indicate heavy smoking, however, include the smell of smoke on clothing or hair, brown discoloration of index and middle finger, discolored teeth, and thickened or ridged fingernails. Most smokers have changes in lung sounds, such as wheezing or scattered rhonchi that clear with coughing.

Nursing Diagnosis. Ineffective individual coping is the most direct nursing diagnosis related to stress, in which the woman is unable to manage internal or environmental stressors adequately due to inadequate resources (physical, psychological, behavioral). Some maturational factors contributing to ineffective coping include career choices and pressures, childbearing and marital problems, retirement, and aging. Situational factors may include sensory overload (work environment, effects of

Assessment Tool

Stress Assessment

I. Personal Information

Age   Marital status
Children   Relatives/friends
Living arrangements   Work
Health state   Limitations/disabilities
Financial state

II. Stressors   Events that have been experienced in the last 12 months. How impor-
Life events   tant (rank: little to great)

	Check if happened	How important
Relationship change	—	—
Career change	—	—
Illness/death	—	—
Personal illness	—	—
Work problems	—	—
Financial problems	—	—
Family problems	—	—
Legal problems	—	—
Health/body changes	—	—
Psychological stress	—	—

Life conditions   Reasonably consistent patterns in life: Describe usual situation related
to each of these that is important.

Living space
Family relations
Employment/career
Financial state
Health state
Recreation/activities
Spiritual values

Coping strategies   Usual ways used to cope with stress. Describe how well these work.
Eat/drink more/less
Use alcohol or other drugs
Sleep more/less
Exercise more/less
Use relaxation technique
Smoke more
Avoid problem/pretend not there
Clarify/set goals
Time management/efficiency
Make changes in job, relations
Pray, meditate, seek spiritual help
Analyze/understand conflicts
Talk with spouse, friends
More recreation/activities
Block out feelings
Desensitize fears, aversions
Seek new relations
Enter therapy/support group
Other

urban living) and inadequate psychological resources (poor self-esteem, helplessness, lack of motivation).

Other nursing diagnoses potentially related to stress include sleep pattern disturbance; alterations in thought processes; anxiety; fear; powerlessness; disturbance in self-concept; impaired communication; and alterations in parenting.

Planning and Intervention. Nursing care focuses on assisting the woman to identify and interpret her stressors and the responses to them. Once this is done, the goal is to reduce or reinterpret stress so it becomes feasible for the woman to cope effectively. Using counseling and teaching skills, the nurse may assist the client in any of these areas: problem solving, decision making, exploration of alternative behaviors and strategies, drawing on other internal and external resources, analyzing usual ways of coping, assessing what works and what does not, and learning specific stress reduction techniques.

In the work setting, nurses can identify and evaluate stressors affecting women and develop recommendations or programs for stress management. Some approaches could be flexible time, child-care programs, educational campaigns, stress reduction workshops, health screening and promotion, time management, conflict management, family problem solving, personal growth groups, fitness programs, stop-smoking programs, assertiveness training, and support groups. When serious problems are identified, such as alcohol or drug abuse, referrals to substance abuse programs are indicated. Psychotherapy or other emotional counseling can be recommended for severe emotional problems.

Many approaches to stress reduction can be used. To obtain maximum benefit, these techniques should be used regularly. Three common approaches are briefly described here.

Progressive relaxation uses tensing and relaxing of muscle groups progressively throughout the body to attain a state of deep relaxation. Beginning in a sitting or lying position, the woman takes a few deep breaths, then progressively tenses and relaxes toes, feet, calves, knees, thighs, buttocks, stomach, lower back, chest, upper back, shoulders, arms and hands, neck, face, eyes, and forehead. Next, the entire body is tensed and relaxed, followed by a few deep breaths and a period of stillness.

Guided imagery has the client focus on images that create a relaxed state. Sitting or lying in a comfortable position, the women closes her eyes and takes several deep breaths. Then she creates a mental image of a scene that she finds satisfying and peaceful, such as a beach, stream, meadow, mountain, or forest. She imagines smells, sounds, textures, colors, and any other aspects of the situation that produce a good feeling. Some

advise this image be written, polished, and put on audiotape. It is then played back for relaxation.

Meditation is an approach to quiet the mind and focus on the deep inner silence or peace. A quiet place is needed, and the woman sits comfortably. She may select a word or sound to chant, a symbol or object to gaze at, or music to focus the mind. Meditation is continued for 15 to 20 minutes, with a passive attitude that accepts thoughts and distractions, then gently refocuses attention on the meditation object.

Evaluation. The first indication of positive action occurs when the woman identifies stressors and her responses to them. She then chooses an approach and follows the techniques to reduce her stress. She reports better sleep and the ability to think more clearly. Depending on her situation, her enhancement of parenting abilities is manifest in both her speech and her actions, or she takes definite steps to overcome her feelings of powerlessness in the workplace and faces her anxieties and fears.

■ FAMILY VIOLENCE AGAINST WOMEN

Family violence is an area of growing national concern. Spouse abuse and battering are social problems affecting every stratum of society and are the most common but least reported forms of violence in the United States. An estimated 4 to 6 million women are battered annually, and 50% to 60% of all women are abused at some time during their marriages, much of which is unreported or concealed in divorce statistics.[37,38] Battery is the single largest cause of injury to women in the United States; 21% of women who use emergency department services seek care for battery. Nearly half of all rapes of women over 30 years of age are part of the battering process.[39]

The serious immediate effects of battering include severe injury or death. About one fourth of all murders are domestic, and, of these, 50% are spouse killings. About one third of female homicide victims are killed by their husbands or boyfriends; a much smaller proportion of men are killed in domestic violence. One fourth of women are abused while pregnant, and 13% of wife-abuse incidents also include child abuse.[40] Long-term effects include continued neglect or abuse of children, perpetuation of patterns of family violence, serious psychopathology, family disruption, and criminal and civil proceedings.

The battered woman is repeatedly subjected to physical or psychological behavior by a man to force her to do what he wants, without regard for her rights. Physical violence usually refers to hitting, punching, or shoving. Nonphysical abuse can include verbal attacks and insults, emotional deprivation, social isolation, economic deprivation, intellectual derision and ridicule, sexual exploitation, and home imprisonment.[41,42] The abusive man intends to cause injury and pain and does not expect retaliation. The woman usually is afraid of the man's greater strength and ability to inflict injury and has no effective ways of defending herself.

Factors Contributing to Spouse Abuse

Conceptual frameworks to explain the causes and dynamics of abuse encompass individual, cultural, social, and political factors. Personality characteristics, stress, poor impulse control, conflict, intergenerational violence cycles, and male domination are identified as contributing factors in various frameworks.

Socialization to abuse and sex role conditioning frameworks propose that children who witness or experience battering are more likely to become batterers, if male, or victims, if female. The cycle of family violence is transmitted from generation to generation. The sex role expectations that women are inferior and dependent and that men are independent and aggressive support a relationship of submission and control.

Family systems and functional theories provide a framework that explains family violence from the perspectives of roles of family members, patterns of relationships, and functional characteristics. Major problems in family systems contribute to abuse, including status incompatibility (overadequate wife–inadequate husband), regulation of intimacy and distance, management of jealousy and loyalty, and issues around control and power. The internalization of neurotic (toxic) shame through identification with shame-based family models provides an explanation of rage as a cover-up for shame. Rage used as a defense against shame can lead to various forms of psychological abuse (criticism, blame, judgmentalism, contempt, arrogance, patronizing) or can result in violence, revenge, or vindictiveness when the person acquires a position of power.[43]

Feminist theory views abuse of women as an expression of male domination manifested within the family that is reinforced by social institutions, economic structures, and sexist division of labor. Patriarchal social values and organization encourage machismo, providing cultural support for male violence precipitated by stress and frustration. The root cause of physical violence is the batterer's need for dominance and control, which is central in the oppression of women.[44,45]

Other factors that contribute to family violence include cultural tolerance based on beliefs in the privacy of the family, institutional indifference with little legal action against batterer's women's economic insecurity due to less educational and job opportunities, and religious traditions that support women's inferiority and uphold men's rights to exercise control of the family.

Characteristics of Battered Women and Battering Men

Common characteristics found in various studies describe abused women as having low self-esteem, believing myths about battering relationships, being traditionalists, believing in the stereotypical feminine role in the home, accepting responsibility for the batterer's actions, feeling guilt, denying their terror and anger, and voicing severe psychophysiological complaints. Characteristics of battering men include having low self-esteem, believing myths about battering relationships, believing in male dominance and the stereotypical masculine role in the family, blaming others for their actions, not believing violent behavior should have negative consequences, and using drinking, sex, and battering to cope with stresses and enhance self-esteem. Several characteristics are the same for abused and abuser, suggesting a basis for their symbiotic relationship (see Myths About Battering Relationships).[46]

Most couples experiencing marital violence share characteristics. These include a high incidence of alcohol abuse, absent or weak religious affiliation, recurrent verbal disputes, low socioeconomic and educational status, prior exposure to family violence, and adherence to rigid, traditional sex roles.[47]

Battered women often attribute their abuse to personal deficiencies. With traditional family and sex role perspectives, they value family unity and believe it is their responsibility to keep the man happy and make the marriage work. If this does not occur, they feel they have failed as women and deserve to be punished. They believe the man's accusations that they are bad wives and inadequate mothers. Over years of being given this message, they internalize it into their low self-esteem and worthlessness. Believing they deserve beating, they become hopeless and depressed.

Battering men usually have a pattern of using violence to solve problems. They have an underlying sense of inadequacy, inferiority, and insecurity; frequently, they also have lower educational and occupational levels than their wives. Assumptions fostered by the culture about male superiority are contradicted by their inability to handle frustrations at work or home, feelings of socioeconomic inferiority, and sense that they cannot achieve their goals. Many men feel undeserving of their wives, yet they blame and punish them. This

Myths About Battering Relationships

Myth	Research Data
Battering occurs only in a small percentage of couples	Battering occurs in 50–60% of marriages, only 10% of women report abuse
Battering occurs only in lower socioeconomic groups	Spouse abuse occurs in middle and upper class families, all age and racial groups; lower class families have a higher incidence of abuse
Battered women invite or provoke abuse	Abuse is triggered by trivial events, silence or distancing by women, alcohol and drug use, and the batterer's loss of control
Alcohol and drug use cause battering	Abuse is associated with alcohol or drugs, but these are excuses for violence or ways to shift the blame—they reduce inhibitions and impulse control and enhance violent tendencies
Battered women can leave abusive relationships if they so choose	Women often are financially dependent, value marriage, and feel responsible, believe family problems are their fault, think their children need a father, are isolated from family and friends, fear more violent retaliation if they leave, have no place to go and few resources
Batterers and battered women cannot change	Both can learn new behaviors and ways of coping with appropriate help; women can develop self-worth and assertion, and relate to men in adaptive ways; men can rechannel aggression, verbalize feelings, restructure their views of women to respect their rights

ambivalence is expressed by alternating episodes of violent eruptions and remorse, contrition and attention. Although they accept the machismo image and often have underlying rage, these men seem childlike, dependent, and needy of nurturing when not angry.

Cycles of Family Violence

Family violence generally follows cycles, which occur over weeks or months. Tension builds over minor conflicts or disagreements, with the woman becoming compliant, passive, or withdrawn to avoid or deflect the man's anger. The man senses her anger and interprets lack of action as weakness, which further exacerbates his aggressiveness. Tension continues to build over incidents, eventually exploding into acute battering that often is triggered by an unrelated event. Common precipitants are arguments over spending money, jealousy by the husband over slights, sexual problems, drinking or drug use, conflicts over childrearing, the husband's unemployment, or pregnancy. The battering phase usually lasts 2 to 24 hours, although it could be a week or more. After severe beating, the woman usually does not seek care at once, experiencing a state of shock or

disbelief and minimizing the injuries. Fear and helplessness may prevent the woman from seeking help. In the final phase, relief is felt by both, and the man often expresses extreme love and kindness and is contrite over his behavior. He may promise it will never happen again and may give her gifts. The woman wants to believe him and to think that this is his real nature and that he will change his abusive behavior.[48]

The cycle repeats itself over the years. Violence usually begins early in marriage, and many women remain for 6 to 7 years in a violent home situation, especially if they have small children. Most women leave the man two to four times and return before they permanently end the relationship. The longer the woman waits to take action, the more entrenched the family dynamics become. Unhealthy interaction patterns are reinforced, with each partner knowing how to hurt the other emotionally. As months and years pass, the woman withdraws from other relatives, friends, and neighbors. She is reluctant to be seen with injuries and is fearful or embarrassed to talk about the beatings, and the husband is possessive and jealous of all outside relations. Social isolation increases with growing helplessness and powerlessness. Accepting abuse and pain as a part of life, the women often develops serious emotional and somatic problems, such as paralyzing anxiety, nightmares, depression, tremors, sweating, alcohol and drug abuse, hypertension, ulcers, and paranoia.

Assessment. Women experiencing family violence are often difficult to identify because they wish to conceal their problems. Risk for battering is increased in women with a history of alcohol or drug abuse, child abuse, or prior spouse abuse in another marriage. Other signs that could indicate a violent family situation include neglected grooming and appearance; depression manifest by fatigue, somatic complaints, or feelings of hopelessness; expressions of helplessness and powerlessness; and an unequal decision-making structure typified by the authoritarian male and submissive, passive female. Women who do not have a network of relatives and friends whom they see regularly and from whom they receive support may be at increased risk for abuse.

When a woman is seen in the clinic or office and reports an injury, or the nurse notices bruising or other injuries, certain cues of abuse can be sought. The woman may have an inappropriate explanation for the injury (fell down stairs, ran into the door). The site and types of injuries tend to be typical, including bruises, abrasions, or contusions of the head, eyes, back of neck, throat, chest, breasts, abdomen, or genitals. Usually the injuries are multiple, in contrast to single or dual sites on extremities (ankles, wrists, feet, hands) in nonabusive injuries. A period of time (days to weeks) may have elapsed before injuries are reported, whereas nonabusive injuries usually are reported promptly. The abused woman is often hesitant or evasive in providing details on how the injury occurred, and her affect may be inappropriate (avoiding eye contact, embarrassment, fright, disorientation, depression). If her husband is present, she may appear anxious and glance at him or seek approval to answer questions. He may be reluctant to leave her alone with the nurse, may interject answers to questions, or may demand to be present.

Often the nurse must build a trusting relationship with the woman before abuse can be disclosed. The nurse needs to convey unconditional acceptance, understanding, sensitivity, and positive regard for the woman. A conditional statement may open the door for discussing abuse, with the nurse saying, "Many women are physically hurt by their husbands (partners). Has this ever happened to you?" If the woman reveals abuse, this may be accompanied by a flood of emotion with crying and pouring out details of years of abuse. The nurse must listen empathetically and convey emotional support without judgment.

Nursing Diagnosis. Abuse trauma related to family violence would be an appropriate nursing diagnosis that would most directly identify the problem. Several other nursing diagnoses might also be appropriate, such as ineffective family coping, in which the family demon-strates destructive behavior in response to an inability to manage stressors because of inadequate psychological or behavioral resources. Fear related to threat of injury or death, powerlessness related to personal and interpersonal characteristics, disturbance in self-concept related to abusive dynamics, and social isolation related to extreme anxiety, depression, or paranoia could be diagnoses. Rape trauma syndrome also could apply, even within the context of marriage or a continued relationship. This is defined as forced, violent sexual assault against the woman's will and without her consent and includes an acute phase of disorganization of the victim's and family's life-style. Other nursing diagnoses are related to the physical trauma and medical treatment of injuries.

Planning and Intervention. Counseling, support, reassurance, and education are used by nurses throughout the care of battered women. Empathetic listening and acceptance provide the environment in which the woman can express, examine, and work through her situation. She will be facing choices among "unacceptable" alternatives, none of which seems a perfect solution. The nurse must be understanding of her ambivalence toward the batterer; the woman would not remain in a cycle of violence unless there were powerful ties to her spouse. During this process, the nurse identifies and clarifies myths and misunderstandings. The woman's capacity to change, to make and follow through with decisions, and to clarify her values and beliefs is constantly supported. This helps the woman increase self-esteem and explore self-beliefs that keep her caught in the cycle of violence, such as guilt, powerlessness, and self-blame.

The battered woman has three basic alternatives: leave the relationship (with threat of homicide, child custody battles, loss of material support); stay and hope that the man will change through counseling, therapy, or legal intervention (data show change is unlikely, and risk of abuse or death continues); or stay and resign herself to no change (risk of abuse or death continues). No alternative seems perfect, yet the woman must choose and make her own decision. Nurses can become frustrated at indecision or the choice to remain in the relationship and will need to assess their own feelings about the process of helping battered women (see box). Rescuing the battered woman is impossible, and the cycle will not stop until she takes the initiative. The woman needs to reestablish a sense of control over her life and feel safe enough to function. The nurse assists this process by building a trusting relationship, allowing expression of fear, providing empathy no matter how terrible the story becomes, and extending dignity by exhibiting a regard for the woman's worth.

The nurse informs battered women of services available in the community, especially women's shelters and safe houses. Physical safety is a central concern.

The woman also needs to learn of her legal rights and the processes of law enforcement that can protect her from battering. If she decides to leave, she should be advised to take the children (if any) to protect them from abuse and to make obtaining custody easier, and to bring extra clothing, important documents, money, and emergency supplies. If the woman decides not to leave, she needs to know that resources are available and that the nurse continues to view her with respect and to offer a supportive relationship.

Nursing intervention may include assisting treatment of the battering man. Group therapy for couples with violent relationships is becoming more available. These groups focus on helping the couple to appreciate similarities between their concerns and problems, obtain support and feedback on adaptive and maladaptive behaviors, learn and practice new behaviors, and improve self-esteem. Because of the diverse factors associated with family violence, each partner may need to be treated separately in the initial phases.

Couples therapy may be effective when the woman is protected from further violence and the man is motivated to seek help. This situation usually occurs when the batterer no longer has access to the woman. Because both are involved in creating and sustaining their relationship, couples therapy allows exploration of the dynamics and roles played in the relationship. Therapeutic strategies are different for couples with abusive problems, and essential components are the control of the batterer's anger, cessation of violence, and learning nonfighting techniques for handling conflict (Fig. 47-2). Couples can be taught to control their violent interactions, and new adaptive behaviors can be learned. Violence resists change, however, without modification of external circumstances, which may be difficult when socioeconomic or educational factors are present.

When the battering man refuses therapy, or when couples or group therapy is unsuccessful, the woman again must face the choice of leaving or staying in the abusive relationship. Breaking the symbiosis with the battering spouse is often extremely difficult. The nurse works toward increased autonomy through use of "I am" statements, values clarification, grief therapy, and support for independent decisions. The woman is aided to identify her strengths and resources and to build on these. Support groups, individual counseling, and psychotherapy can be recommended. The nurse must remember that leaving a violent family situation is a long process, taking on average about 4 to 7 years. Most women who enter a shelter return home. Abused women often need rehabilitation that takes years, as they slowly gain ego strength and self-esteem. The nurse contributes to this process by effective counseling and support at every contact with a battered woman.

Evaluation. Recovery from the trauma of abuse is a long process. Even though the client may make progress in her steps toward autonomy, there may be periods of backsliding. These are part of the process.

When the woman seeks safety or acknowledges she needs help, she has made a first step. Another sign of progress is that she trusts the nurse enough to express her fears. She identifies her strengths and resources and builds on them; she explores and clarifies her values and beliefs as part of her acknowledgment of who she is. She indicates she has attained knowledge and un-

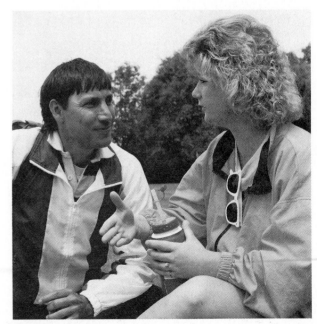

■ *Figure 47–2*

Couples in battering relationships can learn nonfighting techniques for handling conflict through therapy.

derstands her legal rights by acting on them. She makes choices from unacceptable alternatives and follows through with her decisions. As she progresses through these steps, she establishes a sense of control over her life and feels safe enough to function.

■ REFERENCES

1. Hein K: The first pelvic examination and common gynecological problems in adolescent girls. Women Health 9(2/3):47–63, Summer/Fall 1984
2. Isaacs JH: Physician breast examination and breast self examination. Clin Obstet Gynecol 32(4):761–767, December 1989
3. Cooper RA: Mammography. Clin Obstet Gynecol 32(4): 768–785, December 1989
4. Humphrey LJ: Medical management of the fibrocystic breast. In The Fibrocystic Breast. Boston, Tufts University Press, 1983
5. Lynch HT, Watson P, Lynch JF: Epidemiology and risk factors. Clin Obstet Gynecol 32(4):750–760, December 1989
6. Hales D: Genetic time bombs. Family Circle Magazine, pp 42–46, February 1, 1991
7. Mackay J, Steel CM, Elder PA, et al: Allele loss on short arm of chromosome 17 in breast cancers. Lancet 2:1384, 1988
8. Rosenberg AL, Schwartz JF, Feig SA: Clinically occult breast lesions: Localization and significance. Radiology 162:167, 1987
9. Berman RL: Current perspectives in gynecology. Ciba Clin Symp 37(1):2–29, 1985
10. American College of Obstetricians and Gynecologists: Report of task force on routine cancer screening. Washington, DC, American College of Obstetricians and Gynecologists, 1989
11. American Cancer Society: Guidelines for the cancer-related checkup: Recommendations and rationale. CA 30:195–230, 1980
12. Shy K, Chu J, Mandelson M, et al: Papanicolaou smear screening interval and risk of cervical cancer. Obstet Gynecol 74(6):838–843, December 1989
13. Boyce JG, Fruchter RG, Romanzi L, et al: The fallacy of the screening interval for cervical smears. Obstet Gynecol 76(4):637–632, October 1990
14. Baldwin KA, Goodwin K: The Papanicolaou smear. J Nurs Midwif 30(6):327–332, November/December 1985
15. Kneisl C, Ames S: Adult health nursing. Menlo Park, CA, Addison-Wesley, 1986
16. Schneider A, Shah K: The role of vitamins in the etiology of cervical neoplasia: An epidemiological review. Arch Obstet Gynecol 246:1–13, 1989
17. Romney SL, Duttagupta C, Basu J, et al: Plasma vitamin C and uterine cervical dysplasia. Am J Obstet Gynecol 151:976–980, 1985
18. zur Hausen H: Intracellular surveillance of persisting viral infections: Human genital cancer results from deficient cellular control of papilomavirus genome expression. Lancet 2:489–491, 1986
19. Koonings PP, Campbell K, Mishell DR, et al: Relative frequency of primary ovarian neoplasms: A 10-year review. Obstet Gynecol 74(6):921–926, December 1989
20. Sargis N: Detecting ovarian cancer: A challenge for nursing assessment. Oncol Nurs Forum 10(2):48–52, Spring 1983
21. Lazarus R, Launier R: Stress-related transactions between person and environment. In Pervin LA, Lewis M (eds): Perspectives in Interactional Psychology. New York, Plenum Press, 1978
22. Bowles C, Dam-Rabolt M: Stress response and coping patterns. In Griffith-Kennedy J (ed): Contemporary Women's Health: A Nursing Advocacy Approach, pp 126–154. Menlo Park, CA, Addison-Wesley, 1986
23. Women: The road ahead. Time Magazine (Special Issue) 136(19):10–14, 50–52, Fall 1990
24. Wysocki LM, Ossler C: Women, work and health: Issues of importance to the occupational health nurse. Occup Health Nurs 31(11):18–23, 56–61, November 1983
25. Married or single. University of California, Berkeley, Wellness Letter 2(9):1, June 1986
26. Posner I, Lester D, Leitner L: Stress in nurses and other working females. Psychol Rep 54(1):210, February 1984
27. Kirschstein RL: Research on women's health. Am J Public Health 81(3):291–293, March 1991
28. Vicary JR, Mansfield PK, Cohn MD, et al: Substance use among women in the workplace. Occup Health Nurs 33(10):491–495, 527–530, October 1985
29. Wilsnack SC, Klassen AD, Schur BE, et al: Predicting onset and chronicity of women's problem drinking: A five-year longitudinal analysis. Am J Public Health 81(3):305–317, March 1991.
30. Baron JA, Greenberg RE: Cigarette smoking and neoplasms of the female reproductive tract and breast. Semin Reproduct Endocrinol 7(4):335–343, November 1989
31. Mayberry RM: Cigarette smoking, herpes simplex virus type 2 infection, and cervical abnormalities. Am J Public Health 75(6):676–678, June 1985
32. Yeh J, Barbieri RL: Effects of smoking on steroid production, metabolism, and estrogen-related disease. Semin Reproduct Endocrinol 7(4):326–334, November 1989
33. Baron JA, La Vecchia C, Levi F: The antiestrogenic effect of cigarette smoking in women. Am J Obstet Gynecol 162(2):502–514, February 1990
34. Jones CJ, Schiffman MH, Kurman R, et al: Elevated nicotine levels in cervical lavages from passive smokers. Am J Public Health 81(3):378–379, March 1991
35. Charbonneau L: Smoking or health: How long can nurses ignore the facts? Can Nurse 81(7):27–32, August 1985
36. Pirie PL, Murray DM, Luepker RV: Gender differences in cigarette smoking and quitting in a cohort of young adults. Am J Public Health 81(3):324–327, March 1991
37. Pitts D: Women and violence. Crossroads 3(1):1–2, Fall 1990. Rohnert Park, CA, Sonoma State University Women's Resource Center.

38. Amundson MJ: Intervening with launching-stage families and spouse abuse. In Leahey M, Wright LM (eds): Families and Psychosocial Problems, pp 229–249. Springhouse, PA, Springhouse, 1987

39. Greany GD: Is she a battered woman? A guide for emergency response. Am J Nurs 84(6):724–727, 1984

40. O'Reilly J: Wife beating: The silent crime. Time Magazine 122(10):23–26, 1983

41. Walker LE: Battered women, psychology, and public policy. Am Psychol 39(10):1178–1182, 1984

42. Germain CP: Sheltering abused women: A nursing perspective. J Psychosoc Nurs Mental Health Serv 22(9): 24–31, 1984

43. Bradshaw J: Healing the Shame that Binds You. Deerfield Beach, FL, Health Communications, 1988

44. Breines W, Gordon L: The new scholarship on family violence. Signs 8(3):490–531, 1983

45. Campbell J, Humphreys J: Nursing Care of Victims of Family Violence. Reston, VA, Prentice Hall, 1984

46. Reeder S: Ethical Dilemmas for Health Providers in Cases of Spousal Abuse. Paper presented at conference on Bridging the Gaps in Women's Health Care, October 1983, San Antonio, TX

47. Pahl J (ed): Private Violence and Public Policy. London, Routledge and Kegan Paul, 1985

48. Griffith-Kennedy J: Abuse and battering. In Griffith-Kennedy J (ed): Contemporary Women's Health: A Nursing Advocacy Approach, pp 198–220. Menlo Park, CA, Addison-Wesley, 1986

■ SUGGESTED READING

Burgess S: DES daughters: Fighting fear with facts. Am J Nurs 85(6):639–640, June 1985

Coleman E (ed): Chemical Dependency and Intimacy Dysfunction. New York, Haworth Press, 1987

Egan RL: Breast Imaging: Diagnosis and Morphology of Breast Disease. Philadelphia, WB Saunders, 1988

Fillmore KM: Women's drinking across the adult life course as compared to men's. Br J Addict 82:801–811, 1987

Fiore MC, Novotny TE, Pierce JP, et al: Trends in cigarette smoking in the United States: The changing influence of gender and race. JAMA 261:49–55, 1989

Hellberg D, Nilsson S, Haley NJ, et al: Smoking and cervical intraepithelial neoplasia: Nicotine and cotinine in serum and cervical mucus in smokers and nonsmokers. Am J Obstet Gynecol 158:910–913, 1988

Klassen AD, Wilsnack SC: Sexual experience and drinking among women in a US national survey. Arch Sex Behav 15:363–392, 1986

Lynch HT, Watson P, Conway T, et al: Breast cancer family history as a risk factor for early onset breast cancer. Breast Cancer Res Treat 11:263, 1988

Makue DM, Fried VM, Kleinman JC: National trends in the use of preventive health care for women. Am J Public Health 79:21–26, 1989

Orlandi MA: Gender differences in smoking cessation. Women Health 11:237–251, 1987

Mamon JA, Zapka JG: Improving frequency and proficiency of breast self-examination: Effectiveness of an education program. Am J Public Health 75(6):618–624, June 1985

Slattery ML, Robison LM, Schuman KL, et al: Cigarette smoking and exposure to passive smoke are risk factors for cervical cancer. JAMA 261:1593–1598, 1989

Stern PN, Harris CC: Women's health and the self-care paradox: A model to guide self-care readiness. Health Care Women Int 6(1–3):151–163, 1985

Verbrugge IM: Role burdens and physical health of women and men. Women Health 11:47–77, 1986

Wabrek AJ, Gunn JL: Sexual and psychological implications of gynecologic malignancy. JOGN Nurs 13(6):371–376, November/December 1984

48

Nursing Care in Menstrual and Bleeding Disorders

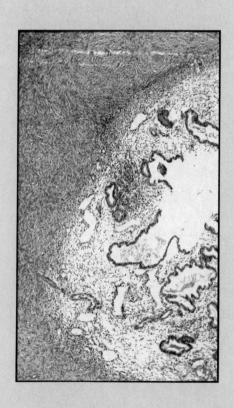

Women may experience alterations in menstrual patterns at various times during the reproductive years. Problems related to menstrual or other uterine bleeding are common, and may include increased or decreased cyclic flow, irregular bleeding patterns, absence of menses (amenorrhea), discomfort or pain associated with menstrual cycles, infections, and natural or induced hypoestrogenic states. Maternity nurses find many occasions when clients in the hospital and in clinics express concerns about menstruation or irregular bleeding not associated with pregnancy. It is important that nurses providing care to women be familiar with common menstrual variations and disorders, and be able to undertake appropriate assessment and nursing care.

■ VARIATIONS IN MENSTRUAL PATTERNS

The normal anatomy and physiology of menstruation are discussed in Chapter 8. There is wide variation in menstrual patterns within the normal range. The mean lengths of menstrual cycles range from a low of 27 days to a high of 29.5 days, but women with normal hormone profiles and regular menstrual cycles may have cycle lengths between 24 and 35 days.[1] The first half of the menstrual cycle (including menstrual, follicular, and periovulatory phases) has a mean length of 14.8 days, with a range of 9 to 23 days. The second half of the cycle (the luteal phase, from ovulation to onset of menses) has a mean length of 13.3 days, with a range of 9 to 20 days.[2] At either extreme, only about 1% of women have very short or very long cycles.

The menstrual phase, during which the endometrium is shed and menstrual bleeding occurs, averages about 5 to 6 days in length. Women with normal, regular cycles may have only 2 to 3 days or as many as 8 to 9 days of bleeding. The amount of menstrual blood loss also varies considerably, ranging from 30 to 100 ml per menses. The average amount of iron lost during menses is 0.5 to 1 mg daily. A regular pattern of menstrual bleeding with decreased amount of flow is termed *hypomenorrhea*, and one with increased amount of flow is termed *hypermenorrhea*.

The menstrual cycle is controlled by multiple complex interactions between the endocrine, nervous, and humoral systems. These interactions involve the hypothalamic–pituitary axis, the ovaries, and the uterus and are mediated by gonadotropic neurohormones. Endocrine cyclicity is the consequence of feedback interplay between the hypothalamic–pituitary complex and the ovaries. Gonadotropin-releasing hormone (Gn-RH)

from the hypothalamus acts on gonadotrope cells in the anterior pituitary, probably by modifying their permeability to ions.[3] Gn-RH induces the gonadotropes to synthesize and secrete FSH (follicle-stimulating hormone) and LH (luteinizing hormone) into the general circulation. FSH and LH are secreted in parallel, even during the LH surge, so the different ovarian responses to these glycoprotein hormones are thought attributable to the quantity and quality of specific membrane receptor cells in the ovary, rather than to secretion ratios of the hormones. As FSH and LH have identical alpha subunits, their ovarian membrane receptor specificity is determined by differences in their beta subunits.[2]

The steroid hormones estradiol and progesterone (secreted by the ovaries) react with nuclear receptors in the interior of target cells. They randomly dissociate from their serum-binding proteins (albumin, sex hormone, and corticosteroid-binding globulins) and diffuse in and out of virtually all body cells. These steroids tend to accumulate primarily in the ovaries, uterus, cervix, vagina, and breasts inducing a variety of responses. Estradiol is especially known for its regulation of endometrial and follicular development and promotion of the midcycle LH surge. Progesterone is best known for its maintenance of the endometrial lining, and feedback inhibition of gonadotropin secretions from the hypothalamic–pituitary complex.

The immunoglobulin content of cervical mucus and vaginal fluid varies during the menstrual cycle, although not in parallel. Cervical mucus IgG levels are lowest at the time of ovulation, whereas vaginal fluid IgG levels are low from ovulation through the luteal phase. Vaginal fluid IgG is relatively high in the postmenstrual and early proliferative phases, and IgA levels are lowest in the luteal phase. The preovulatory and luteal phase levels of IgG and IgA are lower in vaginal fluid than in cervical mucus, whereas these levels are comparable in the ovulatory phase.[4]

Many other metabolic changes occur in association with the menstrual cycle. The basal metabolic rate (BMR) is lowest about 1 week before ovulation, then increases to 8% to 16% during the luteal phase. This produces the subtle temperature changes useful in predicting and detecting ovulation (see Chaps. 11 and 13). Plasma electrolytes vary during the cycle, with sodium levels low during the luteal phase and magnesium levels low at ovulation and highest during menstruation. Zinc is elevated during the menstrual and follicular phases; data on calcium levels are inconsistent. Plasma urea and uric acid, and colloid osmotic pressure in the plasma and interstitial fluid are significantly lower during the luteal phase. Urinary bradykininase activity also decreases during the luteal phase.[2]

Numerous psychological and cognitive-perceptive changes have been related to various phases of the menstrual cycle. Information processing appears to be

Research Highlight

Relaxation Response Helps PMS

Stress appears to exacerbate the symptoms of PMS, including negative life events and daily stressors, which have been related to increased severity of premenstrual negative affect, pain and water retention. Increased physiological responsivity to stress during the luteal phase contributes to PMS symptomatology. The relaxation response is a physiological process elicited by sitting quietly with eyes closed, focusing attention on a repetitive mental activity, and ignoring distracting thoughts. It produces lower heart and respiratory rate, blood pressure, and oxygen consumption; and more alpha and theta activity on EEG. These changes are compatible with decreased sympathetic nervous system arousal and decreased end-organ responsivity to norepinephrine.

The purpose of this study was to determine whether daily practice of the relaxation response would reduce the severity of physical and emotional premenstrual symptoms. Subjects were menstruating women with regular cycles, not breast-feeding or using oral contraceptives, who had not experienced a major traumatic life event or psychiatric illness in the past 6 months, and were not taking prescription medications. Those who exhibited an appropriately high level of premenstrual only symptoms after a 2-month screening phase were eligible for the study. A sample of 46 women was randomly assigned to one of three groups: daily symptom charting only, symptom charting plus reading leisure material, and symptom charting plus relaxation response practiced for 15 to 20 minutes twice daily. Subjects were followed over 5 months and administered the Holmes and Rahe Life Stress Inventory at the end of the study.

The relaxation response group showed significantly greater improvement (58%) than the charting only (17%) and reading groups (27%) for physical symptoms measured daily, and emotional symptoms and symptoms of social withdrawal measured retrospectively. The reading group had more improvement than the charting only group. Women with more severe symptoms showed greatest improvement.

Regular practice of the relaxation response is an effective treatment for physical and emotional premenstrual symptoms. Nurses can include teaching this simple method of relaxation to their clients as an approach to decreasing PMS symptoms and promoting comfort and well-being.

Goodale IL, Domar AD, Benson H: Alleviation of premenstrual syndrome symptoms with the relaxation reponse. Obstet Gynecol 75(4): 649–655, April 1990

---

faster during the periovulatory phase.[5] Sleep-related breathing patterns and auditory brain stem response do not vary across the menstrual cycle. There are significantly greater food cravings and food intake increases during the luteal phase, probably as a consequence of increased BMR. Thirst does not appear to increase at this time. A slight but significant increase in body weight occurs during the luteal phase, probably due to water retention. Variations in mood and feeling state are reported by many women in the late luteal or premenstrual phase, usually involving less positive affect, more reactivity, and greater depressiveness. Lower frustration tolerance with increased irritability is also associated with the premenstrual phase.

Effects of Cigarette Smoking

Women who smoke cigarettes are relatively estrogen-deficient. Smoking affects the hypothalamus, pituitary and adrenal glands, ovaries, and other glands controlling steroid production and metabolism. Nicotine has been found to decrease LH release directly, increase circulating cortisol levels, and inhibit adrenal enzymes. Carbon monoxide or polycyclic aromatic hydrocarbons in smoke may affect activity of enzymes involved in gonadotropin hormone metabolism and may be directly toxic to ovarian follicles.[6] Serum levels of estrogen and estradiol in smokers are 50% lower than those in nonsmokers. Possible mechanisms for this include decreased production of estrogens, alterations in estrogen metabolism, and increase in circulating androgens.

Women who smoke have more symptoms related to estrogen deficiency, such as irregular menses, menopausal symptoms, and hirsutism. Infertility is more common among smokers, probably due to fallopian tube dysfunction. Smokers generally have menopause 1 to 1.5 years earlier than nonsmokers, with an apparent dose–effect relationship (earlier menopause in heavier smokers). Smokers also have an increased incidence of osteoporotic fractures, especially of the hip and spine. Bone mass falls at a higher rate in smokers, and postmenopausal women who smoke have lower bone mineral content.[6]

Because of the antiestrogenic effects of smoke, there are beneficial effects on some diseases caused by estrogen excess. Smokers have a decreased risk of endometrial hyperplasia and have half the risk for endometrial cancer of nonsmokers. Smokers have fewer uterine fibroids, less endometriosis, and less benign breast disease. Smoking does not appear to affect risk of breast cancer.[6,7]

■ NURSING ASSESSMENT

Clients reporting menstrual concerns or bleeding problems are assessed by taking a menstrual and reproductive history, a history of the bleeding problem, and a personal and family health history. Often the history provides the most significant data for determining both the nursing and medical diagnosis, especially for menstrual problems in which the findings on physical examination are normal. The physical examination focuses on a speculum and bimanual pelvic examination, with specimens and diagnostic tests as indicated.

Menstrual History and Assessment of Bleeding Pattern

The menstrual history establishes the woman's usual pattern associated with the menstrual cycle. This provides a baseline from which to evaluate her current symptoms. The nurse must determine what the client means by "bleeding," including the onset, duration, frequency, and intervals between the usual bleeding episodes. Some women do not distinguish between light spotting and frank bleeding, and mistake intermenstrual bleeding for their menstrual period.

The amount of bleeding must be assessed, and this may be difficult. The nurse asks if the bleeding is enough to use a pad or tampon, how often the pad or tampon is changed, and how saturated it is when changed. The number and degree of saturation of pads ar tampons used over a set time period, such as 4 hours, can give some idea of the extent of bleeding (see Chap. 28 for estimation of pad saturation). Women vary in patterns of changing pads or tampons, of course, and in their estimations of time and saturation.

Associated symptoms provide additional diagnostic cues. The patterns of pain or discomfort in relation to bleeding are important: Does pain occur before or after onset of bleeding? Does it continue or cease when bleeding begins? The nurse can assess the severity of pain by asking how much it affects life-style and daily activities. With severe pain, the client may lie down or go to bed and be unable to continue activities. Less severe pain affects activities to varying degrees. The client is asked to describe the character of the pain; such descriptors as aching, cramping, sharp, shooting, burning, or piercing may be used.

The presence of foul-smelling vaginal discharge or a foul smell to blood may indicate infection, especially when fever also occurs. If the client experiences urinary discomfort or burning, the nurse must carefully assess whether the blood comes from the vagina or the urinary meatus. Other areas to check include sudden changes in weight, recent major stress or life changes, severe dieting, drug use, signs of pregnancy, other illness, and contraceptive use. To gain perspective, the client should be asked if she has ever experienced these symptoms before and, if so, when and what was done. Factors that relieve the symptoms, or make them worse, can help in assessment.

Physical Examination

The pelvic examination provides data on the condition of the perineum, vagina, cervix, uterus and adnexa, urethra, and rectum. Some women may mistake bleeding from hemorrhoids or the urinary meatus as coming from the vagina. If blood is present in the vagina, it may originate from vaginal, cervical, or uterine structures. Careful inspection may reveal vaginal lacerations or inflammation, or cervical polyps, infection, or lesions.

Bimanual examination may reveal uterine enlargement, tenderness, or masses; nodules on the rectovaginal septum, ligaments, or cul-de-sac; or adnexal masses, fullness, or tenderness. Combined with data from the history, pelvic findings can affirm the diagnosis. Specimens of vaginal or cervical discharge should be taken for culture or microscopic examination, and Pap smears should be done if indicated. The nurse may perform or assist in the pelvic examination, depending on skills and expertise (see Chap. 19 for pelvic examination technique).

Diagnostic Tests

In addition to a Pap smear and vaginal and cervical smears, other diagnostic tests might be indicated. When there is concern about the extent of blood loss, a hematocrit and hemoglobin, complete blood count and differential, serum iron and iron-binding capacity would be appropriate. To locate nongynecological sources of blood loss, a stool guaiac or urinalysis may be done.

Assessment Tool

Menstrual History

Menarche
  Age menses began _____
  Menstrual pattern first few years:
    Regularity of cycles _____
    Cramping or pain _____
    Length and character of flow _____
  Preparation for menses (extent, who informed her, circumstances)

_____
_____
_____

  Reaction to menarche (feelings, attitudes)

_____
_____
_____

Menstrual cycle characteristics
  Length of cycles (regular, irregular)

_____
_____

  Length and character of flow (how many days, amount of blood, clots)

_____
_____

  Discomfort or pain with menses:
    When pain begins (days, hours before flow; with onset of flow)

_____
_____

    How long pain lasts (hours, days) _____
    Severity of pain (extent of interference with activities, debility)

_____
_____

    Medications or remedies used, effectiveness

_____
_____

  Use of tampons, pads, sponges, etc.

_____
_____

Premenstrual symptoms
  Onset of symptoms (days or hours preceding menstrual flow) _____
  Progression of symptoms (worse, better, when they end) _____
  Types of symptoms and relative severity

_____
_____

  Factors associated with symptoms (food, rest, activity)

_____
_____

  Medical treatment or self-treatment, results

_____
_____

(continued)

Assessment Tool (continued)

Interference with work or daily activities
_____
_____

Effects on spouse, family
_____
_____

Attitudes toward menstruation
  Feelings about menstruation (positive, negative) _____
  Feelings about menstrual symptoms _____
  Perception of relation between menstrual symptoms and woman's status
_____

Feelings about important others' responses to menstrual behaviors
_____
_____

Beliefs about effects of menstrual symptoms on women's cognitive or functional abilities
_____
_____

Knowledge about menstruation
  Physiology of menstrual cycle _____
  Psychology of menstruation _____
  Social constructs related to menstruation _____
  Dysmenorrhea (cause, symptoms, treatment) _____
  PMS (cause, symptoms, treatment) _____

Pregnancy tests are often indicated, because early threatened abortion is a major cause of uterine bleeding. To test for infections as a source of bleeding, a gonorrhea culture or *Chlamydia* culture may be done. Sonography is often used to assess uterine contents and pelvic masses.

■ NURSING DIAGNOSIS

The nursing diagnosis is generally related to the medical (pathophysiological) diagnosis and the client's responses to her condition and symptoms. High Risk for Complications (cancer, anemia, infection, dysplasia, endometriosis, shock) is a nursing diagnosis applicable to almost all bleeding problems. One major focus of nursing care is to detect and prevent such complications.

For many menstrual and bleeding problems, Alteration in Comfort: Pain is an appropriate diagnosis because of the cramping that is a common symptom. Sex-

ual Dysfunction related to painful intercourse, fears about injury, or infertility could occur. Self-Concept Disturbance may occur if the woman experiences negative feelings about her body because of the bleeding problem, or if her role performance is adversely affected. Anxiety and Fear related to the unpredictable nature of the disease or uncertainty of outcomes is a possible nursing diagnosis.

Knowledge Deficits are common nursing diagnoses, related to the pathophysiological condition, myths and misunderstandings, signs and symptoms of complications, medical treatment, needs for nutrition and rest, and nonpharmaceutical therapies. Self-care deficits may be present when the woman does not have the knowledge or skills to take actions that might prevent, improve, or remedy the symptoms or problem. In chronic or serious conditions that can affect life-style or daily activities significantly, there is the High Risk for Ineffective Individual and Family Coping, spiritual distress, and hopelessness.

Nursing diagnoses for specific menstrual and bleeding problems are included in the following sections.

■ NURSING PLANNING AND INTERVENTION

Nursing care for women experiencing menstrual alterations or bleeding problems focuses on alleviating knowledge deficits and assisting the client to understand the cause, course of the disease or condition, treatment regimens, and anticipated outcomes. Self-care is encouraged whenever activities related to diet, rest, stress reduction, and health behaviors can affect the condition or improve symptoms. Anxiety and fear are reduced through providing emotional support, a caring relationship in which feelings can be expressed, empathic listening, and realistic reassurance. Self-concept disturbances or sexual dysfunction may be improved by providing reliable information, clarifying misconceptions, encouraging expression of feelings and views of the self, and teaching about resources within the self and environment to aid in coping.

Additional key points in assessment, diagnosis, and nursing care are discussed for several common menstrual and bleeding disorders. Age-specific causes of bleeding are listed in Table 48-1.

■ EVALUATION

Nursing intervention is evaluated by observing for changes in the client's behavior, level of knowledge and self-care skills, and self-perspectives and attitudes. Indicators of successful intervention occur when the client can express a clear understanding of the causes, treatment, and outcomes for the menstrual pattern alteration or bleeding problem. Self-care interventions are effective when the client knows measures she can take to maximize recovery and maintain health, and to prevent recurrence of problems or complications, and demonstrates intention or takes actions.

Utilizing family and community resources, effective coping patterns, and expressing a positive attitude about her ability to handle the problem indicate successful interventions. When serious or chronic problems are present, nursing care is effective when the client can express her fears and concerns, develop plans for integrating changes into her life-style, and seek assistance appropriately from family, health providers, and the community.

■ DYSFUNCTIONAL UTERINE BLEEDING

Dysfunctional uterine bleeding (DUB) can manifest as abnormally heavy, irregular, or light bleeding. Most problems are caused by endocrine disruptions that prevent the normal cyclic changes in the endometrium from occurring. DUB can be a chronic problem contributing to iron deficiency anemia, or it can be an acute hemorrhagic episode with enough blood loss to cause hypovolemic shock.

TABLE 48–1. COMMON CAUSES OF GYNECOLOGICAL BLEEDING

Age 5–13	Age 14–25	Age 25–35	Age 35–45	Age 45+ (postmenopausal)
Foreign bodies	Pregnancy	Pregnancy	Pregnancy	Estrogen therapy
Self-inflicted lacerations	Oral contraceptives or IUD	Oral contraceptives or IUD	Anovulation	Endometrial hyperplasia or polyps
Vaginitis (nonspecific)	Cervical eversion or cervicitis	Cervical eversion or cervicitis	Endometrial hyperplasia	Endometrial carcinoma
Rule out urinary tract infection and rectal bleeding	Anovulation	Cervical polyps	Uterine myoma	Uterine myoma
	Vaginal lacerations or infections	Anovulation	Adenomyosis	Coital injuries related to atrophy
	Foreign bodies	Vaginal lacerations or infections	Endometriosis	
	Cervical polyps	Foreign bodies	Endometrial carcinoma	
		Uterine myoma	Oral contraceptives or IUD	
		Endometrial hyperplasia	Cervical polyps	
		Endometriosis		

Menorrhagia

Menorrhagia is excessive menstrual flow, usually lasting longer than 7 to 8 days with blood loss of more than 80 to 100 ml. It is one of the most common gynecological problems, occurring in 15% to 20% of otherwise healthy women.[8] Excessive menses can have both endocrine and organic causes. The most common cause is inadequate steroid hormone support for the endometrium. Constant estrogen stimulation to the uterine lining produces an endometrial overgrowth. Once overgrowth has occurred, sporadic and dyscoordinate loss of the endometrium occurs, resulting in either prolonged bleeding or shorter than usual episodic menstruation. Medical treatment is by administration of progestin or estrogen–progestin therapy, which regulates the hormone balance, controls heavy bleeding and reestablishes menstrual cyclicity, usually in 3 to 6 months.[9]

Another common endocrinological cause of menorrhagia includes anovulation. Anovulation may result from pituitary adenoma, which produces excess prolactin and disrupts the hypothalamic–pituitary axis. Polycystic ovarian syndrome also causes anovulation related to abnormal gonadotropic secretion and excess androgen activity.

Heavy bleeding commonly occurs in association with the use of contraceptives. There is a 10% incidence of significant increase in menstrual flow with an intrauterine device (IUD). After discontinuing oral contraceptives, women may experience increased flow. Women occasionally have an episode of heavy bleeding while taking oral contraceptives. With persistent menorrhagia, IUD removal or changing oral contraceptives is usually necessary.

Endometrial infections can cause heavy menstrual bleeding because of disturbance of clotting mechanisms. Increased risk for pelvic infections has been associated with cigarette smoking[10] and cervicitis.[11] Menses are usually painful, and the blood may be foul smelling. The woman may have fever, uterine tenderness and enlargement, and mucopurulent cervical discharge. When the tubes or ovaries are involved in pelvic infections, there may be adnexal fullness, masses, or tenderness. When pelvic inflammatory disease (PID) is suspected, cultures are taken for *Neisseria gonorrhoeae* and *Chlamydia* organisms, and a white blood cell count with differential is ordered. PID is treated with antibiotics and, if severe, may require hospitalization.

Organic causes of heavy menstrual bleeding include various cervical and uterine lesions, including leiomyomas (fibroids), polyps, endometrial hyperplasia, and malignancies. Leiomyomas usually are detected by palpating an enlarged or irregularly shaped uterus. Polyps and hyperplasias occur more frequently in perimenopause, and usually have intermenstrual bleeding also.

These lesions must undergo tissue diagnosis because of their symptomatic overlap with malignancies.

Systemic disease may cause excessive menstrual bleeding, although the incidence is small. Blood dyscrasias, liver and renal disease occasionally cause menorrhagia. Obesity may lead to anovulation, eventually resulting in menorrhagia. Various drugs may also disrupt normal menstrual patterns, causing menorrhagia (i.e., chemotherapy, anticoagulants, steroid hormones, neuroleptics, major tranquilizers).

Oligomenorrhea

Short, scant menstrual flow may result from endocrine dysfunctions. Menstrual flow may be light, or the woman may have spotting for 1 to 2 days. Short cycles (17–20 days) may indicate *anovulation*. Women under 30 years old with consistent anovulatory cycles are more prone to infertility and are at increased risk for endometrial carcinoma. With normal physical examination and documentation of ovulation (by menstrual calendar, basal body temperature chart, and cervical mucus observation), this menstrual pattern is probably normal variant. If cycles are anovulatory, further work-up is needed for potential infertility. (Chap. 13 discusses managing infertility.)

Oral contraceptives often cause light menses because they create a relative estrogen deficiency or have an androgenic influence on the endometrium. If other symptoms of estrogen deficiency are not present, this is considered a benign side-effect. Unless the woman is troubled by oligomenorrhea, there is no cause for concern.

Cervical stenosis may cause light menses with dark brown spotting and cramping. The cervical os may appear occluded on pelvic examination, or it may not admit a sound. Medical treatment often includes progressive cervical dilatation.

Decreased menstrual flow also may be due to *severe weight loss* diets and inadequate protein. Eating disorders may underlie this problem (anorexia, bulimia). Heavy use of *marijuana* can decrease menstrual flow by inhibiting normal estrogen function.[12] Such problems are suspected when physical examination is normal and history does not indicate other causes.

Endometriosis

About 1% to 7% of women in the United States experience endometriosis, a condition in which endometrial tissue is present in the pelvic peritoneum. Endometriosis results from retrograde menstruation, which causes tiny fragments of normal endometrium to take up residence in the lower peritoneal cavity. The most common sites for endometrial implants are the posterior cul-de-sac, ovaries, bladder serosa, fallopian tubes, and large bowel. Women with longer menstrual flow (>8 days) and shorter cycles (<27 days) are at greater risk for endometriosis. The condition is estrogen-dependent, occurs in women age 15 to 44, and is rarely seen before puberty or after menopause. Frequent aerobic exercise is protective against endometriosis, because this decreases the rate of estrogen production.[13]

The symptoms of endometriosis include painful menses and other pelvic pain, cul-de-sac nodularity, adnexal mass, or infertility. Many women have pain with bowel movements during menses, and pain with deep penetration during intercourse. Often there is heavy menstrual bleeding associated with pain that increases over time. On physical examination, the uterus frequently is retroverted and fixed in position, nodules are found on the rectovaginal septum and cul-de-sac, and there is uterosacral ligament tenderness. The diagnosis is confirmed by direct laparoscopic visualization of lesions, which typically appear as bluish-red blebs or dark power burns.[14]

Medical treatment includes medications for pain relief (nonsteroidal anti-inflammatory drugs) and to suppress estrogen production (oral contraceptives, danazol, nafarelin). Surgical therapy may be done to remove adhesions, or laser surgery may be used to ablate lesions. Occasionally, hysterectomy with oophorectomy is performed. Endometriosis is the second most common reason for hysterectomy, accounting for about 19% of operations.[15]

Intermenstrual Bleeding

Bleeding or spotting between menses is often a sign of an organic problem, although there may be functional causes. Midcycle spotting (mittelstaining) is light pink spotting that lasts a few hours to a day and is associated with ovulation. This functional condition is caused by a relative estrogen dip at midcycle just before ovulation. Some women may experience occasional and periodic midcycle spotting. When the history and physical examination are negative, other signs of ovulation help confirm the diagnosis. Usually no medical treatment is needed, although small doses of estrogen around the time of ovulation can prevent the spotting.

Vaginitis or cervicitis may cause intermenstrual spotting or light bleeding. These conditions often are associated with increased discharge, itching, spotting after intercourse, or discomfort with intercourse. Pelvic examination may reveal increased vaginal discharge, erythema, cervical discharge, polyp, or inflammation. When vaginitis is diagnosed, medical treatment is specific for the organism (see Chap. 35).

Irregular intermenstrual bleeding may be an early sign of cytological changes caused by diethylstilbestrol (DES), especially when this occurs in adolescents and young adults. Pap smears and colposcopy are needed for thorough evaluation.

Foreign bodies are another cause of intermenstrual spotting that does not follow a pattern. These are more frequent in young girls and adolescents, although it is not uncommon for women to forget a tampon or diaphragm in the vagina for several days. Associated symptoms include lower abdominal cramping, increased foul-smelling vaginal discharge, and pressure. The foreign body can usually be seen on speculum examination, when it can be removed.

When the cause of irregular genital bleeding is not evident from the history or examination, trauma must be considered. Sexual abuse is a common problem in both female children and adult women and is one of the most frequent causes of genital trauma. Sensitive questioning in a supportive, accepting atmosphere may be necessary to obtain a history of abuse. Nursing diagnoses and nursing care are discussed in Chapter 47. Other causes of trauma may be scratching, falls, and lacerations from using tampon or diaphragm inserters.

Oral contraceptives cause a type of breakthrough bleeding that may occur at any time in the menstrual cycle, is usually not cyclic and regular, but can be recurrent. The amount of bleeding ranges from light spotting to frank, heavy bleeding and may last from a few hours to several days. Ordinarily, there is little or no pain or cramping. Breakthrough bleeding occurs when endometrial sloughing is incomplete during withdrawal menses, and areas build up with varying thickness until the estrogen levels provided by the oral contraceptive are not enough to maintain the endometrium.

Pregnancy must always be considered as a possible cause of intermenstrual bleeding in women of childbearing age. Even those using contraceptives must be evaluated for pregnancy due to contraceptive failure and misuse. Some women continue to have light bleeding at the time their menses would be due, even though they are pregnant.

Endometrial hyperplasia related to hormone imbalances is a frequent cause of sudden, heavy bleeding without a cyclic pattern, particularly in women approaching the cessation of ovarian function. The aging ovary fails to produce estrogen and progesterone with smooth cyclic release in sufficient quantities, and ovulation becomes erratic. Adequate progesterone is necessary to regulate endometrial breakdown during the menstrual phase. When estrogen influences the endometrium in the absence of sufficient progesterone, the endometrium continues to proliferate and grow in thickness. During menses, the endometrium is incompletely sloughed, leading to irregular areas of thick buildup. When the hormone levels no longer support this hyperplastic endometrium, sudden bleeding occurs that can be extremely heavy, with large clots, and can last up to 2 weeks.

When diagnostic tests show endometrial hyperplasia, treatment may be surgery (dilation and curettage [D&C]) or hormone therapy. Frequently, a progestational drug is used, such as medroxyprogesterone acetate (Provera), during the last part of the menstrual cycle to regulate endometrial breakdown and control bleeding. Acute bleeding episodes can be stopped by administering progesterone or estrogen in high doses, followed by an oral contraceptive or estrogen–progesterone combination to control subsequent menstrual bleeding. Careful monitoring of response to treatment is necessary for irregular bleeding in premenopausal women, because of the risk of cancer.

Nursing Assessment

A good history is necessary to identify the character of the bleeding and associated factors. The date of onset of bleeding, how many days bleeding occurred, and how this relates to the woman's menstrual cycle are established as accurately as possible. The character and amount of bleeding are ascertained; the nurse must encourage specific estimations of amount based on tampon or pad use. The nurse asks about presence of clots, tissue, and the odor of the bloody discharge. The usual pattern of discomfort, pain, cramping, or associated symptoms is explored.

The nurse assists with the pelvic examination. Diagnostic tests are usually done, including a Pap smear, vaginal or cervical cultures or smears for microscopic examination. Colposcopy, endometrial or endocervical biopsy may be performed depending on the suspected problem. Sonography or computed tomography may be ordered when pelvic masses are identified.

Nursing Diagnosis and Intervention

Common nursing diagnoses for dysfunctional uterine bleeding include Alterations in Comfort (pain), Knowledge Deficits, Anxiety and Fear, and High Risk for Complications. Nursing care includes education about the condition and medical treatment, information about comfort measures and analgesic medications, and evaluation for complications, as well as teaching the client about identifying and preventing complications. Measures to alleviate pain, such as medications, relaxation, or heat or cold therapy, are explained by the nurse, and the client is taught correct procedures. Sexual dysfunctions related to bleeding problems are identified, and appropriate counseling or referral is provided.

Ineffective Individual or Family Coping, and Disturbance in Self-Concept might occur with persistent or more serious conditions. Education, counseling, and support are provided to assist the client and family understand the condition and its implications. Fear, Ineffective Coping, and Self-Concept Disturbances may be related to the threat of cancer or permanent conditions affecting reproductive roles (infertility, sterility). The nurse provides support through the medical diagnostic process, encourages expression of feelings and communication, and assists in developing effective coping strategies.

Alteration in Nutrition, Ineffective Individual Coping, Disturbance in Self-Concept, and Alteration in Thought Processes are potential diagnoses when bleeding patterns are affected by eating disorders. Interventions are complex and long-term.

■ AMENORRHEA

The absence of menses, or skipping periods, is a common problem among women during the reproductive years. Primary amenorrhea occurs when a girl reaches 16 years of age and has never menstruated. The most frequent causes are structural, congenital, and endocrine abnormalities, such as gonadal dysgenesis, imperforate hymen, absent vagina or uterus, androgen insensitivity syndrome, prepubertal ovarian failure, congenital adrenal hyperplasia, and hypopituitarism.

Although most girls in the United States menstruate by age 12½ to 13 years, menarche may occur much later. The early signs of sexual maturation, breast buds and pubic hair, usually occur about 2 years before onset of menses. If these appear by age 14, investigation of amenorrhea can be delayed until after age 16. Body weight is a significant factor influencing onset of puberty. Most girls weigh about 90 lb when menses begin, so heavy girls usually menstruate earlier than thin girls. A critical weight for initiation and maintenance of menstruation has been considered to be 17% to 20% body fat; however, regular menstrual cycles occur in female athletes with as little as 13.7% body fat.[16]

Secondary amenorrhea occurs when a previously menstruating woman ceases to menstruate; the causes may be organic or functional. *Pregnancy* is probably the most common cause of secondary amenorrhea in women aged 16 to 45. *Oral contraceptives* frequently cause women to skip one or more menses, particularly low-dose estrogen and progestin-only pills. A variety of causes contribute to amenorrhea related to low levels of gonadotropin and estrogen secretion, including stress, weight loss, anorexia nervosa, exercise, and hypothalamic and pituitary lesions.

The most common causes of chronic anovulation secondary to CNS–hypothalamic–pituitary disorders are

---

Causes of Amenorrhea

Abnormalities of the Reproductive Tract

Congenital absence of ovaries or vagina

Complete testicular feminization

Transverse vaginal septum

Imperforate hymen

Intrauterine adhesions (Asherman's syndrome)

Cervical stenosis

Estrogen Present

Chronic anovulation due to feedback disorders:
Polycystic ovaries
Adrenal hyperplasia
Thyroid disorders
Cushing's disease
Ovarian tumors
Adrenal tumors

Estrogen Absent

Gonadal failure:
Gonadal dysgenesis
Premature ovarian failure
Resistant ovary syndrome
Enzymatic defects

Chronic anovulation due to CNS–hypothalamic–
pituitary disorders:
Functional
Stress
Weight loss
Anorexia nervosa
Exercise
Nonfunctional
Pituitary disorders
Tumors
Trauma
Radiation

---

functional, related to stress and other psychological factors. Low or normal gonadotropin levels result from alteration in Gn-RH secretion by the hypothalamus. A hypoestrogenic state results, in which the endometrium does not build up adequately to produce menses. The primary treatment includes counseling directed toward the causes and management of stress. Oral contraceptives or estrogen may be given to initiate hormonal cycling, or Gn-RH therapy may be given to encourage adequate endometrial buildup.

Ovarian cysts may cause amenorrhea, the most common types including follicular and corpus luteum cysts. When the graafian follicle fails to rupture, it may continue to increase in size and secrete estrogen. The ovary may be enlarged to 6 to 8 cm. Because ovulation does not occur, the luteal phase is not entered and the endometrium continues to proliferate under estrogen influence. Usually these cysts resolve spontaneously in several weeks, and menstruation is restored. Oral contraceptives may be used for one to two cycles to cause involution of the cyst. In corpus luteum dysfunction, progesterone continues to be secreted and the secretory endometrium is maintained, similar to early pregnancy. These cysts also tend to regress spontaneously, and regular cycles are restored in a few weeks.

Organic causes of secondary amenorrhea include tumors, infections, or cysts, which compress or destroy the hypothalamus; pituitary necrosis (Sheehan's syndrome); hyperthyroidism; galactorrhea; hyperprolactinemia; adrenal virilization; intrauterine synechiae (Asherman's syndrome); polycystic ovarian syndrome (Stein-Leventhal); Cushing's syndrome; and premature ovarian failure (menopause before age 40). Various drugs may also induce amenorrhea, including estrogen therapy, general anesthesia, phenothiazines, reserpine, MAO inhibitors, opioids, and histamine receptor antagonists.

After an examination to exclude anatomical abnormalities and pregnancy, medical management includes serum prolactin levels. Progestin is administered to evaluate estrogen status, usually medroxyprogesterone acetate for 5 days. Women with normal prolactin levels who have withdrawal bleeding after receiving the progestin challenge are diagnosed chronic anovulation with estrogen present. Women who do not bleed usually have elevated prolactin levels and are diagnosed with estrogen absent disorder. Further testing is done to evaluate the thyroid (TSH levels) and pituitary (computed tomography, MRI), and serum FSH is measured. Low FSH with normal thyroid and pituitary examinations is classified as chronic anovulation with estrogen absent, usually due to functional hypothalamic disorders.[16]

Nursing Assessment

Assessment in primary amenorrhea focuses on degree of secondary sexual development and presence of a normal reproductive tract. For secondary amenorrhea, assessment focuses on the pattern of menses after menarche. It is important to determine if a regular cyclic menstrual pattern was ever established, and how long this pattern lasted. The timing and rate of onset of amenorrhea and any events associated with amenorrhea also are important. History of gynecological procedures or problems is especially noted. For example, a recent D&C or episode of postpartum endometritis provides cues to the cause of secondary amenorrhea. Other common potential causes are examined, including emotional stress, weight loss or gain, altered nutritional patterns, level of exercise activity, and major life events or changes.

The woman's reactions to and approaches to coping with amenorrhea are explored. The meanings it holds for her and her partner and family are important in determining her reactions and coping strategies.

The nurse assists with physical examination, obtaining specimens, and gynecological diagnostic procedures. Signs indicative of genetic or hormonal disorders are noted, such as exophthalmos and thyroid enlargement (hyperthyroidism), moon facies and hirsutism (Cushing's), thinning hair and delayed reflexes (hypothyroidism), and deepening voice, breast atrophy, and temporal baldness (virilizing syndromes).

Nursing Diagnosis and Intervention

Nursing diagnoses often involve an Alteration in Self-Concept because many women view their bodies as functioning abnormally when they experience amenorrhea. There may be Anxiety or Fear about the meanings of the problem and implications about future fertility or femininity. Knowledge Deficits are common, related to the cause, progression, or treatment of the

problem. There may be Sexual Dysfunctions, especially in chronic hypoestrogenic or virilizing conditions.

Nursing care includes education, counseling, reassurance, and increasing options for coping strategies. With serious or permanent disorders, the woman and family may need assistance accepting and integrating the problem and its effects on their lives, and grieving the loss of functions (fertility, menstrual cycles) or threats to well-being (cancer, destructive tumors).

■ MENSTRUAL DISCOMFORT AND PAIN

Discomfort or pain associated with menstruation is a common experience among women. Two clinical syndromes have been identified: dysmenorrhea and premenstrual syndrome (PMS). Dysmenorrhea is characterized by pain that occurs shortly before onset or during menstrual flow, and persists for one to several days of menses. In PMS, symptoms occur in the luteal phase of the menstrual cycle with resolution shortly after onset of menses. Pelvic pathology may be associated with either syndrome, or there may be no apparent organic changes.

Dysmenorrhea

Primary dysmenorrhea occurs without pelvic pathology and is the largest category of menstrual pain. Secondary dysmenorrhea results from organic or pathological causes, such as endometriosis, PID, cervical stenosis, ovarian cysts, uterine myomas, congenital uterine malformations, IUD, or trauma.

Primary dysmenorrhea affects about 50% of postpubescent women. Ten percent of women with primary dysmenorrhea have pain severe enough to incapacitate them for 1 to 3 days each month. Consequences of this incapacity include absenteeism, economic loss, reduced productivity, increased potential for accidents, and reduced work quality. Primary dysmenorrhea occurs most frequently in teenage years and the early twenties, and declines after 30 to 35 years. It occurs more frequently in unmarried than married women, pregnancy and vaginal delivery do not necessarily improve discomfort, and exercise does not have a significant effect on incidence.[17]

The characteristic symptom of primary dysmenorrhea is pain beginning a few hours before or with onset of menses, lasting 48 to 72 hours. The pain is located in the suprapubic region and can be sharp, gripping, cramping, or dull aching. It often is accompanied by

---

Important Causes of Pelvic Pain

Cyclic, Recurrent Menstrual Pain

Dysmenorrhea (primary, secondary)

Endometriosis

Adenomyosis

IUDs

Endometritis or PID

Recurrent Pain Not During Menses

Midcycle ovulation pain (mittelschmerz)

Ovarian cysts (follicular, corpus luteum)

Ovarian or uterine malignancies

Psychogenic pain

Acute, Severe Nonmenstrual Pain

Ectopic pregnancy, actual or pending rupture

Twisted fallopian tube, ovary, or ovarian cyst

Ruptured ovarian cyst

Appendicitis

Acute PID

Acute lower bowel lesions

pelvic fullness or bearing-down sensations that may radiate to the inner thighs and lumbosacral area. Some women experience nausea and vomiting, headache, fatigue, dizziness, faintness, diarrhea, or emotional instability during this time. Almost invariably, dysmenorrhea occurs in ovulatory cycles, usually beginning 6 to 12 months after menarche.

Increased prostaglandin production and release by the endometrium (mainly PGF_{2a}) during menstruation produce incoordinate, spasmodic uterine contractions that cause pain. Women with dysmenorrhea have higher intrauterine pressure during the menstrual period and have double the amount of prostaglandins in their menstrual flow than women without pain. Uterine contractions are more frequent and become uncoordinated or dysrhythmic. With this increased abnormal uterine activity, blood flow is reduced, resulting in uterine ischemia or hypoxia contributing to pain. One type of prostaglandin (PGE_2) and other hormones hypersensitize sensory pain fibers in the uterus to the action of bradykinin and other chemical and physical pain stimuli.[17]

Other mechanisms may be involved in causing dysmenorrhea. Activity of the 5-lipoxygenase pathway is increased in some women with primary dysmenorrhea who do not have increased prostaglandins. This results in increased biosynthesis of leukotrienes, which are potent vasoconstrictors and induce uterine muscle contractions.[18] Circulating vasopressin levels are increased during menses in women with primary dysmenorrhea. With a concomitant increase in oxytocin levels, increased vasopressin causes dysrhythmic uterine contractions that produce uterine hypoxia and ischemia.

There is conflicting information about the impact of the woman's social environment on dysmenorrhea. Women in mental hospitals indicated more menstrual pain when they had less acceptance of the female role, and more pain was reported among college students scoring higher on a masculinity scale. In contrast, femininity scores on a personality inventory were positively correlated with menstrual symptoms in college women and women at a family-planning clinic. Homemakers with no outside career ambitions were found to have more menstrual symptoms, and another study found no association between perimenstrual discomfort and traditional or feminist orientations. Demographic and social characteristics (race, employment status, marital status) have been described as weak correlates of dysmenorrhea, with a negative correlation between dysmenorrhea and income, education, and age. Both negative and positive attitudes associated with menses were correlated with dysmenorrhea; women who felt menstruation should not affect a woman's behavior had less pain, and those who reported greater debilitation during menstruation had more pain.[19]

Medical treatment of primary dysmenorrhea includes oral contraceptives and nonsteroidal anti-inflammatory drugs, which are prostaglandin synthetase inhibitors. A combination estrogen–progestin pill provides relief to 90% or more women with dysmenorrhea. Oral contraceptives reduce menstrual fluid volume through suppression of the endometrium, and suppress ovulation, thus creating an endocrine milieu with low prostaglandin levels. Nonsteroidal anti-inflammatories (e.g., ibuprofen, naproxen, indomethacin) suppress menstrual fluid prostaglandins. They are taken as soon as pain begins after the onset of menstrual flow and continued throughout the first 2 to 3 days of menses.

SECONDARY DYSMENORRHEA

Dysmenorrhea that occurs throughout the duration of the menstrual flow or for more than 2 to 3 days is more likely to be secondary. Women with a history of recurrent PID, irregular menstrual cycles, menorrhagia, IUD use, or infertility are at risk for secondary dysmenorrhea. Age at onset usually is later than in primary dysmenorrhea, except that endometriosis causing secondary dysmenorrhea can occur at or shortly after menarche. Pelvic examination or laparoscopy usually reveals the causes of secondary dysmenorrhea (Table 48-2).

Specific therapy for secondary dysmenorrhea depends on the cause. Women with an IUD can be treated with nonsteroidal anti-inflammatory drugs, because the causes relate to increased prostaglandins. This therapy also is temporarily helpful with uterine myomas, but surgery is the definitive treatment. Antibiotics are given when infections are present, and surgical procedures

---

Characteristic Symptoms of Dysmenorrhea

Onset of pain a few hours before or with menstrual flow

Pain located in suprapubic region, may radiate to inner thighs and lumbosacral area

Character of pain is sharp, gripping, cramping, or dull aching

Pain often accompanied by pelvic fullness or bearing-down sensations

Duration of pain is several hours to about 2 days

Associated symptoms may include:
  Nausea and vomiting
  Headache
  Fatigue
  Dizziness
  Diarrhea
  Emotional instability

TABLE 48-2. CAUSES OF SECONDARY DYSMENORRHEA

Location	Organic Causes
Vagina	Imperforate hymen
	Transverse vaginal septum
Cervix	Cervical stenosis
Uterus	Congenital malformations
	Uterine myomas or polyps
	Endometriosis (adenomyosis)
	Intrauterine adhesions (Asherman's syndrome)
	Intrauterine device (IUD)
Fallopian tubes	Pelvic infammatory disease (PID)
Ovaries	Ovarian cysts or tumors
Peritoneum	Endometriosis
	Pelvic congestion syndrome

are used for anatomical and structural abnormalities. Treatment for endometriosis is discussed above.

Nursing Assessment

Assessment of dysmenorrhea includes a thorough menstrual history and careful exploration of pain and other associated symptoms. It is important to distinguish dysmenorrhea from PMS, because the treatments are different. The amount of disruption in daily activities caused by dysmenorrhea helps assess the severity of pain and debilitating effects of symptoms. The role of stress and anxiety in menstrual pain is complex and may be circular. A life-style and stress history is taken to evaluate the role tension and anxiety may play. The physical examination assists in eliminating significant pathology as the cause of menstrual pain, and the pelvic examination should be normal in primary dysmenorrhea. Diagnostic tests to rule out pathology might include cultures, complete blood count, urinalysis, sedimentation rate, pelvic ultrasonography, laparoscopy, hysteroscopy, and hysterosalpingography.

Nursing Diagnosis and Intervention

Nursing diagnoses related to dysmenorrhea may include Alterations in Comfort (pain), Knowledge Deficits, Ineffective Individual Coping, Alterations in Nutrition, and Disturbance in Self-Concept. Nursing care is based on diagnoses for individual clients. Nursing care for pain can include a number of nonpharmacological approaches. Heat has pain-relieving properties because it causes vasodilation and increased blood flow to the affected area and decreases hypertonic muscle contractions, thus affecting two causes of dysmenorrhea (ischemia, hypertonia). Either dry heat with a heating pad or wet heat in a tub or shower may be effective. Massage or effleurage of the lower abdomen is often therapeutic because it increases the pain threshold by providing a secondary stimulus. Relaxation techniques such as biofeedback, autogenic training, yoga, progressive relaxation, and meditation have been used effectively to relieve menstrual pain.

Knowledge Deficits related to the pathophysiology of dysmenorrhea and psychosocial factors can be alleviated by education and counseling. Many women have heard that dysmenorrhea is a psychosomatic problem and may have had negative experiences in the healthcare system. Nurses can explain how attitudes and beliefs about dysmenorrhea have developed and can correct misinformation and misconceptions by discussing current research and understandings of the problem. Women can be assisted to find ways to prevent or minimize menstrual discomfort. Exercise that tones muscles and increases circulation can allay ischemia. Swimming is excellent for building muscle tone, and other aerobic exercises also can be helpful. Getting adequate rest seems to reduce menstrual pain for some women. Sleep needs often are increased during menstruation, and increased sleep time can relieve tension.

Alterations in Nutrition with less intake of B vitamins (particularly B_6) than needed may contribute to dysmenorrhea. The B vitamins increase protein utilization and help relieve fatigue, tension, and depression. Premenstrually, carbohydrate metabolism may be altered, with mild glucose intolerance and hypoglycemia. A diet high in protein and complex carbohydrates, taken in small frequent amounts, should provide relief for hypoglycemia symptoms.

Women experiencing Disturbance in Self-Concept have negative feelings about or views of themselves related to menstrual pain. They may have one or more days of significant debility, which contributes to lower self-esteem and less effective role performance. Women may have internalized social myths and prejudices surrounding menstrual discomfort and may feel less worthy in comparison to men. Nursing care focuses on helping these clients to formulate more positive attitudes toward menstruation and toward themselves as normal, healthy women. They need reassurance that their attitudes toward femininity and women's roles are not the cause of dysmenorrhea. Explanations of menstrual physiology and psychology can help correct misconceptions. Planning to anticipate and prepare for days when functioning is decreased can help the woman feel more in control. Finding effective methods of pain relief, if possible, can help improve self-concept disturbances.

Ineffective Individual Coping may result when menstrual pain causes additional stress and the woman has inadequate resources to handle her stressors. The woman may feel overwhelmed, may withdraw and become noncommunicative, may become irritable and defensive, and may be prone to accidents. Usually other factors in the woman's life help create a situation in which she is unable to respond effectively; dysmenorrhea is one of many difficulties. Nursing care seeks to identify sources of stress and assist the woman to find ways to remove, reduce, or alleviate causes of stress. Any measures to reduce menstrual pain are helpful. In addition, there may be a need for individual or family therapy, social agency referrals, motivational and values-clarification techniques, and increasing the woman's social and family networks. Problems with dysmenorrhea often increase at important transition points in maturation, such as leaving home, making career choices, getting married, having children, and launching children.

Premenstrual Syndrome (PMS)

PMS is one of the most common disorders of women during the reproductive years, affecting 30% to 40% of American women.[20] PMS has emerged as a complex of physical, behavioral, and emotional symptoms that occur on a recurrent cyclic basis. Although PMS has been studied since 1930 and the term was coined by Dalton in 1953, much is still unknown about etiology.

The accepted clinical definition for PMS includes:

1. Symptoms occur during the luteal phase of the menstrual cycle and resolve within 1 to 2 days after onset of menses; they are recurrent to some degree month after month.
2. There is a symptom-free period of at least 1 week during the follicular phase of the cycle.
3. Symptoms are severe enough to interfere with some aspects of life-style.[20–22]

Guidelines developed by the National Institute of Mental Health (NIMH) for diagnosing PMS include at least a 30% increase in symptom severity in the 6 days before onset of menses, when compared to days 5 to 10 of the cycle. This increase in symptoms must occur in at least two consecutive months.[23]

Symptoms usually begin to appear about 4 to 10 days before menses. As many as 150 different recurrent symptoms have been associated with PMS.[24,25] The most frequently reported PMS symptoms are tension states such as anxiety, nervousness, irritability, frustration, agitation, and argumentativeness. Edema and fluid retention and depression or lowered self-esteem are experienced by many women with PMS. Less frequent

are food cravings, fatigue, headache, painful breasts, and crying. Feelings of panic and loss of control or violent acts and child battering have been reported by a small number of women. Increased accidents and injuries and suicidal ideation are infrequent symptoms. Although women report subjective decreases in work performance, various studies have not found objective alterations in cognition and motor performance during the premenstrual phase.[26]

The relationship between PMS and psychological symptoms such as depression, anxiety, irritability, confusion, and lethargy is not clear. Although edema probably affects these symptoms, the causal paths and networks among factors are complex. The anticipation of symptoms that are unpleasant and disruptive may cause women to feel anxious and depressed, rather than these resulting from a direct physiological effect of PMS. Negative attitudes toward menstruation have been correlated with menstrual symptoms and may augment physiological mechanisms to increase symptomatology. In a study of cognitive processing and abilities, women with PMS showed no significant difference from controls without PMS, although the PMS women subjectively reported decreased functioning. Women with PMS did not show the characteristic cognitive changes associated with clinical depression (depressive memory recall, slower performance, greater distractibility, decreased problem solving).[27]

Characteristic Symptoms of PMS

Onset of symptoms 4 to 10 days before menstrual flow

Recurrent, cyclic symptoms affecting all or many menstrual cycles

Multiple somatic, behavioral, and emotional symptoms that tend to be a typical complex for each individual woman

Symptoms improve after onset of menstrual flow

More common PMS symptoms include:
Fluid retention and peripheral edema
Anxiety, nervousness
Irritability, frustration
Agitation, argumentativeness
Depression, lowered self-esteem
Impaired concentration, being accident prone
Food or sweet or salt craving, hunger, eating binges
Fatigue, lethargy
Headaches, dizziness
Painful breasts, abdominal bloating, pelvic cramping
Crying, emotional instability
Feelings of panic or loss of control

CAUSES OF PMS

The precise etiology of PMS is unknown, although a number of theories have been proposed. PMS probably results from complex interactions between ovarian steroid hormones, endogenous opioid peptides, central neurotransmitters, prostaglandins, and peripheral autonomic and endocrine systems.[20] Imbalances between estrogen (excess) and progesterone (deficiency) have been implicated, especially because of the luteal clustering of symptoms. However, studies have not supported this theory, finding no differences in a number of gonadotropic hormones between women with and without PMS.[21]

Prostaglandin excess or deficiency has been proposed, but the exact balance among prostaglandins that might cause PMS symptoms has not been demonstrated. Two opposite treatment methods, one that increases prostaglandin production (evening primrose oil, which has gamma-linolenic acid) and one that inhibits its action (mefenamic acid) have both been effective under certain circumstances. Reduced prostaglandin levels occur in both the follicular and luteal phase in PMS sufferers and may predispose to symptoms.[20,21]

Endogenous opioid peptides (endorphins, enkephalins, dynorphins), which normally increase in peripheral and central concentrations during the luteal phase, have been found lower in women with PMS during the luteal phase.[28,29] Endorphins affect mood, thus PMS symptoms could be an opiate withdrawal syndrome. Estrogens tend to increase endorphin levels, and women with PMS appear to be functionally hypoestrogenic, experiencing vasomotor symptoms that are physiologically identical with menopausal hot flashes.[30] Data are suggestive of an important role for β-endorphins in the etiology of PMS.

Nutritional deficiencies have been proposed as a cause of PMS, because many women with PMS report cravings for specific types of food or may consume less vitamins and minerals. Lower magnesium levels in red blood cells were found in women with PMS.[31] Another study found no changes in plasma concentrations of magnesium, zinc, vitamin A, vitamin E, thiamine, or pyridoxine in PMS patients compared to controls.[32] There is lack of strong evidence to support nutritional causes for PMS.

MEDICAL THERAPY

Many approaches to treatment have been used; none is uniformly successful. Progesterone has been the most commonly prescribed therapy for PMS for several decades, but clinical trials have failed to demonstrate its superiority over placebos.[20,21] Oral micronized progesterone was recently found more effective than placebos for some symptoms, perhaps by way of a sedative effect or elevation of β-endorphins.[33] Diuretics have been widely used with varying results. Thiazide diuretics and spironolactone have achieved symptom relief, particularly related to fluid retention.

Oral contraceptives have not been documented to treat PMS effectively, but studies were on older medications with high estrogen levels. Newer low-dose and multiphasic pills have not been evaluated; a small subset of PMS patients may respond to these oral contraceptives if other contraindications, such as smoking, are absent. Gonadotropin-releasing hormone (Gn-RH) agonists (leuprolide, naferalin) were found in a small study to improve physical and mental symptoms of PMS, but these medications are intended only for short-term use due to osteoporosis risk with prolonged use.[21]

The prostaglandin inhibitor mefenamic acid taken in large doses throughout the luteal phase relieves many PMS symptoms. It is most effective in women who have dysmenorrhea associated with PMS. Evening primrose oil (Efamol), a prostaglandin precursor that increases prostaglandin synthesis, also reduced PMS symptoms in 62% of women compared to 40% who improved with placebo.[34,35]

Other medical approaches to treating PMS include danazol (effective symptom relief but major side-effects), clonidine and verapamil (especially for anxiety and irritability), and alprazolam (Xanax), which decreases anxiety and improves depression.

Nursing Assessment

Assessment includes a thorough history (menstrual, reproductive, sexual, family, medical, psychiatric, social, and occupational) and detailed information about diet, alcohol and drug use, medications, exercise, cultural and religious practices. Specific history is focused on the onset and progression of menstrual symptoms, as well as the woman's attitudes and responses over time. This includes the age at onset of PMS, duration and precipitating factors, circumstances surrounding the onset and severity of symptoms, enumeration of symptoms, and timing and interval of symptoms. The nurse explores the effectiveness of self-help measures that have been used and medically prescribed treatments. Effects of PMS on self-esteem, body image, self-concept, and relationships are assessed. The general health history provides information about other problems that could contribute to or be confused with PMS.

As part of the assessment, the client fills out a symptom calendar for 2 to 3 months, noting carefully the timing, type, and severity of each premenstrual symptom (Fig. 48-1). Because there are so many different PMS symptoms, assessment is individualized and self-assessment is particularly important. The client needs to identify which symptoms are most frequent

Client Education

Self-Care for PMS

Women with PMS often can reduce symptoms through self-care measures appropriate to their symptom complex:

Fluid retention (breast tenderness, abdominal bloating, peripheral edema):
  Cook without salt or avoid salting cooked foods
  Use fresh or frozen vegetables instead of canned
  Eliminate foods high in sodium (pickles, potato chips, pork, catsup, sauces, prepared soups and other foods, soy sauce)
  Drink 1 quart of water daily
  Use natural diuretics (teas, cranberry and grapefruit juice)

Depression, irritability, mood swings
  Get adequate sleep (at least 7–8 hours per night; more may be needed)
  Get regular exercise (walk about 2 miles/day, swim, bicycle)
  Use multivitamin and multimineral supplements daily
  Be sure to take at least 100 mg of vitmain B_6 per day or eat foods high in B_6 (corn, whole wheat, yeast, tomatoes, sunflower seeds, peanuts)
  Increase calcium, magnesium, and chromium
  Develop support systems (friends, spouse, women's group) for expressing feelings
  Use relaxation techniques (yoga, autogenic training, progressive relaxation, biofeedback, visualization, imagery, meditation)

Headaches and hypoglycemia-type symptoms
  Avoid sweets and refined carbohydrates
  Eat diet high in protein and complex carbohydrates
  Eat several small meals per day
  Avoid caffeine, chocolate, xanthine derivatives
  Do not skip meals
  Snack on fresh fruit or vegetables

and most troublesome, so therapies can be focused on these.

The physical examination seeks evidence of pathology or abnormalities that might be related to symptoms, with particular attention in the pelvic examination to uterine or ovarian enlargement, signs of endometriosis, and structural abnormalities of the reproductive tract.

Nursing Diagnosis and Intervention

Nursing diagnoses related to PMS include Alteration in Comfort (pain), Anxiety and Fear, Ineffective Individual or Family Coping, Fluid Volume Excess, Knowledge Deficit, Alteration in Nutrition, Disturbance in Self-Concept, and Sexual Dysfunction.

The goals of nursing intervention for PMS are to promote a healthy life-style, to alleviate symptoms, and to enhance coping. Treatment for PMS varies according to which symptoms are most disturbing to the client. The most effective nursing therapies include dietary, life-style, and behavioral adjustments; between 36% and 75% of women with PMS have obtained significant symptomatic relief from these.[36] Relaxation techniques are useful in managing discomfort; they also affect PMS symptoms of irritability, depression, and anxiety (nursing diagnosis of anxiety and fear).

Knowledge Deficit is treated by teaching clients about the physiology and psychology of PMS and by clarifying myths or misconceptions about its social and psychological origins and impacts. Public education focused on preadolescents should give young girls accurate information about the menstrual cycle and such problems as dysmenorrhea and PMS. Classes in community clinics, family associations, and women's groups can further educate the public.

Alterations in Nutrition, either by deficits or excesses, may be important factors in PMS symptomatology. Caffeine, chocolate, and other xanthine deriv-

NAME _____   MENSES _____

Date																																				
Day of cycle	1	2	3	4	5	6	7	8	9	10	11	12	13	14	15	16	17	18	19	20	21	22	23	24	25	26	27	28	29	30	31	32	33	34	35	36
Menstruation																																				
Nervous tension																																				
Mood swings																																				
Irritability																																				
Anxiety																																				
Depression																																				
Crying																																				
Forgetfulness																																				
Confusion																																				
Insomnia																																				
Increased naps																																				
Avoid activities																																				
Feel clumsy																																				
Fatigue																																				
Breast tenderness																																				
Abdominal bloating																																				
Swelling—legs, hands																																				
Headaches																																				
Migraine headaches																																				
Hot flushes																																				
Abdominal cramps																																				
General aches																																				
Food cravings—salt																																				
sweets																																				
Skin problems																																				
Weight																																				
BBT																																					

GRADING OF MENSES
1 Light
2 Moderate
3 Heavy
4 Heavy with clots

GRADING OF SYMPTOMS
0 None
1 Mild—does not interfere with activities
2 Moderate—interferes with activities
3 Severe—disabling; unable to function

■ *Figure 48–1*
Menstrual symptom diary.

atives should be eliminated because of their tendency to increase irritability, insomnia, mood changes, and depression. Red meat and fat intake should be reduced; intake of complex carbohydrates, vegetables, whole grains, legumes, and fiber should be increased. Salt and other forms of sodium should be reduced, especially 7 to 9 days before menstruation, when fluid retention occurs. Use of alcohol and tobacco should be curtailed. Adequate fluids and natural diuretics (cranberry or grapefruit juice) are important.

Hypoglycemia-type symptoms (fatigue, headache, dizziness, food cravings) are relieved by avoiding sweets and refined carbohydrates and by eating a diet high in protein and complex carbohydrates. Frequent small meals keep blood glucose levels more stable.

Vitamin B_6 (pyridoxine), a coenzyme in synthesis of certain neurotransmitters, is often recommended to reduce irritability and depression. In large doses (>1 g/ day) it can cause peripheral neuropathy. Data on effectiveness of vitamin B_6 are contradictory. Other vitamins and minerals (calcium, magnesium, chromium, tryptophan, vitamins A and E) have been used, but no convincing data support their effectiveness.[21]

Exercise on a regular basis can reduce stress and cramping and helps relieve depression and moodiness by increasing blood levels of endorphins. Relaxation techniques are effective for reducing both physical and emotional symptoms.[36] When these therapies improve PMS symptoms, alterations in self-concept related to the effects of PMS on work and daily activities are remedied.

Negative attitudes toward menstruation can be changed by education and counseling, which may lead to improved self-concept. Women's group therapy has been effective in correcting stereotypes and providing positive feminine models. The supportive relationships developed in groups, and the sharing of experiences and techniques to alleviate symptoms, help improve self-concept and coping strategies.[26]

Ineffective Individual Coping related to exaggerated self-expectations ("superwoman syndrome") can be improved with counseling to make life-style adjustments that respect needs and accept realistic limitations without feelings of unworthiness. Setting aside time for relaxation or pursuing hobbies is important. Some women need to learn limit setting and more effective sharing of responsibilities with family and coworkers. They may benefit from self-management practices that enable them to put off decisions or prepare ahead for important events that will fall in the premenstrual phase.[37]

With Ineffective Family Coping when PMS causes significant debility to the mother and wife, providing relief for severe PMS symptoms can aid the process of recovery. As the woman is better able to carry out daily activities, emotional reactions and attitudes often improve. When patterns of family interaction have developed that are dysfunctional, family therapy may be necessary to restore communications and functions. Education about PMS is an important nursing contribution to enhancing family function, because it promotes understanding and helps the family to become involved in treatment strategies. Sexual problems related to PMS may be simply avoidance of intercourse premenstrually, which is treatable by reducing PMS symptoms. More complex sexual dysfunctions need referral to sexual therapy.

Evaluation

The effectiveness of nursing care is evaluated by observing for desired changes in client attitudes and behaviors. With PMS, the client reports symptom improvement with successful therapy. Discussions with the client about attitudes toward menstruation and PMS

or use of attitude scales provide data about change in these areas. The client's ability to perform work and family roles and her perceived levels of stress premenstrually provide an indication of how effective the therapeutic program has been.

■ TOXIC SHOCK SYNDROME

Toxic shock syndrome (TSS) is a multisystem infectious disease caused by toxin-producing strains of *Staphylococcus aureus*. The toxin enters the bloodstream through microulcerations in the vaginal or cervical mucosa usually caused by tampons. Almost all cases of TSS have occurred in women, 98% of whom were menstruating and most of whom used vaginal tampons continuously throughout menstruation.[38]

Young women ages 15 to 24 who use tampons are at greatest risk for TSS. The infection develops from *S. aureus* harbored in the vagina. While the majority of women have antibodies to *S. aureus*, only a small number ever develop TSS. High levels of estradiol appear to inhibit toxin production; TSS incidence is greater during menstruation and postpartum when estradiol levels are reduced.[39] Although any tampon could cause TSS, superabsorbent tampons are particularly implicated because they are retained longer vaginally, dry the vaginal mucosa more leading to abrasions, and contain more oxygen to promote bacterial growth.[40]

TSS can be a serious, life-threatening systemic disease with acute, dramatic onset progressing rapidly to hypotensive shock and moribund state. Severe TSS is characterized by the abrupt onset of high fever, vomiting, and diarrhea. These may be accompanied by a sore throat, myalgia, headache, and confusion. Within 24 to 48 hours, the condition may progress to hypotension and shock. A fine, erythematous maculopapular rash develops that resembles sunburn, and the skin begins to desquamate about 10 days later. The acute phase of TSS lasts 4 to 5 days, and convalescence takes place over 1 to 2 weeks.

Laboratory tests show elevated SGOT, SGPT, BUN, creatinine, WBC, and bilirubin, with decreased platelets. Blood, throat, and CSF cultures are negative for other diseases, as is serology. TSS must be distinguished from diseases with similar rashes, such as Rocky Mountain spotted fever, measles, and scarlet fever.

Medical Treatment

Hospitalization is required for most cases of TSS, especially those with severe symptoms. Medical treatment

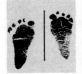

Nursing Care Plan

The Woman with Premenstrual Syndrome (PMS)

Nursing Goals

1. Woman identifies symptoms of PMS and assesses symptom patterns and associated factors.
2. Woman initiates actions to reduce symptoms and debility from PMS.
3. Woman learns and implements self-care to prevent and minimize effects of PMS.
4. Woman seeks appropriate care for family or sexual problems associated with PMS.

Assessment	*Potential Nursing Diagnosis*	*Planning and Intervention*	*Evaluation*
Menstrual history Menarche, menstrual patterns, reactions, preparation Menstrual cycle character and symptoms Attitudes toward menstruation Knowledge about menstruation	Knowledge deficit related to menstrual physiology and psychology	Teach menstrual physiology and psychology Clarify myths, misconceptions Provide information and data on social and psychological factors	Client describes correct understanding of menstrual physiology and psychology; myths and misunderstandings are cleared
Physical and pelvic examination negative for pathology	Alteration in self-concept related to negative attitudes and perceptions toward menstruation	Provide education and counseling about menstruation as normal female functioning Reduce PMS symptoms Suggest group therapy to build positive attitudes and correct social stereotypes	Client accepts normality of menstruation and symptoms Client states positive attitudes and corrects former stereotypes
Specific PMS symptoms Pain, cramping	Alteration in comfort: pain	Prescribe mild analgesics (acetylsalicylic acid, acetaminophen) Apply dry or moist heat Teach relaxation techniques Stress regular exercise	Client says pain and cramping are decreased
Fluid retention: Breast tenderness Abdominal bloating Peripheral edema Weight gain	Fluid volume excess Alteration in nutrition: more sodium than body requirements	Reduce or avoid sodium in foods Drink 1 quart of water daily Use natural diuretics (teas, cranberry and grapefruit juice)	Client states she has less bloating and her symptoms are improved
Depression, irritability, mood swings, frustration, impaired concentration, nervousness, anxiety, emotional instability	Alteration in nutrition: more xanthines than body requirements	Eliminate or reduce caffeine, chocolate, other xanthines; increase vitamin B_6, calcium, magnesium	Client adopts nutritional patterns and feels better

(continued)

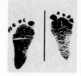

Nursing Care Plan (continued)

Assessment	Potential Nursing Diagnosis	Planning and Intervention	Evaluation
		Stress regular exercise	Client develops coping strategies and performs daily activities more effectively
		Teach relaxation techniques	
	Ineffective individual coping related to PMS symptoms and stress	Counsel on life-style adjustments, limit setting, self-management practices	
Headaches Hypoglycemia-like symptoms: fatigue, dizziness, food cravings, hunger	Alteration in nutrition: less than body requirements for protein and complex carbohydrates; more for simple carbohydrates	Avoid sweets and simple or refined carbohydrates	Client adopts new nutritional patterns and feels better
		Eat diet high in protein and complex carbohydrates	
		Eat several small meals each day	
		Do not skip meals	
		Snack on fresh fruit or vegetables	
Family conflicts or sexual problems	Ineffective family coping related to effects of PMS symptoms on communications and functions	Provide relief of PMS symptoms	Family communicates well, copes more effectively, and redistributes functions
		Provide education and counseling of family about menstrual physiology and psychology; PMS causes and symptoms	
		Teach effective communication techniques to family	
		Involve family in care (diet, exercise, relaxation, rest)	
		Refer for family therapy	
	Sexual dysfunction	Provide relief of PMS symptoms	Couple establishes a satisfying sexual relationship
		Provide education and counseling on sexual response and patterns	Couple makes accommodations to premenstrual problems.
		Refer for sexual counseling for more complex sexual problems	

includes intravenous fluid replacement, cardiorespiratory support, maintenance of blood pressure, and antibiotic therapy for penicillinase-producing *S. aureus*. Electrolytes may be supplemented, and occasionally renal dialysis is needed. Pulmonary and peripheral edema and ascites may result from extravasation of fluids and need intensive management.

Prognosis and recovery are related to severity of the disease and complications. The leading causes of mortality are respiratory failure, uncontrollable hypo-

---

CDC Case Definition for Toxic Shock Syndrome (1982)

Fever (temperature > 38.8°C)

Rash (diffuse erythematous macular)

Desquamation (10 days after onset, mainly of palms and soles)

Hypotension (including orthostatic syncope or dizziness)

Involvement of three or more systems:
  Gastrointestinal (vomiting, diarrhea)
  Muscular (severe myalgias, creatinine phosphokinase > 3 times normal)
  Renal (blood urea nitrogen or creatinine > 2 times normal, >5 WBCs per high-power field without urinary tract infection)
  Hepatic (SGOT, SGPT, total bilirubin > 2 times normal)
  Hematological (platelets < 100,000)
  Central nervous system (disorientation, altered sensorium, headache)
  Respiratory (adult respiratory distress syndrome)

Differentiation from similar-appearing infectious diseases (Rocky Mountain spotted fever, leptospirosis, measles, streptococcal scarlet fever)

Negative blood, throat, and cerebrospinal fluid cultures for other pathogens

---

tension, and disseminated intravascular coagulation (DIC). Infection may recur, especially with the next menstrual period, depending on effectiveness of antibiotic therapy.

Nursing Assessment

To prevent TSS, nurses can assess tampon use practices in their clients, especially extended use. Leaving diaphragms or sponge in the vagina for more than 6 hours after intercourse also increases risk. Nurses must be alert to early signs of TSS, which may resemble upper respiratory infections. When TSS has occurred, the nurse assesses the client's responses to medical therapy, and her abilities to cope emotionally with the impact of this illness. Family responses and adaptations to the illness experience are also assessed.

Nursing Diagnosis and Intervention

During the acute phase of TSS, nursing diagnoses may include Alterations in Tissue Perfusion, Ineffective Breathing Patterns, Decreased Cardiac Output, Impaired

Gas Exchange, Fluid Volume Deficit/Excess, and Self-Care Deficit. Nursing care implements life-supportive and monitoring measures of the medical treatment regimen. Potential complications must be identified early so effective treatment can be initiated. Preventive measures include adequate ventilation, repositioning and ambulation to decrease risk of pneumonia and clotting disorders.

Alterations in Comfort may be related to pain, dehydration, and equipment (e.g., nasogastric [NG] tube, IV, catheter). Nursing care includes administering pain medications and providing comfort measures such as positioning, moisturizing lip creams, mouth care, and ice chips to relieve the dry oral mucosa. Supportive care is provided for alterations in bowel and urinary elimination. Fear, Anxiety, or Powerlessness are potential diagnoses, and the nurse should encourage the client to express feelings and reactions to the illness. As recovery progresses, the client is assisted to perform appropriate self-care to regain some mastery over the body.

Knowledge Deficits related to the illness process, treatment, and prevention of TSS are common. Nurses educate women about how to prevent TSS, especially avoiding high absorbency tampons and prolonged use. Women who have experienced TSS should use other products, such as sanitary pads, and need teaching about early recognition of symptoms. Disturbances in Self-Concept that may result from serious illness often require counseling or psychotherapy.

Evaluation

As an outcome of effective nursing care, women will understand the cause of TSS, and change tampon and contraceptive practices that increase risk. Women who develop TSS will recognize the illness early, seek medical care promptly, and avoid complications.

■ MENOPAUSE

Up to age 40, about 90% of women have regular menstrual cycles, but only 10% have regular cycles continuing to age 50.[41] Menopause, defined as the age of the last menstrual period, occurs at the average age of 50 years, with a range usually between 48 and 52 years. Decline in function of the hypothalamic–pituitary–ovarian system occurs over about 10 years, but is most marked during the 1 to 2 years before cessation of menses. The physiology of menopause is discussed in Chapter 8.

Client Education

Guide for Safe Use of Tampons

Use tampons during time of moderate to heavy flow; change every 1 to 3 hours.

Avoid tampons during times of light flow (beginning, end of menses), when vaginal walls are drier.

Reduce tampon use at night; substitute pads.

Avoid using superabsorbent tampons.

See a health-care professional at once when wearing tampons and these symptoms develop: high fever, vomiting, diarrhea.

See a health-care professional as soon as possible when wearing tampons and these symptoms develop: weakness, skin rash, sore throat, flulike myalgias.

Discontinue tampon use at once if any of the above symptoms develop while wearing a tampon.

Women with a history of TSS should preferably avoid tampons entirely, certainly for 3 to 4 months after acute infection and until cultures for *S. aureus* are negative.

The most common symptoms experienced during the perimenopausal period are hot flashes and faintness, thinning of the vaginal mucosa, and decreased vaginal lubrication. These are related to decreased estrogen and vasomotor instability. Rapid dilation or constriction of vasculature result in sudden sensations of heat, often accompanied by sweating and flushed skin. Some women have brief experiences of being cold all over. Decreased estrogen produces atrophic changes of the labia and vaginal mucosa, often resulting in dryness and irritation, making intercourse uncomfortable.

Menopause in Western cultures has traditionally been associated with varying degrees of emotional instability. As the woman's childbearing years come to an end, she faces a developmental transition and enters a new phase of life. In cultures that value youth and reproductive capacity in women, menopause signifies loss of a socially valued status and may result in depressive symptoms. In other cultures in which older women have heightened social status (e.g., American Indian), menopause is not associated with negative reactions. When menopause is viewed as a natural process and not a disease or deficiency state, most women pass through this transition with little difficulty.[42,43] There appears to be no consistent relationship between biochemical or physiological changes and the woman's behavioral symptomatology.[44]

Abnormal Perimenopausal Vaginal Bleeding

The incidence of dysfunctional vaginal bleeding increases as women approach the end of menses. In peri-menopausal women, hormonal disorders cause most abnormal vaginal bleeding, although other causes such as inflammatory and neoplastic lesions, endometriosis, ovarian tumors and cysts, endocrine disorders, pregnancy, blood disorders, and medications must not be overlooked.

In 40- to 50-year-old women without organic lesions, dysfunctional uterine bleeding is usually due to anovulation, which increases significantly after age 40. Anovulatory cycles in this age group result most often from decreased sensitivity of the oocytes to FSH and LH stimulation. The two common ovarian responses include a persistent ovarian follicle and endometrial hyperplasia, both of which eventually result in bleeding, which may be heavy and irregular.[41]

The assessment and treatment of dysfunctional uterine bleeding has been discussed earlier. Endometrial cancer is an increasing concern as women become older, especially among perimenopausal women with abnormal bleeding and postmenopausal women with any bleeding.

Osteopenia and Osteoporosis

With aging, there is a generalized and progressive loss of both trabecular and cortical bone. *Osteopenia* refers to a condition in which bone mass is substantially lower than the mean level of peak bone mass, and *osteoporosis* is an absolute decrease in the amount of bone to a level below that required for mechanical support.[45,46] The usual manifestation of osteoporosis is fracture with little or no trauma. About 1.5 million fractures are caused by osteoporosis each year in the United States. The lifetime risk for hip fractures in white women is 15%, and about one third of women over age 65 will have a vertebral fracture. Hip fractures carry a poor prognosis, leading to death in 12% to 20% of cases and permanent disability in about 75%.[45]

There are three stages of bone mass change over the life span. The first stage is building of bone and leads to attainment of peak bone mass. After closure of the growth plate about age 20, radial growth continues for another 10 to 15 years. Most of the bone mass is acquired by age 20 to 30. The second stage consists of a slow, age-dependent loss of bone. It begins around age 40 for cortical bone, and age 45 to 50 for trabecular bone. This process continues into extreme old age and is probably similar in both women and men. In women, there is a third stage of transient accelerated postmenopausal bone loss due to decreased estrogen. This is superimposed on the slow stage of bone loss and results in disproportionately more trabecular bone than cortical bone loss.

The amount of bone lost during the last two stages is not well defined, but it is estimated that the slow phase produces a loss of 25% each from trabecular and cortical bone, and the accelerated phase causes women to lose an additional 10% from trabecular and 25% from cortical components. Women, overall, can lose 35% of their cortical bone and 50% of their trabecular bone during a lifetime; men lose about two thirds these amounts.[46,47]

Bone remodeling is a continuous process, in which osteoblasts build bone and osteoclasts resorb it, under the control of calcitriol (vitamin D), calcitonin, parathyroid hormone, and bone-produced proteins. The entire cycle takes 90 days, with about 5% of bone surface being remodeled at any given time. During age-related bone loss, there is a remodeling imbalance with an increase in resorption over formation. This results in increased bone turnover leading to bone loss. In the slow, age-dependent stage, there is gradual thinning of the trabeculae and bone cortex. In the accelerated, postmenopausal stage, there is loss of structural trabeculae and greater trabecular perforation.[45,48]

Osteoporosis is classified into two types. Type I (postmenopausal osteoporosis) affects women within 15 to 20 years after menopause and mainly affects trabecular bone. It may result in fractures of the vertebrae, distal forearm (Colles' fracture), and distal ankle. Vertebral fractures are the crush type and cause pain and deformation. Type II (age-related osteoporosis) occurs in men and woman age 70 or older, but is twice as common in women. It usually results in hip and vertebral fractures, but may affect the humerus, tibia, and pelvis. Vertebral fractures are the multiple wedge type, leading to dorsal kyphosis (dowager's hump).

Predisposing factors for osteopenia and osteoporosis are summarized in the box, Risk Factors for Osteoporosis. Some risk factors are potentially changeable; oth-

ers are not (e.g., sex, race [Asian or white], age, small frame, low body weight). The changeable factors such as cigarette smoking, heavy alcohol use, and sedentary life-style are also risk factors for multiple other diseases. Two specific risk factors are menopause and low-calcium diet.

Medical Treatment

Hormone replacement therapy with estrogen, alone or combined with progestin, is widely used to treat changes associated with menopause, including hot flashes, vag-

---

Risk Factors for Osteoporosis

Factors Not Subject to Alteration

White or Asian

Female sex

Positive family history

Short stature

Small bone structure

Thin or lean body configuration

Postmenopausal status

Advanced age

Behavioral Factors That Can Be Changed

Sedentary life-style

Low calcium intake

Cigarette smoking

Alcohol abuse

High caffeine intake

High protein intake

High phosphate intake

Diseases and Medications

Hyperthyroidism

Cushing's disease

Acromegaly

Hypogonadism

Malabsorption syndromes

Anorexia nervosa

Osteogenesis imperfecta

Hyperparathyroidism

Multiple myeloma

Type 1 diabetes

Chronic corticosteroid therapy

Long-term heparin therapy

inal and urinary tract atrophy, skin changes, and mood changes. Estrogen protects against osteoporosis, as demonstrated in several well-controlled clinical studies.[49] Receptors for estrogen have been found in human bone cells, supporting the theory that estrogen has a direct effect on osteoblast activity as well as reducing osteoclastic resorption.[50,51] An indirect benefit of estrogen therapy may be a protective effect against coronary artery disease, promoting a favorable lipid profile.

Parenteral salmon calcitonin, sodium fluoride, and intranasal calcitonin have been used, but are limited by route of administration, safety, and lack of proved efficacy. Intermittent cyclical therapy with etidronate, an organic bisphosphonate compound, has been found to increase spinal bone mass significantly and reduce the incidence of new vertebral fractures in women with postmenopausal osteoporosis.[52]

Nursing Assessment

The nurse has an important role in identifying risk factors for osteopenia and osteoporosis. The major risk factors are well-documented (see box, Risk Factors for Osteoporosis), and many exert their effects over long time periods. Assessment of dietary habits should begin in preadolescence, with attention to adequate calcium and limited amounts of protein and phosphates. Use of caffeine, cigarettes, and alcohol are assessed frequently through the woman's life, because these affect health in multiple ways and are amenable to intervention. Activity level is important from childhood on in maximizing bone density and preventing bone loss.

Physical examination focuses on the woman's age, race, stature, bone structure, and weight. Obese women have increased supplies of estrogen, even after menopause. The risk of osteoporosis is low among African-American women, who have heavier bone structure and greater mass than white or Asian women. Signs of endocrine or systemic disorders are noted, and further diagnostic testing is undertaken.

Tests for bone mass (bone densitometry) are frequently used to identify women with osteopenia and to assess the extent of osteoporosis. Single or dual photon absorptiometry are most commonly used for spinal and proximal femur measurements. Quantitative computed tomography (QCT) is best suited to measure trabecular bone in the spine, but is expensive and has high radiation exposure. Ultrasound examination of the patella holds promise of being a low-risk and inexpensive tool for identifying osteoporosis risk.[53]

Nursing Diagnosis and Intervention

Nursing diagnoses related to osteoporosis may include High Risk for Injury (fractures, complications), Altera-

tions in Comfort: Pain, Impaired Physical Mobility due to fractures, and Activity Intolerance related to fractures or deformities. Alterations in Nutrition: Less Than Body Requirements for calcium may be a factor that increases the risk of osteopenia. Knowledge Deficits related to causes, prevention, and treatment of osteoporosis are common.

Nursing intervention emphasizes the prevention of osteopenia and minimization of bone loss with aging and menopause. Primary prevention includes nursing actions to assist women in achieving maximal peak bone mass during the years of skeletal maturation. Education and counseling focus on diet and exercise from preadolescence through old age, with the goal of ensuring good calcium intake and limiting protein, phosphates, and substances known to affect bone metabolism (caffeine, cigarettes, alcohol). Regular weight-bearing exercise habits are encouraged and modified according to life cycle needs. Dangers of sedentary life-styles and substance use are emphasized.

Knowledge deficits are reduced by teaching women the major risk factors for osteoporosis and by identifying those factors important in their family and personal histories. Women at higher risk are encouraged to undertake preventive actions as early as possible and to have regular medical monitoring, including bone densitometry. The risks and benefits of estrogen or hormone therapy are discussed, and therapy should be individualized according to the client needs, desires, and individual symptom and risk profile. Calcium supplementation is recommended for women with marginal dietary calcium intake, and sodium intake should be limited because sodium promotes increased urinary excretion of calcium.

Evaluation

Outcomes of effective nursing care include increased knowledge about prevention and treatment of osteoporosis, and behavior changes to reduce risk by maximizing bone mass deposition and minimizing bone loss. Women with increased risk factors will seek medical care and assistance to modify their risks whenever possible. The result of effective interventions will be fewer fractures due to osteoporosis, which reduces suffering and disability in older women and promotes healthier aging.

■ REFERENCES

1. Johannison E, Landgren BM, Rohr HP et al: Endometrial morphology and peripheral hormone levels in women with regular menstrual cycles. Fertil Steril 48: 401, 1987

2. Espey LL, Intissar ABH: Characteristics and control of the normal menstrual cycle. Obstet Gynecol Clin North Am 17(2):275–298, June 1990

3. Hodgen GD: Neuroendocrinology of the normal menstrual cycle. J Reprod Med 34:68, 1989

4. Usala SJ, Usala FO, Haciski R et al: IgG and IgA content of vaginal fluid during the menstrual cycle. J Reprod Med 43(4):292–294, 1989

5. Ho HZ, Gilger JW, Brink TM: Effects of menstrual cycle on spatial information-processes. Percept Motor Skills 63:743, 1986

6. Baron JA, La Vecchia C, Levi F: The antiestrogenic effect of cigarette smoking in women. Am J Obstet Gynecol 162(2):502–514, February 1990

7. Yeh J, Barbieri RL: Effects of smoking on steroid production, metabolism, and estrogen-related disease. Sem Reprod Endocrin 7(4):326–334, November 1989

8. Long CA, Gast MJ: Menorrhagia. Obstet Gynecol Clin North Am 17(2):343–359, June 1990

9. Mattox JH: Abnormal uterine bleeding. In Willson JR, Carrington ER (eds): Obstetrics and Gynecology, 8th ed. St Louis, CV Mosby, 1987

10. Marchbanks PA, Lee NC, Peterson HB: Cigarette smoking as a risk factor for pelvic inflammatory disease. Am J Obstet Gynecol 162(3):639–644, March 1990

11. Keith LG, Creinin M, Method MW: Cervicitis as an antecedent to pelvic infection: A review. Int J Fertil 34(2):109–119, 1989

12. Anderson PO, McGuire GG: Delta-9-tetrahydrocannabinol as an antiemetic. Am J Hosp Pharm 38:641, May 1981

13. Barbieri RL: Etiology and epidemiology of endometriosis. Am J Obstet Gynecol 162(2):565–567, February 1990

14. Adamson GD: Diagnosis and clinical presentation of endometriosis. Am J Obstet Gynecol 162(2):568–569, February 1990

15. Bachman GA: Hysterectomy: A critical review. J Reprod Med 35(9):839–862, September 1990

16. Doody KM, Carr BR: Amenorrhea. Obstet Gynecol Clin North Am 17(2):361–367, June 1990

17. Dawood MY: Dysmenorrhea. Clin Obstet Gynecol 33(1):168–178, March 1990

18. Demers LM, Hahn DW, McGuire JL: Newer concepts in dysmenorrhea research: Leukotrienes and calcium channel blockers. In Dawood MY, McGuire JL, Demers LM (eds): Premenstrual Syndrome and Dysmenorrhea. Baltimore, Urban and Schwartzenberg, 1985

19. Brown MA, Woods NF: Correlates of dysmenorrhea: A challenge to past stereotypes. JOGN Nurs 13(4):256–265 July/August 1984

20. Smith S, Schiff I: The premenstrual syndrome—diagnosis and management. Fertil Steril 52(4):527–543, October 1989

21. Chihal HJ: Premenstrual syndrome: An update for the clinician. Obstet Gynecol Clin North Am 17(2):457–479, June 1990

22. Hsia LSY, Log MH: Premenstrual syndrome: Current concepts in diagnosis and management. J Nurse Midwifery 35(6):351–357, November/December 1990

23. Anderson M, Severino SK, Hurt SW et al: Premenstrual syndrome research: Using the NIMH guidelines. J Clin Psychol 49:484–486, 1988

24. Brown MA, Zimmer PA: Personal and family impact of premenstrual symptoms. JOGN Nurs 15(1):31–38, January/February 1986

25. Rupp SL: Premenstrual syndrome. NAACOG Update Series, Lesson 15, Vol 2, p 43. Princeton, NJ, Continuing Professional Education Center, 1985

26. Coyne CM, Woods NF, Mitchell ES: Premenstrual tension syndrome. JOGN Nurs 14(6):446–454, November/December 1985

27. Rapkin AJ, Chang LC, Reading AE: Mood and cognitive style in premenstrual syndrome. Obstet Gynecol 74(4):644–649, October 1989

28. Tulenheimo A, Laafikainen T, Salminen K: Plasma β-endorphin immunoreactivity in premenstrual tension. Br J Obstet Gynaecol 94:26, 1987

29. Facchinetti F, Martignoni E, Petraglia F et al: Premenstrual fall of plasma β-endorphin in patients with premenstrual syndrome. Fertil Steril 47:570, 1987

30. Casper RF, Graves GR, Reid RL: Objective measurement of hot flushes associated with the premenstrual syndrome. Fertil Steril 47:341 1987

31. Abraham GE: Nutritional factors in the etiology of the premenstrual syndromes. J Reprod Med 28:446, 1983

32. Mira M, Stewart PM, Abraham SF: Vitamin and trace element status in premenstrual syndrome. Am J Clin Nutr 47:636, 1988

33. Dennerstein L, Spencer-Gardner C, Gotts G et al: Progesterone and premenstrual syndrome: A double-blind crossover trial. Br Med J 290:1617, 1985

34. Mira M, McNeil D, Fraser I et al: Mefanamic acid in the treatment of premenstrual syndrome. Obstet Gynecol 68:395, 1986

35. Puloakka J, Makarainen L, Viinikka L et al: Biochemical and clinical effects of treating the premenstrual syndrome with prostaglandin synthesis precursors. J Reprod Med 30:149, 1985

36. Goodale IL, Domar AD, Benson H: Alleviation of premenstrual syndrome symptoms with the relaxation response. Obstet Gynecol 75(4):649–655, April 1990

37. Frank EP: What are nurses doing to help PMS patients? Am J Nurs 86(2):136–140, February 1986

38. Nichols DH, Evrard JR (eds): Ambulatory Gynecology. Philadelphia, Harper & Row, 1985

39. Connell EB: Which contraceptives don't cause TSS? Contemp OB/GYN 26:127, October 1985

40. Wager GP: Toxic shock syndrome. Am J Obstet Gynecol 146(1):93–102, May 1983

41. Nesse RE: Abnormal vaginal bleeding in perimenopausal women. Am Fam Physician 40(1):185–192, July 1989

42. McCrea FB: The politics of menopause: The "discovery" of a deficiency disease. Social Problems 31(1):111–123, 1983

43. Kaufert PA: Anthropology and menopause: The development of a theoretical framework. Maturitas 4:181–193, 1982

44. Voda AM, George T: Menopause. In Werley HH, Fitzpatrick J (eds): Ann Rev Nurs 4:55–75, 1986

45. Riggs BL: Overview of osteoporosis. West J Med 154:63–77, January 1991

46. Watts NB: Prevention of osteoporosis: The role of primary physicians. J Fam Pract 32(3):261–263, 1991

47. Riggs BL, Melton LJ: Medical progress series: Involutional osteoporosis. N Engl J Med 314:1676, 1986

48. Lufkin EG, Ory SJ: Estrogen replacement therapy for the prevention of osteoporosis. Am Fam Physician 40(3):205–212, September 1989

49. Lichtman R: Perimenopausal hormone replacement therapy: Review of the literature. J Nurse Midwifery 36(1):30–48, January/February 1991

50. Eriksen EF, Colvard DS, Gerg NJ et al: Evidence of estrogen receptors in normal human osteoblast-like cells. Science 241:84–86, 1988

51. Komm BS, Terpening CM, Benz DJ et al: Estrogen binding, receptor mRNA, and biologic response in osteoblast-like osteosarcoma cells. Science 241:81–84, 1988

52. Watts NB, Harris ST, Genant HK et al: Intermittant cyclical etidronate treatment of postmenopausal osteoporosis. N Engl J Med 323(2):73–125, July 1990

53. Bourguet CC, Hamrick GA, Gilchrist VJ: The prevalence of osteoporosis risk factors and physician intervention. J Fam Pract 32(3):265–271, 1991

■ SUGGESTED READINGS

Clark-Coller T: Dysfunctional uterine bleeding and amenorrhea: Differential diagnosia and management. J Nurse Midwifery 36(1):49–62, January/February 1991

Connel A: Abnormal uterine bleeding. Nurse Pract 14:40–57, 1989

Dawood MY: Nonsteroidal anti-inflammatory drugs and changing attitudes toward dysmenorrhea. Am J Med 84:23 (Suppl 5A), 1988

Dawood MY, McGuire JL, Demers LM (eds): Premenstrual Syndrome and Dysmenorrhea. Baltimore, Urban and Schwarzenberg, 1985

Dawson-Hughes B, Dallal GE, Krall EA et al: A controlled trial of the effect of calcium supplementation on bone density in postmenopausal women. N Engl J Med 323:878–883, 1990

Douglas LW, Greisman B: Early hypothyroidism in patients with menorrhagia. Am J Obstet Gynecol 160:673, 1989

Gelfand MM, Ferenczy A: A prospective 1-year study of estrogen and progestin in postmenpausal women: Effects on the endometrium. Obstet Gynecol 74:398–402, 1989

Hargrove JT, Maxson WS, Wentz AC et al: Menopausal hormone replacement therapy with continuous daily oral micronized estradiol and progesterone. Obstet Gynecol 73:606–612, 1989

Heaney RP, Avioli OV, Chesnut CH et al: Osteoporotic bone fragility. Detection by ultrasound transmission velocity. JAMA 261:2986–2990, 1989

Heidrich F, Thopson RS: Osteoporosis prevention: Strategies applicable for general populations. J Fam Pract 25:33–39, 1987

Henzl MR, Kwei L: Efficacy and safety of nafarelin in the treatment of endometriosis. Am J Obstet Gynecol 162(2):570–574, February 1990

Kendall KE, Schnurr PP: The effects of vitamin B_6 supplementation of premenstrual symptoms. Obstet Gynecol 70:145, 1987

Larson EB, Bruce RA: Exercise and aging. Ann Intern Med 105:783–785, 1986

Mishell DR (ed): Menopause: Physiology and Pharmacology. Chicago, Year Book Medical, 1987

Neighbours LE, Clelland J, Jackson JR et al: Transcutaneous electrical nerve stimulation for pain relief in primary dysmenorrhea. Clin J Pain 3:17, 1987

Prior JC, Vigna Y, Sciarretta D et al: Conditioning exercise decreases premenstrual symptoms: A prospective, controlled 6-month trial. Fertil Steril 47:402, 1987

Riggs BL, Melton JL (eds): Osteoporosis: Etiology, Diagnosis, and Management. New York, Raven Press, 1988

Santiesteban AJ, Burnham TL, George KL et al: Primary spasmodic dysmenorrhea: The use of TENS on accupuncture points. Am J Acupuncture 13:35, 1985

Storm T, Thamsborog G, Steiniche T et al: The effect of intermittent cyclical etidronate therapy on bone mass and fracture in women with postmenopausal osteoporosis. N Engl J Med 322:1265–1271, 1990

Wasnich RD, Davis JW, Ross PD: Appropriate clinical application of bone density measurements. J Am Med Wom Assoc 45:99–102, 1990

Weinstein L: Efficacy of a continuous estrogen–progestin regimen in the menopausal patient. Obstet Gynecol 69:929–932, 1987

Woods NF, Most A, Longenecker GD: Major life events, daily stressors, and perimenstrual symptoms. Nurs Res 34:263–267, 1985

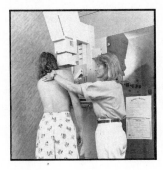

Unit IX
Assessment and Management of Women's Health Promotion

MULTIPLE CHOICE

1. The areas of gynecology most often encountered by the maternity nurse are
   A. Growth and development needs including adolescence and menopause
   B. Health promotion
   C. Common gynecologic problems including menstrual problems and minor infections
   D. Infertility problems and Rh/ABO incompatibilities
   Select the number corresponding to the correct letter or letters.
   1. B and C
   2. A, C, and D
   3. All but A
   4. All but D _____

2. An important component of the gynecologic health history is
   A. A professional demeanor while taking the history
   B. A thorough history, including sexual activity, taken each time the patient is seen
   C. A review of periodic screening procedures for early detection of gynecological problems
   D. A thorough assessment of the client's emotional status _____

3. The most critical screening procedures for women include
   A. Height, weight, and blood pressure
   B. Breast examination
   C. Mammography
   D. Pap smear
   E. Hemoglobin/hematocrit
   F. Pelvic examination
   G. Rectal examination
   H. Stool guaiac
   Select the number corresponding to the correct letter or letters.
   1. All but A
   2. All but C and H
   3. All but G
   4. All but E and H
   5. All but H _____

4. The reasons why a client may not follow health-related advice given by a nurse include
   A. Lack of autonomy in health-seeking behavior
   B. A nonsupportive family
   C. A nontherapeutic relationship with the nurse
   D. An empathic relationship with the physician
   Select the number corresponding to the correct letter or letters.
   1. All but A
   2. B and C
   3. All but D
   4. All but B _____

5. The two most common breast cancers are
   A. Intervillous hyperplasia
   B. Fibroadenoma
   C. Adenocarcinomas
   D. Intraductal papillomas
   E. Ductal carcinomas
   Select the number corresponding to the correct letter or letters.
   1. A and D
   2. B and E
   3. C and D
   4. C and E _____

6. The diagnosis of osteoporosis can be made by
   A. Periodic height and weight measurements only
   B. CAT scan only
   C. Blood test
   D. Clinical signs
   E. Diagnostic radiographic tests
   Select the number corresponding to the correct letter or letters.
   1. B
   2. A and C
   3. D and E
   4. E only _____

7. Recurrent heavy menses over months and years in women 30 to 45 years of age are *most often* due to
   A. Myomata
   B. PMS
   C. Adenomyosis
   D. STDs
   E. Intervillous carcinoma

Select the number corresponding to the correct letter or letters.
1. A and D
2. A and C
3. C and E
4. B and D
5. All of the above ____

8. Very short menstrual cycles may indicate
A. Anemia
B. Improper birth control pill dosage
C. Anovulation
D. Infertility ____

9. The most common cause of secondary amenorrhea in women 16 to 45 years of age is
A. Ovarian cysts
B. STD
C. Pregnancy
D. Hypopituitarism
E. Endometrial hyperplasia ____

10. Which of the following drugs are used in the treatment of dysmenorrhea?
A. Acetaminophen
B. Aspirin
C. Low dose combination birth control pills
D. Naproxen
E. Mefenamic acid
F. Ibuprofen
Select the number corresponding to the correct letter or letters.
1. All of the above
2. All but B and C
3. All but D and E
4. All but C
5. All but F ____

11. The *most frequently* reported PMS symptoms are
A. Food cravings
B. Anxiety, nervousness, agitation
C. Painful breasts
D. Irritability, argumentativeness
E. Headache
F. Frustration
G. Child battering
Select the number corresponding to the correct letter or letters.
1. A, B, C
2. D, F, G
3. B, D, F
4. C, D, E
5. A, C, E ____

12. Which of the following are the *most frequent* reasons why women seek gynecological care?
A. STD
B. Vaginal discharge
C. Perineal lesions

D. Itching
E. Intercycle spotting
Select the number corresponding to the correct letter or letters.
1. A, B, C
2. A, C, E
3. A and C
4. B and E
5. B and D ____

13. Which of the following can be the cause(s) of toxic shock syndrome?
A. Cervical cap
B. Vaginal sprays
C. Tampons
D. Diaphragm left in place for several days
E. Infrequent bathing
F. Multiple sex partners
Select the number corresponding to the correct letter or letters.
1. All of the above
2. A, B, C
3. B, C, E
4. A, C, D
5. A and C
6. C and F ____

14. The most prevalent sexually transmitted disease in the United States today is
A. Trichomonas vaginitis
B. Neisseria gonorrhoeae
C. Gardnerella vaginitis
D. Chlamydia trachomatis
E. AIDS
F. Genital herpes ____

15. Common organisms isolated in pelvic inflammatory disease include
A. Bacteroides
B. Mycoplasma hominis
C. Peptococcus
D. Neisseria gonorrhoeae
E. Peptostreptococcus
F. Chlamydia trachomatis
Select the number corresponding to the correct letter or letters.
1. B, D, F
2. A, C, E
3. All but E and F
4. All but C and E
5. All but A
6. All of the above ____

16. Toxic shock syndrome (TSS) is caused by the organism
A. Chlamydia trachomatis
B. Mycoplasma hominis

C. Peptostreptococcus
D. Staphylococcus aureus
E. Neisseria gonorrhoeae   _____

17. The leading causes of mortality in toxic shock syndrome are
A. Hypervolemia
B. Respiratory failure
C. PID

D. Uncontrollable hypotension
E. DIC

Select the number corresponding to the correct letter or letters.
1. A, C, D
2. C, D, E
3. B, D, E
4. All but C
5. All but C and E
6. All of the above   _____

Appendices

A. THE PREGNANT PATIENT'S BILL OF RIGHTS

B. MILESTONES IN MATERNAL–INFANT HEALTH: UNITED STATES

C. PRENATAL AND POSTPARTUM EXERCISES

Conditioned Relaxation

Tense–Release Relaxation

Imagery Exercises

Neuromuscular Control– "Partner Feedback Relaxation"

Prenatal Exercises

Postpartum Exercises

D. UNIVERSAL PRECAUTIONS FOR PREVENTION OF TRANSMISSION OF HIV, HEPATITIS B VIRUS, AND OTHER BLOODBORNE PATHOGENS IN HEALTH-CARE SETTINGS

Body Fluids to Which Universal Precautions Apply

Body Fluids to Which Universal Precautions Do Not Apply

Precautions for Other Body Fluids in Special Settings

Use of Protective Barriers

E. DRUG USE DURING BREAST-FEEDING

F. CONVERSION TABLE FOR WEIGHTS OF NEWBORN

G. AID FOR VISUALIZATION OF CERVICAL DILATATION

H. RESOURCES FOR MATERNAL-CARE NURSES

Abortion

Alternative Lifestyles

Breast-Feeding

Childbirth Alternatives

Family Planning

Fertility and Infertility

Genetic Counseling

Parenting and Abuse

Professional Organizations

Public Health Organizations

Rape

Sex Education

Sexual Therapy

Sexuality

Sexually Transmitted Diseases

Substance Abuse

I. NANDA LIST OF APPROVED NURSING DIAGNOSES

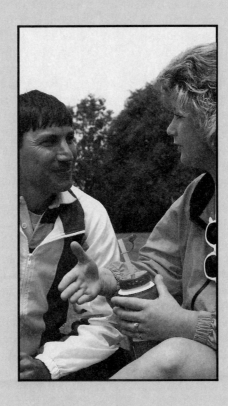

A	*The Pregnant Patient's Bill of Rights*

American parents are becoming increasingly aware that health professionals do not always have scientific data to support common American obstetric practices and that many of these practices are carried out primarily because they are part of medical and hospital tradition. In the last 40 years, many artificial practices have been introduced that have changed childbirth from a physiological event to a very complicated medical procedure in which all kinds of drugs are used and procedures carried out, sometimes unnecessarily, and many of them potentially damaging for the baby and even for the mother. A growing body of research makes it alarmingly clear that every aspect of traditional American hospital care during labor and delivery must now be questioned as to its possible effect on the future well-being of both the obstetric patient and her unborn child.

One in every 35 children born in the United States today will eventually be diagnosed as retarded; one in every 10 to 17 children has been found to have some form of brain dysfunction or learning disability requiring special treatment. Such statistics are not confined to the lower socioeconomic group but cut across all segments of American society.

New concerns are being raised by childbearing women because no one knows what degree of oxygen depletion, head compression, or traction by forceps the unborn or newborn infant can tolerate before that child sustains permanent brain damage or dysfunction. The recent findings regarding the cancer-related drug diethylstilbestrol have alerted the public to the fact that neither the approval of a drug by the U.S. Food and Drug Administration nor the fact that a drug is prescribed by a physician guarantees that a drug or medication is safe for the mother or her unborn child. In fact, the American Academy of Pediatrics Committee on Drugs has recently stated that no drug, whether prescription or over-the-counter, has been proven safe for the unborn child.

The pregnant patient has the right to participate in decisions involving her well-being and that of her unborn child, unless there is a clear-cut medical emergency that prevents her participation. In addition to the rights set forth in the American Hospital Association's "Patient's Bill of Rights" (which has also been adopted by the New York City Department of Health) the pregnant patient, because she represents *two* patients rather than one, should be recognized as having the additional rights listed below.

1. *The pregnant patient has the right*, prior to the administration of any drug or procedure, to be informed by the health professional caring for her of any potential direct or indirect effects, risks, or hazards to herself or her unborn or newborn infant which may result from the use of a drug or procedure prescribed for or administered to her during pregnancy, labor, birth, or lactation.

2. *The pregnant patient has the right*, prior to the proposed therapy, to be informed, not only of the benefits, risks, and hazards of the proposed therapy but also of known alternative therapy, such as available childbirth education classes, which could help to prepare the pregnant patient physically and mentally to cope with the discomfort or stress of pregnancy and the experience of childbirth, thereby reducing or eliminating her need for drugs and obstetric intervention. She should be offered such information early in her pregnancy in order that she may make a reasoned decision.

3. *The pregnant patient has the right*, prior to the administration of any drug, to be informed by the health professional who is prescribing or administering the drug to her that any drug she receives during pregnancy, labor, and birth, no matter how or when the drug is taken or administered, may adversely affect her unborn baby, directly or indirectly, and that there is no drug or chemical that has been proven safe for the unborn child.

4. *The pregnant patient has the right*, if cesarean section is anticipated, to be informed prior to the administration of any drug, and preferably prior to the hospitalization, that minimizing her and, in turn, her baby's intake of nonessential preoperative medicine will benefit her baby.

5. *The pregnant patient has the right*, prior to the administration of a drug or procedure, to be informed if there is NO properly controlled follow-up research that has established the safety of the drug or procedure with regard to its direct or indirect effects on the physiological, mental, and neurological development of the child exposed, via the mother, to the drug or procedure during pregnancy, labor, birth, or lactation (this would apply to virtually all drugs and the vast majority of obstetric procedures).

6. *The pregnant patient has the right*, prior to the administration of any drug, to be informed of the brand name and generic name of the drug in order that she may advise the health professional of any past adverse reaction to the drug.

7. *The pregnant patient has the right* to determine for herself, without pressure from her attendant,

whether she will accept the risks inherent in the proposed therapy or refuse a drug or procedure.

8. *The pregnant patient has the right* to know the name and qualifications of the individual administering a medication or procedure to her during labor or birth.

9. *The pregnant patient has the right* to be informed, prior to the administration of any procedure, whether that procedure is being administered to her for her or her baby's benefit (medically indicated) or as an elective procedure (for convenience or teaching purposes).

10. *The pregnant patient has the right* to be accompanied during the stress of labor and birth by someone she cares for, and to whom she looks for emotional comfort and encouragement.

11. *The pregnant patient has the right* after appropriate medical consultation to choose a position for labor and for birth which is least stressful to her baby and to herself.

12. *The obstetric patient has the right* to have her baby cared for at her bedside if her baby is normal and to feed her baby according to her baby's needs rather than according to the hospital regimen.

13. *The obstetric patient has the right* to be informed in writing of the name of the person who actually delivered her baby and the professional qualifications of that person. This information should also be on the birth certificate.

14. *The obstetric patient has the right* to be informed if there is any known or indicated aspect of her or her baby's care or condition that may cause her or her baby later difficulty or problems.

15. *The obstetric patient has the right* to have her and her baby's hospital medical records complete, accurate, and legible and to have their records, including Nurses' Notes, retained by the hospital until the child reaches at least the age of majority, or, alternatively, to have the records offered to her before they are destroyed.

16. *The obstetric patient*, both during and after her hospital stay, *has the right* to have access to her complete hospital medical records, including Nurses' Notes, and to receive a copy upon payment of a reasonable fee and without incurring the expense of retaining an attorney.

It is the obstetric patient and her baby, not the health professional, who must sustain any trauma or injury resulting from the use of a drug or obstetric procedure. The observation of the rights listed above will not only permit the obstetric patient to participate in the decisions involving her and her baby's health care, but will help to protect the health professional and the hospital against litigation arising from resentment or misunderstanding on the part of the mother.

(Reprinted by permission of the Committee on Patient's Rights, Box 1900, New York, N.Y. 10001.)

1876. The beginning of child-welfare legislation in the United States was the act passed by the New York State Legislature, granting to the *Society for the Prevention of Cruelty to Children* a charter that gave it wide power in the protection of child life.

1900. The *United States Census Bureau* was made a permanent organization. Up to this time, vital statistics were considered to be of so little importance in the United States that as soon as the population was tabulated and classified, the bureau was disbanded, to be reestablished and reorganized every 10 years.

1908. The *Division of Child Hygiene* was established in New York City, the first in the United States, and it was important enough to be recognized nationally. Josephine Baker, M.D., was appointed chief. This was a pioneer achievement, and the methods that evolved had no precedent.

1909. The *American Association for the Study and Prevention of Infant Mortality* was organized and held its first meeting in New Haven, Connecticut. This committee was composed of both professional and lay members and devoted itself entirely to problems connected with child life, particularly to studying and trying to correct the high mortality. At this time there were no records of births or deaths, and the causes of deaths were unknown.

The work of this organization was profoundly significant. In 1918, its expanding activities caused it to change its name to the *American Child Hygiene Association,* and in 1923, the name was changed to the *American Child Health Association.* In 1935, after having contributed to every angle of this pioneer work, the association was disbanded.

1915. The *Birth Registration Area* was established by a federal act. The information is compiled in a uniform manner, giving the birth and the death statistics on which our information on mortality rates is based.

1919. The *American Committee on Maternal Welfare* was founded to stimulate medical cooperation with public and private agencies to protect the lives and health of mothers and infants and to teach principles and practice of personal hygiene and health to parents, physicians, nurses, and others dealing with the problems of maternity. The Committee was incorporated as a nonprofit organization in 1934 for the purpose of studying the maternal mortality rate in the United States and to publish the *Bulletin of Maternal and Child Health.*

1921. The *Sheppard–Towner Bill* was passed by Congress; it was an act for the promotion of the welfare and hygiene of mothers and infants to be administered by the United States Children's Bureau. This bill was introduced in the 65th Congress by Congresswoman Jeanette Rankin of New Jersey. It was reported out of committee favorably but failed to pass.

In the 67th Congress, the bill was again introduced by Senator Sheppard and Congressman Towner and, after much agitation, finally passed—an epoch in child-welfare legislation.

Because of this legislation, there was created at once, in the states that did not already have them, departments that now are quite uniformly labeled Divisions of Bureaus of Maternal and Child Health.

1944. The *Public Health Service Act* brought together all existing laws affecting the public-health service. In addition, the act revised existing laws, provided authority for grants, and authorized expansion of the federal–state cooperative public-health programs that had bearing on maternal and child health programs. This act was to have a great indirect influence on the care of mothers and infants because of its provisions funding research and education of personnel needed in these areas.

1946. The *World Health Organization,* an agency of the United Nations, became a reality. The object of the organization is "the attainment of the highest possible level of health of all the peoples."

1962. The *National Institute of Child Health and Human Development* was authorized. The goal of this Institute was support of research and training in special health problems and needs of mothers and children. This Institute also conducts and supports research in the basic sciences relating to the processes of human growth and development, including prenatal development.

1964. The *Nurse Training Act,* one of the amendments of the Public Health Act, was an indirect aid to maternal and infant care. This act authorized grants for the expansion and improvement of nurse training, assistance to nursing students, scholarship grants to schools of nursing, and the establishment of a National Advisory Council on Nurse Training.

1965. *Amendments to the Social Security Act* provided for a new 5-year program of special project grants for comprehensive health care and services for school and preschool children, particularly in low-income family areas. These amendments also increased the authorization for money to support maternal and child health service programs.

PKU testing became mandatory for all infants in the states of Illinois and Michigan, thus setting a precedent for other states.

1966. The *Department of Health, Education, and Wel-*

fare (DHEW) issued a policy statement on birth control that stated that the Department would support, on request, health programs making family-planning information and services available. Due to this unique statement, federally supported family-planning programs have since slowly begun to evolve.

The *Federal Food, Drug and Cosmetic Act* was instituted on June 14, 1966. This legislation required labeling of ingredients of food represented for special dietary use. Infant foods, particularly, were specified.

The *Child Protection Act of 1966* banned the sale of toys and children's articles containing hazardous substances, regardless of labeling.

1967. *Medicaid* programs were increasing among the states to provide health care for low-income families. Care during pregnancy and child care were included.

1968. *Head Start* programs provided educational opportunities for underprivileged children of preschool age. These programs are often associated with nutritional and health screening programs.

1969. The *National Center for Family Planning* was established under the Health Services and Mental Health Administration, DHEW, to serve as a clearinghouse for information about contraception.

1973. The *United States Supreme Court* struck down almost all state statutes prohibiting or restricting abortion, leaving the abortion decision to the woman and her physician during the first 3 months of pregnancy; after this time the state could regulate abortion procedures only in the interest of maternal health. Essentially, the decision to abort became the right of the individual woman, with the state unable to interfere in her choice except to ensure that the abortion be performed under safe conditions.

National Center on Child Abuse and Neglect was established in DHEW's Office of Child Development to act as a clearinghouse on information about child abuse. A *National commission* was formed to study the role of the federal government in this area and the adequacy of state laws. Funds were made available to regional child-abuse prevention and treatment demonstration programs.

1975. The *National Advisory Council on Maternal Infant and Fetal Nutrition* was established. Annual reports submitted to the President and Congress make continuing recommendations for administrative and legislative changes in programs aimed at low-income individuals at nutritional risk (PL 94–105).

The *WIC* program (Special Supplemental Food Program for Women, Infants, and Children) was intended to provide low-income families with supplemental foods and nutrition education through local agencies, as an adjunct to good health during critical times of growth and development.

1976. The *Early and Periodic Screening, Diagnostic and Treatment* program (EPSDT) provided Medicaid-eligible children with regular health screening and treatment through federal funding.

1977. The *Child Health Assessment Act* (CHAA) extended the early and periodic screening program (EPSDT) to broaden eligibility and to require that treatment be given for conditions discovered during assessment, with exceptions of mental retardation, mental health, developmental problems, and dental care. This legislation also expanded and improved community-health centers.

1979. By this year *all 50 states had enacted laws* requiring every child to be immunized as a condition of entry into school.

1980. The *Children's Bureau* was disbanded after 68 years of significant contributions to the welfare of United States children. This is viewed by many as evidence of weakening of child advocacy in America.

1981. Congress authorized *Medicaid payments for services of nurse–midwives,* making this alternate care available to many women who previously lacked access.

Conditioned Relaxation

Directions: Lie or sit in a comfortable position with pillows for support. Someone may read this to you while you learn to relax or this may be read while recording on an audio cassette. Pause in the reading 3 seconds at each . . . and 6 seconds between paragraphs. Practice 3 to 5 times per week.

Take a few slow, deep breaths . . . Inhale . . . Exhale . . . Inhale . . . Exhale . . .

Focus your attention on your breathing throughout this exercise, and recognize how easily slow, deep breathing alone can help to produce relaxation. Let your body breathe itself, according to its own natural rhythm . . . Slowly and deeply . . .

Now let's begin the exercise with what we call a "cleansing breath," a special message that tells the body we are ready to enter a state of deep relaxation. The cleansing breath is taken as follows . . . Exhale . . . Take a deep breath in through your nose . . . Then blow it out through your mouth.

You may notice a kind of "tingling" sensation when you take the cleansing breath. Whatever you feel is a signal or message to your body that will become associated with relaxation, so that as you practice this exercise over and over again, simply taking the cleansing breath alone will produce the same degree of relaxation that you'll be able to get by completing the entire exercise.

Breathe slowly and deeply . . . As you concentrate your attention on your breathing, focus your eyes on an imaginary spot in the center of your forehead . . . Look at the spot as if you are trying to see it from the inside of your head . . . Raise your eyes way up so as to stare at that spot from the inside of your head. Concentrate your attention on it . . . The more you are able to concentrate on the spot, the better your relaxation response will be . . .

As you continue to focus your attention on the spot, you might notice that your eyelids have become quite tense . . . That's fine, because what we want to do is to teach your body the difference between tension and relaxation. Your eyelids are controlled by some of the smallest muscles in your body, and they become easily tired and fatigued as they become more and more tense. When I count to three, we'll demonstrate the difference between tension and relaxation by allowing your eyelids to close gently, allowing the feelings of tension to melt away quickly.

One . . . Two . . . Three . . . Close your eyelids firmly but not too tightly, and as they close, sense a soothing feeling or relaxation radiate all around your eyes . . . the top of your eyes . . . the bottom . . . the sides . . . the front and back . . .

Breathe slowly and deeply . . . Feel the relaxation in your eyes and how nice it feels . . . Let these feelings of gentle relaxation radiate all around your eyes and out to your forehead . . . to your scalp . . . all around the back of your head . . . to your ears and temples . . . to your cheeks and nose . . . to your mouth and chin . . . and around to your jaw . . . As you feel all the tension flow out of your face and the area around your mouth, relax your jaw muscles . . . As you do so, let your jaw gently open slightly so that all the tension can smoothly flow away . . .

Remember your breathing, slowly and deeply . . . Relax the muscles in your neck . . . As you do so, feel all the tension flow away from the muscles in the back of your neck . . . Let this nice, gentle feeling of relaxation now radiate down into your shoulders . . . Feel the heaviness of your shoulders as the shoulder muscles gently relax . . . This is one of the most important areas of the body to relax because we all tend to store a lot of tension in our necks and shoulders . . . Feel all the tension flow away, and sense the nice, gentle feeling of deep relaxation . . .

Remember your breathing, slowly and deeply . . . Let this feeling of relaxation now radiate down your arms . . . to your elbows . . . forearms . . . wrists . . . and hands . . . Spend a moment to relax each of your fingers . . . your thumb, index finger, middle finger, ring finger, little finger . . . As your hands and arms completely and gently relax, you may notice feelings of warmth and heaviness . . . Some people report pulsations or tingly sensations . . . Some can even sense their heartbeat in their fingertips . . . Others report even magnetic or pulling sensations . . . Whatever you experience is your own body's way of expressing relaxation . . . Remember, you cannot *force* yourself to relax, you can only *allow* yourself to relax . . . Trust your body . . . It knows what to do . . .

Remember your breathing, slowly and deeply . . . Relax your chest . . . and abdomen . . . and let this feeling of relaxation radiate around your sides and ribs, as waves of relaxation cross your shoulder blades to meet at your upper back . . . middle back . . . and lower back . . . Feel all the muscles on either side of your spine softly relax . . . Let this feeling of gentle relaxation now radiate down into your pelvic area . . .

to your buttocks . . . sphincter muscle . . . genitals . . . Feel your whole pelvic area open up and gently relax . . . Relax your thighs . . . knees . . . calves . . . ankles . . . and feet . . . Spend a moment to relax each toe . . . your big toe, second toe, third toe, fourth toe, and little toe . . . Breathe slowly and deeply . . . Relax and enjoy it . . .

Now that your body is gently relaxed and quiet, take a moment, starting from the top of your head working down, to check lightly to see how much relaxation you have obtained . . .

If there is any part of your body that is not yet fully relaxed and comfortable, simply inhale a deep breath and send it into that area, bringing soothing, relaxing, nourishing, healing oxygen into every cell of that area, comforting and relaxing it . . . As you exhale, imagine blowing out, right through your skin, any tension, tightness, pain, or discomfort in that area. Again, as you inhale, bring relaxing, healing oxygen into every cell of that area, and as you exhale, blow away, right through the skin, any tension or discomfort.

In this way you can send your breath to relax any part of your body which is not yet as fully relaxed and comfortable as it can be . . . Breathe slowly and deeply, and with each breath, allow yourself to become twice as relaxed as you were before . . . Inhale . . . Exhale . . . Twice as relaxed . . . Inhale . . . Exhale . . . Twice as relaxed . . .

When you find yourself quiet and fully relaxed, take a moment to enjoy it . . . Sense the gentle warmth and feeling of well-being all through your body . . . If any extraneous thoughts try to interfere, simply allow them to pass through and out of you . . . Ignore them and go back to your breathing, slowly and deeply . . . Slowly and deeply . . . Enjoy this nice state of gentle relaxation . . .

Remember your breathing, slowly and deeply . . . When you end this exercise, you may be surprised to notice that you feel not only relaxed and comfortable, but energized with such a powerful sense of well-being that you will easily be able to meet any demands that arise . . . To end the exercise, tell yourself that you can reach this nice gentle state of Conditioned Relaxation any time you wish by simply taking the cleansing breath . . . Reinforce that cleansing breath by concluding the exercise with it . . . Exhale . . . Inhale deeply through your nose . . . Blow out through the mouth . . . And be well . . .

(Adapted from Bresler DE: Free Yourself from Pain, pp 261–263. New York, Simon & Schuster, 1979.)

Tense–Release Relaxation

Assume a comfortable position, making sure that all your limbs are supported and slightly bent. Start to become aware of your breathing, slowing down and relaxing more on each exhaled breath. Allow your eyes to close . . .

Wrinkle your forehead, lifting your eyebrows as high as you can, and hold for a few seconds. Release and feel the tension flowing from your forehead and scalp . . . Now close your eyes tightly and wrinkle your nose. Hold it for a few seconds, and let go. Feel the tension flowing out of your face . . . Purse your lips and clench your teeth together. Hold for a few seconds. Now release the tension, and feel your jaw drop and your tongue rest loosely in your mouth . . . Push your head down toward your chest and hold for a few seconds. Relax . . .

Now shrug your shoulders up toward your ears, and hold for a few seconds. As you release, feel the tension leaving your neck and upper back . . .

Clench your fists tightly, and feel the tension in your hands. Hold. Now release the tension, and allow your hands to relax . . . Now tense your arms all the way to the shoulders. Hold for a few seconds and relax . . . Hold. Now release the tension and allow your hands to relax . . . Now tense your arms all the way to the shoulders. Hold for a few seconds and relax . . .

Arch your back for a few seconds. Now release . . . Tighten your abdominal muscles and hold for a few seconds. Let go . . . Now tense your buttocks, Hold, and release . . . Tighten your feet, pulling your toes up toward your knees. Hold for a moment. Relax your feet . . . Tense your legs all the way up from your feet to your hips. Hold for a few seconds. Now relax, and feel the tension flowing out of your feet . . .

Breathe slowly, releasing any residual tension on each exhaled breath. Bring your attention to any part of your body that feels tight or uncomfortable, and release it, tensing first if necessary . . . Take time to enjoy this relaxed state, noting the relaxation in your muscles now that you have let go of all tension. Your muscles feel limp and heavy, warm and comfortable . . . Enjoy this good feeling for a few minutes. When you are ready to get up, stretch your arms and legs, take a deep breath, and open your eyes. Always get up slowly so you don't become "dizzy."

From Lieberman A: Easing Labor Pain. Garden City, NY, Doubleday and Co, 1987.)

Imagery Exercises

- Imagine that you are lying on a billowy cloud, moving gently through space. Feel the texture of the cloud as it buoys you up and its slow rocking motion. If colors come into your mind, let yourself be surrounded by them. Be held aloft and carried, or simply rest weightless, as you choose. Let yourself be lulled, as if you were in a hammock. Continue to breathe deeply, as your breath becomes one with the breath of the cloud.

- Imagine that you are floating on your back in water, staring up at the immense, harmonious blue of a cloudless sky. You may be in a lake, or on the ocean, or lying on a lily pad in a pond. You choose the place. Imagine how it feels to be held and gently moved by the natural flow of water. Let your breath be one with the motion of the water, and fill your eyes with the blue of the sky. See nothing else. If sounds come to you, let them flood your ears. Continue to breathe deeply as you float suspended.

- Imagine that you are lying in the cool, high grasses of a fresh green meadow, with a lilting spring breeze rushing over you. In your own hollowed-out hiding place the grass bends down and brushes you, caressing you with long blades that are almost like cool water. Feel the motion of the meadow as it ripples with the wind, a rhythm that is one with the long, peaceful motion of your own relaxed breath. Let yourself be calmed by the sparkling sound of the nearby brook, running full with the first rains of spring.

(Bogin M: The Path to Pain Control, pp 214–215. Boston, Houghton-Mifflin, 1982.)

Neuromuscular Control— "Partner Feedback Relaxation"

Directions: Choose a comfortable position with pillows for support. The emphasis is always on the relaxation, not on the tensing or how quickly the woman can respond. Relax to touch as well as to verbal instructions so these can be conditioned for labor. Breathe comfortably throughout the exercise. The woman learns what relaxation really feels like by partner feedback. She practices how to relax muscles while others are tense like it will be in labor. Practice together for 5 minutes daily.

Verbal Cue by Partner	Action by Woman	Partner's Role
1. Contract your right leg	Tense right thigh and calf; flex ankle	Look over rest of body for obvious signs of tension; lift left leg gently under knee to check relaxation; check both arms; turn head gently side to side to check relaxation of neck
	Focus gaze on one spot to enhance concentration	
	Think about the feeling of tension in the right leg and of relaxation in the rest of the body	Where tension is detected, stroke and give cue, "Relax" or "Release"
Relax your right leg	Relax completely	Stroke right leg; lift gently under right knee to detect tension
2. Contract your left leg	As above	As above
Relax your left leg	As above	As above
3. Contract your left arm	Make a fist; tense entire arm and lift slightly off the floor	Check rest of body for signs of tension; lift right arm gently by hand, swing freely from shoulder; lift knees slightly; observe face; turn head gently side to side to detect neck tension; stroke to signal its release
	Focus gaze on one spot to enhance concentration	
	Think about the feeling of tension in the left arm and of relaxation in the rest of the body	
Relax your left arm	Relax completely	Stroke left arm and shoulder
		Lift left arm gently by hand; swing from shoulder
4. Contract your right arm	As above	As above
Relax your right arm	As above	As above
5. Contract your left arm and right leg	As above	As above
Relax only your left arm	Relax arm	As above
	Keep leg tense	
Relax your right leg	Relax completely	As above

(The previous chart is a combination of two sources—Birth Guide. West Los Angeles ASPO Certified Childbirth Educators, 1990; and Hassid P: Textbook for Childbirth Educators, 3rd ed. Philadelphia, JB Lippincott, 1987.)

Continue on with contracting: left arm and left leg, right arm and left leg, buttocks, neck—make up your own!

Prenatal Exercises

Do each exercise twice at first, progressing at your own pace to five times. The sequence can be repeated in reverse order. Relax and breathe deeply between each exercise.

1. ABDOMINAL-TIGHTENING ON OUTWARD BREATH

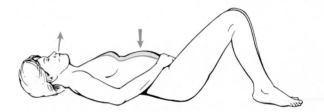

Position: Lying on back or side, knees bent. Place hands on abdominal area below ribs (for the learning process; they can be removed later).

Action: Take a deep complete breath in through the nose, feeling the nostrils widen slightly. Breathing through the nose warms and filters the air. Keep the ribs as still as you can, and let the abdominal wall expand upward. Then, lips slightly parted, blow the air out through the mouth slowly but forcibly, pulling in your abdominal muscles all the while until you feel you have completely emptied your lungs. It's like sustaining a note while blowing a trumpet or singing.

Progression: Other positions, such as sitting or standing. Avoid taking too many deep breaths in succession—you may get dizzy. Deep breathing is very important in pregnancy and the early postpartum phase, but at other times this exercise can be done as simple abdominal muscle contractions on normal outward breath in standing, sitting, or other positions. A rocking chair is ideal!

2. PELVIC FLOOR EXERCISE

Position: Lying down on back, side, or front. (On the front is the most comfortable position postpartum if you have had stitches.) Legs apart and chest relaxed for normal breathing.

Action: Draw up the pelvic floor, feel the additional squeeze from the sides as the sphincters are tightened and the inside passages become tense. Concentrate particularly on the front portion of the pelvic floor—the master sphincter surrounding the vagina and urethra. Place one hand over the pubic bones and think about tightening the birth canal as high as the level of your hand.

Hold for 2 to 3 seconds and then completely relax. Note the sensation as the pelvic floor lets down loosely. Try to slacken it a little more, releasing any residual tension. (This is what you must be able to do during delivery.) Release your jaw, too.

Do only two or three in succession before resting
for a couple of minutes, and always end with a
contraction to return the muscle floor to its supportive resting state. You can provide effective exercise of the muscle by doing this frequently, 50
times or more a day, in a series of five, holding
each contraction for 5 seconds.

3. FOOT-BENDING AND FOOT-STRETCHING

The movement of frequent foot-bending and -stretching
and ankle-rotating provides a venous pump to assist
the return of blood from the lower legs, and will minimize varicosities and swelling of the ankles. Cramps,
which often occur from lack of exercise, may be relieved.

Position: Sitting or lying. In either position, legs can
be relaxed over a pillow or the feet can be elevated. At other times, rest foot on the opposite
knee. (This makes it easier to see your feet late in
pregnancy!) It's also a good way to put on socks
or pantyhose. Sitting with the legs out straight
provides additional stretch of the calf muscles.

Action: Bend the ankle as far as you can, pulling your
toes up toward you, thus stretching the calf muscles; then point the foot downward, making an
arch. Do this several times and take a short rest
before repeating. If pointing the foot results in
cramps, just stretch up . . . relax . . . stretch up.

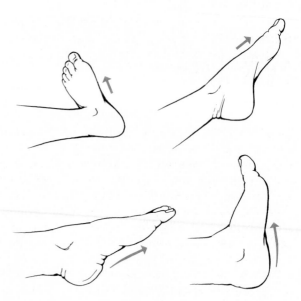

4. ANKLE-ROTATING

Position: As for above Exercise and any time you're
off your feet.

Action: Make large slow circles with each foot, first in
a clockwise, then in a counterclockwise direction.

5. PELVIC-TILTING

Position: Lying on the back with the knees bent is
the easiest starting position for learning the basic
front-to-back action, which is important in the
childbearing year. In late pregnancy, however,
the weight of the uterus compresses the major
blood vessels in this position, so if you experience
discomfort or feel faint, practice this in one of the
other recommended positions.

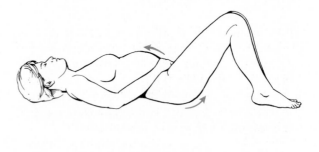

Action: Roll the pelvis back by flattening the lower
back down on the floor. Then make an extra effort. Contract the abdominal muscles on outward
breath and tighten the buttock muscles, too. Additional strong contraction of the muscles is necessary to make this an active strengthening exercise, not just a semipassive movement. To
encourage more action in the lower abdominal
muscles, place a hand just above the pubic bones

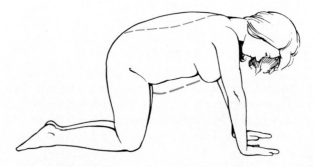

so you can feel the muscles working. Hold the position for 3 seconds and then relax. Keep breathing! Make sure that you do not raise your buttocks at all or shift your shoulders. Do not rock the pelvis upward as this will force the curve in the lower back. *Always emphasize the flattening of the hollow* and add as much additional abdominal wall retraction as you can. Postpartum, think about "making yourself thin" from front to back.

Progression: When you feel that you understand the correct movement, try it standing, side-lying, sitting or on all-fours.

6. STRAIGHT CURL-UP

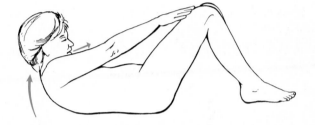

If you are well into the last trimester and have not been exercising the abdominal muscles, save the curl-ups for your postpartum program. If you cannot readily perform a movement, then you must not exert undue strain. In any case, during the last few weeks of pregnancy the size of the baby gets in the way. The other exercises will maintain existing strength at this time and can be done with ease and comfort.

Prenatal: This exercise is for early starters. If you are well into the last trimester and cannot readily perform these movements, then do not try. If the recti muscles have parted, from this pregnancy or a previous one, postpone this exercise and concentrate on supporting the muscles and raising just the head at first (see Chapter 17).

Postpartum: Always check the midline of your abdominal wall before doing this exercise. If the recti muscles have separated more than three fingers' width, support them as described in chapter 17; this is actually a progression of the same exercise.

Position: Lying on the back with knees bent, pelvis tilted back.

Action: Bring your chin onto your chest. As you breathe out, fold forward without any jerking or hinging movement. Come up just as far as the back naturally bends with the waist still down on the surface. This is about 8 inches or an angle of 45°.

Slowly return to the starting position; don't drop back. The arms are held outstretched in front at first, to aid the trunk.

Postpartum Exercises

Commence within 24 hours; repeat each exercise twice to start, progressing at your own pace through the phases. Relax and breathe deeply between each exercise.

The sequence can be repeated in reverse order. Do the exercises at least twice daily.

Phase I

1. Abdominal-Tightening on Outward Breath (See prenatal exercises)
2. Pelvic Floor Exercise (See prenatal exercises)
3. Foot-Bending and Foot-Stretching (See prenatal exercises)
4. Ankle-Rotating (See prenatal exercises)
5. Pelvic-Tilting (See prenatal exercises)

Add Phase II

7. LEG-SLIDING

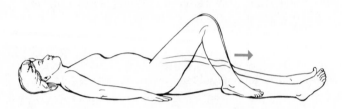

Position: Lying on back, knees bent, pelvis tilted backward, and lumbar spine flattened. Keep breathing normally throughout.

Action: Hold the position of corrected pelvic tilt as, sliding the heels, you slowly stretch the legs out straight. If the abdominals are unable to keep the back flat, draw the knees back up again, one at a time, to the point where the spine began to arch. Work in this range until your abdominals maintain a flattened back with the legs outstretched.

Add Phase III

8. STRAIGHT CURL-UP
(SEE PRENATAL EXERCISES)

9. DIAGONAL CURL-UP

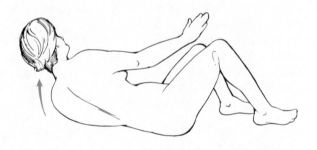

If there is a separation of the recti muscles (see pages 346 and 347), postpone this exercise until the condition has been corrected.

Prenatal: This exercise is also for early starters, although it is a little easier than the straight curl-up since you move obliquely and have more help from other muscles in the corset. If you are in the last trimester and cannot perform this movement with ease and comfort, then do not try.

Position: Lying on the back with knees bent.

Action: Bring your chin onto your chest. As you breathe out, fold forward reaching with your outstretched arms to the outside of the left knee. Slowly return back to the starting position. Repeat the movement to the right knee.

(All exercises and illustrations are from Noble E: Essential Exercises for the Childbearing Year. Boston, Houghton-Mifflin, 1988.)

D	*Universal Precautions for Prevention of Transmission of HIV, Hepatitis B Virus, and Other Bloodborne Pathogens in Health-Care Settings*

Body Fluids to Which Universal Precautions Apply

Universal precautions apply to blood and to other body fluids containing visible blood. Occupational transmission of HIV and HBV to health-care workers by blood is documented. Blood is the single most important source of HIV, HBV, and other bloodborne pathogens in the occupational setting. Infection control efforts for HIV, HBV, and other bloodborne pathogens must focus on preventing exposures to blood as well as on delivering HBV immunization.

Universal precautions also apply to semen and vaginal secretions. Although both of these fluids have been implicated in the sexual transmission of HIV and HBV, they have not been implicated in occupational transmission from patient to health-care worker. This observation is not unexpected, because exposure to semen in the usual health-care setting is limited, and the routine practice of wearing gloves for performing vaginal examinations protects health-care workers from exposure to potentially infectious vaginal secretions.

Universal precautions also apply to tissues and to the following fluids: cerebrospinal fluid (CSF), synovial fluid, pleural fluid, peritoneal fluid, pericardial fluid, and amniotic fluid. The risk of transmission of HIV and HBV from these fluids is unknown; epidemiologic studies in the health-care and community settings are currently inadequate to assess the potential risk to health-care workers from occupational exposures to them. However, HIV has been isolated from CSF, synovial, and amniotic fluid, and HBsAg has been detected in synovial fluid, amniotic fluid, and peritoneal fluid.

Body Fluids to Which Universal Precautions Do Not Apply

Universal precautions do not apply to feces, nasal secretions, sputum, sweat, tears, urine, and vomitus unless they contain visible blood. The risk of transmission of HIV and HBV from these fluids and materials is extremely low or nonexistent. HIV has been isolated and HBsAg has been demonstrated in some of these fluids; however, epidemiologic studies in the health-care and community settings have not implicated these fluids or materials in the transmission of HIV and HBV infections. Some of the above fluids and excretions represent a potential source for nosocomial and community-acquired infections with other pathogens and recommendations for preventing the transmission of non-bloodborne pathogens have been published.

Precautions for Other Body Fluids in Special Settings

Human breast milk has been implicated in perinatal transmission of HIV, and HBsAg has been found in the milk of mothers infected with HBV. However, occupational exposure to human breast milk has not been implicated in the transmission of HIV nor HBV infection to health-care workers. Moreover, the health-care worker will not have the same type of intensive exposure to breast milk as the nursing neonate. Whereas universal precautions do not apply to human breast milk, gloves may be worn by health-care workers in situations where exposures to breast milk might be frequent, for example, in breast milk banking.

Saliva of some persons infected with HBV has been shown to contain HBV-DNA at concentrations 1:1,000 to 1:10,000 of that found in the infected person's serum. HBsAg-positive saliva has been shown to be infectious when injected into experimental animals and in human bite exposures. However, HBsAg-positive saliva has not been shown to be infectious when applied to oral mucous membranes in experimental primate studies or through contamination of musical instruments or cardiopulmonary resuscitation dummies used by HBV carriers. Epidemiologic studies of nonsexual household contacts of HIV-infected patients, including several small series in which HIV transmission failed to occur after bites or after percutaneous inoculation or contamination of cuts and open wounds with saliva from HIV-infected patients, suggest that the potential for salivary transmission of HIV is remote. One case report from Germany has suggested the possibility of transmission of HIV in a household setting from an infected child to a sibling through a human bite. The bite did not break the skin or result in bleeding. Because the date of seroconversion to HIV was not known for either child in this case, evidence for the role of saliva in the transmission of virus is unclear. Another case report suggested the possibility of transmission of HIV from husband to wife by contact with saliva during kissing. However, follow-up studies did not confirm HIV infection in the wife.

Universal precautions do not apply to saliva. General infection control practices already in existence—including the use of gloves for digital examination of mucous membranes and endotracheal suctioning and handwashing after exposure to saliva—should further minimize the minute risk, if any, for salivary transmission of HIV and HBV. Gloves need not be worn when feeding patients and when wiping saliva from skin.

Special precautions, however, are recommended for dentistry. Occupationally acquired infection with HBV in dental workers has been documented, and two possible cases of occupationally acquired HIV infection involving dentists have been reported. During dental procedures, contamination of saliva with blood is predictable, trauma to health-care workers' hands is common, and blood splattering may occur. Infection control precautions for dentistry minimize the potential for nonintact skin and mucous membrane contact of dental health-care workers to blood-contaminated saliva of patients. In addition, the use of gloves for oral examinations and treatment in the dental setting also may protect the patient's oral mucous membranes from exposures to blood, which may occur from breaks in the skin of dental workers' hands.

Use of Protective Barriers

Protective barriers reduce the risk of exposure of the health-care worker's skin or mucous membranes to potentially infective materials. For universal precautions, protective barriers reduce the risk of exposure to blood, body fluids containing visible blood, and other fluids to which universal precautions apply. Examples of protective barriers include gloves, gowns, masks, and protective eyewear. Gloves should reduce the incidence of contamination of hands, but they cannot prevent penetrating injuries due to needles or other sharp instruments. Masks and protective eyewear or face shields should reduce the incidence of contamination of mucous membranes of the mouth, nose, and eyes.

Universal precautions are intended to supplement rather than replace recommendations for routine infection control, such as handwashing and using gloves to prevent gross microbial contamination of hands. Because specifying the types of barriers needed for every possible clinical situation is impractical, some judgment must be exercised.

The risk of nosocomial transmission of HIV, HBV, and other bloodborne pathogens can be minimized if health-care workers use the following general guidelines.*

1. Take care to prevent injuries when using needles, scalpels, and other sharp instruments or devices; when handling sharp instruments after procedures; when cleaning used instruments; and when disposing of used needles. Do not recap used needles by hand; do not remove used needles from disposable syringes by hand; and do not bend, break, or otherwise manipulate used needles by hand. Place used disposable syringes and needles, scalpel blades, and other sharp items in puncture resistant containers for disposal. Locate the puncture-resistant containers as close to the use area as is practical.
2. Use protective barriers to prevent exposure to blood, body fluids containing visible blood, and other fluids to which universal precautions apply. The type of protective barrier(s) should be appropriate for the procedure being performed and the type of exposure anticipated.
3. Immediately and thoroughly wash hands and other skin surfaces that are contaminated with blood, body fluids containing visible blood, or other body fluids to which universal precautions apply.

From *Centers for Disease Control*: Morbidity and Mortality Weekly Report 37(24):377–388, June 24, 1988.

* The August 1987 publication should be consulted for general information and specific recommendations not addressed in this update.

E   *Drug Use During Breast-Feeding**

Drug or Agent	Contra-indicated	R$_x$ With Caution	No Apparent Harm	Insufficient Information	Comment
Analgesics					
Acetaminophen			X		
Aspirin			X		
Propoxyphene (Darvon)			X		
Anticoagulants					
Ethyl biscoumacetate	X				Bleeding infant
Phenindione	X				Bleeding infant
Heparin			X		No passage into milk
Warfarin Na (Coumadin)			X		
Bishydroxycoumarin (Dicumarol)		X			
Anticonvulsants					
Phenobarbital			X		Low levels in infant
Primadone (Mysoline)			X		? Drowsiness
Carbamazepine				X	Significant infant levels; no reported effects
Diphenylhydantoin (Phenytoin, Dilantin)			X		Low levels in infant, methemoglobin, one case
Antihistamines					
Diphenhydramine (Benadryl)			X		Small amounts excreted
Trimeprazine (Temaril)			X		Small amounts excreted
Tripelennamine (Pyribenzamine)			X		Small amounts excreted
Anti-infective Agents					
Aminoglycosides (Kanamycin, gentamicin)			X		Significant excretion in milk; not absorbed
Chloramphenicol	X				Bone marrow depression; gastrointestinal and behavioral effects
Penicillins			X		Possible sensitization
Sulfonamides		X			Hemolysis, G-6-PD deficiency, bilirubin displacement
Tetracyclines			X		Limited absorption by infant
Nalidixic acid		X			Hemolysis
Nitrofurantoin		X			Possible G-6-PD hemolysis
Metronidazole (Flagyl)		X			Low absorption but potentially toxic
Isoniazid		X			High levels in milk, possible toxicity
Pyramethamine	X				Vomiting, marrow suppression, convulsions
Chloraquine			X		Not excreted
Quinine		X			Thrombocytopenia
Anti-inflammatory					
Aspirin			X		
Indomethacin		X			Seizures, one case

(continued)

E					*Drug Use During Breast-Feeding** (continued)

Drug or Agent	Contra-indicated	R$_x$ With Caution	No Apparent Harm	Insufficient Information	Comment
Phenylbutazone		X			Low levels, ? blood dyscrasia
Gold	X				Found in baby; nephritis, hepatitis, hematologic changes
Steroids				X	Low levels with prednisone and prednisolone
Antineoplastic					
Cyclophosphamide	X				Neutropenia
Methotrexate	X				Very small excretion
Antithyroid					
Radioactive iodine	X				Thyroid suppression
Propylthiouracil	X				Thyroid suppression
Bronchodilators					
Aminophylline			X		Irritability, one case
Iodides	X				Thyroid suppression
Sympathomimetics				X	Inhalers probably safe
Cardiovascular Agents					
Digoxin			X		Insignificant levels
Propanolol			X		Insignificant levels
Reserpine	X				Nasal stuffiness, lethargy
Guanethidine (Ismelin)			X		Insignificant levels
Methyldopa (Aldomet)				X	
Cathartics					
Anthroquinones (Cascara, danthron)	X				Diarrhea, cramps
Aloe, senna		X			Safe in moderate dosage
Bulk agents, softeners			X		
Contraceptives, Oral†					
Diethylstilbestrol	X				Possible vaginal cancer
Depo-provera		X			May affect lactation
Norethisterone		X			May affect lactation
Ethinyl estradiol		X			May affect lactation
Diuretics					
Chlorthalidone				X	Low levels, but may accumulate
Thiazides		X			May affect lactation; low levels in milk
Spironolactone			X		Insignificant levels
Ergot Alkaloids					
Bromocriptine	X				Lactation suppressed
Ergot	X				Vomiting, diarrhea, seizures
Ergotamine				X	

(continued)

E	**Drug Use During Breast-Feeding*** (continued)

Drug or Agent	Contra-indicated	R$_x$ With Caution	No Apparent Harm	Insufficient Information	Comment
Ergonovine	X				Brief postpartum course may be safe
Methylergonovine	X				Brief postpartum course may be safe
Hormones					
Corticosteroids				X	Low levels with short-term prednisone or prednisolone
Sex hormones (see above, Contraceptives, Oral)					
Thyroid (T$_3$ or T$_4$)			X		Excreted in milk; may mask hypothyroid infant
Insulin			X		Not absorbed
ACTH			X		Not absorbed
Epinephrine			X		Not absorbed
Narcotics					
Codeine			X		
Meperidine (Demerol)				X	In usual doses
Morphine			X		Low infant levels on usual dosage
Heroin	X				Addiction withdrawal in infants
Methadone		X			Minimal levels
Psychotherapeutic Drugs					
Lithium	X				High levels in milk
Phenothiazines		X			Drowsiness; chronic effects uncertain
Tricyclic antidepressants				X	Low levels; effects uncertain
Diazepam (Valium)	X				Lethargy, weight loss, EEG changes
Meprobamate (Equanil)	X				High levels in milk
Chlordiazepoxide (Librium)			X		Low levels in milk
Radiopharmaceuticals					
^{131}I	X				72 hr, no breast-feeding
Technetium (99M Tc)	X				48 hr, no breast-feeding
^{131}I albumin	X				10 days, no breast-feeding
Sedatives-Hypnotics					
Barbiturates		X			Short-acting, less depressant
Chloral hydrate		X			Drowsiness
Bromides	X				Depression, rash
Diazepam (Valium)	X				Depression, weight loss
Flurazepam				X	Chemically related to diazepam
Nitrazepam				X	
Social-Recreational Drugs					
Alcohol			X		Milk levels equal plasma, moderate consumption apparently safe, high levels inhibit lactation

(continued)

| E | *Drug Use During Breast-Feeding** (continued) | | | | |

Drug or Agent	Contra-indicated	R$_x$ With Caution	No Apparent Harm	Insufficient Information	Comment
Caffeine			X		Jitteriness with very high intakes
Nicotine			X		Low levels in milk
Marijuana			X		Minimal passage in milk
Miscellaneous					
Atropine		X			May cause constipation or inhibit lactation
Dihydrotachysterol		X			Renal calcification in animals

* Drug use during breast-feeding remains controversial.
† Controversy in literature; long-term effects uncertain; one case of gynecomastia.
(Avery GB [ed]: Neonatology, 3rd ed. Philadelphia, JB Lippincott, 1987.)

F	*Conversion Table for Weights of Newborn*

(Gram equivalents for pounds and ounces)

For example, to find weight in pounds and ounces of baby weighing 3315 grams, glance down columns to figure nearest 3315 = 3317. Refer to number at top for pounds and number to far left for ounces = 7 pounds, 5 ounces.

Pounds→ Ounces↓	3	4	5	6	7	8	9	10
0	1361	1814	2268	2722	3175	3629	4082	4536
1	1389	1843	2296	2750	3203	3657	4111	4564
2	1417	1871	2325	2778	3232	3685	4139	4593
3	1446	1899	2353	2807	3260	3714	4167	4621
4	1474	1928	2381	2835	3289	3742	4196	4649
5	1503	1956	2410	2863	3317	3770	4224	4678
6	1531	1984	2438	2892	3345	3799	4252	4706
7	1559	2013	2466	2920	3374	3827	4281	4734
8	1588	2041	2495	2948	3402	3856	4309	4763
9	1616	2070	2523	2977	3430	3884	4338	4791
10	1644	2098	2551	3005	3459	3912	4366	4819
11	1673	2126	2580	3033	3487	3941	4394	4848
12	1701	2155	2608	3062	3515	3969	4423	4876
13	1729	2183	2637	3090	3544	3997	4451	4904
14	1758	2211	2665	3118	3572	4026	4479	4933
15	1786	2240	2693	3147	3600	4054	4508	4961

Or, to convert grams into pounds and *decimals* of a pound, multiply weight in grams by .0022. Thus, $3317 \times .0022$ = 7.2974 (*i.e*, 7.3 pounds, or 7 pounds, 5 ounces).

To convert pounds and ounces into grams, multiply the pounds by 453.6 and the ounces by 28.4 and add the two products. Thus, to convert 7 pounds, 5 ounces, $7 \times 453.6 = 3175$; $5 \times 28.4 = 142$; $3175 + 142 = 3317$ grams.

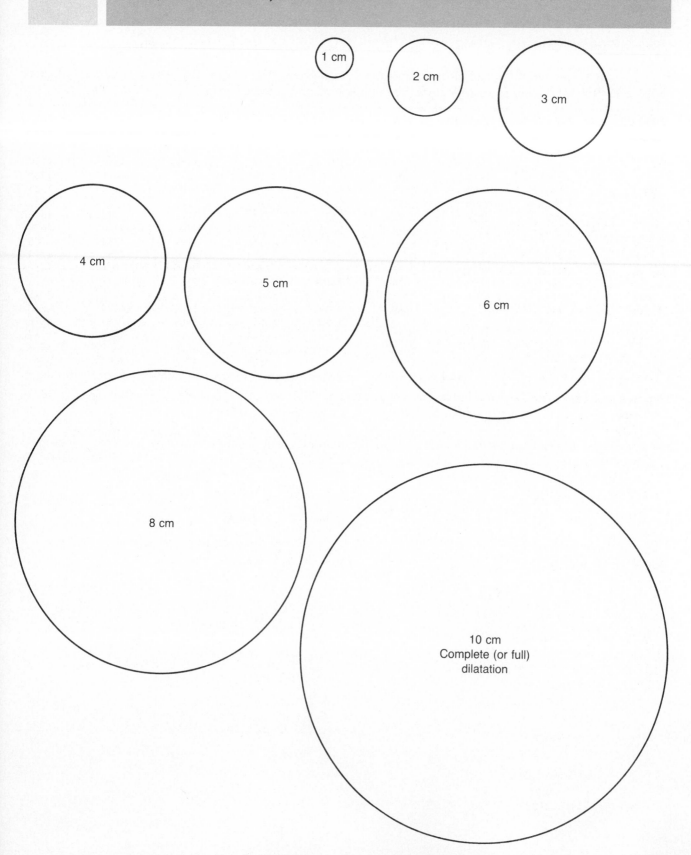

G   *Aid for Visualization of Cervical Dilatation*

H *Resources for Maternal-Care Nurses*

Abortion

PRO CHOICE

National Abortion Rights Action League
1424 K St, NW
Washington, DC 20005

PRO LIFE

National Right to Life Committee
419 7th St, NW
Washington, DC 20045

Alternative Lifestyles

National Gay Task Force
80 Fifth Ave, Suite 1601
New York, NY 10011

Parents and Friends of Gays and Lesbians
PO Box 24565
Los Angeles, CA 90025

or

5715 16th St, NW
Washington, DC 20011

JOURNALS

Alternative Lifestyles
Human Sciences Press
72 Fifth Ave
New York, NY 10011

Journal of Homosexuality
Haworth Press
28 East 22nd St
New York, NY 10010

Breast-Feeding

LaLeche International, Inc.
9616 Minneapolis Ave
Franklin Park, IL 60123

Childbirth Alternatives

American Academy of Husband-Coached Childbirth
PO Box 5224
Sherman Oaks, CA 91413

American College of Home Obstetrics
PO Box 25
River Forest, IL 60305

American Society of Childbirth Educators
PO Box 16159
7113 Lynwood Dr
Tampa, FL 33687

American Society for Psychoprophylaxis in Obstetrics
West 96th St
New York, NY 10025

Caesarean/Support, Education, and Concern
23 Cedar St
Cambridge, MA 02140

Childbirth Education Foundation
PO Box 37
Apalachin, NY 13732

Childbirth Without Pain Education Association
20134 Snowden
Detroit, MI 48235

Informed Homebirth
PO Box 788
Boulder, CO 80306

Maternity Center Association, Inc.
48 East 92nd St
New York, NY 10028

Family Planning

Association for Voluntary Sterilization
122 E 42nd St
New York, NY 10168

Planned Parenthood
1220 19th St, NW
Washington, DC 20036

Zero Population Growth
1346 Connecticut Ave, NW
Washington, DC 20036

Fertility and Infertility

American Fertility Foundation
1608 13th Ave, S, Suite 101
Birmingham, AL 35205

Association for Voluntary Sterilization, Inc
708 Third Ave
New York, NY 10164

Fertility Research Foundation
1430 Second Ave, Suite 103
New York, NY 10021

Surrogate Parenting Associates, Inc
Suite 222, Doctor's Office Building
250 E Liberty St
Louisville, KY 40205

Test-tube Fertilization
Eastern Virginia Medical School
Norfolk General Hospital
The Howard and Georgeanna Jones Institute for
    Reproductive Medicine
304 Medical Tower
Norfolk, VA 23507

Genetic Counseling

National Genetics Foundation
555 W 57th St
New York, NY 10019

Parenting and Abuse

American Association for Marriage and Family Therapy
1717 K St, NW, Suite 407
Washington, DC 20006

Association of Planned Parenthood Professionals
810 Seventh Ave
New York, NY 10019

Department of Health, Education and Welfare
National Center on Child Abuse and Neglect
US Children's Bureau
Office of Child Development
PO Box 1182
Washington, DC 20013

Grief Institute
PO Box 623
Englewood, CO 80151

National Center for the Prevention and Treatment of
    Child Abuse and Neglect
Department of Pediatrics
University of Colorado Medical Center
1205 Oneida St
Denver, CO 80220
    (National Child Protection Newsletter)

National Committee for Prevention of Child Abuse
Suite 510
111 East Wacker Dr
Chicago, IL 60601

National Foundation for Sudden Infant Death, Inc
1501 Broadway
New York, NY 10036

Parenting Materials Information Center
Southwest Educational Development Laboratory
211 E 7th St
Austin, TX 78701

Parents Anonymous
2810 Artesia Blvd
Redondo Beach, CA 90278

Parents of Premature and High Risk Infants International
33 W 42nd St, Suite 1227
New York, NY 10036

Parents Without Partners
7910 Woodmont Ave
Washington, DC 20014

Single Mothers by Choice
501 12th St
Brooklyn, NY 11215

JOURNALS

Family Relations
National Council on Family Relations
1219 University Ave, SE
Minneapolis, MN 55414

Journal of Marriage and the Family
National Council on Family Relations
1219 University Ave, SE
Minneapolis, MN 55414

Professional Organizations

American Association for Maternal and Child Health
233 Prospect, P-209
La Jolla, CA 92037

American College of Nurse-Midwives
1522 K St, NW, Suite 1120
Washington, DC 20005

American College of Obstetricians and Gynecologists
600 Maryland Ave, SW, Suite 300
Washington, DC 20024

American Foundation for Maternal and Child Health
30 Beekman Pl
New York, NY 10022

Maternity Center Association
48 E 92nd St
New York, NY 10028

Public Health Organizations

American Public Health Association
1015 15th St, NW
Washington, DC 20005

American Red Cross
18th and E Sts, NW
Washington, DC 20006

Centers for Disease Control
Atlanta, GA 30333

Medic Alert Foundation
PO Box 1009
Turlock, CA 95380

National Institutes of Health
Bethesda, MD 20014

Project HOPE Health Sciences Education Center
Millwood, VA 22646

Rape

National Center for Prevention and Control of Rape
5600 Fishers Land
Rockville, MD 20857

Sex Education

Council for Sex Information and Education
Box 23088
Washington, DC 20024

Sex Information and Education Council of the United
States
80 Fifth Ave, Suite 801
New York, NY 10011

Sexual Therapy

American Association of Sex Educators, Counselors, and
Therapists
11 Dupont Circle, Suite 220
Washington, DC 20036

Center for Marital and Sexual Studies
5199 East Pacific Coast Hwy
Long Beach, CA 90804

Masters and Johnson Institute
24 South Kings Highway
St Louis, MO 63108

Loyola Sexual Dysfunction Clinic
Loyola University Hospital
2160 S 1st Ave
Maywood, IL 60153

Society for Sex Therapy
% Barry McCarthy, PhD
Department of Psychology
The American University
Washington, DC 20016

Sexuality

Sex and Disability Unit
Human Sexuality Program
University of California
814 Mission St, 2nd Floor
San Francisco, CA 94103

JOURNAL

Sexuality and Disability
Human Sciences Press
72 Fifth Ave
New York, NY 10011

Sexually Transmitted Diseases

American Social Health Association
260 Sheridan Rd
Palo Alto, CA 94306

Centers for Disease Control
Technical Information Services
Bureau of State Services
Atlanta, GA 30333

Herpes Resource Information
Box 100
Palo Alto, CA 94302

National AIDS Hotline
1-800-342-2437

National VD Hotline
1-800-227-8922
(in California, 1-800-982-5883)

Substance Abuse

Alcoholics Anonymous
PO Box 459, Grand Central Station
New York, NY 10017

National Clearinghouse for Alcohol Information
Box 2345
Rockville, MD

National Clearinghouse for Drug Abuse Information
5454 Wisconsin Ave
Chevy Chase, MD 20015

I

NANDA List of Approved Nursing Diagnoses
(in Alphabetical Order)

Activity Intolerance
Activity Intolerance, High Risk for
Adjustment, Impaired
Airway Clearance, Ineffective
Anxiety
Aspiration, High Risk for
Body Image Disturbance
Body Temperature, High Risk for Altered
Breastfeeding, Effective
Breastfeeding, Ineffective
Breathing Pattern, Ineffective
Communication, Impaired Verbal
Constipation
Constipation, Colonic
Constipation, Perceived
Decisional Conflict (Specify)
Decreased Cardiac Output
Defensive Coping
Denial, Ineffective
Diarrhea
Disuse Syndrome, High Risk for
Diversional Activity Deficit
Dysreflexia
Family Coping, Compromised, Ineffective
Family Coping, Disabling, Ineffective
Family Coping: Potential for Growth
Family Processes, Altered
Fatigue
Fear
Fluid Volume Deficit
Fluid Volume Deficit, High Risk for
Fluid Volume Excess
Gas Exchange, Impaired
Grieving, Anticipatory
Grieving, Dysfunctional
Growth and Development, Altered
Health Maintenance, Altered
Health Seeking Behaviors (Specify)
Home Maintenance Management, Impaired
Hopelessness
Hyperthermia
Hypothermia
Incontinence, Bowel
Incontinence, Functional
Incontinence, Reflex
Incontinence, Stress
Incontinence, Total
Incontinence, Urge
Individual Coping, Ineffective
Infection, High Risk for
Injury, High Risk for
Knowledge Deficit (Specify)

Noncompliance (Specify)
Nutrition: Less than Body Requirements, Altered
Nutrition: More than Body Requirements, Altered
Nutrition: Potential for more than Body Requirements, Altered
Oral Mucous Membrane, Altered
Pain
Pain, Chronic
Parental Role Conflict
Parenting, Altered
Parenting, High Risk for Altered
Personal Identity Disturbance
Physical Mobility, Impaired
Poisoning, High Risk for
Post-Trauma Response
Powerlessness
Protection, Altered
Rape-Trauma Syndrome
Rape-Trauma Syndrome: Compound Reaction
Rape-Trauma Syndrome: Silent Reaction
Role Performance, Altered
Self-Care Deficit, Bathing/Hygiene
Self-Care Deficit, Feeding
Self-Care Deficit, Dressing/Grooming
Self-Care Deficit, Toileting
Self-Esteem, Chronic Low
Self-Esteem, Situational Low
Self-Esteem Disturbance
Sensory/Perceptual Alterations (Specify) (Visual, auditory, kinesthetic, gustatory, tactile, olfactory)
Sexual Dysfunction
Sexuality Patterns, Altered
Skin Integrity, Impaired
Skin Integrity, High Risk for Impaired
Sleep Pattern Disturbance
Social Interaction, Impaired
Social Isolation
Spiritual Distress (Distress of the Human Spirit)
Suffocation, High Risk for
Swallowing, Impaired
Thermoregulation, Ineffective
Thought Processes, Altered
Tissue Integrity, Impaired
Tissue Perfusion, Altered (Specify Type) (Renal, cerebral, cardiopulmonary, gastrointestinal, peripheral)
Trauma, High Risk for
Unilateral Neglect
Urinary Elimination, Altered
Urinary Retention
Violence, High Risk for: Self-directed or directed at others

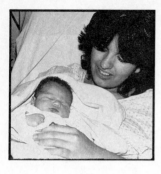

Glossary

ABC. Abbreviation for *alternate birth center*.

abdominal. Belonging to or relating to the abdomen.

a. delivery. Delivery of the child by abdominal section. See *cesarean section*.

a. gestation. Ectopic pregnancy occurring in the cavity of the abdomen.

a. lifting. The lifting of the abdominal wall with the hands to reduce abdominal pressure on the uterus during a contraction in labor.

a. pregnancy. See *a. gestation*.

abduction. The drawing or pulling away (of a part of the body) from the median axis.

ablatio placentae. Premature separation of the normally implanted placenta.

abortion. The termination of pregnancy at any time before the fetus has attained a stage of viability (i.e., before it is capable of extrauterine existence).

complete a. An abortion in which all the products of conception are passed and identified.

criminal a. An abortion performed illegally.

habitual a. An abortion that occurs in the third pregnancy or in subsequent pregnancies.

incomplete a. An abortion in which some but not all the products of conception are passed.

induced a. An abortion that is produced deliberately and intentionally.

inevitable a. The condition that precedes an abortion that will proceed naturally. Vaginal bleeding is profuse, the membranes may have ruptured, and the cervix may have become dilated.

missed a. The condition in which the embryo has died and subsequently the products of conception are retained in the uterus.

spontaneous a. An abortion that starts of its own accord; commonly called a miscarriage.

therapeutic a. An interruption of pregnancy before the 20th week, performed for medical reasons.

threatened a. The condition in which vaginal bleeding or spotting occurs in early pregnancy and the cervix is not dilated. The symptoms may subside and the pregnancy may proceed to full term.

abruptio placentae. Premature separation of a normally implanted placenta. The separation may be complete or partial and very often is considered a medical emergency.

acidosis. A condition resulting in an increase in hydrogen ion concentration causing a lowering of blood pH below 7.35.

metabolic a. Increase in hydrogen ion concentration caused by increased abnormal metabolism (too many acids produced), renal malfunction (acids not being excreted), or excessive loss of base (diarrhea).

acinus cell. Pl. *acini cells*. Milk-secreting cell contained in a lobule of the breast.

acquired immune deficiency syndrome. A new syndrome characterized by the occurrence in previously healthy individuals of *Pneumocystis carinii* pneumonia or other opportunistic infections or the rare malignancy Kaposi's sarcoma. Abnormal T-cell mechanisms are found in victims of this disease.

acrocyanosis. Cyanosis of the extremities, especially of the hands and feet, seen in the newborn for the first few hours after birth.

acromion. An outward extension of the spine of the scapula, used to explain presentation of the fetus.

acrosome. The caplike structure at the head of a sperm cell that contains enzymes believed to play an important role in the entrance of the sperm cell into the ovum.

adduction. The drawing or pulling (of a part of the body) toward the median axis.

adenoma. An epithelial tumor, usually benign, with a glandlike structure.

adnexa. Appendages.

a. uterine. The fallopian tubes and ovaries.

adolescence. The period of life beginning at puberty, when the secondary sex characteristics begin to develop and the capacity for reproduction is reached, and ending with adulthood.

adrenocorticotropic hormone (ACTH). Pituitary hormone that stimulates the adrenal cortex.

afferent. Centripetal; bringing toward a central part, as afferent nerves convey stimuli to the central nervous system.

afibrinogenemia. Lack of fibrinogen in the blood.

afterbirth. The structures cast off after the expulsion of the fetus, including the membranes and the placenta with the attached umbilical cord; the secundines.

afterpains. Those pains, more or less severe, after expulsion of the afterbirth, which result from the contractile efforts of the uterus to return to its normal condition.

agalactia. Absence or failure of the secretion of milk.

albuminuria. The presence of albumin in the urine.

alert inactivity period. Time at which the infant's eyes are open and limb movements are quiet.

alkalosis. A condition resulting from the loss of base, or depletion of acid without comparable loss of base, from body fluids.

allantois. A tubular diverticulum of the posterior part of the yolk sac of the embryo. It passes into the body stalk through which it is accompanied by the allantoic (umbilical) blood vessel, thus taking part in the formation of the umbilical cord; later, it fuses with the chorion and helps to form the placenta.

allele. One of two or more alternate genes that occur at a particular locus of a chromosome which decide alternate inherited characteristics.

alternate birth center (ABC). An organization of a hospital or a free-standing labor and delivery area that provides a homelike atmosphere. It has liberal policies regarding the presence of family and friends, labor practices, no separation of parents and infant, and early discharge.

amenorrhea. Absence or suppression of the menstrual discharge.

amniocentesis. The perforation, by use of a needle, through the abdominal wall into the uterus to obtain a sample of amniotic fluid, for the purpose of fetal genetic or fetal maturity diagnosis.

amnion. The most internal of the fetal membranes, containing the waters that surround the fetus *in utero*.

amnioscope. An instrument for examination of the fetus and amniotic fluid by passage through the maternal abdominal wall into the amniotic cavity, thus permitting direct visualization.

amniotic. Pertaining to the amnion.
   a. fluid. The clear fluid that is 98% water contained in the amnion. This fluid provides protection to the fetus, keeps the temperature constant, and provides some nourishment to the fetus. Also called *liquor amnii*.
   a.f. embolism. The blocking of a maternal artery with amniotic fluid forced into it by strong uterine contractions.
   a. sac. The "bag of membrane" containing the fetus before delivery.

amniotomy. The artificial rupture of the amniotic sac to induce labor.

analgesic. Drug that relieves pain, used during labor.

analogue. A chemical compound with a structure similar to that of another but differing from it with respect to a certain component. It may have similar or opposite action metabolically.

androgen. Any hormonal substance that possesses masculinizing activities, such as the testis hormone.

android. The term adopted for the male type of pelvis.

andrology. The scientific study of the male constitution and diseases, especially male reproductive problems.

anemia. A condition of the blood in which there is a deficiency in the red blood cells per unit volume, in the quantity of hemoglobin, or in the total volume.

anencephaly. A congenital deformity characterized by absence of the cerebrum, cerebellum, and flat bones of the skull.

anesthesia. The loss of sensation or feeling, especially the feeling of pain.

anomaly. An organ or structure that is malformed or in some way abnormal with reference to form, structure, or position.

anorexia. The loss of appetite.

anovular. Not accompanied with the discharge of an ovum; said of cyclic uterine bleeding.

anoxia. Oxygen deficiency; any condition of absence of tissue oxidation.

antenatal. Occurring or formed before birth.

antepartal. Before labor and delivery or childbirth; prenatal.

anthropoid pelvis. See *pelvis, anthropoid*.

antibody. Any of the body immunoglobulins that interact with antigens, neutralize toxins, and agglutinate bacteria or cells.

Apgar scoring system. A system for appraising the condition of a newborn on the basis of heart rate, respiratory effort, muscle tone, reflex irritability, and color. The maximum score is 10. The evaluation is done at 60 seconds after birth, then again at 5 minutes and at 10 minutes if the neonate is unstable.

apnea. Cessation of aspirations for more than 10 seconds associated with generalized cyanosis.

arachnodactyly. A hereditary metabolic disorder characterized by abnormally long and slender fingers and toes. Also called Marfan's syndrome.

areola. The ring of pigment surrounding the nipple.
   secondary a. A circle of faint color sometimes seen just outside the original areola about the fifth month of pregnancy.

arousal. Period when the infant moves from sleep state or drowsiness to awakeness or crying.

arrhythmia. Variation from the normal heartbeat rhythm.

articulation. The fastening together of the various bones of the skeleton in their natural situation; a joint. The articulations of the bones of the body are divided into two principal groups—*synarthroses*, immovable articulations, and *diarthroses*, movable articulations.

artificial feeding. Feeding an infant by bottle rather than at the mother's breast.

artificial insemination. The introduction of semen into the cervix or vagina by artificial means.

artificial menopause. The cessation of menstruation by artificial means such as surgery or irradiation.

Aschheim–Zondek test. See *test, Aschheim–Zondek*.

asexual. Having no sex or functional sexual organs.

Asherman's syndrome. See *syndrome, Asherman's*.

asphyxia. Suspended animation; anoxia and carbon dioxide retention resulting from failure of respiration.
   a. neonatorum. "Asphyxia of the newborn"; deficient respiration in newborn babies. Also called *neonatal asphyxia*.

asthma. A condition marked by recurring attacks of spasmodic dyspnea with wheezing. May be caused by allergies, vigorous exercise, psychological stress, and so on.

atelectasis. The incomplete expansion of a lung or the collapse of a lung.

atonic. Lacking the tone or strength that is normally present.

atresia. Absence of a normally patent passageway.

atrial septal defect. A congenital cardiac anomaly in which there is an abnormal opening between the right and left atria of the heart.

attitude. A posture or position of the body. In obstetrics, the relation of the fetal parts to each other in the uterus. The basic attitude is either flexion or extension.

auscultation. The act of listening for sounds within the body. Used to ascertain the fetal heart.

autosome. Any of the 22 ordinary paired chromosomes as distinguished from the two sex chromosomes.

axis. A line about which any revolving body turns.

pelvic a. The curved line that passes through the centers of all the anteroposterior diameters of the pelvis.

azoospermia. The absence of spermatozoa in the semen.

back labor. A condition that occurs in one fourth of all labors when the position of the fetus is such that the back of the head is directed to the mother's back or turned toward her sacrum. Extreme discomfort is felt by the mother as labor progresses.

bag of waters. The membranes that enclose the liquor amnii of the fetus. See *amniotic sac.*

ballottement. Literally means tossing. A term used in examination when the fetus can be pushed about in the pregnant uterus.

Bandl's ring. A groove on the uterus at the upper level of the fully developed lower uterine segment; visible on the abdomen after hard labor as a transverse or slightly slanting depression between the umbilicus and the pubis. Shows overstretching of lower uterine segment. Resembles a full bladder.

Barr body. The persistent mass of the material of the inactivated X chromosome in cells of normal females. Also called *sex chromatin.*

Bartholin's glands. Glands situated one on each side of the vaginal canal opening into the groove between the hymen and the labia minora.

basal body temperature (BBT). The resting temperature taken in the morning before arising or performing any activity. Characteristic changes in BBT that usually occur in fertile women are used to identify the time ovulation has occurred.

bearing down. Reflex effort by the mother to help with the uterine contractions.

bicornate uterus. Having two horns that, in the embryo, failed to attain complete fusion.

bilirubin. The principal pigment of the bile, reddish yellow in color.

bilirubinemia. The presence of bilirubin in the blood.

bimanual. Performed with or relating to both hands.

b. palpation. Examination of the pelvic organs of a woman by placing one hand on the abdomen and the fingers of the other in the vagina.

biparietal diameter. Largest transverse diameter of the fetal head.

birthing room. A room with homelike decor in which the family labors, delivers, and recovers.

bisexuality. The experiencing of sexual eroticism and genital intimacy with partners of both sexes.

blastocyst. The product of conception after the morula stage and before the embryonic stage.

blastoderm. The outer layer of cells of a fertilized ovum in the blastula stage.

b. vesicle. Hollow space within the morula formed by the rearrangement of cells, and by proliferation.

blastula. The fertilized ovum in the stage in which the cells are arranged in a hollow ball.

body image. The way one pictures one's body.

boggy. Inadequately contracted and having a spongy rather than firm feeling, descriptive of the postdelivery uterus.

bonding. The process by which the human infant becomes attached to his parents.

bony pelvis. Ring of bone containing the sacrum, the coccyx, and two innominate bones.

brachial palsy. See *palsy, brachial.*

Bracht maneuver. See *maneuver, Bracht.*

bradycardia. Slowness of the heartbeat below normal.

brain growth spurt period. A period of accelerated growth and vulnerability to environmental events.

Braxton Hicks contractions. Uterine contractions, occurring periodically during pregnancy, thereby enlarging the uterus to accommodate the growing fetus. During the third trimester, they are felt as a painless hardening or tightening of the uterus. They can become painful and are often difficult to differentiate from labor. Also called *B. H. sign.*

B. H. version. One of the types of operation designed to turn the baby from an undesirable position to a desired one.

breakthrough bleeding. Vaginal spotting or bleeding that occurs between menstrual periods, due to failure of oral contraceptive to support the endometrium adequately.

breast milk jaundice. A condition that occasionally occurs due to a substance in breast milk that inhibits the conjugation of bilirubin. May be treated by temporary or permanent cessation of breast-feeding.

breech. Nates or buttocks.

b. delivery. Labor and delivery marked by breech presentations.

bregma. The point on the surface of the skull at the junction of the coronal and sagittal sutures.

brim. The edge of the superior strait or inlet of the pelvis.

broad ligament. Fibrous sheath covered by peritoneum extending from each side of the uterus to the lateral wall of the pelvis.

bronchopulmonary dysplasia. A chronic lung disease in infants believed to be associated with oxygen toxicity. It is often preceded by severe respiratory distress syndrome and treatment in a high-oxygen environment.

cachexia. Weight loss and wasting associated with systemic illness.

caked breast. See *engorgement.*

Candida albicans. A yeastlike fungus that causes infections in the human being, commonly involving the mucous membranes of the mouth and vagina. During pregnancy, women are more susceptible to candidal infections due to the changed pH of the vagina and increased glycogen in vaginal cells.

candidiasis. A vaginal infection caused by *Candida albicans* with characteristic increased discharge and pruritus.

capacitation. The process by which a spermatozoon is conditioned to fertilize an ovum after it is exposed to the female reproductive tract.

caput. 1. The head, consisting of the cranium, or skull, and the face. 2. Any prominent object, such as the head.

c. succedaneum. An edematous swelling that sometimes appears on the presenting head of the fetus during labor.

carcinogen. A chemical or other substance that can induce or promote cancer.

cardiac anomalies. Anomalies that result from congenital heart defects. These include transposition of the great vessels, atrial septal defect, patent ductus arteriosus, ventricular septal defect, coarctation of the aorta, the tetralogy of Fallot, and others.

catamenia. See *menses.*

catheterization. The use of tubular instrument for withdrawing fluids from (or introducing into) a body cavity, especially the bladder through the urethra for the withdrawal of urine.

caudal. The term applied to analgesia or anesthesia resulting from the introduction of the suitable analgesic or anesthetic solution into the caudal canal (nonclosure of the laminae of the last sacral vertebra).

caul. A portion of the amniotic sac that occasionally envelops the child's head at birth.

cellulitis. Inflammation of cellular tissue.

cephalhematoma. A tumor or swelling between the cranium and the periosteum caused by an effusion of blood.

cephalic. Belonging to the head.

    c. presentation. Presentation of any part of the fetal head in labor.

cephalopelvic disproportion (CPD). A condition in which the fetal head is disproportionately large for passage through the maternal pelvis.

cerclage. Encircling of a part with a wire, metal band, or suture, as for correction of an incompetent cervix.

cerebral palsy. See *palsy, cerebral.*

cerebroside lipidosis. See *disease, Gaucher's.*

cervical mucus. The secretion of the mucous membrane of the cervix.

cervical dilation. See *dilation, cervical.*

cervix. Neckline part; the lower and narrow end of the uterus, between the os and the body of the organ.

cesarean delivery. Delivery of the fetus by an incision through the abdominal wall and the wall of the uterus.

    classical c.d. A cesarean delivery that involves a vertical incision in the abdomen over the fundus and baby and then a vertical incision into the upper uterine segment.

    extraperitoneal c.d. A cesarean section performed when intrauterine infection is present. The incision is low, and the bladder must be dissected off the uterus.

    low-segment c.d. A cesarean delivery in which the incision is made into the lower uterine segment, either transversely or vertically.

Chadwick's sign. The violet color on the mucous membrane of the vagina just below the urethral orifice, seen after the fourth week of pregnancy.

change of life. See *climacteric.*

Chlamydia trachomatis. An organism responsible for a spectrum of diseases including cervicitis, urethritis, acute salpingitis, and endometritis.

chloasma. Pl. *chloasmata.* A cutaneous affliction which exhibits spots and patches of a yellowish brown color. The term cloasma is a vague one and is applied to various kinds of pigmentary discoloration of the skin.

    c. gravidarum, c. uterinum. Chloasma occurring during pregnancy.

chorioamnionitis. An intrauterine infection involving mononuclear and polymorphonuclear leukocytic infiltration of the fetal membranes and amniotic fluid.

chorion. The outermost membrane of the growing zygote, or fertilized ovum, which serves as a protective and nutritive covering.

chorionic villus. Pl. *villi.* One of the villi growing in tufts on the external surface of the chorion.

chromosomal sex. The determination of the sex of an individual by the configuration of chromosomes in his cells (i.e., XY is the male configuration, and XX is the female configuration).

chromosome. One of several small, dark-staining and more or less rod-shaped bodies that appear in the nucleus of the cell at the time of cell divisions and particularly in mitosis.

chromosome disorder. Abnormality of chromosome number or structure.

cilium. Pl. *cilia.* One of the hairlike projections of a structure such as the fallopian tube. The cilia of the fallopian tube beat in such a manner as to direct any overlying fluid in the direction of the uterine cavity. Thus, the cilia are partially responsible for the transportation of an ovum along the tube.

circumcision. The removal of all or part of the prepuce, or foreskin, of the penis.

cleavage. The series of cell divisions that occur during the development of a fertilized ovum into an embryo when the structure remains the same size while the cleavage cells become smaller and smaller.

cleft lip. Congenital incomplete closure of the lip.

cleft palate. Congenital fissure of the palate and the roof of the mouth.

climacteric. A particular epoch of the ordinary term of life at which the body undergoes a considerable change, especially the menopause or "change of life."

climax. See *orgasm.*

clitoris. A small, elongated, erectile body situated at the anterior part of the vulva. An organ of the female homologous with the penis of the male.

clonus. A series of rapid, rhythmic contractions of a muscle occurring involuntarily in response to stretching of the muscle.

clubfoot. A congenitally deformed foot. See *talipes equinovarus.*

coarctation of the aorta. A congenital cardiac anomaly in which there is a constriction of the aorta, causing narrowing of the lumen. This partially obstructs blood flow, creating increased left ventricular pressure and work load.

coccyx. The bone at the caudal end of the spine. In a child the coccyx consists of four or five separate vertebrae; in an adult these bones are fused into one.

cognition. The reasoning, logic, intentional thought, problem-solving, thinking ability of the infant.

coitus. Sexual intercourse, copulation.

    c. interruptus. The practice of withdrawal as a means of contraception. The penis is withdrawn from the vagina before ejaculation.

colostrum. The thin, yellow fluid, high in protein and inorganic salts, that is secreted from the breasts during the last weeks of pregnancy and the 3 days after delivery before milk is produced.

c. corpuscles. Large granular cells found in colostrum.

colporrhaphy. 1. The operation of suturing the vagina. 2. The operation of denuding and suturing the vaginal wall for the purpose of narrowing the vagina.

colposcope. A viewing instrument designed for close examination of the tissues of the cervix, similar to a low-magnification microscope with binocular vision.

colpotomy. Any surgical cutting operation upon the vagina.

commissure. A site of union of corresponding parts.

compliance, lung. Degree of distensibility of the lung's elastic tissue.

conception. The impregnation of the female ovum by the spermatozoon of the male, whence results a new being.

conceptus. Products of conception.

condom. A sheath worn over the penis during sexual intercourse to prevent sperm from entering the vagina.

condyloma. Pl. *condylomata.* A wartlike excrescence near the anus or the vulva; the flat, moist papule of secondary syphilis.

confinement. Term applied to childbirth and the lying-in period.

congenital. Born with a person; existing from or from before birth, as, for example, congenital disease, a disease originating in the fetus before birth.

congenital anomaly. Abnormality present at birth.

conjugate. The anteroposterior diameter of the pelvic inlet.

conjunctivitis. Inflammation of the conjunctiva, the membrane lining the eyelids, generally associated with a discharge.

constipation. The infrequent or difficult passage of feces.

contraception. The prevention of conception or impregnation.

contracted pelvis. See *pelvis, contracted.*

contraction. The intermittent shortening of a muscle, especially the uterus during labor in order to expel the contents.

convulsion. An involuntary and violent contraction of voluntary muscles.

Coombs' test. A test used to detect sensitized red blood cells in erythroblastosis fetalis.

indirect C.t. Determination of Rh-positive antibodies in maternal blood.

direct C.t. Determination of maternal Rh-positive antibodies in fetal cord blood.

cor pulmonale. Heart disease secondary to disease of the lungs or lung blood vessels; a type of heart failure.

corona radiata. The layer of follicular cells arranged in a radial pattern that envelop the zona pellucida of the ovum.

coronal. Belonging to, or relating to, the crown of the head.

c. suture. The suture formed by the union of the frontal bone with the two parietal bones.

corpus albicans. The white fibrous tissue that replaces the corpus luteum in the ovary as it shrinks in the last stages of pregnancy.

corpus luteum. The yellow mass found in the graafian follicle after the ovum has been expelled.

cotyledon. Any one of the subdivisions of the uterine surface of the placenta.

Couvelaire uterus. A severe uterine condition seen in some cases of placental separation, when coagulation is impaired and there is extensive bleeding into the uterine muscle.

Cowper's gland. One of two glands located at the base of the prostate gland and on either side of the membranous urethra that produce a mucinous substance that lubricates the urethra and coats its surface.

CPD. Abbreviation for cephalopelvic disproportion.

cramp. A painful contraction of a muscle.

creatinine. The end product of metabolism, found in muscle and blood and excreted in the urine.

criminal abortion. See *abortion, criminal.*

crowning. The phase in the second stage of labor when a large part of the top of the fetal head is visible in the vaginal opening. The anus is open, and the perineum is distended.

cul-de-sac. [Fr.] A pouch or sac having only one end open.

Douglas' c. A sac or recess formed by a fold of the peritoneum dipping down between the rectum and the uterus. Also called *pouch of Douglas and rectouterine pouch.*

culdoscopy. A visual examination of the organs of a female pelvis with an endoscope.

cumulus oophorus. A loosely arranged solid mass of cells surrounding the ovum in the ovarian follicle.

curanderas. f.; **curanderos** m. Mexican-American folk healer.

curettage. [Fr.] The removal of substances from the wall of a cavity, especially the uterine cavity, with a spoon-shaped instrument called a curet.

cyanosis. A bluish discoloration of the skin or mucous membranes as a result of an excessive concentration of hemoglobin that is not combined with oxygen in the blood.

cyesis. Pregnancy.

cystitis. An infection or inflammation of the urinary bladder.

cystocele. The pouching downward of the bladder through the vaginal wall.

cytomegalic inclusion disease. See *disease, cytomegalic inclusion.*

cytomegalovirus. A herpesvirus that produces unique large cells bearing intranuclear inclusions.

D & C. Abbreviation for dilatation and curettage.

D & E. Abbreviation for dilatation and evacuation.

decidua. The endometrium of a pregnant uterus, which, except for the deepest layer, is shed during childbirth.

d. basalis. The part of the decidua directly underneath the chorionic vesicle and attached to the myometrium, the main muscular mass of the uterus.

decrement. Decrease; also the stage of decline.

delivery. [Fr., *délivrer*, to free, to deliver.] 1. The expulsion of a child by the mother, or its extraction by the obstetric practitioner. 2. The removal of a part from the body, for example, *delivery* of the placenta.

deoxyribonucleic acid (DNA). Chemical forming the genetic code; it occurs as a double-stranded helix within chromosomes.

descent. Passage of the presenting part of the fetus into and through the birth canal; it begins at the onset of labor and proceeds during effacement and dilatation of the cervix.

detumescence. The subsidence of swelling, congestion, or turgor; the period in which the organ or passage decreases in size and returns to its original state.

diabetes or **diabetes mellitus.** An endocrine disorder that involves disruption of normal carbohydrate metabolism caused by a deficiency of insulin. Because there is a significant change in the course of diabetes when pregnancy intervenes, close supervision of the prenatal care of a diabetic gravida is required.

 gestational d. Diabetes initially diagnosed during pregnancy, due to glucose intolerance.

diagonal conjugate measurement. The chief internal pelvic measurement made to determine the actual diameter of the pelvic passage. It is the distance between the sacral promontory and the lower margin of the symphysis pubis.

diamniotic dichorionic twins. See *twins, diamniotic dichorionic.*

diamniotic monochorionic twins. See *twins, diamniotic monochorionic.*

diaphragm. 1. The partition separating the abdominal and thoracic cavities made of muscle and membrane. 2. A contraceptive device made of rubber that is inserted in the vagina to act like a cap over the cervix. To be effective, the device is used with spermicidal cream or jelly.

diaphragmatic. Pertaining to the diaphragm.

 d. hernia. A defect in the development of the diaphragm, which allows the abdominal organs to herniate into the thoracic cavity.

 d. paralysis. A condition resulting from injury to the phrenic nerve during a difficult breech delivery. The paralysis is usually one sided, with irregular thoracic respirations, no abdominal movement on inspiration on the affected side, and cyanosis.

diarrhea. Abnormally frequent and liquid fecal discharges.

diastasis recti. Separation of the abdominal recti muscles, which may occur during pregnancy because of stretching of the abdominal wall.

Dick-Read approach to childbirth. The approach that is based on the understanding that fear of pain produces muscular tension, which produces pain and greater fear. This approach includes an educational program to teach physiological processes of labor, exercise to improve muscle tone, and techniques to assist in relaxation and prevent the fear–tension–pain mechanism. Also called *Read method of childbirth preparation.*

dilatation and curettage (D & C). A method of emptying the contents of the uterus by using cervical dilatation and curettage. The technique is widely used for first-trimester abortions.

dilatation and evacuation (D & E). See *suction curettage.*

dilation. The act of dilating or stretching.

 cervical d. The opening of the cervix to accommodate the birth of the fetus.

dimorphism. The manifestation in the same species of two forms, such as male and female; refers to both bodily form and appearance and to sex differences in behavior and language.

disease. Any departure from health of a structure, organ, or system.

 cytomegalic inclusion d. A disease caused by a group of species specific herpes virus, that inhabit the human salivary glands.

 Gaucher's d. A lipidosis in which the fatty accumulation in the body is largely kerasin. In the infant form, it is characterized by yellow pigmentation of the skin and marked impairment of the central nervous system. It is also known as *cerebroside lipidosis* and is a hereditary defect of the metabolism.

 hemolytic d. Anemia in a fetus or newborn caused by antibodies that are transmitted from the mother due to the incompatibility between the blood group of the mother and her child.

 Hurler's d. (gargoylism). A hereditary disorder caused by an enzyme deficiency. It is characterized by gargoylelike features of the head (depressed bridge of the nose, large prominent tongue, and widely spaced teeth), dwarf structure, short neck, broad short hands, severe mental retardation, blindness, deafness, and cardiovascular defects.

 hyaline membrane d. (HMD). A disease of premature infants characterized by the formation of a translucent membrane in the respiratory passages and the incapacity of the lungs to expand adequately. Also known as respiratory distress syndrome (RDS).

 Niemann–Pick d. A lipidosis characterized by brownish yellow discoloration of the skin and nervous system involvement. It is a hereditary disease and is also known as *sphingomyelin lipidosis.*

 Tay–Sachs d. A hereditary metabolic disorder also known as *ganglioside lipidosis.* It is characterized by a degeneration of brain cells and a red spot on each retina, and eventually by dementia, blindness, paralysis, and death.

 venereal d. One of a number of infectious diseases that are transmitted through sexual contact and may be localized or systemic. Common types are gonorrhea, syphilis, condylomata (venereal warts), and herpes simplex type II.

 Wilson–Mikity d. See *pulmonary dysmaturity.*

disseminated intravascular coagulation. An acquired disorder in which there is acceleration of thrombi formation and also increasing fibrinolytic activity resulting in hemorrhage. The disorder can be either chronic or acute. In obstetrics it is usually acute and considered a medical emergency.

diuresis. An increased excretion of urine.

diuretic. An agent that promotes urine excretion.

dizygotic. Pertaining to or proceeding from two zygotes (ova).

d. twins. See *twins, dizygotic.*

Döderlein's bacillus. The large gram-positive bacterium occurring in the normal vaginal secretion.

dominant inheritance. The acquiring of a characteristic by transmission in a gene from parents to their offspring regardless of the state of the corresponding allele.

Doppler. Device used to monitor fetal heart rate by ultrasound.

Douglas' cul-de-sac. See *cul-de-sac, Douglas.*

Down's syndrome. See *syndrome, Down's.*

ductus. A duct.

d. arteriosus. "Arterial duct," a blood vessel peculiar to the fetus, communicating directly between the pulmonary artery and the aorta.

d. venosus. "Venous duct," a blood vessel peculiar to the fetus, establishing a direct communication between the umbilical vein and the inferior vena cava.

Duncan mechanism. The position of the placenta, with the maternal surface outermost; to be born edgewise.

dyscrasia. A diseased condition.

dysmenorrhea. Painful menstruation.

dyspareunia. Painful intercourse, which can result from penetration, frictional movement, and deep thrusting.

dysplasia. Abnormality of the development of cells or a part.

dyspnea. Labored breathing.

dystocia. Difficult, slow, or painful birth or delivery. It is distinguished as maternal or fetal (i.e., the difficulty is due to some deformity on the part of the mother or on the part of the child).

d., placental. Difficulty in delivering the placenta.

eclampsia. A severe complication occurring in pregnancy or the early puerperium, characterized by hypertension, edema, albuminuria, convulsions, and coma.

ectocervix. The outer portion of the cervix visible on examination.

ectoderm. The outer layer of cells of the primitive embryo.

ectopic. Out of place.

e. gestation. Gestation in which the fetus is out of its normal place in the cavity of the uterus. It includes gestations in the interstitial portion of the tube or in a rudimentary horn of the uterus (cornual pregnancy) and cervical pregnancy, as well as tubal, abdominal, and ovarian pregnancies. Also known as *ectopic pregnancy* and *extrauterine pregnancy.*

e. pregnancy. Same as *ectopic gestation.*

ectropion. Eversion of an edge or margin, as of the columnar epithelium of the endocervical canal onto the ectocervix. The tissue appears darker pink-red and bumpy compared with the smooth pink squamous epithelium of the ectocervix.

EDC. Abbreviation for *expected date of confinement.*

edema. Abnormal swelling due to large amounts of fluid in the tissues.

effacement. Obliteration. In obstetrics, refers to thinning and shortening of the cervix.

efferent. Centrifugal; conveying away from a center, as efferent nerves convey stimuli to the peripheral nervous system.

effleurage. [Fr.] A rubbing movement, as in massage.

ejaculation. A sudden act of expulsion, as of semen.

electronic fetal monitor. A system for monitoring fetal heart rate and uterine activity by electrically operated instruments.

embolism. The sudden blocking of an artery or vein by a blood clot or other obstruction that was brought there by the blood current.

embolus. A clot or other obstruction brought to a vein or artery by the blood from a larger vessel.

embryo. The product of conception *in utero* from the third through the fifth week of gestation; after that length of time it is called the fetus.

embryonic disc. The flattish portion of a fertilized ovum in which the first traces of an embryo are seen.

empathy. The projection of one's own consciousness into that of another. Empathy may be distinguished from sympathy in that the former state includes relative freedom from emotional involvement.

encephalopathy. Any degenerative brain disease.

endocervical. Pertaining to the interior of the cervix of the uterus.

endocervix. 1. The mucous membrane lining of the cervical canal. 2. The region of the opening of the cervix into the uterine cavity.

endometriosis. Pathologic condition in which normal tissue that lines the uterus (endometrial tissue) grows outside of the uterus, often around the fallopian tubes, contributing to infertility.

endometritis. Inflammation of the endometrium.

endometrium. The mucous membrane that lines the uterus.

endorphin. An opiatelike substance produced by the body.

endoscope. An instrument used for viewing the interior of a hollow organ, as the bladder.

endotracheal intubation. The insertion of a tube into the trachea to be used to administer anesthesia, maintain an airway, or ventilate the lungs.

enema. A liquid injected into the rectum.

en face. [Fr.] The position in which the mother's face is rotated so that her eyes and those of her infant meet fully.

engagement. 1. In clinical obstetrics, applies to the entrance of the presenting part into the superior pelvic strait and the beginning of the descent through the pelvic canal. 2. Also relating to parent-infant interaction: behaviors designed to induce and sustain social interchanges.

engorgement. Hyperemia; local congestion; excessive fullness of any organ or passage. In obstetrics, refers to an exaggeration of normal venous and lymph stasis of the breasts, which occurs in relation to lactation.

enhancement. The developmentally optimal level of stimulation.

entoderm. The innermost layer of cells of the primitive embryo.

environment. The animate and inanimate components of the infant's world.

enzygotic. Developed from the same fertilized ovum.

epididymis. Pl. *epididymides*. A part of the canal system of the testes, made up of numerous seminiferous tubules. Its long coiled duct provides for storage, transit, and maturation of spermatozoa.

epidural anesthesia. Anesthesia produced by injecting between the vertebral spines and beneath the ligamentum flavum into the extradural space. It is used in obstetric anesthesia to alleviate maternal pain with minimal danger to the infant. It requires the expertise that is afforded a surgical patient.

epinephrine. A chemical hormone that is secreted by the adrenal medulla. It is released in response to hypoglycemia. This chemical is injected in infants of diabetic mothers to treat hypoglycemia.

episiotomy. Surgical incision of the vulvar orifice for obstetric purposes.

epispadias. A congenital anomaly in which the urethra opens on the dorsal surface of the penis. In severe cases, the upper wall of the urethra may be absent.

Epstein's pearls. Small white cysts on the hard palate or gums of the newborn. They are not abnormal.

Erb's paralysis. Partial paralysis of the brachial plexus, affecting various muscles of the arm and the chest wall.

erectile. Capable of becoming rigid and elevated, such as erectile tissue, found in the penis, clitoris, and nipples.

ergonovine. An alkaloid of ergot and a powerful oxytocic. May be administered intravenously, orally, or intramuscularly. This drug will cause an elevation of blood pressure.

ergot. A drug having the remarkable property of exciting powerfully the contractile force of the uterus, and chiefly used for this purpose, but its long-continued use is highly dangerous. Usually given in the fluid extract.

erotic. Pertaining to sensuousness or sensual arousal.

erythema toxicum. A blotchy rash that may appear in the first few days of life. It develops more frequently on the back, shoulders, and buttocks. No treatment is necessary and it will disappear in a day or so. It is also called *"newborn rash."*

erythroblastosis fetalis. A severe hemolytic disease of the newborn usually due to Rh incompatibility.

esophageal atresia. A congenital defect in which the esophagus ends in a blind pouch rather than a continuous tube to the stomach. It is characterized by excessive drooling, gagging, coughing, vomiting when fed, cyanosis, and dyspnea. The condition is corrected by surgery.

estradiol. An estrogen produced in ovarian follicles. It inhibits the release of follicle-stimulating hormones prior to ovulation.

estrogen. The generic term for the female sex hormones. It is a steroid hormone produced primarily by the ovaries but also by the adrenal cortex. It is responsible for the development of secondary sex characteristics and the cyclic nature of female reproductive physiology.

expected date of confinement (EDC). The calculated date for the birth of the fetus.

external rotation. In childbirth, a change in the position of the fetus following the birth of the head during which the shoulders are born.

extraction, vacuum. In assisted childbirth, the use of a metal cup applied to the fetal head by creating a vacuum between it and the head to assist in the delivery of a fetus. Traction is exerted by means of a short chain attached to the cup, with a handle at its far end.

extraperitoneal. Situated or occurring outside the peritoneal cavity.

extrauterine. Outside of the uterus.
   e. pregnancy. See *ectopic gestation*.

face presentation. A less common head presentation in which the fetal face is presented in labor.

facies. Pl. *facies*. [L.] A term used in anatomy to refer to the front of the head from forehead to chin.

fallopian. [Relating to G. *Fallopius*, a celebrated Italian anatomist of the 16th century.]
   f. tubes. The oviducts—two canals extending from the sides of the fundus uteri.

false labor. A condition in the latter weeks of some pregnancies in which irregular uterine contractions are felt but the cervix is not affected.

false pelvis. See *pelvis, false*.

family-centered care. Maternity care that takes into account other members of the family, particularly fathers and children, in prenatal, intrapartum, and postpartum care of pregnant women.

fecundation. The act of impregnating or the state of being impregnated; the fertilization of the ovum by means of the male seminal element.

fecundity. The ability to produce offspring in large numbers in a short period of time.

ferning. A fernlike pattern seen microscopically when cervical mucus is viewed under the microscope. The specimen is taken from the cervical area, usually obtained during a sterile speculum examination. The pattern confirms the presence of estrogen at midcycle in the menstruating woman. It also documents the rupture of amniotic fluid in the pregnant woman.

fertility. The ability to produce offspring; power of reproduction.
   f. awareness. The development of familiarity with the bodily signs of impending ovulation and bodily signs after ovulation, which enables a woman to anticipate her fertile period and its ending.
   f. rate. The number of births per 1000 women aged 15 through 44 years.

fertilization. The fusion of the spermatozoon with the ovum; it marks the beginning of pregnancy.

fetal. Pertaining to a fetus.
   f. acidosis. A condition of a fetus resulting in the accumulation of acids or depletion of alkaline reserve in the blood and body tissues.
   f. alcohol syndrome. See *syndrome, f. alcohol*.
   f. bradycardia. Slowness of the fetal heartbeat.
   f. distress. A condition of fetal difficulty *in utero* that can occur during either the antenatal or the intrapartum period. Signs are a fetal tachycardia, decrease in

variability, and repetitive late or severe variable decelerations.

f. habitus. The attitude of the fetus, or the relation of the fetal parts to each other.

f. heart rate (FHR). The heart rate of the fetus. Normally, it can be heard about the middle of pregnancy and may vary between 120 to 160 beats per minute.

f. heart tones (FHT). The sounds of a fetal heart as heard by auscultation.

fetoscope. 1. A head stethoscope designed especially for listening to fetal heart tones. 2. An endoscope for viewing a fetus.

fetus. The baby *in utero* from the end of the fifth week of gestation until birth.

FHR. See *fetal heart rate.*

FHT. See *fetal heart tones.*

fibrinogenopenia. Decreased fibrinogen in the blood.

fibroid. See *myoma.*

fimbria. A fringe; especially the fringelike end of the fallopian tube.

fissure. A cleft or groove, which may be normal or abnormal. Anal fissures are painful linear ulcers at the margin of the anus.

fistula. An abnormal passage between two internal organs or between an organ and the surface of the body.

fixation. A sustained gaze on one point.

flaring of nostrils. Widening of nostrils during inspiration; a sign of respiratory distress.

flatulence. An excess amount of gas in the stomach or intestines.

flexion. The act of bending. In obstetrics, the process in the mechanism of labor referring to the bending of the fetal head so that the chin is in contact with the chest, thus presenting the smallest anteroposterior diameter to the pelvis.

foam, contraceptive. A spermicidal preparation that is inserted vaginally prior to intercourse to prevent conception. Its effectiveness is enhanced when it is used with a diaphragm.

folic acid. One of the vitamins of the B complex that is essential for growth and necessary to the proper formation of blood in the body.

follicle. A sac or pouchlike cavity.

follicle-stimulating hormone (FSH). A gonadotropic hormone secreted by the anterior pituitary, which stimulates the development of graafian follicles.

fontanel. The diamond-shaped space between the frontal and two parietal bones in very young infants. This is called the *anterior f.* and is the familiar "soft spot" just above a baby's forehead. A small, triangular one (*posterior f.*) is between the occipital and parietal bones.

footling breech. A breech presentation in which one or both feet or the knees extend below the buttocks. It is also known as incomplete breech presentation.

foramen. A hole, opening, aperture, or orifice—especially one through a bone.

f. ovale. An opening situated in the partition that separates the right and left auricles of the heart in the fetus.

forceps. A two-bladed instrument with a handle used for grasping tissues or sterile dressings in surgery. In obstet-

rics, one of several kinds of instruments used for assisting in the delivery of an infant after the cervix is dilated and the vertex of the fetal head is engaged.

foreskin. The prepuce—the fold of skin covering the glans penis.

fornix. Pl. *fornices.* An arch; any vaulted surface.

f. of the vagina. The angle of reflection of the vaginal mucous membrane onto the cervix uteri.

fourchette. [Fr., "fork."] The posterior angle or commissure of the labia majora.

frenulum linguae. A sharp, thin ridge of tissue that arises in the midline from the base of the tongue and is attached to its undersurface for varying distances. Depending upon this distance of attachment, it restrains the movement of the tongue. Also called *lingual frenum.*

frenum. A fold of mucous membrane that checks, curbs, or restrains the movements of a part.

lingual f. See *frenulum linguae.*

Friedman's curve. A graph designed to describe and record progress during labor.

Friedman's test. See *test, Friedman's.*

FSH. Abbreviation for *follicle-stimulating hormone.*

fundus. The upper rounded portion of the uterus between the points of insertion of the fallopian tubes.

funic souffle. A soft, blowing sound, synchronous with the fetal heart sounds and supposed to be produced in the umbilical cord.

funis. A cord—especially the umbilical cord.

galactagogue. 1. Causing the flow of milk. 2. Any drug that causes the flow of milk to increase.

galactorrhea. Prolonged and abnormal lactation, often profuse.

galactosemia. An inherited autosomal recessive disorder of galactose metabolism.

gamete. A sexual cell; a mature germ cell, as an unfertilized egg or a mature sperm cell.

Gamper method of childbirth preparation. One of a number of methods employed by parents for handling the discomforts of labor.

ganglioside lipidosis. See *disease, Tay–Sachs.*

gargoylism. See *disease, Hurler's.*

gastroenteritis. Inflammation of the stomach and intestines.

gastroschisis. An abdominal wall defect at the base of the umbilical stalk.

gastrostomy. Creation of an artificial opening into the stomach through the abdominal wall, used for feeding purposes.

gastrula. The early embryonic stage that follows the blastula; the cuplike stage with two layers of cells.

gate control theory. A theory proposed in 1965 by Melzack and Wall to explain the neurophysical mechanism underlying the sensation of pain.

Gaucher's disease. See *disease, Gaucher's.*

gavage feeding. Forced feeding, as through a tube into the stomach.

gender identity. The sameness, unity, and persistence of one's individuality as male or female, or ambivalent, especially as experienced in self-awareness and behavior. Gender identity is the private experience of gender role.

gender role. Everything one says and does to indicate to others or the self the degree to which one is male or female, or ambivalent. It includes but is not restricted to sexual arousal and response. Gender role is the public expression of gender identity.

gene. A hereditary germinal factor in the chromosome that carries on a hereditary transmissible character.

genetic anomaly. A marked deviation from the expected standard as a result of an inherited defect.

genetic counseling. A process in which individuals or families are given information that is needed to understand a hereditary disorder.

genetics. The study of heredity.

genital herpes. A viral skin disease of the genitals marked by groups of vesicles 3 mm to 6 mm in diameter.

genitalia. The reproductive organs.

genotype. An individual's entire hereditary constitution.

gestation. The condition of pregnancy; pregnancy; gravidity.

gestational age. The age of the product of conception between fertilization and birth.

glomerular endotheliosis. Overgrowth of the endothelium in the glomerulus.

glucose tolerance test (GTT). See *test, glucose tolerance.*

glycosuria. The presence of glucose (sugar) in the urine.

gonad. A gamete-producing gland; an ovary or testis.

gonadal sex. The sex of an individual determined by the presence of either testes or ovaries as gonads, or in the case of a true hermaphrodite, the presence of gonads of both sexes.

gonadotropin. A substance produced by the anterior pituitary and placenta that has an affinity for or a stimulating effect on the gonads.

gonorrhea. A disease spread by sexual contact that affects the mucosa of the genital tract. The disease may be asymptomatic in women, except for a vaginal discharge. It can produce puerperal infection if present in the cervix at the time of delivery. The infection can infect the infant's eyes at birth.

gonorrheal conjunctivitis. A severe form of conjunctivitis caused by the bacteria of gonorrhea.

gonorrheal salpingitis. An infection of the fallopian tube caused by the gonorrhea bacteria. It may cause a narrowing of the fallopian tube, which may subsequently prevent the passage of a fertilized ovum down the tube, resulting in a tubal pregnancy.

Goodell's sign. Softening of the cervix, a probable sign of pregnancy.

gossypol. A derivative of cottonseed oil that has male contraceptive actions by suppressing sperm production and affecting sperm structure and mobility.

graafian follicles or vesicles. Small spherical bodies in the ovaries, each containing an ovum.

grasp reflex. See *reflex, grasp.*

gravid. Pregnant.

gravida. A pregnant woman.

GTT. Abbreviation for *glucose tolerance test.*

Guthrie method in PKU. A method of diagnosing PKU. It is a blood test in which one or two drops of blood may be taken from an infant's heel; then the blood is tested to determine the phenylalanine level.

gynecoid pelvis. See *pelvis, gynecoid.*

gynecology. The branch of medicine that studies and treats women's diseases, especially of the genital tract.

Haase's rule. A method for calculating the length of an embryo or fetus. During the first 5 months, the number of months should be squared to approximate the length in centimeters (e.g., second month of pregnancy, the fetus is about 4 cm in length). After the fifth month, the number of months should be multiplied by 5.

Harvard pump. A constant infusion pump used to administer oxytocin in labor.

HCG. Abbreviation for *human chorionic gonadotropin.*

Health Systems Agency (HSA). A regional agency within a state that has primary responsibility for health planning and development of health services, manpower, and facilities to meet the needs of its service areas.

Hegar's sign. Softening of the lower uterine segment; a sign of pregnancy.

hematocrit. The volume percentage of red blood corpuscles in whole blood. Formerly, it meant the procedure used to determine this number; now it is the result of that determination.

hematoma. A tumor caused by effused blood. Continued bleeding from lacerations or an episiotomy can cause vaginal or vulvar hematomas in postpartum patients.

hemoglobinopathy. A disorder of the blood resulting from a genetically caused altered molecular structure of hemoglobin.

hemolytic disease. See *disease, hemolytic.*

hemophilia. An inherited condition that is due to a deficiency in a coagulation factor in the blood. It is characterized by subcutaneous and intramuscular hemorrhages, bleeding from the mouth, gum, lips, and tongue, and blood in the urine. It affects males but is transmitted by females.

hemorrhage. Bleeding.

hemorrhagic diathesis. A predisposition to abnormal bleeding.

hemorrhoid. A varicose dilatation of a vein in the rectal area. It may occur around the anus or internally, higher in the rectum.

heparin. An anticoagulant mucopolysaccharide acid.

hepatitis. Inflammation of the liver.

hermaphroditism. A congenital condition of ambiguity of reproductive structures so that the sex of the individual is not clearly defined as exclusively male or female. The condition is named for Hermes and Aphrodite, the Greek god and goddess of love.

hernia. The protrusion of an organ through an abnormal opening in the wall of the cavity that contains it.

diaphragmatic h. See *diaphragmatic hernia.*

umbilical h. The protrusion of the intestines through a rupture at the navel. In an infant, the condition usually disappears spontaneously by 1 year of age.

herpesvirus. A group of viruses characterized by the formation of small vesicles in clusters. The infection may be nongenital or genital (sexually transmitted).

heterosexuality. The selection of partners of the opposite sex for sexual eroticism and genital intimacy; the predominant mode of sexual partner preference.

high risk. Pertaining to an individual, especially an infant, whose medical and physical history, or that of his parents, indicates that the likelihood is great for his having physiological problems.

hip dysplasia. A hereditary condition involving dislocation with partial or complete loss of contact between the femoral head and the cup-shaped cavity on the lateral surface of the hip bone.

histology. The branch of anatomy that deals with the study of the minute structure, composition, and function of the tissues.

HMD. Abbreviation for *hyaline membrane disease.*

HMG. Abbreviation for *human menopausal gonadotropin.*

Homan's sign. An indication of thrombophlebitis if with leg extended and foot flexed, pain and tenderness are produced in the calf.

homologous. Corresponding in structure or origin; derived from the same source.

homosexuality. The selection of partners of the same sex for sexual eroticism and genital intimacy. There are many degrees of its expression.

hormonal sex. The sex of an individual determined by the preponderance of either estrogen (female) or testosterone (male) sex hormones.

hormone. A chemical substance produced in an organ, which, being carried to an associated organ by the bloodstream, excites in the latter organ a functional activity.

HPL. Abbreviation for *human placental lactogen.*

HSA. Abbreviation for *health systems agency.*

human chorionic gonadotropin (HCG). A hormone secreted by the placenta that prolongs the life of the corpus luteum. It is excreted in the mother's urine and makes possible the standard tests for pregnancy.

human menopausal gonadotropin (HMG). A hormone excreted in the urine of postmenopausal women that has the property of stimulating growth and maturity of ovarian follicles.

human placental lactogen (HPL). A hormone secreted by the placenta that influences somatic growth and facilitates preparation of the breasts for lactation.

Hurler's disease. (gargoylism). See *disease, Hurler's.*

hyaline membrane disease (HMD). See *disease, hyaline membrane.*

hydatidiform mole. Transformation and proliferation of the chorionic villi into grapelike cysts, characterized by poorly vascularized and edematous villi.

hydramnios. An excessive amount of amniotic fluid.

hydrocephalus. An excessive accumulation of cerebrospinal fluid in the ventricles of the brain with consequent enlargement of the cranium.

hydrops fetalis. Characteristics of infants having experienced severe Rh hemolytic disease edema, severe pallor, and cardiac decompensation.

hymen. A membranous fold that partially or wholly occludes the external orifice of the vagina, especially in the virgin.

hyperalimentation. The ingestion of more than adequate amounts of nutrients.

hyperbilirubinemia. The presence of excessive amounts of bilirubin in the blood, which may lead to jaundice.

hyperemesis gravidarum. Pernicious vomiting of pregnancy. This condition is present when vomiting is excessive, continues beyond the fourth month, and causes a marked loss of weight and acetonuria.

hyperemia. An excess of blood in a part.

hyperestrogenic. Pertaining to a state of exaggerated estrogen response created by high levels of estrogen secretion.

hypernatremia. Excessive amounts of sodium in the blood.

hyperplasia. Abnormal multiplication or increase in the number of cells in the normal arrangement in tissue.

hypertension. Persistent high blood pressure, especially arterial blood pressure.

    pregnancy-induced h. (PIH). A diagnostic label used to describe the syndrome of hypertension, edema, and proteinuria evident in certain pregnant women. Preeclampsia and eclampsia are two categories of PIH.

hypertonic. 1. Having high osmotic pressure. 2. Having abnormally high muscle tone.

    h. saline. A concentrated salt solution, as is instilled into the amniotic fluid for a mid-trimester abortion.

    h. uterine dysfunction. An abnormality in the functioning of the uterus to propel the fetus through the birth canal. Uterine action is incoordinate; although there is constant tension in the muscle, the contractions are of poor quality.

hyperventilation. The condition that results from rapid and deep breathing and is marked by confusion, dizziness, numbness, and muscular cramps.

hypnosis. An artificially induced state of extreme suggestibility in which the patient is insensible to outside impressions.

hypocalcemia. Reduction of blood calcium below normal.

hypofibrinogenemia. Deficiency of fibrinogen in the blood.

hypogalactia. Deficiency in the secretion of milk.

hypoglycemia. An abnormally diminished content of glucose in the blood.

hypoprothrombinemia prophylaxis. The administration of vitamin K, intramuscularly, to a newborn as a preventive measure against neonatal hemorrhagic disease.

hypospadias. A developmental anomaly in which the urethra opens on the underside of the penis.

hypotension. Abnormally low blood pressure.

hypothalamus. A specialized structure within the brain located just above the pituitary that regulates and controls a number of autonomic activities, including the release of gonadotropic hormones by the pituitary gland.

hypothermic reaction. A reaction of low body temperature of the mother after delivery.

hypotonic uterine dysfunction. An abnormality in the functioning of the uterus to propel the fetus through the birth canal in which contractions decrease in strength and the tone of the uterine muscles is less than usual.

hypovolemia. An abnormally decreased volume of liquid (plasma) circulating in the body.

hypoxia. Insufficient oxygen to support normal metabolic requirements.

intrauterine h. A condition of hypoxia in the fetus that can be determined in labor by indicators such as meconium-stained amniotic fluid, abnormal fetal heart rate, and fetal acidosis.

hysterectomy. The surgical removal of the uterus by cutting either through the abdominal wall or through the vagina.

hysterosalpingography. The making of a record by x-ray of the uterus and uterine tubes after injecting them with opaque material.

hysterotomy. A method of mid-trimester abortion involving an incision into the uterus by a surgical procedure. Also called *minicesarean section*.

icterus neonatorum. The jaundice of a newborn.

identification. The process whereby an individual likens himself to another person.

IDM. Abbreviation for *infant of a diabetic mother*.

iliopectineal line. The linea terminalis.

ilium. Pl. *ilia*. The upper and largest portion of the hip bone.

imperforate anus. An abnormal closing of the anus.

implantation. Process by which the conceptus attaches to the uterine wall and penetrates both the uterine endometrium and the maternal circulatory system.

impotence. A male sexual dysfunction involving impairment of erection; an inability to attain or sustain an erection and have intercourse in 25% of the attempts.

impregnation. The act of becoming pregnant. See *fertilization*.

inborn error of metabolism. Hereditary lack of enzyme required for normal metabolism to occur.

incompetent cervical os. A mechanical defect in the cervix, which causes late habitual abortion or preterm labor.

incomplete abortion. See *abortion, incomplete*.

incontinence. Inability to control the excretion of urine or feces.

increment. That by which anything is increased.

induced abortion. See *abortion, induced*.

induration. The process or quality of hardening.

inertia. Inactivity; inability to move spontaneously. Sluggishness of uterine contractions during labor.

inevitable abortion. See *abortion, inevitable*.

infant. A baby; a child under 2 years of age.

i. mortality rate. The number of infant deaths per 1000 live births.

infertility. The condition of being unfruitful or barren; sterility.

inlet. The upper limit of the pelvic cavity (brim).

intercourse. A mutual exchange, especially sexually; coitus.

internal rotation. The process in the delivery of a baby in which the fetal head is rotated so that it enters the pelvis in the transverse position and exits in the anteroposterior position.

interstitial pregnancy. An ectopic pregnancy that develops in that portion of the tube that passes through the uterine wall.

interval minilaparotomy. A sterilization technique in which a small incision is made below the pubic hair line for tubal ligation.

interval of fertility. Those days during the menstrual cycle during which a woman can conceive, determined by considering the life span of both ova and sperm and the cyclic variability. It ranges from about 8 to 15 days in duration.

intracranial hemorrhage. Bleeding within the cranium. When it occurs in a newborn as a result of a long labor or difficult delivery, it is extremely grave. Also called *subdural hematoma*.

intrauterine. Inside the uterus.

i. device (IUD). A small, flexible appliance that is inserted into the uterine cavity to prevent conception. It may be in various shapes (spirals, loops, rings) and of various materials (plastic tubing, nylon thread, stainless steel).

i. growth retardation (IUGR). The condition of an infant born at 40 weeks' gestation and weighing less than 2500 g (or below the tenth percentile for weight or length).

i. hypoxia. See *hypoxia, intrauterine*.

i. parabiosis. The joining of fetal twins anatomically and physiologically.

introitus. A term applied to the opening of the vagina.

in utero. Inside the uterus.

inversion. A turning upside down, inside out, or end for end.

i. of the uterus. The state of the womb being turned inside out, caused by violently drawing away the placenta before it is detached by the natural process of labor.

inverted nipple. A nipple that recedes rather than becoming erect.

in vitro **fertilization.** A system of impregnation in which ova are extracted from a woman, fertilized in a test tube, and implanted in the uterus.

involution. 1. A rolling or pushing inward. 2. A retrograde process of change that is the reverse of evolution; particularly applied to the return of the uterus to its normal size and condition after parturition.

ischial tuberosity. A protuberance on either side of the ischium.

ischium. The posterior and inferior bone of the pelvis, distinct and separate in the fetus and the infant, or the corresponding part of the hip bone in the adult.

isotonic. Having the same osmotic pressure, especially a salt solution having the same osmotic pressure as blood.

IUD. Abbreviation for *intrauterine device*.

IUGR. Abbreviation for *intrauterine growth retardation*.

jaundice. A condition characterized by hyperbilirubinemia and yellowness in the skin, eyes, and mucous membranes.

jelly. A soft substance that is coherent, tremulous, and more or less transparent.

    contraceptive j. A spermicidal preparation that is inserted vaginally prior to intercourse to prevent conception. Its effectiveness is enhanced when it is used with a diaphragm.

    j. of Wharton. See *Wharton's jelly.*

kalemia. The presence of potassium in the blood.

karyotype. The chromosome makeup of the nucleus of a human cell; also, the photomicrograph of chromosomes arranged in an organized way.

Kegel's exercise. The tightening and relaxing of the pubococcygeal muscle. It aids in toning the vagina, strengthening the perineum, preventing hemorrhoids, and controlling stress incontinence of urine.

kernicterus. The accumulation of unconjugated bilirubin in brain cells resulting in neurologic impairment.

ketamine. A dissociative intravenous analgesic that, used in proper doses during labor, is associated with a minimal newborn depression, no appreciable effects on uterine activity, and few bad dreams or hallucinations.

ketoacidosis. Acidosis due to accumulation of ketone bodies from incomplete metabolism of fatty acids.

Klinefelter's syndrome. See *syndrome, Klinefelter's.*

labia. The nominative plural of *labium*. Lips or liplike structures.

    l. majora. The folds of skin containing fat and covered with hair that form each side of the vulva.

    l. minora. The nymphae, or folds of delicate skin inside the labia majora.

labor. Parturition; the series of processes by which the products of conception are expelled from the mother's body.

laceration. Tearing of vulvar, vaginal, and sometimes rectal tissue during childbirth.

lack of arousal. A female sexual dysfunction formerly called frigidity. It involves failure to respond adequately with congestion and lubrication even with appropriate sexual stimulation.

lactation. The act or period of giving milk; the secretion of milk; the time or period of secreting milk.

lactosuria. The presence of lactose in the urine, a condition common during lactation.

LaLeche League. An organization that holds classes about breast-feeding for women either before or after the baby is born.

Lamaze method of delivery. The most widely used prepared childbirth method in the United States. It uses an individualized approach with classes for both parents in the anatomy and neuromuscular activity of the reproductive system, breathing techniques in labor, and exercises. Sometimes other subjects such as nutrition, hygiene, and child care are taught. Also called *psychoprophylactic method of prepared childbirth.*

lambdoid. Having the shape of the Greek letter λ (lambda).

l. suture. The suture between the occipital and two parietal bones.

laminaria. A genus of seaweeds. Also, a small stick of hygroscopic material that absorbs moisture rapidly and expands. It is used to begin initial dilation of the cervix prior to abortion.

lanugo. The fine hair on the body of the fetus. The fine, downy hair found on nearly all parts of the body except the palms of the hands and the soles of the feet.

laparoscopy. The introduction of a slender, long surgical instrument (the laparoscope) into the abdominal cavity through very small incisions, not involving actual opening of the abdominal cavity. This procedure is often used for female sterilization.

laparotomy. Surgical entry into the abdominal cavity.

large for gestational age (LGA). Pertaining to an infant born at 36 weeks' gestation and weighing 3500 g (about the 90th percentile for weight). LGA infants are immature but overgrown and are typical of diabetic mothers.

layette. The complete outfit of clothing for a newborn.

Leboyer method of delivery. A method of delivery based on theories of a French obstetrician, Frederick Leboyer. The method avoids harsh, sudden sensory stimulation of the newborn by providing him a quiet, dimly lit delivery room and warm bath to make birth less of a traumatic event.

Leopold's maneuver. See *maneuver, Leopold's.*

Let-down reflex. See *reflex, let-down.*

leukorrhea. A whitish discharge from the female genital organs.

LGA. Abbreviation for *large for gestational age.*

LH. Abbreviation for *luteinizing hormone.*

LHRF. Abbreviation for *luteinizing hormone releasing factor.*

lie. Lie of the fetus. It is the relation of the long axis of the fetus to that of the mother. It is either longitudinal or transverse.

ligation. The binding or tying of a vessel with a substance such as string or catgut.

    tubal l. The sterilization of a woman by surgically interrupting her fallopian tubes to prevent ova from being transported to the uterus and to prevent sperm from fertilizing the ovum. The method may involve ligation, crushing, burning, coagulating, or embedding the ends of the tubes.

lightening. The sensation of decreased abdominal distention produced by the descent of the uterus into the pelvic cavity, which occurs from 2 to 3 weeks before the onset of labor.

linea. Pl. *lineae.* A line or thread.

    l. alba. The central tendinous line extending from the pubic bone to the ensiform cartilage.

    l. nigra. A dark line appearing on the abdomen and extending from the pubis toward the umbilicus—considered one of the signs of pregnancy.

    l. terminalis. The oblique ridge on the inner surface of the ilium, continued on the pubis, which separates the tube from the false pelvis. Formerly called the iliopectineal line.

lingua.   Tongue.

l. frenata.   Tongue-tie.

lipid.   One of a group of fats in the body that is easily stored and serves as a source of fuel, is an important part of cells, and serves other useful functions. It may be a fatty acid, neutral fat, wax, or steroid.

lipidosis.   A disorder of cellular lipid metabolism that involves abnormal accumulation of lipid. The lipidoses include Tay–Sachs disease, Niemann–Pick disease, and Gaucher's disease.

liquor.   A liquid.

l. amnii.   The fluid contained within the amnion in which the fetus floats. See *amniotic fluid*.

Listeria monocytogenes.   A gram-positive bacillus that causes upper respiratory tract disease, septicemia, encephalitic disease, and perinatal infections associated with abortion and stillbirth.

lithotomy.   The surgical incision of an organ or duct, especially the bladder.

l. position.   The bodily posture of a patient lying down with hips and knees flexed and thighs abducted and rotated.

lochia.   The discharge from the genital canal during the first or second week following delivery.

low birth weight.   The weight of an infant at birth of 2500 g or less.

L/S ratio.   The ratio of lecithin to sphingomyelin in the amniotic fluid. It increases suddenly at 35 to 36 weeks' gestation and indicates pulmonary maturity.

lumbar sympathetic block.   The blocking of neuropathways of pain by injecting a local anesthetic at L2. It abolishes pain in the uterus only.

lunar month.   A period of 4 weeks. Because a lunar month usually corresponds to the length of the menstrual cycle, it is often used for calculating fetal development.

luteinizing hormone (LH).   A hormone released by the pituitary gland to bring about the final ripening of the graafian follicle and ovulation.

l. h. releasing factor (LHRF).   A substance secreted by the hypothalamus that causes the pituitary gland to release luteinizing hormone.

luteolysis.   The destruction of the corpus luteum through the dissolution of cellular structure. Thus, luteolysis interferes with the function of the corpus luteum in progesterone secretion.

lysozyme.   A crystalline, basic protein present in many body fluids that functions as an antibacterial enzyme.

maneuver.   A planned process involving dexterity; in obstetrics, a procedure used by an obstetrician in assisting manually in delivery.

Bracht m.   A method of assisting with the delivery of the aftercoming head in a breech delivery. The back is gently arched to the mother's abdomen when the scapulae are seen. The arms then tend to deliver spontaneously. Suprapubic pressure is applied to assist descent of the head into the pelvis, and the suspended body continues to be brought slowly to the mother's abdomen. The face and occiput should then deliver spontaneously.

Leopold's m.   Four maneuvers for diagnosing the fetal position by external palpation of the mother's abdomen.

Mauriceau–Smellie–Veit m.   A method of assisting with the delivery of the aftercoming head in a breech delivery. Two fingers of the left hand are placed firmly over the mandibles to flex the head. The right hand is placed over the back, with the fingers over the shoulders to guide the shoulders and head. The torso is elevated slowly with flexion of the head maintained by the maxillary pressure. Suprapubic pressure is applied by an assistant during these maneuvers to aid the descent of the head into the pelvis, and eventually with the suprapubic and maxillary pressure, the occiput is delivered.

Ortolani's m.   A diagnostic procedure performed on the newborn to determine congenital hip dysplasia.

Ritgen m.   Delivery of the infant's head by lifting the head upward and forward through the vulva, between contractions, by pressing with the tips of the fingers upon the perineum behind the anus.

Sellick's m.   A technique in which pressure is applied to the ring of cartilage at the lower part of the larynx to prevent aspiration of gastric contents during anesthesia induction.

manual rotation.   A maneuver used to turn the fetal head by hand from a transverse to an anteroposterior position to facilitate delivery.

Marfan's syndrome.   See *arachnodactyly*.

marginal sinus rupture.   A disorder of placental attachment, a mild type of abruptio placentae in which slight separation occurs at the edge of the placenta in the region of the marginal sinus of the mother.

mask of pregnancy.   See *chloasma*.

mastitis.   Inflammation of the breast.

masturbation.   Self-stimulation of the genitals in men or women, usually to attain orgasm.

maternal infant bonding.   See *bonding*.

maternity clinical specialist.   A nurse at the master's level with expertise in adaptational and physiological problems in maternity care.

maternity nurse practitioner.   A specialty nurse practitioner who provides prenatal care for uncomplicated pregnancies, postpartum care, contraception counseling, and management of minor problems. Also called *OB-GYN nurse practitioner*.

maturation.   In biology, a process of cell division during which the number of chromosomes in the germ cells is reduced to one half the number characteristic of the species.

Mauriceau–Smellie–Veit maneuver.   See *maneuver, Mauriceau–Smellie–Veit*.

McDonald technique.   A simple technique for cerclage that involves placing a nonabsorbable suture around the cervix high on the cervical mucosa.

McDonald's measurement.   Measurement of the height of the uterine fundus with a tape measure; the distance from symphysis pubis to fundus.

meatus. A passage; an opening leading to a canal, duct, or cavity.

m. urinarius. The external orifice of the urethra.

mechanism. The manner of combinations that subserve a common function. In obstetrics refers to labor and delivery.

meconium. The dark green or black substance found in the large intestine of the fetus or newly born infant.

meiosis. The special method for cell division that a sex cell undergoes through which it is matured and its genetic material, or chromosomes, is prepared for fertilization.

menarche. The establishment or the beginning of the menstrual function.

Mendelian disorder. A genetic disorder that follows the inheritance patterns described by Mendel (i.e., dominant, recessive).

meningomyelocele. A malformation that accompanies spina bifida when the membranes covering the spinal cord as well as the cord bulge through the opening in the spine.

menopause. The period at which menstruation ceases; the "change of life."

menorrhagia. Excessive uterine bleeding occurring at the regular time of menstrual flow.

menses. [Pl. of Latin *mensis*, month.] The periodic monthly discharge of blood from the uterus; the catamenia.

menstrual extraction. The aspiration of the endometrium performed in very early pregnancy without cervical dilatation using a small cannula and syringe or other low-pressure suction.

menstruation. The cyclic, physiologic uterine bleeding that normally recurs at approximately 4-week intervals, in the absence of pregnancy, during the reproductive period.

mentum. The chin.

mesoderm. The middle layer of cells derived from the primitive embryo.

metritis. Inflammation of the uterus.

metrorrhagia. Uterine bleeding that occurs at irregular intervals; the amount of flow is usually average.

microcephaly. Abnormal smallness of the head, usually accompanied by mental retardation.

micropill. An oral contraceptive that contains a lower dosage (50 mcg or less) of estrogen than the standard pill.

micturition. Urination.

midwifery. The practice of assisting at childbirth. See *nurse–midwife.*

migration. In obstetrics refers to the passage of the ovum from the ovary to the uterus.

milia. Plural of milium.

milium. A small white nodule of the skin, usually caused by clogged sebaceous glands or hair follicles.

milk ejection reflex. See *reflex, milk ejection.*

milk-leg. Phlebitis of the femoral vein, occasionally following delivery.

milk let-down. See *reflex, milk ejection.*

minicesarean section. See *hysterotomy.*

minipill. An oral contraceptive that contains only progestin and no estrogen.

miscarriage. Lay term for abortion.

missed abortion. See *abortion, missed.*

mittelschmerz. Painful discomfort sometimes experienced during ovulation or in the middle of the menstrual cycle.

molding. The shaping of the baby's head so as to adjust itself to the size and shape of the birth canal.

mongolian spots. Gray-blue pigmented areas seen on some infants, especially those with dark skins. These have no relationship to mongolism and disappear spontaneously later.

monilial infection. An infection caused by a genus of fungi formerly called *Monilia,* now called *Candida.* Examples are thrush and monilial vaginitis.

monoamniotic monochorionic twins. See *twins, monoamniotic monochorionic.*

monotrophy. The principle, stated by Bowlby in 1958, that the structure of the attachment process is such that parents become attached to only one infant at a time.

monozygotic. Pertaining to or derived from one zygote.

m. twins. See *twins, monozygotic.*

mons veneris. The eminence in the upper and anterior part of the pubes of women.

Montgomery's tubercles. Small, nodular follicles or glands on the areolae around the nipples.

morning-after pill. A method of contraception not in general use. The postcoital pill, diethylstilbestrol (DES) is a synthetic estrogen with severe side-effects including nausea, vomiting, and headache. It is used only in emergency situations, such as rape, because it has been shown to cause vaginal cancer in some offspring of mothers who took it.

morning sickness. A symptom of pregnancy in some women, characterized by waves of nausea and sometimes vomiting. It usually occurs in the early part of the day and subsides in a few hours. It may appear 2 weeks after the first missed menstrual period and subside 6 or 8 weeks later.

Moro reflex. See *reflex, Moro.*

morphological sex. The sex of an individual as determined by the body shape and characteristic with appropriate secondary sex characteristics. In the case of a true hermaphrodite, the individual has a mixture of the body and secondary sex characteristics of both sexes.

morula. The fertilized ovum at the 16-cell stage 3 days after conception. It is traveling from the fallopian tube into the uterine cavity prior to implantation.

mother–baby couple care. An organization of postpartum units that includes rooming-in or satellite nurseries, with the same nurse caring for mother and baby.

mucous membrane. The lining of a body cavity or passageway that is connected to the exterior and is protected by a slimy substance it secretes called mucus.

mucous plug. A plug that closes the cervical canal during pregnancy. It is made of mucous secretions of the cervix.

mucus-trap suction. Suction using a catheter with a mucus trap; used to aspirate the newborn without the mucus being drawn into the nurse's mouth.

multigravida. A woman who has been pregnant several times, or many times.

multipara. A woman who has borne several, or many, children.

multiple pregnancy. The condition in which two or more embryos develop in the uterus at the same time.

mutagen. A chemical or substance that causes a change in gene structure or alteration of genetic information.

mutation. A change in gene or chromosome in gametes that may be transmitted to offspring.

myoma. Pl. *myomata*. A uterine tumor made up of muscular elements; a benign tumor of the uterine muscle. Also called a *fibroid*.

myomotomy. An incision into a myoma.

myotonia. Increased muscle tension and tone; increased contractility of muscles.

myxedema. A condition characterized by a dry, waxy type of swelling, with abnormal deposits of the glycoprotein mucin, in the skin. The facial changes are often associated with hypothyroidism.

Nägele's rule. A method of calculating the expected date of confinement. The date is calculated by subtracting 3 calendar months from the first day of the last menstrual period and adding 7 days.

natal. Pertaining to birth.

natural childbirth. See *prepared childbirth*.

natural method of birth control. An approach to contraception that relies upon identification of the fertile period and avoidance of intercourse during this time. Such a method may involve predicting ovulation by use of a menstrual calendar, identifying changes in cervical mucus, or identifying when ovulation has occurred using a basal body temperature chart, or a combination of these. Some couples use other contraceptive methods during the fertile period rather than avoid intercourse.

nausea. An unpleasant feeling vaguely in the area of the upper abdomen that often culminates in vomiting.

navel. The umbilicus.

necrotizing enterocolitis (NEC). An acute inflammatory bowel disorder that occurs primarily in preterm or low-birth-weight neonates.

neonatal. Pertaining to the newborn, usually considered the first 4 weeks of life.

> **n. asphyxia.** Respiratory failure in a newborn; also called *asphyxia neonatorum*.

> **n. period.** The period from birth through the 28th day of life.

neonate. The infant from birth through the first 28 days of life.

neonatology. The study of the diagnosis and treatment of disorders of the newborn.

nephropathy. Any disease of the kidneys.

neural tube defect. Congenital malformation that involves defects of the spinal column caused by failure of the neural tube to close during embryonic development.

neurohormonal. Pertaining to both a nerve or nerves and a hormone.

nevus. A natural mark or blemish; a mole; a circumscribed deposit of pigmentary matter in the skin present at birth (birthmark).

nidation. The implantation of the fertilized ovum in the endometrium of the pregnant uterus.

Niemann–Pick disease. See *disease, Niemann-Pick*.

nocturnal ejaculation. An orgasm with ejaculation of seminal fluid that occurs during sleep particularly in adolescent boys. Also called *"wet dreams."*

nonorgasm. A female sexual dysfunction in which sexual arousal with congestion and lubrication occurs but orgasm is inhibited.

nonviable fetus. A fetus that is incapable of surviving outside the uterus.

norm. Rule, generally for behavior.

nuclear family. A family group that consists of the father, mother, and children.

nulligravida. A woman who has never been pregnant.

nullipara. A woman who has not borne children.

nurse–midwife. A registered nurse who has completed a recognized program of study and clinical experience leading to a certificate in nurse–midwifery.

nurse practitioner. A registered nurse with additional preparation in physical and psychosocial assessment, who provides primary-care management for patients with common acute and chronic illnesses and developmental needs.

OB-GYN nurse practitioner. See *maternity nurse practitioner*.

obstetrics. The branch of medicine that is concerned with the management of women during pregnancy, childbirth, and the puerperium.

occipitobregmatic. Pertaining to the occiput (the back part of the head) and the bregma (junction of the coronal and sagittal sutures).

OCT. Abbreviation for *oxytocin challenge test*.

oligohydramnios. Deficiency of amniotic fluid.

oligospermia. Deficiency in the number of sperm cells in the semen.

oliguria. Suppression of urinary excretion.

omphalic. Pertaining to the umbilicus.

omphalocele. Congenital herniation of the abdominal viscera through a defect in the abdominal wall at the umbilicus.

oocyesis. Ovarian pregnancy.

oocyte. A developing egg cell in one of two stages. A primary oocyte develops from an oogonium, which subsequently divides into a secondary oocyte and a polar body. Ovulation follows, and the mature ovum and a second polar body develop.

oophorectomy. The surgical removal of an ovary or ovaries.

ophthalmia neonatorum. Acute purulent conjunctivitis of the newborn, usually due to gonorrheal infection.

oral contraceptive. A conception preventive taken by mouth.

organogenesis. The beginning and development of organs.

orgasm. The culmination of sexual excitement. Also called *climax*.

orgasmic platform. The thickened area of congested tissue that builds up in and surrounds the lower third of the vagina during high levels of sexual arousal and just preceding orgasm.

Ortolani's maneuver. See *maneuver, Ortolani's*.

os. Any opening in the body, but particularly the cervical opening.

osmolality. A property of a solution that depends on the concentration of the substance dissolved per unit of solvent.

ova. Plural of ovum.

ovary. The sexual gland of the female in which the ova are developed. There are two ovaries, one at each side of the pelvis.

overstimulation. The presence of sensory input when an infant is not receptive to it.

ovulation. The growth and discharge of an unimpregnated ovum, usually coincident with the menstrual period.

ovum. The female reproductive cell. The human ovum is a round cell about $1/120$ of an inch in diameter, developed in the ovary.

oxytocic. 1. Accelerating parturition. 2. A medicine that accelerates parturition.

oxytocin. A hormone produced by the hypothalamus that stimulates contraction of the uterus, used to induce or intensify labor.

o. challenge test. See *test, oxytocin challenge*.

pain. A localized sensation of hurt. In clinical practice, it can be defined as whatever the experiencing person says it is, existing whenever he says it does.

p. intensity. The severity of the pain sensation.

p. tolerance. The intensity or duration of pain that the patient is willing to endure without making further efforts to relieve it.

palpation. The act of feeling with the hands and fingers portions of the body for purposes of diagnosis.

palsy. A synonym for paralysis, used in connection with certain special forms.

Bell's p. Peripheral facial paralysis due to lesion of the facial nerve, resulting in characteristic distortion of the face.

brachial p. Paralysis of an arm.

cerebral p. A motor and speech disorder resulting from an injury to the brain at birth or earlier.

Erb's p. The upper-arm type of brachial birth palsy.

Papanicolaou smear. Cytology test of cervical cells used as a screening for cervical cancer.

para. The term used to refer to past pregnancies that have produced an infant that has been viable, whether the infant is alive at birth or not.

paracervical block. The blocking of neuropathways of pain by injecting a local anesthetic into the parametrium at sites in the cervix. It abolishes pain in the uterus only.

parametritis. Inflammation of the parametrium. Also called *pelvic cellulitis*.

parametrium. The fibrous subserous coat of the supravag-

inal portion of the uterus, extending laterally between the layers of the broad ligaments.

parenteral feeding. Feeding by routes other than through the alimentary canal, such as intravenously.

parity. The condition of a woman with respect to her having borne children.

parovarian. Pertaining to the residual structure in the broad ligament between the ovary and the fallopian tube.

parturient. Bringing forth; pertaining to childbearing. A woman in childbirth.

parturition. The act or process of giving birth to a child.

patent ductus arteriosus. A congenital cardiac anomaly in which the vascular connection between the pulmonary artery and aorta, which is open during fetal life, does not close after birth as it should, causing the recirculation of arterial blood through the lungs.

patulous. Spreading somewhat widely apart; open.

pedigree. A record of an individual's ancestors. In genetics, it is used for analyzing Mendelian traits.

pelvic. Pertaining to the pelvis.

p. axis. See *axis, pelvic*.

p. cellulitis. See *parametritis*.

p. congestion. Excessive accumulation of blood in the pelvic region.

p. inlet. Inlet to the true pelvis.

pelvic inflammatory disease (PID). Infection of the pelvic organs often caused by the presence of an IUD or venereal disease.

pelvimeter. An instrument for measuring the diameters and capacity of the pelvis.

pelvimetry. The measurement of the dimensions and capacity of the pelvis.

pelvis. The lower part of the body bounded by the two hip bones, the sacrum, and the coccyx.

android p. One of the four main types of female pelvis, generally characterized as resembling the pelvis of a male and having a wedge-shaped inlet and narrow anterior segment.

anthropoid p. One of the four main types of female pelvis, generally characterized by a long anteroposterior diameter of the inlet.

contracted p. A pelvis that measures 1 cm to 3 cm shorter than normal in any important diameter.

false p. The part of the pelvis superior to a plane passing through the linea terminalis.

gynecoid p. The most prevalent of the four main types of female pelvis, having a rounded oval shape.

platypelloid p. One of the four main types of female pelvis, having a flattened pelvic inlet.

true p. The part of the pelvis inferior to a plane passing through the linea terminalis.

penis. The male organ of copulation.

perinatal. Pertaining to the time before and after birth; variously defined as beginning at conception through the 28th day of life or conception through the first year of life.

perineorrhaphy. Suture of the perineum; the operation for the repair of lacerations of the perineum.

perineotomy. A surgical incision through the perineum.

perineum. The area between the vagina and the rectum.

periodic breathing. A common pattern of periods of apnea of 10 seconds or less noted in premature infants.

peritoneoscopy. Direct visualization of the tubes and ovaries with an endoscope.

peritoneum. A strong serous membrane investing the inner surface of the abdominal walls and the viscera of the abdomen.

peritonitis. Inflammation of the peritoneum.

phenylketonuria (PKU). An inborn error of metabolism resulting in a deficiency in liver enzyme. It may be detected by blood or urine tests. Early treatment will prevent mental retardation.

phimosis. Tightness of the foreskin.

phlebitis. Inflammation of a vein.

phocomelia. A developmental anomaly characterized by total absence or stunting of the arms or legs.

phospholipid. Any lipid that contains phosphorus; the major form of lipid in all cell membranes.

phototherapy. The use of light to treat a disease, especially the use of intense fluorescent light to reduce serum bilirubin in the treatment of hyperbilirubinemia.

physiologic jaundice. Mild icterus neonatorum lasting a few days.

pica. The abnormal intake of specific substances such as clay dirt, cornstarch, or plaster. It may characterize the behavior of malnourished children or pregnant women.

Pitocin. A proprietary solution of oxytocin.

PKU. Abbreviation for *phenylketonuria.*

placenta. The circular, flat, vascular structure in the impregnated uterus forming the principal medium of communication between the mother and the fetus.

    ablatio p. See *abruptio placentae.*

    abruptio p. Premature separation of the normally implanted placenta.

    p. accreta. A condition in which one or more cotyledons of the placenta are abnormally adherent to the uterine wall, making separation of the placenta difficult or impossible.

    previa p. A placenta that is implanted in the lower uterine segment so that it adjoins or covers the internal os of the cervix.

platypelloid pelvis. See *pelvis, platypelloid.*

plexus. A network or tangle, such as a network of veins, lymphatic vessels, or nerves.

polycythemia. An increased red blood cell volume.

polydactyly. A developmental anomaly characterized by extra digits on the hands or feet.

polygalactia. Excessive secretion of milk.

polyhydramnios. Hydramnios.

position. The situation of the fetus in the pelvis; determined by the relation of some arbitrarily chosen portion of the fetus to the right or the left side of the mother's pelvis. Thus, each presentation has either a right or left position.

postasphyxia encephalopathy. One of various central nervous system symptoms caused by injury resulting from episodes of perinatal asphyxia.

postcoital test. See *test, postcoital.*

postmaturity. Overdevelopment, as of a postmature infant who was born after pregnancy has progressed beyond full term.

postnatal. Occurring after birth, referring to the infant.

postpartum. After delivery or childbirth, referring to the mother.

    p. hemorrhage. Loss of 500 ml or more of blood from the uterus after completion of the third stage of labor.

    p. period. The period occurring after childbirth, referring to the mother.

post-term infant. An infant born after the onset of the 42nd week of gestation.

PPM. Abbreviation for *psychoprophylactic method of prepared childbirth.*

precipitate delivery. A delivery that occurs with undue rapidity (less than 3 hours) and usually without the benefit of asepsis.

preeclampsia. A disorder encountered during pregnancy or early in the puerperium, characterized by hypertension, edema, and albuminuria.

pregnancy. [Latin, *praeg'nans,* literally "previous to bringing forth."] The state of being with young or with child. The normal duration of pregnancy in the human female is 280 days, or 10 lunar months, or 9 calendar months. See also *abdominal p., ectopic p., interstitial p., multiple p., tubal p.*

premature infant. An infant that weighs 2500 g or less at birth.

premature ejaculation. A male sexual dysfunction in which difficulty is met in controlling orgasm for a sufficient period of time to enable his partner to attain sexual satisfaction.

premature infant. An infant born before the 37th week of gestation, regardless of weight; preterm infant.

premature rupture of membranes. Rupture of the amniotic sac before the onset of uterine contractions.

prematurity. Underdevelopment, as of a premature infant.

premenstrual tension. A syndrome sometimes experienced during the 10 days preceding menstruation. It is characterized by irritability, insomnia, headache, pain in the breasts, abdominal distention, nausea, anorexia, constipation, emotional instability, and urinary frequency.

prepared childbirth. The methods by which parents actively participate in childbirth. Some approaches include the concepts and techniques of Dick–Read, Lamaze, and Bradley. Also called *natural childbirth.*

prepuce. The fold of skin that covers the glans penis in the male.

    p. of the clitoris. The fold of mucous membrane that covers the glans clitoris.

presentation. Term used to designate that part of the fetus nearest the internal os, or that part that is felt by the examiner's hand when doing the vaginal examination.

presumptive signs of pregnancy. Signs that strongly suggest that a healthy woman is pregnant. These include menstrual suppression, nausea, vomiting, frequency of micturition, tenderness and other changes of breasts, "quickening," Chadwick's sign, pigmentation of the skin, and abdominal striae.

preterm infant. See *premature infant.*

primigravida. Pl. *primigravidas.* A woman who is pregnant for the first time.

primipara. Pl. *primiparas.* A woman who has given birth to her first child.

probable signs of pregnancy. Signs that the likelihood of pregnancy is great. These include enlargement of the abdomen, changes in the size, shape, and consistency of the uterus, fetal outline felt by palpation, changes in the cervix, Braxton Hicks contractions, and a positive pregnancy test.

prodromal. Premonitory; indicating the approach of a disease.

p. labor. The latent or early phase in which there is some effacement and slow dilatation of the cervix. It lasts perhaps an average of 8½ hours in a nullipara.

progesterone. The pure hormone contained in the corpora lutea whose function is to prepare the endometrium for the reception and development of the fertilized ovum.

progestin. Any of the synthetic progesterone preparations that are used in oral contraceptives. The common types include norethynodrel, norethindrone, ethynodiol diacetate, and norgestrel.

prolactin. A proteohormone from the anterior pituitary that stimulates lactation in the mammary glands.

prolan. Zondek's term for the gonadotropic principle of human-pregnancy urine, responsible for the biologic pregnancy tests.

prolapse of umbilical cord. Delivery of the umbilical cord in labor prior to the delivery of the fetus.

promontory. A small projection; a prominence.

p. of the sacrum. The superior or projecting portion of the sacrum when *in situ* in the pelvis, at the junction of the sacrum and the last lumbar vertebra.

prostaglandin. Any of a group of fatty acids found in semen, which are effective abortifacients at any stage of pregnancy. These are the most common agents for inducing mid-trimester abortion through instillation into the amniotic fluid.

prostate gland. A gland in the male that surrounds the neck of the bladder and urethra.

proteinuria. The presence of protein in the urine.

pruritus. Intense itching, usually referring to the genital area.

pseudocyesis. An apparent condition of pregnancy; the woman really believes she is pregnant when, as a matter of fact, she is not.

psychogenic sexual stimuli. Stimuli processed through the higher brain centers that cause sexual arousal. These include sensory stimuli such as sight, sound, taste, smell, and touch, and cognitive events such as thoughts, fantasies, memories, and images.

psychophysiology. The interaction between psychological and physiological processes, that is, between higher mental processes and the responses of muscles, glands, and organs.

psychoprophylactic method of prepared childbirth (PPM). See *Lamaze method of delivery.*

psychosexual method of childbirth. A method of childbirth preparation developed by Sheila Kitzinger based on a method using sensory memory and the Stanislavsky method of acting. Sexuality is seen as part of the larger whole encompassing family relationships, birth, cuddling, and feeding.

puberty. The age at which the generative organs become functionally active.

pubic. Belonging to the pubis.

pubiotomy. The operation of cutting through the pubic bone lateral to the median line.

pubis. The os pubis or pubic bone forming the front of the pelvis.

pudenda. [L.] The plural of pudendum.

pudendal. Relating to the pudenda.

p. block. The blocking of neuropathways of pain by injecting a local anesthetic into the pudendal nerve. It abolishes pain in the vagina and perineum.

pudendum. [Latin, *pudere,* to have shame or modesty.] The external genital parts of either sex, but especially of the female.

puerperal fever. Infection, accompanied by fever, which develops in a wound to the birth canal during delivery.

puerperium. The period elapsing between the termination of labor and the return of the uterus to its normal condition, about 6 weeks.

pulmonary dysmaturity. An insidious disease of premature infants beginning with mild respiratory symptoms after the first week of life. The cause is thought to be collapse of the bronchial tree, with partial airway obstruction following aspiration of small amounts of milk as a result of a poorly developed gag reflex. Also known as *Wilson–Mikity disease.*

pyelonephritis. Inflammation of the kidney due to bacterial infection. In pregnancy, hormonal and anatomical changes cause narrowing of the lower ureter and dilation of the upper ureter and renal pelvis, thus increasing the risk of infection.

pyloric stenosis. A congenital anomaly manifested in an infant from the first to the second or third week by projectile vomiting 30 minutes after feeding. Surgery removes a stricture of the pylorus that is the cause.

quickening. The mother's first perception of the movements of the fetus.

rabbit test. See *test, Friedman's.*

radioimmunoassay test. See *test, radioimmunoassay.*

RDS. Abbreviation for *respiratory distress syndrome.* See *disease, hyaline membrane.*

Read method of childbirth preparation. See *Dick–Read approach to childbirth.*

reanastomosis. The reestablishing of a connection between vessels, such as surgically reconnecting the severed vas deferens or fallopian tubes following sterilization. The purpose of this surgery is to reestablish fertility, but success rates are variable.

recessive inheritance. The acquisition of a characteristic from both parents that is the result of an allele that must be carried by both members of a pair of homologous chromosomes.

rectocele. The protrusion by hernia of a part of the rectum into the vagina.

reflex. An involuntary activity.

grasp r. The reflex present at birth in an infant's hands and feet causing the fingers and toes to curl around an object placed touching them.

let-down r. See *milk ejection r.*

milk ejection r. The activation of a process by which contractions of the myoepithelial cells in a mother's breast propel milk along the duct into the lactiferous sinuses. Also called *let-down reflex* and *milk let-down.*

Moro r. See *startle r.*

rooting r. The tendency of an infant to open his mouth and turn toward an object that is gently stroking his cheek or the corner of his mouth.

startle r. The reflex that is present from birth to age 3 months that indicates an awareness of equilibrium by a symmetrical drawing up of legs and grasping of arms in response to a sudden jarring of his crib or clothes. Also known as *Moro reflex.*

stepping r. The reflex that is present at birth but disappears soon after that causes an infant to make little stepping or prancing movements when he is held upright with his feet touching a surface.

sucking r. The reflex in infants to suck anything that comes in contact with their lips. It seems to be a great need for the first 2 months of life, is present while sleeping, and need not be nutritive.

swallowing r. The reflex present at birth to swallow food that an infant sucks into his mouth.

tonic neck r. The tendency of an infant while lying on his back to turn his head to one side and extend the arm and leg on that side, flexing the arm and leg on the other side.

reflexogenic sexual stimulus. A direct stimulation of an erogenous area that causes sexual arousal in a reflexive, or automatic, manner.

respiratory distress syndrome (RDS). See *disease, hyaline membrane.*

resuscitation. The restoring to life of a patient who is apparently dead or dying.

retinal vein thrombosis. The presence of an obstruction caused by an aggregation of blood factors in the retinal vein. This clotting disorder may be partially the result of the use of oral contraceptives.

retraction ring. Physiologic area of constriction at the junction of the upper, or contracting, portion and the lower, or dilating, portion of the uterus; Bandl's ring is pathologic constriction of the retraction ring.

retroflexion. The bending backward of an organ on its axis, specifically the tipping backward of a uterus upon itself.

retrolental fibroplasia. An acquired disease of a premature infant resulting in eye injury as a result of continuous oxygen therapy in high concentration.

retroversion. The tipping backward of an entire organ; in the case of retroversion of the uterus, the turning back of the entire uterus in relation to the pelvic axis.

Rh. Abbreviation for *Rhesus*, a type of monkey. This term is used for a property of human blood cells, because of its relationship to a similar property in the blood cells of Rhesus monkeys.

Rh factor. A term applied to an inherited antigen in the human blood.

RhoGAM. A preparation of anti-Rh antibodies administered by injection to unsensitized Rh-negative women following childbirth or abortion, to prevent the development of endogenous antibodies that could later lead to erythroblastosis fetalis (Rh disease of the fetus) in a subsequent pregnancy.

rhythm method. A birth control method relying upon abstinence from sexual intercourse before, during, and after the period of time the ovum is capable of being fertilized.

Ritgen maneuver. See *maneuver, Ritgen.*

roentgenogram. A record of the internal structure of a body by the use of x-ray photography.

role complementarity. The learning of roles in pairs.

role differentiation. The process by which roles are structured and delineated.

rollover test. See *test, rollover.*

rooming-in. The hospital practice in which postpartum mothers have their infants in their rooms all the time, except for necessary examinations or procedures.

rooting reflex. See *reflex, rooting.*

rotation. The turning on an axis; specifically, in labor, the turning of the fetal head through a right angle so that the longest diameter of the head corresponds to the longest diameter of the pelvic outlet.

rubella. German measles.

r. syndrome. See *syndrome, rubella.*

Rubin's test. See *test, Rubin's.*

rupture of the membranes. The breaking of the amniotic sac, which may occur spontaneously and be the first indication of approaching labor. If the membranes have not ruptured previously, they must be broken before the fetal head is delivered to prevent aspiration of fluid when the infant takes its first breath.

sacral promontory. The marked projection in the pelvis formed by the junction of the last lumbar vertebra and the sacrum.

sacrococcygeal articulation. The joint or juncture of the sacrum and coccyx.

sacroiliac articulation. The two joints or junctures of the sacrum and the ilium on either side of the pelvis.

sacrum. A triangular wedge-shaped bone, consisting of five vertebrae fused together, which serves as the back part of the pelvis.

saddle block. The blocking of neuropathways of pain by injecting a local anesthetic into the subarachnoid space in the spine. A *true saddle block* blocks pain in the perineum. A *modified saddle block* abolishes both uterine and perineal discomfort.

Saf-T-Coil. One of the commonly used intrauterine devices.

salpingitis. Inflammation of the fallopian tubes.

scarf sign. A test to assess infant maturity. The infant's arms are drawn across the neck and as far across the opposite shoulder as possible. In the premature infant there is less resistance and greater draping (or scarf) effect; the elbow will reach near or across the midline. In the full-term infant, the elbow will not reach the midline.

Schultze's mechanism. The expulsion of the placenta with the fetal surfaces presenting.

sebum. The secretions of the sebaceous glands of the skin; a thick, semifluid substance composed of fat and epithelial cell debris.

secondary areola. See *areola, secondary.*

secundines. The afterbirth; the placenta and membranes expelled after the birth of a child.

segmentation. The process of division by which the fertilized ovum multiplies before differentiation into layers occurs.

Sellick's maneuver. See *maneuver, Sellick's.*

semen. 1. A seed. 2. The fluid secreted by the male reproductive organs.

sensory modalities. The areas of sensation: vision, touch, hearing, taste, smell, and movement.

separation of the placenta. Detachment of the placenta from the wall of the uterus.

sex chromatin. See *Barr body.*

sex chromosome. One of two chromosomes in human cells that are associated with the determination of the sex of the individual. A male cell normally contains one X and one Y chromosome, and a female cell contains two X chromosomes.

sex-linked inheritance trait. An inheritance trait in which the gene is carried on the X chromosome and is expressed in the male offspring. (Males do not possess another X chromosome to offset the effects of the X chromosome that carries the gene.)

sexologist. A specialist in the area of human sexuality; one engaged in sex research or particularly learned in the physiological, behavioral, or psychoemotional aspects of sexuality.

sex role. The public expression of gender identity; all actions used to convey one's maleness or femaleness.

sex therapy. A short-term therapy aimed at relief of the sexual symptom, which uses systematically structured sexual experiencing with conjoint therapeutic sessions. It is designed to modify immediate obstacles to sexual functioning, although intrapsychic and transactional conflicts are also dealt with to some extent.

sexual dysfunction. A psychosomatic disorder that makes it impossible for an individual to have or enjoy intercourse. There is inadequate sexual response involving both vasocongestive and orgasmic components either together or separately. See also *impotence, premature ejaculation, vaginismus, lack of arousal, nonorgasm,* and *dyspareunia.*

sexuality. The complex of emotions, attitudes, preferences, and behaviors related to the individual's expression of the sexual self and eroticism. Components of sexuality include the individual's genetic, hormonal, gonadal, and morphologic sex gender identity, sex role, and sexual partner preference.

sexually transmitted diseases (STD). A variety of diseases usually transmitted by direct sexual contact with an infected individual.

SGA. Abbreviation for *small for gestational age.*

Shake test. See *test, Shake.*

Shirodkar technique. A technique for cerclage that involves elevating the vaginal mucous membrane and tying some material (i.e. suture) around the internal os of the cervix. The vaginal mucosa is then restored to its original position and sutured.

shoulder dystocia. A serious complication in the birth of an oversized infant whose unusually large shoulders arrest at either the pelvic brim or the outlet.

shoulder presentation. A serious complication of birth in which the infant lies crosswise in the uterus instead of longitudinally. The risk of perinatal mortality is reduced by a cesarean delivery.

show. Popularly, the blood-tinged mucus discharged from the vagina before or during labor.

sickle cell anemia. A hereditary, genetically determined hemolytic anemia. It is generally manifest before childbearing, and crises may occur in the nonpregnant as well as pregnant state. One must consider not only the impact of pregnancy in precipitating crises in a patient with sickle cell anemia but also the genetic outlook and limited life expectancy of the patient.

sitz bath. A treatment for perineal or perianal discomfort in which the patient sits for 20 minutes three to four times per day in very warm water that may have astringents or solutions added.

Skene's gland. One of two glands just within the meatus of the female urethra; regarded as the homologue of the prostate gland in the male.

smegma. A thick cheesy secretion found under the prepuce and in the region of the clitoris and the labia minora.

small for gestational age (SGA). Pertaining to infants whose weight falls below the tenth percentile for their gestational age. These infants have experienced growth retardation during the prenatal period and may be born close to term but weigh less than 2500 g.

socialization. The process by which an individual learns society's expectations for behavior.

souffle. A soft, blowing auscultatory sound.

   funic s. A soft hissing sound, synchronous with the fetal heart sounds produced by blood being transported through the umbilical vessels.

   placental s. A soft blowing sound caused by the blood flow in the placenta and synchronous with the maternal pulse.

   uterine s. Soft blowing sound caused by the blood flow in the arteries of the uterus and synchronous with the maternal pulse.

spermatocyte. A developing sperm cell in one of two stages. A primary spermatocyte develops from a spermatogonium and subsequently divides into two secondary spermatocytes. Each spermatocyte divides into two spermatids.

spermatogenesis. The process of forming spermatozoa.

spermatogonium. Pl. *spermatogonia.* The undivided male germ cell that develops in the seminiferous tubes. Each will eventually develop into four spermatozoa.

spermatozoon. Pl. *spermatozoa.* A mature male germ cell; the mobile microscopic sexual element that resembles in shape an elongated tadpole.

spermicide. An agent that destroys spermatozoa; used as a contraceptive.

sphingomyelin lipidosis. See *disease, Niemann–Pick.*

spina bifida. A rather common malformation due to the congenital absence of one or more vertebral arches, usually at the lower part of the spine.

spinal anesthesia. Relief of pain by injecting a local anesthetic into the subarachnoid space in the spine.

spontaneous rupture of the membranes. Rupture of the amniotic sac without medical interference.

spotting. Spotting of blood from the vagina between periods.

startle reflex. See *reflex, startle.*

station. Measurement of the fetal descent into the bony pelvis in relationship to the ischial spines.

stenosis. The narrowing of a duct or canal. See *pyloric stenosis.*

stepping reflex. See *reflex, stepping.*

sterilization. 1. A process of eliminating microbial viability. 2. A permanent method of contraception; process by which an individual is made incapable of reproduction.

steroid hormones. Sex hormones and hormones of the adrenal cortex.

stilbestrol. Diethylstilbestrol, an estrogenic compound.

stillborn. Born dead.

stimulus. Any environmental event that activates a reaction in one of the senses.

striae gravidarum. Shining, reddish lines upon the abdomen, thighs, and breasts during pregnancy.

subdural hematoma. A hemorrhage under the tough outer covering (periosteum) of the skull or cranium.

subinvolution. Failure of a part to return to its normal size and condition after enlargement from functional activity, as subinvolution of the uterus, which exists when normal involution of the puerperal uterus is retarded.

succedaneum. See *caput.*

sucking reflex. See *reflex, sucking.*

suction curettage. A method of first-trimester abortion using cervical dilation and suction evacuation of uterine contents. Also known as *dilatation and evacuation (D&E).*

supine hypotensive syndrome. A condition in which the blood pressure is lowered and bradycardia occurs when the pregnant woman is in the supine position. Caused by compression of the inferior vena cava by the pregnant uterus.

suppository, contraceptive. A suppository containing a spermicide that is inserted in the vagina prior to intercourse for purposes of contraception.

suprapubic. Located above the pubic area; slightly above the symphysis pubis in the midlower abdomen.

surfactant. A mixture of the secretions of the lungs and air passages that reduces the surface tension of pulmonary fluids and thus contributes to the elastic properties of lung tissue.

swallowing reflex. See *reflex, swallowing.*

symphysis. The union of bones by means of an intervening substance; a variety of synarthrosis.

   s. pubis. "Symphysis of the pubis." The pubic articulation or union of the pubic bones, which are connected with each other by interarticular cartilage.

symptothermal method. Combination of the ovulation, or Billings, method (based on symptoms that provide clues as to when ovulation is occurring) and the BBT method. This approach tends to improve effectiveness of the fertility awareness approach to birth control. It also decreases the number of days on which a couple is permitted to have sexual intercourse.

synchondrosis. A union of bones by means of a fibrous or elastic cartilage.

syncope. A temporary loss of consciousness, a faint.

syndrome. A set of symptoms characterizing a particular state of abnormality or illness.

   adrenogenital s. A hyperfunction of the adrenal cortex. It is manifested by virilism in the female at birth and precocious sexual development in the male 3 or 4 years after birth.

   Asherman's s. Amenorrhea due to adhesions within the uterine cavity, usually as a result of postpartum or postabortal infection or pelvic tuberculosis.

   Down's s. A chromosomal abnormality characterized by slanting eyes set close together; narrow palpebral fissures; flat nose; protruding large fissured tongue; small head and flat occiput; broad pudgy neck; short, thick hands with simian creases on the palms; defective mentality; underdeveloped muscles, loose joints, and heart and alimentary tract abnormalities. The syndrome may be inherited, although its incidence increases with maternal age. Also called *trisomy 21* and, formerly, *mongolism.*

   fetal alcohol s. A congenital anomaly resulting from maternal alcohol intake above 3 oz of absolute alcohol per day. It is characterized by typical craniofacial and limb defects, cardiovascular defects, intrauterine growth retardation, and developmental delay. No *safe* alcohol limit has been determined.

   Klinefelter's s. A genetic defect characterized by variable degrees of masculinization, small testes, or uncertain genitalia.

   Marfan's s. See *arachnodactyly.*

   respiratory distress s. See *disease, hyaline membrane.*

   rubella s. A congenital syndrome caused by a rubella infection suffered by the mother during the first 16 weeks of pregnancy. It is characterized by varying combinations of cardiac anomalies, eye defects, developmental ear defects, encephalitis, immunologic defects, jaundice, osteomyelitis, pneumonitis, and other problems.

   Turner's s. A genetic defect characterized by undifferentiated gonads, short stature, and other abnormalities, which may include webbing of the neck, low posterior hairline, and cardiac defects.

synergistic. Acting together in a way that one agent enhances the effect of the other, and their combined effect is greater than the sum of their individual effects.

syphilis. A serious contagious venereal disease that is transmitted by direct intimate contact or congenitally. It is divided into three stages (primary, secondary, and tertiary) that have different characteristics, lesions being apparent in the primary and secondary stages. It is treatable with penicillin.

talipes equinovarus. The typical clubfoot. Its elements are equinus or plantar flexion of the foot at the ankle, varus or inversion deformity of the heel, and forefoot adduction.

Tay–Sachs disease. See *disease, Tay–Sachs.*

TENS. Abbreviation for *transcutaneous electric nerve stimulation.*

teratogen. A chemical or substance that interferes with fetal development after conception.

teratogenic. Tending to produce anomalies of formation or physical defects in an embryo or fetus.

test. An examination, trial, or method of assessment.

Aschheim–Zondek t. A test for the diagnosis of pregnancy. Repeated injections of small quantities of urine voided during the first weeks of pregnancy produce in infantile mice, within 100 hours, (1) minute intrafollicular ovarian hemorrhage and (2) the development of lutein cells.

Friedman's t. A modification of the Aschheim–Zondek test for pregnancy; the urine of early pregnancy is injected in 4-ml doses intravenously twice daily for 2 days into an unmated mature rabbit. If, at the end of this time, the ovaries of the rabbit contain fresh corpora lutea or hemorrhagic corpora, the test is positive.

glucose tolerance t. (GTT). A test of carbohydrate metabolism in which 100 g of glucose is given orally while fasting; blood sugar should return to normal in 2 to 2½ hours. It is a test for diabetes.

Nonstress t. A test providing information about fetal well-being, by using the external fetal monitor and evaluating the fetal heart rate for accelerations from the baseline rate.

oxytocin challenge/contraction stress t. A test providing information about uteroplacental function, by using the external fetal monitor and evaluating the fetal heart rate in response to either spontaneous or induced uterine contractions.

postcoital t. A test of the cervical mucus within 12 hours following intercourse. It permits evaluation of placement of spermatozoa, the quality of cervical secretions, and their ability to support the life of spermatozoa.

rabbit t. See *Friedman's test.*

radioimmunoassay t. A test of blood serum for pregnancy. It is very accurate from the eighth day after fertilization.

rollover t. A simple test for preeclampsia in which the diastolic blood pressure is recorded with the patient in a lateral recumbent position, then on her back. A positive result is indicated if diastolic blood pressure increases by 20 mm Hg or more.

Rubin's t. A test for evaluating tubal function using uterotubal insufflation with carbon dioxide. If the manometer registers no higher than 100 mm Hg, the tubes are patent. If it rises to 200 mm Hg, the tubes are completely occluded.

Shake t. The foam stability test to measure precisely the L/S ratio in the fetus. It is relatively simple and quick. The test depends on the ability of the surfactant in the amniotic fluid when mixed with ethanol to generate stable foam at the air–liquid interface.

testes. Two male reproduction glands, located in the scrotum, that produce testosterone, the male hormone, and spermatozoa, the male reproductive cells.

testicle. One of the two glands contained in the male scrotum.

testosterone. The principal male sex hormone produced in the testes in response to the luteinizing hormone. It is believed to be responsible for regulating spermatogenesis, male characteristics, and maintaining muscle mass and bone tissue in the adult.

tetralogy of Fallot. A combination of four congenital cardiac anomalies including ventricular septal defect, pulmonary stenosis, overriding aorta, and hypertrophy of the right ventricle.

β-thalassemia disease. A hemolytic anemia caused by diminished synthesis of beta chains of hemoglobin.

theoretical effectiveness of a contraceptive method. The maximum effectiveness of a contraceptive method in preventing pregnancy under ideal conditions and when it is completely understood.

thermacogenesis. The elevating of body temperature by the action of a drug.

thermoregulation, neonatal. Regulation of body heat. Pertains particularly to the newborn's ability to regulate his temperature.

thrombocytopenia. A decrease in the number of platelets in circulating blood.

thromboembolic disorder. A disorder involving the obstruction of a blood vessel with thrombotic material brought by the blood to the site from its origin.

thromboembolism. The blocking of a blood vessel with a thrombus that has broken loose from its site of formation.

thrombophlebitis. A condition in which inflammation of the wall of a vein has preceded the formation of a thrombus.

thrombus. A coagulation of blood elements, often causing an obstruction at the point of formation.

thrush. An infection caused by the fungus *Candida albicans,* characterized by whitish plaques in the mouth.

toco-. Combining form meaning parturition or childbirth.

tocodynamometer. An instrument that measures the expulsive force of uterine contractions in childbirth.

tocolytic drug. A drug used to suppress preterm labor, usually by inhibiting uterine contractions.

tomography. The recording of internal body images in a particular plane by using an x-ray source.

tongue-tie. A condition in which the attachment of the thin ridge of tissue in the middle of the base of the tongue (the frenulum linguae) extends far forward causing a concavity at the tip of the tongue on its upper surface. Also called *lingua frenata.*

tonic neck reflex. See *reflex, tonic neck.*

toxoplasmosis. A congenital disease characterized by lesions of the central nervous system, which may lead to blindness, brain defects, and death.

transcutaneous electric nerve stimulation. The use of a mild electric current through the skin to relieve pain.

transplacental. Crossing the placenta, especially the exchange of hormones, nutrients, waste products, and drugs between the mother and fetus.

transposition of the great vessels. A congenital cardiac anomaly in which the aorta originates from the right ventricle rather than the left, and the pulmonary artery originates from the left ventricle rather than the right.

transverse arrest. An abnormal fetal position in which rotation of the head is incomplete and the head is stopped in the transverse position.

Trendelenburg's position.   A position in which a patient lies on his back with his head tilted downward 15° to 40° with the bed at an angle at his knees.

Treponema pallidum.   A genus of spirochetes responsible for causing syphilis.

Trichomonas.   A genus of parasitic flagellate protozoa.
   t. vaginalis.   A species sometimes found in the vagina.
   t. vaginitis.   A vaginal infection caused by *Trichomonas vaginalis* with characteristic increased discharge and pruritus, or itching.

trimester.   One of three periods into which pregnancy is divided. Specific things happen in each trimester.

trisomy.   A chromosomal abnormality in which a particular chromosome is in triplicate rather than the usual pair.
   t. 21.   See *syndrome, Down's.*

trophoblast.   The peripheral cells of the blastocyst, which attach the fertilized ovum to the uterine wall and become the placenta and the membranes around the embryo/fetus.

true pelvis.   See *pelvis, true.*

tubal ligation.   See *ligation, tubal.*

tubal pregnancy.   An ectopic pregnancy in which the fertilized ovum is embedded in one of the fallopian tubes rather than the wall of the uterus.

tuberischii.   Pertaining to the ischial tuberosities, the protuberances at the sides of the pelvic outlet.

Turner's syndrome.   See *syndrome, Turner's.*

twins.   Two offspring produced in the same pregnancy.
   diamniotic dichorionic t.   Twins that develop within separate amniotic sacs and have separate chorions.
   diamniotic monochorionic t.   Twins that develop within separate amniotic sacs and have one chorion.
   dizygotic t.   Twins that develop from separate zygotes, or fertilized ova; dichorionic twins; fraternal twins.
   monoamniotic monochorionic t.   Twins that develop within the same amniotic sac and have one chorion.
   monozygotic t.   Twins that develop from the same zygote; monochorionic twins; identical twins.

ultrasound.   The use of sound waves to visualize outlines of structures within the body. Used for fetal assessment because it poses a minimal risk.

umbilical.   Pertaining to the umbilicus.
   u. arteries.   The two arteries that accompany and form part of the umbilical cord.
   u. catheterization.   A method of inserting a catheter into the umbilicus of a high-risk neonate to provide a route for parenteral feeding, exchange transfusion, or obtaining blood samples.
   u. cord.   [Latin, *funis umbilicalis.*] The cord connecting the placenta with the umbilicus of the fetus and at the close of gestation principally made up of the two umbilical arteries and the umbilical vein, encased in a mass of gelatinous tissue called "Wharton's jelly."
   u. hernia.   Hernia at or near the umbilicus.
   u. vein.   Forms a part of the umbilical cord.

umbilicus.   [L.] The navel; the cicatrix or scar that marks the attachment of the umbilical cord to the placenta.

ureter.   The tube through which urine passes from the kidney to the bladder.

use effectiveness of a contraceptive method.   The effectiveness of a contraceptive method under actual conditions of use, in which some people use it correctly and others use it carelessly or incorrectly.

uterine souffle.   See *souffle, uterine.*

uterotubal insufflation.   A procedure used in Rubin's test involving the introduction of carbon dioxide into the uterus by way of a cannula. If one or both tubes are patent, the carbon dioxide flows through the uterus and tubes into the peritoneal cavity. When the patient sits up, the carbon dioxide rises to the diaphragm, causing pain in the shoulder referred there by way of the phrenic nerve.

uterus.   The hollow muscular organ in the female designed for the lodgement and nourishment of the fetus during its development until birth.

vacuum aspiration.   A method used for first-trimester abortions in which the contents of the uterus are removed by applying a vacuum through a hollow curet or cannula inserted into the uterus.

vacuum extraction.   See *extraction, vacuum.*

vagina.   [Latin, a sheath.] The canal in the female, extending from the vulva to the cervix of the uterus.

vaginismus.   A female sexual dysfunction that involves a painful spasm of the vagina preventing penetration.

vaginitis.   An infection involving the mucous membrane of the vagina, commonly associated with increased malodorous discharge, itching, and burning.
   trichomonas v.   See *trichomonas vaginitis.*

varicosity.   The condition of a vein that is unnaturally and permanently distended.

vasectomy.   The surgical interruption and ligation of the vas deferens, the spermatic duct, to prevent sperm from being in the ejaculate. It is the method of male sterilization.

vasocongestion.   Excessive accumulation of blood in the blood vessels.

venereal disease.   See *disease, venereal.*

venous stasis.   Stoppage or diminution of the flow of blood in the veins.

venous thrombosis.   The presence of a thrombus in a vein.

ventricular septal defect.   A congenital cardiac anomaly in which there is an abnormal opening between the right and left ventricles.

vernix caseosa.   "Cheesy varnish." The layer of fatty matter that covers the skin of the fetus.

version.   The act of turning; specifically, a turning of the fetus in the uterus so as to change the presenting part and bring it into more favorable position for delivery.

vertex.   The summit or top of anything. In anatomy, the top or crown of the head.
   v. presentation.   Presentation of the vertex of the fetus in labor.

vestibule.   A triangular space between the labia minora; the urinary meatus and the vagina open into it.

viable. A term signifying "able or likely to live;" applied to the condition of the child at birth.

villus. Pl. *villi.* A small vascular process or protrusion growing on a mucous surface, such as the chorionic villi seen in tufts on the chorion of the early embryo.

vulva. The external genitals of the female.

weaning. The discontinuance of breast-feeding of an infant and the substitution of other forms of nourishment.

Wharton's jelly. [Thomas *Wharton,* English anatomist, died 1673.] The jellylike mucous tissue composing the bulk of the umbilical cord.

Wilson–Mikity disease. See *pulmonary dysmaturity.*

witches' milk. A milky fluid secreted from the breast of the newly born.

withdrawal. The practice of retracting the penis from the vagina in intercourse prior to ejaculation, used as a method of contraception.

womb. The uterus.

Wright method. A method of childbirth preparation based on psychoprophylaxis but using less active breathing than the Lamaze method.

x-ray pelvimetry. The measurement of pelvic size by x-rays. Although it is the most accurate method of measuring the pelvis, the exposure to x-rays precludes its regular use.

Zatuchni–Andros prognostic index. A system to evaluate the feasibility of vaginal delivery in breech presentations.

zona pellucida. A transparent belt; translucent or shining through.

zygote. A cell resulting from the fusion of two gametes.

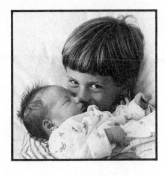

Answers for the Study Aids

Answers to Conference Materials are not included in this section because of their content. Some answers are given for discussion questions, while in other cases text page references are given.

Unit I
Nursing, Family Health, and Reproduction

Multiple Choice

1. A
2. C
3. B

Unit II
Biophysical Aspects of Human Reproduction

Multiple Choice

1. B	12. C	26. B
2. C	13. A	27. A
3. A. 4	14. C	28. D
B. 4	15. C	29. C
C. 1	16. B	30. B
D. 3	17. C	31. C
4. C	18. D	32. C
5. A. 2	19. D	33. B
B. 3	20. 2	34. A
6. B	21. A	35. 1
7. D	22. C	36. 4
8. A	23. B	37. B
9. B	24. C	38. C
10. B	25. A	39. B
11. A		

Unit III
Assessment and Management in Sexuality and Reproduction

Multiple Choice

1. 3	5. A	9. D
2. B	6. C	10. A
3. B	7. B	11. A
4. A	8. B	12. I

13. C	17. A	21. 2
14. B	18. B	22. 4
15. C	19. C	23. 3
16. 3	20. 2	24. 2

Discussion

21. The nurse must attain a level of personal comfort with sexuality through increasing information and knowledge through books, articles, workshops, or classes. The nurse must develop attitudes and values that are tolerant of diverse sexual practices through values clarification activities and discussion of sexual practices.

22. A sexual history includes a description of the problem and its onset and course, the client's ideas about causes, prior treatment and outcomes, and expectations or goals for current therapy. During pregnancy, attitudes and beliefs about sex and pregnancy, understanding of physiological and emotional changes, and physiological status of the pregnancy are added.

23. Common dysfunctional sexual problems during pregnancy include changes in sex drive, dyspareunia, avoidance of sex, and male erectile dysfunction.

24. General principles in response to children's questions about sex include short answers with simple explanations, matter-of-fact tone, use of accurate terms and explanations for anatomy and physiology, calm replies with straightforward explanation of meanings of obscene words, and reinforcing and clarifying as the child seeks more information.

25. Teenager unable to assume responsibilities of motherhood; using pregnancy to alleviate doubts about femininity but not psychologically capable of caring for child; unmarried women who feel they need support of a partner for childrearing; marital conflicts and pending breakup; poor physical or mental health; interference with important life goals; risk of congenital or hereditary defects.

26. There are few negative psychological reactions when professional staff have positive attitudes and are accepting; women who are separated, di-

vorced, or widowed have higher rates of psychiatric admissions; children of mothers denied abortion had higher rates of illness and poorer grades in school despite similar birth histories and intelligence levels.

Unit IV
Assessment and Management in the Antepartum Period

Multiple Choice

1. 2	15. 4	29. 2
2. C	16. C	30. 4
3. A	17. B	31. 2
4. B	18. D	32. A
5. D	19. D	33. 4
6. D	20. 1	34. 2
7. B	21. 3	35. 4
8. 2	22. 4	36. 4
9. C	23. B	37. 1
10. B	24. B	38. B
11. 3	25. 4	39. 3
12. B and C	26. 3	40. 3
13. D	27. A	41. 3
14. A, B, C, E, F	28. B	

Discussion

42. Regular exercise increases energy, decreases fatigue, decreases backache, strengthens abdominal muscles, enhances circulation, and increases flexibility, stamina, and endurance. Recovery after birth may be quicker for fit women. Exercises include swimming and brisk walking (especially good for women exercising for the first time). Other exercises the nurse can recommend are included in the Appendix.
43. See Table 19-2, Occupations Commonly Held by Women Working in Industry and Potential Occupational Hazards.
44. Nipple rolling, nipple stretching, nipple cups for inverted nipples.

Unit V
Assessment and Management in the Intrapartum Period

Multiple Choice

1. A	C. 2	8. 4
2. Situation No. 1: 3	D. 2	9. 2
Situation No. 2: 2	4. C	10. 3
Situation No. 3: 2	5. 3	11. B
3. A. 2	6. 4	12. 4
B. 3	7. C	13. 3

14. 3	19. 2	22. A
15. 3	20. A	23. D
16. C	21. A. 1	24. D
17. 3	B. 3	25. A
18. 5	C. 2	

Completion

26. A. Every client
    B. Every client
    C. Per order
    D. Every client
    E. Every client
    F. Per order
27. A. LOT
    B. LOA
    C. LOP
    D. LSP
    E. RMA
28. A. Complete or full dilatation
    B. 100% effacement
    C. Boggy uterus or atony
    D. Episiotomy
    E. Engagement
29. A. Diagonal conjugate
    B. True conjugate
    C. Bi-ischial
30. A. B
    B. A
    C. C
31. C

Unit VI
Assessment and Management in the Postpartum Period

Multiple Choice

1. 3	6. C	10. A
2. 1	7. 2	11. A
3. 1	8. C	12. C
4. 4	9. C	13. D
5. 1		

Discussion

14. During pregnancy, *estrogen* and *progesterone* exert an inhibitory effect on lactation. Following delivery of the placenta, the main source of these two hormones, the inhibitory effect is removed. The anterior pituitary continues to secrete *prolactin*, which stimulates secretion by the mammary alveolar cells.
15. There appears to be a sensitive period in the first minutes and hours after birth when it seems to be important for the mother and father to have close

contact with their infant to enhance later optimal development.

Unit VII
Assessment and Management of High Risk Maternal Conditions

Multiple Choice

1. 1	B. 1	23. C
2. 1	C. 3	24. D
3. 3	14. 2	25. B
4. 4	15. 2	26. C
5. 2	16. 2	27. B
6. 3	17. 3	28. D
7. 3	18. 2	29. 3
8. A	19. 2	30. A
9. A	20. 3	31. 4
10. 2	21. 3	32. 4
11. A. 1	22. A. 3	33. 3
B. 2	B. 1	34. A
C. 3	C. 2	35. 2
12. 4	D. 4	36. 3
13. A. 2		

Discussion

37. Elevated temperature (38.4°C, or 101°F)
Lassitude or malaise
Chills or a chilly sensation
Loss of appetite
38. Peritonitis is an infection of the peritoneum that may be localized to the pelvis or generalized. Parametritis is an infection of the loose fibroareolar pelvic connective tissue. Both of these conditions may be caused by a puerperal infection that extends by way of the lymphatics of the uterine wall.
39. Pain
Fever
Swelling of the affected leg (edema)

Unit VIII
Assessment and Management of High Risk Perinatal Conditions

Multiple Choice

1. 4	7. A	13. 1
2. 2	8. D	14. 1
3. A	9. 4	15. 1
4. 3	10. 4	16. 1
5. B	11. 3	17. 2
6. 2	12. 2	

Unit IX
Assessment and Management of Women's Health Promotion

Multiple Choice

1. 4	7. 2	13. 4
2. C	8. C	14. D
3. 5	9. C	15. 6
4. 3	10. 1	16. D
5. 4	11. 3	17. 3
6. 3	12. 5	

Index

Numbers followed by an f indicate a figure; t following a page number indicates tabular material.

Photo Credits

The following sources are gratefully acknowledged for the use of the photographs found on the chapter opening pages specified:

Tracy Baldwin—pages 303, 350
Tracy Baldwin, Booth Maternity Center—page 319
Carnegie Institute of Washington, Department of Embryology, Davis Division—page 143
The Children's Hospital of Philadelphia—page 1168
Friend and Denny, Medichrome—page 998
Hewlett-Packard Company—page 15
Lyn Jones—pages 75, 454, 466, 681
Media Services, Sonoma State University—pages 287, 387
L. Moskowitz, Medichrome—page 1258
Osteopathic Hospital of Maine, Portland, Maine—page 973
Barbara Proud—pages 171, 217, 237, 507, 871, 1227
Sexually Transmitted Diseases—page 846
Kathy Sloan—pages 3, 24, 32, 44, 58, 119, 537, 561, 592, 607, 641, 707, 728, 820, 1024, 1082
St. Anne's Maternity Home—page 895
University of Pennsylvania—pages 89, 1047, 1112

ISBN 0-397-54813-3

90000

9 780397 548132